Fourth Edition

Surgery of the Stomach and Duodenum

EDITED BY

Lloyd M. Nyhus, M.D., F.A.C.S.

Warren H. Cole Professor and Head, Department of Surgery, University of Illinois College of Medicine at Chicago; Surgeon-in-Chief, University of Illinois Hospital, Chicago, Illinois

Christopher Wastell, M.S., F.R.C.S.

Professor of Surgery, Charing Cross and Westminster Medical School, London University; Honorary Consultant Surgeon to Westminster and St. Stephen's Hospitals, London, England

Foreword by Martin Allgöwer, M.D.

Professor of Surgery, University of Basel, Kantonsspital, Basel, Switzerland

Little, Brown and Company

Boston / Toronto

Fourth Edition

Library of Congress Catalog Card No. 85-82481

ISBN 0-316-61740-7

Printed in the United States of America

MV

Contents

Contributing Authors

J. Alexander-Williams, M.D., Ch.M., F.R.C.S., F.A.C.S.
Consultant Surgeon, General Hospital; Senior Clinical Lecturer, University of Birmingham, Birmingham, England
Chapter 25

Helene P. Ayres, B.A.
Editor, Department of Surgery, Ohio State University College of Medicine, Columbus, Ohio
Chapter 18

Jamil Bahnini, M.D.
Chief Resident, Faculty of Medicine, Louis Pasteur University and Department of General and Digestive Surgery, Centre Hospitalier Universitaire de Hautepierre, Strasbourg, France
Chapter 1: Special Comment

J. H. Baron, D.M., F.R.C.P.
Senior Lecturer and Consultant, Departments of Surgery and Medicine, Royal Postgraduate Medical School and Hammersmith Hospital; Subdean, St. Mary's Hospital Medical School, London, England
Chapter 4

Clarence J. Berne, M.D.
Professor Emeritus and Former Chairman, Department of Surgery, University of Southern California School of Medicine, Los Angeles, California
Chapter 16

S. R. Bloom, M.A., M.D., D.Sc., F.R.C.P.
Professor of Medicine, Royal Postgraduate Medical School; Consultant Physician, Hammersmith Hospital, London, England
Chapter 3: Part II

C. Thomas Bombeck, M.D.
Professor of Surgery, University of Illinois College of Medicine at Chicago; Chief, Surgical Gastroenterology, University of Illinois Hospital, Chicago, Illinois
Chapter 22

Bobby C. Brown, M.D.
Pathologist, The Piedmont Hospital, Atlanta, Georgia
Chapter 26

David C. Carter, M.D., F.R.C.S.
St. Mungo Professor of Surgery, University of Glasgow; Consultant Surgeon, University Department of Surgery, Royal Infirmary, Glasgow, Scotland
Chapter 3: Part II: Special Comment

Jameson L. Chassin, M.D.
Professor of Clinical Surgery, New York University School of Medicine, New York; Director of Surgery, Booth Memorial Hospital, Flushing, New York
Chapter 28

Robert E. Condon, M.D., M.S., F.A.C.S.
Ausman Professor and Chairman, Department of Surgery, Medical College of Wisconsin, Milwaukee, Wisconsin
Chapter 21

Clarence Dennis, M.D., Ph.D.
Professor of Surgery, State University of New York at Stony Brook Health Sciences Center School of Medicine, Stony Brook; Staff Surgeon and Associate Chief of Staff for Research and Development, Veterans Administration Medical Center, Northport, New York
Chapter 1; Chapter 1: Special Comment

Philip E. Donahue, M.D.
Associate Professor of Surgery, University of Illinois College of Medicine at Chicago; Chief of General Surgery, Veterans Administration (West Side) Hospital, Chicago, Illinois
Chapter 5: Special Comment; Chapter 15

Herbert L. Duthie, M.D., Ch.M.
Provost, Welsh National School of Medicine, Cardiff; Consultant Surgeon, South Glamorgan Health Authority, Wales
Chapter 9: Special Comment

Harold Ellis, F.R.C.S.
Professor of Surgery, Westminster Medical School; Chairman of Surgery, Westminster Hospital, London, England
Chapter 17

Richard G. Fiddian-Green, M.D.
Professor and Chairman, Division of General Surgery, University of Massachusetts Medical Center, Worcester, Massachusetts
Chapter 7

J. W. L. Fielding, M.D., Ch.B., F.R.C.S.
Senior Lecturer in Surgery, University of Birmingham; Honorary Consultant Surgeon, Queen Elizabeth Hospital, Birmingham, England
Chapter 25

L. P. Fielding, M.B., F.R.C.S.
Clinical Professor of Surgery, Yale University School of Medicine, New Haven; Chief of Surgery, St. Mary's Hospital, Waterbury, Connecticut
Chapter 10

Robert L. Goodale, M.D., Ph.D.
Associate Professor of Surgery, University of Minnesota Medical School, Minneapolis, Minnesota
Chapter 5

Stephen W. Gray, Ph.D.
Professor of Anatomy, Emory University School of Medicine; Scientific Staff, Emory University Hospital, Atlanta, Georgia
Chapter 26

A. Gerson Greenburg, M.D., Ph.D.
Professor of Surgery, University of California, San Diego, School of Medicine; Acting Chief, Surgical Service, Veterans Administration Hospital, San Diego, California
Chapter 12: Special Comment

Charles A. Griffith, M.D., F.A.C.S.
Clinical Associate Professor of Surgery, University of Washington School of Medicine, Seattle; Honorary Staff, Overlake Hospital, Bellevue, Washington
Chapters 2, 12

Ulf Haglund, M.D.
Associate Professor of Surgery, University of Lund, Mälmo; Consultant Surgeon, Mälmo General Hospital, Mälmo, Sweden
Chapter 3: Part I

John Lynwood Herrington, Jr., M.D.
Professor of Clinical Surgery, Vanderbilt University School of Medicine; Attending Surgeon, St. Thomas Hospital, Nashville, Tennessee
Chapters 14, 20

F. K. Holle, M.D.
Professor of Surgery, University of Munich Policlinic; Director, Department of Surgery, University of Munich Policlinic, Munich, West Germany
Chapter 13: Special Comment

Louis F. Hollender, M.D., D^res/h.c.
Professor of Surgery, Faculty of Medicine, Louis Pasteur University; Chief, Department of General and Digestive Surgery, Centre Hospitalier Universitaire de Hautepierre, Strasbourg, France
Chapter 1: Special Comment

A. H. Hölscher, M.D.
Department of Surgery, Technical University of Munich; Department of Surgery, Klinikum rechts der Isar, Munich, West Germany
Chapter 9

Jerry M. Jesseph, M.D.
Resident, Department of Surgery, Indiana University School of Medicine and Indiana University Hospital, Indianapolis, Indiana
Chapter 30

†John E. Jesseph, M.D.
Professor and Chairman, Department of Surgery, Indiana University School of Medicine; Attending Surgeon and Chairman, Department of Surgery, Indiana University Hospital, Indianapolis, Indiana
Chapter 30

Stephen N. Joffe, M.D., F.R.C.S., F.A.C.S.
Professor of Surgery, University of Cincinnati College of Medicine, Cincinnati, Ohio
Chapter 13: Special Comment

Alan G. Johnson, M.Chir., F.R.C.S.
Professor of Surgery, University of Sheffield; Honorary Consultant Surgeon, Royal Hallamshire Hospital, Sheffield, South Yorks, United Kingdom
Chapter 11

Terence Kennedy, M.D., M.S., F.R.C.S.
Honorary Lecturer of Surgery, The Queens University; Consultant Surgeon, Royal Victoria Hospital, Belfast, Northern Ireland
Chapter 20: Special Comment

John G. Kral, M.D., Ph.D.
Associate Professor of Surgery, Columbia University College of Physicians and Surgeons; Attending Surgeon and Director, Division of Surgical Metabolism, St. Luke's-Roosevelt Hospital Center, New York, New York
Chapter 29: Special Comment

Edward E. Mason, M.D., Ph.D.
Professor and Chairman of General Surgery, University of Iowa College of Medicine; Surgeon, University of Iowa Hospitals and Clinics, Iowa City, Iowa
Chapter 29

John D. Mullins, M.D.
Chief Resident in Surgery, The Piedmont Hospital, Atlanta, Georgia
Chapter 26

Ronald Lee Nichols, M.D.
Henderson Professor of Surgery, Professor of Microbiology and Immunology, Tulane University School of Medicine, New Orleans, Louisiana
Chapter 24

Lloyd M. Nyhus, M.D., F.A.C.S.
Warren H. Cole Professor and Head, Department of Surgery, University of Illinois College of Medicine at Chicago; Surgeon-in-Chief, University of Illinois Hospital, Chicago, Illinois
Chapters 15, 19; Appendix A

Minoru Oi, M.D.
Emeritus Professor of Surgery, Jikei University School of Medicine, Tokyo; Honorary President, Tokyo Kosei Nenkin Hospital, Tokyo, Japan
Chapter 10: Special Comment

Lars Olbe, M.D.
Associate Professor of Surgery, University of Gothenburg; Senior Surgeon, Department of Surgery II, Sahlgren Hospital, Gothenburg, Sweden
Chapter 3: Part I

John F. O'Leary, M.D.
Surgical Fellow, University of Minnesota Medical School, Minneapolis, Minnesota
Chapter 5

J. M. Polak, D.Sc., M.D., M.R.C. Path.
Reader in Histochemistry, Royal Postgraduate Medical School, London, England
Chapter 3: Part II

†Deceased.

Wallace P. Ritchie, Jr., M.D., Ph.D.
Professor and Chairman, Department of Surgery, Temple University School of Medicine; Attending Surgeon, Temple University Hospital, Philadelphia, Pennsylvania
Chapter 23

Leonard Rosoff, Sr., M.D.
Professor Emeritus and Former Chairman of the Department of Surgery, University of Southern California School of Medicine; Former Director of Surgery, Los Angeles County-University of Southern California Medical Center, Los Angeles, California
Chapter 16

Jack Rudick, M.D.
Clinical Professor of Surgery, Mount Sinai School of Medicine of the City University of New York; Attending Surgeon, The Mount Sinai Hospital, New York, New York
Chapter 8

Witold Rudowski, M.D.
Professor of Surgery, Director and Head, Department of Surgery, Research Institute of Hematology and Blood Transfusion, Warsaw, Poland
Chapter 1: Special Comment

G. R. Sagor, M.B., F.R.C.S.
Consultant Surgeon, Department of Surgery, St. Albans City Hospital, St. Albans, United Kingdom
Chapter 3: Part II

Richard P. Saik, M.D.
Associate Professor of Surgery, University of California, San Diego, School of Medicine; Staff Physician, Surgical Service, Veterans Administration Hospital, San Diego, California
Chapter 12: Special Comment

John L. Sawyers, M.D.
Professor and Chairman, Department of Surgery, Vanderbilt University School of Medicine; Surgeon-in-Chief, Vanderbilt University Hospital, Nashville, Tennessee
Chapter 14, 20

Charles M. Sheaff, M.D., Ph.D.
Assistant Professor of Surgery, University of Illinois College of Medicine; Attending Surgeon, Department of General Surgery, Cook County Hospital, Chicago, Illinois
Chapter 19

J. R. Siewert, M.D.
Professor of Surgery, Technical University of Munich; Director, Department of Surgery, Klinikum rechts der Isar, Munich, West Germany
Chapter 9

Bernard Sigel, M.D.
Professor and Chairman, Department of the Medical College of Pennsylvania; Chief of Surgery, Medical College of Pennsylvania Hospital, Philadelphia, Pennsylvania
Chapter 18: Special Comment

John E. Skandalakis, M.D., Ph.D., F.A.C.S.
Chris Carlos Professor of Surgical Anatomy and Technique, Departments of Surgery and Anatomy, Emory University School of Medicine; Senior Attending Surgeon, The Piedmont Hospital, Atlanta, Georgia
Chapter 26

Lewis Spitz, M.B., Ch.B., Ph.D., F.R.C.S.
Nuffield Professor of Paediatric Surgery, Institute of Child Health, University of London; Honorary Consultant Surgeon, The Hospital for Sick Children, London, England
Chapter 27

William E. Strodel, M.D.
Assistant Professor of Surgery, University of Michigan Medical School; Attending Surgeon, Department of Surgery, Veterans Administration Hospital, Ann Arbor, Michigan
Chapter 7

Stephen B. Vogel, M.D.
Associate Professor of Surgery, University of Florida College of Medicine, Gainesville, Florida
Chapter 7: Special Comment

†Owen H. Wangensteen, M.D.
Regents' Professor of Surgery, University of Minnesota Medical School; Chairman Emeritus, Department of Surgery, University of Minnesota Hospitals, Minneapolis, Minnesota
Chapter 1

Sarah D. Wangensteen, B.A.
Senior Medical Historian Emerita, Department of Medical History, University of Minnesota Medical School, Minneapolis, Minnesota
Chapter 1

†Deceased.

Christopher Wastell, M.S., F.R.C.S.
Professor of Surgery, Charing Cross and Westminster Medical School, London University; Honorary Consultant Surgeon to Westminster and St. Stephen's Hospitals, London, England
Chapters 10, 13

Richard Whitehead, F.R.C.P.A.
Professor of Pathology, Flinders University of South Australia School of Medicine; Head, Department of Pathology, Flinders Medical Centre, Bedford Park, South Australia
Chapter 6

Robert M. Zollinger, M.D.
Regents' Professor and Chairman Emeritus, Department of Surgery, Ohio State University College of Medicine, Columbus, Ohio
Chapter 18

Foreword

It is a real privilege to make some introductory comments about *Surgery of the Stomach and Duodenum,* particularly in light of the proud fact that this monumental work, once pioneered by Henry Harkins and so ably continued by its present editors, has come to its fourth edition. The editorship by "general surgeons at heart" strengthens our belief that surgery of the alimentary tract will remain, I hope forever, the backbone of general surgery.

There is an obvious problem! Should the surgeon be the only responsible partner for the patient from symptoms to diagnosis and finally to operation? Should the surgeon, on the contrary, honor the traditional "separation of authority" by sharing responsibility with a gastroenterologist? Both types of management appear valid, provided that a critical quality control of diagnostic and therapeutic procedures safeguards the interests of the patient. Surgeons are not newcomers to the various techniques of endoscopy and should never be considered trespassers into the gastroenterologists' field. A common interest and responsibility in these procedures would appear to be the most satisfactory attitude of both surgeons and gastroenterologists. It is of more than symbolic importance that the division of diagnostic techniques in this volume has a mixed authorship of gastroenterologists and surgeons.

The various aspects of peptic ulcer disease are dealt with extensively in this book. In light of the fascinating results with "vagolytic drugs" and various surgical vagotomies, one cannot help feeling that "vagal autosabotage" (primarily at night?) is paramount among the pathogenic factors. In fact, diminution of gastric secretion to "acid on demand" by adequate reduction of vagal activity seems the most logical approach to therapy. While medication may successfully overcome this "vagal dysfunction," it does not cure the disease and therefore does not prevent recurrence in a high percentage of patients who discontinue their medication. Complete surgical denervation of the parietal cell mass seems to be most effective in curing the disease permanently. There is no doubt, however, that certain structural variances with regard to location and mass of the parietal cells, so succinctly discussed in the two contributions by Griffith, are able to interfere in some pyloric and prepyloric ulcers with the permanent success of vagotomy. This book does away with all traditional and modern "monomanias" in dealing with ulcer disease.

Nyhus and Wastell have succeeded in bringing together a group of authors who give a wealth of information to the surgeon and also to the gastroenterologist. Without any doubt this book will help them to be more valid and knowledgeable partners in advising and treating patients suffering from gastroduodenal disease of any kind.

Martin Allgöwer

Preface

In the 30 years since the conception of the first edition of this volume, major changes have occurred in the field of gastric and duodenal surgery. These changes encompass our understanding of basic pathophysiology, the incidence of disease, approaches to medical and surgical therapy, and the final results of this treatment. Indeed, due to early success of medical treatment of the duodenal ulcer with H-2 receptor blockers and the marked decrease of the need for operative intervention, the purpose of producing another book on this subject might be questioned. The need is greater now than before. Surgical house officers of the past gained much of their technical experience performing operations on the stomach and duodenum. The paucity of similar experience today suggests a real need for a ready reference. Further, there are diseases of the stomach and duodenum other than peptic ulcer that continue to perplex the diagnostician—physician or surgeon. We hope this comprehensive presentation includes most, if not all, of these entities. Returning to the subject of peptic ulcer, it is only by proper application of the surgical principles outlined in this book that patients with duodenal and gastric ulcer can be cured. Few patients are cured by other means of therapy.

The fourth edition remains true to the first three in basic format. Fundamental concepts are presented by authorities in the field. The Special Comment sections, which proved to be innovations for the book publishing field, have been expanded. Many chapters have been completely rewritten, and all have been updated. Completely new material on upper gastrointestinal endoscopy, duodenal reflux syndrome, selective vagotomy plus suprapyloric antrectomy, bacteriology of the stomach, stapling in esophageal and gastric surgery, and the surgical treatment of obesity has been added. Two popular sections of previous editions, an author index and a chapter and appendix on the editors' personal operative techniques have again been included.

We continue to believe that *Surgery of the Stomach and Duodenum*, Fourth Edition, will be valuable to a broad spectrum of persons interested in the subject. We hope that scientists, house staff personnel, candidates for surgical examinations, gastroenterologists, and the world of surgery in general will find areas of interest here.

The editors express their appreciation to Curtis Vouwie of Little, Brown and Company for his patience, advice, and understanding, and to Cynthia Baron for an outstanding job of supervising the copyediting and editorial production of the book. Dr. Nyhus is particularly indebted to Catherine Judge, Publications Editor, Department of Surgery, University of Illinois College of Medicine at Chicago, for the many difficult tasks that she performed in the development of this book. Prof. Wastell extends his thanks to Lyn Judd for her help in typing and retyping manuscripts in addition to carrying out the other duties of a busy secretary.

L. M. N.
C. W.

I

History and Basic Science

Drug Notice

The contributors, the editors, and the publishers have made every effort to ensure the accuracy and appropriateness of the drug dosages presented in this textbook. The medications described do not necessarily have specific approval by the Food and Drug Administration for use in the diseases and dosages for which they are recommended. The package insert for each drug should be consulted for use and dosage as approved by the FDA. Because standards for usage change, it is advisable to keep abreast of revised recommendations, particularly those concerning new drugs.

1

History of Gastric Surgery: Glimpses into Its Early and More Recent Past

Owen H. Wangensteen
Sarah D. Wangensteen
Clarence Dennis

Surgical Antecedents to Abdominal Surgery

Evolution of surgery of the body cavities, the abdomen, thorax, and cranium, was slow; owing primarily to the great hazard of infection, it had to await the development of prophylactic surgical antisepsis. Alexander Monro I, in two successive papers (1737, 1752), reported a mortality for amputation at the Royal Infirmary in Edinburgh of 8 percent, a figure not improved on until the waning decades of the nineteenth century. Monro cited "little circumstances" as the responsible factor in the achievement of the Edinburgh staff. Perusal of his publications indicates he placed considerable emphasis on careful hemostasis, leaving the long strands of ligature on vessels within the wound, which he did not close completely. Cutting ligatures of blood vessels on the knot, often credited to William Lawrence (1815), was described by Lancelot Haire of the Haslar Naval Hospital in 1786. However, attention to cleanliness, not cited by Monro, must have been the most important desideratum in the Edinburgh accomplishment.

Claude Pouteau of Lyons (1760) reported 120 instances of perineal lithotomy for the removal of vesical calculi, with three deaths (a mortality of 2.5 percent), a record not bettered in the nineteenth century by world-famous urologists. Pouteau was a fine surgical anatomist and respected the prostatic fascia enveloping the rich prostatic plexus of vessels, first named as an anatomical entity by G. S. Pattison (1820),[1] then of the University of Maryland. Pouteau also was an ardent advocate of surgical cleanliness.

These surgical procedures, however, were extracavitary operations, in which it was possible to allow the wound to remain open. Vincent v. Kern (1826), Robert Liston (1841), and A. Burow (1859) all followed the practice of leaving amputation wounds open, undoubt-

[1]Often erroneously credited to the French surgeon-anatomist C. Denonvilliers, who redescribed the prostatic fascia in a Paris dissertation of 1837.

Supported by grants from the Margaret W. Harmon, the Alice M. O'Brien, and the Ralph and Marian Falk Research Funds.

edly a factor in their ability to perform amputation with modest mortalities.[2]

Acceptance of prophylactic surgical antisepsis, urged by Ignacz P. Semmelweis (1847)[3] and his Vienna colleagues, notably v. Hebra, Skoda, Haller, and Rokitansky, unfortunately was long delayed by traditional opposition to innovation. W. W. Keen (1898) placed the beginnings of general acceptance of prophylactic surgical antisepsis in the year 1876;[4] William S. Halsted (1904) placed it in 1878; however, leading American surgeons, including Samuel D. Gross, were still repudiating Listerian practices during the first and second official meetings of the American Surgical Association in 1882 and 1883. Joseph Lister's chief emphasis was on placement of antiseptics (phenol) into wounds. He did not scrub his hands with soap and water and then with an antiseptic solution, as had Semmelweis. In fact, only after retirement in 1892 from his professorship at King's College, London, did Lister capitulate to prophylactic surgical antisepsis.

The first surgeon to adopt Semmelweis's practices was Alfred Hegar,[5] a gynecologist in Freiburg. He was able to report (1876–1877) 15 successive successful ovariotomies by total commitment to the doctrine of prophylactic surgical antisepsis advocated by Semmelweis.

We are inclined to place general acceptance of prophylactic surgical antisepsis in 1885, a year that demarcated collapse of resistance to Lister and was accompanied by announcements of success attending high standards of surgical cleanliness. Lawson Tait (1886), a keen controversialist, though rejecting Listerian methods completely, was able to report 139 consecutive successful ovariotomies observing only strict surgical cleanliness.

The influence of Louis Pasteur and Lister on the advance of surgery was great. Lister even cited Pasteur as his model; however, Lister followed the traditional method of placing antiseptics into wounds, a practice dating back to biblical times. Pasteur, on the contrary, employed heat and sterile filters to preserve the sterility of his test fluids, finally putting to rest, with the help of the physicist John Tyndall, the doctrine of spontaneous generation. The cleric Lazaro Spallanzani (1767) had virtually destroyed the theory a century earlier, but the work of Tyndall in support of Pasteur's view that unclean air was responsible for contamination of flasks containing sterile fluid resolved the issue. Tyndall (1881) showed that clean air devoid of particulate matter (bacteria) did not diffract light rays as did foul air.

Surgical Anesthesia

All of surgery took a great leap forward with the introduction of ether anesthesia, first publicly demonstrated at the Massachusetts General Hospital on October 16, 1846. Several observers as long ago as 1800, notably the chemist Humphry Davy (1800), had the phenomenon of anesthesia for the relief of pain during surgical procedures within their grasp but failed to appreciate the potential importance of their observations. Frolics with both ether and nitrous oxide date back to the beginning of the nineteenth century. Crawford W. Long of Georgia had employed ether anesthesia surgically as early as 1842 in a number of operations but failed to publish until 1849. J. Y. Simpson of Edinburgh invoked use of chloroform for anesthesia in 1847, which was in vogue for a long period of time but is rarely used today because of the hazards encountered in prolonged administration.

[2]It will surprise the modern-day student of wounds to learn that Zimmerman and Veith (1967) joined Allbutt (1905) and Garrison (1922) in condemning open treatment of contaminated wounds, which has gained universal approval of all military surgeons since World War I (1917). (L. M. Zimmerman and I. Veith, *Great Ideas in the History of Surgery,* New York: Dover, 1967, pp. 75, 101; F. H. Allbutt, *The Historical Relations of Medicine and Surgery to the End of the Sixteenth Century,* London: Macmillan, 1905, p. 52; F. H. Garrison, *Introduction to the History of Medicine,* Philadelphia: Saunders, 1922, p. 148.)

[3]Semmelweis summarized his observations and experience in the prevention of puerperal fever in his magnificent monograph of 1861, today a collector's item.

[4]Keen (1898) said that surgery of the alimentary tract really began with the publication of a St. Petersburg inaugural dissertation in 1875 by Tschertneisky-Barischewsky, who operated on 35 dogs, resecting short segments of the small intestine, with 29 recoveries.

[5]Hegar (1882) was the first biographer of Semmelweis.

Gastric Cancer

BILLROTH AND GASTRIC RESECTION FOR CANCER

Theodor Billroth (1829–1894) was the strong man of the Third Vienna Medical Faculty (Fig. 1-1A). Believing that a technique could be developed for excision of gastric cancer, he sent his younger associates, Carl Gussenbauer and Alexander v. Winiwarter, to the laboratory to work out a technique of gastric resection on dogs in June, 1874 (Fig. 1-1B, C). There they developed what has subsequently come to be known as the Billroth I operation.

Only two of their seven dogs survived for a long period of time. When sacrificed eight months after the operation, one dog had two anastomotic neostomal ulcers. Two of the seven dogs died of suture leakage.

As a corollary to their study, Gussenbauer and Winiwarter examined the postmortem protocols of the Vienna Pathological Institute for the years 1817–1873 and came up with the remarkable circumstance that of 542 pyloric carcinomas, 223 (41 percent) presented no suggestion of distant metastases, an occurrence favorable to consideration of resection for gastric cancer. In approximately 43 percent, at postmortem examination the tumor was found to be movable.[6]

Billroth, one of the greatest surgical teachers of all time, had studied under Bernhard v. Langenbeck in Berlin. He had wrestled with the thought of becoming a pathologist but considered the broader, more challenging life of the surgeon, accompanied by its greater emoluments, to be a more promising life for him, and he therefore resisted offers of professorships in pathology. In 1860 Billroth became Professor of Surgery at the University of Zürich, Switzerland, where for seven years he had a record of achievement in directing an enterprising surgical clinic. In 1867 Billroth left Zürich to become Professor of Surgery at the University of Vienna and Chief of the 2nd Surgical Service. Here Billroth spent the remainder of his professional life (1867–1894), declining to become his teacher's successor in Berlin when Langenbeck retired in 1882. In both Zürich and Vienna, Billroth was greatly appreciated by his colleagues and developed strong and lasting friendships with many. In 1886 Billroth lamented the separation of operative and tutorial functions of the surgical teacher. Even so, he obviously continued the tradition of combining both functions in the surgical arena, as may be seen in a well-known painting (Fig. 1-2).

Despite his great breadth of knowledge of surgery and allied sciences, Billroth was slow in accepting Listerian practices that had emanated from Glasgow (1867), Edinburgh (1870–1877), and London (1877–1893). Lister (1827–1912) and Billroth (1829–1894) were, in fact, contemporaries. Lister's professorial career terminated at King's College Hospital in London in 1892, and his practice as an active surgeon ended there in 1893. Lister's life as a scientist culminated in 1896 in his Presidential Address before the British Association for the Advancement of Science, even though an occasional paper issued from his pen as late as 1908.

Having spent a quarter of a century in Vienna, Billroth certainly should have known the name of Semmelweis. Similarly, Hegar's great success (1876–1877) in employing Semmelweis's technique (1847, 1861) of prophylactic surgical antisepsis should have been familiar to all Vienna surgeons of Billroth's period. After a number of Lister's papers on antiseptic surgical practices had appeared in print, Billroth sent a succession of young surgeons from his Vienna clinic to Lister at the Royal Infirmary at Edinburgh and to King's College Hospital in London, where Lister had gone in 1877.

By 1881, when Billroth operated on Therese Heller for a gastric cancer, he had become a convert to surgical antisepsis. This famous operation was carried out on January 29, 1881. The historic paper appeared in print in the *Wiener Medizinische Wochenschrift* six days

[6]Gussenbauer became professor at Liege, then went to Prague before succeeding Billroth at the University of Vienna on the latter's death in 1894. Winiwarter, after the Vienna period, lived in Liege, became a Belgian citizen, and was active on the Allied side in World War I, a circumstance very disturbing to his former Austrian and German colleagues.

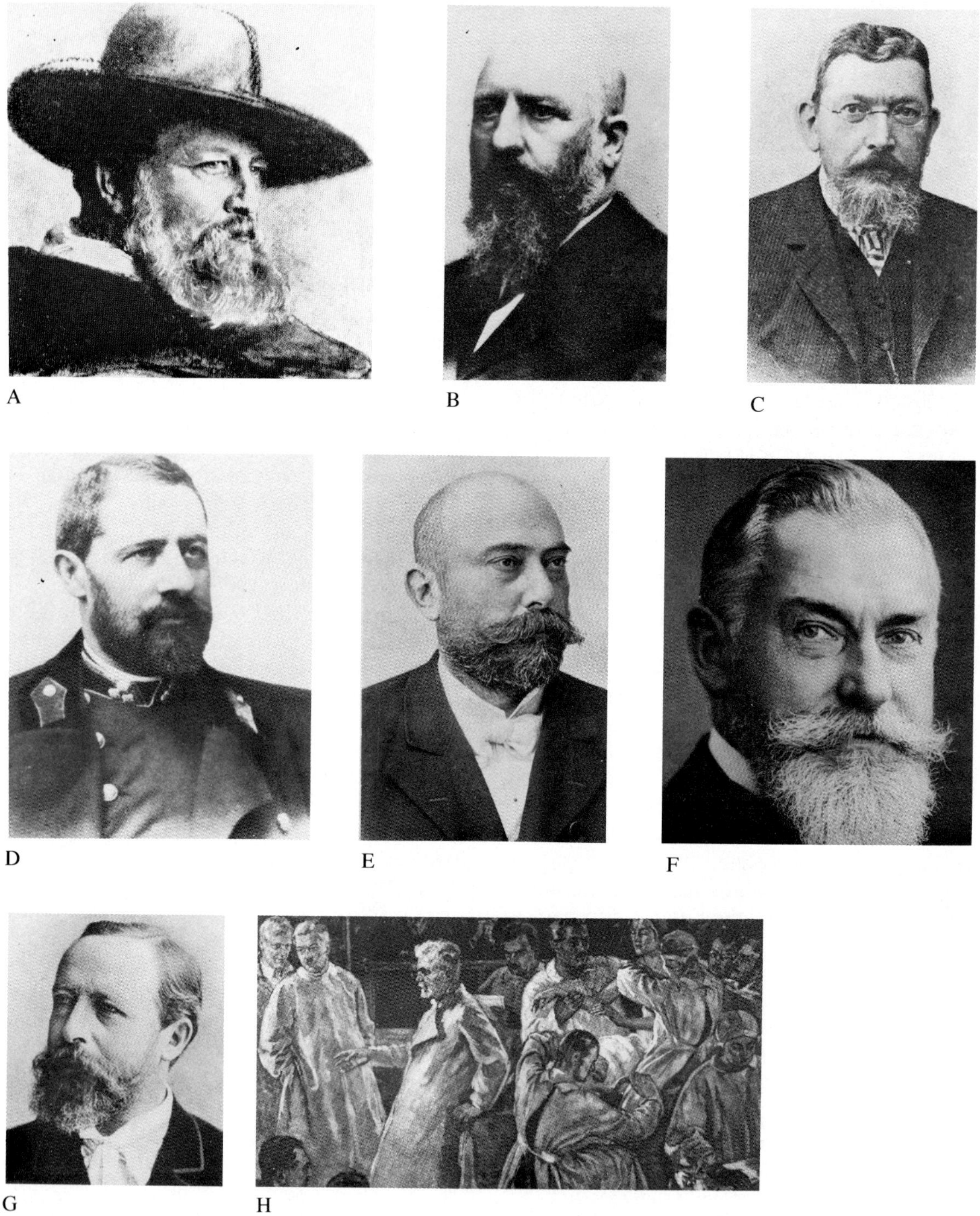

Fig. 1-1. Billroth and his Vienna School of Surgeons. (A) Theodor Billroth (1829–1894). (B) Carl Gussenbauer (1842–1903), Billroth's successor in 1894. (C) Alexander v. Winiwarter (1848–1917), with Gussenbauer, established the prototype of Billroth's gastrectomy. (D) Anton v. Wölfler (1850–1917), author of gastrojejunostomy. (E) Karl Nicoladoni (1847–1902), suggested a drainage procedure to Wölfler. Although Nicoladoni did not work with Billroth, he was a student of Wölfler, thus the connection. (F) Vincenz v. Czerny (1842–1916), who declined an offer to succeed Billroth. (G) Johann v. Mikulicz-Radecki (1850–1905). Billroth's greatest pupil. (H) Anton v. Eiselsberg (1860–1939), last of Billroth's famous Vienna pupils.

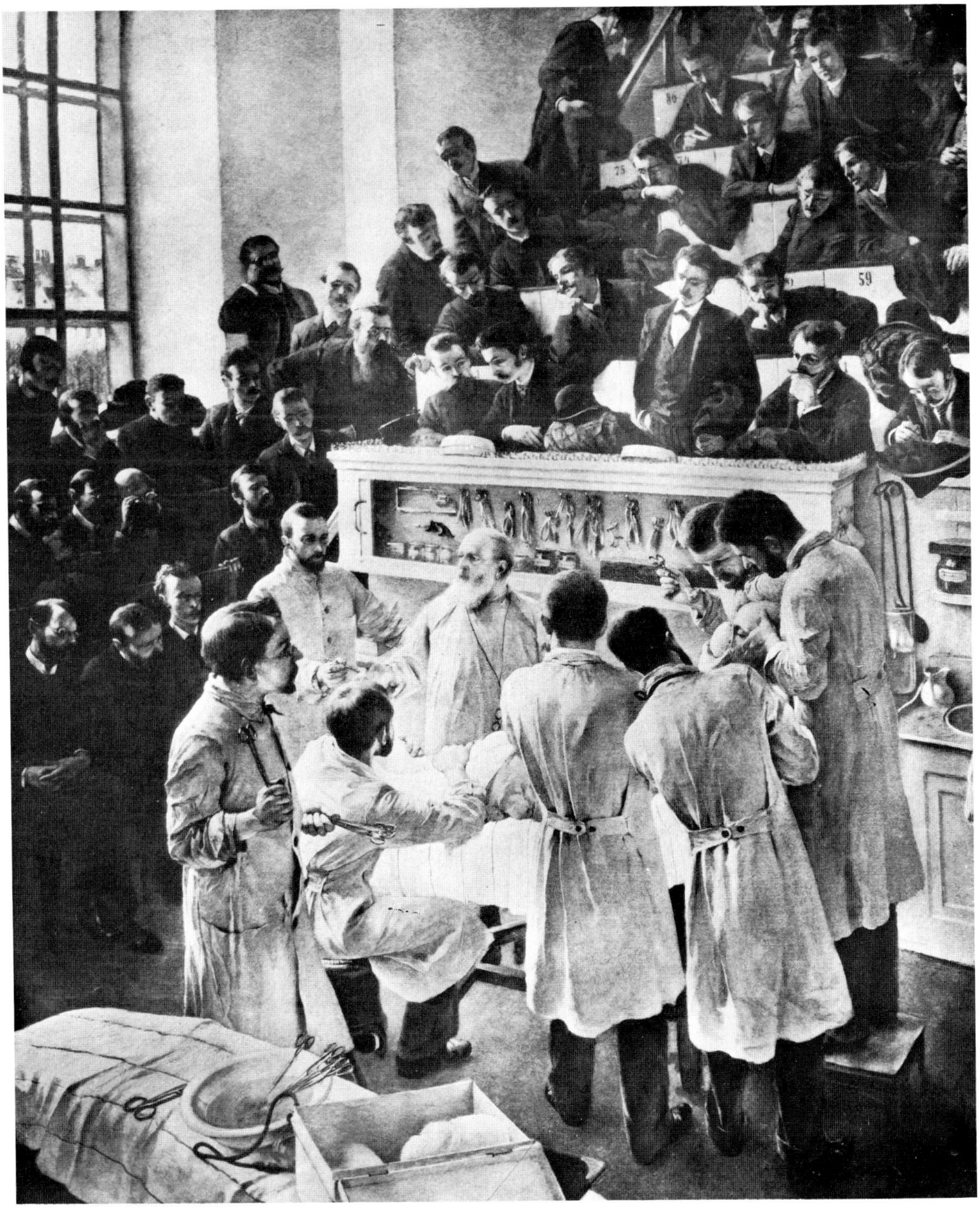

Fig. 1-2. Billroth in his new surgical amphitheater at Allgemeines Krankenhaus in 1889.

later, February 4, 1881, in a letter addressed to the editor, L. Wittelshöfer. Obviously Billroth appreciated the importance of the achievement, but his famous patient survived for only a few months.

Billroth actually was not the first to undertake resection for gastric cancer. He was preceded by Jules E. Péan of Paris (1879)[7] and Ludwik Rydygier of Culm, Poland (1880),[8] both of whom operated unsuccessfully. It is generally believed that their patients died of peritonitis from gastric leakage at the site of anastomosis, probably because the number of sutures was inadequate. Both Péan and Rydygier had used catgut sutures for the anastomoses, which were gastroduodenostomies. Herbert Ziegler (1949) reports that a surgeon in Arras, France, was the first, in 1878, to undertake gastric resection in humans, a circumstance that Ziegler says is not documented.

Billroth's operation (1881) was on Therese Heller, a 43-year-old Vienna housewife. The hospital record, as reviewed by Ziegler (1949), indicates that an hour was consumed in washing out the patient's stomach with 1½ liters of water until the returns were clear. The operation was performed under chloroform anesthesia with antiseptic precautions but without the use of carbolic acid spray.

Billroth made a right transverse incision 11 cm in length, crossing the midline[9] directly over the palpable tumor. The abdominal wall was very thin. Carbolized silk was employed for ligatures and suture. A few hazelnut-sized mesenteric lymph node metastases were found, one of which on microscopic section proved to be a medullary type of cancer. Billroth divided the duodenum 1.5 cm distal to the tumor mass through normal tissue, employing sterile cloths and sponges to protect the wound edges from contamination on opening the stomach. He approximated the edges in the lower segment of the divided stomach and made a gastroduodenal anastomosis at the lesser curvature. The sutures included the entire gastric wall except the mucosa, with similar inclusion on the duodenal side. The sutures were tied after the approximated wound edges were inverted. Billroth employed 21 sutures to approximate the edges of the gastric wound not included in the anastomosis and 33 interrupted sutures for the duodenogastric anastomosis.

Ziegler states that Billroth's patient suffered some postoperative collapse the next day; her pulse was 110 and her temperature 38.4° C (101° F). The highest postoperative temperature was 39° C (102° F). By the third postoperative day, the patient was doing extremely well and eating. When the dressing was changed on the sixth postoperative day, the wound exhibited no evidence of suppuration, and the majority of the cutaneous sutures were removed. Some fever persisted for 14 days, owing, it was believed, to a small sacral decubitus ulcer. On the 20th of February, 22 days after the operation, the patient asked for dismissal. She continued to do well for some time and survived the operation a little less than four months.

The patient died of obvious recurrence on May 24, 1881. Dr. Zemann, an assistant of Richard Heschl (Rokitansky's successor), did the autopsy, apparently in the house where the patient died. The residual gastric specimen was removed. It is reproduced from a sketch by Ziegler (Fig. 1-3).

Anton v. Wölfler (Fig. 1-1D), a pupil of Billroth, had already published a brief paper (1881), entitled "Professor Billroth's Gastric Resections for Pyloric Cancer," before Therese Heller died. Wölfler's publication was translated into Italian, Russian, and English, by which time four gastric resections for cancer had been done in Billroth's clinic. Within 11 months following Billroth's first operation, says Ziegler, 21 such operations had

[7]Péan's operation, performed April 9, 1879, lasted 2½ hours. A 5-inch long incision was made just to the left of the umbilicus. The patient was transfused twice during the postoperative period, once with 50 ml of blood and on another occasion with 80 ml. He died on the fifth day while preparations were being made for a third transfusion. Autopsy was denied. The possibility that the patient died from the transfusions cannot be excluded; this was 40 years before the establishment of blood groups made transfusion practicable. (*Gaz. Hôp.* [Paris] 52:473, 1879.)

[8]Rydygier's original Polish account (1880) appeared in a German translation in 1881. (*Dtsch. Z. Chir.* 14:252, 1881; see also *Dtsch. Ges. Chir.* 10:28, 1881.)

[9]A. v. Eiselsberg reported that Billroth subsequently used the midline vertical incision in such operations. (*Wien. Med. Wochenschr.* 86:122, 1936.)

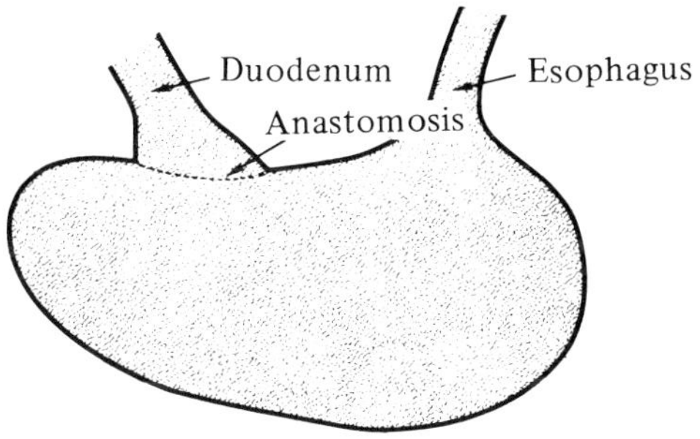

Fig. 1-3. Sketch of postmortem specimen of Therese Heller's residual stomach, upon which Billroth performed his first resection for gastric cancer. (Resketched from Ziegler, *Krebsartz* 4:49, 1949.)

been performed, several of them in Billroth's clinic. Only three of these patients survived for some period of time, all of whom had been operated on in Billroth's clinic, one by Billroth and the other two by Wölfler and Vincenz v. Czerny (Fig. 1-1F).[10] During the same period, Billroth had four operative failures. By 1890, said Ziegler, 41 gastric resections had been done for cancer in the Billroth Clinic, with 19 operative successes. In 1896 Hans Haberkant of Danzig reported that a total of 257 resections for gastric cancer had been performed, with a mortality of 54.4 percent, which was obviously not very encouraging.

TOTAL GASTRECTOMY FOR CANCER

The first successful total gastrectomy for cancer was performed by the Swiss surgeon Carl Schlatter (1897), who anastomosed the divided esophagus end-to-side to the jejunum. C. B. Brigham (1898) also excised the entire stomach, the patient surviving for an astonishingly long period of time. J. L. Herrington (1969) wrote, "It has been authenticated that the patient survived for 18 years and died of unrelated causes." This was a most unusual, miraclelike result; survival beyond three years after total gastrectomy is indeed extraordinary because of depletion of vitamin B_{12} stores in the liver.[11]

MERREM'S EXPERIMENTAL PYLORECTOMY

Daniel Merrem (1810) published a Latin account of his observations on experimental surgery in animals, including pylorectomy. He operated on three dogs, two of which survived for variable periods of time. Merrem acquired his M.D. degree from the University of Marburg in 1810 and in 1812 became General Staff Surgeon in the Westphalian Army Corps, concerned with sanitary measures in the field. He participated in the Franco-Russian campaign, returning to Germany after Napoleon's rout on the flight from Moscow.

The distinguished American medical historian Owsei Temkin has provided a translation (1957) of Merrem's description of the operation on one of the dogs that survived for 23 days. Merrem removed only 0.635 cm of the duodenum and of the stomach on either side of the pyloric sphincter, obviously a very limited resection. In effecting the anastomosis, Merrem placed three sutures ½ inch from the edge of the divided stomach, and did the same on the duodenal side.

RECOGNITION OF GASTRIC CANCER

High school students just before World War I, in their elementary course in German, read Theodor Storm, author of *Immensee*. Storm died of gastric cancer in 1888. One of his last poetical works was "Beginn des Endes," a poem that expressed well the conventional sequence of events in patients with gastric cancer. Said Storm in his poem, "It is a prick, it

[10]Eiselsberg wrote that Wölfler notified Billroth, who was away on vacation, that another patient with gastric cancer had been admitted to the clinic shortly after Billroth's first success. Should he operate or await Billroth's return? Replied Billroth, "If the patient is a woman, go ahead." Eiselsberg's inference was that Billroth believed that women tolerated peritoneal infection better than men. (*Wien. Med. Wochenschr.* 86:122, 1936.)

[11]Only since W. B. Castle's identification of the "gastric intrinsic factor" (*Am. J. Med. Sci.* 178:748, 1929) and the availability of vitamin B_{12} has it been possible to keep totally gastrectomized patients alive for periods of up to 30 years. A total gastrectomy demands that the excised stomach have a short segment of the esophagus at the proximal end and a similar duodenal segment at the site of distal section. Employing this criterion, a number of so-called total gastrectomies in the literature qualify only as nearly total gastric excisions.

is nothing; it is too late!" Translation of Storm's poem reads as follows:[12]

Beginning of the End

'Tis but a prick, 'tis scarce a pain,
  Just felt, to which no name you give:
Henceforth it speaks again—again,
  Uneasy now you have to live.

If to complain you try—of what?
  You cannot put it into speech:
Within you say, "Indeed 'tis naught!"
  Henceforth it holds fast like a leech.

So seldom strange your world does grow,
  And quickly are you stript of hope,
Until at last you really know
  That with Death's shaft you cannot cope.

It is certain that early diagnosis is the key to success in the management of all visceral cancers, including cancer of the stomach, colon, and rectum. All statistical studies provide factual evidence of the importance of early diagnosis to achieve any suggestion of success in operating for gastric cancer.

When O. H. Wangensteen succeeded to the chairmanship of the Department of Surgery of the University of Minnesota (January 1, 1930), there was not a single instance of a five-year cure following operation for gastric cancer on the records of the University Hospitals. Every experienced surgeon comes to know that his or her achievement with gastric cancer depends almost solely on having the opportunity to operate when the lesion is limited to the stomach. Most surgeons of that generation, unfortunately, were dealing with late-stage cases. Surgeons were then completely dependent on radiologists for detection of gastric cancer. Unfortunately, very few, including the most skilled American roentgenologists of the stomach, were able to detect mucosal lesions, though they had genuine expertise in finding ulcerative lesions burrowing into the gastric wall and also in recognizing polypoid lesions extending into the lumen of the stomach.

Whereas Johann v. Mikulicz Radecki (Fig. 1-1G) had employed esophagoscopy and gastroscopy with rigid instruments in the early 1880s, it remained for Rudolf Schindler (1932) to develop a flexible gastroscope. Nevertheless, frequent recourse to gastroscopy, even in the best clinics in the United States, has been, in the main, a fairly recent development, to which the very flexible Olympic fiberscope has made a significant contribution.[13]

In November, 1966, during the International Cancer Conference in Tokyo, Wangensteen had the opportunity to witness, in Professor Komei Nakayama's Surgical Clinic at the Women's Medical College in Tokyo, the Japanese radiographers' manner of detecting early gastric cancers. With the patient erect, 200 cc of air was injected into the stomach through a nasal catheter. Then a very modest amount of barium, not more than a few ounces, was swallowed by the patient, and the fluoroscopist, in broad daylight, carried out an examination of about 45 minutes, rotating the patient in many positions and taking as many as 40 films. What the radiographer saw was delineated on a nearby television screen.

On completion of the examination, the films were immediately inspected, and gastroscopy and biopsy were done if a suspicious lesion was noted. As many as 20 gastroscopies were being performed per day in well-organized Japanese gastroenterology clinics. During the same period (1966) in the University of Minnesota Hospitals, perhaps as many as two or three gastroscopies were done in a week.

During this visit to Japan, David State and Wangensteen attended a conference on gastric cancer in Nagoya and saw several impressive presentations of materials accumulated by Japanese oncologists including pathologists, radiographers, gastroscopists, and surgeons. Their cooperation was very noticeable and was obviously a telling factor in the ability of Japanese surgeons to detect and operate on mucosal gastric cancers in the early stage, achieving five-year survival rates of 25 percent among all patients with gastric cancer reporting for study—an accomplishment that

[12]Translated for O. H. Wangensteen by Elizabeth Nissen in 1947.

[13]We no longer see perforation of the cervical esophagus attending esophagoscopy and gastroscopy, which occurred not infrequently with the use of earlier, more rigid instruments.

exceeds the performance of experienced gastric surgeons everywhere.

Many were bewildered by the fact that the Japanese had achieved recognition of early mucosal gastric cancers that had defied American radiographers and surgeons. In the ensuing discussion, State proposed the establishment of an international panel for the appraisal and assessment of the Japanese findings, a suggestion accepted by the Japanese panelists with the polite, impenetrable smile of the afternoon Japanese teahouse. Wangensteen took home the large and well-illustrated tome on gastric cancer by M. Kuru (1967), Director of the Japanese Imperial Tokyo Cancer Institute, and showed it to colleagues in the Department of Pathology at Minnesota. They informed him that, without exception, the instances of early mucosal gastric cancers illustrated in Kuru's book were definitely cancer and not simple gastritis. This represented an extraordinary and significant development to Wangensteen (1968), who could only wish he had the opportunity to relive his long experience in attempting to achieve a better record with gastric cancer.[14] As did many surgeons of that day, he lamented having the misfortune of being far too long on the wrong side of the cancer "woodpile." Fresh cases were piling in daily, but the surgeons failed to recognize them.

A high index of suspicion in the clinician's mind has been and continues to be an important factor in the recognition of all malignant tumors. Wangensteen stressed over the years the importance of an achlorhydric response to histamine in the recognition of gastric cancer; as a consequence of this policy, he continued to receive greetings in the Christmas holiday season from patients in whom near-total or total gastrectomy was done for gastric cancer 25 to 30 and more years before. If a patient has abdominal pain, a demonstrable gastric defect, and achlorhydria, no competent physician would advise delay; over the years, however, Wangensteen's chief role as a consultant had often been to suggest that the patient have a gastric analysis under histamine stimulation. Unfortunately, this simple expedient is too often neglected and a gastric defect is merely watched when it should be submitted to gastroscopic biopsy or immediate resection.

The Swedish radiographer Sølve Welin of Malmö, employing air-contrast studies in the detection of lesions of the colon, a method very similar to that in current practice with Japanese radiographers, stated in 1955 that he could detect lesions 5 mm in diameter. Welin put considerably more air into the colon than the Japanese radiographers placed in the stomach but used far less barium in the examination than most of his American counterparts.

The technique that Welin used in the colon with such great success in the detection of tiny mucosal lesions should be invoked also by all radiographers for the early detection of mucosal gastric cancer. For oncoming American surgeons of the alimentary tract, the air-contrast studies of Welin and Japanese radiographers should be of the greatest help in bringing patients with gastric and colon cancer to operation early, thus providing an opportunity for greater achievement with the problem, which was denied gastric surgeons of earlier days.

David W. Gelfand of Detroit (1975) reported an experience of 2000 examinations in the Japanese style of air-barium contrast x-ray studies of the stomach; he found the method far more sensitive in the detection of small lesions than conventional radiography.

EARLY DETECTION ATTITUDE

In a comprehensive tract on gastric cancer, William H. Welch (1885) wrote quite discouragingly on surgical treatment of the lesion. He reported that no instances of recovery following operation for gastric cancer had been recorded, even though Billroth's operative success "made a great sensation in the medical world." The longest survival time after operation was only one and a half years, probably Wölfler's patient. He indicated, nevertheless,

[14]Over the nine-year period 1950–1958 at the University of Minnesota's Department of Surgery, the best achievement of five-year symptomless survival was 17 percent of all gastric cancer patients who came for diagnosis and treatment. (*Am. J. Surg.* 115:7, 1968.)

that though the promise was not great, surgery was the only hope.

Fifteen years later William Osler and Thomas McCrae (1900) wrote a small monograph on cancer of the stomach. They had nothing to report concerning the results of surgery but said it was the only hope. In 1916 Frank Smithies and Albert Ochsner addressed the same problem in a large monograph in which Ochsner dealt primarily with operative techniques of managing gastric cancer (1916) but had very little to say concerning results.

On the occasion of the International Conference on Cancer held in London in August, 1928, which Wangensteen had the pleasure of attending as a representative of the University of Minnesota, King George V, through his advisors, said, "I note with interest that your object is research, both into the cure and causes of cancer. No doubt, in the last resort the discovery of the cause is the only certain and absolute means of cure. But I am glad you have not ignored the practical side of the problem. Remembering the thousands of sufferers from cancer, I feel that if your discussions lead to advance in diagnosis, treatment, or even palliation of disease, this Conference will have justified itself and earned the gratitude of mankind." Events of the intervening half century suggest that those well-chosen words of King George V were indeed prophetic.

Professor N. Friedreich (1874) of Heidelberg had reported cure of a patient treated with ingestion of a decoction of condurango. The remedy apparently emanated from Ecuador, and the Surgeon General of the Navy, Dr. W. S. W. Ruschenberger, was sent to Quito to assess the situation. He reported in a 28-page monograph (1873) that there was much testimony but little evidence that condurango cured gastric cancer. Undoubtedly, Friedrich had confused gastric ulcer with cancer.[15]

In the second edition of this monograph, *Surgery of the Stomach and Duodenum* (1969), Wolfgang Denk reported (p. 23) that Billroth had performed 34 resections for gastric cancer, with a hospital mortality of 48.1 percent. During the period from October, 1889 to October, 1894, the mortality for gastric resections, said Denk, had been lowered to 29.4 percent at the Billroth Clinic.

DECREASED INCIDENCE

Since 1940 there has been a significant decrease in the incidence and mortality of gastric cancer. At one time cancer of the stomach was the leading cause of death from cancer in the United States. In more recent years, the most frequent cause of death from cancer has been cancer of the colon and rectum, which takes approximately fifty thousand lives annually. A similar drop in the incidence of gastric cancer has been observed in the Scandinavian countries. It still continues to be very prevalent in Chile, Iceland, Hungary, and Japan. What etiological factors are involved in the observed decrease in the Scandinavian countries and in the United States remains an enigma.

HOPELESS ATTITUDE TOWARD GASTRIC CANCER NOW OBSOLETE

No discussion of chronic gastric ulcer is complete without considering the possibility that the lesion might be malignant. A panel discussion on the management of gastric ulcer was held in late October, 1954 at the Walter Reed General Hospital, one of the great military hospitals of the world. In the ensuing discussion, E. D. Palmer, a well-known American gastroenterologist, stated, "I do not think a patient with cancer of the stomach should be operated upon unless there is a complication, such as obstruction." We hope such therapeutic nihilism concerning the curability of gastric cancer is now extinct.

The discussion just alluded to took place 70 years after Welch (1885) appraised the unpromising role of surgery in dealing with gastric cancer yet recognized that surgery was the only hope for patients afflicted with the lesion. Survey of a 22-year experience (1936–1958) with gastric cancer at the University of

[15]Wangensteen first learned of the use of decoction of condurango as a treatment for gastric cancer while a student in the Medical Outpatient Department at the University of Minnesota in the early 1920s. Dr. C. B. Wright, an accomplished internist with a special interest in the alimentary canal, customarily prescribed condurango for patients with gastric cancer and sent them home with the advice to return in six months.

Minnesota Hospitals disclosed that 183 patients undergoing resection for gastric cancer were alive and free from disease 5 to 20 years after operation—to be sure, a very modest accomplishment.

Today, with far better techniques of early recognition and the disappearance of therapeutic skeptics, a greatly improved achievement in dealing with gastric cancer is a foregone conclusion. Early diagnosis and adequate gastrectomy accompanied by proper regional lymphadenectomy provide the best assurances of a satisfying outcome. Better anesthesia, recognition of the electrolyte and fluid needs of patients, finer techniques of gastrointestinal anastomoses, and use of inlying nasogastric duodenal suction tubes are also important factors in bringing about this dramatic improvement in mortality in operations for gastric cancer. Nevertheless, the mortality continues to be considerably higher than in similar operations for peptic ulcer.

EVOLUTION OF GASTRIC ANASTOMOSES

Billroth's first gastric resection was a gastroduodenal anastomosis with partial closure of the aboral gastric segment. Observance of leaks at the lesser curvature in the anastomosis led to its being called the *Jammer Ecke* ("crying corner"), a technical matter that has long since been overcome by surgeons. Billroth subsequently closed the proximal end of the divided stomach completely and added a gastrojejunostomy, an operation that Wölfler had performed in September, 1881 for an obstructing gastric cancer that he regarded as unresectable. Karl Nicoladoni, who assisted at the operation, made the suggestion of performing the drainage procedure to Wölfler during the operation (Fig. 1-1E).

There was a period extending up to the early 1940s when surgeons continued to debate whether gastrojejunal anastomoses should be isoperistaltic or retroperistaltic, anterior or retrocolic; whether the afferent jejunal loop should be long or short; and whether the entire width of the divided stomach should be employed in the anastomosis. A long list of distinguished names emerged with suggestions of additional variants in the technique.[16]

More gastric surgeons today favor the Hofmeister partial closure of the oral segment of the divided stomach rather than the Reichel-Pólya anastomosis, which united the entire width of the divided stomach to the jejunum. William J. Mayo made the work of the Budapest surgeon Eugen Pólya known to American surgeons (Fig. 1-4A, E). William Mayo, who with his brother Charles developed one of the world's great surgical clinics, was a pioneer in gastric cancer surgery in America. He died of gastric cancer at age 78.

In our view, the only important desideratum is that the anastomosis be at least as wide as the diameter of the smallest participating component in the union. The jejunum at the level of the ligament of Treitz varies normally between 4 and 4.5 cm in diameter (Fig. 1-5).

All anastomoses are, in effect, end-to-end unions; patency of the afferent inlet and the efferent outlet, with closure of the intervening gastric and jejunal walls, constitutes the only important technical consideration. The debates throughout more than half a century over the observed vicious circle (1885–1942) relate almost solely to the surgeon's desire to escape iatrogenic obstructions, which were attributed to a variety of unrelated causes. On observing the experimental studies of Clarence Dennis on the use of the closed anastomosis in the Department of Surgery at Minnesota, Wangensteen became a convert in 1939 to closed anastomoses, employing a one-layer closure with interrupted sutures of fine silk inverting not less than 5 mm nor more than 7.5 mm of the adjacent walls of the lumina to be approximated. This simple guide served to point up the circumstance that overinversion was the sole cause of efferent outlet obstruction in gastrojejunal anastomoses, an observation confirmed by an experience of more than two decades in making such anas-

[16]Courvoisier (1883), v. Hacker (1885), Krönlein (1888), Jaboulay (1892), Kocher (1893), Braun (1893), Roux (1897), Shoemaker (1911), Devine (1925), and Bancroft (1932) deserve mention as having described variants of gastrojejunal anastomoses. (See John M. Waugh and Robert T. Hood, Jr., Gastric operations: A historic review, *Q. Rev. Surg. Gynecol. Obstet.* 10:201, 1953, and 11:1, 1954.)

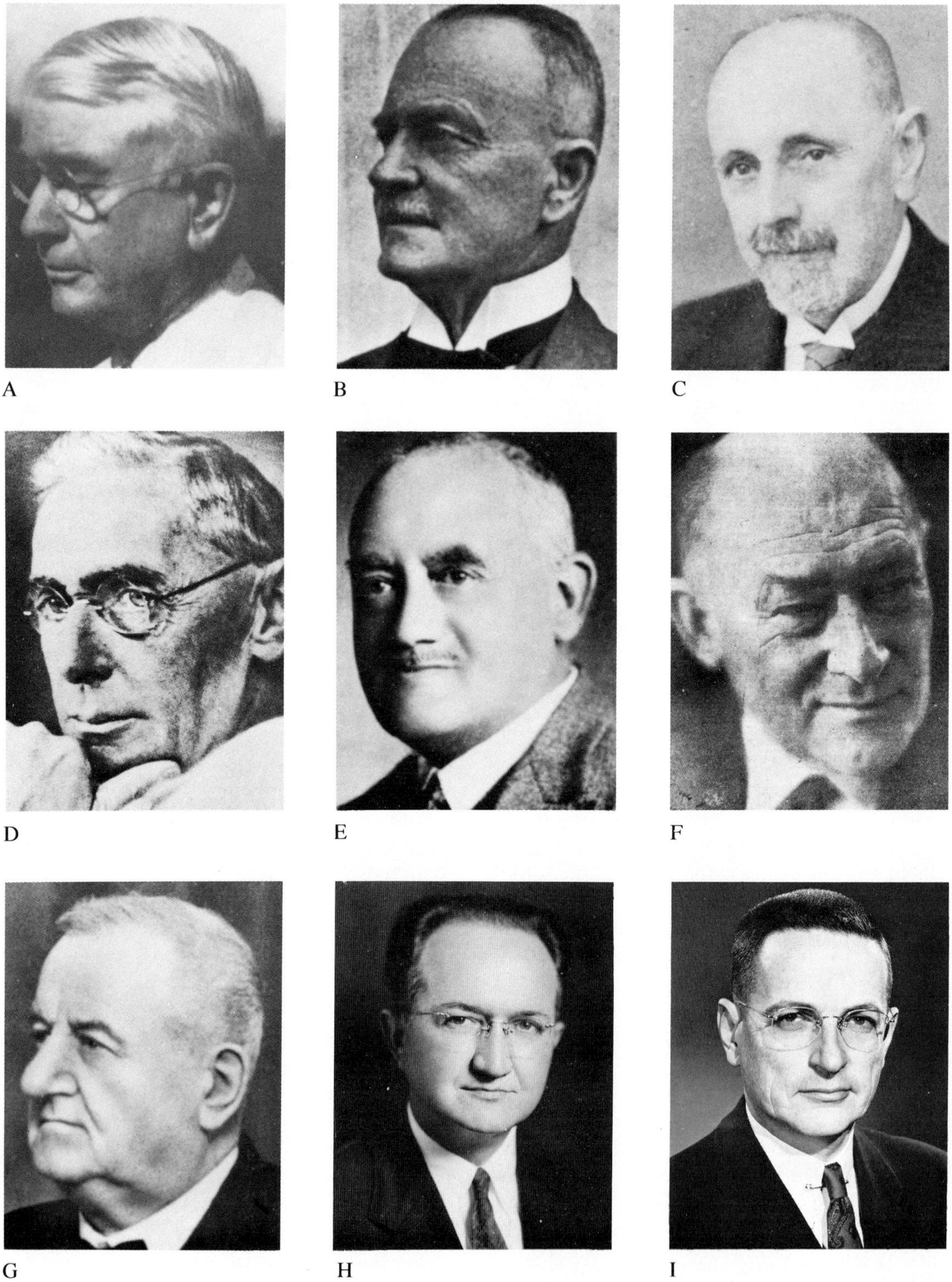

Fig. 1-4. Other illustrious gastric surgeons. (A) William J. Mayo (1861–1939), America's pioneer gastric cancer surgeon. (B) Eugen Enderlen (1863–1940), distinguished for significant experiments on peptic ulcer. (C) Hans Finsterer (1874–1955), who advanced surgery for peptic ulcer by continual evaluation of his own surgical results. (D) Hans v. Haberer (1875–1958), keenest exponent of the Billroth I operation for many years. (E) Eugen Pólya (1876–1944), distinguished Hungarian gastric surgeon and patriot. (F) André Latarjet (1876–1947), first among gastric surgeons

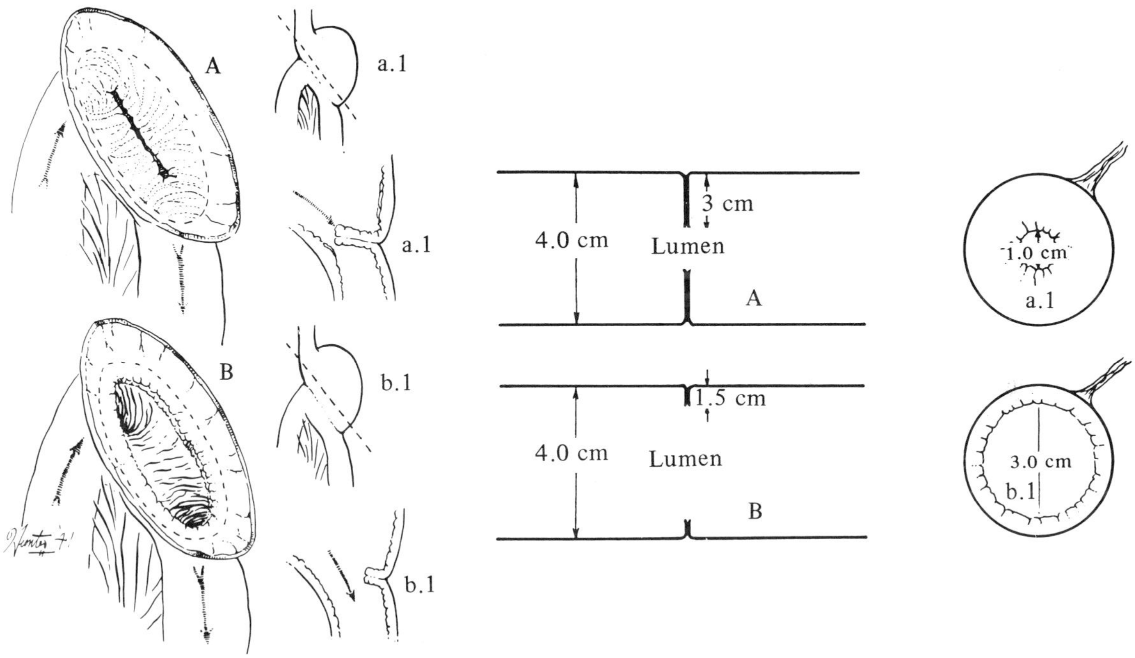

Fig. 1-5. (A) Hofmeister gastrojejunal anastomosis, indicating that the conventional gastrojejunal three-row suture inversion of the 1930s could readily obstruct the efferent outlet. Preservation of a patulous afferent inlet and of the efferent outlet is assured by the one-row suture inversion. (B) Compromise of the lumen in end-to-end jejunal anastomosis. The single one-layer closure, with minimal inversion (0.5–0.75 cm), ensures a patulous lumen. (From O. H. Wangensteen, *Intestinal Obstructions* (3d ed.), 1955, pp. 328–329. Courtesy of Charles C Thomas, Publisher, Springfield, Ill.)

to recognize that complemental gastrojejunostomy could convert vagotomy failure to success. (G) Swiss surgeon Eugen Bircher (1882–1956), first to perform selective vagotomy for peptic ulcer. (H) Lester R. Dragstedt (1893–1975), illustrious experimentalist and keen exponent of vagotomy for duodenal ulcer. (I) Henry N. Harkins (1905–1967), led the renaissance in the use of the Billroth I anastomosis (gastroduodenostomy) and demonstrated the feasibility of selective and highly selective methods of vagotomy.

tomoses without incurring any instances of outlet obstruction, which had plagued gastric surgeons for decades. Certainly the conventional three-row gastrointestinal sutures of four decades ago are now only a matter of history, reflecting the slowness of the learning process.[17]

Arthur Allen and Claude Welch (1941), great Boston gastric surgeons of that era, indicated that obstruction of the efferent stoma occurred frequently in patients undergoing gastrojejunal anastomoses at the Massachusetts General Hospital and that secondary op-

[17]Wangensteen relates: "Shortly after the end of World War II, I was visited by Paul Banzet, a distinguished gastric surgeon from Paris. I took him to the operating room, where my then Senior Resident, Yoshio Sako, was doing a Billroth II resection for duodenal ulcer. Within the hour our visitor was back in my office, protesting the single-layer closure of the divided duodenum and of the gastrojejunal anastomosis. Said he, 'Why, I use five rows of sutures to invert the duodenal stump.' I replied, 'What good are the other four if the first inversion is inadequate?' After all, adequate inversion is a major desideratum in all gastrointestinal suturing."

erations to relieve persistent stomal obstruction of the efferent outlet were necessary in 5.3 percent of the overall group of patients undergoing such operations.

Surgeons need to be more mindful of the architecture of all anastomoses of tubular structures. The experience of this clinic over the 1939–1967 period suggests very definitely that stomal obstruction is not observed if the luminal diameter of the smallest participating component, the jejunum, is not compromised.

Importance of the Submucous Coat in Gastrointestinal Surgery

Students of the problem of intestinal anastomoses often credit Halsted with the discovery of the importance of including the strong submucous coat of the intestine in the performance of intestinal suture and anastomoses. However, Antoine Lembert (1826) apparently included the entire thickness of the intestinal wall in making such anastomoses, for he indicated that the sutures were extruded into the intestinal lumen. Halsted (1887), on the basis of a few beautifully executed experiments, rightfully pointed out that such is not good practice—that sutures penetrating the intestinal lumen produce bending or kinking of the intestine accompanied by serosal adhesions, probably suggesting leakage through the needle tract to the peritoneal surface. Halsted and others have observed that sutures extending into the lumen of the intestine are extruded into the intestine. Conversely, Halsted observed in his experiments that when the suture needle includes the submucosa but does not enter the intestinal lumen, the sutures remain in place and are not extruded either to the peritoneal surface or into the lumen of the intestine.[18] Inasmuch as the mucosal blood vessels lie in the submucosa, we use pallor of the serosal intestinal surface over the needle point to determine whether the suture needle has included the submucosa; also, increased tissue resistance to the needle provides additional evidence.

Incision for Extended Gastrectomy

In his first gastrectomy, Billroth used an upper transverse incision but in subsequent operations elected a vertical incision. For high-lying lesions, some surgeons make the approach through a left thoracoabdominal incision. Wangensteen found the vertical extrapleural sternal-split incision, shown in Figure 1-6, to provide excellent exposure of the upper abdomen and the lower reaches of the thoracic esophagus.

Cancers high on the gastric lesser curvature mandate total gastrectomy. The Roux-en-Y anastomosis (Fig. 1-7A), precluding intraesophageal regurgitation, is to be preferred to the end-to-side esophagojejunal anastomosis (Fig. 1-7B), even though an enteroanastomosis is provided. An adequate lymphadenectomy is an integral part of a satisfactory operation for gastric cancer.

Peptic Ulcer

Techniques of gastric surgery for the relief of peptic ulcer are direct outgrowths of operations devised by Billroth and his associates for gastric cancer. When Rydygier (1882) performed a successful Billroth I resection for a benign pyloric ulcer, the editor of *Zentralblatt für Chirurgie* commented, "Hoffentlich auch letzte." ("Hopefully, also the last.") Shortly thereafter, in the hands of French and German surgeons, gastric surgery for peptic ulcer became popular.

DERIVATION OF THE DESIGNATION "PEPTIC ULCER"

Tables 1-1, 1-2, and 1-3 provide information on the progress of knowledge concerning gastric secretion derived from experiment and observation. What elements in gastric juice are responsible for its solvent action was long a matter of speculation.

[18] Peter D. Olch, long an ardent student of Halsted and his important contributions to the literature, observed that the National Library of Medicine's copy of Samuel D. Gross's monograph, *Experimental and Critical Inquiry into the Nature and Treatment of Wounds of the Intestine* (1843), had a marginal notation in Halsted's handwriting (pages 4 and 5) that read "copy," obviously a note to his secretary. Gross had pointed out that the submucosa is the strongest coat of the intestine; his publication antedated elective abdominal surgery by four decades. In his treatise of 1887 on intestinal suture, Halsted does not include a reference to Gross's observation; he does, however, allude to Lembert.

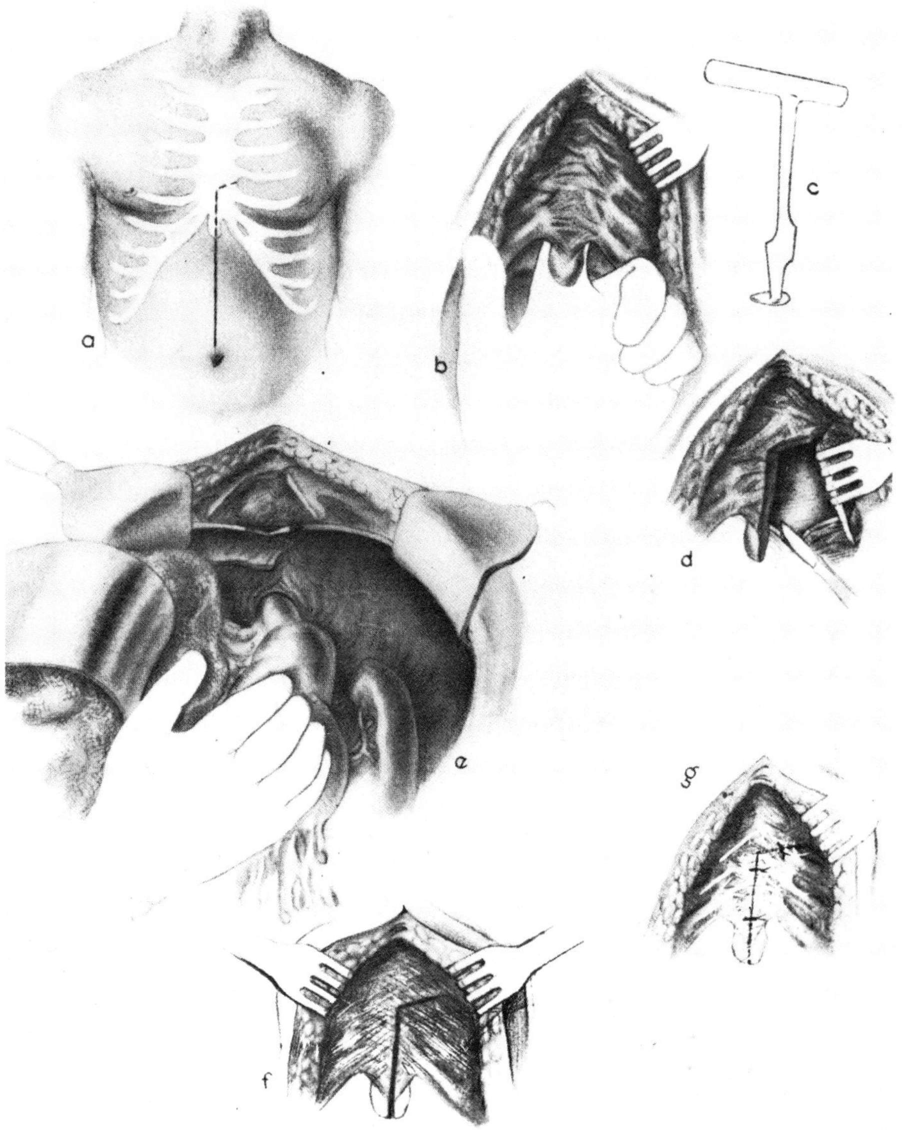

Fig. 1-6. Exposure provided by sternal-split incision for total gastrectomy. (From O. H. Wangensteen, *Rev. Gastroenterol.* 20:611,1953.)

L'Académie Royale des Sciences proposed in 1823 a prize for a series of chemical and physiological experiments pointing up the nature of digestion. In 1825 the Royal Commission, consisting of some of the greatest contemporary French scientists—Magendie, Gay-Lussac, Cuvier, Duméril, and Thenard, announced that no prize would be awarded but that two papers submitted would receive honorable mention and an award of 1500 French francs each. First cited was the entry of the French investigators, F. Leuret and J. L. Lassaigne; the second paper was that of F. Tiedemann and L. Gmelin of Heidelberg, which had been submitted by title, without the names of the authors. Interestingly, the French authors found the acid in the gastric juice to be lactic; Tiedemann and Gmelin had correctly concluded it was hydrochloric acid (HCl). When

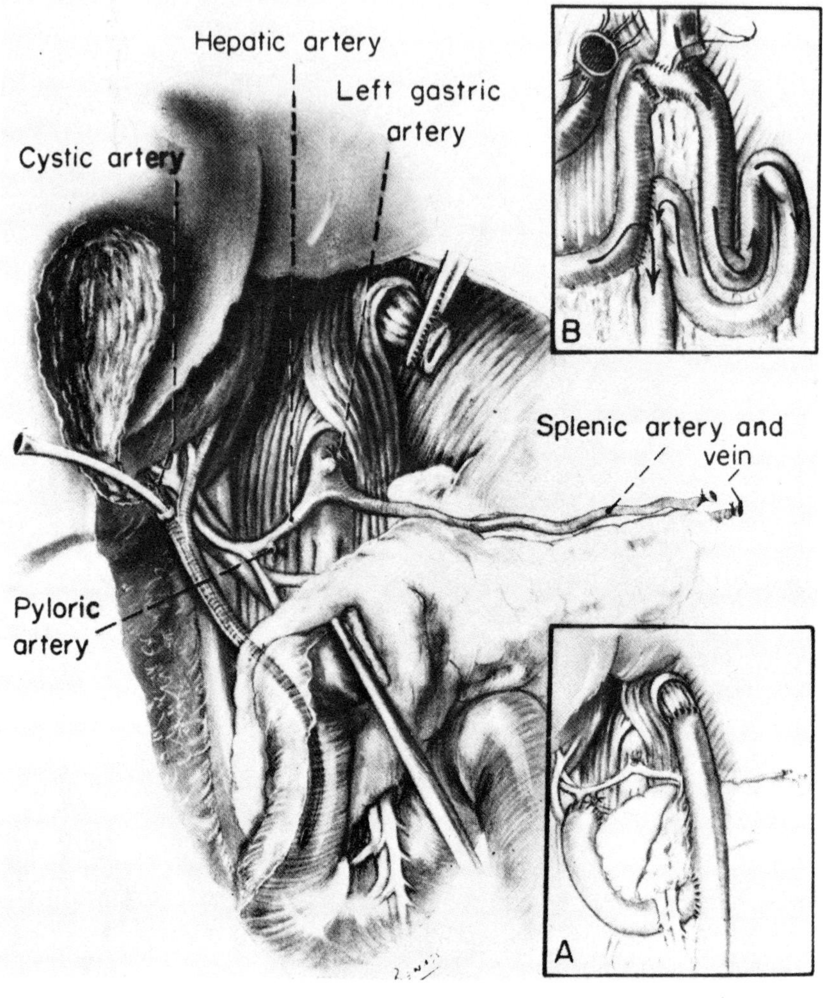

Fig. 1-7. Total gastrectomy and completed lymph-node dissection. The Roux-en-Y anastomosis (A) is preferable to the end-to-end or end-to-side esophagojejunal anastomosis (B).

the decision of the commission was announced, the German authors declined both the honorable mention and the money, indicating that their results would have been verified if the commissioners had repeated the experiments, as they properly should have done. This was certainly not the first nor the last time that a royal or other commission had come up with a judgment that time proved wrong.

In his elegant small monograph (1833) William Beaumont recognized the presence of a ferment in the gastric juice, conclusion no. 24, among his 51 summating observations (Fig. 1-8A). The conclusion reads: "It [gastric juice] contains free *Muriatic Acid* and some other chemical principles." Beaumont made this "clairvoyant" deduction by noting the difference between the digestive power of the gastric juice in Alexis St. Martin's stomach and that of collected gastric juice, kept in a beaker at room temperature, in which weighed amounts of food were submerged. Beaumont determined in every experiment the exact temperature of Alexis' stomach (usually in the area of 38° C [100° F]), whereas the temperature on the shelves of the laboratory, where

Table 1-1. Experiments on gastric digestion

Author	Date of publication	Method of experiment	Findings and conclusions
Tyson	1683	Snake	Corrosive menstruum
Vallisnieri	1713	Ostrich	Gastric juice, the active agent in digestion
Réaumur	1752	Sponges and spheres in birds, dog, sheep	Disproved trituration; established solvent power of gastric juice
Stevens	1777	Perforated spheres: humans, dog, sheep	Stomach secretes powerful solvent
Spallanzani	1780	Sponges, metal tubes: fish, birds, cat, dog, humans	Digestion performed by gastric juice
Hunter	1786	Fish, lizards, frogs	Powerful digestive ferment Thesis of "living principle"
Young	1803	Snake, frog, humans	Powerful digestive menstruum; supported Hunter's "living principle"
Beaumont	1825 1833	Alexis St. Martin	Solvent power of gastric juice for food and chemical agents
Flourens	1832	Sheep, rabbits	Living animals are digested when placed in stomach
Schwann	1836	In vitro studies	Pepsin
Bernard	1855	Gastric fistula, dog	Disproved "living principle"
Pavy	1856	Gastric fistula, dog	Confirmed Bernard's findings

Source: Data from O. H. Wangensteen, Claude Bernard's Work on Digestion. In F. Grande and M. B. Visscher (Eds.), *Claude Bernard and Experimental Medicine*. Cambridge, Mass.: Schenkman, 1967. P. 63. Reproduced by permission of the publisher.

the collected juice was kept, was usually between 1° C and 4.5° C (30° F and 40° F).

Beaumont's conclusion no. 25 is probably equally important: Free HCl is absent in the empty stomach; its secretion is provoked by the presence of food. Gastric physiologists were slow to appreciate fully this important observation of Beaumont, a circumstance responsible for designating the gastric acid of the empty stomach as lactic or phosphoric acid. The presence of free HCl in an empty stomach suggests the patient may have a duodenal ulcer.

Johannes Müller and Theodor Schwann (1836), on reading Beaumont's monograph, boiled a sample of gastric juice and noted it had lost its proteolytic quality, thus verifying Beaumont's conclusion that gastric juice contained "chemical principles" other than HCl. Schwann called the ferment *pepsin,* adding that Hippocrates had employed the term *pepsis* for the "cooking" activity of the stomach on food.

Claude Bernard decided in 1853 at age 40 to give up a career in clinical surgery to become one of the first professional physiologists (Fig. 1-8B).[19] He disproved the "living principle" of John Hunter by immersing a frog in the gastric fistula of a dog, demonstrating that peptic digestion of the living frog's legs did occur.

Interestingly enough, Lester Dragstedt, the greatest among surgical students of peptic ulcer, suggested in 1936 that the qualifying word *peptic* be deleted in describing ulcer and that the term used should be *acid ulcer* (Fig. 1-4H). In a simple experiment performed in this laboratory by Enrique Sanchez and asso-

[19]Bernard's superb anatomical dissections alerted his teacher, Francis Magendie, to his great promise as an investigator. Copies of Bernard's *Operative Surgery,* written with Charles Huette in 1856, were issued to all military surgeons of the Union Army in the American Civil War (1861–1865).

Table 1-2. Experiments on the nature of gastric secretion

Author	Date of publication	Method of experiment	Findings and conclusions
Réaumur	1752	Birds, dogs, sheep	Changes blue litmus paper red
Hunter	1772	Humans	Weak acid
	1786	Humans	Uncertain
Spallanzani	1780	Birds, fish, dogs, humans	Occasionally but not usually acid; varies with type of food
Magendie	1817	Dogs	Lactic acid
Prout	1824	Animals and humans	Hydrochloric acid
Children	1824	Humans	Hydrochloric acid (confirmed Prout)
Leuret and Lassaigne	1825	Dogs	Lactic acid
Tiedemann and Gmelin	1826	Dogs	Hydrochloric acid
Beaumont	1833	Humans (gastric fistula)	Hydrochloric acid; chemical principle
Braconnot	1835	Dogs (juice collected on sponges)	Hydrochloric acid
Blondlot	1843	Dog (gastric fistula)	Phosphoric acid
Bernard	1844	Dogs	Lactic acid
Bidder and Schmidt	1852	Dogs and sheep	Hydrochloric acid
Smith	1856	Alexis St. Martin	Lactic acid
Pavy	1856	Rabbits, dogs, humans	Hydrochloric acid
Holmes	1861	Inference	Findings favor lactic acid

Source: Data from O. H. Wangensteen, Claude Bernard's Work on Digestion. In F. Grande and M. B. Visscher (Eds.), *Claude Bernard and Experimental Medicine*. Cambridge, Mass.: Schenkman, 1967. Pp. 66–68. Reproduced by permission of the publisher.

Table 1-3. Physiological milestones in the study of gastric secretion

Author	Date	Discovery
Klemensiewicz	1875	Isolated antral pouch
Heidenhain	1878, 1879	Denervated gastric pouch
Pavlov	1897	Innervated gastric pouch
Sokolov	1904	Acid antral inhibition
Edkins	1906	Antral influence (gastrin)
Popielski	1920	Histamine found to be powerful gastric secretory stimulant
Mann et al.	1923	Duodenoileal drainage
Smidt	1923, 1924	Antral exclusion provokes hypersecretion
Lim et al.	1925	Denervated isolated stomach
Dragstedt	1930	Innervated total stomach
Code, Varco	1940	Histamine in beeswax
Dragstedt et al.	1951	Transplantation antrum to colon
Griffith, Harkins	1957	Modified vagotomy
Gregory, Tracy	1961	Purification of gastrin
Gregory et al.	1964	Structure of gastrin

Source: Data from O. H. Wangensteen, Claude Bernard's Work on Digestion. In F. Grande and M. B. Visscher (Eds.), *Claude Bernard and Experimental Medicine*. Cambridge, Mass.: Schenkman, 1967. Pp. 73–74. Reproduced by permission of the publisher.

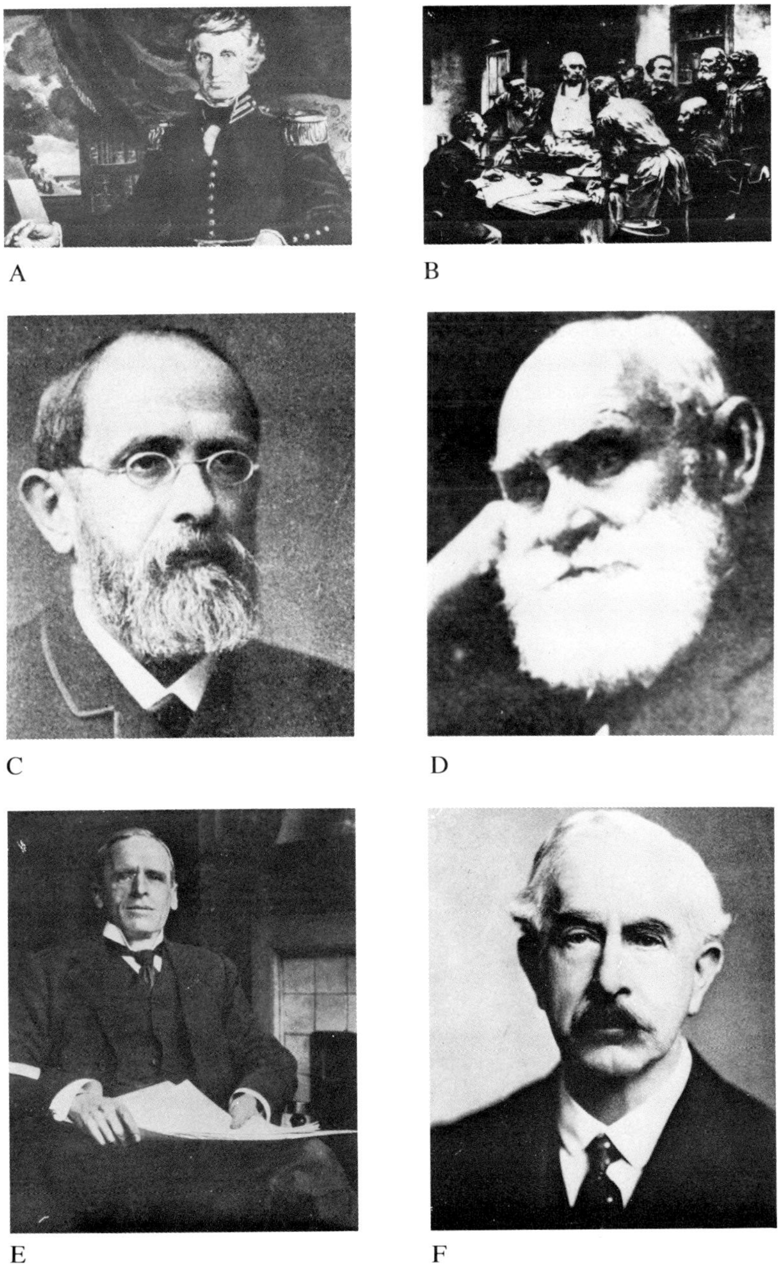

Fig. 1-8. Nineteenth-century gastric physiologists. (A) William Beaumont (1785–1853), whose experiments in remote American Army posts promoted understanding of gastric digestion and secretion. (B) Claude Bernard (1813–1878), first professional French physiologist, and associates. (C) Rudolf Heidenhain (1834–1897), innovator of the denervated isolated gastric pouch. (D) Ivan Pavlov (1849–1936), the greatest physiologist of digestion. (E) Ernest Starling (1866–1927), distinguished English physiologist, discoverer of secretin. (F) John Edkins (1863–1940), who discovered gastrin.

ciates (1948), it was observed that excision of the acid- and pepsin-secreting area of the stomach attending complemental pyloric obstruction failed to produce esophageal perforation in dogs on administration of histamine. Donald Ferguson and his associates (1950), in the same laboratory, observed that perfusion of the cat's esophagus with gastric juice obtained from patients with duodenal ulcer caused perforation quite regularly within 2 hours and occasionally within 20 minutes, whereas irrigation of the cat's esophagus with 0.10N HCl caused only slight reddening. Wangensteen, H. D. Root, and associates (1958) subsequently demonstrated that cooled gastric juice, on the contrary, exhibited no proteolytic effect on the esophageal mucosa. Obviously, the designation *peptic ulcer* must be retained.

EARLY EXPERIMENTAL VAGOTOMY STUDIES

The discovery of the influence of vagal denervation on gastric secretion has a long history dating back to Benjamin Brodie (1814), who observed that the mucosa of the empty stomach appeared dry a few hours after bilateral vagal section. Friedrich Bidder and Carl Schmidt (1852) noted that the sight and smell of food excited gastric secretion. Moritz Schiff (1867) showed that dogs could remain in good health and nutrition after bilateral subdiaphragmatic vagal section. The creation of an isolated denervated pouch by Rudolf Heidenhain (1878) of Breslau and an innervated pouch by Ivan Pavlov (1887–1904) lent tremendous impetus to the study of gastric secretion (Fig. 1-8C, D). In the canine experiments in which he developed the isolated, denervated gastric pouch, Heidenhain employed Listerian antiseptic practices. Heidenhain died of a perforated ulcer.

PAVLOV'S WORK ON GASTRIC SECRETION

The work of Pavlov and his physiological school in gastric physiology, which won Pavlov the Nobel Prize in 1904, is the finest in the literature. He was a master experimentalist; his work is reminiscent of Beaumont's incisive and important studies of the gastric fistula of St. Martin.

Pavlov and Mme. Schumova-Simanovskaja (1890) published their results on the effect of vagotomy and cervical esophagostomy on secretion from isolated innervated canine gastric pouches. Intramediastinal transection of the right vagus trunk was performed through the neck, dividing the vagal trunk beyond the recurrent laryngeal nerve. The left vagus was completely sectioned in the neck.

The Russian authors validated the thesis that gastric secretion on sight, smell, and chewing of food is vagally incited and sustained. In his early experiments, Pavlov's dogs survived only a few days. N. P. Jurgens of Pavlov's laboratory (1892) performed bilateral subdiaphragmatic section of the vagi and noted that the effects, previously reported by Pavlov in acute experiments, were still in evidence nine and a half months later.

In a critical experiment Ernest H. Starling, discoverer of secretin, demonstrated that the exocrine secretion of the pancreas is primarily hormonal in origin (Fig. 1-8E).[20] When Pavlov repeated the experiment in his own laboratory, he verified Starling's observation and abandoned his creative work in gastroenterology, beginning his studies of conditioned reflexes. Starling's pupil, John Edkins, discovered the antral hormone gastrin in 1906, the importance of which was long denied by physiologists (Fig. 1-8F). The surgeon W. Heneage Ogilvie (1936, 1938) established the importance of the antrum for gastric secretion, and the Liverpool physiologist R. A. Gregory (1962) was able to confirm Edkins' findings. Donald R. Kemp (1973) of Melbourne, Australia, performed an important study evaluating the completeness of vagotomy through canine experiments of the effects of progressive vagal section on gastric acid.

Before the turn of the century there was a well-established rationale for the performance of vagotomy for peptic ulcer. The role of acid peptic juice in the genesis of peptic ulcer had long been recognized by clinicians. Karl

[20]See Carleton B. Chapman, Ernest Henry Starling, the clinician's physiologist, *Ann. Hist. Med.* 57(Suppl. 2):1, 1962.

Schwarz (1910) said, "No acid, no ulcer," an expression that has come to be dogma for clinicians; but, as has already been pointed out, the digestive power of gastric juice is completely dependent on the presence of pepsin with active proteolytic power.

CLINICAL VAGOTOMY STUDIES

In the second decade of this century, European surgeons began invoking division of the vagus nerves both above and below the diaphragm for a variety of conditions with gastric symptoms. Eugen Bircher (1920) mentioned 20 patients with varying gastric symptoms on whom he had performed incomplete vagotomy beneath the diaphragm (Fig. 1-4G). In 1931 he stated that most of the patients on whom he had performed subdiaphragmatic vagotomy in 1919 remained well.

Bircher (1925) described a type of selective vagotomy of the gastric fundus, probably the first suggestion of employment of selective clinical vagotomy. Certain it is that truncal vagotomy and large gastric resections for peptic ulcer are unphysiological procedures. The surprising thing is that this type of vagotomy is not more often followed by manifestations of dysfunction. Limitation of the vagal denervation to the acid- and pepsin-secreting area of the stomach, as currently done in many clinics, would appear to be a far more physiological operation.

It seems strange indeed that almost 40 years intervened between Bircher's first trial with selective vagotomy and today's refinements of the procedure. Had the hand of the surgeon been less influenced by empiricism and more by the sophisticated and precise approach of Pavlov, selective vagotomy as a clinical procedure for peptic ulcer would undoubtedly have been invoked long ago.

The important work of André Latarjet of Lyons (1922–1924) deserves attention (Fig. 1-4F). He and several German-speaking European surgeons employed vagotomy for a number of clinical conditions, performing the procedure both above and below the diaphragm. Latarjet, observing that bilateral division of the major vagal trunks interfered with gastric emptying, added a gastrojejunostomy to correct the situation. Of the 24 patients operated on, 6 had duodenal ulcer.

A group of surgeons at the Mt. Sinai Hospital in New York, including Eugene Klein, employed partial section of the vagus nerves as a complement to gastric resection in the 1930s. They observed that the incidence of achlorhydria following such procedures was greater than that attending gastric resection alone.

The important work of Dragstedt and his associates (1943–1952) established definitely the important role of vagotomy in depressing gastric secretion in patients with duodenal ulcer. Dragstedt's first procedure was a supradiaphragmatic truncal vagotomy, but like Latarjet, he found that an accompanying gastrojejunostomy was necessary to relieve gastric retention, thus mandating the abdominal approach. A fortunate circumstance in highly selective vagotomy of the acid- and pepsin-secreting area is that gastric emptying apparently is not interfered with, and a complementary drainage operation is usually unnecessary.

Surgeons have learned from long experience that well-controlled clinical trials, such as those that John Goligher and his associates conducted at Leeds, are necessary to reaffirm suggestions pointed up by experimental data. It too often happens that there is some overlooked item with a direct bearing on the issue.

It should be of more than passing interest to all medical persons that a committee of the American Gastroenterological Association (1952) had divided opinions of the merit of vagotomy for duodenal ulcer. It was actually A. V. Pollock (1952), then a surgical tutor at Leeds, who saved the day for vagotomy. In a careful follow-up study of 589 patients operated on for ulcer, in the Yorkshire area of England, Pollock found that neostomal ulcer was observed in only 3 percent—an encouraging sequel to the doubts expressed by the committee regarding the promise of vagotomy.

OPERATIONS FOR GASTRIC ULCER

Because of the possibility of cancer lurking in the "bed" of chronic gastric ulcer, most surgeons prefer to excise the defect, even though it lies high on the lesser curvature. A number of surgeons, basing their reasoning on the analogy of gastric resection for duodenal ulcer, perform the Madlener operation (1923), resecting the stomach beyond the ulcer, leaving the high-lying gastric ulcer on the lesser curvature in situ. Dragstedt was partial to the Madlener operation for high-lying gastric ulcers, but Wangensteen heard him say in discussion that twice in his experience the ulcer left behind proved to be cancer. Wangensteen did not find it technically difficult to excise a paraesophageal gastric ulcer. With adequate exposure, the excision leaves a functional goosenecklike esophagogastric juncture.

In the early decades of this century, excision of gastric ulcer was a commonly accepted procedure. In many instances, the excision extended almost to the greater curvature, creating problems of gastric emptying. William Mayo (1911) made an important contribution to excision for chronic gastric ulcer of the lesser curvature by adding a complemental gastrojejunostomy. Undoubtedly, an extended V-shaped excision is frequently tantamount to preantral transverse gastric section with consequent impaired gastric emptying, owing to vagal section to the antrum.

A few American surgeons in recent years have suggested vagotomy plus gastrojejunostomy for chronic gastric ulcer. When it is agreed that operation is indicated for persistent gastric ulcer, most surgeons today excise the ulcer. Every experienced gastric surgeon has seen instances in which only a drainage operation was performed and the gastric defect eventually proved to be cancer.

GASTROJEJUNOSTOMY AND PYLOROPLASTY FOR DUODENAL ULCER

The Heineke-Mikulicz pyloroplasty has an interesting derivation. W. H. Heineke performed the first successful pyloroplasty in 1886; it was described by F. Fronmüller in a thesis. Priority is usually credited to the Italian surgeon Pietro Loreta (1882). Loreta, however, did not do a conventional pyloroplasty, as may be noted in T. Holmes' (1885) lengthy review of Loreta's four cases in the *British Medical Journal*. Loreta made an antral incision 3 cm proximal to and above the pylorus; then he dilated the obstructed pylorus with his finger. Holmes reports that all four of Loreta's patients did well.

Mikulicz (1887) reported a successful pylorectomy for pyloric stenosis. A year later, however, the patient still experienced symptoms. Simultaneously, Mikulicz reported the instance of a female factory worker, age 17, for whom he did a pyloroplasty for a bleeding duodenal ulcer. A deep crater extending 2 cm into the pancreas was present at operation. The patient died of hemorrhage; obviously, a gastric resection should have been done.

Richard Lewisohn (1925) reported a 34 percent incidence of neostomal ulcer after gastrojejunostomy at the New York Mt. Sinai Hospital. Whereas many European surgeons had abandoned gastrojejunostomy in favor of gastric resection by then, it was still the popular operation for duodenal ulcer in this country. William Mayo (1924) said, "I hold no brief for gastroenterostomy," yet he went on to report 94 percent satisfactory results attending gastrojejunostomy performed for duodenal ulcer. Donald Balfour (1930) reported satisfactory relief of symptoms in 87 percent of his patients who had undergone gastrojejunostomy for duodenal ulcer and complete relief in 68 percent. Hemorrhage was the most frequent complication in those who failed to obtain relief.

In the same issue of the *Annals of Surgery*, E. Starr Judd (1930) reported on his technique of pyloroplasty and concomitant excision of duodenal ulcer. He indicated that gastrojejunostomy "will probably remain the popular operation for duodenal ulcer." The Heineke-Mikulicz pyloroplasty was first performed at the Mayo Clinic for duodenal ulcer in 1896 and was done together with excision of the ulcer in 1902. Transverse pyloroplasty with excision of the ulcer, Judd believed, could be done in approximately 50 percent of patients with duodenal ulcer needing operation, with satisfactory results in 90 percent.[21]

[21]The passing of gastrojejunostomy as a standard operation for ulcer was noted by Wangensteen in 1942 (*J. Lancet* 62:415, 1942).

H. Schmilinsky (1918), acting on the belief that gastrojejunostomy was a good operation for duodenal ulcer, effected total intragastric regurgitation by dividing the jejunum beyond the ligament of Treitz and anastomosing the proximal end of the divided jejunum to the gastric fundus; the distal jejunal end was united to the antrum, creating what the author described as an internal pharmacy. The operation was a complete failure because it provoked a profound and continuous stimulus for the gastrin phase of gastric secretion, attended regularly by a high incidence of neostomal ulcer; nevertheless, the operation is periodically rediscovered. Schmilinsky never retracted his support of the operation; his thesis was that if some intragastric regurgitation was good, as in the conventional gastrojejunostomy, complete reflux of bile, pancreatic juice, and succus entericus into the stomach was better.

Gastrojejunostomy with complemental truncal vagotomy was, for a long period of time, Dragstedt's preferred operation for duodenal ulcer. J. A. Weinberg's (1956) favorable report on vagotomy and a complemental pyloroplasty, with an 8 percent incidence of recurrence, brought that drainage procedure into general use. Lord Moynihan (1932), a predecessor of Goligher in the professorship at Leeds, considered gastric resection too radical an operation to perform for duodenal ulcer. He much preferred either gastrojejunostomy or gastroduodenostomy. Of his last 1000 patients, Moynihan said he had lost only 1 patient and that the incidence of neostomal ulcer was 1.8 percent. The follow-up at Leeds obviously is better today.

NEOSTOMAL ULCER AFTER BILLROTH RESECTIONS FOR DUODENAL ULCER

Billroth I Resections

For a long period of time, Hans v. Haberer was the keenest exponent of the Billroth I operation for duodenal ulcer (Fig. 1-4D). However, by 1939 he had abandoned it, finding that neostomal ulcer attended his Billroth I resections with unexpected frequency. Haberer's advice was ignored, however, and surgeons had to rediscover the ulcer-provoking quality of the Billroth I operation for duodenal ulcer. Sixteen years later, N. B. Ordahl and associates (1955) indicated that the observed recurrence in men at a Boston veterans hospital was 18 percent. Goligher (1956) in essence corroborated Ordahl's findings, reporting a 17 percent incidence of neostomal ulcer in patients with duodenal ulcer undergoing a Billroth I resection. S. Wallensten (1957), then of Örebro, Sweden, experienced a recurrence rate of 11 percent under similar circumstances. Hans Finsterer, a pupil of Hochenegg (Anton v. Eiselsberg's counterpart), because of his important work is evaluating features of gastric resection that spelled success or failure, acceded to a professorship at the University of Vienna at age 61 (Fig. 1-4C).

In an important paper D. H. Stern and J. H. Walsh (1973) provided what appears to be a cogent reason for the more frequent occurrence of neostomal ulcer attending the Billroth I resection. These authors observed after antral excision that food, on entering the duodenum in Billroth I resections, stimulates gastrin release, a phenomenon not observed in Billroth II resections, in which the food bypasses the duodenum and enters the jejunum directly. Their inference is that the proximal reaches of the duodenum also secrete gastrin.

Billroth I gastrectomy for the treatment of duodenal ulcer is infrequently performed today. Vagotomy plus antrectomy ad modum Billroth I, however, as championed by Henry N. Harkins (Fig. 1-4I), has taken an important position in this treatment, with a reported recurrence rate of ulcer of only 0.5 percent. Similarly, the Billroth I gastrectomy performed without vagotomy is the operation of choice for benign gastric ulcer.

Billroth II Resections

The highest recorded incidence of recurrence after Billroth II resections was reported in 1965 by William Scott and associates W. G. Rhea and D. A. Killen from the Vanderbilt Clinic. They indicated an observed recurrence rate of 24 percent in their clinic 10 years after such operations for duodenal ulcer. In a subsequent publication Scott indicated that in the literature the overall recurrence rate attending Billroth II resections for duodenal ulcer without complemental vagotomy was about 8 percent. In later publications Scott has not alluded to the Vanderbilt 24 percent recurrence rate mentioned in the 1965 paper.

Today, very few surgeons perform any type of gastric resection for duodenal ulcer without doing a complemental vagotomy. By these standards, segmental resection would appear to bear up quite satisfactorily with both Billroth I and II operations for duodenal ulcer. In a collective review, Leslie Wise and Walter Ballinger (1974) suggested that the incidences of neostomal ulcer attending vagotomy operations and Billroth I and II resections for duodenal ulcer are not far apart, a surprising finding especially in the light of the experience of Haberer (1939), Ordahl (1955), and others shortly thereafter with the Billroth I resection.

THE ANTRAL EXCLUSION OPERATION

This operation was devised in 1895 by Eiselsberg for inoperable gastric cancer (Fig. 1-1H). He divided the stomach proximal to the cancer and made a terminolateral gastrojejunal anastomosis. Interestingly enough, among the 16 patients in his initial report, there were 2 with peptic ulcer. In 1913 Haberer expressed misgivings about the acceptability of antral exclusion in gastric resection for duodenal ulcer, and by 1921 he had abandoned pyloric exclusion operations completely. H. Smidt (1924) of Jena described the tremendous increase in acid peptic secretion attending pyloric exclusion, thus establishing definitely the rationale for failure of the procedure. Eugen Enderlen and L. Zukschwerdt (1931), both of Heidelberg, confirmed Smidt's earlier findings (Fig. 1-4B).[22] Dragstedt and his associates (1951) have provided additional confirmation of this occurrence.

In a dog that was fed meat, Smidt observed an 82 percent increase in gastric secretory responses after the antral operation. Smidt also sketched a similar but less striking occurrence in dogs with antral exclusion fed milk or bread.[23]

Two papers of Ogilvie, reporting his clinical experience employing Billroth I gastric resections with and without antral exclusion, served to inform surgeons that antral exclusion was not a satisfactory operation for duodenal ulcer. R. Wilmanns (1926) indicated that when the antral and pyloric mucosa was excised in antral exclusion, combined with an adequate Billroth II resection, the results were as good as in the conventional Billroth II resection for duodenal ulcer, a finding confirmed by R. F. Rauch (1952).

William Waddell and M. K. Bartlett (1957) made an effort to resurrect the antral exclusion operation, combining it with the truncal vagotomy. The work of L. R. Sauvage and Henry Harkins (1953) and of William D. Kelly (1955) provides convincing evidence that a complementary vagotomy, added to antral exclusion, fails to protect against neostomal ulcer. The various physiological mechanisms for the failure of antral exclusion were presented by Nyhus (1960).

SEGMENTAL GASTRIC RESECTION

Segmental gastric resection was introduced by Mikulicz (1897) for peptic ulcer of the lesser curvature. He described it, gave the operation its name, and abandoned it all within the same year. In 1909 the procedure was taken up by both Bernard Riedel of Jena and Erwin Payr of Leipzig. Wangensteen adopted the procedure in 1948 for difficult duodenal ulcers that had perforated into the hepatoduodenal ligment.[24] He learned that the reason the operation had failed in the hands of the European surgeons was that the stomach failed to empty satisfactorily after transverse preantral section. Simple innovation of a complemental pyloroplasty solved that part of the problem.

Among 35 patients with duodenal ulcer in whom 85 percent of the acid- and pepsin-secreting area was excised, radiographic suggestion of an asymptomatic recurrence

[22]Enderlen was a superb clinical surgeon who worked actively in an experimental laboratory in immediate juxtaposition to his operating suite. He trained several gastric surgeons, including Hotz, v. Redwitz, and Zukschwerdt.

[23]Wangensteen met the author of these experiments in Guleke's surgical clinic in Jena in the spring of 1928.

[24]See *JAMA* 149:18, 1952.

was observed in 1 patient; reoperation was not necessary. Because symptoms of severe dumping were observed in many of these patients, the extent of the gastric resection was diminished. A 25 percent segmental gastric resection proved ineffective. A compromise was then made, resulting in a 50 percent segmental resection. Henry Sosin and Victor Gilbertsen, in a careful 1969 follow-up study for the second edition of this monograph (pp. 529–38), showed that the incidence of recurrence attending this type of segmental resection was approximately 8 percent. Sosin added vagotomy to segmental resection in another series of 85 patients, but the incidence of recurrence remained the same. In only half of the recurrences was surgical correction necessary.

Whereas complemental vagotomy combined with either of the Billroth procedures regularly decreases the observed incidence of neostomal ulcer, Sosin (1969) observed that it fails to improve the situation in segmental resection for duodenal ulcer, an occurrence that remains unexplained. One might reasonably have anticipated some lessening of the recurrence rate attending employment of complemental vagotomy in segmental gastric resection. It may well be that truncal vagotomy and preantral transverse section of the stomach cause delay in emptying, a possibility not yet adequately explored.

For gastric ulcer, a 50 percent segmental resection of the acid- and pepsin-secreting area accompanied by a pyloroplasty has been uniformly successful. Segmental resection is a satisfactory operation for gastric ulcer. A complemental pyloroplasty is, of course, mandatory. Tetsuo Maki (1967) has shown that when the antrum is divided no more than 1.5 cm proximal to the pylorus a concomitant pyloroplasty is unnecessary. Maki and associates (1975) have affirmed this view in a follow-up study.

SURGICAL CLOSURE OF PEPTIC ULCER PERFORATION

Hermann Kriege (1892) reported the first successful closure of a perforated gastric ulcer, high on the anterior wall of the gastric fundus. Approximately 20 hours intervened between the time of perforation and the interference of Kriege's superior, Professor Huessner, not because the entity was unrecognized but because Heussner was otherwise occupied. Henry P. Dean of London (1894) is often credited with the first successful closure of a duodenal ulcer, as the title of his paper would suggest. However, perusal of the case history reveals the patient suffered an intestinal adhesive obstruction during recovery, a complication that proved fatal.[25]

GASTRIC RESECTION FOR PEPTIC ULCER PERFORATION

Haberer (1919), an early advocate of gastric resection, reported two successful instances of operation for acutely perforated peptic ulcer; in one of these a pyloric exclusion was performed, a procedure that Haberer abandoned shortly thereafter because of the high incidence of recurrent ulcer.

A. Odelberg of Stockholm (1927) reported 20 cases in which he performed primary resection for perforated ulcer, with 1 death. Serge Yudin (1929–1937) of Moscow was a strong supporter of primary gastric resection for early perforation, as was Michael DeBakey (1940). In the second edition of this monograph (1969), DeBakey and G. L. Jordan suggested that primary resection be done only for patients with a prior history of peptic ulcer, emphasizing the important role of youth and early surgical intervention as criteria for primary resection.

That recurrent ulcer attends mere closure of the perforation in approximately one-third of instances is generally recognized. Even so, Wangensteen favored the simplest procedure. One does not give a drowning man a swimming lesson but drags him to shore.

Of the various complications attending peptic ulcer, hemorrhage commands by far the highest mortality. Until an effective antipeptic agent is discovered, it is unlikely that massive gastric hemorrhage can be adequately dealt with by other than surgical means. Intraperi-

[25] At autopsy, a perforation was found at the site where the tight band occluded the intestine, not an uncommon complication in acute adhesive obstruction when unrelieved, since the band cuts into the intestine with a sawlike action.

toneal injections of vasopressin (Pitressin) have been used with success, as have intra-arterial injections through a femoral catheter inserted directly into the left gastric artery, but these measures are at best palliative, and rebleeding often recurs. The retarding effect of gastric cooling on intragastric digestion in canine experiments suggested the innovation of continuous cooling of the entire stomach through a gastric balloon, a procedure initiated in Wangensteen's clinic in 1958 for patients with massive hemorrhage from duodenal ulcer. Although not effective in all instances, it did prove to be a useful method for the arrest of massive gastric hemorrhage from acid-peptic ulcer.

Gastric Miscellany

THE ZOLLINGER-ELLISON SYNDROME

This entity deserves mention in a chapter devoted to the history of gastric surgery even though it will be dealt with at length in another segment of this monograph. At the 1955 session of the American Surgical Association, the University of Ohio surgeons Robert M. Zollinger and Edwin H. Ellison startled that august body by narrating successful results of therapy for what many experienced gastric surgeons had come to believe were instances of intractable duodenal ulcer. The authors reported instances in which a favorable response had attended excision of an unsuspected pancreatic tumor that stimulated gastric secretion. R. A. Strøm (1952) of Norway and the British surgeons Frank Forty and G. M. Barrett (1952) had reported somewhat similar instances. The observations of Zollinger and Ellison are unique in that they opened up a whole new area of investigation. The Liverpool physiologists R. A. Gregory and Hilda J. Tracy (1963) succeeded in extracting a gastrinlike hormone from a pancreatic tumor that had given rise to surprisingly large volumes of gastric secretion and maximal gastric acidity; they also extracted a similar hormone from antral hog mucosa. Stanley R. Friesen (1967) demonstrated that in the presence of malignant pancreatic tumor with metastases causing the Zollinger-Ellison syndrome, total gastrectomy not infrequently brought about disappearance of metastases. It would appear that gastric antral, duodenal, and upper jejunal mucosa also partake of the qualities of an endocrine organ, as was forcefully brought out by James C. Thompson (1975) in the Galveston Symposium on gastrointestinal hormones.

GASTRIC WOUNDS

Recovery from a gastric fistula resulting from a spear wound in a hunting accident in Bohemia was reported by Johann Schenck in the last decades of the sixteenth century. The patient kept the fistula reasonably dry with linen cloths. Several similar events in which many of the victims survived were described by a succession of observers in the seventeenth and eighteenth centuries.

Nolleson *le fils* (1767) reported the case of a Palatinate soldier, Rumpf by name, who was cut by a saber in the left hypochondrium and conveyed to a hospital in what appeared to be a "nearly hopeless state." Nolleson sutured the wound in the stomach and dressed the external wound with wine, in which measure he was aided by Delblanc, the surgeon on duty that day at the hospital. The wounded man was bled nine times in the next three days, and his wound was dressed with vulnerary agents; even so, he recovered.

GASTROTOMY FOR REMOVAL OF FOREIGN BODIES

Oswald Croll (1609) reported the instance of a peasant knife-swallower in Prague who loved to startle audiences by withdrawing a concealed knife from his gullet after quaffing a stein of beer. His technique was to pass a 9-inch-long knife, handle first, down the esophagus, grasping it firmly by the blade.

The circumstance occasioning Croll's report occurred in 1602; the knife descended into the lower esophagus beyond the subject's reach, and when the beer was swallowed, the knife slid into his stomach. There it remained for seven weeks and two days until successfully withdrawn through an incision by the barber-surgeon Florian Matthis of Bradenburg, undoubtedly one of the first to remove a foreign body by gastrotomy. Croll saw the peasant after his recovery. (The knife was among the scientific curios in the collection of Emperor Rudolf II.)

The case of Andreas Grünheide, living 7 miles from Königsberg, is recounted by Daniel Becker (1640), a consultant.[26] Grünheide awoke one morning feeling nauseated. In an attempt to provoke vomiting, he tickled his throat with the shaft of his knife; the blade slipped from his fingers and the knife receded into the distal reaches of the esophagus, from whence he was unable to retrieve it. He stood in the inverted posture with his head on the ground, but without effect. He then drank some Landsberg beer and the knife slipped into his stomach. Becker brought the patient to Königsberg and summoned the whole "Collegius Medicus" to deliberate over the situation. It was decided to remove the knife from the stomach by incision, "which procedure should be done before the dog-days." The operation was performed on July 9, 1635, by Daniel Schwabe, a wound and lithotomy surgeon, in the presence of Becker and other local physicians.

The patient was bound to a board, and the site of the incision was marked with charcoal. An incision was made over the point of the knife, which was then removed. The patient joyfully announced that it was his knife. The gastric wound closed shut immediately on withdrawal of the knife, but nevertheless was reinforced with a few sutures. The King of Poland, Ladislaus IV, came to Königsberg to see the knife, the patient, and his wound. Later, the knife was sent to the king, at his request. Grünheide recovered completely, returned to his farm work, and was married in 1641.

The Königsberg account is listed by B. Credé (1886) as the first of 26 instances in which a foreign body was removed from the stomach; the other 25 were all in the nineteenth century. Most of the patients were salvaged by surgical intervention.

Huard and Imbault-Huart (1971) describe a previously unpublished instance of gastrotomy occurring in 1819.[27] In 1818 a 24-year-old Frenchwoman inserted a silver fork into her throat to induce vomiting. The fork slid from her fingers and descended into the stomach. For about five months she was symptomless, but then periods of distress developed and a tender small mass could be felt. A consultation was held including the well-known Montpellier surgeon Jacques Delpech, who determined that gastrotomy was the only recourse. On May 1, 1819, the abdomen was opened by Cayroche of Mende, while three servants restrained the patient. The fork was exposed, and its prongs were found embedded in the gastric wall. When disengaged, it was readily removed. The patient recovered.

GASTROSTOMY STUDIES ON PATIENTS WITH GASTRIC FISTULAS

Jacob Helm of Vienna, apparently the first to study gastric digestion in a patient, published an account of his research in 1803. Mrs. Theresia Perzin, age 56, suffered gastric perforation that led to a persistent gastric fistula. Over five years, Helm made observations of his patient's stomach that confirmed Spallanzani's earlier experiments with a number of animals, demonstrating the digestive power of gastric juice. Helm's observations, therefore, contributed essentially no new information.

Beaumont's studies (1833) of Alexis St. Martin, who suffered a persistent gastric fistula from a shotgun blast at close range in 1822, by contrast, contributed important new information. Beaumont correctly concluded that "chemical principles" other than HCl were present in the gastric juice, and that during fasting, the stomach did not secrete. Several observers since Beaumont, notably Otto Gruenewaldt (1853), have utilized the opportunity to study gastric digestion in patients with external gastric fistulas. In this century,

[26]Becker ("Beckher" in some accounts) included a letter of 1607 giving a report of the Prague knife-swallower by a consultant and a picture of the Königsberg patient, showing the knife and wound. A review of the Königsberg case, with reproductions of several paintings of the event, has been presented by D. C. Schechter and Henry Swan (*Surgery* 51:814, 1962).

[27]Cayroche's report of the operation was found by Huard and Imbault-Huart in the Archives of the Société de la Faculté de Médecine de Paris.

the studies of A. J. Carlson (1912–1915) on his fistulous subject, Fred Vlcek, and those of Stewart Wolf and Harold Wolff on Tom Little (1943) are best known.

GASTROSTOMY

The Paris physiologist Pierre Flourens (1832) studied digestion in sheep by opening the rumen, reticulum, and omasum in successive experiments. He was interested in the phenomenon of rumination in quadrupeds and detected forceful gastric contractions on his finger when it was introduced into the various pouches. He noted too that vagotomy inhibited these contractions, whereas division of the lower thoracic spinal cord did not.

Nicolas Blondlot of Nancy had assisted the physician H. Braconnot (1835) in recovering gastric juice from dogs that had swallowed sponges with attached strings (see Table 1-2). In 1843 he performed gastrostomies on dogs to continue the studies. He wrapped omentum around the stomach and brought out a tentlike gastric segment through the rectus muscles of the abdominal wall to minimize leaking from the fistula.

It is to be noted (Table 1-2) that Braconnot concluded that gastric juice contained HCl, whereas Blondlot concluded that gastric acid was phosphoric. Beaumont (1833) had recognized that Alexis' stomach needed the stimulus of food to excite secretion, a circumstance more appreciated today.

Karl Bardeleben (1849) made canine gastric fistulas a few years after Blondlot's contribution. Bardeleben performed a two-stage cervical esophagostomy, dividing the esophagus completely to exclude entry of saliva into the stomach. Despite this novel approach, Bardeleben made no significant contribution to the physiology of gastric secretion.

The Russian physiologist W. Bassow (1843) performed gastrostomies on dogs to explore the promise of the operation for clinical purposes.

The first to perform a gastrostomy on a person was the French surgeon Charles Sédillot (1849), though C. A. Egeberg, a Norwegian surgeon of Rigshospitalet, had made the suggestion of performing gastrostomy at the May 8, 1837, meeting of the Christiana Medical Society. The patient concerned was a hospital employee, Ole Olesen, age 36, who had difficulty in swallowing.

A. Verneuil (1876) performed the first successful gastrostomy on a boy of 17 with a lye stricture of the esophagus. The Paris physiologist Charles Richet (1878) performed many studies of gastric secretion on Verneuil's young subject. It remained, however, for Heidenhain (1878) and Pavlov (1887–1900), with the device of the isolated canine gastric pouch, to add significantly to the important studies of Beaumont that had been done a half century earlier.

K. Lennander (1908) reported the use of gastrostomy for relief of acute gastric dilatation attending perforation of peptic ulcer.

CONGENITAL HYPERTROPHIC PYLORIC STENOSIS

Conrad Ramstedt[28] performed a successful extramucosal pyloromyotomy for congenital hypertrophic pyloric stenosis on August 23, 1911, and another on June 18, 1912. He was a practicing surgeon in Münster who continued to operate quite regularly until failing vision persuaded him to retire at age 80. Ramstedt cited W. Weber of Dresden as his predecessor in the operation. Weber had reported two successful cases in 1910; however, he attempted to cover the prolapsed mucosa with the serosal surface of the divided muscle, a maneuver Ramstedt also tried, but rejected, employing instead adjacent omentum for the purpose. H. Dufour and P. Fredet (1908) reported successful instances of extramucosal myotomy but in which the surgeon Fredet closed the longitudinal incision transversely, imitating the closure of the open Heineke-Mikulicz pyloroplasty. In fact many surgeons allude to the procedure as the Fredet-Ramstedt operation. Wangensteen spent the school year 1927–1928 abroad and was surprised to note that even then, gastrojejunostomy was more frequently performed in Germany than Ramstedt's extra-

[28]Spelled *Rammstedt* in some citations.

mucosal pyloromyotomy for congenital hypertrophic pyloric stenosis. Today, accomplished pediatric surgeons have reported large series of patients with this challenging entity without hospital mortality. The important roles in this accomplishment of E. J. Donovan of the Columbia Presbyterian Center, New York, and of Robert Gross of Boston, deserve special mention. Donovan (1937) reported 243 operations with 1 death (a 0.41 percent mortality). Gross (1953) reported that the mortality of the Children's Hospital in Boston since 1940 had been under 1 percent.

CONGENITAL TRACHEOESOPHAGEAL ATRESIA

Although many earlier attempts were made to correct this defect, the first salvage of an infant with esophageal atresia and a fistula from the trachea to the distal blind esophageal segment was accomplished at the University of Minnesota by N. Logan Leven (1941) in 1939 and 1940. He recognized three goals: prevention of regurgitation of swallowed saliva and consequent aspiration pneumonia; division of the fistula to prevent reflux of gastrostomy feedings into the trachea through the fistula; and restoration of esophageal continuity. He approached the first two goals in three stages. On November 29, 1939, he performed a feeding gastrostomy, passing the catheter into the duodenum to lessen the risk of regurgitation to the trachea through the distal esophagus. On January 5, 1940, the fistula was ligated extrapleurally, and on March 27, 1940, a cervical esophagostomy was done to prevent accumulation of oral secretions from spilling into the trachea. Some years later Richard L. Varco used a segment of jejunum to restore continuity. The patient was alive and well in 1983.

Cameron Haight and H. A. Towsley lauded Leven's accomplishment and undertook to correct all the abnormalities of a tracheoesophageal fistula in the initial operation. They were first successful on March 15, 1941. Although only one of their first nine attempts resulted in long-term survival, this advance opened the way to the regular successes observed today.

OPERATIONS FOR CARDIOSPASM (MEGAESOPHAGUS)

An unusual esophagogastric condition for which surgeons have devised adequate operative procedures is megaesophagus. Mikulicz (1904) advised dilatation for the lesion and coined the term *cardiospasm.*

In 1910 W. Wendel of Vienna did an open cardioplasty of the Heineke-Mikulicz variety, followed in turn by Hans Heyrovsky (1913), also of Vienna, who made a transdiaphragmatic lateral anastomosis between the gastric fundus and the dilated esophagus. E. Heller (1913) of Leipzig,[29] made both an anterior and a posterior extramucosal vertical incision through the cardiac sphincter area, an operation that still survives in the form of a single anterior incision. Wangensteen (1951), conscious of the great sensitivity of the esophageal mucosa to injury by gastric juice, predicted failure of anastomotic procedures of the Wendel-Heyrovsky and Gröndahl (1916) variety and proposed, for patients with a huge megaesophagus, excision of the entire acid- and pepsin-secreting area of the stomach, anastomosing the gastric antrum to the esophagus. The operation proved quite successful in most of the seven instances in which it was performed. The esophagus of one patient accommodated 3 liters of barium. Whereas patients swallow quite satisfactorily after the Heller operation, dilatation of the esophagus persists. On the contrary, considerable reduction in the diameter of the megaesophagus regularly attends excision of the acid- and pepsin-secreting area. An unexpected finding attending the operation was supervention of a megaloblastic anemia owing to loss of vitamin B_{12} absorption, a finding previously known for total gastrectomy and satisfactorily combatted by intramuscular injections of vitamin B_{12}, as noted by W. D. Kelly and associates (1954) and L. D. MacLean and R. D. Sundberg (1956).

[29]Wangensteen visited Heller at St. George's Krankenhaus in Leipzig in the spring of 1928. He was using deep blue drapes in operations to avoid the glare of the conventional white. Moynihan introduced green drapes for that purpose in 1915. (See *Lancet* 2:214, 1915.)

ORGAN SUSPENSION

Moynihan devoted 20 pages of his 1926 text to visceral prolapse and suspension of organs, including the stomach. The two chief exponents of the procedures were Thorskild Rovsing (1913) of Copenhagen and Robert Coffey (1923) of Portland, Oregon. It is surprising to note Moynihan's enthusiasm for such operations, which were commonplace in the early decades of this century. The procedures that survived the longest were renal and uterine suspensions. In September, 1927, Wangensteen spent a few days visiting hospitals in Copenhagen including the Rikshospitalet where Rovsing worked. At the end of a long day of making complete ward rounds with the senior surgical resident, Suermont, he remarked, "You have not shown me a single instance of organ suspension." After a brief period of suspense, Suermont replied, "The professor has been dead six months."

A few months later, a distinguished Swedish surgeon came for a brief visit to the University of Minnesota Hospitals. One morning he examined the posted operating list. The gynecologists had five uterine suspensions listed. Said he, "I have practiced surgery in Stockholm for more than a quarter of a century. I have never seen such an operation performed."

Surgery is at a disadvantage in trying to deal effectively with the force of gravity in overcoming organ prolapse. We believe that many operations for hemorrhoids, apart from bleeding prolapse and an acutely thrombosed external pile, are unnecessary. Henry Smith (1823–1894), a King's College surgeon, often said, "Hemorrhoids are a magnificent source of income."[30] We are reassured by some surgical colleagues that hemorrhoidectomy too is becoming a less frequent operation.

It would be possible to trace the history of gastric surgery up to today, but that is, after all, the mission of all the rest of this volume.

[30]Professor Henry Smith is quoted by H. Willoughby in *King's and Some King's Men,* London: Oxford University Press, 1935, p. 212. (O. H. Wangensteen, Remarks on unnecessary operations, *Am. J. Gastroenterol.* 22:202, 1954.)

References

GASTRIC CANCER

Allen, A. W., and Welch, C. E. Jejunostomy for the relief of malfunctioning gastroenterostomy stoma. *Surgery* 9:163, 1941.

Andren, L., Srieberg, S., and Welin, S. Roentgen diagnosis of small polyps in the colon and rectum. *Acta Radiol.* 43:201, 1955.

Billroth, T. Offenes Schreiben an Herrn Dr. L. Wittelshöfer. *Wien. Med. Wochenschr.* 31:161, 1881.

Brigham, C. B. Case of removal of entire stomach for carcinoma: Esophagoduodenostomy; recovery. *Boston Med. Surg. J.* 138:415, 1898.

Burow, A. Ueber die Ursache der häufigen Todesfälle nach Amputationen. *Dtsch. Klin.* 11:207, 217, 1859.

Friedreich, N. Ein Fall von Magenkrebs. *Berlin Klin. Wochenschr.* 11:1, 1874.

Gelfand, D. W. The double-contrast upper gastrointestinal examination in the Japanese style. *Am. J. Gastroenterol.* 63:216, 1975.

George V. Quoted in O. H. Wangensteen, *Cancer of the Esophagus and the Stomach* (2d ed.). New York: American Cancer Society, 1956. P. 137.

Gussenbauer, C., and Winiwarter, A. Die partielle Magenresection. Eine experimentelle operative Studie. *Arch. Klin. Chir.* 19:347, 1876.

Haberkant, H. Ueber die bis jetzt erzielten unmittelbaren und weiteren Erfolge der verschiedenen Operationen am Magen. *Arch. Klin. Chir.* 51:484, 1896.

Haire, L. Remarks on Mr. Lucas's practical observations on amputation. *Lond. Med. J.* 7:377, 1786.

Halsted, W. S. Circular suture of the intestine. *Am. J. Med. Sci.* 94:436, 1887.

Halsted, W. S. The training of the Surgeon (Annual Address in Medicine, Yale University, 1904). In W. C. Burket (Ed.), *Surgical Papers,* Vol. 2. Baltimore: Johns Hopkins Press, 1924. P. 529.

Hegar, A. Zur Ovariotomie. *Volkmann's Sammlung Klin. Vorträge,* No. 109, Gynäkologie, no. 36, 1876–1877. P. 811.

Hegar, A. Ignaz Philipp Semmelweiss, sein Leben und seine Lehre. Freiburg and Tübingen: J. C. B. Mohr, 1882.

Herrington, J. L., Jr. Remedial Operations Following Gastric Resection. In H. N. Harkins and L. M. Nyhus (Eds.), *Surgery of the Stomach and Duodenum* (2d ed.). Boston: Little, Brown, 1969. P. 751.

Keen, W. W. The Cartwright lectures on the surgery of the stomach: Gastrolysis, gastrotomy, and gastrostomy. *N.Y. Med. J.* 67:629, 1898.

Kern, V. *Ueber die Handlungsweise bei Absetzung der Glieder* (2d ed.). Vienna: Mechitaristen, 1826. Pp. 30–35.

Kuru, M. *Atlas of Early Carcinoma of the Stomach*. Tokyo: Nakayama-Shoten, 1967.

Lawrence, W. A new method of tying the arteries in aneurism, amputation, and other surgical operations. *Medchir. Trans.* 6:156, 1815.

Lembert, A. Mémoire sur l'entéroraphie avec la description d'un procédé nouveau pour pratiquer cette opération chirurgicale. *Rep. Gén. Anat. Physiol. Pathol.* 2:100, 1826.

Lister, J. On the Interdependence of Science and the Healing Art (Presidential Address to the British Association for the Advancement of Science, 1896). In H. C. Cameron and W. W. Cheyne (Eds.), *The Collected Papers of Joseph Baron Lister,* Vol. 2. Oxford: Clarendon Press, 1909. P. 489.

Liston, R. Results of amputations at University-College Hospital, London. *Medchir. Trans.* 24:155, 1841.

Long, C. W. An account of the first use of sulphuric ether by inhalation as an anaesthetic in surgical operations. *South. Med. Surg. J.* 5:705, 1849.

Merrem, D. K. T. *Animadversiones quaedam chirurgicae experimentis in animalibus factis illustratae*. Giessen: Tasché & Müller, 1810.

Monro I, A. Remarks on the amputations of the larger extremities. *Med. Essays Observations* (Edinb.) 4:342, 1737; 4:276, 1752.

Osler, W., and McCrae, T. *Cancer of the Stomach, A Clinical Study*. Philadelphia: Blakiston, 1900. P. 152.

Palmer, E. D. Discussion. *Am. J. Gastroenterol.* 24:361, 1955.

Pattison, G. S. Experimental observations on the operation of lithotomy, with the description of a fascia of the prostate gland. *Am. Med. Recorder* 3:1, 1820.

Pouteau, C. *Mélanges de chirurgie*. Lyons: Regnault, 1760. P. 198.

Ruschenberger, W. S. W. *A Report on the Origin and Therapeutic Properties of Condurango*. Washington, D.C.: U.S. Navy Department, 1873.

Schindler, R. Ein völlig ungefährliches, flexibles Gastroskop. *Münch. Med. Wschr.* 79:1268, 1932.

Schlatter, C. Vollständiger Entfernung des Magens, Oesophagoenterostomie, beim Menschen. *Beitr. Klin. Chir.* 19:757, 1897.

Semmelweis, I. P. Höchst wichtige Erfahrungen über die Aetiologic der in Gebäranstalten epidemischen Puerperalfieber. *Z. k. k. Ges. Aerzte Wien* 4:242, 1847; 5:64, 1849.

Semmelweis, I. P. *Die Aetiologie, der Begriff und die Prophylaxis des Kindbettfiebers*. Budapest, Vienna, Leipzig: Hartleben, 1861.

Simpson, J. Y. Discovery of a new anaesthetic agent, more efficient than sulphuric ether. *Lond. Med. Gaz.* 5:934, 1847.

Smithies, F., and Ochsner, A. J. *Cancer of the Stomach*. Philadelphia: Saunders, 1916. Pp. 417–471.

Spallanzani, L. *Saggio die osservazioni microscopiche relative al sistema della generazione*. Modena, 1767.

Tait, L. One hundred and thirty-nine consecutive ovariotomies performed between January 1st, 1884, and December 31st, 1885, without a death. *Br. Med. J.* 1:921, 1886.

Temkin, O. Merrem's youthful dream. *Bull. Hist. Med.* 31:29, 1957. Postscript. *Bull Hist. Med.* 34:74, 1960.

Tyndall, J. *Essays on the Floating-Matter of the Air in Relation to Putrefaction and Infection*. London: Longmans, Green, 1881.

Wangensteen, O. H. *Cancer of the Esophagus and Stomach* (2d ed.). New York: American Cancer Society, 1956.

Wangensteen, O. H., and Sosin, H. How can the outlook in alimentary tract cancer be improved? *Am. J. Surg.* 115:7, 1968.

Welch, W. H. Cancer of the Stomach. In W. Pepper, *System of Practical Medicine by American Authors*. Philadelphia: Lea Bros., 1885. P. 575.

Wölfler, A. Gastro-Enterostomie. *Zentralbl. Chir.* 8:705, 1881.

Wölfler, A. *Ueber die von Herrn Professor Billroth Ausgeführten Resectionen des carcinomatösen Pylorus*. Vienna: Braumüller, 1881.

Ziegler, H. Billroths erste Magenresektion. *Krebsarzt* 4:49, 1949.

PEPTIC ULCER

American Gastroenterological Association, Committee on Study of Vagotomy and Gastric Resection for Peptic Ulcer, S. M. Jordan, Chairman. Report. *Gastroenterology* 22:297, 493, 1952.

Balfour, D. C. Results of gastroenterostomy for ulcer of the duodenum and stomach. *Ann. Surg.* 92:558, 1930.

Beaumont, W. *Experiments and Observations on the Gastric Juice, and the Physiology of Digestion*. Plattsburgh, N.Y.: F. P. Allen, 1833.

Bidder, F. H., and Schmidt, C. *Die Verdauungssäfte und der Stoffwechsel*. Mitau, Leipzig: Reyher, 1852.

Bircher, E. Die Resektion von Aesten der N. Vagus zur Behandlung gastrischer Affektionen. *Schweiz. Med. Wochenschr.* 50:519, 1920.

Bircher, E. *Die Technik der Magenchirurgie*. Stuttgart: Enke, 1925. Pp. 20–25.

Bircher, E. Die Behandlung gastrischer Affektionen durch Eingriffe am N. vagus und sympathicus. *Arch. Klin. Chir.* 167:463, 1931.

Brodie, B. C. Experiments and observations on the influence of the nerves of the eighth pair on the secretions of the stomach. *Philos. Trans.* 104:102, 1814.

Dean, H. P. A case of perforation of a chronic ulcer of the duodenum successfully treated by excision. Death two months later from acute intestinal obstruction by a band. *Br. Med. J.* 1:1014, 1894.

DeBakey, M. E. Acute perforated gastroduodenal ulceration. *Surgery* 8:852, 1028, 1940.

DeBakey, M. E., and Jordan, G. L., Jr. Gastrectomy for Perforated Ulcer. In H. N. Harkins and L. M. Nyhus (Eds.), *Surgery of the Stomach and Duodenum* (2d ed.). Boston: Little, Brown, 1969. P. 834.

Dennis, C. Oblique, aseptic end-to-end intestinal anastomosis. *Surgery* 5:548, 1939.

Dragstedt, L. R. Acid ulcer. *Surg. Gynecol. Obstet.* 62:118, 1936.

Dragstedt, L. R., Oberhelman, H. A., Jr., and Smith, C. A. Experimental hyperfunction of gastric antrum with ulcer formation. *Ann. Surg.* 134:332, 1951.

Dragstedt, L. R., and Owens, F. M. Supradiaphragmatic section of the vagus nerves in treatment of duodenal ulcer. *Proc. Soc. Exp. Biol. Med.* 53:152, 1943.

Eiselsberg, A. Über Ausschaltung inoperabler Pylorus-strikturen nebst Bemerkungen über die Jejunostomie. *Arch. Klin. Chir.* 50:919, 1895.

Enderlen, E., and Zukschwerdt, L. Erregung der Magensaftsekretion nach Resektion des Antrum. *Dtsch. Z. Chir.* 232:290, 1931.

Ferguson, D. J., Sanchez-Palomera, E., Sako, Y., et al. Studies on experimental esophagitis. *Surgery* 28:1022, 1950.

Forty, F., and Barrett, G. M. Peptic ulceration of third part of the duodenum associated with islet-cell tumors of the pancreas. *Br. J. Surg.* 40:60, 1952.

Friesen, S. R. Effect of total gastrectomy on the Zollinger-Ellison tumor: Observations by second-look procedures. *Surgery* 62:609, 1967.

Fronmüller, F. *Operation der Pylorusstenose* (Erlangen dissertation). Fürth: Schröder, 1886.

Goligher, J. C., Moir, P. J., and Rigley, J. H. Billroth I and Pólya operations for duodenal ulcer—A comparison. *Lancet* 2:220, 1956.

Gregory, R. A. Gastric Secretion. In A. N. Smith (Ed.), *Symposium on the Surgical Physiology of the Gastro-intestinal Tract*. Edinburgh: Morrison and Gibb, 1962. P. 57.

Gregory, R. A., and Tracy, H. J. Constitution and properties of two gastrins extracted from hog antral mucosa. *J. Physiol.* (Lond.) 169:18P, 1963.

Griffith, C. A., and Harkins, H. N. Partial gastric vagotomy: An experimental study. *Gastroenterology* 32:96, 1957.

Haberer, H. Ulcus pepticum jejuni postoperativum. *Dtsch Gesellsch. Chir.* 42:68, 1913.

Haberer, H. Zur Therapie akuter Geschwürsperforationen des Magens und Duodenums in die freie Bauchhöhle. *Wien. Klin. Wochenschr.* 32:413, 1919.

Haberer, H. Bedeutung des Pylorus für das Zustandekommen des postoperativen jejunalulcus. *Arch. Klin. Chir.* 117:50, 1921.

Haberer, H. Meine Korrekturoperationen bei Eingriffen am Magen und Duodenum. *Arch. Klin. Chir.* 196:304, 1939.

Heidenhain, R. P. H. Ueber die Pepsinbildung in den Pylorusdrüsen. *Pflügers Arch. Gesamte Physiol.* 18:169, 1878.

Holmes, T. Review. *Br. Med. J.* 1:372, 1885.

Judd, E. S., and Hazeltine, M. E. The results of operations for excision of ulcer of the duodenum. *Ann. Surg.* 92:563, 1930.

Jurgens, N. P. Sur la sécrétion stomacale chez les chiens ayant subi la section sousdiaphragmatique des nerfs pneumogastriques. *Archs. Sci. Biol.* (St. Petersb.) 1:323, 1892.

Kelly, W. D. Influence of anatomical relationships of gastric antrum on gastric secretion and gastrojejunal ulcer. Ph.D. Dissertation, University of Minnesota, 1955. Table II.

Kemp, D. R. A histological and functional study of the gastric mucosal innervation in the dog. *Aust. N. Z. J. Surg.* 43:288, 1973.

Klein, E. Left vagus section and partial gastrectomy for duodenal ulcer with hyperacidity. *Ann. Surg.* 90:65, 1929.

Kriege, H. Ein Fall von einem Frei in die Bauchhöhle perforirten Magengeschwür. Laparotomie. Naht der Perforationsstelle. Heilung. *Berl. Klin. Wochenschr.* 29:1244, 1280, 1892.

Latarjet, A. Résection des nerfs de l'estomac. Technique opératoire. Résultats cliniques. *Bull. Acad. Natl. Méd.* (Paris) 87:681, 1922.

Latarjet, A., and Wertheimer, P. Quelques résultats

de l'énervation gastrique. *Presse Méd.* 2:993, 1923.
Lewisohn, R. The frequency of gastrojejunal ulcers. *Surg. Gynecol. Obstet.* 40:70, 1925.
Loreta, P. Intorno alla divulsione digitale del pilore. *Mem. Reale Accad. Sci. Ist. Bologna* 4:353, 1882.
Madlener, M. Über Pylorektomie bei pylorusfernem Magengeschwür. *Zentralbl. Chir.* 50:1313, 1923.
Maki, T., Shiratori, T., Hatafuku, T., et al. Pylorus-preserving gastrectomy as an improved operation for gastric surgery. *Surgery* 61:838, 1967.
Maki, T., Shiratori, T., Hatafuku, T., et al. Pylorus-preserving gastrectomy for gastric ulcer. *Surgery* 77:92, 1975.
Mayo, W. J. Ulcer of the stomach and duodenum with special reference to the end results. *Ann. Surg.* 54:313, 1911.
Mayo, W. J. Gastroenterostomy. *Surg. Gynecol. Obstet.* 39:241, 1924.
Mikulicz-Radecki, J. Zur operativen Behandlung des stenosirenden Magengeschwürs. *Dtsch. Gesellsch. Chir.* 16:337, 1887.
Mikulicz-Radecki, J. Chirurgische Behandlung des chronischen Magengeschwürs. *Dtsch. Gesellsch. Chir.* 26:31, 1897.
Moynihan, B. G. A. The prognosis of gastric and duodenal ulcer. *Br. Med. J.* 1:1, 1932.
Müller, J., and Schwann, T. Versuche über die künstliche Verdauung der geronnenen Eiweisses. *Arch. Anat. Physiol. Wiss. Med.* 1836. P. 66.
Nyhus, L. M. The role of the antrum in the surgical treatment of peptic ulcer. *Gastroenterology* 38:21, 1960.
Odelberg, A. Primary resection of the stomach in perforating gastric and duodenal ulcers. *Acta Chir. Scand.* 62(Suppl. 8):159, 1927.
Ogilvie, H. Physiology and the surgeon. *Edinb. Med. J.* 43:61, 1936.
Ogilvie, H. Approach to gastric surgery. II. Ulcer of the stomach. *Lancet* 2:295, 1938.
Ordahl, N. B., Ross, R. P., and Baker, D. V., Jr. The failure of partial gastrectomy with gastroduodenostomy in the treatment of duodenal ulcer. *Surgery* 38:158, 1955.
Pavlov, I. P. *The Work of the Digestive Glands* (trans. W. H. Thompson). London: Griffin, 1902.
Pavlov, I. P., and Schumova-Simanovskaja, E. Innervation der Magendrüsen beim Hunde. *Zentralbl. Physiol.* 3:113, 1889.
Payr, E. Erfahrungen über Excision und Resektion bei Magengeschwüren. *Arch. Klin. Chir.* 90:989, 1909.
Pollock, A. V. Vagotomy in the treatment of peptic ulceration. *Lancet* 2:795, 1952.
Rauch, R. F. An evaluation of gastric resection for peptic ulcer. *Surgery* 32:638, 1952.
Rhea, W. G., Jr., Killen, D. A., and Scott, H. W., Jr. Long term results of partial gastric resection without vagotomy in duodenal ulcer disease. *Surg. Gynecol. Obstet.* 120:970, 1965.
Riedel, B. Entfernung des mittleren Abschnittes vom Magen wegen Geschwür. *Dtsch. Med. Wochenschr.* 35:17, 54, 1909.
Rydygier, L. Die erste Magenresection beim Magengeschwür. *Berl. Klin. Wochenschr.* 19:39, 1882.
Rydygier, L. Die erste Magenresektion beim Magengeschwür (review). *Zentralbl. Chir.* 9:198, 1882.
Sanchez, H., Sako, Y., and Wangensteen, O. H. Sensitivity of the esophagus to the acid-pepsin action. *Am. J. Physiol.* 105:476, 1948.
Sauvage, L. R., Schmitz, E. J., Storer, E. H., et al. Physiologic stimulatory mechanisms of gastric secretion and peptic ulceration. *Surg. Gynecol. Obstet.* 96:127, 1953.
Schiff, M. *Leçons sur la physiologie de la digestion,* Vol. 1. Florence, Turin: Loescher, 1867. P. 36.
Schindler, R. Ein völlig ungefährliches, flexibles Gastroskop. *Münch. Med. Wschr.* 79:1268, 1932.
Schmilinsky, H. Die Einleitung der gesamten Duodenalsäfte in den Magen (innere Apotheke). *Zentralbl. Chir.* 45:416, 1918.
Schwann, T. Ueber das Wesen des Verdauungsprocesses. *Arch. Anat. Physiol. Wiss. Med.* 1836. P. 90.
Schwarz, K. Ueber penetrierende Magenund Jejunalgeschwür. *Beitr. Klin. Chir.* 67:96, 1910.
Smidt, H. Experimentelle Studien . . . nach der Pylorusausschaltung. . . . *Arch. Klin. Chir.* 125:26, 1923.
Smidt, H. Über Magenresektionen und Magenchemismus. *Arch. Klin. Chir.* 130:307, 1924.
Stern, D. H., and Walsh, J. H. Gastrin release in postoperative ulcer patients: Evidence for release of duodenal gastrin. *Gastroenterology* 64:363, 1973.
Strøm, R. A. Case of peptic ulcer and insuloma. *Acta Chir. Scand.* 104:252, 1952.
Thompson, J. C. (Ed.). *Gastrointestinal Hormones: A Symposium.* Austin, Texas: University of Texas Press, 1975.
Tiedemann, F., and Gmelin, L. *Recherches expérimentales, physiologiques et chimiques sur la digestion.* Paris: Baillière, 1827. Pp. xviii–xxi.

Waddell, W. R., and Bartlett, M. K. Antral exclusion with vagotomy for duodenal ulcer. *Ann. Surg.* 146:3, 1957.

Wallensten, S. Gastric resection for peptic ulcer: Billroth I versus Billroth II. *Surgery* 41:341, 1957.

Wangensteen, O. H. Aseptic gastric resection. I. A method of aseptic anastomosis adaptable to any segment of the alimentary canal (esophagus, stomach, small or large intestine). II. Including preliminary description of subtotal excision of the acid-secreting area for ulcer. *Surg. Gynecol. Obstet.* 70:59, 1940.

Wangensteen, O. H. The Cause and Prevention of Stomal Obstruction in Gastrojejunal Anastomosis. In *Medico-surgical Tributes to Harold Brunn.* Berkeley: University of California Press, 1942. P. 551.

Wangensteen, O. H., Root, H. D., Jensen, C. B., et al. Gastric hypothermia: Its clinical use in massive hematemesis. *Surgery* 44:265, 1958.

Weinberg, J. A., Stempein, S. J., Movius, H. J., et al. Vagotomy and pyloroplasty in the treatment of duodenal ulcer. *Am. J. Surg.* 92:202, 1956.

Wilmanns, R. Resectio praepylorica bei ulcus duodeni. *Zentralbl. Chir.* 53:1874, 1926.

Wise, L., and Ballinger, W. F. The elective surgical treatment of chronic duodenal ulcer: A critical review. *Surgery* 76:811, 1974.

Yudine, S. A propos du traitement des ulcères perforés de l'estomac et du duodenum. *Bull. Soc. Natl. Chir.* (Paris) 55(2):1233, 1929.

Yudine, S. Etude sur les ulcères gastriques et duodénaux perforés. *J. Int. Chir.* 4:219, 1939.

Zollinger, R. M., and Ellison, E. H. Primary peptic ulcerations of the jejunum associated with islet cell tumors of the pancreas. *Ann. Surg.* 142:709, 1955.

GASTRIC MISCELLANY

Bardeleben, K. Beiträge zur Lehre von der Verdauung. *Arch. Physiol. Heilkunde* 8:1, 1849.

Bassow, W. Voie artificielle dans l'estomac des animaux. *Bull. Soc. Imp. Natl. Moscou* 16:315, 1843.

Beaumont, W. *Experiments and Observations on the Gastric Juice, and the Physiology of Digestion.* Plattsburgh, N.Y.: F. P. Allen, 1833.

Becker, D. *Cultrivori prussiaci curatio singularis.* Leyden: Maire, 1640. Pp. 17, 122.

Blondlot, N. *Traité analytique de la digestion considérée particulièrement dans l'homme et dans les animaux vertébrés.* Paris: Fortin, Masson, 1843.

Braconnot, H. Expériences chimiques sur le suc gastrique. *Ann. Chimie Physiol.* 59:348, 1835.

Carlson, A. J. Contributions to the physiology of the stomach. *Am. J. Physiol.* Vols. 31–38, 1912–15.

Coffey, R. C. *Gastro-enteroptosis.* New York: Appleton, 1923. P. 218.

Credé, B. Gastrotomie wegen Fremdkörper. *Arch. Klin. Chir.* 33:574, 1886.

Croll, O. *Basilica chymica . . . .* Frankfurt: 1609. Pp. 64–65.

Donovan, E. J. Congenital hypertrophic pyloric stenosis in infancy. *J.A.M.A.* 109:558, 1937.

Dufour, H., and Fredet, P. La sténose hypertrophique du pylore . . . et son traitement chirurgicale. *Rev. Chir.* (Paris) 37:208, 1908.

Egeberg, C. A. Om behandlingen af impenetrable Stricturer i Madröret (Oesophagus). *Norsk Mag. Laegevidenskaben* 2:97, 1841.

Flourens, P. Expériences sur le mécanisme de la rumination. *Ann. Sci. Nat.* (Paris) 27:34, 291, 1832.

Gröndahl, N. B. Cardioplastik ved Cardiospasmus. *Nord. Med. Ark.* 49:236, 1916.

Gross, R. E. *Surgery of Infancy and Childhood.* Philadelphia: Saunders, 1953, P. 143.

Gruenewaldt, O. Succi gastrici humani indoles physica et chemica, ope fistulae stomachalis indagata (dissertation). Dorpat: 1853.

Haight, C., and Towsley, H. A. Congenital atresia of the esophagus with tracheoesophageal fistula: Extrapleural ligation of fistula and end-to-end anastomosis of esophageal segments. *Surg. Gynecol. Obstet.* 76:672, 1943.

Heller, E. Extramukoese Cardioplastik beim chronischen Cardiospasmus mit Dilatation des Oesophagus. *Mitt. Grenzgeb. Med. Chir.* 27:414, 1913–14.

Helm, J. *Zwey Krankengeschichten . . . nebst Untersuchung der Verdaulichkeit der Nahrungsmittel . . .* Vienna: Camesinaischen Buchhandlung, 1803.

Heyrovsky, H. Casuistik und Therapie der idiopathischen Dilatation der Speiseröhre, Oesophagogastroanastomose. *Arch. Klin. Chir.* 100:703, 1913.

Huard, P., and Imbault-Huart, M. J. A propos de la taille gastrique au XIXème siècle. *Epistème* 5:45, 1971.

Kelly, W. D., MacLean, L. D., Perry, J. F., et al. A study of patients following total and near-total gastrectomy. *Surgery* 35:964, 1954.

Lennander, K. G. Temporäre Gastrostomie bei Magen- oder Duodenalgeschwüren, besonders bei perforierten Geschwüren. *Dtsch. Z. Chir.* 92:297, 1908.

Leven, N. L. Congenital atresia of the esophagus with tracheoesophageal fistula: Report of successful extrapleural ligation of the fistulous communication and cervical esophagostomy. *J. Thorac. Surg.* 10:648, 1941.

MacLean, L. D., and Sundberg, R. D. Incidence of megaloblastic anemia after gastrectomy. *N. Engl. J. Med.* 254:885, 1956.

Mikulicz-Radecki, J. Zur Pathologie und Therapie des Cardiospasmus. *Dtsch. Med. Wochenschr.* 30:17, 1904.

Moynihan, B. *Abdominal Operations* (4th ed.), Vol. 1. Philadelphia: Saunders, 1926. Pp. 179–98.

Nolleson *le fils*. Sur une plaie d'estomac, guérie par la suture du pelletier. *J. Méd. Chir. Pharm.* 27:595, 1767.

Rammstedt, C. Zur Operation der angeborenen Pylorusstenose. *Med. Klin.* 8:1702, 1912.

Rammstedt, C. Die Operation der angeborenen Pylorusstenose. *Zentralbl. Chir.* 40:3, 1913.

Richet, C. R. Resumé des observations faites sur Marcelin R. . . . atteint de fistule gastrique. *J. Anat. Physiol.* 14:326, 1878.

Rovsing, T. Gastrocoloptosis. *Ann. Surg.* 57:1, 1913.

Schenck, J. *Observationum medicarum, rararum, novarum, admirabilium, et monstrosarum . . . .* Frankfurt: 1609. P. 38.

Sédillot, C. E. Opération de gastro-stomie, pratiquée pour la première fois le 13 novembre 1849. *Gaz. Méd. Strassbourg* 9:366, 1849.

Verneuil, A. A. S. Sur une opération de gastrostomie. *Bull. Acad. Méd.* 5:1016, 1023, 1876.

Wangensteen, O. H. A physiologic operation for mega-esophagus (dystonia, cardiospasm, achalasia). *Ann. Surg.* 134(1):301, 1951.

Weber, W. Ueber eine technische Neuerung bei der Operation der Pylorusstenose des Säuglings. *Berl. Klin. Wochenschr.* 47(1):763, 1910.

Wendel, W. Zur Chirurgie des Oesophagus. *Arch. Klin. Chir.* 93:311, 1910.

Wolf, S., and Wolff, H. G. *Human Gastric Function, an Experimental Study of a Man and His Stomach.* London: Oxford University Press, 1943.

SPECIAL COMMENT

Owen Harding Wangensteen: Surgical Educator

Clarence Dennis

Born of Norwegian Lutheran stock in the farming community of Lake Park, Minnesota, in 1898, Owen H. Wangensteen (Fig. 1-9) became intrigued with medical quandaries while assisting as a boy in the difficult delivery of a litter of pigs. He received his Doctor of Medicine degree from the University of Minnesota in 1922 and served an internship in the University Hospital.

With an avid curiosity and a staunch readiness to challenge authoritarian dicta if they did not match his own observations, he early attracted the attention of Dr. Elias P. Lyon, Dean of the School of Medicine and a dedicated sponsor of the thesis that chairmen of university clinical departments should be true academicians and investigators. Wangensteen has recounted that he did not win a residency in surgery when first sought and that through Dean Lyon he spent a year with Dr. George Fahr, Professor of Medicine and coworker with Willem Einthoven on the electrocardiogram. A fine academician himself, Fahr instilled those patterns of approach to problems in medicine that so characterized Wangensteen throughout his career.

Following his work with Fahr, Wangensteen spent a year doing surgery at the Mayo Clinic arranged by Dean Lyon, and a year as Senior Surgical Resident at the University Hospital in Minneapolis. After a year as Assistant Professor he was given the opportunity by Dean Lyon to spend a year in Europe to enhance his foundation for an academic career. Through Fahr's experience in Berne, Wangensteen went to the clinic of Professor F. DeQuervain, but he spent much of his year as a volunteer assistant to Professor Leon Ascher of the Physiological Institute, an experience that led him to think physiologically and develop the belief that how the organ or organism works is more important than the anatomical structure.

Dean Lyon had been grooming Wangen-

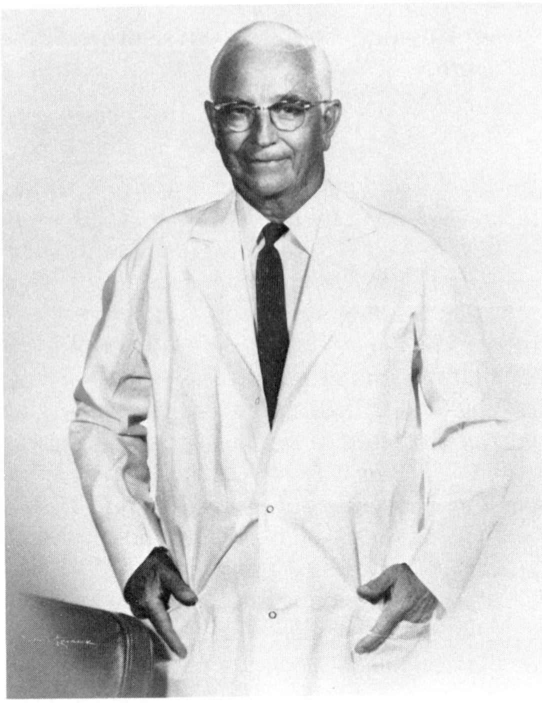

Fig. 1-9. Owen Harding Wangensteen (1898–1981).

steen to be Chairman of the Department of Surgery, especially after Francis Newton visited in 1925 and Mont Reid in 1927, and both had declined the chair in the belief that there could be no future at Minnesota.

Wangensteen was appointed Chairman of the Department of Surgery in 1930, three months before his thirty-second birthday, and to full professorship the following year, and served in these capacities until 1967. At Minnesota, the Department of Surgery was the last major department in the medical school to undergo transformation from a journeyman-style education given primarily by practitioners in the Twin Cities. The transition to an academic department under Wangensteen was a stormy one for him. Having no surgical residents, he took the salaries of the clinical professors to enable him to appoint six surgical fellows. The repercussions from the part-time and volunteer faculty and their supporters were such as to make his position precarious, and preservation of the budding surgical academic department required heavy support. Among the staunch and far-seeing supporters who prevailed in their efforts to save his chairmanship were University President Lotus D. Coffman, Dr. Arthur Strachauer (Wangensteen's predecessor as chairman), Dean Lyon, and Dr. William J. Mayo.

Early in his chairmanship, Wangensteen became intrigued with the frequency with which catheter enterostomies performed for relief in intestinal obstruction led to fistulas. He accepted the problem of intestinal obstruction as a field of study in which he would not compete with anyone locally. This resulted in a monograph for which he was awarded the Samuel D. Gross prize of the city of Philadelphia in 1935. The monograph was refused by publisher after publisher, including W. B. Saunders and Lea & Febiger, until finally it was accepted by Charles C Thomas. Similarly, Wangensteen's initial work on the use of the nasogastric tube in the treatment of small intestinal obstruction was refused by journal after journal, including the *Proceedings of the Society for Experimental Biology and Medicine* and *Surgery, Gynecology and Obstetrics*. This experience led him to join with Alton Ochsner in founding *Surgery*, a journal in which new and unconventional but sound ideas would be welcomed.

During his career Wangensteen published more than nine hundred papers and exerted a tremendous impact on surgical thinking and practice. He contributed in a wide variety of fields and activities, including, in addition to intestinal obstruction, the etiology of appendicitis, the etiology of peptic ulcer, the "second look" for abdominal cancers, and surgery of the stomach; he created the Forum on Fundamental Surgical Problems of the American College of Surgeons.

Wangensteen and his wife, Sarah, co-wrote a historical treatise, *The Rise of Surgery*, in 1978, and he was busily engaged on a projected companion volume, "Schools of Surgery," at the time of his death.

Recognition was heaped on him. Honorary degrees were bestowed on him by the University of Buffalo, the University of Chicago, St. Olaf College, Hamline University, Temple University, the University of Paris, the Royal

Colleges of Surgeons of Edinburgh, of England, and of Ireland, and others; awards and prizes came as well.

At the time of his retirement as "Chief" of the Department of Surgery in 1967, Wangensteen had trained 20 chairpersons of departments of surgery in American medical schools, as well as 30 full professors and 50 more full-time academicians.

In an interview with Dr. K. A. Merendino at the time of his retirement, Wangensteen stated that his most satisfying accomplishments were the achievements of his younger associates. He always believed that he was given a great opportunity without earning it and that he had to work to justify it. Regarding his trainees and fellow faculty members, he stated, "I provided an opportunity for them. In that milieu we probably had one of the finest orchestral bands of surgeons that has been assembled in the twentieth century. That is the nature of my donation to the University of Minnesota, far more important than the money I have raised, and it probably is in essence the nature of my contribution to surgery."

Owen Wangensteen died quickly of coronary occlusion on January 13, 1981. He is mourned by friends and former patients, but he is especially mourned by a veritable army of his trainees, every one of whom is deeply grateful to him.

SPECIAL COMMENT

Jules Emile Péan

Louis F. Hollender
Jamil Bahnini

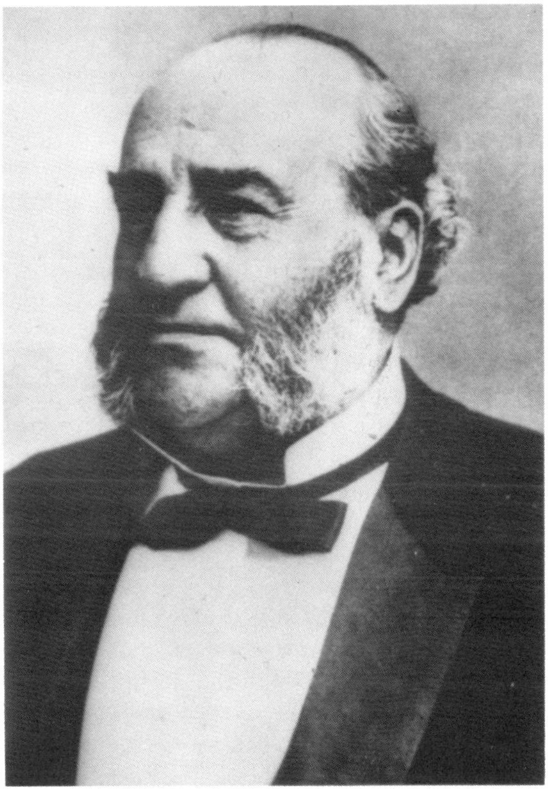

Fig. 1-10. Jules Emile Péan, 1830–1898.

Jules Emile Péan (Fig. 1-10) was born in 1830 at Marboue, near Chateaudun, to a miller's family. He used to say that his beginnings in Paris were hard, but this does not sound true for Péan, whose family probably lived according to the wise, saving principles of the country of Beauce. Péan never had the experience of being a "poor student."

Péan was admitted to the medical school of Paris in 1855. Exhausting work enabled him to obtain several degrees in a short time, but led to such severe illness that he had to retire to Algeria for a year.

Péan received his surgical training and practice with Denonvilliers and Nélaton. In 1868 he was granted a Doctor of Medicine degree in surgery. During his residency Péan shared a warm family life with his two sisters, Rose and Clémentine, who managed the household. Péan often invited his friends for dinner but sometimes worried about his income, which by then was up to 400,000 francs, although he had been a surgeon for just four years.

In 1869 Péan married Miss Giroux De Burzareingues and had three daughters, Juliette, Henriette, and Adrienne. Mrs. Péan well understood that being the wife of the busiest surgeon in Paris was not easy. The sumptuous dinners she used to hold in their magnificent apartment, Vendôme Place, were gatherings of "tout-Paris."

Péan was not attracted to these society gatherings, and he seldom attended the opera. He used to get up early in the morning and start his day's work at the Augustines and Frères-St.-Jean de Dieu surgical clinics, where he visited the patients on whom he had operated. He then would go to the St.-Louis Hospital to operate on and visit patients. After a light lunch he would continue to operate until 3 P.M., when he started his endless consultations, which lasted until long after dinner time.

On July 28, 1865, Péan presented to the Academy the case of a woman he had cured of a huge ovarian cyst. The presentation was a masterstroke. Although the academic papers of the time did not mention anything, it is beyond any doubt that Péan's report gave rise to comment and discussion. Such an operation was not in common use because most surgeons were afraid to open the peritoneal cavity and would leave the cyst to be filled with air. Velpeau, who attended the academic session on that day, had stated years before, in 1856, that ovariectomy was an awful operation and must be avoided, even though a few instances of cysts that had healed were recorded. Actually, Péan followed in the footsteps of Eugène Koeberlé of Strasbourg, whose pioneering work was begun long before, when he reported at the academy instances of successful ovariectomies performed at the St.-Barbe Surgical Clinic. From June, 1862 to October, 1864, Koeberlé operated on more than 120 ovarian cysts and had a 30 percent mortality. That was unexpected and unhoped for.

Péan's teacher, Nélaton, who was an incontestable surgical master, went through a disastrous experience with ovariectomy. He went to London to meet and watch the famous surgeons Baker Brown and Spencer Wells. On his return to Meudon, he tried to perform the ovariectomy procedure he saw in London. All of the 17 women he operated on died.

This failure explains the sensation made by the young, tall, broad-shouldered surgeon who talked in a rough manner and whose name was Péan. Péan got in to the habit of reporting new surgical cases at the academy. From 1860 to 1869 he recorded six successful ovariectomies and a hysterectomy using an abdominal approach. As a result of his fame and glory, jealousy and deep hostility grew in the hearts of Péan's opponents. Péan, however, was such a gifted and talented surgeon that hostility sometimes turned into trusting friendship.

Ricord related the story of an American woman who complained of a great abdominal distention, believed to be an ovarian cyst. Ricord advised her against the operation and, much more, against Péan. Nevertheless, the appeal of forbidden fruit led this young woman to the surgeon of St.-Louis. Péan declared he would operate on her in the presence of Ricord. It was a successful operation, the patient lived, and Ricord became one of Péan's closest friends.

Péan held the surgical art in such veneration that he operated in evening dress, a flamboyant behavior his detractors criticized. He wrapped a towel around his neck, under which his shirtfront remained clean and white. He then rolled up his sleeves and handled the surgical instruments with the utmost care. According to one story, he extracted an ovarian cyst and uterine fibroma without thrusting his powerful hands into the patient's belly.

Péan's dedication, confidence, and skill were the reasons he performed as successfully as Spencer Wells, Atlee, and Koeberlé operations that were considered miracles. Péan was one of the great pioneers in abdominal surgery. In 1867 he performed the first successful splenectomy. It was not planned but occurred during a laparotomy for an ovarian cyst and showed how impulsive and inspired a surgeon Péan was. Péan was particularly concerned with hemostasis—he hated blood. In 1868 he had a special hemostatic clip made by Gueride, the mechanism of which was based on the rack and pinion principle.

In April, 1879 Péan performed the first gastric resection for cancer. Remaining true to his belief that any cancer should be removed, Péan resected the patient's pylorus and restored the continuity of the digestive tract—a pylorectomy for a pyloroduodenal cancer. The patient died on the fifth postoperative day. Billroth did his first gastric resection (pylorectomy) in January, 1881. This operation on a 44-year-old woman with carcinoma of the stomach was the first successful gastrectomy.

Meanwhile Péan was reaching the decisive age of 62 and had to leave the St.-Louis Hospital. He built with his own funds the hospital that bears his name and where he worked for six more years. Péan was elected to the Academy of Medicine on November 22, 1887, after failing to be elected twice before—the first time on April 12, 1882, and the second time, on July 27, 1883. He lost one of the elections to Lannelongue. These failures were a great trial in the life of a man who promoted and developed a wide range of surgical fields, and his surgical colleagues were more than concerned about them. Péan was sensitive about academic honors and was promoted to the rank of Commandeur de la Legion d'Honneur in 1892.

Péan regularly attended the French Surgical Congress. Its 1893 session will never be forgotten. A young, blue-eyed, blond man, about 40 years of age, got up and in a wild and forward manner criticized the transvaginal hysterectomy called the Péan operation. That man was Doyen. Péan, old and weak, stretched to his full height and answered: "Mr. Doyen does not understand at all the principle of my operation. I can add that Mr. Doyen has not yet performed as many successful operations as I have. He is lucky enough to have been born when most discoveries have already been made!"

Péan's life was shaped of honor, celebrity, and rough contention. He never tried to escape from the professional life in which he was so involved, although in his youth he had been interested for a while in painting and drawing. Péan did not experience the decrepitude of old age. On January 25, 1898, he caught cold on his return from a hunting party, held at his castle at Boulayes. He spent a bad night but nevertheless performed a nephrectomy the next day. That was his last operation. He died of severe pneumonia four days later. Péan was buried at the cemetery of Montparnasse after an official funeral.

J. L. Faure said of Péan: "Time that spoilt anything will never wipe out the work of Péan. What makes a work of a man eternal and preserves him from oblivion are not things that bear his name but things that seem to come from the unknown."

SPECIAL COMMENT
Ludwik Rydygier

Witold Rudowski

Ludwik Rydygier, the founder of the Polish Association of Surgeons, was born in Dusocin, district Grudziadz, in the north of Poland on August 21, 1850. In 1869 he graduated from high school in the city of Chelmno on the Vistula River and the same year was admitted to the Medical Faculty of the University of Greifswald, Germany. During his five years of study at the university, Rydygier was the cofounder of the Polish student union *Polonia*. After five years in Greifswald, Rydygier moved to the universities in Berlin and Strasbourg to complete his undergraduate education and training. In the autumn of 1873, Rydygier returned to Greifswald University, where on December 8, 1873 he received his M.B. degree. Almost immediately after graduation, Rydygier started his M.D. dissertation, also at Greifswald, under the direction of Professor Carl Hueter, the head of the department of surgery.

On March 28, 1874, Rydygier was granted an M.D. degree in surgery and obstetrics (Fig. 1-11) after presentation of a 55-page dissertation entitled "Experimentelle Beiträge zur Lehre von der Wirkung von Carbolsäure" (Experimental Investigations on the Effect of Carbolic Acid). It was an important contribution to antiseptic surgery, demonstrating not only the beneficial aspects but also the toxic side effects of carbolic acid. In a short time Rydygier was appointed an assistant surgeon in the Department of Surgery at Greifswald.

In 1878 Rydygier completed another dissertation "Eine neue Methode zur Behandlung der Pseudoarthroses" (A New Method of

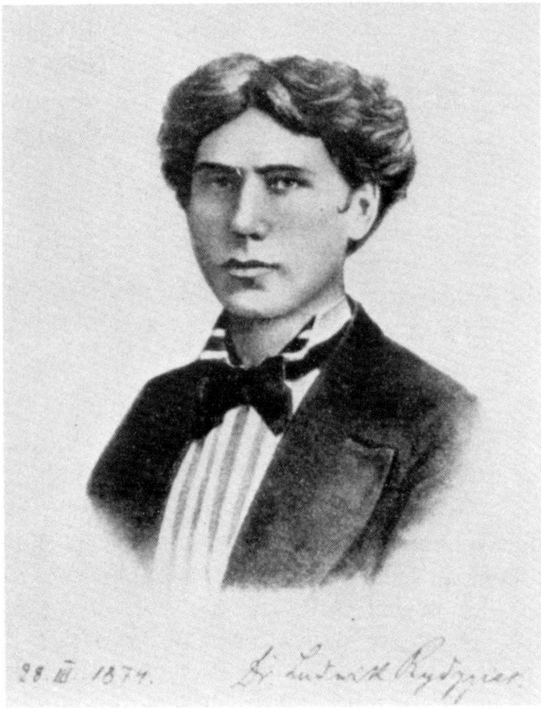

Fig. 1-11. Photograph of Ludwik Rydygier with his signature and the date he received his M.D. degree. (From S. Sokót, *Ludwik Rydygier /1850–1920/*. Warsaw: Polish Medical Publishers, 1961. P. 52.)

Treatment of Pseudoarthroses), which was presented at the Medical College of the University in Jena to obtain the title of *Dozent,* corresponding to associate professor of surgery. He worked for a time in the Department of Surgery at the University of Jena, of which Professor F. J. von Ried was head. In addition to practicing clinical surgery, Rydygier lectured to medical students on various surgical topics, but with particular reference to bone and joint surgery. Rydygier had also visited the university Departments of Surgery in Warsaw and in Vienna, where he watched operations performed by Professor Theodor Billroth.

At the end of 1878 Rydygier returned to Chelmno to start his surgical practice. There he founded a private clinic with 25 beds and specialized in treating general surgical and gynecological problems (Figs. 1-12, 1-13). For the next nine years Rydygier worked in Chelmno, developing a large surgical practice as well as conducting surgical research. Rydygier's surgical activities became so widely known that in 1887 he was invited to take the Chair of Surgery at the Jagiellonian University in Cracow. Rydygier's predecessor at this, the oldest Polish University, was another great surgeon—Jan Mikulicz.

Rydygier was Chairman and Head of the Department of Surgery at the Jagiellonian University until 1897. During these eventful years he was able to create a new department of surgery fitted with the latest equipment. In the academic year 1888–1889, Rydygier was elected a dean of the medical faculty at the Jagiellonian University. In 1889 he organized the First Congress of Polish Surgeons and became the founder of the Polish Association of Surgeons. In 1897 Rydygier moved to Lwow and took the Chair of Surgery at Lwow University. Later he was elected Rector Magnificus of this university for the period 1901–1902 (Fig. 1-14). In 1903 Rydygier received an invitation to become a lecturer in surgery at Charles University in Prague, but he did not accept the appointment, deciding instead to continue his work at Lwow. In his final years, Rydygier contributed greatly to the organization and curriculum of the medical school at the University of Poznan. Rydygier died suddenly on June 23, 1920, in Lwow.

From the very beginning of his surgical practice, it was obvious that Rydygier was an extremely skilled research-oriented surgeon. In his early postgraduate years, he witnessed the rapid progress of gastrointestinal surgery and the beneficial effects of antiseptic, and later, aseptic methods. Rydygier was extremely interested in the promotion of new techniques in surgery of the abdominal organs. His greatest achievements were related to surgery of the stomach.

After a series of animal experiments, Rydygier mastered the technique of partial gastric resection and gastroduodenal anastomosis. On November 16, 1880, in his clinic at Chelmno, Rydygier performed the second,

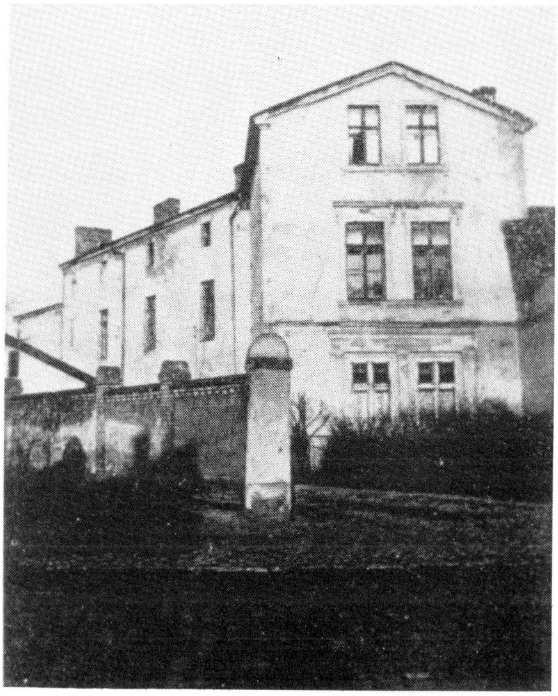

Fig. 1-12. Rydygier's clinic in Chelmno, on the Vistula. (From S. Sokót, *Ludwik Rydygier /1850–1920/*. Warsaw: Polish Medical Publishers, 1961. P. 45.)

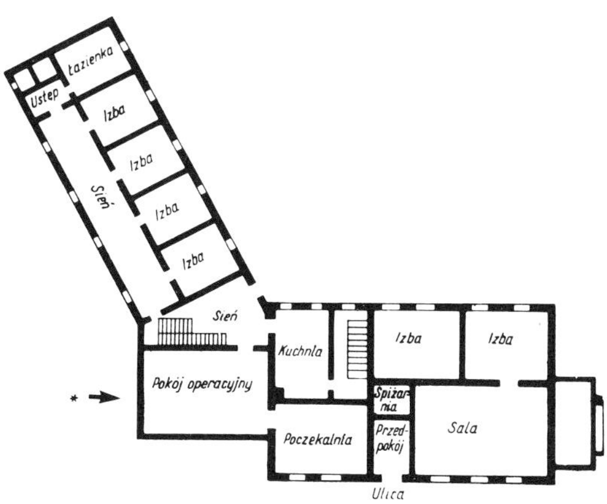

Fig. 1-13. The layout of Rydygier's clinic in Chelmno. Operating theater marked by asterisk. (From S. Sokót, *Ludwik Rydygier /1850–1920/*. Warsaw: Polish Medical Publishers, 1961. P. 42.)

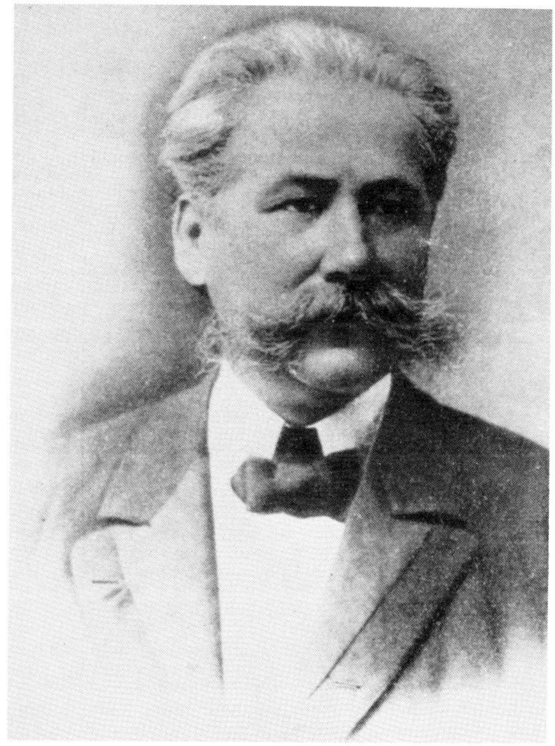

Fig. 1-14. Rydygier at the time he was elected Rector Magnificus of the University of Lwow, 1901. (From S. Sokót, *Ludwik Rydygier /1850–1920/*. Warsaw: Polish Medical Publishers, 1961. P. 84.)

after Péan, partial resection of the prepyloric part of the stomach in a patient with cancer involving the pylorus. He gave an exact and detailed description of the technique of this procedure. Thus it turns out that Billroth was third in the field of gastric resection, not doing his first gastrectomy for cancer until two months after Rydygier had done his. Rydygier is not given proper credit for his pioneering work, particularly in the German literature. But the facts are on record in two articles published in 1881 (Rydygier, L., *Dtsch. Zeitschr. Chir.* 14:252, 1881, and Billroth, Th., *Wien. Med. Wochenschr.* 31:16, 1881).

Rydygier was the first surgeon ever to resect successfully a part of the stomach for ulcer (Fig. 1-15). He performed this operation

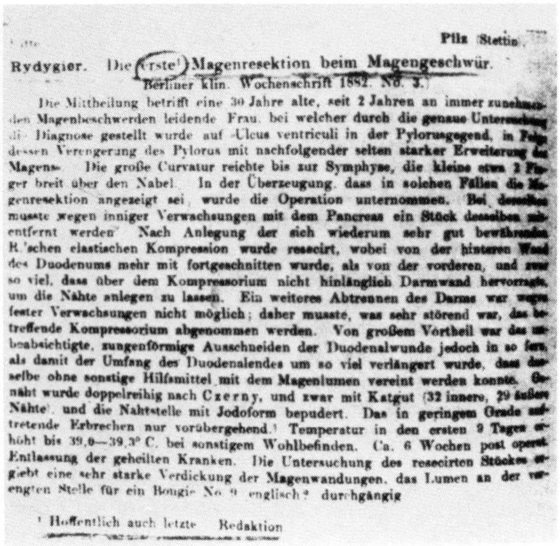

Pilz (Stettin).

Rydygier. Die erste[1] Magenresektion beim Magengeschwür.
(Berliner klin. Wochenschrift 1882. No. 3.)

Die Mittheilung betrifft eine 30 Jahre alte, seit 2 Jahren an immer zunehmenden Magenbeschwerden leidende Frau, bei welcher durch die genaue Untersuchung die Diagnose gestellt wurde auf Ulcus ventriculi in der Pylorusgegend, in Folge dessen Verengerung des Pylorus mit nachfolgender selten starker Erweiterung des Magens. Die große Curvatur reichte bis zur Symphyse, die kleine etwa 2 Finger breit über den Nabel. In der Überzeugung, dass in solchen Fällen die Magenresektion angezeigt sei, wurde die Operation unternommen. Bei derselben musste wegen inniger Verwachsungen mit dem Pancreas ein Stück desselben mitentfernt werden. Nach Anlegung der sich wiederum sehr gut bewährenden R.'schen elastischen Kompression wurde resecirt, wobei von der hinteren Wand des Duodenums mehr mit fortgeschnitten wurde, als von der vorderen, und zwar so viel, dass über dem Kompressorium nicht hinlänglich Darmwand hervorragte, um die Nähte anlegen zu lassen. Ein weiteres Abtrennen des Darms war wegen fester Verwachsungen nicht möglich; daher musste, was sehr störend war, das betreffende Kompressorium abgenommen werden. Von großem Vortheil war das unbeabsichtigte, zungenförmige Ausschneiden der Duodenalwunde jedoch in so fern, als damit der Umfang des Duodenalendes um so viel verlängert wurde, dass dasselbe ohne sonstige Hilfsmittel mit dem Magenlumen vereint werden konnte. Genäht wurde doppelreihig nach Czerny, und zwar mit Katgut (32 innere, 29 äußere Nähte), und die Nahtstelle mit Jodoform bepudert. Das in geringem Grade auftretende Erbrechen nur vorübergehend. Temperatur in den ersten 9 Tagen erhöht bis 39,0—39,3° C. bei sonstigem Wohlbefinden. Ca. 6 Wochen post operat. Entlassung der geheilten Kranken. Die Untersuchung des resecirten Stückes ergiebt eine sehr starke Verdickung der Magenwandungen, das Lumen an der verengten Stelle für ein Bougie No. 9 (englisch?) durchgängig.

[1] Hoffentlich auch letzte. Redaktion.

Fig. 1-15. The abstract of Rydygier's paper on gastric resection in peptic ulcer of the stomach published in *Zentralblatt für Chirurgie*. The words "first gastric resection" are underlined and the footnote from the editorial board reads: "Hoping the last one." (From S. Sokót, *Ludwik Rydygier /1850–1920/*. Warsaw: Polish Medical Publishers, 1961. P. 103.)

on November 21, 1881.[1] Rydygier also established precise indications for operations for pyloric stenosis, bleeding from perforations, and gastric cancer (Fig. 1-16). His later surgical work included the development of new methods for removal of stones from the urinary bladder by the transperitoneal approach; for intracapsular prostatectomy, which prevented injury to the prostatic part of the urethra during operation; for replacement of the resected portions of the urethra by skin grafts; and for surgical care of pseudoarthrosis. Rydygier was one of the first surgeons to resect the gangrenous loop of the intestine in instances of strangulated hernia. In 1895 he described a method of fixation of the mobile spleen in a pocket from the parietal peritoneum. Rydygier recommended an extensive sacral approach in the surgical treatment of rectal cancer.

[1]Rydygier, L. Die erste Magenresection beim Magengeschwur. *Berl. Klin. Wochenschr.* 19:39, 1882.

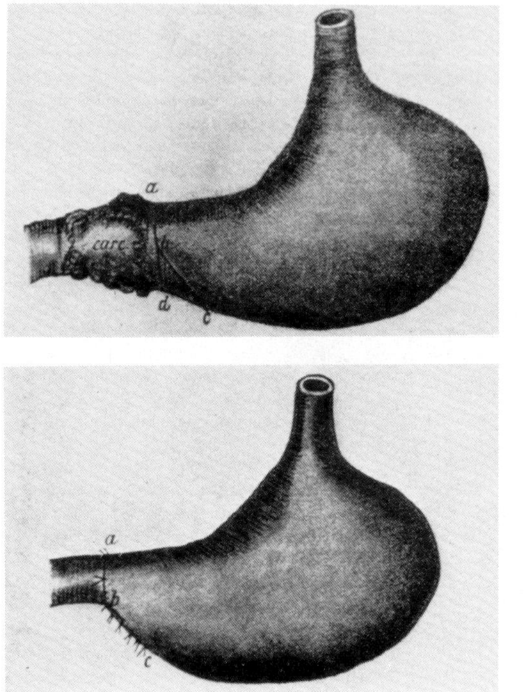

Fig. 1-16. The technique of pyloric resection as practiced by Rydygier with a two-layer gastroduodenal anastomosis. (From S. Sokót, *Ludwik Rydygier /1850–1920/*. Warsaw: Polish Medical Publishers, 1961. P. 102.)

Rydygier also made several attempts to promote and develop vascular surgery. In 1901 he described a new approach to aneurysms of the innominate artery. His hope to suture a wound of the heart was never realized.

Rydygier was an excellent academic teacher, creating the Polish surgical school. His most renowned pupils were Schramm and Ostrowski of Lwow and Krynski and Zaorski of Warsaw. The list of Rydygier's publications contains 200 papers in Polish, German, and French medical journals.

The contributions of Rydygier to the progress of Polish surgery were not limited to new concepts and methods in surgical technique and practice. As mentioned before, Rydygier was the founder and became the honorary president of the Polish Association of Surgeons. This was of particular importance because in the second half of the nineteenth century Poland was unable to share in the rapid and great advances of the rest of the world in surgery. Poland was deprived of her independence and split among three empires. The medical schools closed, and the hospitals were not given financial aid by the various rulers of the empires. Nevertheless, though temporarily expunged from the map of Europe, Poland was still conscious of her own existence, and scientific advances were made by its citizens. One of them was Ludwik Rydygier, who organized regular meetings that attracted surgeons from all three parts of divided Poland. Rydygier's goals were to elevate the level of Polish surgery to world standards, promote surgical education and training, and contribute to the art and science of surgery.

Rydygier always expressed his patriotic attachment to Poland. He remained true in these feelings from early years until the end of his life. By spelling his name in the Polish way, *Rydygier,* he emphasized his Polish origin and nationality. It is beyond any doubt that Rydygier was truly an "ambassador of Polish surgery" at a most difficult time in Polish history.

Suggested Reading

Sokol, S. *Ludwik Rydygier, 1850–1920.* Warsaw: Polish Medical Publishers, 1961.

EDITOR'S COMMENT

We are indebted to Sarah Wangensteen and Clarence Dennis for updating this superb review of the historical aspects of gastric surgery.

The world of surgery was saddened by the news of Dr. Wangensteen's death in 1981. His many contributions, so nicely outlined by Dr. Dennis, will remain an important part of the history of surgery.

Dr. Wangensteen, better known as "the Chief" or "O.H.W." to his students, was no stranger to the subject of gastric surgery. Although he may have written on the subject earlier, the 1935 article quoted by Rosoff and Berne in their chapters of this book gives some indication of his long interest (O. H. Wangensteen, *Minn. Med.* 18:477, 1935).

Dr. Wangensteen became head of the Department of Surgery at the University of Minnesota in 1930 at the age of 31. His retirement from that position in 1967 was the occasion for summing up the accomplishments of those 37 years. Suffice it to indicate that he converted the surgical scene at the University of Minnesota over those years into one of the world's surgical showcases. Most important of all, because of the quantity and quality of the men and women he trained, he has been called the finest surgical educator since William Hunter.

For those interested in more historical aspects of gastrointestinal physiology, a small monograph is available. Lick and Balser of Munich have brought together a wealth of material including many unusual illustrations (R. F. Lick and D. Balser, Die geschichte der angewandten magenphysiologie. *Materia Medica Nordmark: Wissenschaftliches Beiblatts* 60:1, 1967).

Dr. Henry N. Harkins (Fig. 1-41) was the senior editor of *Surgery of the Stomach and Duodenum* during its earlier editions. I believe that he should be credited with the current popularity of gastroduodenal anastomosis following resection of the stomach and with the very basic work he and his colleagues did to show the rationale of selective and highly selective vagotomy. He, too, is credited with developing a superb school of surgery at the University of Washington, Seattle, and with training a number of surgical leaders.

Three contemporary surgeons, Billroth of Austria, Rydygier of Poland, and Péan of France are credited with pioneering work in the field of gastric surgery. Volumes have been written about Billroth, but Péan and Rydygier have not fared as well. Personal contacts with knowledgeable colleagues in France and Poland brought to light the additional information included here in the special comments on Péan and Rydygier. (L. M. N.)

2

Anatomy

Charles A. Griffith

Embryology

The following account is limited to the development of normal adult structures. Space does not permit a detailed explanation of the numerous congenital abnormalities described by others [35] and discussed in Chapter 27.

THE ADULT FOREGUT

The embryological foregut forms the esophagus, stomach, and proximal duodenum. The term *proximal duodenum* refers to the first segment of the duodenum between the pylorus and the head of the pancreas. Like the stomach, the proximal duodenum is attached to the lesser omentum (hepatoduodenal ligament) and greater omentum, and, also like the stomach, the proximal duodenum is freely mobile and expansile. Radiologists call it the *bulb*. The duodenum distal to this proximal segment represents the beginning of the midgut, which is fixed posteriorly to the dorsal body wall, medially to the head of the pancreas, and anteriorly to the hepatic flexure of the colon and mesocolon. Radiologists call this part of the duodenum the *descending portion*, or *duodenal loop*, because it loops around the head of the pancreas. Unlike the bulb, the duodenal loop is fixed, and it is not nearly so expansile.

Rotation

The foregut first appears as a tube lying longitudinally in the cephalocaudal axis. It is suspended by both ventral and dorsal midsagittal mesenteries. The stomach appears as a fusiform dilatation within the foregut. Because the stomach's dorsal mesenteric border grows much more than its ventral border, the stomach rotates on its longitudinal axis 90 degrees to the right. The distal stomach and duodenum then swing up and over to the right upper quadrant. The results of this growth and rotation are as follows: (1) The original right surface of stomach and duodenum faces posteriorly; (2) the original ventral mesenteric border of the stomach faces cephalad and to the right as the lesser curvature, and the ventral mesentery becomes the lesser omentum; and (3) the dorsal mesenteric border faces caudad and to the left as the greater curvature, and the dorsal mesentery becomes the greater omentum.

Lesser Omentum

A primitive ventral mesentery originally suspends the entire gut. The portion suspending the midgut and hindgut disappears, and only the foregut retains its ventral mesentery, which extends distally on the abdominal wall to the umbilicus and on the foregut to the proximal duodenum.

During rotation of the stomach, the liver grows into the ventral mesentery. In the adult state, therefore, the ventral mesentery runs from the lesser curvature to the liver as the lesser omentum, embraces the liver, and then runs to the ventral abdominal wall as the falciform ligament. The free caudal edge of the ventral mesentery between proximal duodenum and liver is the hepatoduodenal ligament (the anterior boundary of the epiploic foramen of Winslow), and the free caudal edge between the liver and abdominal wall is the falciform ligament running to the umbilicus.

Greater Omentum

The primitive dorsal mesentery suspends the entire gut (foregut, midgut, and hindgut). The proximal portion of the dorsal mesentery suspending the foregut is the dorsal mesogastrium. During rotation of the stomach, the dorsal mesogastrium balloons to the left as a large sac called the *omental bursa*. The original right peritoneal surface of the dorsal mesogastrium lines the interior of this sac, and the left surface of dorsal mesogastrium lines the exterior. The anterior wall of the sac contains the spleen and attaches to the greater curvature. The posterior wall contains the pancreas and fuses to the dorsal body wall.

After rotation of the stomach, the anterior wall of the omental sac hangs from the greater curvature (Fig. 2-1A). The posterior wall of the omental sac fuses to the transverse colon and mesocolon (Fig. 2-1B). The inner surfaces of the omental sac then fuse to each other. This fusion starts at the tip of the sac and progresses toward the greater curvature. On the left, fusion stops at the transverse colon (Fig. 2-1C). On the right, fusion continues above the colon (Fig. 2-1D). Thus the adult omentum consists of two parts: (1) the portion extending from the greater curvature to the transverse colon and spleen (gastrocolic and gastrosplenic ligaments) and (2) the portion hanging free from the transverse colon.

Fixation by Peritoneal Fusion

The duodenum follows the stomach's rotation of 90 degrees to the right and migrates with the distal stomach to the right upper quadrant. Accordingly, the original right surface of the duodenum faces posteriorly, and the original dorsal mesenteric border of the proximal and descending duodenum faces to the left. The proximal duodenum remains free and mobile, but the descending portion of the duodenum and the attached head of pancreas fuse to the dorsal body wall and thus become fixed.

SURGICAL APPLICATIONS

Entering the Lesser Peritoneum

The difference between Figure 2-1C and 2-1D illustrates the ease or difficulty one can encounter in entering the lesser peritoneal space through the gastrocolic ligament. Retracting the transverse colon and free omentum inferiorly stretches out the gastrocolic ligament to facilitate its surgical dissection. On the right, the gastrocolic ligament is relatively fixed, fatty, and short. The midcolic vessels lie directly underneath. Incising this six-layered area of gastrocolic ligament is therefore apt to be bloody and hazardous. On the left, however, the two-layered gastrocolic ligament is more mobile and thin. It is also longer; that is, more space exists between stomach and colon. Furthermore, the area immediately inferior to the anastomosis between the right and left gastroepiploic vessels is avascular. Incising the gastrocolic ligament here provides a spacious and bloodless entry into the lesser peritoneal space. A finger inserted into the lesser peritoneal space at this point leads to safe excision of the omentum from the greater curvature by protecting the midcolic vessels distally and the splenic vessels proximally.

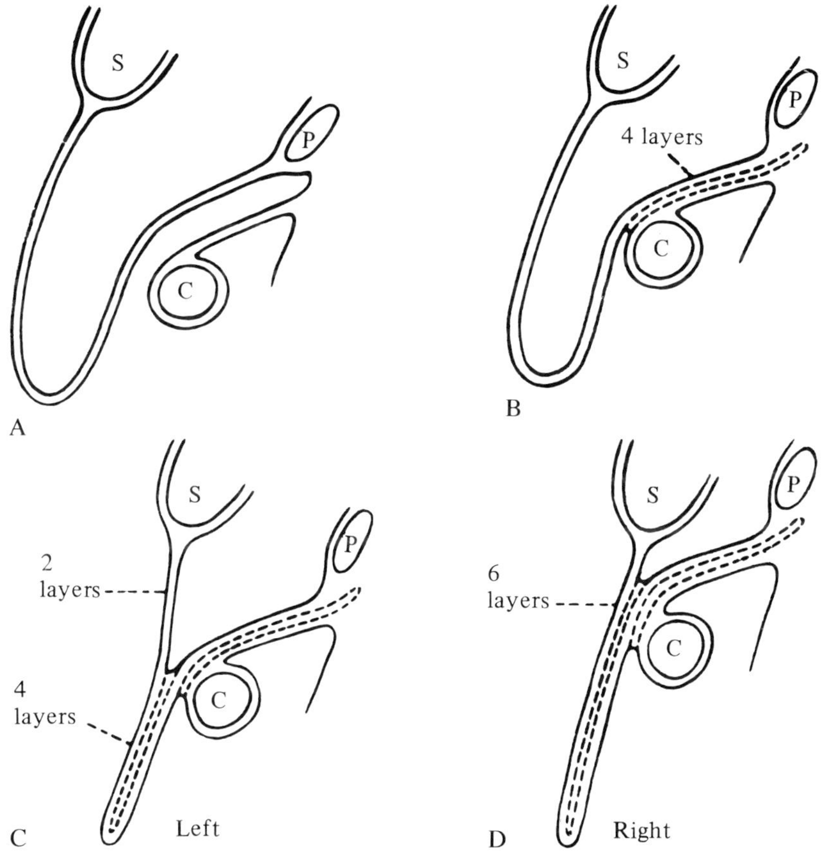

Fig. 2-1. The formation of the greater omentum. (A) After rotation of the stomach and formation of the omental bursa. (B) After fusion of the posterior wall of the omental bursa to the transverse colon and mesocolon. (C, D) After fusion of anterior and posterior walls of omental bursa to form adult omentum on the left side (C) and right side (D). (S = stomach; P = pancreas; C = colon.)

Restoring Embryological Relationships

On the patient's right, the fixed duodenum may be released by incising the peritoneum lateral to the duodenum and then sweeping the duodenum and pancreatic head away from the kidney and inferior vena cava medially to the aorta. This dissection restores embryological relationships for exposure of the posterior pancreatic head and distal common duct and also for mobilization of the duodenum. It is commonly called the Kocher maneuver but, as pointed out by Madden et al. [74], Jourdan and Vautrin performed it well before Kocher.

A similar situation exists on the patient's left, where the posterior layer of omental bursa containing the body and tail of the pancreas fuses with the dorsal body wall. Cutting the posterior peritoneal reflections onto the spleen (splenophrenic, splenorenal, and splenocolic ligaments) and dissecting the spleen and pancreas from the posterior body wall to the aorta also restore embryological relationships.

Splenic Injury

The variable development of the greater omentum results in the absence or presence of various peritoneal folds coursing between the omentum, greater curvature, and spleen. When these folds are present, traction exerted on them by pulling the greater omentum and stomach inferiorly may result in tearing of the splenic capsule and pulp. This accident is probably the most common event necessitating splenectomy during gastric operations; vigilance is required in identifying peritoneal folds when the abdomen is first explored to avoid tearing them and the spleen initially or subsequently during the operation [86].

Mucosa

Figure 2-2A divides the stomach into the traditional gross anatomical areas. However, if we define *fundus* as the stomach's dome, or that part above the esophageal inlet, and define *pylorus* as the part at the pyloric sphincter, then the fundus and pylorus are the only parts of the stomach we can accurately delineate by gross examination. We cannot accurately delineate the cardia, corpus, and antrum, because the stomach's gross configuration does not present any landmarks that allow us to do so.[1] To impart surgical usefulness to Figure 2-2A, histological and physiological studies are necessary (Fig. 2-2B).

MUCOSAL TYPES

Older histological terminology is both confusing and surgically meaningless.[2] To impart more surgical meaning, the four distinct types of mucosa in the adult foregut are divided as follows:

1. *Stratified squamous epithelium* lines the esophagus. Mucous cells underlie the most distal esophageal epithelium.
2. *Parietal mucosa,* which Kay of Glasgow first called the *parietal cell mass* and others the *oxyntic mucosa,* contains the parietal and chief cells that secrete acid and pepsin, respectively. Explanation for the concentrated population of mucous cells in the most proximal parietal mucosa (Fig. 2-2B) is only teleological. Not enough mucus is produced to prevent reflux esophagitis or to obviate the need for excising all of the parietal mucosa in the Zollinger-Ellison syndrome.
3. *Antral mucosa* contains mucous cells and the G cells that secrete gastrin. Chief and parietal cells are scarce to absent. In contrast to the acid surface of the parietal mucosa, the surface of the antral mucosa is neutral or slightly alkaline.
4. *Duodenal mucosa* is characterized by the presence of Brunner's glands, which always extend distally as far as the papilla of Vater and, in most bodies, beyond the papilla but never as far as the jejunum [63]. The alkaline mucus secreted by Brunner's glands provides the proximal duodenum with more resistance to acid-peptic ulceration than the jejunum. This resistance has been used as a point in favor of the Billroth I over the Billroth II anastomosis [42].[3]

MUCOSAL RESISTANCE AND ULCERATION

The esophageal squamous epithelium is the least resistant to acid-pepsin ulceration of the four mucosal types. Following, in order of increasing resistance, are the duodenal mucosa, the antral mucosa, and the parietal mucosa.

Because parietal mucosa is the most resistant to acid-peptic ulceration, gastric ulcer there is rare. Careful histological studies have

[1]The incisura angularis ventriculi on the lesser curvature separates corpus from antrum in textbooks and in the dissecting laboratory, but in the operating room this landmark either cannot be found or can be only vaguely located. Furthermore, the incisura angularis ventriculi may often be confused with peristaltic waves on radiographs. Even when an incisura angularis is thought to be identified, its position changes as the patient changes from an erect to a horizontal position.

[2]*Proper gastric glands, principal gastric glands,* or merely *gastric glands* are names that implicate this mucosa as the main source of the stomach's digestive juice. The term *fundic glands* originates from the fact that these glands were first studied in the gross fundus. This term is confusing because it implies the erroneous concept that these glands are confined to the gross fundus. *Cardiac glands* is another term that considers the corpus together with the fundus as one *cardiac part* of the stomach; thus the stomach has been divided into two parts, the *pyloric* and the *cardiac,* or *fundic,* regions. The word *cardiac* is confusing, however, because it associates this mucosal type with that of the gross cardia. Last, the *pyloric* part of the stomach does not permit distinction between the gross pylorus and the gross antrum. The antral mucosa has been called the *pyloric glands.*

[3]The distal extent of the foregut, or the boundary between the foregut and midgut, is not clearly defined. On the basis of gross anatomy we may consider the distal foregut as the free, mobile, expansile proximal duodenum between the pylorus and the pancreas that is suspended by the hepatoduodenal ligament (the distal limit of the ventral mesentery suspending the foregut). On the basis of histology, we may consider the distal extent of Brunner's glands to mark the limit of the foregut.

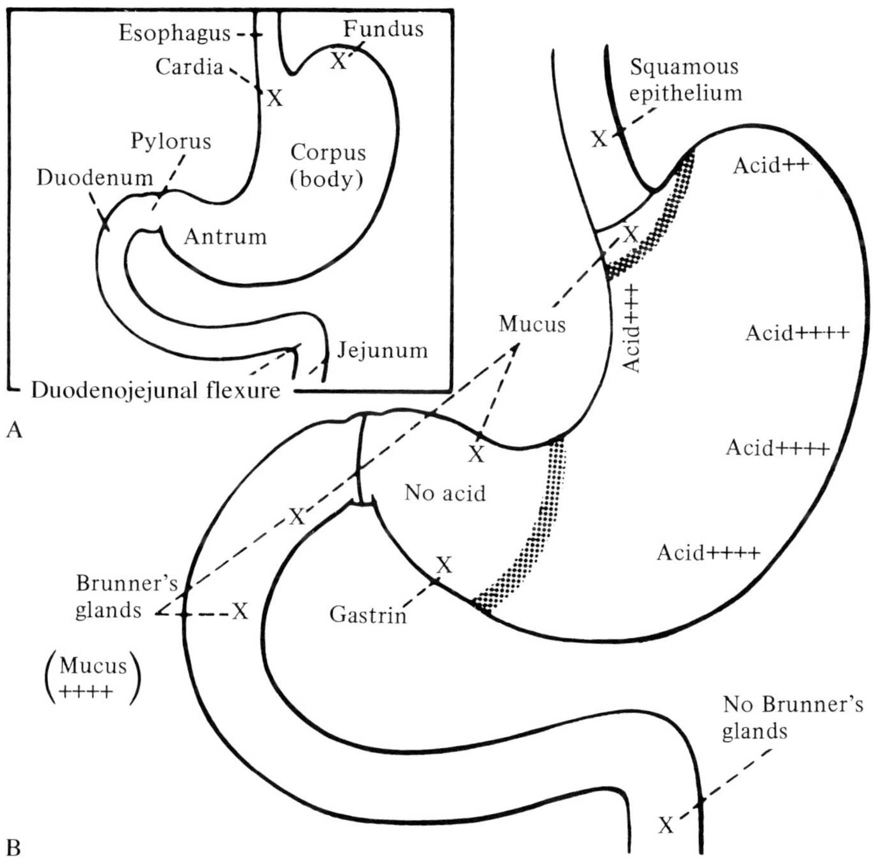

Fig. 2-2. Location of various mucosal types and their secretions in the gross stomach and duodenum. (A) Gross anatomical areas. (B) Secretory areas. Broad lines delineate the proximal and distal extent of the acid area. Concentration of acid cells in the fundus is about half of, and along the lesser curvature is about three-fourths of, the maximal concentration of acid cells in the corpus [13]. For reasons of simplicity, this diagram does not indicate the variation in distance from the antral-parietal mucosal border to the pylorus.

shown that gastric ulcers in the parietal area occur either in ectopic islands of antral mucosa within the parietal mucosa or in parietal mucosa that has become "intestinalized" or "antralized" by injury from duodenal reflux [19]. The surfaces of both the ectopic islands of antral mucosa and the "antralized" parietal mucosa are neutral or alkaline [18, 20, 89].

MUCOSAL JUNCTIONS

In normal stomachs the boundaries delineating the four types of mucosa may be demonstrated quite sharply and distinctly. However, the demonstration requires painstaking and meticulous methods of pinning the fresh stomach out on a flat surface, cutting microscopic sections in the proper longitudinal axis, and plotting the microscopic differences on a map of the gross stomach.

Mucosal Esophagogastric Junction

The mucosal esophagogastric junction is readily seen as a sharp line on the gross mucosal surface. Microscopic sections through this junction reveal an abrupt transition from stratified squamous epithelium to gastric mucosa with mucous glands underlying both types of epithelium.

Antral-Parietal Mucosal Junction
No gross anatomical landmarks exist to locate the antral-parietal mucosal border. As shown in Figure 2-3, however, the border usually lies in the general area where the rugal folds of the corpus flatten out onto the smooth surface of the antrum [62]. Microscopic sections reveal that the parietal mucosa gives way to the antral mucosa either abruptly or gradually in a zone of transition that rarely exceeds 1 cm. The antral-parietal border can also be clearly demonstrated by topical Congo red [84, 85] or intravenous neutral red [97]. The distance from this border to the pylorus varies considerably.

Mucosal Gastroduodenal Junction
The mucosal gastroduodenal junction usually is within the pyloric sphincter but may be either immediately proximal or immediately distal to it [62, 92]. Although the gastroduodenal junction may be seen on close inspection to be a straight or dentate line, this junction is not nearly so obvious as the gross esophagogastric junction. However, microscopic sections always reveal a sharp transition from antral to duodenal mucosa.

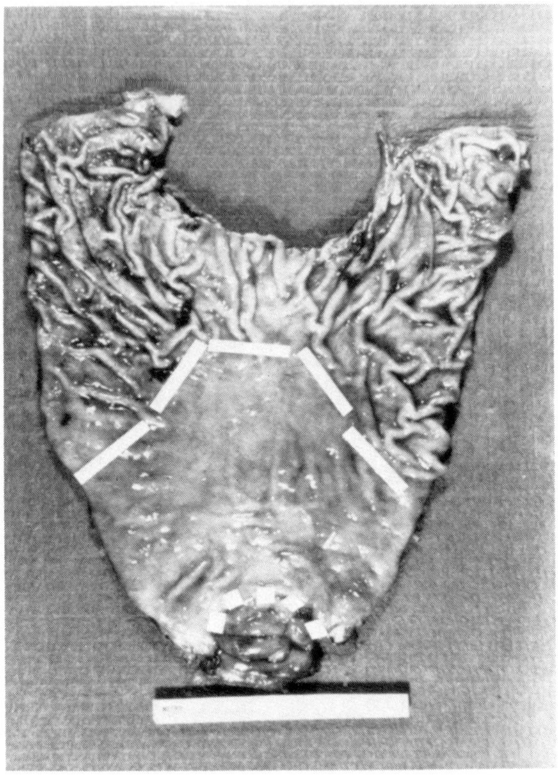

Fig. 2-3. Mucosal surface of a gastric specimen opened along the greater curvature after hemigastrectomy. The mucosa of the corpus is thrown into rugal folds; the mucosa of the antrum is flat.

Surgical Applications
MUCOSAL JUNCTIONS AND PEPTIC ULCER. Oi et al. [89–93] showed that ulcers occur adjacent to mucosal junctions. Reflux esophagitis and ulceration are most severe immediately proximal to the esophagogastric junction. With the unusual exception of postbulbar ulcer, duodenal ulcers occur just distal to the gastroduodenal junction. Gastric ulcers most commonly occur immediately distal to the antral-parietal mucosal junction or, as Capper showed [18, 20], the antralized parietal-mucosal junction. Thus peptic ulcers occur at, or adjacent to, junctions where the pH of the mucosal surface changes, and always on the alkaline side of the junction.

PYLORIC ULCER: DUODENAL OR GASTRIC? The antral-duodenal mucosal junction usually lies within the pyloric channel but may lie proximal or distal to it. In the first instance, the pyloric channel ulcer is duodenal; in the second, the ulcer is gastric. This histological differentiation may or may not explain the unique intractability of pyloric ulcer. Perhaps pylorospasm offers a better explanation.

PREPYLORIC DUODENAL ULCER. In the unusual to rare patient, the antral-duodenal mucosal boder lies as far as 2 cm proximal to the pylorus [63, 92]. In these patients a prepyloric ulcer may therefore be duodenal rather than gastric.

HIGH AND LOW GASTRIC ULCERS. The usual location of the antral-parietal mucosal border in the distal part of the middle third of the stomach explains the usual location of gastric ulcers. However, the location of the antral-

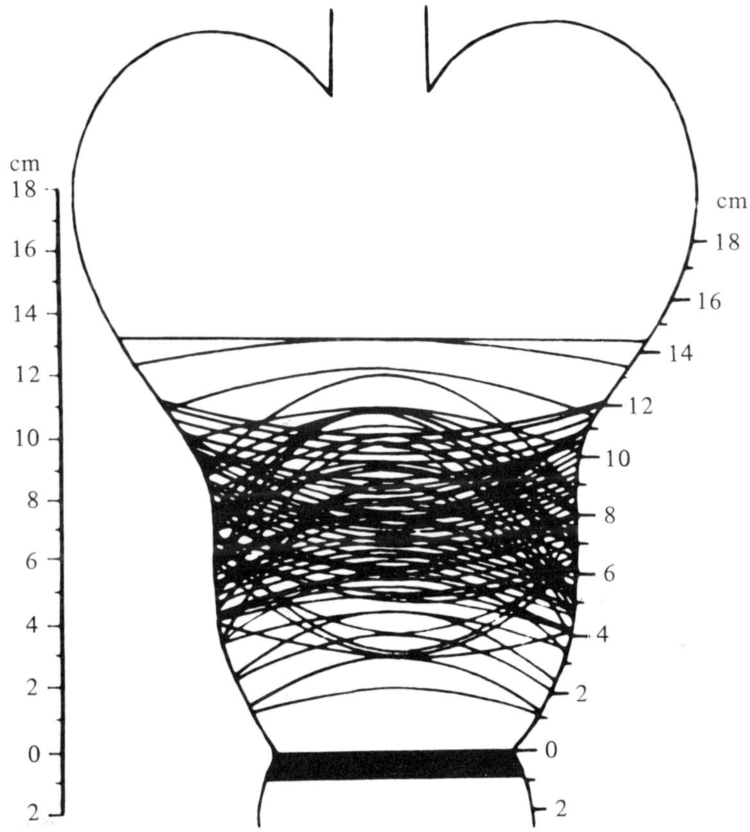

Fig. 2-4. Variable locations of the antral-parietal borders in 100 stomachs without ulcer opened along the greater curve and laid flat. The lines were drawn from measurements in centimeters from the pylorus on both the greater and lesser curves. The convex lines represent the antral-parietal mucosal borders. The concave lines represent the border of the circular muscle bundle (see the section in this chapter, Musculature). Most gastric ulcers occur in the area where the convex and concave lines overlap. Note the most distal antral-parietal borders, which preclude completeness of the distal part of a parietal vagotomy, as do short nerves of Latarjet in Fig. 2-7. (From Oi et al. [89]. Reproduced with courtesy of The Williams & Wilkins Company.)

parietal border varies considerably (Fig. 2-4). When located in the proximal third of the stomach, accompanied by antralization of the parietal mucosa, the ulcer is high—in the unusual to rare instance as high as the cardia. In contrast, when the antral-parietal border is low, the ulcer is prepyloric (or, in Oi's terminology, "juxtapyloric"). Prepyloric ulcers are much more commonly gastric than duodenal.

THE ANTRAL CELL MASS. In most patients with gastric ulcer and in patients without ulcer but with dyspepsia of gastritis due to duodenal reflux through an incompetent pylorus [19], the antral cell mass is relatively large and the parietal cell mass small. The converse generally holds true in patients with duodenal ulcer [25]. The occurrence of an extremely small antral cell mass (Fig. 2-4) assumes surgical importance when selective vagotomy of the parietal mucosa is done.

Musculature

For practical surgical purposes, the three gastric muscles—outer longitudinal, middle circular, inner oblique—are fused and compose one muscular layer. But when we remove the mucosa and submucosa from this layer and view the oblique and circular muscles from within, we see specific anatomical variations that Oi et al. [89] have related to the formation of gastric ulcer.

MUSCLE BORDERS

The inner oblique muscle is absent along the lesser curvature. Its fibers nearest to the lesser curvature run parallel to this curve in the anterior and posterior walls of the stomach. The thickest fibers of the middle circular muscle that run across the lesser curvature have been called the circular muscle bundle. As the antral-parietal mucosal border varies in location, so the border of the circular muscle bundle varies. Gastric ulcers occur on the lesser curvature in the area void of the oblique muscle and proximal to the circular muscle bundle. Furthermore, gastric ulcers occur most commonly when the circular muscle border underlies the antral-parietal mucosal border. When these two borders are not in proximity to each other, gastric ulcer is rare but gastritis is not. Thus Oi et al. entitled their work "A possible dual control mechanism in the origin of peptic ulcer" [89]; the paper proposes the theses of mucosal sensitivity and of the kinetic strain of muscular activity (Fig. 2-4).

This dual control also influences the formation of duodenal ulcer just distal to the pylorus. The pyloric sphincter consists of a thickening of the middle circular muscle; with the rare exceptions previously described, this sphincteric border underlies the antral-duodenal mucosal border.

THE PYLORUS

When the pylorus was not readily located because of edema or fibrosis, Mayo [75] would describe its identification by a vein that is quite constant. This vein has been called the pyloric vein of Mayo.

The middle circular muscle thickens *gradually* to form the pyloric sphincter. This thickening ends *abruptly* on the duodenal side. Also, the circular muscle fibers of the pyloric sphincter converge on the lesser curvature to form a *torus* [117].

SURGICAL APPLICATIONS

To preserve gastric muscle, and with it the gastric reservoir, Kirk [56] took advantage of the plane between muscle and submucosa to perform his mucosal antrectomy with pyloroplasty. To preserve pyloric function as well, I have performed suprapyloric mucosal antrectomy [3]. Reconstruction after these procedures emphasizes the nicety of the two-layered anastomosis—namely, the suturing of mucosa and submucosa to mucosa and submucosa as one inner layer, and of muscle to muscle as one outer layer. When applied to gastroduodenostomy and gastroenterostomy, this anastomotic technique minimizes inversion at the stoma and also reduces the chance of postoperative hemorrhage from the submucosal plexus.

Seaman [107] described hyperplasia of the pyloric torus as a flattening of the canal on roentgenogram and a palpable nodule at operation. It is postulated that hyperplasia of the torus may precede adult hypertrophic pyloric stenosis.

The abrupt ending of the pyloric thickening on the duodenal side, in contrast to its gradual beginning on the gastric side, explains the error of entering the duodenal lumen during pyloromyotomy for infantile hypertrophic pyloric stenosis.

Sympathetic Nerves

Preganglionic efferent fibers destined for the stomach and duodenum leave the spinal cord (fifth or sixth to ninth or tenth thoracic segments), traverse their respective sympathetic ganglia without synapse, and unite to join the greater splanchnic nerves. On reaching the celiac ganglia by way of the greater splanchnics, the preganglionic fibers form a synapse with the postganglionic fibers that go to the stomach and proximal duodenum by way of the various branches of the celiac artery. The afferent system consists of a single neuron that returns along the same pathways. In addition to these sympathetic fibers, the canine abdominal vagi contain adrenergic fibers arising primarily from the stellate ganglia [1].

SURGICAL APPLICATIONS

Results of thoracolumbar sympathectomy and vagotomy have established the afferent sympathetic fibers as the pathways for the perception of visceral pain. Although complete vagotomy affords immediate relief of pain from duodenal ulcer left in situ, the pain may be reproduced if, as repeatedly demonstrated by Dragstedt, dilute acid is instilled through the nasogastric tube. Furthermore, in patients with complete vagotomy determined by negative insulin tests but with recurrent ulcer caused by gastric stasis or ulcerogenic pancreatic tumor, the pain of recurrent ulcer is perceived. In contrast, patients with thoracolumbar sympathectomy for hypertension may not perceive the pain of peptic ulcer until perforation incites the somatic pain of peritonitis.

The stomach and duodenum receive most of their sympathetic innervation from the seventh and eighth thoracic spinal segments. The pain of peptic ulcer is therefore most commonly perceived in the seventh and eighth thoracic dermatomes (the epigastrium). Higher (fifth and sixth) or lower (ninth and tenth) thoracic segments, however, may also contribute many fibers to the stomach and duodenum. Thus we encounter a few patients with peptic ulcer who complain of pain in the lower thorax and others whose pain is around the umbilicus. The observations by Kimura [55] of visceral pain during abdominal operations under local anesthesia confirmed the localization of referred pain to the specific dermatomes.

Parasympathetic Nerves

So far as is known, the vagus nerves are the sole source of parasympathetic innervation of the foregut and midgut. The existence of a splanchnic parasympathetic system from the thoracolumbar spinal segments in humans is only conjectural. Whereas the sympathetic system innervates the entire embryological gut, the vagal system innervates only the foregut and midgut; the sacral parasympathetic system innervates the hindgut. The boundary between the midgut and hindgut is at the splenic flexure of the colon. At this boundary vagal innervation ends and sacral innervation begins; also at this boundary the superior mesenteric artery ends and the inferior mesenteric artery begins.

Preganglionic efferent vagal fibers reach the foregut directly close to the midgut, traverse various autonomic ganglia without synapse, and accompany the arterial supply to the liver, biliary tract, pancreas, and intestine. The preganglionic fibers synapse with the postganglionic fibers in the intramural plexuses of the gut.

THE VAGI FROM THORAX TO ABDOMEN

When we consider the vagi in terms of systemic anatomy, we learn anatomical constants. In contrast, when we consider the vagi in terms of regional anatomy at the diaphragmatic esophageal hiatus, we see a maze of variations.

Systemic Anatomy: The Constants

Below each pulmonary hilus, the *left and right vagus nerves* descend on either side of the esophagus and, in the lower thorax, branch and communicate with each other as the *esophageal plexus* around the esophagus. Depending on the variable number of branches that each vagus nerve contributes to form this plexus, the complexity of the plexus varies from body to body. The branches of the esophageal plexus then unite to form *two, and only two, vagal trunks*—one *anterior* and the other *posterior* to the esophagus. The anterior vagal trunk divides into the *anterior gastric* and *hepatic vagal divisions*. The posterior trunk divides into the *posterior gastric and celiac vagal divisions*.

Regional Anatomy: The Variations at the Hiatus

The diaphragm has no embryological relationship with the vagal system. Thus we see that the vagal system descends through the hiatus in the form of any one of its three components. One must identify the specific component of the vagal system at hand; the notion of variable numbers of multiple nerves is surgically useless (Fig. 2-5).

Another cause of variations at the hiatus is the embryological rotation of the stomach. Before rotation the vagal trunks lie on each side of the esophagus, and their gastric divisions descend along each side of the stomach's lesser curvature. The gastric divisions rotate with the stomach and, after rotation, lie in constant positions at the gastric cardia and along the lesser curvature. At the higher level of the hiatus, well away from the effect of rotation, the vagal trunks may not rotate completely with the stomach and therefore assume variable positions in adults (Fig. 2-6).

THE ABDOMINAL VAGI

The most recent and most thorough anatomical study with a review of older studies [77, 82, 83] was reported by Shandalakis and his associates [112]. Their description and illustrations are remarkably similar to the findings of my dissections supervised by Dr. Robert Johnson when he was Professor of Anatomy at the University of Washington. The following account is taken from the anatomical concept taught by Dr. Johnson.

The anterior vagi are conceived in terms of three components: (1) the *hepatic division,* (2) the *pyloric nerve* of McCrea [77], and (3) the *anterior gastric division.* The last was termed the *principal* or *greater anterior gastric nerve* by Latarjet [64, 65] and his student Wertheimer [119]; it is now commonly called the *nerve of Latarjet.* The pyloric nerve of McCrea is more often absent than present. When absent, its pyloric fibers are most commonly a part of the hepatic division and descend to the pylorus (and distal antrum and proximal duodenum) within the hepatoduodenal ligament, usually in company with the right gastric artery. In its classic position the pyloric nerve runs within the lesser omentum midway between the hepatic and anterior gastric divisions to the distal antrum and pylorus. In a lower position the nerve of McCrea runs just above and parallel to the nerve of Latarjet. In this pattern Loeweneck [72] called McCrea's pyloric nerve the "antral nerve," and others have referred to the "double nerve of Loeweneck." Finally, the nerves of McCrea and Latarjet may be incorporated into one nerve, which runs all the way to the pylorus and, rarely, onto the proximal duodenum (Fig. 2-7).

The hepatic division is constant from the standpoint that it can always be seen within the stretched-out lesser omentum just beneath the undersurface of the liver in contrast against the dark background of the caudate lobe of the liver. Usually as a few small fibers in parallel, *the hepatic vagi accompany the vestige of the left hepatic artery from the left gastric artery (or with this aberrant left hepatic artery when it is present)* within the lesser omentum to the hepatic plexus, which is an autonomic plexus enmeshing the hepatic ducts and arteries in the hilus of the liver.

The posterior vagi consist of the *posterior gastric division* (posterior nerve of Latarjet) and the *celiac division.* No specific posterior pyloric nerve exists. Although the posterior nerve of Latarjet reaches the distal antrum in a few bodies, it is usually shorter and has fewer gastric branches than the anterior nerve. Aside from these differences, the posterior gastric nerve may be conceived as the counterpart of the anterior nerve.

The celiac division is constant in two respects. First, it is the largest of the four truncal divisions and may be conceived of as the continuation of the posterior trunk. Second, it always descends within the pancreaticoduodenal fold as one large fiber to the celiac and superior mesenteric autonomic plexuses. Two variations are of surgical importance. The first concerns its variable positions within the pancreaticoduodenal fold. Second, as the posterior trunk–celiac division, some or all of the posterior gastric vagi may arise just above the celiac plexus and accompany the left gastric artery to the stomach [48] (Fig. 2-8).

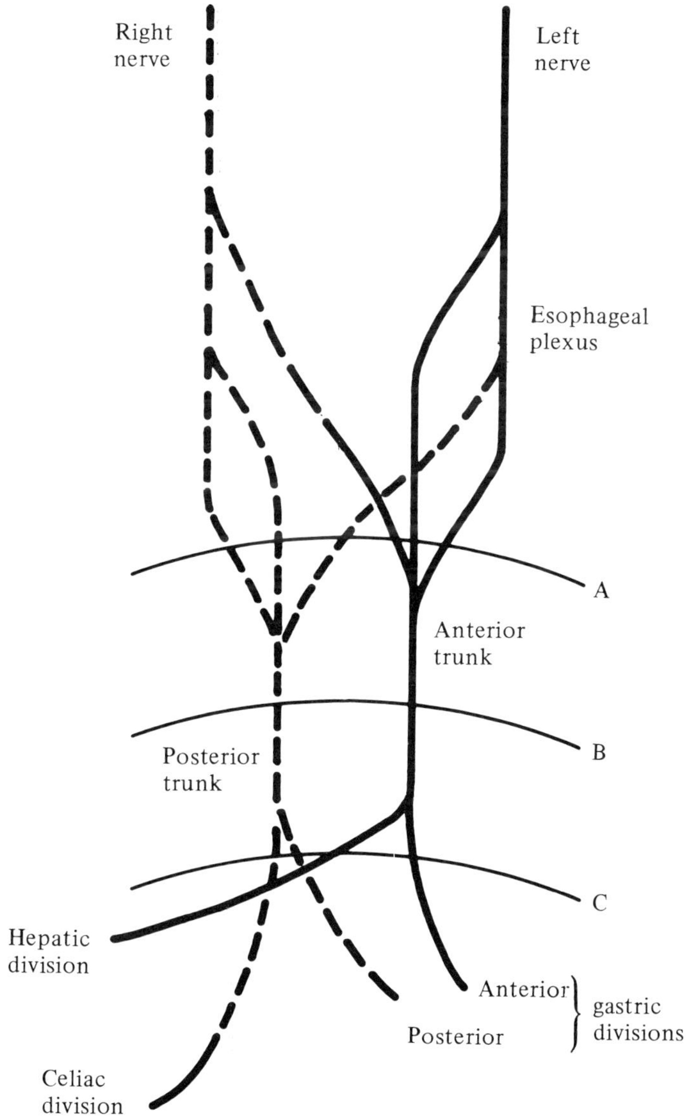

Fig. 2-5. The three constant components of the vagal system—the esophageal plexus, the two trunks, and the four truncal divisions. Pseudovariations result when this system is diagramed. (A) "Multiple nerves" at the hiatus. (B) Two trunks at the hiatus. (C) "Multiple nerves" at the hiatus. (From Griffith [38]. By permission of W. B. Saunders Company.)

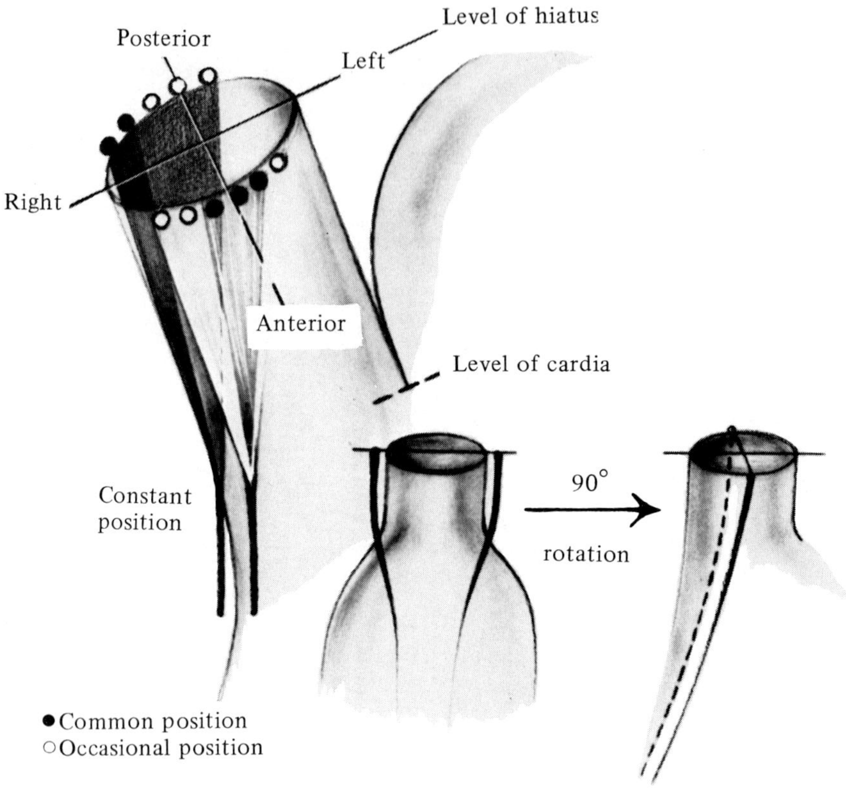

Fig. 2-6. Effect of embryological rotation of the stomach on the ultimate positions of the vagal trunks and gastric truncal divisions in adults. At the level of the distal esophagus and gastric cardia, the positions of the gastric truncal divisions are constant. At the level of the esophageal hiatus, the positions of the vagal trunks are variable. Not diagrammed are the variable positions of the vagi away from the esophagus at the hiatus. The anterior trunk, or an esophageal plexus branch contributing to it, may lie closer to the left anterior aspect of the hiatal ring than to the esophagus. The posterior trunk, or a contributing esophageal plexus branch, most commonly lies closer to the aorta and right diaphragmatic crus than to the esophagus. (From Griffith [38]. By permission of W. B. Saunders Company.)

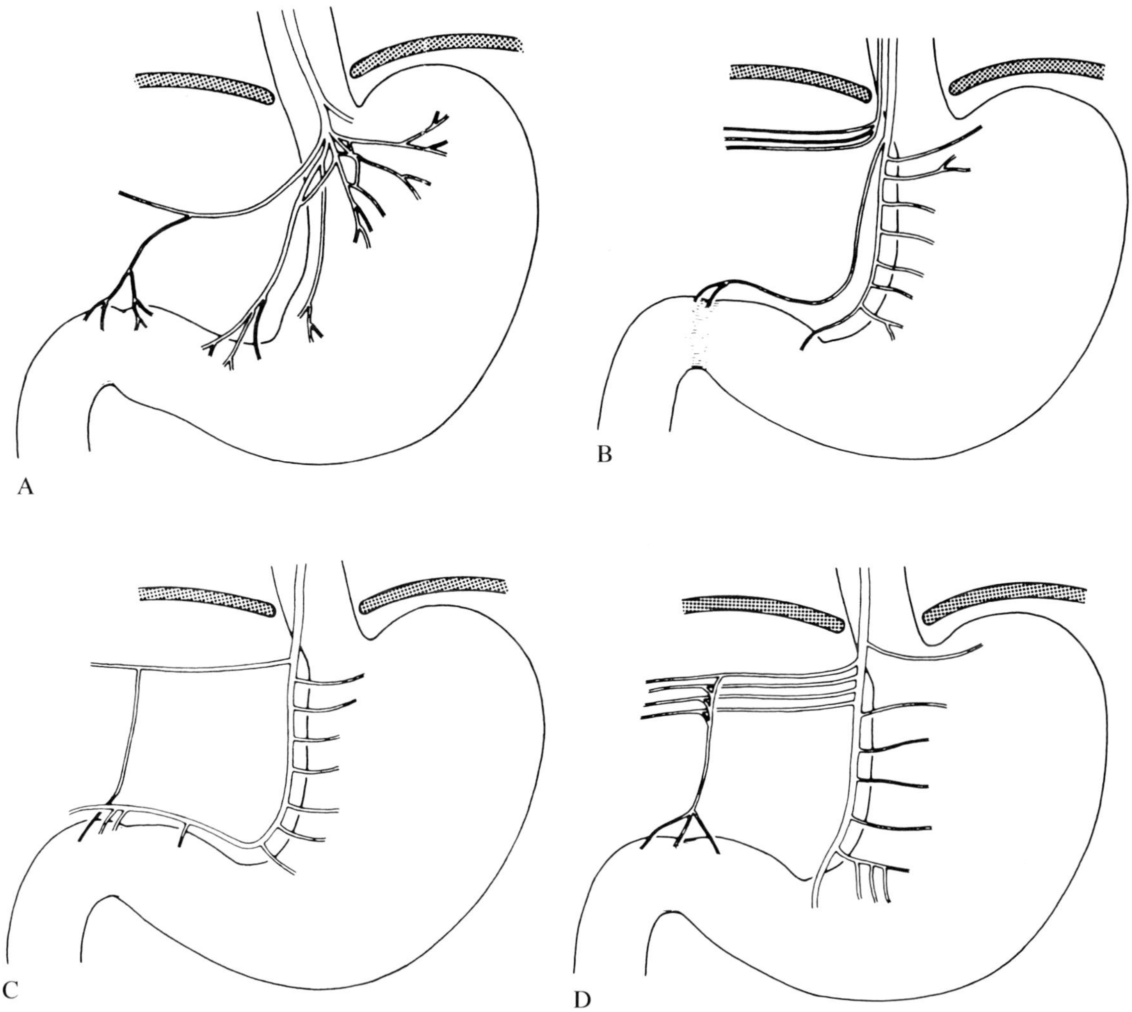

Fig. 2-7. Variations of the anterior vagi. (A) The pyloric nerve of McCrea and the hepatic division are incorporated into one nerve proximally, and divide into one hepatic nerve and one pyloric nerve distally. This diagram is modified from McCrea's original sketch. (B) The pyloric nerve of McCrea is distinct and separate from both the hepatic division and the nerve of Latarjet. Its position in the lesser omentum varies. The hepatic division consists of multiple fibers. None descends to the pylorus. (C) The pyloric nerve of McCrea is grossly absent but is incorporated within the anterior nerve of Latarjet to form one long nerve. There is no crow's foot. Supplemental pyloric fibers descend from the hepatic division. (D) The pyloric nerve of McCrea is incorporated entirely within the hepatic division. Although it is not apparent in these diagrams, this last variation accounts for significantly short nerves of Latarjet. (From Skandalakis et al. [112]. Reproduced by courtesy of J. B. Lippincott Company.)

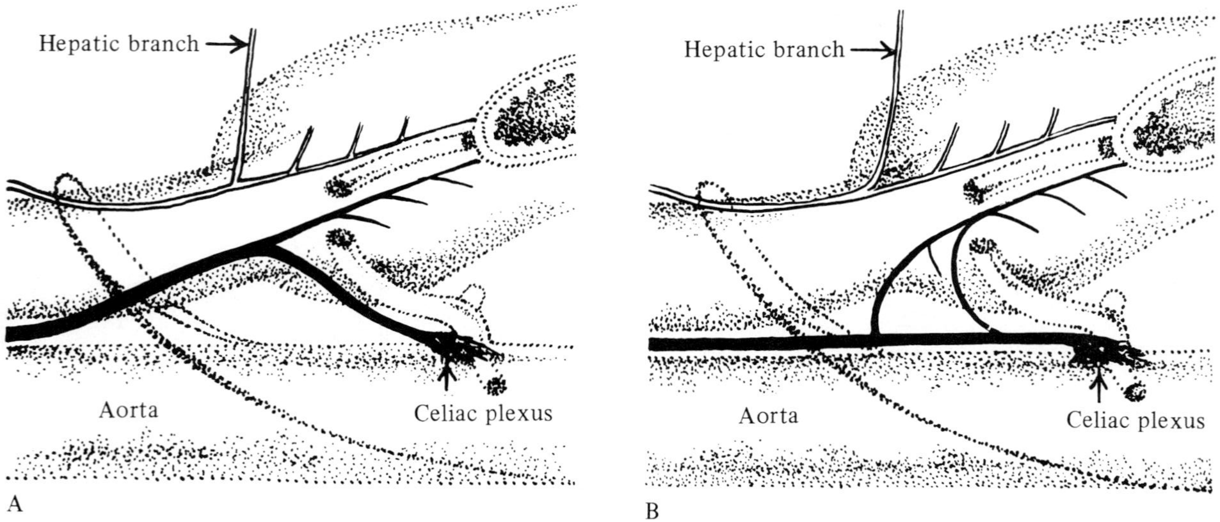

Fig. 2-8. The celiac vagi. (A) Usual course of the celiac vagal division along the left gastric artery. (B) Occasionally the celiac division runs adjacent to the diaphragmatic crura and aorta. Note the posterior gastric vagi accompanying the left gastric artery to the stomach, as described by Jackson [48]. (From Griffith [37].)

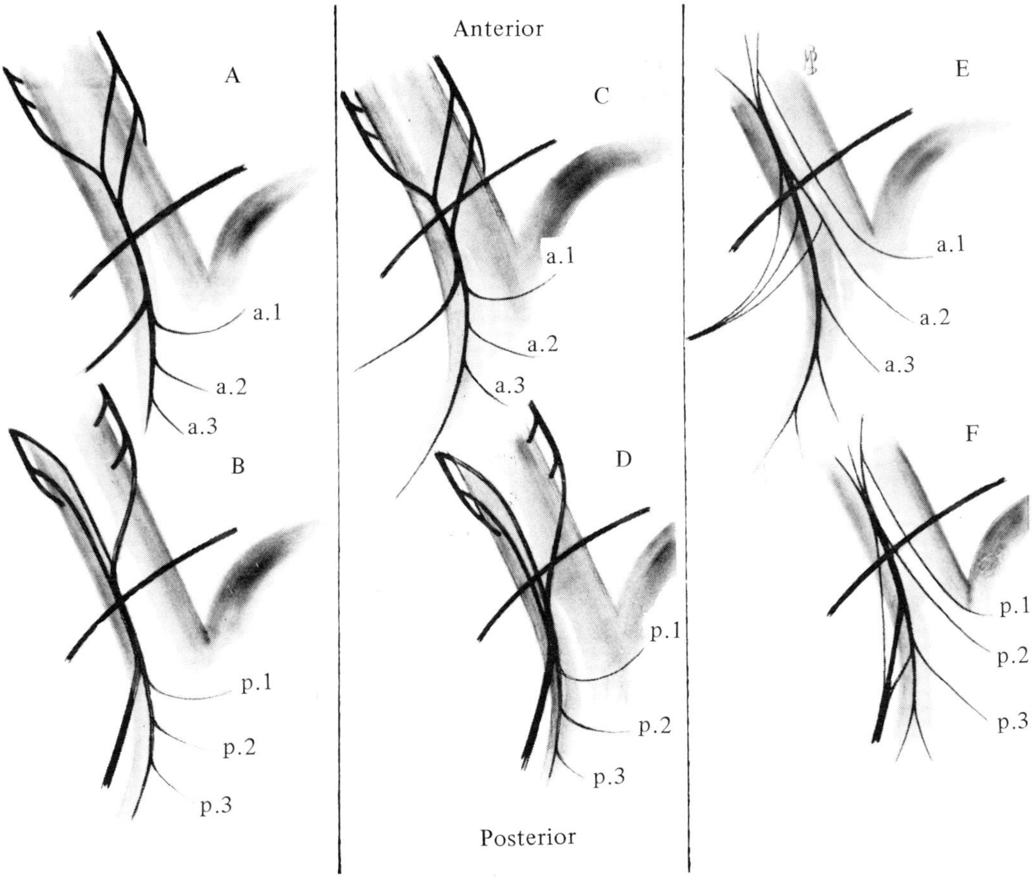

Fig. 2-9. Variations of the proximal gastric vagi. The peripheral distribution is constant, but the level of origin varies from the level of the gastric cardia to levels above the diaphragm. The origin also varies from the gastric truncal divisions to the trunks to the esophageal plexus. The diaphragm is interposed to show the same variations as diagramed in Fig. 2-5. (From Griffith [38]. Reproduced by courtesy of W. B. Saunders Company.)

The Proximal Gastric Vagi

The end branches to the proximal fundus have variable origins. In some bodies the most proximal gastric branches arise from the nerves of Latarjet at or just above the gastric cardia. In other bodies the most proximal branches arise from the trunks well above the cardia, and even from the esophageal plexus above the hiatus (Fig. 2-9). The branch labeled "p.1" in Figure 2-9 is Grassi's criminal nerve [34]. Although this branch has received particular attention, other branches are equally important. These branches often lie within or deep to the esophageal fascia propria and rarely if ever within the esophageal muscularis [37, 38, 111]. Fibers within the esophageal muscle innervate the esophagus and not the stomach.

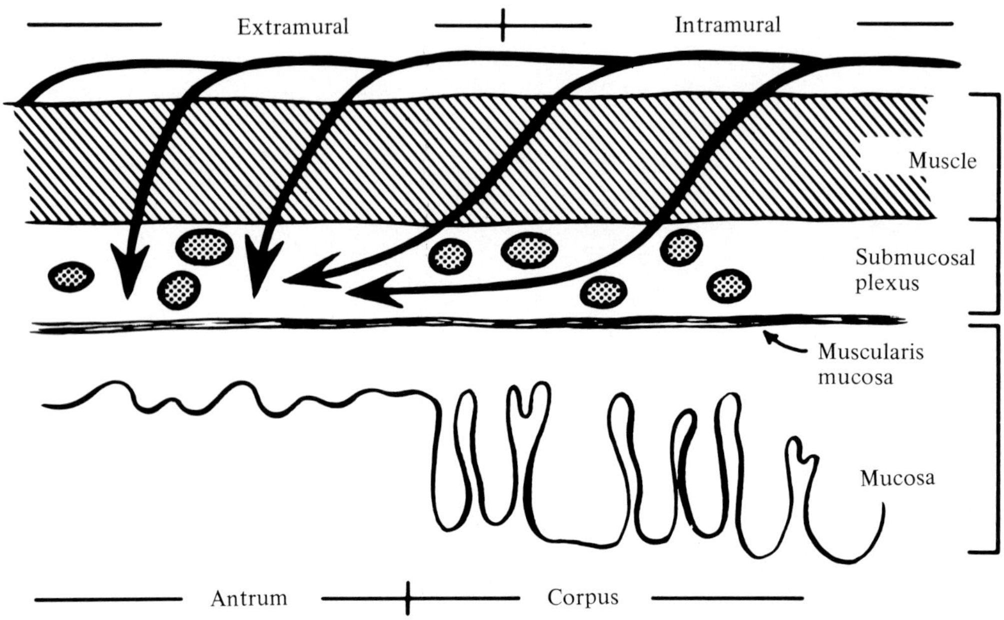

Fig. 2-10. Vagal pathways to the antral mucosa. The extramural supply comes from end branches of the nerve of Latarjet. The intramural supply comes from more proximal branches of the nerve of Latarjet. (From Legros and Griffith [69]. Reproduced by courtesy of C. V. Mosby Company.)

Segmental Innervation of the Stomach

The development of the method of electrical vagal stimulation in the presence of circulating neutral red by my research associate, Pritchard, enabled us to demonstrate the anatomical distribution of vagal fibers to the parietal mucosa [97]. The fibers from each left and right vagus nerve are distributed diffusely throughout the parietal mucosa as a result of their intermingling with each other in the esophageal plexus. At the level of this plexus, however, innervation becomes segmental. Each branch of the esophageal plexus innervates a segment of parietal mucosa via the vagal trunk to which it contributes. The anterior and posterior gastric divisions from the anterior and posterior trunks innervate the anterior and posterior mucosal surfaces, respectively. And each terminal branch from the gastric divisions (nerves of Latarjet) innervates its own small segment of parietal mucosa. Furthermore, by correlating the amount of innervated mucosa with the amount of the contractile response of the stomach, we showed that each end branch innervates its own small segment of muscle [54]. Thus the demonstration of segmental innervation of both the parietal mucosa and gastric muscle indicates that the innervation of the whole stomach is segmental. This segmental pattern of innervation is the same in dogs [97], cats [40], rats [8], and humans.

The method using neutral red did not permit visualization of the exact pattern of innervation of the antral mucosa. But this method did permit demonstration of two distinct anatomical routes for innervation of the antrum [69]. The *extramural route* is from the end branches of the nerves of Latarjet. The *intramural route* is from more proximal branches of the nerves of Latarjet that run in the submucosa beneath the parietal mucosa to the antral mucosa (Fig. 2-10).

Innervation of the Midgut

The peripheral distribution of the hepatic and celiac divisions cannot be demonstrated by gross anatomical dissections. It is impossible to trace all hepatic fibers through the hepatic autonomic plexus. (The "adventitial" tissue removed from the cystic and common ducts to demonstrate the junction of these ducts during cholecystectomy contains many ganglia of the hepatic plexus.) Similarly, it is impossible to trace all celiac fibers through the celiac and superior mesenteric plexuses. However, by physiological methods of visceral motility, we have shown that electrical stimulation of the hepatic division elicits contraction of the gallbladder and proximal duodenum; stimulation of the celiac division elicits contraction of the entire midgut except the gallbladder. Stimulation of the hepatic and celiac divisions elicits no gastric response [114]. There is also strong evidence that both the hepatic and celiac vagi (ventral anlage) are supplied by the hepatic division, and the body and tail (dorsal anlage), by the celiac division. Figure 2-11 shows the distribution of the hepatic and celiac vagi. This diagram is based on my own studies and those of others [58, 81, 82, 84 103–105].

SURGICAL APPLICATIONS

Terminology

It is appropriate in a chapter on anatomy to use terms that have anatomical meaning. For example, I coined the term *total abdominal vagotomy* to describe the anatomical fact that Dragstedt cut all abdominal vagi [36]. When this *total vagotomy* is complete, the stomach and entire midgut are denervated; when incomplete, the incompleteness may involve not only the gastric component but also the hepatic and celiac components. The term *truncal vagotomy* is anatomically correct only when the surgeon cuts the two trunks; it is incorrect when the surgeon cuts multiple fibers of the esophageal plexus or multiple fibers of the truncal divisions (see Fig. 2-5). Furthermore, as discussed in a succeeding section, the word *truncal* perpetuates the anatomical misconception that was and is directly responsible for the problem of incomplete vagotomy. For the purpose of comparison to total vagotomy, I used the term *gastric vagotomy* to describe a vagotomy confined to the stomach with preservation of the hepatic and celiac vagi. Although this term is anatomically correct, it conflicted with Dragstedt's terminology because he often referred to his total vagotomy as a gastric vagotomy.

For these reasons, the word *selective* was added to the term *gastric vagotomy,* and the surgical term *selective vagotomy* has since taken precedence over the anatomical term *gastric vagotomy*. We initially called the third type of vagotomy a *partial gastric vagotomy* [43], which is anatomically correct but not precise. Of more importance, the term *partial gastric* was heresy in the days of the all-or-none fallacy, which held that a vagotomy of only a part of the stomach was impossible. After Kay of Glasgow coined the term *parietal cell mass,* we used the term *selective vagotomy of the parietal cell mass* [3]. This term described precisely what we did in dogs but, because of its verbosity, I now use the shorter term *parietal vagotomy*. The original goal of complete denervation of the parietal mucosa remains. As described in a later section, however, this goal cannot be attained in all patients because of anatomical variations.

Whereas the words *total* and *parietal* have anatomical meaning, the word *selective* does not and, furthermore, may be confused with the phrase *highly selective*. It may therefore be more fitting, if anatomical terminology is ever accepted, to abandon the word *selective* and return to the anatomically correct term *gastric vagotomy*. Until that time, I shall use the word *selective*. Finally, from the standpoint of another consideration, all three types of vagotomy cut preganglionic fibers, and all cells in the entire gastrointestinal tract are innervated directly by postganglionic cells.[4]

[4]All the other synonyms are recognized, particularly *selective proximal vagotomy* (SPV), preferred by Holle who, with Hart, was the first to report its use in humans (but with pyloroplasty). The terms *highly selective vagotomy* (HSV) of Johnston and *parietal cell vagotomy* (PCV) of our coinvestigator Amdrup were applied coincidentally and independently without drainage for the original purpose of preventing dumping. The term *proximal gastric vagotomy,* chosen by a poll and preferred by the editors, is quite similar to our original *partial gastric vagotomy,* but does clarify that our *partial* is the proximal part of the stom-

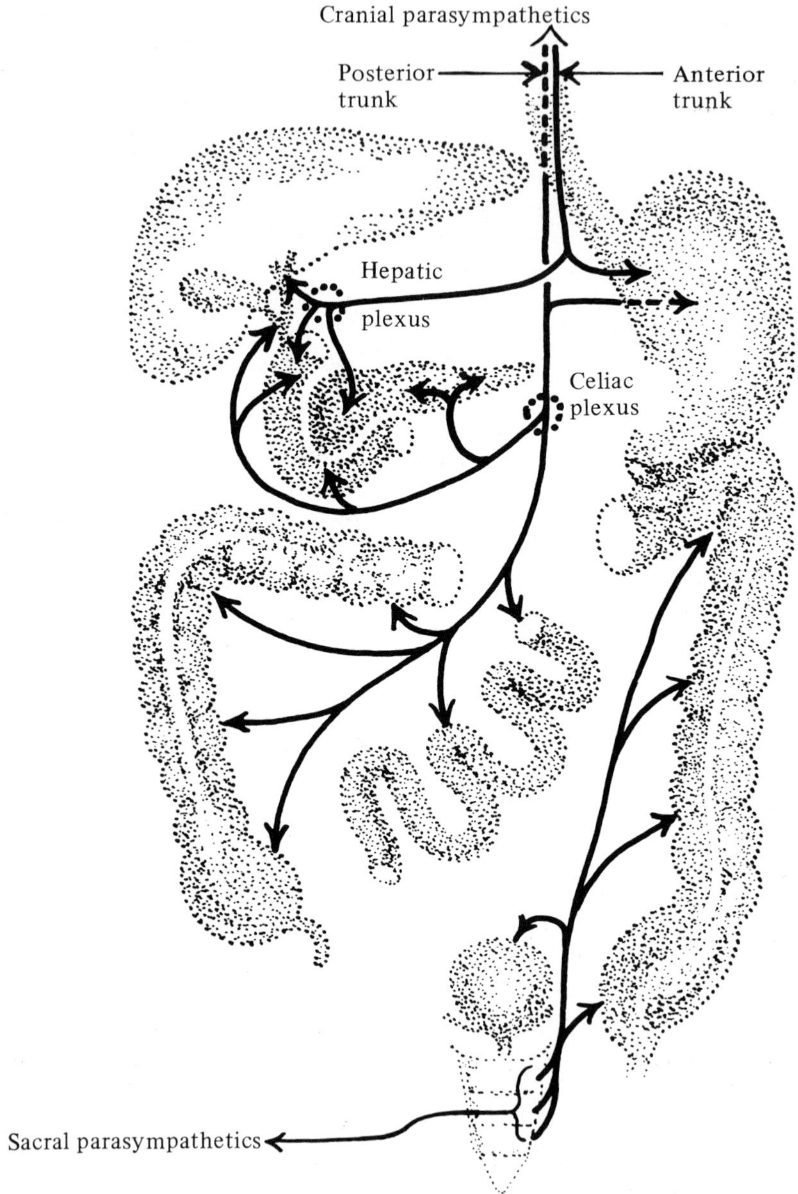

Fig. 2-11. Distribution of the hepatic and celiac vagi. Preganglionic celiac vagal fibers reach the midgut in company with the superior mesenteric artery and its branches. (From Griffith [37].)

The Problem of Incomplete Vagotomy and Its Solution

When Dragstedt devised his vagotomy by means of many canine experiments, he divided the vagal system at the diaphragmatic esophageal hiatus, where, in dogs, the system almost invariably and conveniently exists as the two and only two trunks. When he applied this technique to humans, he found the variations illustrated in Figures 2-5 and 2-6. Thus did the problem of incomplete vagotomy arise. In an attempt to solve this problem, many regional anatomical studies of the vagi at the hiatus were done. These studies reported the existence of two trunks at the hiatus in about 75 percent of bodies; the other 25 percent had variable numbers of multiple nerves (the esophageal plexus of the truncal divisions) in variable positions. In translating these anatomical findings to the surgical dissection confined to the hiatus, the surgeon could not know (and still cannot know) how many nerves there were or where they were. Dragstedt wrote [28]: "The percentage of incomplete vagotomies steadily decreases as the surgeon gains experience, but is not eliminated by present techniques, and this constitutes the chief weakness in this method of surgical therapy." Or, as put more succinctly by one of Dragstedt's leading disciples, Woodward [121]: "The major disadvantage is the unavoidably rather high incidence of incomplete vagotomy."

This unavoidable incidence of incomplete vagotomy with the hiatal technique occurs not because of failure to transect a tiny fiber closely applied to the encircled esophagus but because of failure to encircle, and bring into the surgical field, one or more large vagal fibers (Figs. 2-12, 2-13, upper arrow).

As illustrated by the lower arrows in Figures 2-12 and 2-13, the solution to the problem of incomplete vagotomy requires that we lower our sights from the hiatus to the most distal esophagus and gastric cardia, which is the one and only area where all gastric vagi gather to innervate the stomach. Also in this area are three landmarks that are always present—the cardioesophageal angle of His, the hepatic division, and the celiac division. These landmarks guide the encircling finger to include all gastric vagi with anatomical certainty. The technique of this encirclement is described in Chapter 12. After the encirclement, either selective or total vagotomy may be done.

ANATOMICAL TYPES OF INCOMPLETE VAGOTOMY. In our early studies on segmental innervation of the stomach [97], we learned that the various anatomical types of incomplete vagotomy that occur in the clinical situation resulted in areas of innervated mucosa that varied considerably in size. These findings suggested different secretory and ulcerogenic potentials. For example, if a vagal trunk is left intact at the hiatus, the entire ipsilateral wall of the stomach remains innervated. Or, if a large esophageal plexus branch contributing to that trunk is left intact, two-thirds or three-fourths of the ipsilateral wall remains innervated. In contrast, if one of the end branches of high origin to the fundus is left intact (e.g., "a.1" in Fig. 2-9E), only a small, corresponding segment in the fundus remains innervated. The difference between an intact trunk and an intact fundic branch is illustrated in Figure 2-14.

THE VARIABLE ADEQUACY OF INCOMPLETE VAGOTOMY. We compared the two types of incomplete vagotomy in Figure 2-14 with secretory tests and experimental ulcers in Shay rats. With an intact trunk, the secretory potential was virtually unchanged, and experimental ulcers developed. This type of incomplete vagotomy was termed *inadequate* because it affords inadequate protection against ulceration. With an intact fundic branch, secretion was reduced almost as much as by a complete vagotomy and no ulcers developed. This type of incomplete vagotomy was termed *adequate* because it affords adequate protection against ulceration [66].

The foregoing remarks are not meant to imply that slipshod techniques are satisfactory if

---

ach. Both are referred to as PGV, however, which raises a final point. All of the synonyms are verbose and encourage the use of acronyms, which are readily understood locally but often misunderstood nationally and internationally unless repeatedly defined.

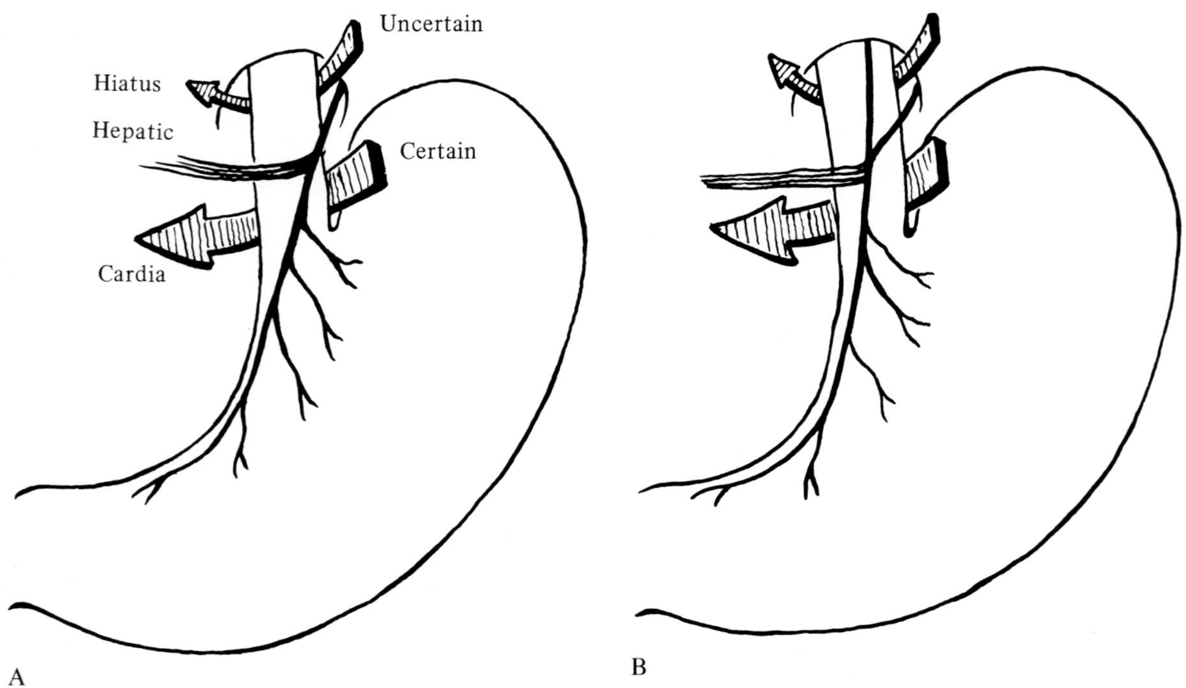

Fig. 2-12. Encirclement of the anterior vagi. At the hiatus the anterior trunk (A) or a branch of the esophageal plexus contributing to the anterior trunk (B) may lie well to the left of the patient's esophagus. Failure to encircle the trunk (A) should lead to a continued search for it. However, the encirclement of a branch of the esophageal plexus may dissuade further search, and the remaining branch is overlooked (B). In contrast to this uncertain encirclement at the hiatus, the encirclement of all gastric vagi at the cardia is certain. (From Griffith [40]. In R. Maingot [Ed.], *Abdominal Surgery* [6th ed.], 1974. Courtesy of Appleton-Century-Crofts, Publishing Division of Prentice-Hall, Inc., New York.)

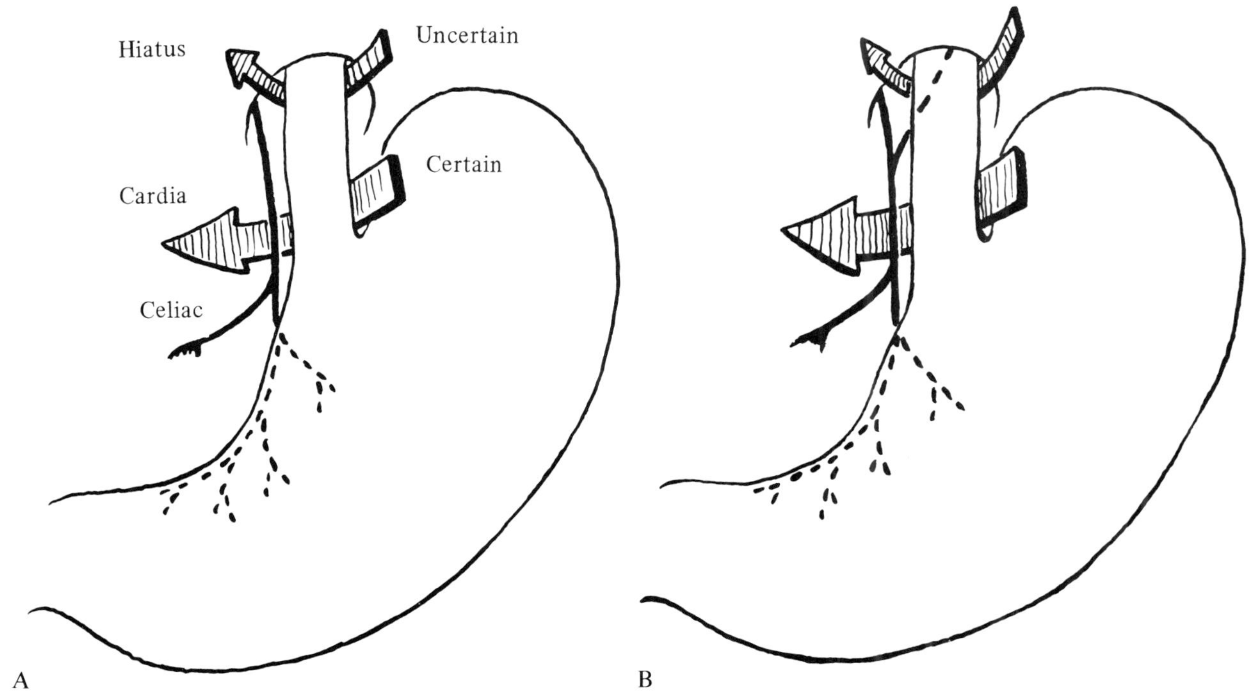

Fig. 2-13. Encirclement of the posterior vagi. At the hiatus the posterior trunk (A) or a branch of the esophageal plexus contributing to the posterior trunk (B) may lie well posterior to the esophagus in an extremely dorsal position adjacent to the right diaphragmatic crus, and it continues in this extremely dorsal position as the celiac division to the celiac autonomic plexus (see Fig. 2-6). In this circumstance the posterior trunk (A) or a contributing branch of the esophageal plexus (B) may be excluded from the encirclement at the hiatus, but at the gastric cardia may always be included by virtue of the fact that at the lower level of the cardia the celiac vagal division may always be positively identified by palpating its course to the celiac plexus. (From Griffith [40]. In R. Maingot [Ed.], *Abdominal Surgery* [6th ed.], 1974. Courtesy of Appleton-Century-Crofts, Publishing Division of Prentice-Hall, Inc., New York.)

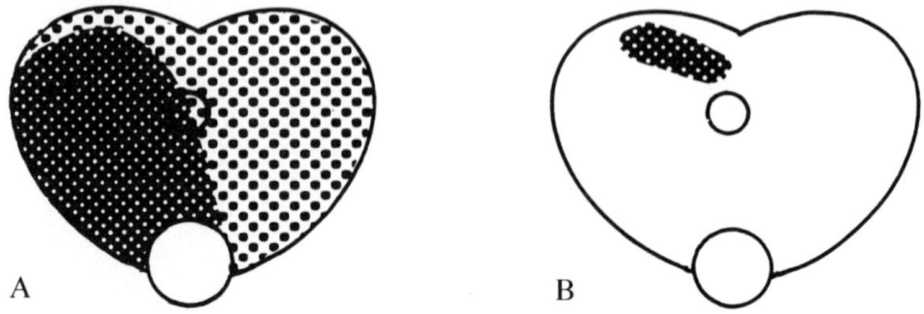

Fig. 2-14. Variable adequacy of incomplete vagotomy according to anatomical type. (A) With an intact vagal trunk, the ipsilateral wall of the stomach remains innervated and continues to secrete *(dark shading)*. The contralateral wall also secretes *(light shading)* because of the vagal release of gastrin. (B) With an intact terminal branch to the fundus, only a small area of mucosa remains innervated with a correspondingly and markedly reduced secretion. (From Pritchart et al. [97]. By permission of *Surgery, Gynecology & Obstetrics*.)

incomplete but adequate vagotomy is the result. The goal remains an all-out effort to accomplish a complete vagotomy. However, these experimental findings form the basis for the well-known clinical finding that only some and not all incomplete vagotomies cause recurrent ulcer. This circumstance is discussed additionally when the revised anatomical basis for interpreting the insulin test is presented.

The Permanence of Adequacy

The anatomical concept of adequacy is clinically meaningless if an adequate vagotomy becomes inadequate by reinnervation. Of principal concern is the process of *sprouting*, which can occur only if vagotomy is incomplete. Intact fibrils at the cellular level in the residually innervated mucosa send out sprouts that reinnervate cells in the adjacent denervated mucosa [87]. We found that sprouting was quite limited and relatively ineffectual. The residually innervated areas increased only slightly in size, and the secretory and ulcerogenic potential was virtually unchanged [52, 53, 70]. Thus an adequate vagotomy remains permanently adequate (Fig. 2-15).

Another concern is vagal reinnervation by *restoration of continuity of divided nerve ends*. Dragstedt's group put the quietus on this type of reinnervation with their classic experiment reported in 1950; they obtained permanently complete vagotomy (up to four years [26]) by merely crushing rather than dividing the vagal trunks, and concluded that the potential for functional restoration of divided nerves is nil [30]. As far as I know, no one has disproved their conclusion. Specifically, no one has correlated any restoration of continuity of divided vagal fibers with a resultant return of increased gastric secretion in either animals or humans. The anatomical concept of adequacy of vagotomy and its permanence is given additional support by a revised interpretation of the insulin test.[5]

[5]In personal letters Dr. Dragstedt wrote: ". . . the secretory fibers in the vagus nerves to the stomach do not regenerate after division any more than do the motor fibers to the laryngeal muscles after division of the recurrent laryngeal nerve. In both cases preganglionic fibers are divided. . . . If functional regeneration of the vagus nerves were of frequent occurrence, as is for instance regeneration of the divided postganglionic sympathetics, vagotomy would long since have fallen into disrepute" (7 June 1961).

He also wrote: "We have followed many, many patients with persistently negative insulin tests for as long as eleven years. . . . I find it difficult to believe that the nerves rejoin . . ." (18 May 1968). Nevertheless, Dragstedt continued to excise lengthy segments of fibers rather than merely divide them. This practice most probably stemmed from a concern of regeneration when he did his first vagotomies in the early 1940s [29] and remained an unbroken habit throughout the years even though his many observations in animals and humans allayed his initial wariness. Other surgeons followed suit, and the tradition of excising segments of vagal fibers and submitting them for microscopical examination continues.

I concede that this practice may provide some support to the surgeon in a court of law, but not if a knowledgeable attorney points out that the pathologist cannot determine whether the

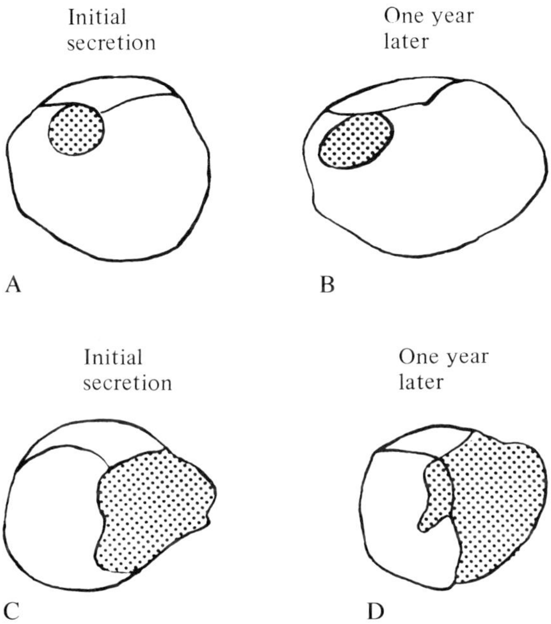

Fig. 2-15. Minimal reinnervation by sprouting. Parietal mucosal surfaces of rats opened along the greater curvature. Rumen and antrum removed. Secretion from areas of residual innervation initially *(left)* and one year after *(right)* an incomplete vagotomy of an intact branch to the fundus (A) and an incomplete vagotomy of an intact trunk (B). The minimal increase in size of the area innervated by the one fundic branch (A) appears insignificant. The area innervated by the one trunk (B) has extended across the lesser curvature as a result of sprouting. (From Jones and Griffith [52]. Reproduced by courtesy of J. B. Lippincott Company.)

Revised Criteria for the Insulin Test

When Hollander devised his criteria for interpreting his insulin test, he thought vagotomy obeyed the law of all or none and assumed there were "no degrees of vagality" [49]. He therefore interpreted his results only as negative or positive. This interpretation is still used in many centers, despite the fact that it denies the occurrence of various types of incomplete vagotomy with variable degrees of adequacy. We compared the insulin responses of an intact trunk with an intact fundic branch. As shown in Figure 2-16, there are indeed variable degrees of vagality [67]. Consequently, as proposed by Ross and Kay [102], positive insulin responses are classified as adequate or inadequate. The former response is typically small and delayed (Fig. 2-16C) and indicates adequate protection against recurrent ulcer; the latter is large and early (Fig. 2-16B) and indicates inadequate protection against recurrence. These two examples of incomplete vagotomy in Figure 2-16 represent the extremes of adequacy and inadequacy, and do not include the shades of gray in between. However, these revised criteria have proved to work quite well in differentiating the incomplete vagotomy that causes recurrence from that which does not [10, 11, 39, 41, 102], and therefore are much more useful than Hollander's original criteria.

Failure to differentiate the adequate from the inadequate response perpetuates the all-or-none fallacy and hinders recognition of causes for recurrence other than incomplete vagotomy. If the adequate responses are included with the inadequate responses as one group, the results lead to the misinterpretation that all recurrences associated with positive tests are caused by incomplete vagotomy. A recurrence associated with a small, delayed adequate response requires search for another cause of recurrence. Demonstrating the adequacy of a vagotomy by the various secretory tests and the K test [61] avoids the futile effort of completing an incomplete but adequate vagotomy and indicates the need for other measures, e.g., in patients with persistent hypersecretion from antral hyperfunction with or without G-cell hyperplasia or in patients with secondary gastric ulceration from duodenal reflux [41].

vagi are gastric or hepatic or celiac fibers and, more important, cannot determine whether *all* of the patient's gastric vagi are under the microscope. But I do not abide with the statement that the "completeness of vagotomy was confirmed by microscopical study" in reports of experimental studies. The ability to perform a complete vagotomy comes from gross anatomical and not histological knowledge. And the various intraoperative tests are best used only to supplement anatomical knowledge and not to replace it. The tests may be abandoned after this knowledge is learned and the surgical skill to apply it is acquired. These views are based on hard data and results, but are not generally accepted.

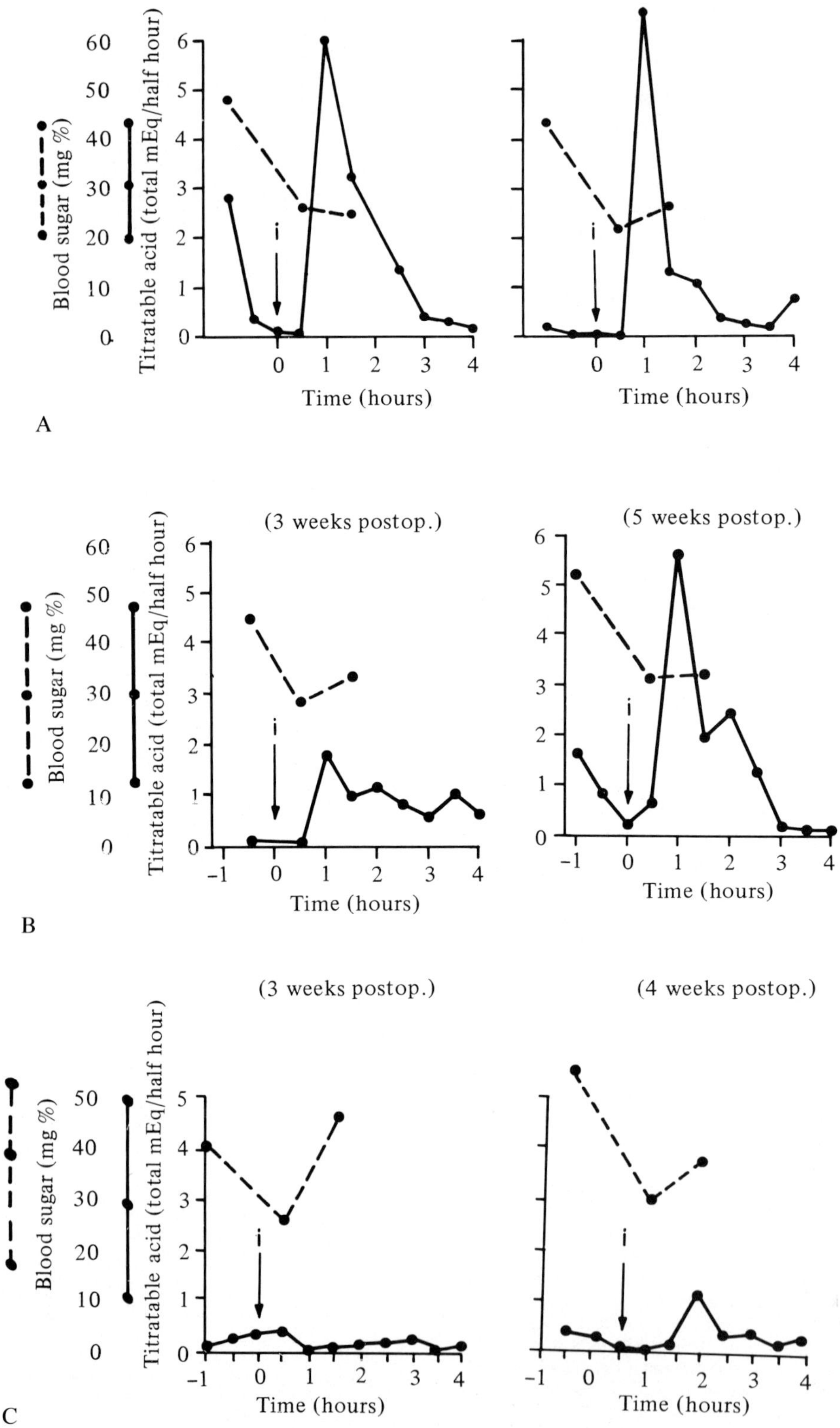
Blood sugar (mg %)
Titratable acid (total mEq/half hour)
Time (hours)
A
(3 weeks postop.)
(5 weeks postop.)
B
(3 weeks postop.)
(4 weeks postop.)
C

Return of Secretion by Recovery
Dragstedt [30] wrote, ". . . a negative insulin reaction immediately after operation, followed by a positive reaction from six weeks to three months subsequently, does not mean that the vagus nerves have regenerated but rather that traumatized vagus nerves that have not been divided have recovered from the trauma and are able to convey secretory nerve impulses." Whether this *rapid return of secretion* is caused by recovery of the nerves only or of the whole organism is moot, but Dragstedt's point is confirmed by the findings in Figure 2-16. Recovery from an adequate vagotomy can convert an initially negative insulin response to a small and delayed positive response in the *short term* (Fig. 2-16C), but in the *long term* additional conversion from a negative or adequate response to a large and early inadequate response does not occur [10, 11, 39, 41, 102]. In contrast, recovery from an inadequate vagotomy can convert an initial and relatively small response to a large and early inadequate response with virtually complete return of secretion (Fig. 2-16B). Unfortunately, confusion exists because the latter type of recovery has been, and still is, misinterpreted as evidence for reinnervation.[6]

[6]Before segmental innervation of the stomach was known, it was assumed that the vagal fibers in a branch of the esophageal plexus, for example, were distributed to the stomach in a shotgun pattern; it was also assumed that, after an incomplete vagotomy of one intact branch of the esophageal plexus, the islands of residual innervation in the shotgun pattern could reinnervate the rest of the denervated stomach by sprouting [86, 87]. Clark [21] studied an incomplete vagotomy of one intact esophageal plexus branch in cats and noted complete return of gastric motility in four to six weeks. He attributed the return of function to vagal reinnervation by sprouting. Clark's findings attracted considerable attention at the time (1964), and in some circles his experiment is still quoted. However, now that vagal innervation of the stomach is known to be segmental, it is also known that Clark's incomplete vagotomy was inadequate at the outset [66, 67, 70] and that the rapid return of function represented recovery rather than reinnervation.

The Anatomical Basis for Parietal and Selective Vagotomy
Both Dragstedt [26] and Hollander [46] rejected our initial experiments [43] because, at that time, they and all other physiologists and surgeons believed that vagotomy obeyed the law of all or none. This law, as expressed by Dragstedt [27], held that any single fiber remaining after an incomplete vagotomy "appears to be able to activate the entire glandular apparatus, acting presumably through the submucosal plexus of Meissner." It therefore followed that the intact vagal fibers to the antrum after parietal vagotomy would activate the corpus and fundus. Dragstedt and Hollander also objected to selective vagotomy and postulated that intact hepatic and celiac vagal fibers might reach the stomach by circuitous pathways through their respective autonomic plexuses. Their objections deterred clinical trial of parietal (but not selective) vagotomy and necessitated additional experiments.

Using methods of both motility and secretion, we showed that the hepatic and celiac vagi do not innervate the stomach and therefore that selective vagotomy provides a complete gastric vagotomy [39, 43, 114]. Disproving the law of all or none was much more difficult. Finally, after some 10 years of fruitless effort, and as previously described [97], we proved that vagal innervation of the stomach is segmental. Although this finding showed that the parietal mucosa could be selectively vagotomized, the question arose whether the residually innervated antral mucosa could reinnervate the denervated parietal mucosa by sprouting. Long-term experiments showed that this type of reinnervation is probably insignificant (see Fig. 2-15). These findings led to the final experiments [3] that prompted our coinvestigator Amdrup to start

Fig. 2-16. Results of insulin tests. (A) Two insulin tests before vagotomy in a dog. The responses are large and occur early. (B) Two insulin tests after incomplete vagotomy of one intact trunk. At three weeks *(left)* the response is small, but at five weeks *(right)* the response has recovered to equal the preoperative response. (C) Two insulin tests after an incomplete vagotomy of one intact branch to a small area of mucosa in the fundus. At three weeks *(left)* the insulin test is negative, but at four weeks *(right)* a small and delayed response is apparent.

a clinical trial after his return to Denmark in 1969.

Dissection of the Distal Esophagus for Parietal, Selective, and Total Vagotomy

Just as Dragstedt repeatedly emphasized a thorough dissection of the esophagus at or above the hiatus in search of small vagal fibers to complete his total vagotomy, so must we thoroughly dissect the distal esophagus to complete parietal and selective vagotomy (and also total vagotomy when it is done at the distal esophagus). The goal is transection of each and every fiber that may arise from the trunks or esophageal plexus above the surgical field and descend to the proximal stomach (Fig. 2-9E, F). I have described an adequate dissection in terms of mobilizing and baring enough of the distal esophagus so that it can be seen in its entire circumference and palpated with at least two encircling fingers [38]. The late Harold Burge [17] did the same dissection to encircle the distal esophagus with his electrode and ensure the completeness of vagotomy (the Burge test).

In more recent years it has become popular to think in terms of "skeletonizing the esophagus for 5 to 7 cm" (which permits encirclement with two fingers or Burge's electrode). The fibers in question may lie within or deep to the esophageal fascia propria but not deep within the esophageal muscle. The latter fibers innervate the esophagus and not the stomach [37, 38, 111]. To accomplish a complete vagotomy, therefore, the esophagus need not be circumcised or perforated (or transected in experimental animals). The completed dissection is illustrated in Figure 12-14. Failure to complete this dissection has resulted in unacceptably high rates of recurrent ulcer after all three types of vagotomy, but particularly after parietal vagotomy [44, 60].

Incomplete Vagotomy of the Distal Parietal Mucosa After Parietal Vagotomy

The preceding considerations of the esophageal dissection concern the *proximal* extent of parietal vagotomy, which, even though complete, does not prevent recurrence [5]. This section considers the *distal* extent of parietal vagotomy, which concerns two anatomical variations—the variable extent of the parietal mucosa distally and the variable lengths of the anterior nerve of Latarjet. The former is diagramed in Figure 2-4. As noted in this diagram, if the vagotomy is extended to a point on the lesser curvature 6 cm from the pylorus (which is about as far as one can go and still preserve enough antral motility to prevent gastric stasis), denervation of the distal parietal mucosa will be complete in most patients. In other patients the vagotomy of the distal parietal mucosa is incomplete, but the area of incompleteness is not large enough to cause recurrence, and the vagotomy is therefore adequate. In smaller numbers of patients, perhaps 5 percent or less, the parietal mucosa extends to distances 4, 3, and even less than 2 cm from the pylorus. In these patients with a correspondingly and extremely small area of antral mucosa, the area of the residually innervated distal parietal mucosa may be large enough for the incomplete vagotomy to be inadequate. Both Allgöwer [2] and I have seen extremely small antra with topical Congo red. Amdrup [5] has seen the same with the pH electrode, which he still uses. In addition, Allgöwer and Amdrup have seen dense populations of parietal cells in some antra removed for recurrence. Amdrup has become reluctant to perform parietal vagotomy in the presence of a small antrum.

With regard to the variable length of the anterior nerve of Latarjet (see Fig. 2-7), at one extreme is the nerve that contains all the pyloric fibers from the hepatic division and the nerve of McCrea, and runs all the way to and beyond the pylorus. At the other extreme is the considerably shorter nerve that contains no pyloric fibers, which, in these instances, are carried in either or both the hepatic division and nerve of McCrea. These short nerves of Latarjet barely reach the 6 cm point from the pylorus and, in a few bodies, end well proximal to this point [111, 112]. In the study by Andersen's group, the shortest nerve of Latarjet ended a measured 8.5 cm from the pyloric ring [88].

Thus there is no correlation between the distal extent of the anterior nerve of Latarjet and the distal extent of the parietal mucosa [96]. The patients of concern are those who have extremely small antra and extremely short nerves of Latarjet, and who therefore have sizable areas of residual innervation in the distal parietal mucosa after parietal vagotomy. Insulin tests in these patients indicate incomplete vagotomy but do not localize the area of incompleteness. If the so-called K test [61] were used universally, the areas of incompleteness in the distal parietal mucosa would be seen and more fully appreciated.

The terminal branches of the anterior nerve of Latarjet on the lesser curvature have been termed the "crow's foot," and have been used as a landmark for the distal extent of parietal vagotomy. Although not all that constant, the crow's foot landmark has proved quite workable in most patients.[7]

Return of Secretion by Reinnervation (Sprouting)

Up to this point I have stated that sprouting is probably insignificant, and that an incomplete but adequate vagotomy remains permanently adequate. These conclusions are derived from our experiments with small areas of residually innervated mucosa in the small stomachs of small animals, and must be modified when applied to the correspondingly larger areas of residually innervated mucosa in the larger stomachs of humans. The larger the area of residual innervation, the larger is its circumference and, in turn, the larger is the eventual area of residual innervation after sprouting. (Fig. 2-15 shows that more mucosa is reinnervated after an incomplete vagotomy of an intact trunk than of an intact fundic branch.)

Accordingly, reinnervation by sprouting may well explain the gradual increase in gastric secretion *over the long term* in some patients with an adequate vagotomy but not in patients with a complete gastric vagotomy. Although this increase in secretion is never enough to approach the level of preoperative secretion, it may be just enough to tip the scales toward recurrence in the unusual patient. This consideration applies particularly to patients with parietal vagotomy.

Three specific anatomical areas are of concern. The first, common to all types of vagotomy, is the area innervated by an intact fundic branch (see Fig. 2-14). Second, and unique to parietal vagotomy, is the antral mucosa. As illustrated in Figure 2-10, parietal vagotomy transects the intramural route of innervation and preserves the extramural route. Sprouting from the innervated extramural fibrils reinnervates some or all of the denervated intramural fibrils. The importance of this is unknown, but it is known that the innervated antrum has considerably more secretory potential than the denervated antrum [3, 110]. Third, and also unique to parietal vagotomy, is the most distal area of the parietal mucosa. If denervated, it may be reinnervated by sprouting from the innervated antral mucosa. If residually innervated but the vagotomy is adequate (see Fig. 2-4), the size of the innervated area increases slightly by sprouting. And as previously discussed with reference to Figure 2-4, the size of the residually innervated area in the distal parietal mucosa may be large enough to constitute a *potentially* inadequate vagotomy at the outset in about 5 percent of instances. (The word *potentially* is used because we do not yet know what the incidence *actually* is.)[8]

[7]Payne [94] introduced the term crow's foot to Seattle surgeons to describe the pattern of the terminal branches of the descending left gastric artery along the lesser curvature, and made the point that during gastric resection antral mucosa is rarely found proximal to this crow's foot. In 1967, while watching Hart of Holle's department perform a parietal vagotomy in Munich, I asked him how far he extended his dissection distally. Hart pointed to the general area where the descending left gastric artery and the nerve of Latarjet terminate. When I acknowledged his answer and referred to the area as the crow's foot, Hart thought I meant the end branches of the nerve of Latarjet. He was amused by the term and used it repeatedly to a large audience of German surgeons on closed circuit television. Thus did Payne's arterial crow's foot become the neural crow's foot. (From my point of view, the former still looks more like a crow's foot than the latter. The most proximal of the terminal arterial branches usually ascends to resemble the spur; the two or three distal branches are the claws.)

[8]Most recently Joffe's group [51] found signs of reinnervation by electron microscopy in rats after parietal vagotomy, with rapid return of secretion. These findings are in marked contrast to our studies in rats; we found minimal reinnervation (see Fig. 2-15) and virtually no return of secretion after adequate vagotomy [52, 53]. From personal communications [50] it may be concluded that Joffe's findings of reinnervation are most probably caused by sprouting and not restoration of continuity of divided nerves. The latter seems impossible through the imbrication of the anterior and posterior gastric walls constructed over the lesser curvature to prevent necrotic perforation in humans.

Hepatic and Celiac Vagotomy
Low-lying hepatic vagal fibers (see Fig. 2-7) may be partially or completely transected during a gastric resection that extends high on the lesser curve. Similarly, the celiac division in its position adjacent to the main left gastric artery (see Fig. 2-8) may be divided when this artery is ligated and transected. Accidental and unrecognized hepatic and celiac vagotomy may account for some sequelae (see Chap. 12) not readily explained by the gastric resection per se. Conversely, the incidence of incomplete hepatic and incomplete celiac vagotomy is as high or higher than the incidence of incomplete gastric vagotomy when total vagotomy is done at the hiatus. But because there are no tests for the completeness of either hepatic or celiac vagotomy, the incidence of complete or incomplete hepatic or celiac vagotomy is unknown. This is but one of perhaps many reasons for the variable occurrence of the sequelae of hepatic and celiac vagotomy in series of allegedly complete total vagotomy.

Arteries

Figure 2-17 is a diagram of the usual arterial pattern supplying the stomach and duodenum. Like many similar diagrams, this figure neglects two important considerations: (1) the extensive intramural anastomoses (submucosal plexus), and (2) the frequent variations in origin and distribution of the main arteries [78, 79, 80, 81]. The literature has repeatedly emphasized arterial variations pertinent to hazards in operations on the biliary tract, but has not extensively covered gastric operations. Accordingly, this section stresses arterial variations relative to gastric operations. (The appearance of an unusual variation on an arteriogram is striking, in fact so striking that it may be given a new name. As far as I know, arteriography has not revealed any "new" variations unknown to older generations of anatomists. However, any and all "discoveries" are certainly advantageous to surgeons.)

SUBMUCOSAL PLEXUS
The stomach receives its blood supply through its two mesenteric borders (the lesser and greater curvatures). The right and left gastric arteries run within the lesser omentum adjacent to the lesser curvature, and the right and left gastroepiploic arteries and vasa brevia run within the greater omentum adjacent to the greater curvature. These arteries supply the stomach by sending off specific anterior and posterior gastric branches that penetrate the stomach's muscular coat anteriorly and posteriorly, close to the lesser and greater curvatures. On reaching the submucosa, these gastric branches ramify extensively throughout the entire submucosa. Maintaining a relatively large caliber, these submucosal ramifications anastomose frequently with each other to form the submucosal plexus, which consists of both the arteries and their venous counterparts. Independent branches from the submucosal plexus supply the mucosa everywhere except in the lesser curvature, which receives delicate branches directly from the right and left gastric arteries.

Surgical Applications
ULCERATION OF THE LESSER CURVATURE. The frequent incidence of gastric ulcer along the lesser curvature was once related to its distinctive circulation [12, 98]. Now, with Oi's dual control mechanism as an explanation [89], this distinctive circulation may be of concern only as a factor for the well-known intractability of many lesser curvature ulcers.

NECROTIC PERFORATION. Of more importance is the occurrence of necrotic perforation along the lesser curvature after its blood supply is interrupted by parietal vagotomy. Although several reported and unreported instances of this frequently fatal complication occurred in the early and mid-1970s, it occurred in our experimental laboratory some 20 years earlier. The first three dogs with parietal vagotomy died of necrotic perforation; the next 10 dogs lived and provided the material for our first report [43]. These three deaths were described in our original manuscript but fell to editorial deletion during the course of

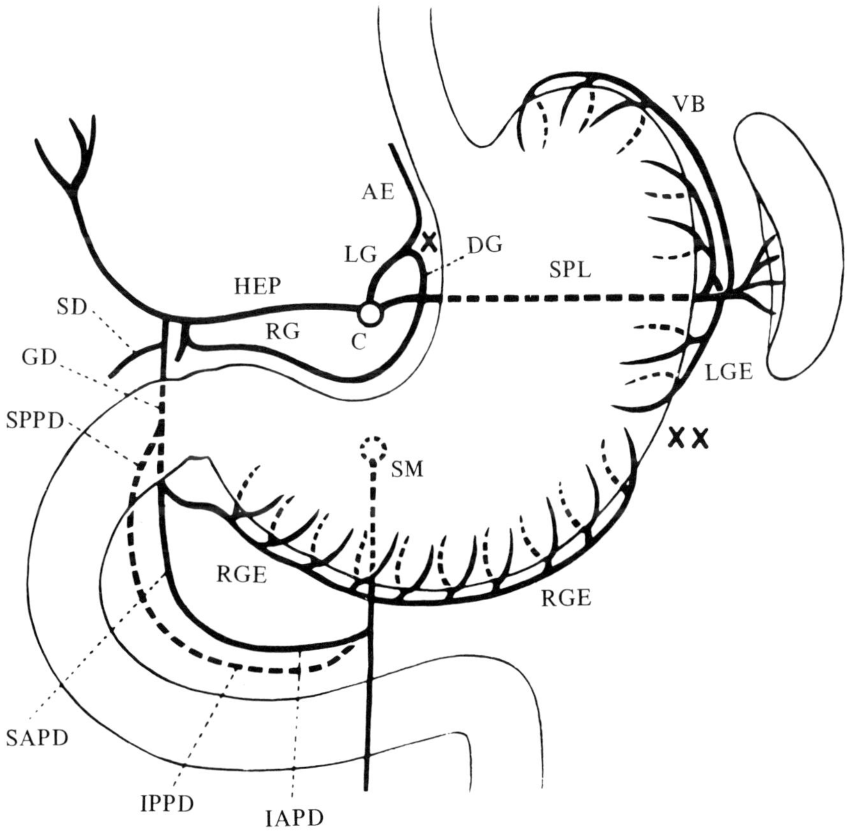

Fig. 2-17. The arterial supply to the stomach and duodenum. (C = celiac; HEP = hepatic; RG = right gastric; GD = gastroduodenal; SD = supraduodenal; SPPD = superior posterior pancreaticoduodenal (retroduodenal); SAPD = superior anterior pancreaticoduodenal; RGE = right gastroepiploic; IAPD = inferior anterior pancreaticoduodenal; IPPD = inferior posterior pancreaticoduodenal; LG = left gastric; AE = ascending esophageal branch; DG = descending gastric branch; SPL = splenic; VB = vasa brevia; LGE = left gastroepiploic; X = bifurcation of left gastric; XX = anastomosis of right gastroepiploic and left gastroepiploic; SM = superior mesenteric.)

rejections by several surgical journals in the United States. The manuscript was eventually accepted for publication by *Gastroenterology.* It is now well known that necrotic perforation is best avoided by imbricating the anterior and posterior gastric walls over the lesser curvature. This unique necrosis was my first experience with failure of the collateral circulation.

COLLATERAL CIRCULATION. The large volume of blood flowing through the submucosal plexus and the abundant anastomoses within the submucosal plexus constitute the collateral circulation that permits extensive devascularization of the stomach without causing necrosis. Brown and Derr [16] demonstrated complete filling of all intramural vessels of the stomach by injecting any of the four major arteries after ligating all other extramural vessels. This finding confirms (1) the futility of controlling hemorrhage from gastric ulcer by ligating extrinsic arteries, (2) the viability of a stomach supplied by only the right gastroepiploic artery (plus or minus the right gastric) and mobilized to the chest or neck for anastomosis, (3) the viability of a gastric remnant supplied by only the left gastroepiploic artery and vasa brevia (after subtotal gastrectomy with ligation of the left gastric), and (4) the viability of a small gastric cuff supplied by only the descending esophageal arteries anastomosing with the submucosal plexus after 90 to 95 percent resection, in which all extrinsic vessels are ligated. Occasionally these procedures tax the capabilities of the submucosal plexus, but only rarely does it fail. Fatal ischemic necrosis of the gastric remnant after gastric resection, for example, is extremely rare, but it can and does occur. This complication may be caused by atherosclerotic occlusion of the vasa brevia and left gastroepiploic artery [47], but more commonly it is caused by insufficient blood descending from the esophagus into the submucosal plexus [32, 106, 113, 115].

HEMORRHAGE. Because of its extensive submucosal plexus, the stomach is the most vascularized segment of the alimentary tract. The gastric mucosa requires a tremendous amount of blood (and energy) to form and secrete gastric juice. The smallest and most superficial erosions can hemorrhage profusely. Surgeons must take every precaution to prevent postoperative hemorrhage from the suture line after incising or transecting the stomach.

ARTERIOVENOUS SHUNTS. The submucosal plexus contains many arteriovenous shunts [9, 109]. Eiseman et al. [31] concluded that vasopressin decreases bleeding from esophageal varices by closing these arteriovenous shunts and thereby lowering portal venous pressure. Peters and Womack [95] showed that the shunts close to supply a maximum of blood to the mucosa for the secretion of gastric juice, and open to divert blood from the mucosa when the mucosa is at rest.

PANCREATICODUODENAL ARCADES

The gastroduodenal artery usually arises from the hepatic artery of its right and left branches and descends in a position dorsal to the most proximal duodenum. Its first branch is the posterosuperior pancreaticoduodenal (or retroduodenal) artery, which descends in close association with the common bile duct (it often spirals around the distal common duct) to the posterior head of the pancreas and posterior duodenum. The retroduodenal artery is relatively large, and its injury by careless duodenal mobilization, common duct exploration, or sphincterotomy can cause brisk hemorrhage. After sending off its retroduodenal branch, the gastroduodenal artery curves anteriorly to run forward and medial to the duodenum, where the head of the pancreas becomes closely attached to the duodenum. The gastroduodenal artery terminates by dividing into the right gastroepiploic and superior anterior pancreaticoduodenal arteries.[9]

The posterosuperior (retroduodenal) and anterior pancreaticoduodenal arteries anastomose with their inferior anterior and posterior pancreaticoduodenal counterparts, which arise from the superior mesenteric artery (or its first jejunal branches, or its aberrant right hepatic branch, when present). The anterior pancreaticoduodenal arcade supplies the anterior head of the pancreas and anterior duodenum with specific pancreatic and duodenal branches. The posterior pancreaticoduodenal arcade supplies the posterior head of the pancreas and posterior duodenum in a similar manner. The superior and inferior pancreaticoduodenal arteries may either branch into two to four vessels or remain as single trunks. In any event, the anastomosis between the superior and inferior vessels is direct and rich.

[9] Where the gastroduodenal artery comes anteriorly from behind the duodenum, it runs medial to the duodenum just above the level of the lesser duodenal papilla (when this papilla is present). In this area, therefore, the gastroduodenal artery is an important landmark when freeing the duodenum from the head of the pancreas (e.g., when removing a penetrating ulcer). Dissecting too far beyond the gastroduodenal artery can disrupt the duct of Santorini (when this duct is present, which it is 70 percent of the time) and cause pancreatic fistula. The gastroduodenal artery divides into its anterior pancreaticoduodenal and gastroepiploic branches at variable levels. When it divides early in its course, the pancreaticoduodenal artery is the landmark for the duct of Santorini; when it divides late, the gastroduodenal artery itself is the landmark [59].

Surgical Applications
This direct and rich anastomosis in the pancreaticoduodenal arcades represents the most important route of collateral circulation between the celiac and superior mesenteric arteries. In only about 1 percent of instances is it lacking, which occurs when the gastroduodenal artery arises from the superior mesenteric. This collateral circulation concerns us in the following respects: (1) It prevents fatal hepatic necrosis after resecting gastric carcinoma by excising the celiac axis and hepatic artery proximal to the origin of the gastroduodenal artery [6, 7, 22, 80]; (2) it is one of several routes to the liver that explain the unpredictable results of ligating the hepatic artery [14, 15, 73, 80, 99, 100, 101]; and (3) it accounts for the futility of ligating the gastroduodenal or superior pancreaticoduodenal arteries to control bleeding from duodenal ulcer, for bleeding will continue from the inferior pancreaticoduodenal arteries.

Another anatomical aspect of hemorrhage from the gastroduodenal or superior pancreaticoduodenal artery concerns a selective decrease in hepatic arterial flow. Blood destined for the liver by way of the hepatic artery is diverted through the gastroduodenal artery and out the ulcer. Thus blood flow to the liver is decreased by the same mechanism as that by which a hole in a garden hose decreases flow out of the nozzle. The result is hepatic anoxia more severe than that caused by the total blood loss per se [71].

CELIAC AXIS
Although the celiac artery usually trifurcates into the hepatic, left gastric, and splenic arteries, any of these three main branches may arise independently from any of the other branches or they may branch independently from the aorta or superior mesenteric artery. Conversely, the superior mesenteric, middle and left colic, and dorsal pancreatic arteries may arise from the celiac axis or from one of its main branches. Thus resecting the celiac axis may entail ligating more than one artery, and, more important, it may interrupt arterial flow to the small intestine, transverse colon, and pancreas if one does not heed the precautions described by Appleby [6].

LEFT GASTRIC ARTERY
As the left gastric artery ascends to the proximal lesser curvature, it may send off a large left hepatic branch just before it reaches the lesser curvature. This left hepatic artery runs within the lesser omentum to the hilus of the liver. Although Michels [81] reported a 25 percent incidence of this left hepatic branch, surgical experience based on seeing and feeling a sizable pulsating artery indicates a lesser incidence. These aberrant left hepatic arteries carry either the entire or partial arterial supply to the left lobe of the liver. *Thus ligating the left gastric artery proximal to the origin of its left hepatic branch (when present) may cause left lobar hepatic necrosis* [33]. To emphasize the occurrence and importance of this left hepatic artery, the French refer to the left gastric as the *hepatogastric* artery.

The occurrence of this aberrant left hepatic artery from the left gastric artery depends on the variable development of an artery which, in the embryo, runs across the lesser omentum to connect the left gastric with the hepatic artery in the hilus of the liver. Occasionally this connecting artery persists, but usually it becomes obliterated. When this artery loses only its connection with the hepatic artery, it persists as a left hepatic from the left gastric. When this artery loses only its connection with the left gastric, it persists as an accessory left gastric from the hepatic. Another source of an accessory left gastric is the splenic artery, which from anywhere along its course occasionally sends a large artery up to the posterior surface of the fundus. (As a result of arteriography, this variation has been called the "posterior gastric artery.")

On reaching the proximal lesser curvature, the left gastric artery bifurcates into an ascending esophageal branch (or branches) and a descending gastric branch, which immediately turns forward and then runs down the lesser curvature. Usually this descending gastric artery divides into anterior and posterior branches, which in turn send off branches to the anterior and posterior aspects of the lesser curvature. As described by Payne [94], the descending left gastric artery, or its anterior descending branch, terminates on the lesser curvature by sending "out a crow's foot type cluster with both distal and proximal ramifications." This arterial crow's foot accompanies the terminal branches of the anterior nerve of Latarjet, which have also been called the crow's foot (see Footnote 7). The arterial crow's foot is not diagramed in Figure 2-17, an error of omission because the arterial crow's foot is quite constant. Furthermore, the anastomosis between the left and right gastric arteries diagramed in Figure 2-17 is also erroneous in view of the occasional necrotic perforation of the lesser curvature after parietal vagotomy.

GASTROEPIPLOIC ARTERIES AND VASA BREVIA

The right gastroepiploic artery usually arises from the gastroduodenal artery, but occasionally it branches from the superior mesenteric. It runs close to the greater curvature within the gastroduodenal artery, but occasionally it branches from the superior mesenteric. It runs close to the greater curvature within the gastrocolic ligament and supplies the stomach with independent gastric branches, each of which divides into anterior and posterior rami that run to the anterior and posterior aspects of the greater curvature, respectively.

The left gastroepiploic artery arises from the main splenic trunk or its terminal branches, runs adjacent to the tail of the pancreas and splenic hilus, and reaches the greater curvature by way of the gastrosplenic ligament. The vasa brevia usually arise from the splenic trunk or its terminal branches also, but occasionally they arise from the left gastroepiploic artery. The vasa brevia run through the gastrosplenic ligament to the greater curvature from the level of the spleen to the cardia; some may reach the esophagus. Gastric branches from the vasa brevia and the left gastroepiploic artery are significantly longer than those from the right gastroepiploic artery and accordingly can be more easily ligated and transected individually in freeing the greater curvature of omentum to remove the stomach or spleen. Besides the vasa brevia and gastric branches of the left gastroepiploic artery, we must also control the main left gastroepiploic trunk itself during splenectomy when this artery runs within, or arises from, the splenic hilus.

The pattern of anastomosis between the right and left gastroepiploic arteries varies from no gross connection outside the stomach to a connection so large that the exact area of anastomosis is difficult to locate. Usually, however, the site of anastomosis is readily apparent.

VASCULAR LANDMARKS FOR DISTAL RESECTION

As previously stated, there are no gross anatomical landmarks on the external surface of the stomach that delineate the proximal extent of the antrum. However, two areas pertain, one on the lesser curvature, where the left gastric artery bifurcates into its ascending esophageal and descending gastric branches, and the other on the greater curvature, where the right and left gastroepiploic arteries anastomose (see Fig. 2-17, points X and XX). When the space indicating the anastomosis of the two gastroepiploic vessels does not exist and point XX is not obvious, point XX can be estimated fairly accurately because the left epiploic artery arises opposite the two distal gastric branches of the left gastroepiploic artery (Fig. 2-18). If the stomach is transected between points X and XX, the resection approximates 50 percent. This "hemigastrectomy" removes all antral mucosa plus a variable amount of parietal mucosa. The specimen shown in Figure 2-3 was removed by these landmarks. A two-thirds to three-fourths subtotal resection starts on the greater curvature proximal to the last three or four gastric branches of the left gastroepiploic artery and proceeds to point X. A "blind antrectomy," i.e., a resection done without demonstrating the antral-parietal mucosal border, may be done with reasonable assurance of removing all antral mucosa by starting on the greater curvature distal to the origin of the last three or four gastric branches of the right gastroepiploic artery, and going to the lesser curvature below point X but above the proximal ramus of the crow's foot of the descending left gastric artery.

The idea of using vascular landmarks stems from the heyday of gastric resection, when complete removal of antral mucosa was considered all-important. Furthermore, in those days the first senior coeditor of this book, the late H. N. Harkins, used planimetry of both the specimen and the in situ remnant as a more accurate method of determining the extent of resection. Now these vascular landmarks are more or less forgotten when we do a vagotomy and leave all or part of the antral mucosa in the acid stream. But we must still consider the importance of the antral mucosa in the duodenal stump after a Billroth II resection, and also in the unusual instance of antral hyperfunction with or without G-cell hyperplasia.

ABDOMINAL ESOPHAGUS

Ascending esophageal branches from the left gastric artery (or, when present, its left hepatic branch or an accessory left gastric) usually constitute the main blood supply of the abdominal esophagus. Only rarely are these branches absent. Usually branches from the left inferior phrenic artery, which vary greatly in origin (2 percent arise from the left gastric), supplement this supply; rarely, the right inferior phrenic artery provides supplemental circulation. Occasionally the highest vasa brevia reaches the esophagus. All these esophageal arteries anastomose, strongly or weakly, with branches descending from the thoracic esophagus [108, 116]. Depending on the volume of these anastomoses and the number of esophageal arteries ligated in a dissection, the viability of the abdominal esophagus plus any small attached gastric remnant may or may not be jeopardized.

PYLORUS AND PROXIMAL DUODENUM

The superior aspect of this segment is supplied by branches of the right gastric and supraduodenal arteries descending within the hepatoduodenal ligament. The right gastric artery usually arises from the hepatic or left hepatic distal to the origin of the gastroduodenal artery. The supraduodenal artery is inconstant. When present, it usually comes from the retroduodenal or gastroduodenal artery. Because of varying arterial patterns supplying the anterosuperior aspect of the duodenum just beyond the pylorus, the vascularity of this specific area may be weak. Mayo [76], Wilkie [120], and Reeves [98] correlated this relative ischemia to frequency of ulcer in this area. However, as in gastric ulcer of the lesser curvature, Oi's dual control mechanism [89] has replaced this thesis. Nevertheless, Mayo's "anaemic spot" may still pertain to intractability. The gastroduodenal artery or its pancreaticoduodenal and right gastroepiploic branches also send specific arteries to the inferior and medial aspect of the pylorus and proximal duodenum by way of the greater omentum. These arteries present variable patterns. These variations, plus a scanty submucosal plexus in the duodenum, may represent an underlying factor in necrosis and leak from a duodenal stump or anastomosis if the duodenum has been freed excessively from its mesenteric attachments.

GREATER OMENTUM

Formation of the omentum by peritoneal fusion (see Fig. 2-1) leads us to an appreciation of its blood supply (Fig. 2-18). Within the splenocolic ligament (i.e., that portion of the gastrocolic and gastrosplenic segment of omentum running from spleen to splenic flexure of colon), the left epiploic branches of the left gastroepiploic artery descend to the omentum. Thus cutting this splenocolic ligament to mobilize the splenic flexure often causes troublesome bleeding from the left epiploic vessels. The left epiploics run within the anterior layer of omentum over the transverse colon into the free omentum, where they sink into its posterior layer. Anastomosing with their counterparts from the right gastroepiploics, the left and right epiploics form the arc of Barkow, which lies within the omentum's posterior layer approximately midway between transverse colon and distal free edge of omentum. The more medial epiploic branches (5 to 15) from the right and left gastroepiploic vessels descend as the anterior epiploics in the anterior layer of omentum to its free distal

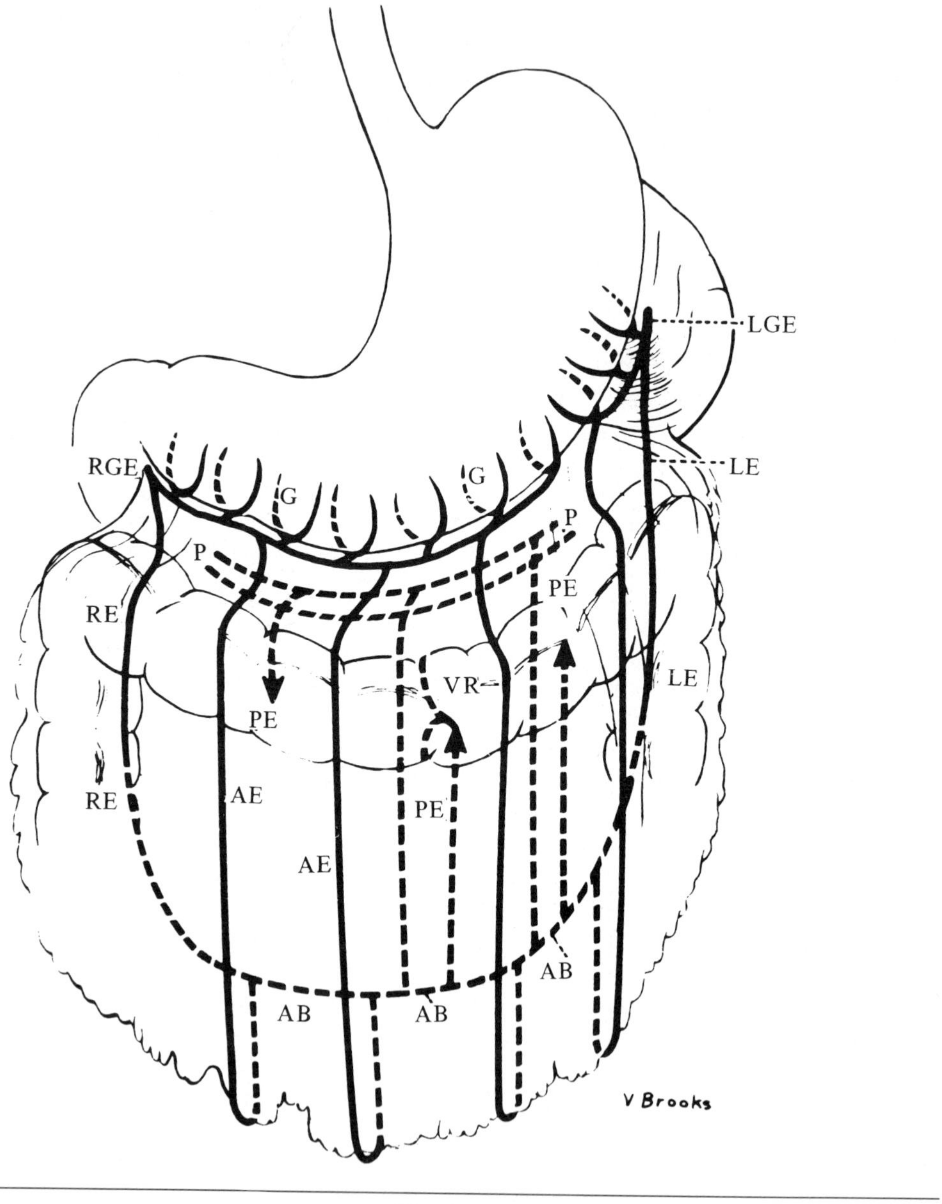

Fig. 2-18. The arterial supply to the greater omentum. (RGE = right gastroepiploic; LGE = left gastroepiploic; RE = right epiploic; LE = left epiploic; AB = arc of Barkow; G = gastric branches; AE = anterior epiploic branches; PE = posterior epiploic branches; P = pancreatic artery; VR = vasa recta of midcolic artery.)

edge, wind around this edge, and ascend in the posterior layer of omentum to enter the arc of Barkow. Pancreatic vessels (transverse or dorsal or great pancreatic) send off posterior epiploic branches into the transverse mesocolon. Some of these posterior epiploics either sink into the transverse colon or anastomose with vasa recta of the midcolic circulation; others continue down the posterior layer of omentum to enter the arc of Barkow.

Surgical Applications

Separating omentum from transverse colon requires incising the posterior layer of omentum and cutting the posterior epiploic vessels therein. Thus the bloodiness of this dissection, often described as avascular, depends on the variable size and number of the posterior epiploics.

Preserving the omentum's viability when separating it from the greater curvature does not require preserving the right gastroepiploic and its omental branches by ligating only the gastric branches (a tedious task). A much easier procedure entails transecting the gastrocolic ligament inferior to the gastroepiploics and ligating the anterior epiploics. On the left, however, only the gastric branches of the left gastroepiploic are ligated; the left epiploics are preserved. On the extreme right, the right gastroepiploic is ligated distal to the origin of the right epiploic, which is also saved. Thus preserving the arc of Barkow prevents omental necrosis. Even after ligating the right epiploic in some instances, the left epiploics and posterior epiploics furnish enough blood to the arc of Barkow to prevent omental necrosis. Only rarely will this technique jeopardize omental viability and necessitate its removal, which was suggested by Kirschner and Garlock as a routine practice [57].

Lymphatics

The anatomy of lymphatic drainage from the stomach is readily understood by realizing that lymphatic flow is the reverse of arterial flow and that lymphatic channels follow the arteries.

INTRINSIC

Lymph originates primarily in the mucosa and drains into the *lymphatic submucosal plexus*, which is associated with the arterial (and venous) submucosal plexus aforementioned. Lymphatic channels drain the submucosal plexus outward through the muscularis into the *subserosal lymphatic plexus*, which is a network of channels just beneath the peritoneum. From this point, lymphatic drainage continues through extrinsic channels.

The lymphatic submucosal plexus is just as rich and extensive as the arterial and venous submucosal plexus. Thus a carcinoma localized to a small area of mucosa may spread all over the stomach in the submucosa. Furthermore, this submucosal plexus anastomoses with a rich submucosal plexus in the esophagus. Thus submucosal invasion of gastric carcinoma into the esophagus is common. Because the duodenum possesses a scanty submucosal plexus, however, submucosal spread into the duodenum is unusual. In contrast, the subserosal plexus of stomach and duodenum anastomoses extensively, and this anastomosis accounts for most instances of duodenal invasion by gastric carcinoma [122, 123].

The abundance of the submucosal and subserosal lymphatics, together with the frequent occurrence of diffuse premalignant mucosal degeneration with multicentric origin of carcinoma [24], represents the anatomical basis for wide resections of stomach, distal esophagus, and proximal duodenum to cure gastric carcinoma.

EXTRINSIC

Extrinsic lymphatic channels[10] follow the arteries (Fig. 2-19). Accordingly, Coller et al. [23] divided the stomach into four zones of lymphatic drainage that correspond to the four zones of anterial supply:

[10]We learn extrinsic lymphatic pathways from four sources: (1) from injecting and dissecting gross lymphatics in cadavers [103] (2) from dissecting lymphatic metastases in specimens of gastric carcinoma [23], (3) from staining lymph nodes by injecting dyes into the stomach during operation [118], and (4) from dissecting at autopsy or "second look" procedures lymph nodes missed at primary surgical resection [8].

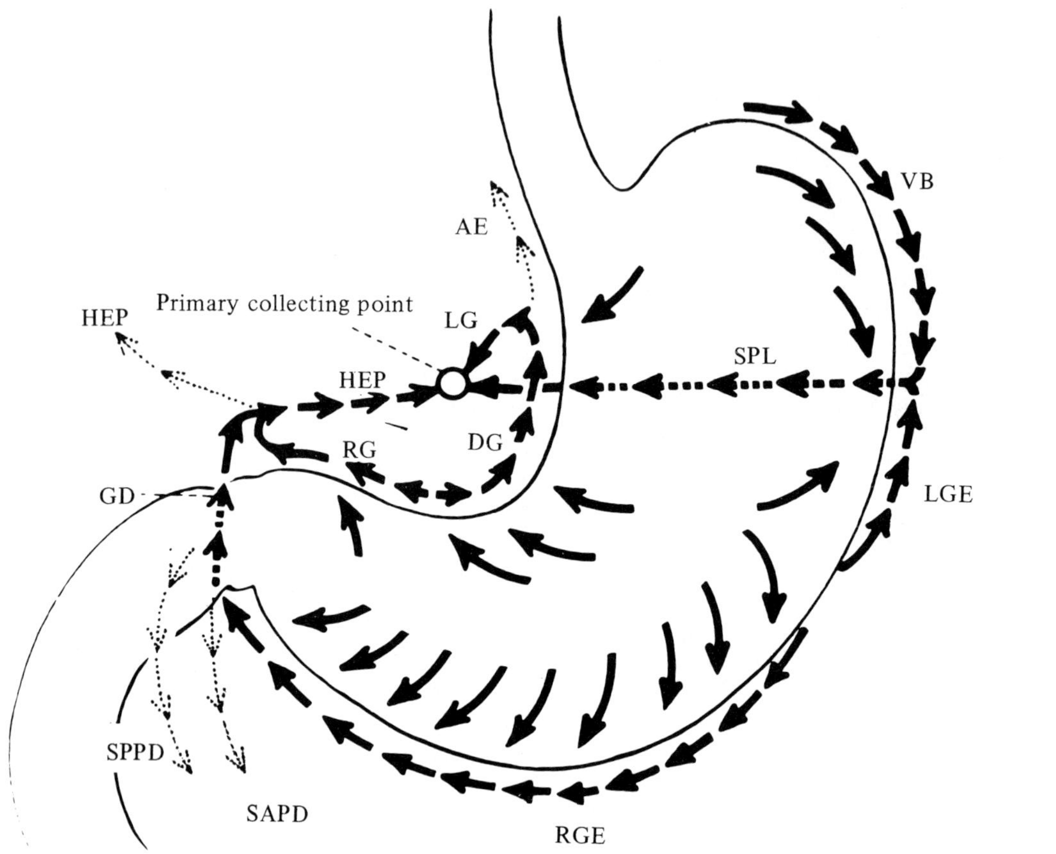

Fig. 2-19. The lymphatic drainage of the stomach. Arrows indicate direction of drainage, which follows the arteries (see Fig. 2-17 for key to abbreviations of arteries). Dotted arrows indicate immediate secondary routes of lymphatic drainage.

1. The area of the stomach supplied by the right gastroepiploic artery drains into lymph nodes in the omentum surrounding the right gastroepiploic vessels and into subpyloric nodes around the gastroduodenal artery. From the subpyloric nodes, primary lymphatic drainage continues up the gastroduodenal artery to the hepatic nodes around the hepatic artery and then along the hepatic artery to celiac nodes surrounding the celiac axis. This lymphatic pathway communicates with two immediate secondary pathways: First, the lymphatics around the gastroduodenal artery communicate with lymphatics of the pancreaticoduodenal arcades; and second, the lymphatics around the hepatic artery communicate with lymphatics associated with the hepatic artery in the hepatoduodenal ligament and hilus of the liver. This is how gastric carcinoma frequently spreads to lymph nodes anterior and posterior to the head of the pancreas and to nodes in the hepatic pedicle [8].
2. The area of the stomach supplied by the vasa brevia and left gastroepiploic artery drains across the gastrosplenic ligament to pancreaticosplenic nodes in the hilus of the spleen adjacent to the tail of the pancreas and then through nodes surrounding the splenic artery to the celiac nodes. (Secondary pathways may follow the most superior

vasa brevia upward to lymphatics adjacent to the abdominal esophagus.)

3. The area of the stomach supplied by the left gastric artery drains to nodes in the lesser omentum surrounding the bifurcation of the left gastric artery and then through nodes along the main trunk of the left gastric artery to the celiac nodes. (The nodes at the bifurcation of the left gastric artery communicate with lymphatics that accompany the ascending esophageal branches to the cardia and abdominal esophagus; these lymphatics represent another, secondary route of drainage.)[11]
4. The area of the stomach supplied by the right gastric artery drains lymph to suprapyloric nodes in the lesser omentum surrounding the right gastric vessels. From these nodes, drainage continues to lymphatics surrounding the hepatic artery, which join the lymphatics draining the right gastroepiploic area along the hepatic artery to the celiac nodes.

The celiac nodes represent the primary collecting point for all four primary pathways draining the stomach. From this point, lymph flows up the periaortic chain and thoracic duct.

Surgical Applications

Evaluating any operative procedure designed to eradicate extrinsic lymphatic metastases necessitates considering primary lymphatic pathways, their immediate secondary routes, and the primary collecting point. On this anatomical basis, carcinoma of the descending colon, for example, presents a relatively easy approach: Removing the left colon and its mesentery to the aorta at the origin of the inferior mesenteric artery excises its primary lymphatics in their entirety and the primary collecting point en bloc. The stomach, however, presents a much more complex anatomical problem. Excising its primary lymphatics and primary collecting point en bloc (in keeping with the principles of en bloc technique) entails removing the celiac artery at the aorta and all its branches supplying the stomach. This would require splenectomy, total pancreatectomy, duodenectomy, and a graft replacing the hepatic artery. Current methods do not entail such radical excision and therefore do not completely excise all the primary lymphatics. I compromise by removing only the parts of the lymphatic drainage that are indicated by the location of the tumor and thus the lymphatics most probably involved. For example, one can easily excise the left gastroepiploic and vasa brevia pathway by removing the spleen and pancreas up to the point of origin of the splenic artery at the aorta. One can also easily excise the left gastric pathway by removing the lesser omentum and the main left gastric trunk up to the point where it meets the aorta (beware of the hepatogastric artery). But one cannot excise the right gastroepiploic and right gastric pathways without taking the hepatic artery, duodenum, and head of the pancreas. Removing the duodenum and head of the pancreas, as advocated by Harvey et al. [45], only partially excises this lymphatic pathway because the hepatic artery is preserved.

One of the reasons for failure of these compromising procedures is the fact that, although cancer localized in any of the four zones generally metastasizes through the lymphatic drainage of that zone, metastasis may occur along other routes. For example, cancer located along the proximal greater curvature (vasa brevia) may metastasize to subpyloric nodes around the gastroduodenal artery, either by diffuse spread through the submucosal plexus or by retrograde flow after metastatic block of primary zonal drainage. Furthermore, none of these compromising procedures excises the primary collecting point en bloc. Appleby [6, 7] has excised the celiac axis to remove the celiac nodes, and in more than 30 patients who underwent resection to cure cancer he found only 4 who did not already have metastasis to celiac nodes. But even this procedure compromises by preserving the pancreaticoduodenal and gastroduodenal vessels,

[11] In the presence of an accessory left gastric artery from hepatic or splenic arteries or an aberrant left hepatic from the left gastric artery, lymphatics may also follow these vessels. These variable arteries and their lymphatic pathways are not diagramed in Figures 2-17 and 2-18.

and accordingly it does not permit en bloc excision of their associated lymphatics draining the right gastroepiploic and right gastric areas.

References

1. Ahlman, B. H. J., Larson, G. M., Bombeck, C. T., et al. Origin of the adrenergic nerve fibers in the subdiaphragmatic vagus in the dog. *Am. J. Surg.* 137:116, 1979.
2. Allgöwer, M. Personal communication, 1979.
3. Amdrup, B. M., and Griffith, C. A. Selective vagotomy of the parietal cell mass. *Ann. Surg.* 170:207, 1969.
4. Amdrup, B. M., and Griffith, C. A. The effects of vagotomy upon biliary function in dogs. *J. Surg. Res.* 10:209, 1970.
5. Amdrup E. Personal communications, 1980, 1982.
6. Appleby, L. H. The coeliac axis in the expansion of the operation for gastric carcinoma. *Cancer* 6:704, 1953.
7. Appleby, L. H. Personal communication, 1959.
8. Arhelger, S. W., Lober, P. H., and Wangensteen, O. H. Dissection of the hepatic pedicle and retropancreaticoduodenal areas for cancer of the stomach. *Surgery* 38:675, 1955.
9. Barlow, T. E., Bentley, F. H., and Walder, D. N. Arteries, veins, and arteriovenous anastomoses in the human stomach. *Surg. Gynecol. Obstet.* 93:657, 1951.
10. Bell, P. R. F. The long-term effect of vagotomy on the maximal acid response to histamine in man. *Gastroenterology* 46:387, 1964.
11. Bell, P. R. F. The insulin test after vagotomy. In T. F. Thompson and I. E. Gillespie (Eds.), *Postgraduate Gastroenterology.* London: Bailliere, Tindall & Cox, 1966. P. 241.
12. Bentley, F. H., and Barlow, T. E. Stomach—vascular supply of in relation to gastric ulcer. In E. R. Carling and J. P. Ross (Eds.), *Surgical Process.* London: Butterworth, 1952.
13. Berger, E. H. The distribution of parietal cells in the stomach: A histotopographic study. *Am. J. Anat.* 54:87, 1934.
14. Berman, J. K., and Fields, D. C. Advanced atrophic cirrhosis: Present status of hepatic, splenic, and left gastric arterial occlusion as an aid in the control of its complications. *Arch. Surg.* 68:432, 1954.
15. Berman, J. K., and Hull, J. E. Hepatic, splenic, and left gastric arterial ligations in advanced portal cirrhosis. *Arch. Surg.* 65:37, 1952.
16. Brown, J. R., and Derr, J. W. Arterial blood supply of human stomach. *Arch. Surg.* 64:616, 1952.
17. Burge, H. W., and Frohm, M. J. N. The technique of bilateral selective vagotomy with the electrical stimulation test. *Br. J. Surg.* 56:452, 1969.
18. Capper, W. M. Factors in the pathogenesis of gastric ulcer. *Ann. R. Coll. Surg. Engl.* 40:21, 1967.
19. Capper, W. M., Airth, G. R., and Kilby, J. O. A test for pyloric regurgitation. *Lancet* 2:621, 1966.
20. Capper, W. M., Butler, T. J., Buckler, K. G., et al. Variation in size of the gastric antrum. *Ann. Surg.* 163:281, 1966.
21. Clark, C. G. Recovery of gastric function after incomplete vagotomy. *Br. J. Surg.* 51:539, 1964.
22. Clarke, J. S. Hepatic necrosis following celiac artery ligation during gastric resection in man. *Arch. Surg.* 71:171, 1955.
23. Coller, F. A., Kay, E. B., and McIntyre, R. S. Regional lymphatic metastases of carcinoma of the stomach. *Arch. Surg.* 43:748, 1941.
24. Collins, W. T., and Gall, E. A. Gastric carcinoma: A multicentric lesion. *Cancer* 5:62, 1952.
25. Cox, A. J., Jr. Stomach size and its relation to chronic peptic ulcer. *Arch. Pathol.* 54:407, 1952.
26. Dragstedt, L. R. Personal communications, 1956, 1961, 1963, 1968.
27. Dragstedt, L. R., Harper, P. V., Tovee, E. B., et al. Section of the nerves to the stomach in the treatment of peptic ulcer. *Ann. Surg.* 126:687, 1947.
28. Dragstedt, L. R., Oberhelman, H. A., Jr., and Woodward, E. R. Physiology of gastric secretion and its relation to the ulcer problem. *JAMA* 147:1615, 1951.
29. Dragstedt, L. R., and Owens, F. M., Jr. Supradiaphragmatic section of vagus nerves in treatment of duodenal ulcer. *Proc. Soc. Exp. Biol. Med.* 53:153, 1943.
30. Dragstedt, L. R., Woodward, E. R., and Camp, E. H. Question of the return of gastric secretion after complete vagotomy. *Arch. Surg.* 61:775, 1950.
31. Eiseman, B., Silen, W., Tyler, P., et al. The portal hypotensive action of Pituitrin. *Surg. Forum* 10:286, 1960.

32. Fell, S. C., Seidenberg, B., and Hurwitt, E. S. Ischemic necrosis of the gastric remnant: An uncommon complication of radical subtotal gastrectomy. *Surgery* 43:490, 1958.
33. Friesen, S. R. The significance of the anomalous origin of the left hepatic artery from the left gastric artery in operations upon the stomach and esophagus. *Am. Surg.* 23:1103, 1967.
34. Grassi, G. Highly selective vagotomy with intraoperative acid secretion of completeness of vagal section. *Surg. Gynecol. Obstet.* 140:259, 1975.
35. Gray, S. W., and Skandalakis, J. E. *Embryology for Surgeons.* Philadelphia: Saunders, 1972.
36. Griffith, C. A. Gastric vagotomy vs. total abdominal vagotomy. *Arch. Surg.* 81:781, 1960.
37. Griffith, C. A. Selective gastric vagotomy. *West. J. Surg. Obstet. Gynecol.* 70:107, 175, 1962.
38. Griffith, C. A. A new anatomic approach to the problem of incomplete vagotomy. *Surg. Clin. North Am.* 44:1239, 1964.
39. Griffith, C. A. Completeness of gastric vagotomy by the selective technic. *Am. J. Dig. Dis.* 12:333, 1967.
40. Griffith, C. A. Types of vagotomy: Preference for the selective procedure. In R. Maingot (Ed.), *Abdominal Operations* (6th ed.). New York: Appleton-Century-Crofts, 1974.
41. Griffith, C. A. Long-term results of selective vagotomy plus pyloroplasty. *Am. J. Surg.* 139:608, 1980.
42. Griffith, C. A., and Harkins, H. N. The role of Brunner's glands in the intrinsic resistance of the duodenum to acid-peptic digestion. *Ann. Surg.* 143:160, 1956.
43. Griffith, C. A., and Harkins, H. N. Partial gastric vagotomy. *Gastroenterology* 32:96, 1957.
44. Hallenbeck, G. A., Gleysteen, J. J., Aldrete, J. S., et al. Proximal gastric vagotomy: Effect of two operative techniques on clinical and gastric secretory results. *Ann. Surg.* 184:435, 1976.
45. Harvey, H. D., Titherington, J. B., Stout, A. P., et al. Gastric carcinoma: Experiences from 1916 to 1949 and present concepts. *Cancer* 4:717, 1951.
46. Hollander, F. Personal communication, 1956.
47. Jackson, P. P. Ischemic necrosis of the proximal gastric remnant following subtotal gastrectomy. *Ann. Surg.* 150:1071, 1959.
48. Jackson, R. G. Anatomy of the vagus nerves in the region of the lower esophagus and the stomach. *Anat. Rec.* 103:1, 1949.
49. Jemerin, E. E., Hollander, F., and Weinstein, V. A. Comparison of insulin and food stimuli for gastric pouches. *Gastroenterology* 1:500, 1943.
50. Joffe, S. N. Personal communications, 1982.
51. Joffe, S. N., Crocket, A., and Doyle, D. Morphologic and functional evidence of reinnervation of the parietal cell mass after parietal vagotomy. *Am. J. Surg.* 143:80, 1982.
52. Jones, W. M., and Griffith, C. A. On the question of vagal reinnervation of the stomach. Part I. *Ann. Surg.* 171:365, 1970.
53. Jones, W. M., and Griffith, C. A. On the question of vagal reinnervation of the stomach. Part II. *Ann. Surg.* 171:369, 1970.
54. Jones, W. M., and Griffith, C. A. Unpublished data, 1970.
55. Kimura, C. Visceral sensation. *Acta Neuroveg.* (Vienna) 28:405, 1966.
56. Kirk, R. M. Mucosal antrectomy with vagotomy in the treatment of duodenal ulcer. *Br. J. Surg.* 52:604, 1965.
57. Kirschner, P. A., and Garlock, J. H. The rationale of routine omentectomy in subtotal gastrectomy. *Surgery* 36:884, 1954.
58. Kjllgren, K. The innervation of the biliary system and the proximal part of the duodenum from a surgical aspect. *Acta Chir. Scand.* 107:230, 1954.
59. Kleitsch, W. P. Anatomy of the pancreas. *Arch. Surg.* 71:795, 1955.
60. Kronborg, O., Jorgensen, P. M., and Holst-Christensen, J. Influence of different techniques of proximal gastric vagotomy upon risk of recurrent duodenal ulcer and gastric acid secretion. *Acta Chir. Scand.* 143:53, 1977.
61. Kusakari, K., Nyhus, L. M., Gillison, E. W., et al. An endoscopic test for completeness of vagotomy. *Arch. Surg.* 105:386, 1972.
62. Landboe-Christensen, E. Extent of the pylorus zone in the human stomach. *Acta Pathol. Microbiol. Scand.* 54(Suppl.):671, 1944.
63. Landboe-Christensen, E. *The Duodenal Glands of Brunner in Man: Their Distribution and Quantity.* London: Humphrey Milford, Oxford University Press, 1944.
64. Latarjet, A. Preliminaire sur l'innervation et l'enervation de l'estomac. *Lyon Med.* 130:166, 1921.
65. Latarjet, A. Resection des nerfs de l'estomac. *Bull. Acad. Natl'l. Med.* (Paris) 87:681, 1922.
66. Legros, G., and Griffith, C. A. The anatomic basis for the variable adequacy of incomplete

vagotomy. Part I. *Ann. Surg.* 168:1030, 1968.

67. Legros, G., and Griffith, C. A. The anatomic basis for the variable adequacy of incomplete vagotomy. Part II. *Ann. Surg.* 168:1035, 1968.
68. Legros, G., and Griffith, C. A. The abdominal vagal system in rats. *J. Surg. Res.* 9:183, 1969.
69. Legros, G., and Griffith, C. A. The anatomic pathways of the vagal fibers to the antral mucosa. *Surgery* 66:751, 1969.
70. Legros, G., and Griffith, C. A. The permanence of adequate incomplete vagotomy. *Surgery* 67:654, 1970.
71. LeVeen, H. H., Mulder, A. G., and Prokop, F. The physiological mechanism for death in massively bleeding peptic ulcer. *Surg. Gynecol. Obstet.* 94:433, 1952.
72. Loeweneck, V. H., Ludinghausen, M. V., and Mepel, W. N. vagus and cholinergisches system am magen des menschen. *Munch. Med. Wochenschr.* 109:1754, 1967.
73. Madden, J. L. Ligation of the hepatic and splenic arteries in the treatment of cirrhosis of the liver. *Surg. Gynecol. Obstet.* 96:594, 1953.
74. Madden, J. L., Kandalaft, S., and Eghrari, M. Mobilization of the duodenum: A surgical maneuver incorrectly credited to Kocher. *Surgery* 63:522, 1968.
75. Mayo, W. J. The contributions of surgery to a better understanding of gastric and duodenal ulcer. *Ann. Surg.* 45:810, 1907.
76. Mayo, W. J. Anaemic spot on the duodenum. *Surg. Gynecol. Obstet.* 6:600, 1908.
77. McCrea, E. D. A. The abdominal distribution of the vagus. *J. Anat.* 59:18, 1924.
78. Michels, N. A. The hepatic, cystic, and retroduodenal arteries and their relations to the biliary ducts. *Ann. Surg.* 133:503, 1951.
79. Michels, N. A. Variational anatomy of the hepatic, cystic, and retroduodenal arteries: A statistical analysis of their origin, distribution, and relations to the biliary ducts in 200 bodies. *Arch. Surg.* 66:20, 1953.
80. Michels, N. A. Collateral arterial pathways to the liver after ligation of the hepatic artery and removal of the celiac axis. *Cancer* 6:708, 1953.
81. Michels, N. A. *Blood Supply and Anatomy of the Upper Abdominal Organs*. Philadelphia: Lippincott, 1955.
82. Mitchell, G. A. G. A macroscopic study of the nerve supply of the stomach. *J. Anat.* 75:50, 1940.
83. Mitchell, G. A. G. Nerve supply of the gastrointestinal tract. *Clin. Symp.* 2:143, 1959.
84. Moe, R. E., and Klopper, P. J. Demonstration of the functional anatomy of the canine gastric antrum. II. Operative techniques not requiring gastrostomy. *Am. J. Surg.* 111:80, 1966.
85. Moe, R. E., Klopper, P. J., and Nyhus, L. M. Demonstration of the functional anatomy of the canine gastric antrum. *Am. J. Surg.* 110:277, 1965.
86. Morgenstern, L. The avoidable complications of splenectomy. *Surg. Gynecol. Obstet.* 145:525, 1977.
87. Murray, J. G. The consequences of injury and disease of nervous tissue. *J. R. Coll. Surg. Edinb.* 4:199, 1959.
88. Nielsen, H. O., Muñoz, J. D., Kronborg, O., et al. The antrum in duodenal ulcer patients: Relationship between antrum size, nerve of Latarjet, gastrin cell quantity, and gastric acid secretion. *Scand. J. Gastroenterol.* 16:491, 1981.
89. Oi, M., Ito, Y., Kumagi, F., Yoshida, K., et al. A possible dual control mechanism in the origin of peptic ulcer. *Gastroenterology* 57:280, 1969.
90. Oi, M., and Oshida, K. The association of esophageal, gastric, and duodenal ulcers. *Gastroenterology* 36:57, 1959.
91. Oi, M., Oshida, K., and Sugimura, S. The location of gastric ulcer. *Gastroenterology* 36:45, 1959.
92. Oi, M., and Sakurai, Y. The location of duodenal ulcer. *Gastroenterology* 36:60, 1959.
93. Oi, M., Tanaka, U., Yoshida, K., et al. Dual control of peptic ulcers by both the gastric mucosa and musculature. *Rev. Surg.* 23:373, 1966.
94. Payne, J. T. The significance of vascular landmarks in gastric resection. *West. J. Surg. Obstet. Gynecol.* 71:161, 1963.
95. Peters, R. M., and Womack, N. A. Hemodynamics of gastric secretion. *Ann. Surg.* 148:537, 1958.
96. Poppen, B., Delin, A., and Sandstedt, B. Parietal cell vagotomy: Localization of the microscopical antral-fundic boundary in relation to the macroscopical. *Acta Chir. Scand.* 142:251, 1976.
97. Pritchard, G. R., Griffith, C. A., and Harkins, H. N. A physiologic demonstration of the anatomic distribution of the vagal system to the stomach. *Surg. Gynecol. Obstet.* 126:791, 1968.
98. Reeves, T. B. A study of the arteries supplying the stomach and duodenum and their relation to ulcer. *Surg. Gynecol. Obstet.* 30:374, 1920.

99. Reinhoff, W. F., Jr. Ligation of the hepatic and splenic arteries in the treatment of portal hypertension with a report of six cases: A preliminary report. *Bull. Johns Hopkins Hosp.* 88:368, 1951.
100. Reinhoff, W. F., Jr., and Woods, A. C., Jr. Ligation of the hepatic and splenic arteries in treatment of cirrhosis with ascites. *JAMA* 152:687, 1953.
101. Rosenbaum, D., and Egbert, J. L. Liver necrosis and death following hepatic artery ligation. *JAMA* 149:1210, 1952.
102. Ross, B., and Kay, A. W. The insulin test after vagotomy. *Gastroenterology* 46:1379, 1964.
103. Rouviere, H. *Anatomy of the Human Lymphatic System.* Ann Arbor, Mich.: Edward Bros., 1938.
104. Royster, H. P., Sloan, A. M., McCain, L. L., et al. The anatomy of the nerves supplying the common duct and proximal duodenum. *Surgery* 26:413, 1949.
105. Ruckley, C. V. A study of the variations of the abdominal vagi. *Br. J. Surg.* 51:569, 1964.
106. Rutter, A. G. Ischemic necrosis of the stomach following subtotal gastrectomy. *Lancet* 2:1021, 1953.
107. Seaman, W. B. Focal hypertrophy of the pyloric muscle-torus hyperplasia. *Am. J. Roentgenol. Radium Ther. Nucl. Med.* 96:388, 1966.
108. Shapiro, A. L., and Robilard, G. L. The esophageal arteries. *Ann. Surg.* 131:171, 1950.
109. Sherman, J. L., and Newman, S. Functioning arteriovenous anastomoses in the stomach and duodenum. *Am. J. Physiol.* 179:279, 1954.
110. Shiina, E., and Griffith, C. A. Selective and total vagotomy without drainage. *Ann. Surg.* 169:326, 1969.
111. Skandalakis, J. E. Personal communication, 1981.
112. Skandalakis, J. E., Gray, W., Saria, R. E., et al. Distribution of the vagus nerve to the stomach. *Am. Surg.* 46:130, 1980.
113. Spencer, F. C. Ischemic necrosis of remaining stomach following subtotal gastrectomy. *Arch. Surg.* 73:844, 1956.
114. Stavney, L. S., Kato, T., Griffith, C. A., et al. A physiologic study of motility changes following selective gastric vagotomy. *J. Surg. Res.* 3:390, 1963.
115. Stuart, J. R., and Jordan, P. H. Unusual complications of subtotal gastric resection. *Arch. Surg.* 74:459, 1957.
116. Swigart, L. V. L., Siekert, R. G., Hambley, W. C., et al. The esophageal arteries. *Surg. Gynecol. Obstet.* 90:234, 1950.
117. Torgensen, J. Muscular build and movements of stomach and duodenal bulb. *Acta Radiol.* (Suppl.):45, 1942.
118. Weinberg, J., and Greaney, E. M. Identification of regional lymph nodes by means of vital staining dye during surgery of gastric cancer. *Surg. Gynecol. Obstet.* 90:561, 1950.
119. Wertheimer, P. L'Innervation et l'enervation gastriques: Etude anatomique, experimentale, et clinique. Lyon: Imprimerie-Express, 1922.
120. Wilkie, D. P. D. The blood supply of the duodenum, with special reference to the supraduodenal artery. *Surg. Gynecol. Obstet.* 13:399, 1911.
121. Woodward, E. R. Peptic ulceration of the stomach and duodenum. *Surg. Clin. North Am.* 39:1195, 1959.
122. Zinninger, M. M. Extension of gastric cancer in the intramural lymphatics and its relation to gastrectomy. *Am. Surg.* 20:920, 1954.
123. Zinninger, M. M., and Collins, W. T. Extension of carcinoma of the stomach into the duodenum and esophagus. *Ann. Surg.* 130:557, 1949.

EDITOR'S COMMENT

There is a wealth of anatomical detail in this presentation. As usual, the more we learn, the more questions arise for further study. The observation that the change from antral gastric mucosa to classical duodenal mucosa is not fixed at a point within or distal to the pylorus becomes important in the evaluation of postoperative results following procedures for channel and prepyloric ulcers. The position of the ulcer in relation to the pylorus and the type of mucosa present were thought to be important to the end result following proximal gastric vagotomy (PGV) (*World J. Surg.* 2:91, 1978). This is not a constant relationship, and the entire thesis is questioned (*Surgery* 94:802, 1983).

I found the details of anatomical variation relating to the nerve of Laterjet in its distal distribution of marked interest. This combined with a wide variety of corpus-antrum mucosal boundaries (proximal or distal) gives one pause as to the practical nature of PGV in denervating sufficient parietal cell mass to cure the ulcer diathesis in a given patient (*Scand. J. Gastroenterol.* 18:465, 1983).

Although vascular factors may be important in the etiology of lesser gastric curvature necrosis following PGV, certainly good operative technique or lack of it may play a role. It is relatively easy to "gouge" unknowingly the lesser curvature musculature with the artery forceps. A diligent search must be made for these technical errors at the completion of each dissection. In addition, reperitonealization and invagination of the lesser curvature of the stomach after PGV is indicated (*Arch. Surg.* 113:207, 1978). (L.M.N.)

3

Physiology

PART I
Gastroduodenal Physiology and Pathophysiology

Lars Olbe and Ulf Haglund

This chapter summarizes basic concepts of gastroduodenal physiology and pathophysiology, no doubt with the inevitable errors that emerge from emphasizing relatively new ideas. Specific topics include mechanisms regulating gastric acid secretion in humans and the barrier function of gastric mucosa. Furthermore, possible differences between persons with normal gastrointestinal tracts and ulcer patients with regard to mechanisms regulating acid secretion are discussed.

Gastric Mucosa and Its Secretory Products

The gastric mucosa consists of a surface layer of mucus-producing columnar cells and coiled, sometimes branched, glands. The glands contain mucous, parietal (oxyntic), chief (peptic), and endocrine cells. At the gastroesophageal junction, the cardiac gland area is several centimeters wide. The glands of the cardiac area contain few parietal and chief cells. It is not known whether the cardiac gland area has any specific endocrine function. In the corpus-fundus region (oxyntic gland area), the mucosa invaginates into gastric pits occupying about one-quarter of the mucosal depth. Three to seven oxyntic glands discharge their contents into each gastric pit. The oxyntic glands contain mucous cells interspersed with parietal cells in the midportion of the glands, chief cells at the base of the glands, and endocrine cells in the basal half of the glands.

The pyloric gland area in the antrum constitutes the aboral 20 percent of the gastric mucosa. A transitional zone, 0.5-2.0 cm wide, separates the oxyntic gland area from the pyloric gland area and contains mixed glands. The glands of the antrum contain mucous cells, very few parietal cells, and endocrine cells. The mucosa of the antrum is the richest source of gastrin in the body. The endocrine cells producing gastrin (G cells) are most abundant in the midportion of the glands. The membrane of the gastrin-containing cell reaches the lumen of the gland, constituting an anatomical basis for postulating a chemical influence on the G cell from the gastric contents and a discharge of gastrin into the gastric contents [179], in addition to the internal secretion of gastrin.

The transitional zone between the pyloric gland area and the oxyntic gland area can often, but by no means always, be roughly localized at the point where the longitudinal folds of the oxyntic gland mucosa merge into the flatter mucosa of the antrum. At the lesser curvature the transitional zone is usually located just above the angle of the stomach, but it can be found anywhere from this point up to a few centimeters from the cardiac gland area, which has to be taken into account when a complete antrectomy is pursued. A more precise localization of the transitional zone during operation requires stimulation of gastric acid secretion and determination of the boundary by an appropriate pH-indicator technique.

The gland cells of the gastric mucosa are continually renewed. A high mitotic rate has been found in cells at the gland necks, known as mucous neck cells. These cells are assumed to be undifferentiated, with a potential of differentiating into either surface mucous cells, with migration toward the surface, or parietal cells or chief cells, with migration toward the base of the glands.

INNERVATION AND BLOOD SUPPLY OF THE GASTRIC MUCOSA

Preganglionic efferent vagal fibers synapse on ganglionic cells in the myenteric (Auerbach) plexus and in the submucosal (Meissner) plexus. Most of the ganglionic cells reveal intense acetylcholinesterase activity [78], suggesting that they are cholinergic. The terminations of the postganglionic fibers in the gastric mucosa have not been conclusively demonstrated. The anatomical basis for direct innervation of the parietal cells and gastrin-containing cells is lacking; there is, however, strong physiological evidence for vagal activation of these structures.

The sympathetic innervation of the stomach is mainly derived from postganglionic adrenergic fibers of the celiac ganglia. These fibers display catecholamine fluorescence and terminate in close contact with the intramural ganglionic cells. There is no evidence that there are adrenergic or serotonin-containing ganglionic cells within the gastric wall. A few adrenergic fibers innervate intramural blood vessels. It therefore seems plausible that activation of the sympathetic nervous system of the stomach influences the gastric functions—apart from blood flow—by modulating the activity of the intramural ganglionic cells. Physiological evidence for such a mechanism has been found in studies on gastric motility [82].

The nervous control of gastrointestinal function utilizes peptidergic nerves in addition to the traditional adrenergic and cholinergic nerve fibers. In these nerves several of the gastrointestinal peptide hormones serve as transmitter substances. Vasoactive intestinal peptide (VIP), substance P, and gastrin are examples of proposed neurotransmitters. It has been shown that the gastric receptive relaxation [113] is a vagal reflex with a nonadrenergic, noncholinergic transmitter substance. Experiments in cats favor the idea that VIP might be a transmitter in this reflex [48]. The exact additional roles of these peptidergic nerves and of the humoral peptide system in gastrointestinal physiology and pathophysiology are under intense investigation.

The arteries penetrating the gastric wall usually split into an extensive, freely anastomosing submucosal plexus from which a remarkably rich capillary network is formed around the gastric glands. Mucosal arteries may also arise directly from the external vascular arcades. According to recent studies using modern techniques, arteriovenous anastomoses do not exist in the stomach [68, 133].

Stimulation of the sympathetic nerves has a vasoconstrictive action, while vagal stimulation has a vasodilatative action that is partly blocked by atropine [113].

All gastric acid secretory stimulants increase the mucosal blood flow. The magnitude of gastric mucosal-submucosal blood flow correlates well with basal and pentagastrin-stimulated acid secretion [68, 75, 94]. Knight et al. [94], measuring gastric mucosal blood flow with a neutral red clearance test, postulated that patients with duodenal ulcer produced more acid than healthy volunteers per unit of mucosal blood flow, the difference disappearing after proximal gastric vagotomy. This difference between duodenal ulcer patients and healthy persons could not be confirmed by others using ^{14}C-aminopyrine clearance [68] or ^{85}krypton elimination techniques [75].

Epinephrine and norepinephrine reduce mucosal blood flow and inhibit acid secretion. Thus the inhibition of acid secretion could be secondary to decreased mucosal blood flow or be caused by a separate adrenergic action. The inhibition of pentagastrin-stimulated acid secretion in the dog by norepinephrine was found to be most likely secondary to a decreased mucosal blood flow, while the inhibition of acid secretion by isoprenaline was found to be independent of a decreased mucosal blood flow [31], showing that separate adrenergic actions on mucosal blood flow and acid secretion can be displayed. An adrenergic stimulant of the β_2 type has produced marked inhibition of gastric acid secretion [54]. The site of action of this pharmacological adrenergic inhibition of gastric acid secretion is unknown.

ELECTROLYTE SECRETION

The electrolytes in gastric juice are a mixture of secretions from parietal and nonparietal cells. The nonparietal cell secretion is a mucus-containing juice that is slightly alkaline because of a bicarbonate concentration of about 25 mmol/L, and it contains sodium, potassium, and chloride in about the same concentrations as are found in the extracellular fluid. In the parietal cells, secretory canaliculi are invaginated from the apical surface. The secretory canaliculi are lined with microvilli, giving a secretory surface of about 1.3 sq m/cu cm. The parietal cells secrete hydrochloric acid and potassium chloride solution in a ratio of about 15:1. The maximal hydrogen ion concentration found in the gastric juice of humans is about 150 mmol/L. The electrolyte composition in the gastric juice depends mainly on the proportions of parietal and nonparietal cell secretion: When the parietal cells are activated, the hydrogen ion concentration in the gastric juice increases while the sodium concentration declines. However, there is also an exchange of sodium for hydrogen ions diffusing back into the gastric mucosa. The exchange does not seem to have a simple 1:1 relationship, and this results in a net gain of solute and fluid in the gastric lumen [18]. Under normal conditions, the exchange of sodium for hydrogen across the mucosa contributes only slightly to the sodium concentration in the gastric juice. However, when the gastric mucosa has been damaged, e.g., by aspirin or duodenal contents containing bile acids, the back-diffusion of hydrogen ions in exchange for sodium is markedly increased.

During acid secretion the metabolism in the parietal cells is mainly aerobic. More than one hydrogen ion is secreted per oxygen molecule. At the same time the mucosa consumes one molecule of carbon dioxide for each hydrogen ion secreted. The mucosa thus expends more carbon dioxide than oxygen during acid secretion. Carbonic anhydrase present in the parietal cells facilitates the hydration of carbon dioxide to form bicarbonate ions. In vitro the histamine-stimulated gastric mucosa still secretes acid after removal of the external supply of carbon dioxide. During this condition, ulcers are formed in the isolated mucosa in the course of 3 to 4 hours [33]. Another example of rapid ulceration is the formulation of stress ulcers by hemorrhagic shock, a phenomenon linked to a marked decrease in gastric mucosal energy metabolism [117].

The bicarbonate formed in the parietal cells is released into the blood. Determination of the excess bicarbonate in the blood during acid secretion was used to estimate gastric acid secretion following a meal in humans, and the results suggested that the acid response reaches the same level as the maximal acid response to histamine [93, 146].

Recently, techniques have been developed that allow the study of acid secretory mechanisms at the parietal cell level using isolated gastric glands [17] or enriched isolated parietal cells [160]. It has been demonstrated in isolated gastric glands that the secretory canaliculi of the parietal cell are the site of formation of acid [16]. The parietal cells contain an adenosine triphosphatase (ATPase) that seems to be specific for these cells. This H^+/K^+ ATPase is located in the microvilli of the secretory canaliculi [147]. H^+/K^+ ATPase is probably executing the final H^+ secretory step. Selective inhibition of H^+/K^+ ATPase can be induced by substituted benzimidazoles. These drugs inhibit basal and stimulated acid secretion *in vivo* and *in vitro* [53, 126], including intracellular stimulation with cyclic adenosine monophosphate (c-AMP). Clinically the substituted benzimidazole omeprazole has been successfully used on a hitherto limited number of peptic ulcer patients and patients with gastrinoma [128].

INTRINSIC FACTOR SECRETION

The intrinsic factor, a mucoprotein secreted by the gastric mucosa, forms a complex with vitamin B_{12}. In the presence of calcium ions, the specific complex facilitates absorption of vitamin B_{12} in the distal ileum. The site of origin of intrinsic factor shows species differences. In the human gastric mucosa, intrinsic factor has been localized to the parietal cells. Intrinsic factor is continuously secreted in amounts exceeding the requirements for normal vitamin B_{12} absorption. As expected, the secretion of intrinsic factor increases whenever gastric acid secretion is stimulated.

PEPSINOGEN SECRETION

The gastroduodenal mucosa secretes pepsinogens that are inactive proenzymes. Below a pH of 5 the pepsinogens are converted to pepsins with a lower molecular weight by an autocatalytic process. The pepsins are responsible for the protease activity. In a neutral or alkaline milieu, the pepsins are irreversibly inactivated.

Seven pepsinogens have been identified in human gastric juice. These pepsinogens are separable into two immunochemically different groups, pepsinogen I and pepsinogen II [148]. Pepsinogens I and II have been localized to the chief cells and mucous neck cells in the corpus-fundus region, and pepsinogen II has also been found in the pyloric gland area and in Brunner's glands [149]. A radioimmunoassay for pepsinogen I in serum has been developed. The serum pepsinogen I levels probably reflect the peptic cell mass and are unchanged by feeding [150]. Gastric pepsinogen secretion for the most part parallels gastric acid secretion [85], which suggests a correlation between the peptic cell mass and the parietal cell mass.

Cholinergic mechanisms, e.g., physiological and pharmacological vagal activation, produce marked pepsinogen secretion. Local application of acid in the stomach stimulates pepsinogen secretion, possibly by a local cholinergic reflex [85]. The gastric acid stimulants histamine and gastrin produce a moderate pepsinogen secretion in humans and a weak pepsinogen secretion in dogs. High doses of gastrin or histamine inhibit vagally stimulated pepsinogen secretion in the dogs [127]. Secretin is unique in stimulating pepsinogen secretion and inhibiting acid secretion [24, 85]. Pepsinogen secretion is inhibited by atropine, prostaglandins, gastric inhibitory polypeptide (GIP), and VIP [66].

MUCUS SECRETION

Gastric mucus is secreted by the surface mucous cells and the mucous cells of the glands. The chemical composition of the mucus varies among species and includes mucoproteins, mucopolysaccharides, and proteins. In humans and pigs the mucoproteins predominate, forming a family of large-sized molecules, all of which are gel-forming and are built up of smaller mucoprotein units joined by interchain disulfide links [1]. Carbohydrate compounds surrounding a protein core constitute the bulk of the mucoproteins and include hexose, hexosamine, fucose, and sialic acid. The structures of the water-soluble mucus and the water-insoluble mucous gel are similar. The mucoproteins are unchanged by pepsin but are precipitated by acidification, probably because of changes in the state of ionization of the mucoproteins [18], to form visible mucus.

Salicylate inhibits mucus biosynthesis. Under normal conditions, small amounts of sulphated compounds, originating mainly from the saliva, are found in the mucus of the gastric juice. Sulphate is taken up to a slight degree in the mucous cells of normal gastric mucosa, but the sulphate uptake is markedly increased in gastritic mucosa that contains intestinal metaplasia [156].

Gastric mucous secretion is stimulated by serotonin and several hormones (gastrin, cholecystokinin, and secretin), but the effect of vagal stimulation on gastric mucous secretion is controversial [116, 180]. Rubbing of the mucosa or local application of acid or hypertonic solutions increases the gastric mucus secretion.

A main function of the gastric mucus is lubrication. It is unknown whether the state of ionization of the mucoproteins affects the diffusion of chemical agents to the glandular cells, e.g., chemicals releasing gastrin from the G cells and chemicals injurious to the mucous cells.

Brunner's glands are localized in the submucosa of the proximal duodenum and extend from the pylorus to the papilla of Vater. The area of Brunner's glands is more resistant to the injurious effects of acid and gastric juice than other parts of the small intestine. Brunner's glands secrete an alkaline mucus containing pepsinogens. The secretion is stimulated by food by way of humoral mechanisms.

The surface epithelium of the proximal duodenum transports bicarbonate to the lumen. This transport is stimulated by prostaglandin E_2 and inhibited by aspirin [57]. The alkalinization produced by the surface epithelium and the Brunner's glands is considered to protect the duodenal surfaces from the aggression induced by acid.

In this connection, the question about a possible defect of acid neutralization in the duodenum of duodenal ulcer patients may be raised. The ratio between the maximal secretions of gastric acid and duodenal bicarbonate is approximately equal in healthy persons and in duodenal ulcer patients. Duodenal ulcer patients are, however, less sensitive to secretin than healthy persons, and they produce a lower bicarbonate response to duodenal acidification than do healthy persons. The reduced sensitivity to secretin and duodenal acidification in duodenal ulcer patients is normalized after gastric vagotomy [20, 190].

GASTRIC MUCOSAL BARRIER

Under normal conditions there is an insignificant movement of hydrogen ions from the gastric lumen into the tissue and an insignificant sequential movement of sodium ions across the mucosa into the gastric lumen. The major part of this barrier probably resides in the surface mucous cells and may thus reflect the integrity of the gastric mucosa. Substances that are soluble in lipids and non-ionized at an acid pH readily penetrate the lipoprotein layer in the apical cell membrane of the surface mucous cells. These substances can reversibly break down the barrier function or destroy the cells.

In addition to the protective role played by the mucous cells themselves, a "mucus-bicarbonate" barrier may be important [189]. According to this theory bicarbonate secreted by the epithelium diffuses through the mucus toward the lumen, while hydrogen ions diffuse in the opposite direction. Thus a pH gradient is created across the unstirred layer of adherent mucus, contributing to the protection of the gastric mucosa.

Substances capable of breaking down the barrier function include exogenous agents, such as ethanol in concentrations above 10 percent, and salicylic and acetylsalicylic acid at an acid pH. Acetylsalicylic acid, having a pH of 3.5, becomes ionized at the intracellular pH and can then exert its toxic effect. This toxic effect may lead to disruption of both the apical membrane of the surface mucous cells and the tight junctions between these cells, causing desquamation and even bleeding erosions. Increased back-diffusion of acid from the lumen into the gastric mucosa and increased gain of sodium ions in the gastric lumen by acetylsalicylic acid have been shown in both dogs and humans [77].

Back-diffusion of acid through the gastric mucosa initiates a series of events in dogs [32]. Gastric motility is strongly stimulated, possibly because of increased cholinergic activity of the gastric intramural plexuses. Secretion of acid and pepsinogen is also stimulated. Histamine is released from the mucosal stores, probably from the mast cells. The mucosal blood flow and the capillary permeability are increased, resulting in mucosal edema. Damage to the surface mucous cells and increased capillary permeability cause a leakage of proteins from the interstitial fluid and the plasma into the gastric lumen. The mucosal blood vessels may be destroyed, producing interstitial hemorrhage or overt bleeding. The last phenomenon is particularly prominent during concomitant cholinergic stimulation, which may explain the effect of anticholinergic therapy or vagotomy on this type of bleeding gastritis in clinical practice.

Detergents are capable of breaking down the gastric mucosal barrier function. Endogenous detergents include bile salts and lysolecithin. Increased back-diffusion of acid into the gastric mucosa has been produced by bile salts and lysolecithin in dogs [32] and by bile salts in humans [76]. Bile salts and lysolecithin are found in the duodenal contents and may regurgitate into the stomach, initiating damage to the gastric mucosal barrier. The damage of the gastric mucosal barrier by bile salts seems related to gastric acid secretion (i.e., damage increases with increasing acidity [142]). Ulceration of the gastric mucosa may thus be a consequence of an attack on the gastric mucosal barrier by endogenous or exogenous agents, allowing entrance of acid into the mucosa. The extent of the damage is probably dependent on both the concentration and duration of such an agent and on the acid secretory level. The back-diffusion of acids is higher in the pyloric gland area than in the oxyntic gland area [76]. Another way of expressing this concept of the pathogenesis of gastric ulceration is to state that gastric ulceration is more dependent on acid absorption than on acid secretion.

It has been generally accepted that most gastric ulcer patients have a hyposecretion of gastric acid, based on the fact that the collected gastric acid output in these patients is lower than in healthy persons. The observed hyposecretion of acid in gastric ulcer patients may be partly dependent on the degree of gastritis in the oxyntic gland area and partly only apparent as a consequence of increased back-diffusion of acid. The back-diffusion of acid in the stomach of humans has been estimated after instillation of isotonic hydrochloric acid in the stomach or by trapping the secreted acid with an intragastric buffer solution during pentagastrin stimulation [28]. The back-diffusion of acid was found to be considerably greater in gastric ulcer patients compared with both healthy persons and duodenal ulcer patients. The difference between the absorbed amounts of acid in seven gastric ulcer patients and nine healthy controls amounted to about 8 mmol/hr. Still higher figures for back-diffusion of acid have been recorded in patients with multiple gastric stress ulcers [76].

Regurgitation of duodenal contents into the stomach is much more common in gastric ulcer patients than in healthy persons [142]. The cause of the frequent regurgitation of duodenal contents into the stomach in gastric ulcer patients has not been established. However, the pylorus of gastric ulcer patients is markedly insensitive to cholecystokinin and secretin [55]. In healthy persons cholecystokinin and secretin increase the pressure in the pylorus. A mean bile salt concentration of 5.3 mmol/L has been found in the gastric juice of gastric ulcer patients after a meal, a figure much higher than that found in healthy persons [142]. This concentration of bile salts significantly increases the back-diffusion of acid in the human stomach [76]. The phospholipase A of pancreatic juice hydrolyzes the lecithin of bile, forming lysolecithin in the duodenum. The reaction is activated by bile acids and trypsins. Phospholipase A of human pancreatic juice has no effect on the gastric mucosal barrier [32]. The lysolecithin concentration in gastric juice collected during the night has been found to be much higher in patients with gastric ulcer than in healthy persons and patients with duodenal ulcers [84]. The lysolecithin concentration found in the gastric juice of gastric ulcer patients is well above that known to be capable of breaking the gastric mucosal barrier in dogs [32].

It is unknown whether there are any substances that facilitate the acid attack on the mucosa of the duodenal bulb and what the mechanism might be.

Gastric Motility and Emptying

The physiology of gastric motor function is rather complex. A few introductory statements may facilitate the interpretation of studies on gastric motor function. The main function of the sphincters, both the lower esophageal and the pyloric, is probably to prevent regurgitation of gastric contents to the esophagus and reflux of duodenal contents into the stomach, respectively. The pylorus is probably of minor importance in the gastric emptying of fluids, serving as the last component in the propulsive motor activity of the antrum. On the other hand, the pylorus, or at least the pylorus and the distal few centimeters of the antrum, seem to have a key role in slowing the gastric emptying of solids by retropulsion of the solids back into the main stomach. The pattern of gastric emptying is different for fluids and solids.

Short gastric contractions can occur in any part of the stomach, although they occur most frequently in the antrum. Visible peristaltic contractions arise in the middle of the corpus region and sweep downward, ending in the pyloric region. In humans a maximal and regular frequency of three contractions per minute appears after a meal. Gastric emptying is mainly regulated by changes in the gastric motor activity and not by changes in the receptive capacity of the duodenum [14]. Gastric emptying of fluids proceeds exponentially, the rate of emptying being proportional to the volume of the gastric contents. It has been claimed that the corpus-fundus area acts as a reservoir and the antrum as a metering pump, and that the rate of emptying is regulated by changes in the stroke volume of the antrum. However, this concept is an oversimplification. In the gastric emptying of solids, the antrum-pylorus region participates by both propulsion and retropulsion [43]. In gastric emptying of fluids, the antrum-pylorus region participates actively to some degree, since the emptying rate is increased after gastric resection [14, 43]. However, the rate of gastric emptying of fluids can still be markedly influenced by the duodenum after a Billroth I resection [14].

Whether the gastric emptying of fluids from the corpus-fundus region is modulated from the duodenum by changes in propulsive motor activity or by changes in relaxation is open to question. Certainly, the corpus-fundus region has a marked capacity to relax, i.e., a capacity to increase its volume without any significant increase of intraluminal pressure. In many studies the short gastric contractions have been determined by an *isometric* technique, i.e., registration of increases of pressure at a constant volume. These pressure waves, often referred to as gastric motility, cannot be differentiated into propulsive and nonpropulsive contractions, and, in addition, the technique does not allow the registration of relaxation. However, an *isotonic* registration of gastric motor activity, i.e., a registration of volume changes in the stomach at a constant intraluminal pressure, does reflect relaxation; at the same time, the short gastric contractions can be determined. With this background it is perhaps easier to accept the fact that gastrin has been reported to increase gastric motility and to inhibit pyloric contraction but also to delay gastric emptying [56].

During the past decade a number of gastrointestinal hormones have been shown to induce effects on the lower esophageal sphincter, the pyloric sphincter, gastric motility, and gastric emptying. However, the physiological importance of these pharmacological effects is, with few exceptions, open to question. Physiological significance of a hormone action cannot be claimed until it has been shown that the action is produced with doses of the exogenous pure hormone equivalent to amounts of the endogenous hormone released under physiological conditions. The action can be direct or augmentative.

LOWER ESOPHAGEAL SPHINCTER

The lower esophageal sphincter is influenced by cholinergic and adrenergic mechanisms. Gastrin increases the lower esophageal sphincter pressure, but the doses required result in a blood concentration of gastrin well above physiological levels. Furthermore, pernicious anemia patients with hypergastrinemia have displayed a normal sphincter pressure [112]. Secretin [29] and glucagon [83] antagonize the gastrin action on the sphincter pressure and in high dosage are capable of reducing the resting sphincter pressure. Whether or not these hormones participate as modulators in the physiological regulation of sphincter pressure remains open to question. Neurotensin in physiological concentrations lowers the sphincter pressure [145]. Prostaglandins can affect the sphincter pressure: in opossums, prostaglandin F (PGF) has increased the lower esophageal sphincter pressure, while prostaglandin E (PGE) has reduced the sphincter pressure [63].

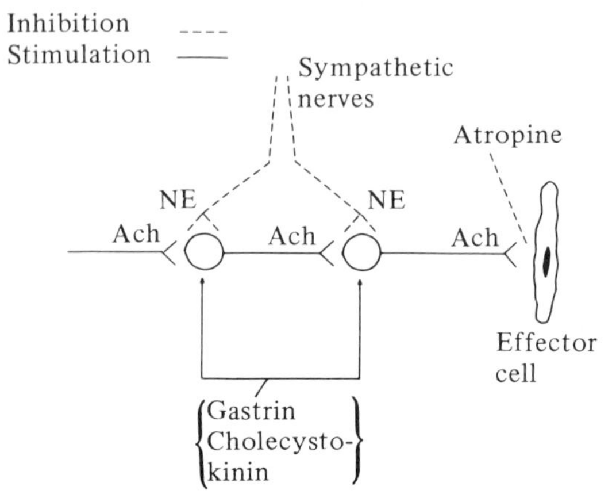

Fig. 3-1. The mode of action of gastrin and cholecystokinin on acetylcholine (Ach) release from Auerbach's plexus, and the interaction of these hormones with norepinephrine (NE) from the sympathetic nervous system. (Modified from Vizi et al. [181].)

STIMULATION OF GASTRIC MOTILITY

Gastric motility is stimulated by activation of cholinergic fibers mainly in the vagal nerves but also in the splanchnic nerves [113]. The electrophysiological properties of these cholinergic vagal fibers are different from the properties of vagal fibers producing relaxation, acid secretion, pepsinogen secretion, and increased blood flow. Distention of the stomach results in increased gastric motility. The distention effect is probably mediated by both nervous and hormonal mechanisms. Reflex stimulation of gastric motility occurs through vagovagal reflexes, but short intramural reflex pathways probably operate similarly to those involved in activation of acid secretion. At least in dogs, distention of the antrum with an antral pH above 1.5 to 2.0 produces a release of gastrin, and this hormone can increase gastric motility.

The closely related hormones gastrin and cholecystokinin can, under appropriate conditions, increase gastric motility. It is possible that the effect of gastrin and cholecystokinin is mediated by stimulation of the ganglionic cells in the Auerbach plexus (Fig. 3-1), resulting in an increased release of acetylcholine [181] and that the last link in the chain of events is a peripheral cholinergic effect. The increased gastric motility produced by gastrin and cholecystokinin is very sensitive to inhibition by atropine.

Motilin is a polypeptide extracted from the duodenal mucosa. It has the property of stimulating gastric motility without any influence on acid secretion [40, 66]. Motilin is made up of 22 amino acids and has a molecular weight of 2700. The amino acid sequence is different from that of other gastrointestinal hormones. The same effect, stimulation of gastric motility without any change of acid secretion, is produced by duodenal alkalinization, which indicates a paired duodenal, pH-dependent humoral mechanism in the control of gastric motility: High duodenal pH results in increased gastric motility mediated by motilin, and low duodenal pH results in decreased gastric motility mediated by secretin and cholecystokinin.

INHIBITION OF GASTRIC MOTILITY

Inhibition of gastric motility can be produced by both nervous and hormonal mechanisms. Stimulation of sympathetic adrenergic fibers with their nerve terminals surrounding the intramural ganglionic cells blocks the ganglionic activation produced by preganglionic vagal stimulation or by gastrin [82, 181]. Inhibition of gastric motility by stimulation of sympathetic adrenergic fibers has been observed only with a background of increased gastric motility produced by vagal stimulation or by gastrin.

Several gastrointestinal hormones or candidate hormones have been reported to inhibit gastric motility: secretin, glucagon, cholecystokinin, GIP, and VIP [66, 112]. Intraduodenal administration of glucose or fat elevates levels of serum GIP. GIP inhibits gastric motility as well as acid secretion. The pattern of release and effect of GIP corresponds to an enterogastrone activity. Vasoactive intestinal peptide has been reported to inhibit gastric motility [112]. Relaxation of the corpus-fundus region of the stomach is produced by stimulation of noncholinergic, nonadrenergic vagal fibers [113]. Experiments on cats have demonstrated that an increase in VIP level in plasma and gastric relaxation are simultaneously induced by direct vagal stimulation or as a reflex effect elicited by esophageal distention [48]. Furthermore, infusion of VIP induces gastric relaxation. Based on these data it has been suggested that VIP is a transmitter in the gastric receptive relaxation reflex.

Activation of the relaxant vagal fibers does not inhibit but rather enhances the short gastric pressure waves activated by cholinergic vagal stimulation. Vagal reflex relaxation can be initiated by touching the mucosa of the pharynx, by distention of the esophagus, and probably by distention of the stomach [81]. After proximal gastric vagotomy, the relaxant function as well as the rhythmic pressure activity was found to be markedly reduced [80]. Intraduodenal administration of glucose or fat in humans produces a marked relaxation of the corpus-fundus region both before and after antrectomy [14]. It seems reasonable to assume that this relaxation effect is involved in the delayed gastric emptying of fluids produced by intraduodenal administration of glucose or fat. To what extent long vagal reflexes from the duodenum and release of duodenal hormones (secretin, enteroglucagon, cholecystokinin, GIP, VIP, and neurotensin) participate in producing gastric relaxation by intraduodenal administration of glucose or fat is open to question.

PYLORIC SPHINCTER

In humans the pyloric pressure increases in response to intraduodenal administration of acid or fat. It has been shown that cholecystokinin and secretin significantly increase the pyloric pressure in humans and that the hormones act additively [56]. At least in the case of cholecystokinin, which produces an increase in pyloric pressure at a dose below 2 units/kg/hr, the effect is probably of physiological importance. Gastrin antagonizes the actions of both cholecystokinin and secretin on the pyloric pressure but at a rather high dosage level. However, duodenal acidification produces a significantly higher pyloric pressure than the combined action of cholecystokinin and secretin, suggesting that reflexes or other hormones are involved in the physiological regulation of pyloric sphincter activity.

GASTRIC EMPTYING

An increase in the rate of gastric emptying of fluids has been produced by gastric distention only and is mainly caused by reflex mechanisms. Delayed emptying of fluids can be initiated by a number of duodenal mechanisms. The mechanisms inhibiting gastric emptying of fluids are activated by intraduodenal administration of hyperosmolal solutions, acid, and fatty acids, particularly those with a chain of 12–18 carbon atoms. The inhibitory mechanisms may be mediated through both reflex pathways and release of inhibitory hormones and may include both active relaxation and inhibition of gastric motility. The inhibition of gastric emptying elicited from the duodenum has been reduced by vagotomy but has been unchanged by section of the splanchnic nerves in animal experiments, indicating participation of vagal reflex pathways and hormonal mechanisms. Cholecystokinin, secretin, and gastrin inhibit the gastric emptying of fluids in the dog [35]. There is reasonable evidence to suggest that the inhibition of gastric emptying by cholecystokinin might be of physiological importance and that inhibition of gastric emptying by gastrin might be a pharmacological effect. The influence of duodenal mechanisms on gastric emptying of solids has been studied to a minor extent.

In most duodenal ulcer patients the gastric emptying of both fluids and solids is abnormally rapid [191]. The effect of duodenal acidification on gastric emptying of fluids in duodenal ulcer patients is surprisingly variable. Some patients show an almost complete inhibition of gastric emptying by duodenal acidification and probably correspond to the patients with marked gastric retention during an ulcer episode, despite the absence of any marked organic obstruction. In many duodenal ulcer patients duodenal acidification increases the rate of gastric emptying of fluids, which is a reversal of the response in healthy persons [191]. The increased rate of gastric emptying of fluids by duodenal acidification in many duodenal ulcer patients may be caused by the abnormally high partial pressure of carbon dioxide in the duodenum that has been found in these patients. The balance between mechanisms stimulating and inhibiting gastric emptying of fluids seems to be very unstable in duodenal ulcer patients. The accelerated gastric emptying of solids in duodenal ulcer patients results in a more rapid loss of buffer from the stomach after meals than occurs in healthy persons. The combination of acid hypersecretion and rapid buffer emptying after a meal in duodenal ulcer patients [58] leads to an abnormally high acidity in the stomach and duodenal bulb. The mean rate of gastric emptying of fluids in gastric ulcer patients is slower than in healthy persons and in duodenal ulcer patients [60].

In dogs resection of the pylorus and a few centimeters of the distal antrum was found to increase slightly the rate of gastric emptying of fluids and increase markedly the rate of gastric emptying of solids [43]. After Billroth I resection in ulcer patients, the rate is still controlled by duodenal inhibitory mechanisms [14]. Proximal gastric vagotomy and vagotomy plus antrectomy in duodenal ulcer patients have been reported to increase initially the rate of gastric emptying of fluids without changing the late phase of emptying of fluids, while both operations delayed gastric emptying of solids [41].

Trophic Effect of Gastrin

There is an abundance of data from animal experiments supporting the trophic effect of gastrin on the gastric mucosa. In patients, the evidence for a trophic action of gastrin on the parietal cells is more indirect.

An unequivocal hyperplasia of the parietal cells has been found in patients with the hypergastrinemic Zollinger-Ellison syndrome [120]. There is evidence supporting the view that gastrin from the antrum may have an important trophic action on the parietal cells of humans. The reported findings of a subnormal number of parietal cells in the gastric remnant after partial gastrectomy presented a weak argument, however, since the preoperative number of parietal cells, as well as the extent and effect of postoperative reflux gastritis, was unknown. On the other hand, antrectomy in duodenal ulcer patients has resulted in a 45 percent reduction of the maximal acid response to pentagastrin with an unchanged sensitivity to pentagastrin (Fig. 3-2) [10]. The effect of antrectomy was equivalent to a noncompetitive inhibition. The effect has been found to be irreversible [27] and can more likely be explained by a diminished functional parietal cell mass. Continuous intravenous infusion of pentagastrin during the first postoperative week has partly and significantly prevented the reduction of the maximal acid response to pentagastrin by antrectomy [13].

Mechanisms Regulating Gastric Acid Secretion

The mechanisms regulating acid secretion at the parietal cell level have been explored using isolated gastric glands or parietal cells or both and indirect determination of acid secretion by the aminopyrine accumulation technique [17]. Human isolated gastric glands were stimulated to about the same degree by db-cAMP and histamine [69]. Carbachol induced a significant

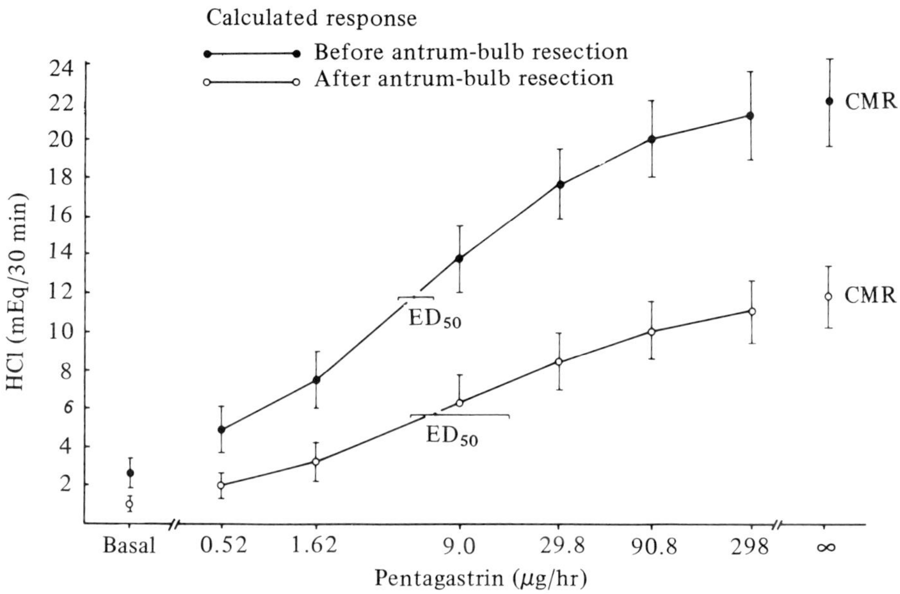

Fig. 3-2. Mean calculated dose-response relation for pentagastrin-stimulated acid secretion in 14 peptic ulcer patients before and after resection of the antrum and duodenal bulb. The calculated data for each patient were obtained by computerized direct least squares fit to the nonlinear form of the Michaelis-Menten equation from the observed data. (CMR = mean calculated maximal response ± SEM; ED_{50} = median dose for half maximal acid response ± one quartile.) (From Bergegårdh et al. [10].)

stimulation but much less pronounced than that induced by histamine, while gastrin had no significant stimulatory effect [69]. Similar results were previously obtained using rabbit gastric isolated glands [15, 16]. Canine parietal cells, however, are maximally stimulated by carbachol. The response to histamine is impressive but less than that induced by carbachol, while gastrin has a weak but statistically significant effect [160, 162].

These three secretagogues have no significant potentiating effect in human isolated glands [69], while such effects have been demonstrated between histamine and gastrin as well as between histamine and carbachol but not by carbachol and gastrin in isolated canine parietal cells [161]. In rabbit isolated glands a potentiation between histamine and carbachol has been demonstrated [15]. Furthermore, specific histamine H_2-receptor blockade by cimetidine blocked the stimulatory effect of histamine dose-dependently but had no effect on the response to carbachol or gastrin. Atropine, on the other hand, caused a parallel displacement of the dose-response curve to carbachol but failed to inhibit the effect of histamine or gastrin [162]. These data support the existence of at least three pharmacological receptors on the parietal cell, a histamine H_2, a muscarinic, and a gastrin receptor. Hypothetically, it has been suggested that the external influence on the parietal cells is maintained through these three receptors, including a permissive action between the effects of activated receptors [161], probably at an intracellular level. Since the effect of cAMP is not influenced by atropine or cimetidine, the level of the permissive action seems to be external to the cAMP level [162].

Regulation of gastric acid secretion in vivo is still more complex. Established and conceivable mechanisms are presented in Table 3-1. Individual stimulating and inhibiting factors are characterized in the following discussion. An important aspect in the physiological regulation of gastric acid secretion is the inter-

Table 3-1. Mechanisms regulating gastric acid secretion

STIMULATION

- I. Cholinergic reflex activation of parietal cell area (influence on transformation of immature proliferative cells into parietal cells?)
  - A. Vagal activation
    - 1. Physiological
      - a. Cephalic (tonus, sham feeding)
      - b. Vagovagal reflex (distention of stomach)
    - 2. Pharmacological
      - a. Insulin-induced hypoglycemia
      - b. 2-Deoxy-D-glucose
  - B. Intramural reflex (distention of parietal cell area)
- II. Chemical activation of parietal cell area by digested protein
- III. Gastrin (trophic effect on parietal cell mucosa)
  - A. Antral gastrin release
    - 1. Vagal activation (cephalic or reflex)
    - 2. Distention (vagovagal and intramural reflexes)
    - 3. Chemical activation from antral lumen (ethanol, amino acids, digested protein)
    - 4. Humoral agents (epinephrine, bombesin)
  - B. Intestinal gastrin release
- IV. Nongastrin intestinal factors
  - A. Cholecystokinin (?)
  - B. Unidentified hormone from jejunum (entero-oxyntin)
- V. Gastric histamine

INHIBITION

- I. Blocked release of antral gastrin into blood
  - A. Acidification of antrum
  - B. Interaction by other hormones (secretin, glucagon, calcitonin)
- II. Acidification of the duodenum
  - A. Hormonal
    - 1. Bulbogastrone
    - 2. Secretin (?)
  - B. Blocked release of duodenal gastrin (?)
  - C. Reflex inhibition
- III. Fatty acids in duodenum release
  - A. Gastric inhibitory polypeptide (GIP)
  - B. Cholecystokinin (?)
  - C. Neurotensin
  - D. Other enterogastrones (?)
- IV. Vagal release of inhibitory hormone (vagogastrone)

action between individual stimulating and inhibiting factors. A noteworthy illustration of the augmentative effect of the combined action of two stimulants is the synergism between the nervous and humoral activation of the parietal cell area. This concept was introduced in 1942 by Uvnäs, who postulated a neurohumoral mechanism for the vagal activation of gastric acid secretion by a synergism between direct vagal action on the acid-secreting glands and the action of vagally released gastrin. Most of the immense amount of data concerning acid secretory mechanisms is derived from animal experiments, those with the dog predominating. Differences between humans and experimental animals will be emphasized throughout the discussion, although the focus is on data obtained in humans.

The parietal cell is assumed to have three main stimulatory receptors: receptors for gastrin, acetylcholine, and histamine. The mutual relations among these receptors are obscure. At least two hormones, secretin and bulbogastrone, seem to block specifically gastrin action on the parietal cell and do not inhibit acid secretion stimulated by histamine or pure cholinergic activation [66, 187]. However, atropine inhibits gastric acid secretion stimulated by both cholinergic activation and gastrin or histamine [102, 110], and the histamine H_2 receptor-blockers inhibit gastric acid secretion stimulated by both histamine and gastrin or cholinergic activation [61, 102, 110, 192].

CHOLINERGIC REFLEX ACTIVATION OF PARIETAL CELL AREA

Vagal Activation

SHAM FEEDING. Physiological vagal activation can be accomplished by sham feeding, i.e., the experimental subject chews and swallows the food in a perfectly normal way, but the food never reaches the stomach. The deviation of food in sham feeding experiments is achieved by an esophagostomy in dogs and can be attained postoperatively in ulcer patients by pushing a wide gastrostomy tube up into the esophagus [96]. A simpler technique of sham feeding, the "chew and spit" technique, can be used in humans [123], but the nasogastric tube will disturb the chewing of food, the food is of course not swallowed in a normal way, and small amounts of food will always reach the stomach. Nevertheless, accurate sham feeding and sham feeding by the chew and spit technique result in a gastric acid response of the same magnitude in humans [96, 114, 168].

In dogs and humans both a direct vagal action on the parietal cell area and gastrin released from the antrum are involved in the gastric acid response to sham feeding.

In humans the release of gastrin by sham feeding is minimal [51, 52, 167, 171]. Direct vagal action on the parietal cell area is undoubtedly of great importance in the gastric acid response to sham feeding. Sham feeding results in no significant acid secretion after proximal gastric vagotomy [52, 97, 130, 171]. The acid response to sham feeding may be used as a test for completeness of vagotomy [106] and is safer and more reliable than the insulin test [172]. After resection of the antrum and duodenal bulb in duodenal ulcer patients, sham feeding still produced a marked acid response [99]. Obviously in humans physiological vagal activation can induce gastric acid secretion without the contribution of vagally released gastrin from the antrum-bulb region, but it is still uncertain whether physiological direct vagal action on the parietal cell area can produce an acid response in the absence of gastrin.

It has often been assumed that vagal excitation of the parietal cells is exerted by a cholinergic transmission, in accordance with the fact that a large dose of atropine completely abolishes the acid response to sham feeding in dogs [121]. A large dose of atropine, however, allows the drug to enter the central nervous system, where it may interrupt a cholinergic transmission in a reflex and consequently eliminate the reflex response totally independently of the peripheral mechanism of transmission. In fact, low increasing doses of an anticholinergic drug that does not penetrate into the brain inhibited the acid response to sham feeding in humans by about 65 percent but did not abolish the acid response [167, 171]. The result suggests that the vagal neurotransmission at the acid-secreting glands is only partially cholinergic and leads to the speculation that some gastrointestinal peptide may act as a peripheral cotransmitter in the vagal nerve.

BASAL VAGAL ACTIVITY. There is strong evidence for a basal vagal activity continuously playing on the parietal cell area. There is, however, no evidence to suggest that vagal hyperactivity is a common characteristic of duodenal ulcer patients [155], although some ulcer patients may have an increased vagal tone [51].

Dragstedt [44], who introduced vagotomy as a routine surgical treatment of duodenal ulcer and contributed extensively to the development of experimental surgery in the study of gastric physiology, considered the main effects of vagotomy to be elimination of the interdigestive cephalic phase of gastric acid secretion and reduced sensitivity of the parietal cells to humoral stimuli. The basal gastric acid secretion is higher in duodenal ulcer patients than in healthy persons and is highest between 5 P.M. and 2 A.M. [119]. The basal gastric acid secretion in duodenal ulcer patients is markedly reduced by all types of vagotomy, including proximal gastric vagotomy, suggesting that direct vagal activation of the parietal cell area contributes considerably to the stimulation of spontaneous acid secretion. Truncal vagotomy in dogs shifts the dose-response curve for gastrin or histamine to the right but does not reduce the maximal acid response to these agents; thus higher doses of gastrin or histamine are needed after vagotomy to obtain the maximal acid responses [47]. Complete truncal vagotomy in humans also shifts the dose-response curve for gastrin to the right [45].

In the duodenal ulcer patient, however, a complete vagotomy, irrespective of type, causes a reduction of about 60 percent of the maximal acid response to histamine or gastrin, and the reduction remains for at least three years. The postvagotomy reduction of the maximal acid response to histamine in ulcer patients is unaffected by increasing the dose of histamine. In the immediately postvagotomy period, however, the maximal acid response to histamine can be completely restored to the prevagotomy level in patients who have undergone antrectomy by subthreshold doses of a cholinergic agent [25]. This finding supports the view that the postvagotomy reduction is caused by elimination of the basal vagal activation of the parietal cell area, which sensitizes the parietal cells to the action of histamine. It is true that six months after proximal gastric vagotomy, the additional injection of a cholinergic drug cannot restore the maximal acid response to pentagastrin to the prevagotomy level [144]. The reason for this discrepancy is unknown.

The effect of antrectomy, which possibly represents withdrawal of the trophic effect of antral gastrin (see the section in this chapter, Trophic Effect of Gastrin), and of subsequent vagotomy on the maximal acid response to histamine in duodenal ulcer patients is shown in Figure 3-3 [26]. The effect of concomitant cholinergic stimulation on the maximal acid response to histamine in the immediate postvagotomy period is shown in Figure 3-4. Subthreshold doses of a cholinergic agent restored the maximal acid response to histamine to the prevagotomy level, but the maximal acid response to histamine could not be increased above postantrectomy level, despite increasing cholinergic stimulation [25].

DISTENTION OF THE STOMACH. Distention of the stomach results in gastric acid secretion through many routes of stimulation: long, probably vagovagal reflex pathways, short intramural reflexes, and gastrin release from the antrum. Distention of the main stomach in antrectomized dogs produced a marked acid response from the main stomach amounting to almost 50 percent of the maximal acid response to histamine, while at the same time producing no acid response from an adjacent vagally denervated gastric pouch [65]. Distention of a totally denervated gastric pouch produced only a very small acid response [64]. These results suggest reflex activation of the parietal cell mucosa by distention through both vagovagal reflex pathways and intramural reflex pathways.

In humans, distention of the corpus-fundus region produces a marked gastric acid response amounting to about 50 percent of the maximal acid response to pentagastrin, and the increase of acid secretion by distention can be abolished by atropinization [67]. Distention of the antrum also elicits a reflex activation of the parietal cell mucosa in ulcer patients [12].

PHARMACOLOGICAL VAGAL ACTIVATION. Pharmacological vagal activation can be elicited by insulin-induced hypoglycemia or by 2-deoxy-D-glucose, which produces intracellular glycopenia. Insulin-induced hypoglycemia has been widely used in experimental studies on vagal activation of gastric acid secretion and is commonly used as a postoperative check on the completeness of vagotomy. It should be emphasized that the gastric acid response to insulin-induced hypoglycemia is dose dependent (the optimal dose in humans is 0.2 IU/kg both in patients not operated on and in patients with incomplete vagotomy [30]) and that insulin-induced hypoglycemia elicits several stimulatory and inhibitory mechanisms involved in the gastric acid response. The stimulatory mechanisms may include direct vagal activation of the parietal cell area, vagal release of antral gastrin, nonvagal release of gastrin, and, possibly, release of other humoral factors. The inhibitory mechanisms may include insulin-potassium-dependent inhibition, acid inhibition of the gastrin mechanism, vagal inhibition of duodenal gastrin release, vagal release of vagogastrone, and, possibly, release of glucagon. Direct vagal activation of the parietal cell area is undoubtedly a dominating mechanism, but the acid response to insulin-induced hypoglycemia is quantitatively dependent on the balance between all stimulatory and inhibitory mechanisms and is therefore somewhat unpredictable and not quite comparable to the acid response elicited by physiological vagal activation.

The outcome of the balance between stimulatory and inhibitory mechanisms is still more unpredictable after vagotomy, when the importance of nonvagal mechanisms is greatly increased against the effect of the remaining vagal fibers. A positive insulin test following vagotomy is not proof of an incomplete vagotomy. As an example, insulin-induced hypoglycemia causes increased blood levels of epinephrine, epinephrine releases gastrin, and, in patients who have undergone vagotomy, in-

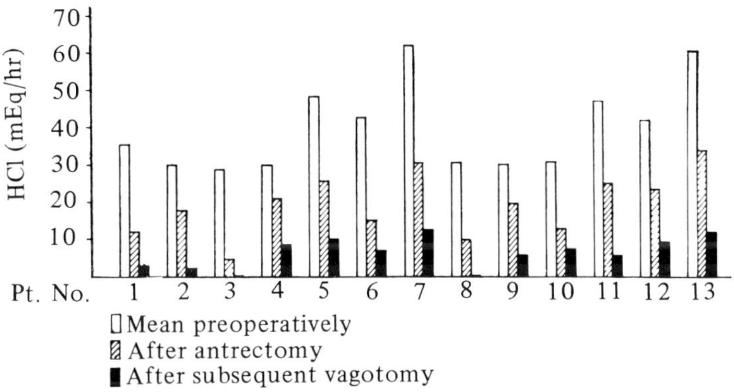

Fig. 3-3. Maximal acid responses to histamine in 13 duodenal ulcer patients preoperatively, after resection of the antrum and duodenal bulb, and after subsequent vagotomy. (From Broomé et al., *Gastroenterology* 52:952. Copyright © 1967, The Williams & Wilkins Co., Baltimore.)

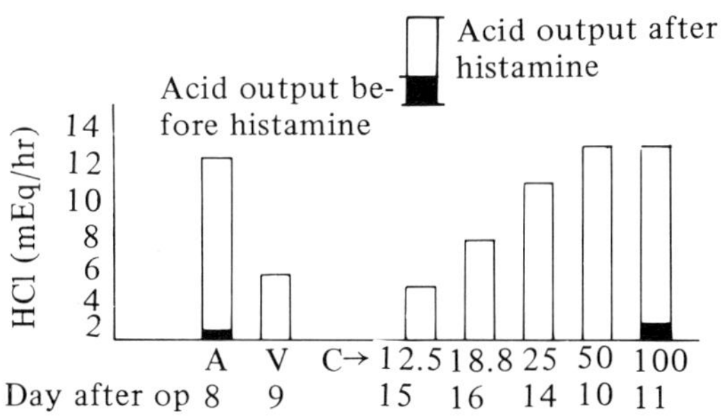

Fig. 3-4. Effects of vagotomy and of carbacholine in the immediate postvagotomy period on the maximal acid response to histamine in a duodenal ulcer patient who had previously undergone antrectomy. (A = after resection of antrum and duodenal bulb; V = after vagotomy; C = dose of carbacholine [μg].)

sulin-induced hypoglycemia always produces serum gastrin increments, irrespective of a gastric acid response to the insulin hypoglycemia. In patients who have undergone vagotomy, a β-adrenergic blockade reduces both the gastrin and the gastric acid responses to insulin-induced hypoglycemia and can in fact convert Hollander tests from positive to negative [107]. In duodenal ulcer patients with vagotomy, insulin-induced hypoglycemia produces an increased gastric acid secretion in from 3 to 30 percent in the immediate postvagotomy period, independently of the type of vagotomy performed [87].

A number of criteria have been proposed to define an unequivocal acid response to insulin-induced hypoglycemia following vagotomy. All proposed criteria have the weak background that the spontaneous variations of basal acid secretion over several hours in patients with vagotomy are unknown. It is probably preferable to give the absolute figures for both basal acid secretion over a prolonged period of time and acid secretion following insulin injection. A positive insulin test following vagotomy has often been interpreted to suggest remaining vagal innervation of the parietal cell mucosa. This interpretation is probably valid for a large and early acid response but is more open to question for a borderline or late gastric acid response. The frequency of positive insulin tests increases with time after vagotomy, reaching to 60 to 90 percent after two to four years [87]. Although an acid response to insulin-induced hypoglycemia is a common finding two to four years after vagotomy, it amounts to only about 10 percent of the preoperative acid response.

Conversion of negative insulin tests into positive insulin tests occurs most often during the first six months after vagotomy [159]. Also, there are significant and successive increases of basal acid secretion and of the maximal acid response to pentagastrin during the first year after vagotomy [87]. Whether the increase of gastric secretion with time after vagotomy is caused by recovery from vagal neurapraxia, partial reinnervation of the parietal cell mucosa, or increased gastrin action on the parietal cells is open to question. If the nerve-sprouting phenomenon occurs in the human stomach after vagotomy, the conditions for vagal reinnervation of the parietal cell mucosa are exceptionally favorable after proximal gastric vagotomy, since part of the stomach, the antrum, is intentionally left vagally innervated.

Intramural Reflex Activation

Grossman has reemphasized the existence and importance of reflex stimulation of gastric acid secretion by gastric distention [64, 65]. A neurophysiological basis for the reflex has been established [34]. In duodenal ulcer patients, graded distention of the corpus-fundus region results in a successively increasing acid response, amounting to 50 percent of the maximal acid response to pentagastrin at a distention volume of 600 ml. The increase of acid secretion in response to distention is completely abolished by atropine. After proximal gastric vagotomy resulting in negative insulin tests, distention of the corpus-fundus region still produces an acid response [67]. The results indicate that distention of the corpus-fundus region in humans produces a cholinergic activation of the parietal cell mucosa through both vagovagal and local intramural reflexes. The interpretation implies that a mechanism for nervous activation of the parietal cell mucosa still remains after vagotomy and can be activated during a meal.

CHEMICAL ACTIVATION OF PARIETAL CELL AREA

It is well known that intragastric instillation of amino acids or peptides stimulates gastric acid secretion by release of gastrin from the antrum. Furthermore, it has been found that these chemical agents also have a direct action on the acid-secreting glands [36]. Liver extract, a peptide solution, glycine, or a control buffer were instilled into denervated fundic pouches of dogs. The fluid later removed from the pouch was titrated back to the initial pH of the stimulating solution. The acid secretion produced by glycine, the peptide solution, and particularly the liver extract significantly exceeded the acid response to the control buffer without evoking any acid secretion from a gastric fistula or any increase in serum gastrin level. With large volumes of liver extract concomitantly distending the denervated fundic pouch, the acid response amounted to 80 percent of the maximal acid response to histamine. The stimulating mechanism was sensitive to pH and resulted in marked gastric acid secretion above a pH of 4.5.

Gastrin

The antrum is the richest source of gastrin. Gastrin has been localized to the G cells by an immunohistochemical technique [115]. In humans the duodenal gastrin concentration is relatively high, almost in the vicinity of the antral gastrin content [122]. The intestinal gastrin concentration was found to be highest in the proximal duodenum of all species studied and diminished rapidly in the distal direction. Small amounts of gastrin can be extracted from the corpus-fundus region of the stomach and from the pancreas. There is evidence for release of gastrin from the human small intestine in response to a meal, since a meal has produced a serum gastrin increment following partial gastrectomy [103, 173]. The serum gastrin increment was more pronounced in patients with additional truncal vagotomy [103] and in patients with a gastroduodenostomy [173], indicating that release of intestinal gastrin is most prominent from the duodenum and is facilitated by vagal denervation of the small intestine.

The predominant gastrin in antral mucosa is G_{17}, which constitutes 80 to 90 percent of the gastrin, while G_{34} is the predominant gastrin in serum [19]. Both the total gastrin concentration and the relative amounts of G_{17} are considerably less in the duodenum than they are in the antrum, with the ratio of G_{17}/G_{34} gradually decreasing toward the distal part of the small intestine [19]. The number of G cells in the antrum of duodenal ulcer patients is usually normal, but the antral gastrin content is significantly higher than it is in healthy persons [5]. The gastrin content in the duodenum and the percentage of G_{34} in the antrum (5 percent) and duodenum (30–40 percent) were similar in duodenal ulcer patients and healthy individuals. In some duodenal ulcer patients with fasting hypergastrinemia, however, a marked G-cell hyperplasia in the antrum has been found, in contrast to the normal number of antral G cells found in gastrinoma patients [137].

It has been suggested that the Zollinger-Ellison syndrome (hypergastrinemia with acid hypersecretion) may occur in two separate entities: gastrinoma and antral G-cell hyperplasia. The antral G-cell hyperplasia patients may be characterized by moderate fasting hypergastrinemia, excessive serum gastrin response to a meal, and no serum gastrin increment in response to secretin or calcium [174]; these patients may represent only a small proportion of the duodenal ulcer population [70]. Apart from an unknown incidence of antral G-cell hyperplasia in duodenal ulcer patients, antral G-cell hyperplasia is also found among hypochlorhydric, hypergastrinemic [104] patients with atrophic gastritis. The hyperplasia is possibly an effect secondary to chronic hypochlorhydria [135]. Somewhat surprisingly, the fasting serum gastrin concentration in duodenal ulcer patients who underwent partial gastrectomy without vagotomy was found to be only slightly lower than in duodenal ulcer patients who did not undergo an operation [99, 163], which indicates that a substantial part of the gastrin in fasting serum originates from the small intestine. In this context it should be observed that the abundance of gastrins of large molecular size in fasting human serum is a controversial subject [141, 194].

RELEASE MECHANISMS

Physiological and Pharmacological Vagal Activation

Physiological vagal activation by sham feeding or pharmacological vagal activation by insulin-induced hypoglycemia results in release of gastrin in both dogs and humans. In the dogs the gastrin release seems to be a mechanism of vagal release from the antrum, since denervation of the antrum has abolished the gastrin response to both stimuli [176]. The effect of vagally released gastrin acting as a single stimulus for acid secretion has been found to be nil, somewhat surprisingly, since sham feeding in dogs with a Heidenhain pouch and with an isolated innervated antral pouch produced a marked rise in serum gastrin level but no acid response from the Heidenhain pouch [176].

The absent acid response to vagally released gastrin may be explained partly by a reduced sensitivity to gastrin of the vagally denervated parietal cell area [47] and partly by concomitant vagal release of an inhibitory humoral agent capable of blocking the action of gastrin. The nature and origin of this agent are uncertain and it has tentatively been named *vagogastrone* [66]. If this inhibitory mechanism were operative in humans, it would contribute to the absent gastric acid response to sham feeding [97, 171] and insulin-induced hypoglycemia that occurs after complete proximal gastric vagotomy.

Studies on vagal release of gastrin in humans have resulted in a more complex picture than the scheme obtained from dog data. Sham feeding in humans results in both a gastric acid response and an increase in serum gastrin level. In earlier studies the gastrin response to sham feeding in duodenal ulcer patients was substantial [99, 114], while in recent studies the gastrin response seemed to be minimal. Sham feeding seems to evoke an increase in serum gastrin concentration of 5–15 pg/ml in both healthy persons and duodenal ulcer patients [51, 52]. This minimal gastrin response to sham feeding has not been detectable in most studies [101, 118, 171]. The gastrin response is almost abolished after resection of the antrum and duodenal bulb [99]. It has not been proved that the gastrin release from the antrum induced by sham feeding in duodenal ulcer patients is vagal, although the gastrin released by sham feeding in the dog certainly is vagally released [176].

A vagal release of gastrin in humans is ad-

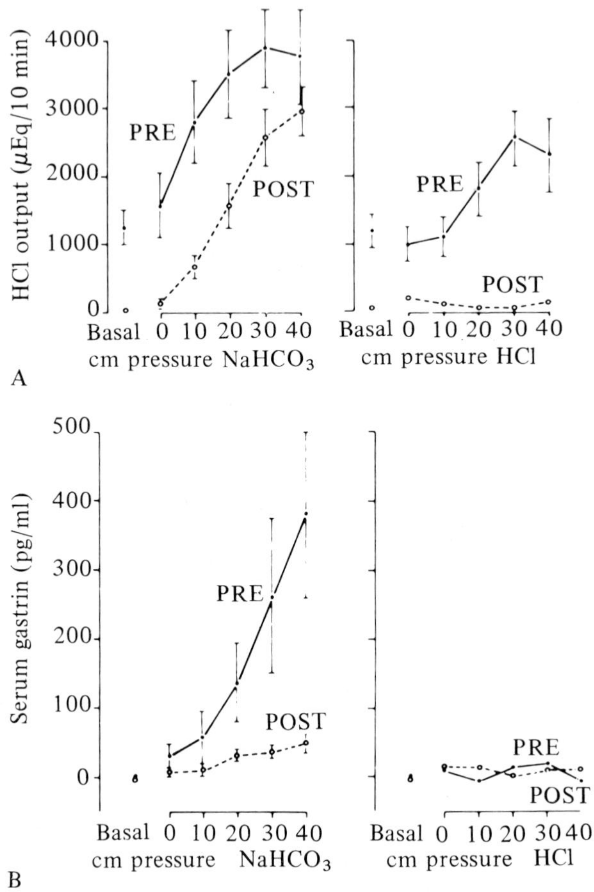

Fig. 3-5. (A) Gastric fistula acid output and (B) serum gastrin increment in response to antral distention with 0.1 mmol $NaHCO_3$ *(left)* and 0.1 mmol HCl *(right)* before and after vagal denervation of the antral pouch in 3 dogs. (From Debas et al., *Gastroenterology* 66: 526. Copyright © 1974, The Williams & Wilkins Co., Baltimore.)

ditionally supported by the finding that sham feeding evoked a substantial gastrin response after pretreatment with anticholinergics [52, 171]. This result suggests a noncholinergic vagal release of gastrin that is normally suppressed by a cholinergic mechanism. A cholinergic inhibition of gastrin release induced by bombesin has in fact been demonstrated [175]. It has been proposed that the noncholinergic vagal transmitter for release of gastrin may be bombesin [154], but it is uncertain how the cholinergic inhibitory mechanism operates.

The peak acid response to sham feeding in duodenal ulcer patients amounts to only 55 percent of the maximal acid response to exogenous gastrin, even under optimal conditions for vagal release of antral gastrin with neutral gastric contents [95]; on the other hand, the peak acid response to sham feeding in dogs is equivalent to the maximal acid response to exogenous gastrin [138]. The minimal gastrin response to sham feeding and the relatively low peak acid response to sham feeding in humans may reflect a vagal inhibitory mechanism that is more efficient in humans than in dogs.

The gastrin release stimulated by insulin-induced hypoglycemia in duodenal ulcer patients is abolished by partial gastrectomy [163]

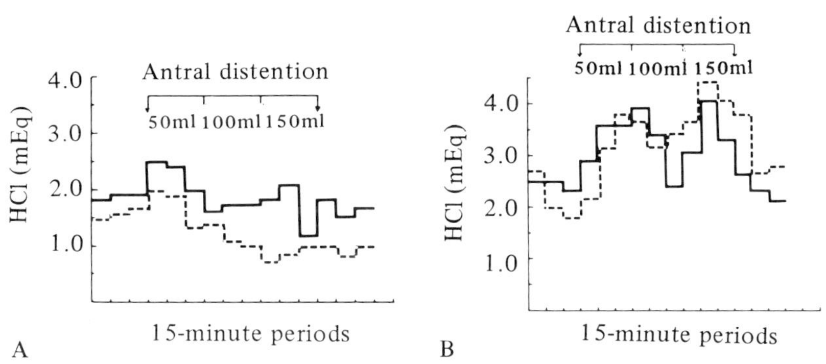

Fig. 3-6. Gastric acid response to graded antral distention with (———) and without (---------) alkaline buffer perfusion of the stomach in (A) 6 healthy persons and (B) 11 patients with active duodenal ulcer. (From Bergegårdh et al. [11].)

and consequently originates from the antrum. However, the gastrin response to insulin-induced hypoglycemia in humans is at least partly nonvagal and noncholinergic. A significant serum gastrin increment in response to insulin hypoglycemia remains after any type of vagotomy, including selective and truncal vagotomy [165] and is probably mediated by epinephrine [107]. Atropinization significantly reduced the gastric acid response to insulin-induced hypoglycemia in humans determined by continuous intragastric titration to pH 5.5 and significantly increased the gastrin response [49]. The remaining serum gastrin increase after atropinization suggests a noncholinergic release of gastrin, and the actual enhancement of gastrin release by atropinization indicates a cholinergic and possibly vagal inhibitory mechanism operative in humans on gastric release.

Gastric and Antral Distention

Graded balloon distention of the antrum in humans under optimal conditions for gastrin release by continuous neutralization of the gastric contents produces no gastric acid response in healthy persons and a slight-to-moderate acid response in ulcer patients [11]. The ulcer patients responding to antral distention with gastric acid secretion showed no concomitant rise in serum gastrin concentration [12] in accord with the observation that gastric distention in healthy persons did not change the serum gastrin levels [153]. The present data suggest that moderate antral distention produces a reflex release of gastrin in dogs, but not in humans, and activates gastric acid secretion through reflex pathways from the antrum to the parietal cell area in dogs and in ulcer patients, but not in healthy persons (Figs. 3-5, 3-6).

Antral Chemical Stimulation

In humans intragastric instillation of chemical stimuli results in release of gastrin and activation of gastric acid secretion. Intragastric instillation of acetylcholine, ethanol, or a meat extract stimulates acid secretion in humans [188], but ethanol seems to be a poor gastrin releaser [9]. Oral administration of calcium carbonate stimulates both gastrin release and gastric acid secretion in humans, while equivalent amounts of sodium bicarbonate have no effect [6]. A protein meal is a more potent stimulus for gastrin release than a carbohydrate or fat meal [59]. The serum gastrin response to a protein meal has usually been found to be greater in duodenal ulcer patients than in healthy persons [141, 178], although wide variations have been observed [58]. The gastric acid response to instillation of a meat extract into the stomach is higher in duodenal ulcer patients than in healthy persons, and the response is significantly correlated to the maximal acid response to histamine [62].

By intragastric titration of the gastric contents to pH 5.5, it has been possible to determine the gastric acid response to a meal in humans [58]. The gastric acid response to a meal in duodenal ulcer patients is larger than the response in healthy persons (Fig. 3-7). A significant difference between the gastric acid responses to a meal in duodenal ulcer patients and those in healthy persons remained after relating the peak acid response to a meal to the maximal acid response to histamine; the relation was 115 percent in duodenal ulcer patients and 85 percent in healthy persons. Only a weak correlation was found between the acid secretory rate and the serum gastrin increase after a meal. The results suggest that the marked gastric acid response to a meal in duodenal ulcer patients is caused partly by a large parietal cell mass and partly by an increased parietal cell responsiveness to a meal. In fact, an increased sensitivity to pentagastrin [74] and endogenous gastrin [108] has been found in duodenal ulcer patients. Duodenal ulcer patients secrete more acid in response to pentagastrin than do healthy persons. If the acid responses to increasing doses of pentagastrin are normalized as a percentage of highest observed response to pentagastrin, there is still a significantly greater response to pentagastrin in duodenal ulcer patients than in healthy persons (Fig. 3-8), which is also reflected in a significantly lower median effective dose of pentagastrin for duodenal ulcer patients [74].

The serum gastrin increase in response to ingestion of meat extract in duodenal ulcer patients is markedly enhanced to a similar degree by proximal gastric vagotomy and by selective gastric vagotomy [79]. The postvagotomy enhancement was found to be less marked in patients who had an additional pyloroplasty. In agreement with the gastrin data is the observation that a gastric acid response to intragastric administration of meat extract in duodenal ulcer patients remained after vagotomy and was found to be as high after proximal gastric vagotomy as after selective gastric vagotomy [73]. The results suggest that the chemically induced gastrin release from the human antrum is independent of the vagal innervation of the antrum.

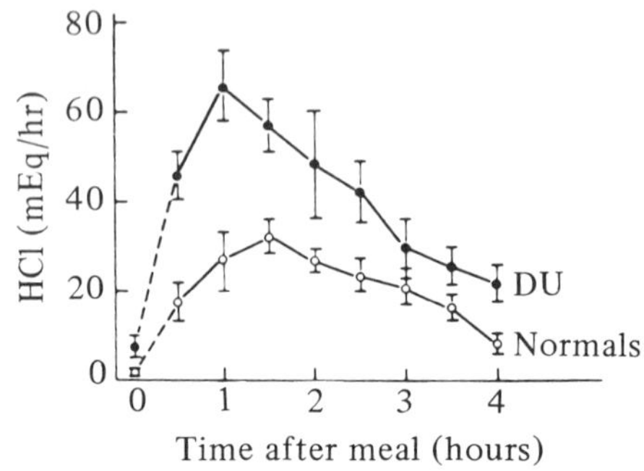

Fig. 3-7. Mean gastric acid responses to a meal in 6 healthy individuals and 7 duodenal ulcer (DU) patients. (From Fordtran and Walsh [58]. Reproduced from *J. Clin. Invest.* 52:645, 1973 by copyright permission of The American Society for Clinical Investigation.)

Release from the Upper Small Intestine

There is substantial evidence that gastrin is released from the upper small intestine, at least in humans. A serum gastrin response to an ordinary meal remains after partial gastrectomy [103], which suggests extragastric gastrin release. The serum gastrin increases in response to a meal were more marked after total gastrectomy and partial gastrectomy with truncal vagotomy than after partial gastrectomy alone [103], which indicates that the vagus nerve exerts an inhibitory influence on the release of gastrin from the small intestine. Such a vagal inhibition of gastrin release is detectable in the small intestine, because vagal release of intestinal gastrin is very small or nonexistent in both dogs and humans [99, 176]. The serum gastrin response to a meal in humans is more marked after partial gastrectomy with gastroduodenostomy plus truncal vagotomy than it is after partial gastrectomy with gastrojejunostomy plus truncal vagotomy [173], which indicates that meal-induced intestinal gastrin release is most prominent from the duodenum.

Two observations have opened the question of still another mechanism for gastrin release in the intestinal phase of gastric acid secretion. In both dogs and humans atropinization enhances the serum gastrin response to a meal [121, 185]. In dogs, atropinization completely eliminates vagally, chemically, and

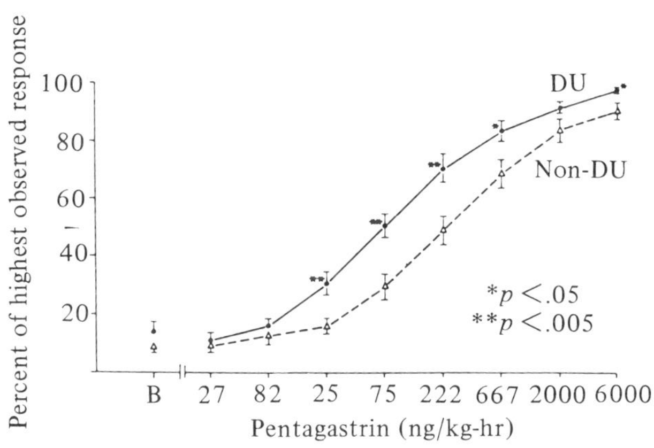

Fig. 3-8. Mean acid output during infusion of graded doses of pentagastrin in 20 healthy persons and 20 duodenal ulcer (DU) patients. (From Isenberg et al. [74]. Reproduced from *J. Clin. Invest.* 55:330, 1975 by copyright permission of The American Society for Clinical Investigation.)

mechanically induced gastrin release from the antrum, and antrectomy completely abolishes the serum gastrin response to a meal [39]. Since the serum gastrin response to a meal remained and was even enhanced in intact dogs after atropinization, either the intestinal gastrin release was markedly facilitated by the atropinization or a substance was liberated from the small intestine by food that in turn released gastrin from the antrum by an atropine-resistant mechanism.

The last hypothesis may explain the surprising observation that local application of acetylcholine in the distal canine duodenum did not change serum gastrin levels, while acetylcholine in the jejunum markedly increased serum gastrin levels [8]. Since the gastrin content of the intestinal mucosa in dogs is very low, with the exception of the proximal duodenum, and, furthermore, since it successively decreases in the distal direction, the observations may indicate liberation of a substance from the jejunum that releases gastrin from the antrum. A new peptide with the property of releasing gastrin from the antrum and stimulating gastric acid secretion has been isolated from the skin of frogs of the *bombina* species. This compound is a tetradecapeptide with no resemblance to gastrin, and it has been named *bombesin*. Injection of bombesin in dogs and humans produced marked serum gastrin increments and gastric acid secretion [21]. In dogs the serum gastrin response to bombesin was inhibited but not abolished by atropinization and was almost abolished by antrectomy.

Epinephrine

Epinephrine has been shown to release gastrin in dogs [72]. Intravenous infusion of epinephrine in low doses (25–75 ng/kg/min) significantly increases serum gastrin levels and gastric acid secretion in humans, and the gastrin and acid responses are completely suppressed by prior administration of a β-adrenergic blocking agent [164]. In a few experiments, larger doses of epinephrine decreased the serum gastrin concentration. The stimulatory doses of epinephrine probably result in the same levels as those obtained after insulin hypoglycemia [164]. The nonvagal release of gastrin from the antrum produced by insulin hypoglycemia and found in patients after vagotomy has therefore been attributed to epinephrine [165].

Inhibition of Gastric Acid Secretion

ANTRAL MECHANISMS

Antral Acidification

The brilliant studies of Dragstedt and his collaborators have unequivocally demonstrated that acidification of the antrum inhibits gastric acid secretion. The only established mechanism by which acidification of the antrum inhibits gastric acid secretion is through blocking release of gastrin into the circulation [109] (Fig. 3-9). The serum gastrin increase following vagal [121], mechanical [37], and chemical [39] stimulation of the antrum is completely abolished by antral acidification. The gastrin release induced by bombesin [21] and epinephrine is possibly more resistant to acidification of the antrum. Gastric acid secretion stimulated by antral gastrin release is maximally inhibited at an antral pH of 1.0–1.5, and the inhibition usually vanishes at an antral pH of about 3.

It has been suggested that the pH in the antrum regulates acid secretion through the interplay between gastrin and somatostatin. At vagal stimulation and low antral pH, the D cells secrete somatostatin, which as a paracrine effect inhibits the G cells from secreting gastrin. At higher pH the somatostatin secretion is blocked and the G cells are free to secrete gastrin [131, 179].

Hormones

Several hormones with the established property of inhibiting gastric acid secretion are also capable of inhibiting gastrin release and have been shown to decrease fasting serum gastrin levels and to reduce the rise in serum gastrin level after a meal. This dual inhibitory effect has been produced by secretin [177], glucagon [71], GIP, and VIP [140], while the effect of calcitonin is controversial [7, 22]. Whether this hormonal inhibition of gastrin release is a purely pharmacological effect or has any physiological importance is unknown.

Reflex Inhibition

Reflex inhibition of gastric acid secretion from the upper gastrointestinal tract is another conceivable inhibitory mechanism. The prerequisites for such a mechanism exist, since afferent vagal discharge has been observed from receptors in the gastric and duodenal mucosa that respond to mechanical stimulation, acidification, or alkalinization [34]. There is evidence for reflex inhibition by duodenal acidification in both dogs and humans, but reflex inhibition by antral acidification has not been demonstrated.

Antral Acidification in Duodenal Ulcer Patients

Acidification of the antrum in duodenal ulcer patients has been shown to reduce basal acid secretion [105] and the gastric acid response to sham feeding [95]. Acidification of the gastric contents, allowing them to pass into the duodenum, evokes both antral and duodenal inhibitory mechanisms. Instillation of acid into the stomach has markedly reduced the high fasting serum gastrin levels in persons with pernicious anemia [193]. Intragastric titration with a stepwise decreasing pH from 5.5 to 1.0 successively inhibited the serum gastrin response and the gastric acid response to a protein hydrolysate meal in duodenal ulcer patients [100]. At an intragastric pH of 1.0, both the serum gastrin response and the gastric acid response to the protein hydrolysate meal were completely abolished. By use of a similar technique, it has been found that the inhibition of the gastric acid response to a protein hydrolysate meal at an intragastric pH of 2.5 was significantly less in duodenal ulcer patients than in healthy persons, indicating a defective acid inhibitory mechanism in duodenal ulcer patients [183, 184].

ANTRAL DISTENTION

Balloon distention of the antrum stimulates acid secretion slightly in duodenal ulcer patients but inhibits basal secretion in healthy persons [11]. Furthermore, in healthy persons antral distention consistently induced an approximately 20 percent reduction of submaximal pentagastrin-stimulated acid secretion [151, 152]. No such inhibition was found in duodenal ulcer patients [151]. The mechanism by which antral distention inhibits pentagastrin-stimulated gastric secretion in healthy persons is unknown.

MECHANISMS ACTIVATED BY DUODENAL ACIDIFICATION

Acidification of the duodenum inhibits gastric acid secretion in both dogs and humans. In

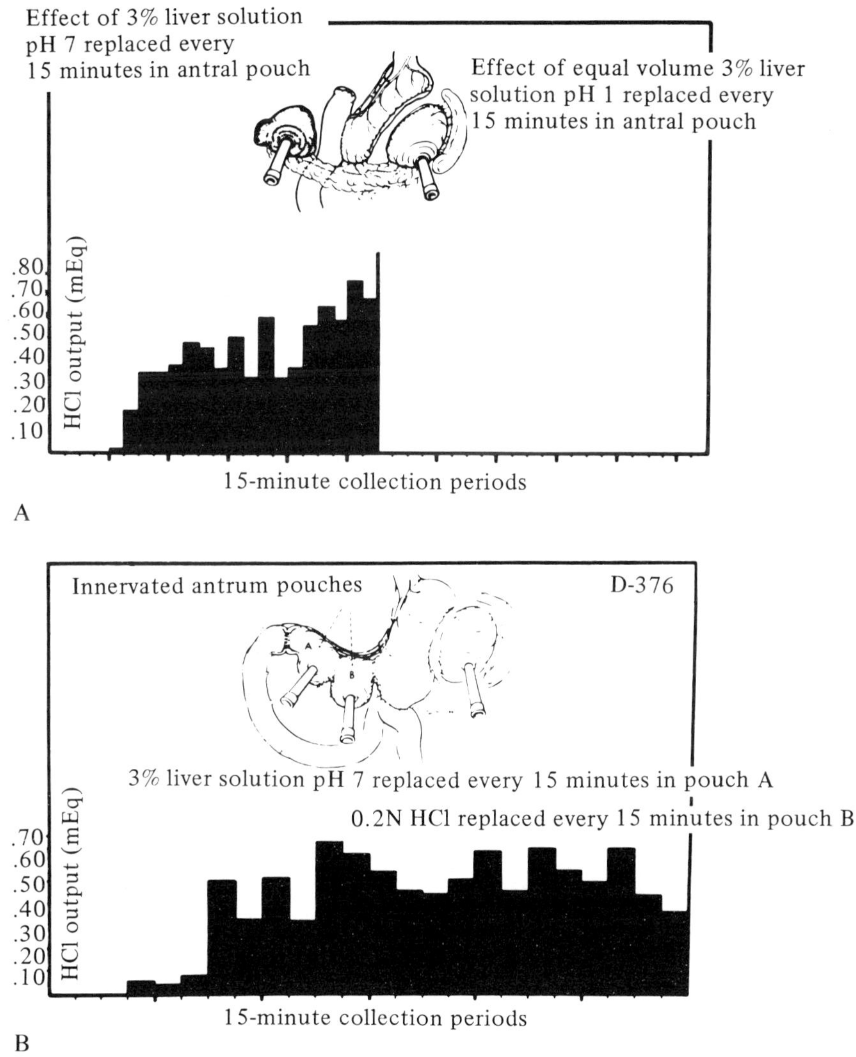

Fig. 3-9. Effect on canine Heidenhain pouch response to mechanical and chemical stimulation of the antrum by acidification of (A) stimulated antral pouch and (B) separate antral pouch. (From Longhi et al. [109]. By permission of the American Physiological Society.)

dogs the major inhibitory mechanism is humoral and is particularly effective against gastrin-stimulated gastric acid secretion [86]. In humans the degree of inhibition produced by duodenal acidification is more variable, and it is controversial whether or not the inhibition is equally pronounced in healthy persons and duodenal ulcer patients [191]. Instillation of large amounts of acid into the human duodenum inhibits both gastrin-stimulated and histamine-stimulated [88] gastric acid secretion.

Acidification of the duodenal bulb in dogs inhibits gastrin-stimulated but not histamine-stimulated acid secretion, even if the duodenal bulb is completely denervated [4, 89]. A successively increasing inhibitory effect has been observed when the pH in the duodenal bulb is decreasing from around 4 to 1. Acidification of an isolated duodenal bulb has markedly reduced pentagastrin-stimulated acid secretion without stimulating pancreatic secretion, while acidification of the duodenum beyond the bulb has produced a brisk pancreatic secretion and concomitantly a very slight inhibition of pentagastrin-stimulated acid secretion [2] (Fig. 3-10), which suggests that the inhibitory humoral agent liberated by acidification of the duodenal bulb is not identical with secretin. The humoral agent has been named *bulbogastrone* [66]. Crude extracts prepared from the mucosa of the duodenal bulb have been shown to inhibit gastric acid secretion [4]. Bulbogastrone seems to block specifically the gastrin action on the parietal cells. Whether bulbogastrone also inhibits gastrin release is unknown.

Acidification of the duodenum releases secretin. There is less plasma secretin increment in response to duodenal acidification in duodenal ulcer patients than in healthy persons [23]. This finding is in accordance with previous observations that duodenal ulcer patients produce a lower pancreatic secretory response to duodenal acidification than do healthy persons [20, 190]. Secretin has the dual pharmacological effect of inhibiting gastric acid secretion and suppressing serum gastrin levels in humans [100]. Since the pH threshold for release of secretin is about 4.5 [86], and since the fasting and postprandial pH in the duodenal bulb is well below this at 2.0–3.5 and the postbulbar pH above 5 [4, 86], it may be questioned whether enough secretin is released by duodenal acidification under physiological conditions to inhibit gastric acid secretion. Small amounts of released secretin may be quite enough for stimulation of pancreatic secretion, because of synergistic cooperation with simultaneously released cholecystokinin, but insufficient to inhibit gastric acid secretion. In fact, exogenous secretin in doses resulting in plasma secretin levels well above those produced by duodenal acidification did not inhibit pentagastrin-stimulated acid secretion in humans [186].

Whether acidification of the duodenum blocks release of duodenal gastrin into the circulation in a manner analogous to the antral inhibitory mechanism is unknown.

Acidification of the distal duodenum inhibits pentagastrin-stimulated acid secretion in healthy persons and duodenal ulcer patients, and this inhibition is not attributed to released secretin, since the resulting plasma secretin levels were shown to be insufficient to inhibit acid secretion [186]. The inhibition was abolished by proximal gastric vagotomy and was therefore presumably caused by an inhibitory vagal reflex. The demonstrated inhibitory reflex mechanism is unlikely to be operating under physiological conditions, but it emphasizes the possible existence of analogous inhibitory reflexes in the antrum and duodenal bulb.

MECHANISMS ACTIVATED BY FAT OR HYPEROSMOLAL SOLUTIONS IN THE SMALL INTESTINE

Fat in an absorbable form or hyperosmolal solutions introduced into the duodenum inhibit gastric acid secretion The inhibition is effective against gastrin-stimulated acid secretion, while the inhibition of histamine-stimulated acid secretion is controversial and may be dependent on the amount of fat or hyperosmolal solutions [86, 92]. The major mechanism is inhibition mediated through one or more humoral agents liberated from the small intestine, traditionally named the enterogastrone effect, although inhibitory reflex mechanisms may contribute.

Neurotensin seems to contribute to the inhibitory effect evoked by fat in the small intestine [91]. The inhibition has been reported to be less pronounced after vagotomy [90, 111], which indicates either partial reflex inhibition or that inhibitory hormonal activity is particularly effective on vagally innervated oxyntic glands.

The gastric inhibitory polypeptide (GIP) is present in the upper small intestine predominantly in the duodenum, with a probable cellular localization to the D_1 cells [134]. Gastric inhibitory polypeptide inhibits gastrin-stimulated and histamine-stimulated gastric acid secretion and suppresses release of gastrin [66, 140]; GIP is released by fat and glucose in the duodenum.

The vasoactive intestinal peptide has been

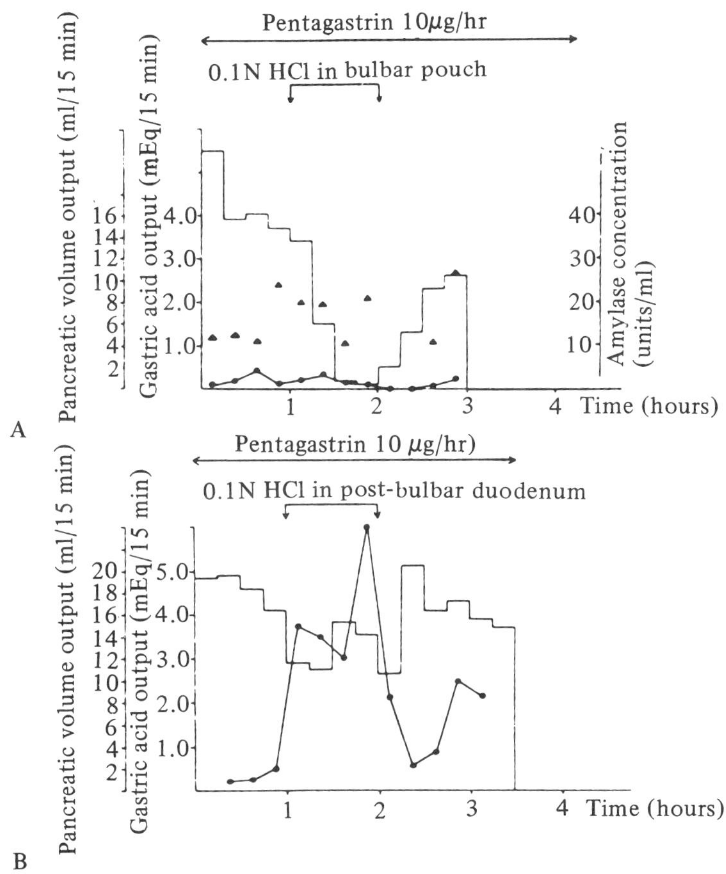

Fig. 3-10. Effect on pentagastrin-stimulated gastric acid secretion and on pancreatic secretion of acidification of (A) isolated duodenal bulb or (B) distal duodenum in a dog with gastric and pancreatic fistulas. (┌┐ = gastric acid output; •—• = pancreatic volume output; ▲ = pancreatic amylase concentration.) (From Andersson [2], *Acta Hepatogastroenterol.* 19:458, 1972.)

found throughout the gastrointestinal tract with a possible cellular localization to the D cells [136]. Vasoactive intestinal peptide inhibits both gastrin-stimulated and histamine-stimulated gastric acid secretion and suppresses release of gastrin [66, 140]. Its physiological importance as an enterogastrone is open to question.

Enteroglucagon has been found in endocrine cells of the mucosa of the small intestine, with the highest quantity in the ileum [23]. Enteroglucagon is released by fat or glucose in the small intestine, and after oral glucose administration it has been found to be particularly high in patients with the dumping syndrome [23]. Enteroglucagon is structurally related to pancreatic glucagon, since enteroglucagon cross-reacts with glucagon antibodies. Glucagon inhibits gastric acid secretion [42] and suppresses the release of gastrin [71]. The role of enteroglucagon as an enterogastrone is unknown.

VAGAL RELEASE OF INHIBITORY HORMONE

It has previously been discussed that vagal activation or vagotomy influences gastric acid secretion and release of gastrin in many ways. In humans any type of vagotomy reduces the maximal acid responses to pentagastrin and histamine to the same extent [87]. As consequences of the decreased acid secretion rate following vagotomy, the acid inhibition of gastrin release is less effective and the serum gastrin response to a meal is hence increased after both proximal gastric vagotomy and other types of vagotomy [79]. Furthermore, the serum gastrin response to a meal has been found to be more pronounced after partial gastrectomy plus truncal vagotomy than after partial gastrectomy alone [103], which indicates that release of intestinal gastrin is under vagal inhibitory control in humans. In addition to the established vagal release of antral gastrin in both dogs and humans [51, 52, 114, 121, 176], there is, at least in dogs, substantial evidence for vagal release of the inhibitory hormone tentatively named *vagogastrone* [66]. Extragastric vagotomy in dogs with a Heidenhain pouch increased the acid response to various doses of pentagastrin but did not change the acid responses to histamine, while extragastric vagotomy had no effect on the acid responses to gastrin and histamine from innervated gastric pouches [166]. Thus the extragastric vagi apparently release an inhibitor that counteracts the action of gastrin at the parietal cell level and is particularly effective in vagally denervated mucosa.

This interpretation is supported by reports that vagal activation by sham feeding inhibits pentagastrin-stimulated acid secretion from Heidenhain pouches and simultaneously augments the pentagastrin-stimulated acid secretion from innervated main stomachs, while Heidenhain pouch responses to histamine are not inhibited [139, 157]. The inhibition remained after extragastric vagotomy [157] and was abolished by truncal vagotomy [139, 157], which indicates that the inhibitor originates from the stomach or possibly the most proximal part of the duodenum.

Vagal release of an inhibitor may explain why sham feeding did not produce any acid response in dogs with a Heidenhain pouch and an isolated antral pouch, despite a marked gastrin increment, while local application of acetylcholine to the antral pouches, resulting in the same serum gastrin increment, did produce acid secretion [176]. This result also indicates that the inhibitor is not released from the antrum by a cholinergic mechanism.

The vagogastrone mechanism exists in humans [169] but is less efficient than in dogs (Fig. 3-11).

PROSTAGLANDINS

Prostaglandins have been isolated from gastrointestinal mucosa and muscle of animals and humans [182]. The physiological importance of prostaglandins in the control of gastrointestinal motility and secretion is unknown; however, the pharmacological effects of certain prostaglandins include changes in gastrointestinal muscle tone and inhibition of gastric acid secretion. Prostaglandins are rapidly metabolized and can be synthesized and degraded in the same tissue. On the hypothetical assumption that prostaglandins participate physiologically in inhibition of gastric acid secretion, it therefore seems reasonable that they may act as local inhibitory regulators rather than as circulating inhibitory hormones. An analogous role is attributed to histamine as a local stimulatory regulator of gastric acid secretion. Vagal electrical stimulation, gastrin, and histamine have been found to increase the release of prostaglandins from intestinal mucosa. By oral administration, synthetic analogues of prostaglandins with a more prolonged degradation have been reported to inhibit markedly gastric acid secretion in humans.

Prostaglandins probably play their major role in gastric pathophysiology not by regulating acid secretion or gastric motor function but by influencing gastric mucosal resistance. Prostaglandins increase gastric bicarbonate secretion. Moreover, the prostaglandins seem to exert a cytoprotective effect [143] and protect the mucosa from damage by absolute alcohol, acid, and boiling water.

Synergism Between Gastric Acid Stimulants

The cephalic phase of gastric acid secretion is produced by the simultaneous and cooperative actions of vagally mediated activation of the parietal cell area and vagally released gas-

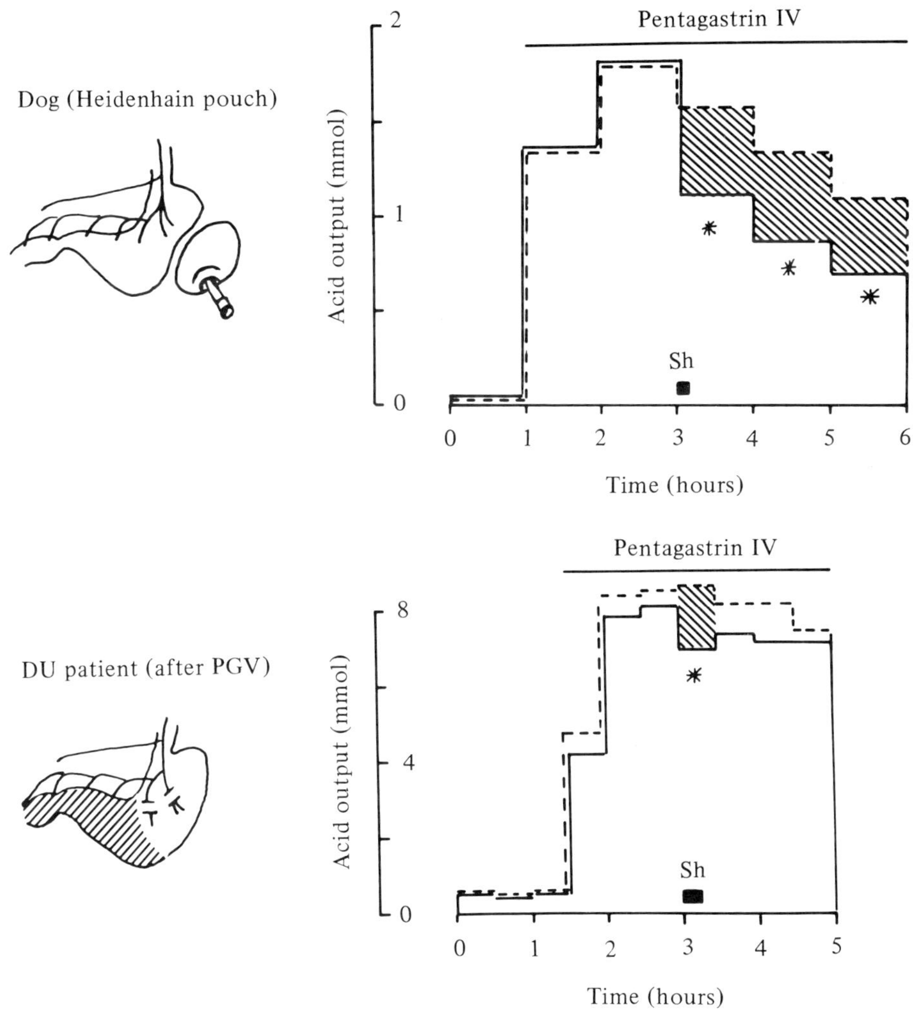

Fig. 3-11. The effect of sham feeding (Sh) on the acid secretion induced by intravenous infusion of a submaximal dose of pentagastrin. *Upper panel:* Mean values (*) from experiments on 4 dogs provided with denervated pouches of the oxyntic gland area (data from Sjödin [157]). *Lower panel:* Mean values (*) from experiments in 7 duodenal ulcer (DU) patients after proximal gastric vagotomy (PGV). (——— = pentagastrin + sham feeding; --------- = pentagastrin (control), *$p < .05$; ▧ = differences in acid output with and without sham feeding.) (From Stenquist [167].)

trin from the antrum. In dogs, vagally released gastrin markedly enhances the action of direct vagal activation of the parietal cell area, an enhancement that can be mimicked by an intravenous infusion of subthreshold doses of exogenous gastrin [124] (Fig. 3-12). The marked augmentative effect of gastrin on direct vagal activation of the oxyntic glands is, however, not a characteristic quality of gastrin but a property shared with other humoral stimuli, e.g., histamine and an unidentified intestinal humoral agent [125] (Fig. 3-13).

In duodenal ulcer patients the vagally released gastrin seems to have only an additive secretory effect on the acid secretion pro-

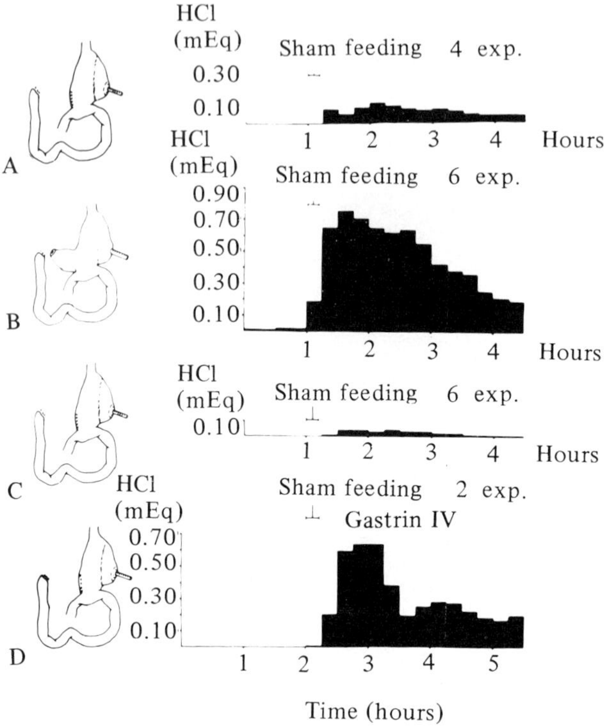

Fig. 3-12. Gastric acid response to sham feeding in a dog with a Pavlov pouch (A), after elimination of acid inhibition from the antrum and duodenum (B), after resection of the antrum and duodenal bulb (C), and after resection of the antrum and duodenal bulb with concomitant intravenous infusion of a subthreshold dose of crude gastrin (D). (From Olbe [124]. Copyright © 1966 by The Regents of California: reprinted by permission of the University of California Press.)

duced by direct vagal activation of the oxyntic glands. After resection of the antrum and duodenal bulb, which eliminates vagally released gastrin in duodenal ulcer patients [99], exogenous gastrin has only an additive secretory effect on the gastric acid response to sham feeding [98] (Fig. 3-14), which suggests that vagally released gastrin is of minor importance in the cephalic phase of acid secretion in duodenal ulcer patients. It is true that antrum and bulb resection markedly reduces the gastric acid response to sham feeding in duodenal ulcer patients, but the main reduction is presumably caused by a functional or morphological decrease in the parietal cell mass, reflected in a corresponding reduction of the maximal acid response to pentagastrin (Fig. 3-14).

In dogs antrectomy either has no effect or enhances the maximal acid response to exogenous gastrin [3]. In humans, or at least in duodenal ulcer patients, the gastrin from the antrum and duodenal bulb seems to have a predominantly trophic effect on the parietal cells, and the vagally released gastrin from the antrum and bulb is of minor importance in the cephalic phase of acid secretion. The converse is true in dogs. The poor acid secretory effect of vagally released gastrin in humans does not by any means exclude a marked synergism between the action of gastrin and the direct vagal activation of the human oxyntic glands, since the fasting serum gastrin concentration in duodenal ulcer patients with partial gastrectomy has been found to be only slightly lower than in duodenal ulcer patients not operated on [99,

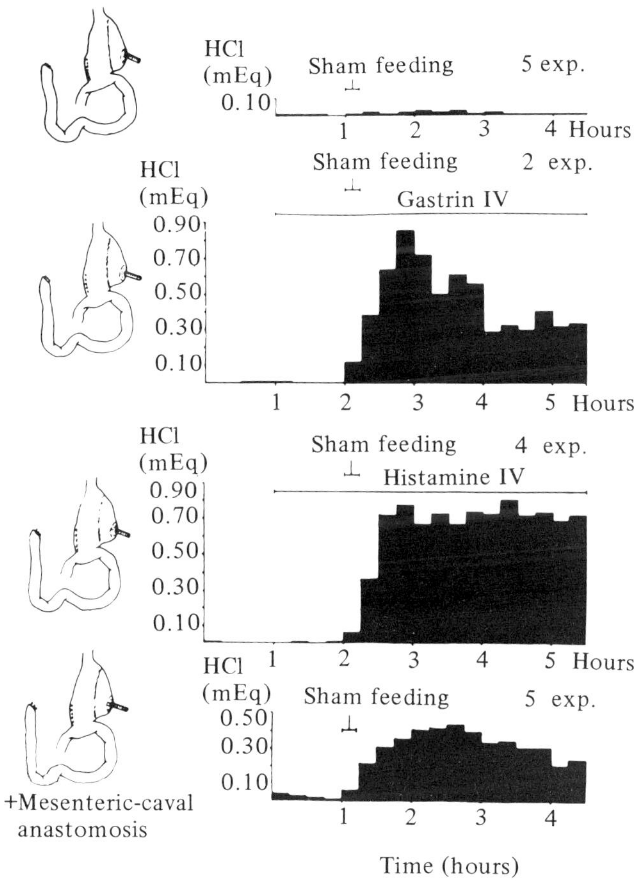

Fig. 3-13. The effect of intravenous infusions of crude gastrin or histamine in subthreshold dosages and of anastomosis of the superior mesenteric vein to the inferior caval vein on the gastric acid response to sham feeding in a dog with resected antrum and duodenal bulb and a Pavlov pouch. (From Olbe [125].)

163]. The possibility of such a synergism is favored by the reports that subthreshold doses of a cholinergic drug potentiate the maximal acid response to histamine in patients who have undergone vagotomy and antrectomy [25] and that subthreshold doses of exogenous gastrin enhance gastric acid responses to insulin-induced hypoglycemia in patients with incomplete vagotomy [46].

In the gastric phase of acid secretion at least three different stimuli activate the secretory process. Digested proteins directly stimulate the oxyntic glands [36]. Reflex activation of the oxyntic glands is produced by gastric distention and is mediated through long reflexes from both the antrum [37] and the corpus-fundus region [65] and through short intramural reflexes in the corpus-fundus region [64]. Gastrin is released by chemical stimulation of distention of the antrum and by an oxyntopyloric distention reflex [38] in dogs, although gastric distention is a poor stimulus for gastrin release in humans [12, 153]. As in the cephalic phase of gastric acid secretion, the distention reflex activation of the oxyntic glands markedly enhances the action of humoral stimuli in dogs [64, 65].

In the intestinal phase of gastric acid secretion, release of intestinal gastrin may contrib-

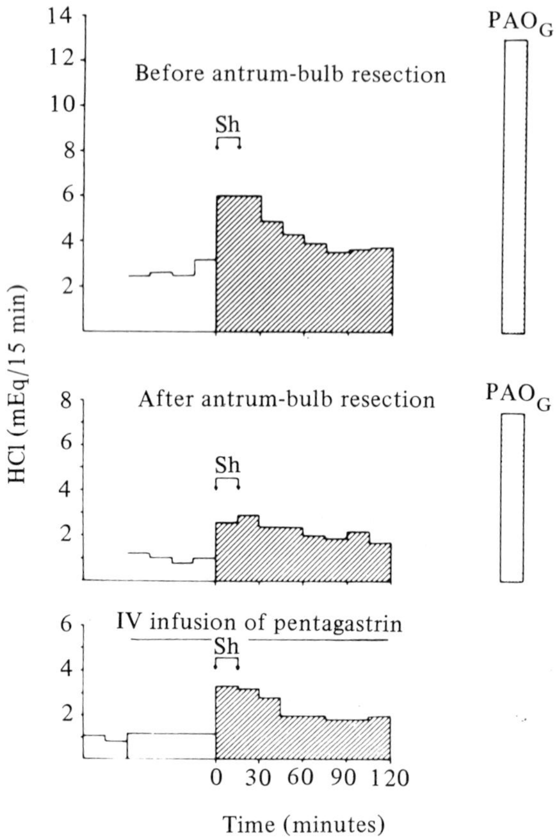

Fig. 3-14. Mean gastric acid responses to sham feeding in 4 duodenal ulcer patients before and after resection of the antrum and duodenal bulb, and after resection with and without concomitant intravenous infusion of pentagastrin in a barely suprathreshold dosage. PAO_G = mean peak acid responses to pentagastrin. (From Knutson and Olbe [98].)

ute in humans [103, 173], but, except for gastrin release from the duodenal bulb, it is probably a minor contributory factor in dogs [39, 158]. At least one nongastrin stimulatory agent is released from the intestine by food [129, 158]. This agent, *entero-oxyntin*, is inactivated to a marked extent by liver passage [129] but has the capacity to augment substantially both the gastrin action on the oxyntic glands [158] and the vagal activation of the oxyntic glands (see Fig. 3-13).

Pathophysiological Characteristics of Ulcer Patients

There are data accumulating supporting the view that peptic ulcer disease is a heterogeneous group of disorders. It is common to summarize the pathophysiology of peptic ulcer disease as an imbalance between aggressive and defensive factors. Gastric ulcer patients often have a normal or subnormal acid secretion, and in these patients a defective mucosal resistance may be most important. Patients with juxtapyloric ulcers are, as a group, hypersecretors of acid. This condition may be caused by an increased parietal cell mass (inherited or caused by excessive trophic effects of gastrin, for example) or by hyperfunctioning cells. Data from isolated gastric glands favor the alternative of an increased number of gastric glands containing a normal number of normally functioning parietal cells per gland [69]. Duodenal ulcer patients are found to have an increased sensitivity to both exogenous [74, 132] and endogenous [108] gastrin. It is therefore not surprising that duodenal ulcer patients have an increased acid response to a meal [58]; hypersecretion in these patients has been attributed to vagal hyperactivity [44]. Using pancreatic polypeptide as an indirect and rough measure of vagal activity, however, no clear differences were found between healthy persons and patients with duodenal ulcer [155].

A defective inhibition of acid secretion is an alternative explanation to hypersecretion. As discussed previously, there is reasonable evidence of a defect in at least three different inhibitory mechanisms in duodenal ulcer patients:

1. Antral distention inhibits gastric secretion in healthy persons but not in duodenal ulcer patients [151, 152].
2. Antral acidification inhibits the acid response to a meal [58, 183, 184] and insulin hypoglycemia [170] less effectively in duodenal ulcer patients.
3. The inhibitory effect of intraduodenal administration of small volumes of fat (20 ml

oleic acid) is significantly weaker in duodenal ulcer patients [90].

References

1. Allen, A., and Snary, D. The structure and function of gastric mucus. *Gut* 13:666, 1972.
2. Andersson, S. Duodenal inhibition of gastric acid secretion. *Acta Hepatogastroenterol.* 19:458, 1972.
3. Andersson, S., and Grossman, M. I. Effect of antrectomy on gastric secretion of acid and pepsin in response to histamine and gastrin in dogs. *Gastroenterology* 49:246, 1965.
4. Andersson, S., Nilsson, G., Sjödin, L., and Uvnäs, B. Mechanism of Duodenal Inhibition of Gastric Acid Secretion. In S. Andersson (Ed.), *Frontiers in Gastrointestinal Hormone Research* (Nobel Symposium 16). Stockholm: Almqvist & Wiksell, 1973. Pp. 223–38.
5. Arnold R., Creutzfeldt, C., Track, N. S., and Creutzfeldt, W. Mucosal gastrin concentration, molecular forms of gastrin, number and ultrastructure of G-cells in patients with duodenal ulcer. *Gut* 17:745, 1976.
6. Barreras, R. F. Calcium and gastric secretion. *Gastroenterology* 64:1168, 1973.
7. Becker, H. D., Reeder, D. D., Scurry, M. T., and Thompson, J. C. Inhibition of gastrin release and gastric secretion by calcitonin in patients with peptic ulcer. *Am. J. Surg.* 127:71, 1974.
8. Becker, H. D., Reeder, D. D., and Thompson, J. C. Direct measurement of gastrin release from duodenum and jejunum in dogs. *Am. J. Physiol.* 227:897, 1974.
9. Becker, H. D., Reeder, D. D., and Thompson, J. C. Gastrin release by ethanol in man and in dogs. *Ann. Surg.* 179:906, 1974.
10. Bergegådh, S., Broman, G., Knutson, U. et al. Gastric acid responses to graded i.v. infusions of pentagastrin and histalog in peptic ulcer patients before and after antrum-bulb resection. *Scand. J. Gastroenterol.* 11:337, 1976.
11. Bergegårdh, S., Knutson, U., and Olbe, L. The effect of intragastric neutralization on the gastric acid response to antral distension in man. *Scand. J. Gastroenterol.* 10:625, 1975.
12. Bergegårdh, S., Nilsson, G., and Olbe, L. The effect of antral distension on acid and plasma gastrin in duodenal ulcer patients. *Scand. J. Gastroenterol.* 11:475, 1976.
13. Bergegårdh, S., and Olbe, L. The effect of long-term postoperative pentagastrin infusion on the maximal acid responses to pentagastrin in patients subjected to antrectomy, *Scand. J. Gastroenterol.* 11:347, 1976.
14. Berger, T. Studies on the gastric emptying mechanism in healthy persons and patients after partial gastrectomy. *Acta Chir. Scand.* 404 (Suppl.), 1969.
15. Berglindh, T. Potentiation by carbachol and aminophylline of histamine and db-cAMP induced parietal cell activity in isolated gastric glands. *Acta Physiol. Scand.* 99:75, 1977.
16. Berglindh, T., Dibona, D. R., Ito, S., and Sachs, G. Probes of parietal cell function. *Am. J. Physiol.* 238:G165, 1980.
17. Berglindh, T., and Öbrink, K.-J. A method for preparing isolated glands from the rabbit gastric mucosa. *Acta Physiol. Scand.* 96:150, 1976.
18. Berkowitz, J. M., and Praissman, M. Use of synthetic membrane models in the study of gastric secretory processes. *Adv. Exp. Med. Biol.* 7:309, 1970.
19. Berson, S. A., and Yalow, R. S. Nature of immunoreactive gastrin extracted from tissues of gastrointestinal tract. *Gastroenterology* 60:215, 1971.
20. Berstad, A., Roland, M., Petersen, H., and Liavåg, I. The pancreatic exocrine secretion in duodenal ulcer patients before and after selective proximal vagotomy of the stomach. *Scand. J. Gastroenterol.* 9:431, 1974.
21. Bertaccini, G., Erspamer, V., Melchiorri, P., and Sopranzi, N. Gastrin release by bombesin in the dog. *Br. J. Pharmacol.* 52:219, 1974.
22. Bieberdorf, F. A., Gray, T. K., Walsh, J. H., and Fordtran, J. S. Effect of calcitonin on meal-stimulated gastric acid secretion and serum gastrin concentration. *Gastroenterology* 66:343, 1974.
23. Bloom, S. R. Radioimmunoassay of intestinal hormones. *Gut* 15:502, 1974.
24. Brooks, A. M., Isenberg, J., and Grossman, M. I. The effect of secretin, glucagon, and duodenal acidification on pepsin secretion in man. *Gastroenterology* 57:159, 1969.
25. Broomé, A. Mechanism of the vagotomy-induced suppression of the maximal acid response to histamine in antrectomized duodenal ulcer patients. *Scand. J. Gastroenterol.* 2:275, 1967.

26. Broomé. A., Bergström. H., and Olbe, L. Maximal acid response to histamine in duodenal ulcer patients subjected to resection of the antrum and duodenal bulb followed by vagotomy. *Gastroenterology* 52:952, 1967.
27. Broomé, A., and Olbe, L. Studies on the mechanism of the antrectomy-induced suppression of the maximal acid response to histamine in duodenal ulcer patients. *Scand. J. Gastroenterol.* 4:281, 1969.
28. Chapman, M. L., Werther, J. L., Rudick, J., and Janowitz, H. D. Pentagastrin infusion–glycine instillation as a measure of acid absorption in the human stomach: Comparison to an instilled acid load. *Gastroenterology* 63:962, 1972.
29. Cohen, S., and Lipshutz, W. Hormonal regulation of human lower esophageal sphincter competence: Interaction of gastrin and secretin. *J. Clin. Invest.* 50:449, 1971.
30. Cowley, D. J., and Baron, J. H. Insulin-stimulated gastric acid secretion after vagotomy in man. *Am. J. Dig. Dis.* 18:544, 1973.
31. Curwain, B. P., and Holten, P. The effects of isoprenaline and noradrenaline on pentagastrin-stimulated gastric acid secretion and mucosal blood flow in the dog. *Br. J. Pharmacol.* 46:225, 1972.
32. Davenport, H. W. Back Diffusion of Acid through the Gastric Mucosa and its Physiological consequences. In G. B. Glass (Ed.), *Progress in Gastroenterology,* Vol. 2. New York: Grune & Stratton, 1970. Pp. 42–56.
33. Davies, R. E., and Longmuir, N. M. Production of ulcers in isolated frog gastric mucosa. *Biochem. J.* 42:621, 1948.
34. Davison, J. S. Response of single vagal afferent fibres to mechanical and chemical stimulation of the gastric and duodenal mucosa in cats. *Q. J. Exp. Physiol.* 57:405, 1972.
35. Debas, H. T., Farooq, O., and Grossman, M. I. Inhibition of gastric emptying is a physiological action of cholecystokinin. *Gastroenterology* 68:1211, 1975.
36. Debas, H. T., and Grossman, M. I. Chemicals bathing oxyntic gland area stimulate acid secretion. *Gastroenterology* 66:836, 1974.
37. Debas, H. T., Konturek, S. J., Walsh, J. H., and Grossman, M. I. Proof of a pyloro-oxyntic reflex for stimulation of acid secretion. *Gastroenterology* 66:526, 1974.
38. Debas, H. T., Walsh, J. H., and Grossman, M. I. Evidence for an oxynto-pyloric reflex for release of gastrin. *Gastroenterology* 66:837, 1974.
39. Debas, H. T., Walsh, J. H., and Grossman, M. I. Mechanisms of Release of Antral Gastrin. In J. C. Thompson and M. I. Grossman (Eds.), *Proceedings of the International Symposium on Gastrointestinal Hormones.* Austin, Tex.: University of Texas Press, 1975. P. 425.
40. Demling, L., and Domschke, W. (Eds.). Proceedings of a symposium on motilin: Origin, chemistry, and actions. *Scand. J. Gastroenterol.* 11(Suppl. 39), 1976.
41. Donovan, I. A., Griffen, D. W., Harding, L. K., and Alexander-Williams, J. Paradoxical gastric emptying after gastric surgery in man. *Br. J. Surg.* 61:916, 1974.
42. Dotevall, G., Kock, N. G., and Walan, A. Inhibition of pentagastrin-induced gastric acid secretion in man by glucagon given intravenously. *Scand. J. Gastroenterol.* 4:713, 1969.
43. Dozois, R. R., Kelly, K. A., and Code, C. F. Effect of distal antrectomy on gastric emptying of liquids and solids. *Gastroenterology* 61:675, 1971.
44. Dragstedt, L. R. Peptic ulcer. *Am. J. Surg.* 117:143, 1969.
45. Elder, J. B., Gillespie, G., Campbell, E. H. G., et al. The effect of vagotomy on the lower part of the acid dose-response curve to pentagastrin in man. *Clin. Sci.* 43:193, 1972.
46. Elder, J. B., Gillespie, G., Gillespie, I. E., et al. The effect of sub-threshold doses of pentagastrin on the acid response to insulin in duodenal ulcer subjects before and after truncal vagotomy. *Clin. Sci.* 43:201, 1972.
47. Emås. S., and Grossman, M. I. Effect of truncal vagotomy on acid and pepsin responses to histamine and gastrin in dogs. *Am. J. Physiol.* 212:1007, 1967.
48. Fahrenkrug, J., Haglund, U., Jodal, M., et al. Nervous release of vasoactive intestinal polypeptide in the gastrointestinal tract of cats: Possible physiological implications. *J. Physiol.* (Lond.) 284:291, 1978.
49. Farooq, O., and Walsh, J. H. Atropine enhances gastrin release produced by insulin hypoglycemia in man. *Gastroenterology* 66:872, 1974.
50. Feldman, M., Dickerman, R. M., McClelland, R. N., et al. Effect of selective proximal vagotomy on food-stimulated gastric acid secretion and gastrin release in patients with duodenal ulcer. *Gastroenterology* 76:926, 1979.
51. Feldman, M., Richardson, C. T., and Ford-

tran, J. S. Effect of sham feeding on gastric acid secretion in healthy subjects and duodenal ulcer patients: Evidence for increased basal vagal tone in some ulcer patients. *Gastroenterology* 79:796, 1980.
52. Feldman, M., Richardson, C. T., Taylor, I. L., and Walsh, J. H. Effect of atropine on vagal release of gastrin and pancreatic polypeptide. *J. Clin. Invest.* 63:294, 1979.
53. Fellenius, E., Berglindh, T., Sachs, G., et al. Substituted benzimidazoles inhibit gastric acid secretion by blocking ($H^+ + K^+$) ATPase. *Nature* 290:159, 1981.
54. Fielding, L. P., Curwain, B. P., Russell, R. C. G., and Bloom, S. R. Evidence for separate actions of an adrenergic B_2 stimulant and a histamine H_2 blocker on the oxyntic and gastrin cells. *Br. J. Surg.* 61:914, 1974.
55. Fisher, R. S., and Cohen, S. Pyloric-sphincter dysfunction in patients with gastric ulcer. *N. Engl. J. Med.* 288:273, 1973.
56. Fisher, R. S., Lipshutz, W., and Cohen, S. The hormonal regulation of pyloric sphincter function. *J. Clin. Invest.* 52:1289, 1973.
57. Flemström, G., and Nylander, O. Stimulation of duodenal epithelial HCO_3-transport in the guinea pig and cat by luminal prostaglandin E_2. *Prostaglandins* 21:47, 1981.
58. Fordtran, J. S., and Walsh, J. H. Gastric acid secretion rate and buffer content of the stomach after eating. *J. Clin. Invest.* 52:645, 1973.
59. Ganguli, P. C. The effect of protein, carbohydrate, and fat on plasma gastrin concentrations in human subjects. *Gut* 11:1061, 1970.
60. George, J. D. Gastric acidity and motility. *Am. J. Dig. Dis.* 13:376, 1968.
61. Gibson, R., Hirschowitz, B. I., and Hutchinson, G. Actions of metiamide, an H_2-histamine receptor antagonist, on gastric H^+ and pepsin secretion in dogs. *Gastroenterology* 67:93, 1974.
62. Giles, G. R., and Clark, C. G. Gastric secretion stimulated by meat extract in man. *Scand. J. Gastroenterol.* 1:159, 1966.
63. Goyal, R. K., Rattan, S., and Hersh, T. Comparison of the effect of prostaglandins E_1, E_2, and A_2, and of hypovolemic hypotension on the lower esophageal sphincter. *Gastroenterology* 65:608, 1973.
64. Grossman, M. I. Stimulation of secretion of acid by distention of denervated fundic pouches in dogs. *Gastroenterology* 41:385, 1961.
65. Grossman, M. I. Secretion of acid and pepsin in response to distention of vagally innervated fundic gland area in dogs. *Gastroenterology* 42:718, 1962.
66. Grossman, M. I., and others. Candidate hormones of the gut. *Gastroenterology* 67:730, 1974.
67. Grötzinger, U., Bergegårdh, S., and Olbe, L. The effect of atropine and proximal gastric vagotomy on the acid response to fundic distention in man. *Gut* 18:303, 1977.
68. Guth, P. H., Bauman, H., Grossman, M. I., et al. Measurement of gastric mucosal blood flow in man. *Gastroenterology* 74:831, 1978.
69. Haglund, U., Elander, B., Fellenius, E., et al. The effects of secretagogues on isolated human gastric gland. *Scand. J. Gastroenterol.* 17:455, 1982.
70. Hansky, J. Antral-gastrin-cell hyperplasia in peptic ulcer disease. *Lancet* 1:1344, 1974.
71. Hansky, J., Soveny, C., and Korman, M. G. The effect of glucagon on serum gastrin. *Gut* 14:457, 1973.
72. Hayes, J. R., Ardill, J., Kennedy, T. L., et al. Stimulation of gastrin release by catecholamines. *Lancet* 1:819, 1972.
73. Humphrey, C. S., Smith, R. B., Lyndon, P. J., and Johnston, D. Effect of truncal vagotomy, selective vagotomy and pyloroplasty, and highly selective vagotomy without drainage on the response to meat extract in man. *Br. J. Surg.* 59:906, 1972.
74. Isenberg, J. I., Maxwell, V., Walsh, J. H., and Grossman, M. I. Increased sensitivity to stimulation of acid secretion by pentagastrin in duodenal ulcer. *J. Clin. Invest.* 55:330, 1975.
75. Ivarsson, L. E., Darle, N., Hultén, L., et al. Gastric blood flow and distribution: The effect of pentagastrin anesthetized in cat and man as studied by an inert gas elimination method. *Scand. J. Gastroenterol.* 17:1037, 1982.
76. Ivey, K. J. Gastric mucosal barrier. *Gastroenterology* 61:247, 1971.
77. Ivey, K. J., Morrison, S., and Gray, C. Effect of salicylates on the gastric mucosal barrier in man. *J. Appl. Physiol.* 33:81, 1972.
78. Jacobowitz, D. Histochemical studies of the autonomic innervation of the gut. *J. Pharmacol. Exp. Ther.* 149:358, 1965.
79. Jaffe, B. M., Clendinnen, B. G., Clarke, R. J., and Alexander-Williams, J. Effect of selective and proximal gastric vagotomy on serum gastrin. *Gastroenterology* 66:944, 1974.
80. Jahnberg, T., Martinsson, J., Hultén, L., and Fasth, S. Dynamic gastric response to expan-

sion before and after vagotomy. *Scand. J. Gastroenterol.* 10:593, 1975.
81. Jansson, G. Extrinsic nervous control of gastric motility. *Acta Physiol. Scand.* 326(Suppl.), 1969.
82. Jansson, G., and Martinson, J. Studies on the ganglionic site of action of sympathetic outflow to the stomach. *Acta Physiol. Scand.* 68:184, 1966.
83. Jennewein, H. M., Waldeck, F., Siewert, R., et al. The interaction of glucagon and pentagastrin on the lower oesophageal sphincter in man and dog. *Gut* 14:861, 1973.
84. Johnson, A. G., and McDermott, S. J. Lysolecithin: A factor in the pathogenesis of gastric ulceration? *Gut* 15:710, 1974.
85. Johnson, L. R. Effect of gastric mucosal acidification on the action of pepsigogues. *Am. J. Physiol.* 225:1411, 1973.
86. Johnson, L. R., and Grossman, M. I. Intestinal hormones as inhibitors of gastric secretion. *Gastroenterology* 60:120, 1971.
87. Johnston, D. Highly selective vagotomy. *Gut* 15:748, 1974.
88. Johnston, D., and Duthie, H. L. Inhibition of histamine-stimulated gastric secretion by acid in the duodenum in man. *Gut* 7:58, 1966.
89. Kaminski, D. L., and Ruwart, M. J. The effect of vagotomy on the canine enterogastrone mechanism. *Surgery* 81:80, 1977.
90. Kihl, B., and Olbe, L. Fat inhibition of gastric acid secretion in duodenal ulcer patients before and after proximal gastric vagotomy. *Gut* 21:1056, 1980.
91. Kihl, B., Rökaeus, Å., Rosell, S., and Olbe, L. Fat inhibition of gastric acid secretion in man and plasma concentrations of neurotensin-like immunoreactivity. *Scand. J. Gastroenterol.* 16:513, 1981.
92. Kihl, B., Rökaeus, A., Rosell, S., and Olbe, L. The effect of intraduodenal instillation of oleic acid on plasma neurotensin-like immunoreactivity and on gastric acid secretion stimulated by betazole and sham feeding in man. *Scand. J. Gastroenterol.* 17:633, 1982.
93. Kivilaakso, E., and Silen, W. Pathogenesis of experimental gastric mucosal injury. *N. Engl. J. Med.* 301:364, 1979.
94. Knight, S. E., McIsaac, R. L., and Fielding, L. P. Comparison of gastric mucosal blood flow (GMBF) in normal subjects and patients with duodenal ulcer. *Br. J. Surg.* 64:824, 1977.
95. Knutson, U., Bergegårdh, S., and Olbe, L. The effect of intragastric pH variations on the gastric acid response to sham feeding in duodenal ulcer patients. *Scand. J. Gastroenterol.* 9:357, 1974.
96. Knutson, U., and Olbe, L. Gastric acid response to sham feeding in duodenal ulcer patients. *Scand. J. Gastroenterol.* 8:513, 1973.
97. Knutson, U., and Olbe, L. The gastric acid response to sham feeding in duodenal ulcer patients after proximal selective vagotomy. *Scand. J. Gastroenterol.* 20(Suppl. 8):16, 1973.
98. Knutson, U., and Olbe, L. The effect of exogenous gastrin on the acid sham feeding response in antrum-bulb-resected duodenal ulcer patients. *Scand. J. Gastroenterol.* 9:231, 1974.
99. Knutson, U., Olbe, L., and Ganguli, P. C. Gastric acid and plasma gastrin responses to sham feeding in duodenal ulcer patients before and after resection of antrum and duodenal bulb. *Scand. J. Gastroenterol.* 9:351, 1974.
100. Konturek, S. J., Biernat, J., and Olesky, J. Serum gastrin and gastric acid responses to meals at various pH levels in man. *Gut* 15:526, 1974.
101. Konturek, S. J., Kwiecien, N., Obtulowiez, E., et al. Cephalic phase of gastric secretion in healthy subjects and duodenal ulcer patients: Role of vagal innervation. *Gut* 20:875, 1979.
102. Konturek, S. J., Tasler, J., Obtulowicz, W., and Rehfeld, J. F. Effect of metiamide, a histamine H_2-receptor antagonist, on mucosal blood flow and serum gastrin level. *Gastroenterology* 66:982, 1974.
103. Korman, M. G., Soveny, C., and Hansky, J. Extragastric gastrin. *Gut* 13:346, 1972.
104. Korman, M. G., Strickland, R. G., and Hansky, J. The functional "G" cell mass in atrophic gastritis. *Gut* 13:340, 1972.
105. Køster, K. H., and Rune, S. J. Antral control of gastric acid secretion. *Lancet* 2:1183, 1963.
106. Kronborg, O., and Andersen, D. Acid response to sham feeding as a test for completeness of vagotomy. *Scand. J. Gastroenterol.* 15:119, 1980.
107. Kronborg, O., Pedersen, T., Stadil, F., and Rehfeld, J. F. The effect of beta-adrenergic blockade upon gastric acid and gastrin secretion during hypoglycemia before and after vagotomy. *Scand. J. Gastroenterol.* 9:173, 1974.
108. Lam, S. K., Isenberg, J. I., Grossman, M. I., et al. Gastric acid secretion is abnormally sensitive to endogenous gastrin release after peptone test meals in duodenal ulcer patients. *J.*

Clin. Invest. 65:555, 1980.
109. Longhi, E. H., Greenlee, H. B., Bravo, J. L. et al. Question of an inhibitory hormone from the gastric antrum. *Am. J. Physiol.* 191:64, 1957.
110. Lundell, L. Elucidation by a H_2-receptor antagonist of the significance of mucosal histamine mobilization in exciting acid secretion. *J. Physiol.* (Lond.) 244:365, 1975.
111. Lyndon, P. J., and Johnston, D. The effect of fat in the duodenum on gastric secretion before and after truncal vagotomy and highly selective vagotomy in man. *Br. J. Surg.* 59:905, 1972.
112. Makhlouf, G. M. The neuroendocrine design of the gut. *Gastroenterology* 67:159, 1974.
113. Martinson, J. Studies on the efferent vagal control of the stomach. *Acta Physiol. Scand.* 255(Suppl.), 1965.
114. Mayer, G., Arnold R., Feurle, G., et al. Influence of feeding and sham feeding upon serum gastrin and gastric acid secretion in control subjects and duodenal ulcer patients. *Scand. J. Gastroenterol.* 9:703, 1974.
115. McGuigan, J., and Grieder, M. H. Correlative immunochemical and light microscopic studies of the gastrin cell of the antral mucosa. *Gastroenterology* 60:223, 1971.
116. Menguy, R. Gastric mucus and the gastric mucous barrier. *Am. J. Surg.* 117:806, 1969.
117. Menguy, R., Desbaillets, L., and Masters, Y. F. Mechanism of stress ulcer: Influence of hypovolemic shock on energy metabolism in the gastric mucosa. *Gastroenterology* 66:46, 1974.
118. Mignon, M. Galmiche, J. P., Accary, J. P., and Bonfils, S. Serum gastrin, gastric acid, and pepsin responses to sham feeding in man. *Gastroenterology* 66:856, 1974.
119. Moore, J. G., and Englert, E., Jr. Circadian rhythm of gastric acid secretion in man. *Nature* 226:1261, 1970.
120. Neuburger, P., Lewin, M., and Bonfils, S. Parietal and chief cell populations in four cases of the Zollinger-Ellison syndrome. *Gastroenterology* 63:937, 1972.
121. Nilsson, G., Simon, J., Yalow, R. S., and Berson, S. A. Plasma gastrin and gastric acid responses to sham feeding and feeding in dogs. *Gastroenterology* 63:51, 1972.
122. Nilsson, G., Yalow, R. S., and Berson, S. A. Distribution of Gastrin in the Gastrointestinal Tract of Human, Dog, Cat, and Hog. In S. Andersson (Ed.), *Frontiers in Gastrointestinal Hormone Research* (Nobel Symposium 16). Stockholm: Almqvist & Wiksell, 1973. Pp. 95–101.
123. Noring, O. Studies on the cephalic phase of gastric secretion in normal subjects and ulcer patients. *Gastroenterology* 18:413, 1951.
124. Olbe, L. Vagal Release of Gastrin. In M. I. Grossman (Ed.), *Gastrin.* Berkeley, Calif.: University of California Press, 1966. Pp. 83–107.
125. Olbe, L. Potentiation of acid sham feeding response in Pavlov pouch dogs by histamine and by mesenteric-caval vein anastomosis. *Acta Physiol. Scand.* 66:473, 1966.
126. Olbe, L., Haglund, U., Leth, R., et al. Effects of substituted benzimidazole (H 149/94) on gastric acid secretion in humans. *Gastroenterology* 83:193, 1982.
127. Olbe, L., Ridley, P. T., and Ulvnäs, B. Effects of gastrin and histamine on vagally induced acid and pepsin secretion in antrectomized dogs. *Acta Physiol. Scand.* 72:492, 1968.
128. Olbe, L., Sachs, G., Carlsson, E., et al. Substituted benzimidazoles: A new approach to control of gastric acid secretion. Symposium of the 7th World Congress of Gastroenterology, Stockholm, 1982.
129. Orloff, M. J., Abbott, A. G., and Rosen, H. Nature of the humoral agent responsible for portacaval shunt–related gastric hypersecretion in man. *Am. J. Surg.* 120:237, 1970.
130. Overgaard Nielsen, H., Bekker, C., Kronborg, O., and Andersen, D. Gastric acid response to sham feeding and pentagastrin before and after parietal cell vagotomy in patients with duodenal ulcer. *Scand. J. Gastroenterol.* 17:133, 1982.
131. Pearse, A. G. E., Polak, J. M., and Bloom, S. R. The newer gut hormones: Cellular sources, physiology, pathology, and clinical aspects. *Gastroenterology* 72:746, 1977.
132. Petersen, H., and Myren, J. Pentagastrin dose-response in peptic ulcer disease. *Scand. J. Gastroenterol.* 10:705, 1975.
133. Piasecki, C. Patterns of blood supply to human gastroduodenal mucosa: A basis for local ischemia. In L. P. Fielding (Ed.), *Gastrointestinal Mucosal Blood Flow.* Edinburgh: Churchill Livingstone, 1980. Pp. 3–16.
134. Polak, J. M., Bloom, S. R., Kuzio, M., et al. Cellular localization of gastric inhibitory polypeptide in the duodenum and jejunum. *Gut* 14:284, 1973.
135. Polak, J., Hoffbrand, A. V., Reed, P.I., et al.

Qualitative and quantitative studies of antral and fundic G. cells in pernicious anaemia. *Scand. J. Gastroenterol.* 8:361, 1973.

136. Polak, J. M., Pearse, A. G. E., Garaud, J.-C., and Bloom, S. R. Cellular localization of a vasoactive intestinal peptide in the mammalian and avian gastrointestinal tract. *Gut* 15:720, 1974.
137. Polak, J. M., Stagg, B., and Pearse, A. G. E. Two types of Zollinger-Ellison syndrome: Immunofluorescent, cytochemical, and ultrastructural studies of the antral and pancreatic gastrin cells in different clinical states. *Gut* 13:501, 1972.
138. Preshaw, R. M. Gastric acid output after sham feeding and during release or infusion of gastrin. *Am. J. Physiol.* 210:1409, 1970.
139. Preshaw, R. M. Inhibition of pentagastrin-stimulated gastric acid output by sham feeding. *Fed. Proc.* 32:410, 1973.
140. Rayford, P. L., Villar, H. V., Reeder, D. D., and Thompson, J. C. Effect of GIP and VIP on gastrin release and gastric secretion. *Physiologist* 17:319, 1974.
141. Rehfeld, J. F., and Stadil, F. Serum gastrin components in normal subjects and duodenal ulcer patients during fasting and feeding. Presented at the 5th World Congress of Gastroenterology, Mexico City, Oct. 13–19, 1974. Abstracts, p. 285.
142. Rhodes, J. Etiology of gastric ulcer. *Gastroenterology* 63:171, 1972.
143. Robert, A. Cytoprotection by prostaglandins. *Gastroenterology* 77:761, 1979.
144. Roland, M., Berstad, A., and Liavåg, I. Acid and pepsin secretion in duodenal ulcer patients in response to graded doses of pentagastrin or pentagastrin and carbocholine before and after proximal gastric vagotomy. *Scand. J. Gastroenterol.* 9:511, 1974.
145. Rosell, S., Thor, K., Rökaeus, Å., et al. Plasma concentration of neurotensin-like immunoreactivity (NTLI) and lower esophageal sphincter (LES) pressure in man following infusion of (Gln^4)-neurotensin. *Acta Physiol. Scand.* 109:369, 1980.
146. Rune, S. J. Comparison of the rates of gastric secretion in man after ingestion of food and after maximal stimulation with histamine. *Gut* 7:344, 1966.
147. Saccomani, G. H., Helander, H. F., Graco, S., et al. Characterizations of gastric mucosal membranes. X. Immunological studies of gastric $H^+ + K^+$ ATPase, *J. Cell. Biol.* 83:271, 1979.
148. Samloff, I. M. Pepsinogens, pepsins, and pepsin inhibitors. *Gastroenterology* 60:586, 1971.
149. Samloff, I. M., and Liebman, W. M. Cellular localization of the group II pepsinogens in human stomach and duodenum. *Gastroenterology* 65:36, 1973.
150. Samloff, I. M., and Liebman, W. M. Radioimmunoassay of group I pepsinogens in serum. *Gastroenterology* 66:494, 1974.
151. Schöön, I.-M., Bergegårdh, S., Grötzinger, U., and Olbe, L. Evidence for a defective inhibition of pentagastrin-stimulated gastric acid secretion by antral distension in the duodenal ulcer patient. *Gastroenterology* 75:363, 1978.
152. Schöön, I.-M., Lundqvist, G., Rehfeld, J., and Olbe, L. A study of the effect of antral distension on gastric acid secretion in man. *Digestion* 21:57, 1981.
153. Schrumpf, E., and Stadaas, J. Effect of gastric distention on motility and plasma gastrin concentration before and after secretin administration. *Scand. J. Gastroenterol.* 9:119, 1974.
154. Schubert, M. L., and Makhlouf, G. M. Regulation of gastrin and somatostatin secretion by intramural neurons: Effect of nicotinic receptor stimulation with dimethyl-phenylpiperazinium. *Gastroenterology* 83:626, 1982.
155. Schwartz, T. W., Stenquist, B., Olbe, L., and Stadil, F. Synchronous oscillations in the basal secretion of pancreatic-polypeptide and gastric acid. *Gastroenterology* 76:14, 1979.
156. Shimamoto, K., Kawai, K., Murakami, K., et al. Autoradiographic studies on the mucin metabolism in human gastric mucosa with special reference to intestinal metaplasia. *Acta Hepatogastroenterol.* 20:490, 1973.
157. Sjödin, L. Inhibition of gastrin-stimulated canine acid secretion by sham-feeding. *Scand. J. Gastroenterol.* 10:73, 1975.
158. Slaff, G. F. Intestinal phase of gastric acid secretion: Augmentation of maximal response of Heidenhain pouch to gastrin *Gastroenterology* 66:656, 1974.
159. Smith, I. S., Gillespie, G., Elder, J. B., et al. Time of conversion of insulin response after vagotomy. *Gastroenterology* 62:912, 1972.
160. Soll, A. H. The actions of secretagogues on oxygen uptake by isolated mammalian parietal cells. *J. Clin. Invest.* 61:370, 1978.
161. Soll, A. H. The interaction of histamine with gastrin and carbamylcholine on oxygen uptake

by isolated mammalian parietal cells. *J. Clin. Invest.* 61:381, 1978.

162. Soll, A. H. Secretagogues stimulation of [^{14}C] aminopyrine accumulation by isolated canine parietal cells. *Am. J. Physiol.* 238:G366, 1980.
163. Stadil, F., and Rehfeld, J. F. Hypoglycemic release of gastrin in man. *Scand. J. Gastroenterol.* 7:509, 1972.
164. Stadil, F., and Rehfeld, J. F. Release of gastrin by epinephrine in man. *Gastroenterology* 65:210, 1973.
165. Stadil, F., and Rehfeld, J. F. Gastrin response to insulin after selective, highly selective, and truncal vagotomy. *Gastroenterology* 66:7, 1974.
166. Stening, G. F., and Grossman, M. I. Gastric acid response to pentagastrin and histamine after extragastric vagotomy in dogs. *Gastroenterology* 59:364, 1970.
167. Stenquist, B. Studies on vagal activation of gastric acid secretion in man. *Acta Physiol. Scand.* (Suppl.):465, 1979.
168. Stenquist, B., Knutson, U., and Olbe, L. Gastric acid responses to adequate and modified sham feeding and to insulin hypoglycaemia in duodenal ulcer patients. *Scand. J. Gastroenterol.* 13:357, 1978.
169. Stenquist, B., Knutson, U., and Olbe, L. The vagogastrone mechanism in man. *Scand. J. Gastroenterol.* 13:895, 1978.
170. Stenquist, B., Knutson, U., Rehnberg, O., and Olbe, L. The effect of intragastric pH variations on the gastric acid response to insulin hypoglycaemia in healthy subjects and duodenal ulcer patients. *Scand. J. Gastroenterol.* 12:169, 1977.
171. Stenquist, B., Rehfeld, J. F., and Olbe, L. Effects of proximal gastric vagotomy and anticholinergics on the acid and gastrin responses to sham feeding in duodenal ulcer patients. *Gut* 20:1020, 1979.
172. Stenquist, B., Rehnberg, O., and Olbe, L. Sham feeding versus insulin as a test for completeness of vagotomy. *Hepato-Gastroenterol* (Suppl.), XI Int. Congr. Gastroenterol. (abstr.), P. 138, 1980.
173. Stern, D. H., and Walsh, J. H. Gastrin release in postoperative ulcer patients: Evidence for release of duodenal gastrin. *Gastroenterology* 64:363, 1973.
174. Straus, E., and Yalow, R. S. Differential diagnosis in hyperchlorhydric hypergastrinemia. *Gastroenterology* 66:867, 1974.
175. Taylor, I. L., Walsh, J. H., Carter, D., et al. Effects of atropine and bethanechol on bombesin-stimulated release of pancreatic polypeptide and gastrin in dog. *Gastroenterology* 77:714, 1979.
176. Tepperman, B. L., Walsh, J. H., and Preshaw, R. M. Effect of antral denervation on gastrin release by sham feeding and insulin hypoglycemia in dogs. *Gastroenterology* 63:973, 1972.
177. Thompson, J. C., Reeder, D. D., Bunchman, H. H., et al. Effect of secretin on circulating gastrin. *Ann. Surg.* 176:384, 1972.
178. Trudeau, W. L., and McGuigan, J. E. Serum gastrin levels in patients with peptic ulcer disease. *Gastroenterology* 59:6, 1970.
179. Uvnäs-Wallensten, K., Eféndić, S., and Luft, R. Vagal release of somatostatin into the antral lumen of cats. *Acta Physiol. Scand.* 99:126, 1977.
180. Vagne, M., and Fargier, M.-C. Effect of pentagastrin and secretin on gastric mucus secretion in conscious cats. *Gastroenterology* 65:757, 1973.
181. Vizi, S. E., Bertaccini, G., Impicciatore, M., and Knoll, J. Evidence that acetylcholine released by gastrin and related polypeptides contributes to their effect on gastrointestinal motility. *Gastroenterology* 64:268, 1973.
182. Waller, S. L. Prostaglandins and the gastrointestinal tract. *Gut* 14:402, 1973.
183. Walsh, J. H., Richardson, C. T., and Fordtran, J. S. Diminished inhibition of acid secretion by low pH in duodenal ulcer (DU) patients. *Clin. Res.* 22:371A, 1974.
184. Walsh, J. H., Richardson, C. T., and Fordtran, J. S. pH dependence of acid secretion and gastrin release in normal and ulcer subjects. *J. Clin. Invest.* 55:462, 1975.
185. Walsh, J. H., Yalow, R. S., and Berson, S. A. The effect of atropine on plasma gastrin response to feeding. *Gastroenterology* 60:16, 1971.
186. Ward, A. S., and Bloom, S. R. The role of secretin in the inhibition of gastric secretion by intraduodenal acid. *Gut* 15:889, 1974.
187. Way, L. W. Effect of secretin on gastric acid secretion in response to cholinergic stimuli. *Gastroenterology* 59:510, 1970.
188. Wilkinson, A. R., Humphrey, C. S., and Johnston, D. Comparison of stimulants of antral release in man. *Br. J. Surg.* 57:383, 1970.
189. Williams, S. E., and Turnberg, L. A. Demonstration of a pH gradient across mucus ad-

herent to rabbit gastric mucosa: Evidence for a "mucus-bicarbonate" barrier. *Gut* 22:94, 1981.
190. Wormsley, K. G. The effect of vagotomy on the human pancreatic response to direct and indirect stimulation. *Scand. J. Gastroenterol.* 7:85, 1972.
191. Wormsley, K. G. The pathophysiology of duodenal ulceration. *Gut* 15:59, 1974.
192. Wyllie, J. H., Ealding, W. D. P., Hesselbo, T., and Black, J. W. Inhibition of gastric secretion in man by metiamide: A new orally active histamine H_2-receptor antagonist. *Gut* 14:424, 1973.
193. Yalow, R. S., and Berson, S. A. Radioimmunoassay of gastrin. *Gastroenterology* 58:1, 1970.
194. Yalow, R. S., and Wu, N. Additional studies on the nature of big big gastrin. *Gastroenterology* 65:19, 1973.

PART II
Peptide Hormones of the Stomach and Duodenum

G. R. Sagor
S. R. Bloom
J. M. Polak

It is now accepted that the gastrointestinal tract, besides its established functions of digestion and absorption, also behaves as an endocrine organ. The concept is relatively new, and has been reinforced over the last decade, with major strides being made in the field because of advances in the technology of protein purification, radioimmunoassay and immunocytochemistry. The advances have been particularly important in studies of the upper gastrointestinal tract. The early concept of the chemical reflex control of gastric acid secretion by gastrin and of pancreaticobiliary function by secretin and cholecystokinin-pancreozymin has been expanded by the discovery of a large number of peptides in the upper gastrointestinal (GI) tract. These hormones not only play a part in the physiology of this area but also may contribute to the pathophysiology of a number of gastrointestinal diseases and to some of the unwanted sequelae of surgical treatment of these problems.

General Concepts

THE INVESTIGATION OF ENDOCRINE CELL MORPHOLOGY

In 1938 Feyrter described the numerous "clear cells" in the mucosa of the GI tract, so designated because they fail to take up conventional stains. The endocrine granules in these cells can be demonstrated on light and ultrastructural microscopy by silver impregnation methods (argentaffin and argyrophil). However, electron microscopy and immunocytochemistry are the most reliable and specific methods of investigating endocrine cell morphology.

Using electron microscopy, two types of endocrine cells have been identified in the mucosa of the GI tracts. The "open" cell is elongated, with basally situated secretory granules. The microvilli of these cells connect with the gut lumen (Fig. 3-15) and presumably act as chemoreceptors to changes in intraluminal content. The "closed" cell does not communicate with the lumen and may secrete its peptide hormone in response to changes in the local tissue environment.

Immunocytochemistry is the use of labeled antibodies as specific reagents for the localization of tissue constituents (antigens) in situ (Fig. 3-16). The technique was devised by Coons, Ledue, and Connolly in 1955. The antibodies, which are normally gamma globulins, are raised by immunizing rabbits or guinea pigs with antigen, which should be pure or synthetic, to ensure as specific an antibody as possible. Nevertheless, the resulting antiserum will not be directed specifically and solely to the injected antigen, and because the donor animal's serum will also contain many natural antibodies that may react with tissue components, a positive-appearing immunoreaction cannot be assumed to be caused by the specific desired antigen-antibody reaction unless stringent controls are carried out. Refinements of the technique are continually taking place. Thus the development of new cross-

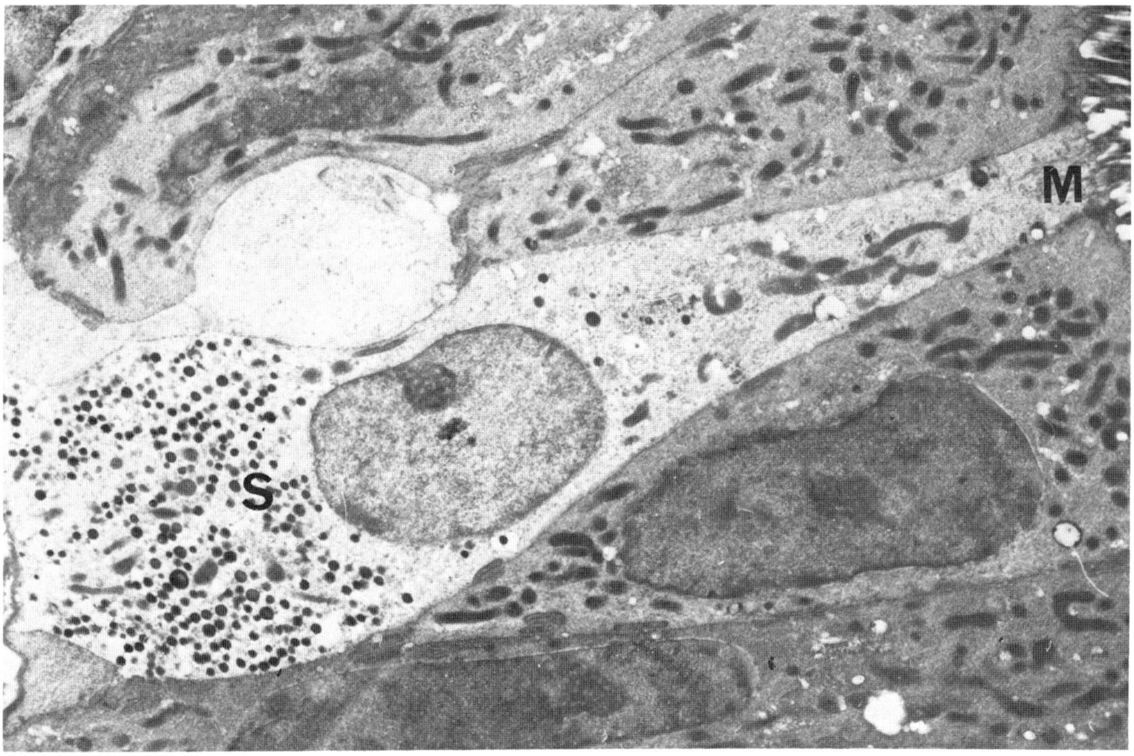

Fig. 3-15. Electron micrograph of an endocrine cell with characteristic secretory granules (S) lying toward the basement membrane and microvilli projecting into the lumen (M). (×6.9K)

linking fixatives has improved tissue fixation, while the problems of crossreaction have been reduced by the production of more specific antibodies. It is now possible to quantify immunostained material on a comparative basis, and estimations can be made of the volume density of an immunostained element compared with the rest of the tissue, and the total population of a particular endocrine cell in a given sample.

Immunocytochemistry is also invaluable in the diagnosis of the endocrine-producing tumors of the pancreas and GI tract (apudomas). Another advance in the field of immunocytochemistry has been the introduction of a new marker for the detection of apudomas or endocrine tumors [55]. Neuron-specific enolase (NSE) is a neural form of the glycolytic enzyme enolase that has been found to be produced by all types of apudomas but not by nonendocrine tumors. Thus apudoma cells can be detected by using antisera to NSE (Fig. 3-17). NSE-like immunoreactivity is also found in all endocrine cells of the GI tract, and in enteric and pancreatic nerves. Immunocytochemical staining for NSE can now be regarded as the best means of identification of the neuroendocrine system of the GI tract in its entirety (Fig. 3-18).

RADIOIMMUNOASSAY

Radioimmunoassay depends on a quantitative interaction between an antigen and its specific antibody. A known amount of antigen labeled with radioactive iodine competes for a specific antibody with an unknown amount of unlabeled antigen in the sample to be investigated. The amount of antigen or peptide in the sample is measured by the ratio of antibody-bound iodinated antigen to unbound antigen. The

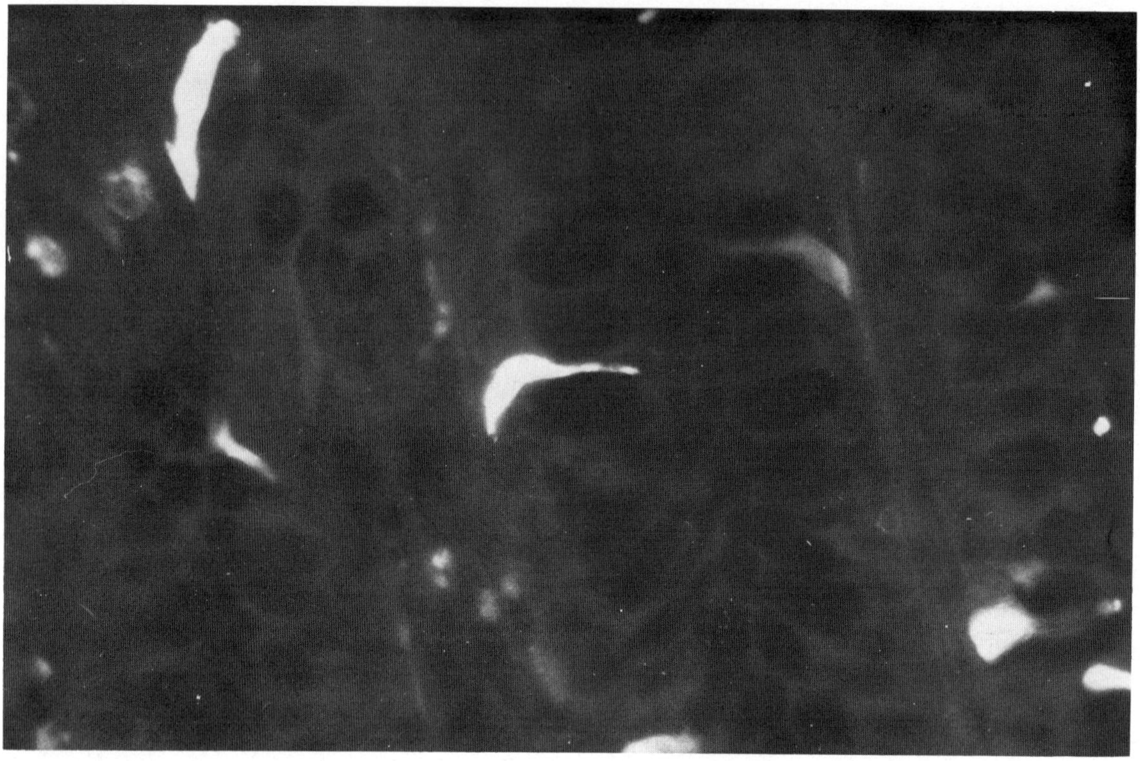

Fig. 3-16. Enteroglucagon immunoreactive cells in the mucosa of the human colon. (×450)

technique was first developed by Berson and Yalow in 1958 and has replaced bioassay for the measurement of the GI peptides.

THE APUD CONCEPT

The clear cells in the pancreas and GI tract mucosa described by Feyrter were thought to produce secretions that acted on neighboring tissues in a paracrine manner. It was later shown [41] that these clear cells had common cytochemical and functional characteristics, and the term *APUD* was coined from the initial letters of some of these characteristics, that is *a*mine content, *p*recursor *u*ptake, and *d*ecarboxylation.

Embryologically the largest group of APUD cells, those of the GI tract and pancreas, are derived from a single region of neuroendocrine-programmed ectoblast. The APUD cells of the central nervous system are neuroectodermal in origin, while other APUD cells are derived from the definitive neural crest. It thus becomes clear that the APUD concept embraces a diffuse neuroendocrine system and that the GI tract may be considered an endocrine organ within this system.

Physiology

The peptides of the GI tract may be divided according to their mode of action (Table 3-2). *Circulating* hormones are released from the endocrine cell into the bloodstream and have their effect on distant receptors. *Paracrine* hormones are released from the endocrine cell into the intercellular fluid and act locally. The third group is composed of *neurotransmitters* which are released from nerve synapses after depolarization and form part of the peptidergic system which is part of the autonomic nervous system. The latter two groups are

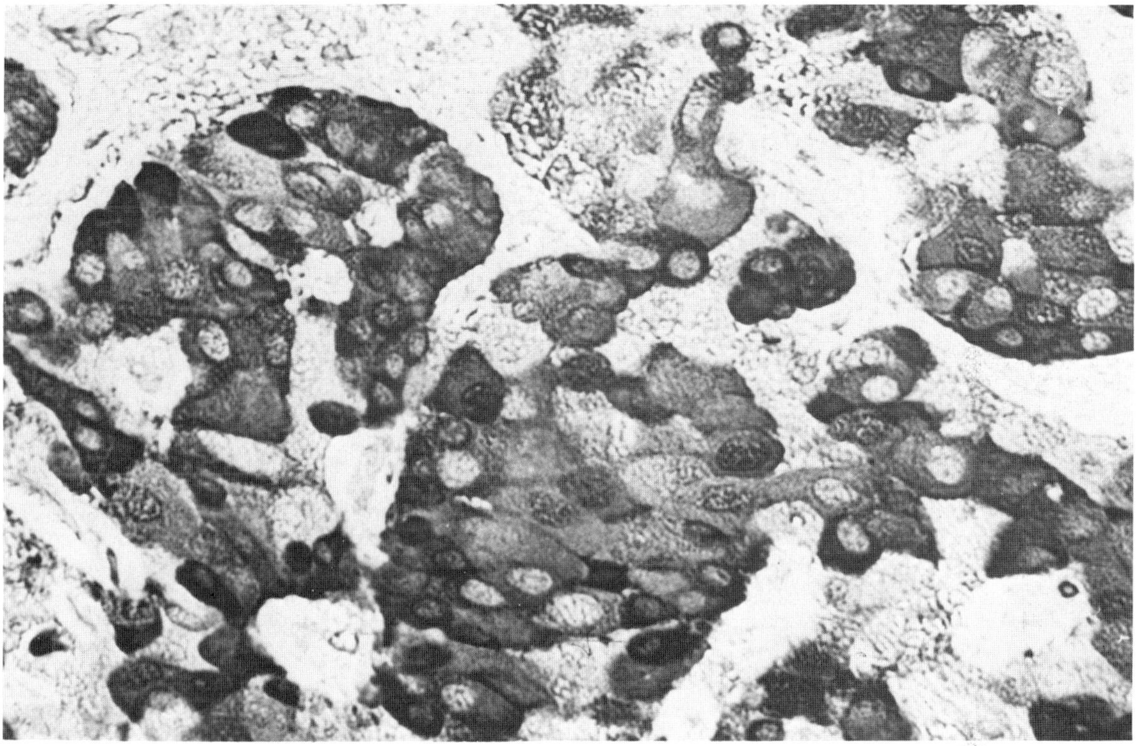

Fig. 3-17. Neuron-specific enolase immunoreactivity in cells of a pancreatic glucagonoma. (×450)

found in the central nervous system as well as the GI tract, and have therefore been grouped as "brain-gut" peptides. While the endocrine cells releasing circulating hormones are found in the mucosa of the GI tract, the peptidergic nerves are found in the submucosa and muscle, often in close contact with the myenteric plexus. Some peptides, such as cholecystokinin, may have more than one mode of action.

GASTRIN

Although Edkins discovered in 1905 that a gastric mucosal extract was capable of stimulating gastric acid secretion, it was only in 1964 that gastrin was isolated and synthesized. Gastrin is produced by the mucosal G cells and has been isolated in three major forms—gastrin-14 (G-14), gastrin-17 (G-17), and gastrin-34 (G-34), or big gastrin. "Big, big gastrin," previously described, is now regarded as an artifact of some gastrin radioimmunoassay systems. All forms of gastrin share a common C-terminal portion and differ only in their chain length. The largest quantities of gastrin are found in the gastric antrum, mainly G-17. Less gastrin is found in the duodenum, with even less in the upper jejunum, mostly G-34. Gastrin-34 is the main form of gastrin circulating in the plasma. Although G-17 is more potent with regard to stimulation of gastric acid secretion, G-34 is less rapidly metabolized; thus the two forms are equally active in this respect. Both histamine and acetylcholine seem to be necessary background influences for the maximum effect of gastrin on the parietal cell.

Gastrin is released by food (mostly amino acids), by vagal stimulation, and after antral distention, which is thought to be mediated by the vagus and local reflexes. While vagal stimulation releases gastrin, an inhibitory effect on the G cells by vagal stimulation can occur un-

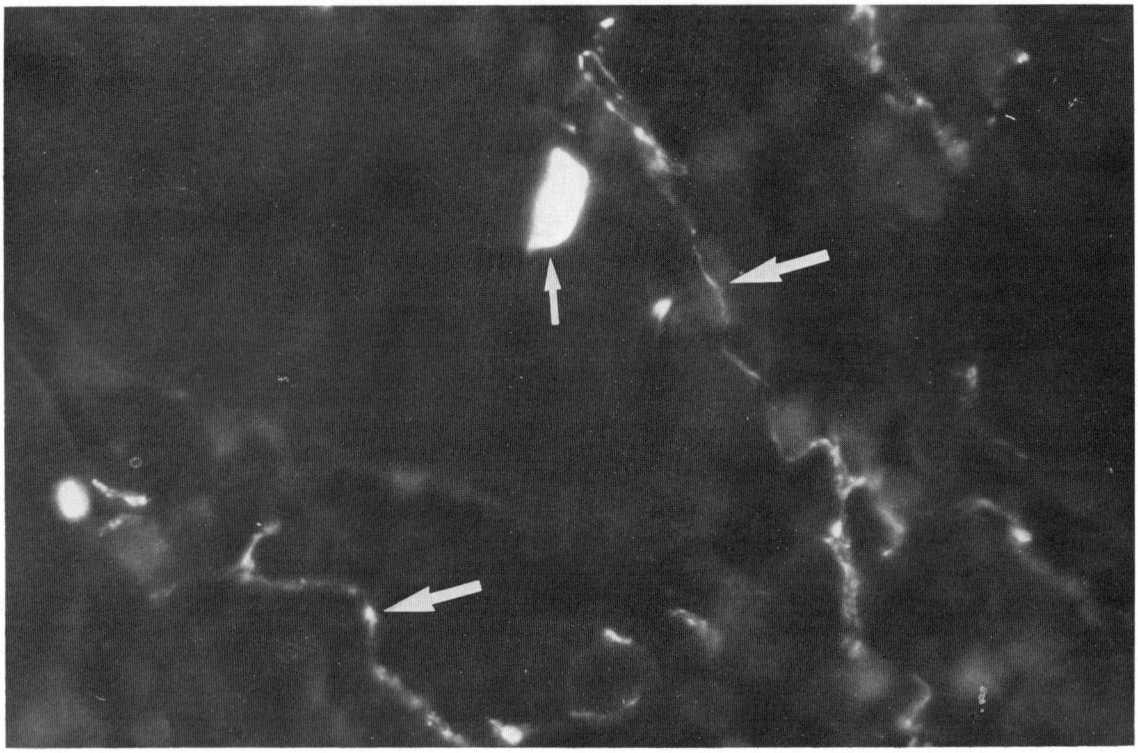

Fig. 3-18. Neuron-specific enolase immunoreactive endocrine cell *(small arrow)* and nerve fibers *(large arrows)* in the feline colonic mucosa. (×450)

Table 3-2. The main peptides

Circulating peptides	Brain-intestinal peptides
Gastrin	Vasoactive intestinal peptide
Secretin	Somatostatin
Cholecystokinin	Neurotensin
Pancreatic polypeptide	Cholecystokinin
Motilin	
Gastric inhibitory peptide	
Enteroglucagon	

der certain circumstances [58]; thus the part played by the vagus nerve in this respect is complex. Gastrin release is inhibited by antral acidification in a negative feedback mechanism, and by certain duodenal hormones, stimulated by the entry of acid and chyme into the duodenum.

While the effect on gastric acid secretion is its main property, gastrin also has a trophic effect on the mucosa of the stomach and duodenum [18, 28]. The possible trophic role of gastrin on the small intestine is in doubt. While some workers have shown a trophic effect of pentagastrin on the small intestine [40], others have failed to confirm this [33, 38].

SECRETIN

Secretin, the first intestinal hormone found, was discovered in 1902 by Bayliss and Starling, heralding the birth of gastrointestinal endocrinology. However, it was not until 1961 that this peptide was isolated.

Secretin is a 27 amino acid peptide, produced by the S cells of the duodenum and upper jejunum. It is released by duodenal acidification (pH <4.5), with only small amounts released postprandially (± 1 pmol/L). Its main action is to stimulate pancreatic bicarbonate secretion, an action requiring potentiation by cholecystokinin and vagal activity.

CHOLECYSTOKININ

Cholecystokinin (CCK), initially discovered in 1928 by Ivy and Oldberg, is a substance in duodenal mucosa that is capable of causing the gallbladder to contract. Harper and Raper in 1943 gave the name *pancreozymin* to a hormone capable of stimulating the pancreas to secrete enzyme-rich juice. It has subsequently been shown that these two substances are identical, and although the term cholecystokinin-pancreozymin has been used, traditionally the name cholecystokinin has been retained for this peptide.

The cell of origin of CCK is the I cell, and the highest concentration is found in the upper jejunum. Cholecystokinin promotes gallbladder concentration and stimulates the exocrine pancreas to secrete enzyme-rich juice. The stimulating effect of secretin on pancreatic bicarbonate production is potentiated by CCK. This peptide is also found in the brain as the C-terminal octapeptide, where it probably acts as a neurotransmitter.

GASTRIC INHIBITORY PEPTIDE

This 42 amino acid peptide is secreted by the K cells found in the duodenum and jejunum. Gastric inhibitory peptide is released postprandially and inhibits gastric acid secretion, although the physiological importance of this action is uncertain. It also stimulates the release of insulin from the pancreas in response to orally ingested glucose. The latter action has prompted its alternative name of *g*lucose-dependent *I*nsulinotrophic *p*olypeptide.

MOTILIN

Motilin is secreted by endocrine cells in the duodenum, jejunum, and to a lesser extent, upper ileum. This peptide is thought to play an important part in adjusting the motor activity of the GI tract. High plasma levels of motilin are found in basal conditions, with ingestion of fat causing a rise, and carbohydrates and proteins causing a fall. Peaks in plasma motilin level occur at the onset of a new interdigestive myoelectrical complex, and infusion of motilin can initiate a new wave of contractions. Motilin also has an effect on gastric emptying, with small increments stimulating and larger rises inhibiting emptying.

VASOACTIVE INTESTINAL PEPTIDE

Vasoactive intestinal peptide (VIP), a 28 amino acid peptide, acts as a paracrine hormone or peptidergic neurotransmitter, rather than as a circulating hormone. In the alimentary tract, VIP is produced in nerve endings and is present throughout the submucosa and muscle layers and within the myenteric plexus, where it is found in large storage granules within these neurons [15]. It has a powerful vasodilatory action, probably by virtue of its ability to relax smooth muscle. Pharmacological doses of VIP inhibit gastric acid production, stimulate the release of pancreatic juice and insulin, and promote glucogenolysis. Besides the GI tract, VIP is found in noncholinergic nonadrenergic nerves in many other tissues and also in all areas of the central nervous system.

SOMATOSTATIN

Somatostatin was originally isolated from the hypothalamus. Besides the central nervous system, it is also found in the gastrointestinal tract, where the greatest concentration is in the gastric antrum and pancreatic islet D cells. It is thought to act as a paracrine hormone or neurotransmitter.

This peptide has a wide range of inhibitory actions. Its original name, *growth hormone–release inhibiting hormone* (GH-RIH), arises from its inhibitory action on the release of growth hormone. It also inhibits the release of gastric acid, which has led to the suggestion that it may be of therapeutic value in the management of acute bleeding ulcers [44]. Other inhibitory actions of somatostatin are on the release of insulin, glucagon, gastrin, secretin, GIP, motilin, neurotensin, and enteroglucagon. Gallbladder contractions, gastric emptying and the secretion of pancreatic juice are also inhibited by this peptide.

BOMBESIN

Bombesin, a 14 amino acid peptide, is found in the GI tract, brain, and lung. In the GI tract it is maximally concentrated in the gastric antrum and upper duodenum, with small amounts found in the pancreas. The actions of bombesin are opposite to those of somatostatin, stimulating intestinal motor activity, gallbladder contractions, pancreatic enzyme secretion, and the release of gastric acid, gastrin, and enteroglucagon.

Gastrointestinal Hormonal Changes in Diseases of the Upper Gastrointestinal Tract

DUODENAL ULCER

Persons with duodenal ulcers secrete increased amounts of acid [4] and have more prolonged acidification of the duodenum [37] than healthy individuals. This is caused in part by increased vagal drive, an increase in parietal cell mass [22], and increased sensitivity of parietal cells to stimuli [26]. However, a number of findings suggest that some of the GI peptides may play a part in the pathophysiology of this condition.

Duodenal ulcer patients have a greater mean G cell count (18 million) than controls (10 million) [46]. Not only are their parietal cells more sensitive to pentagastrin compared with controls [26], but there also appears to be a defective acid inhibitory feedback mechanism on the antral G cells [57]; persons with duodenal ulcer require very high acidity (pH 1) to suppress their meal-stimulated acid and gastrin release. Thus duodenal ulcer patients who are normal secretors have a higher and more sustained postprandial rise in plasma gastrin level, while those who are hypersecretors do not [16].

It has also been suggested that there may be a failure of duodenal inhibition and neutralization of acid in duodenal ulcer. Two peptides, secretin and somatostatin, may be implicated in this defect. Secretin is normally released from the S cells of the duodenal mucosa when the pH falls below 4.5, and it then stimulates the production of bicarbonate from the pancreas. In severe duodenal ulceration there has been shown to be decreased release of secretin after duodenal acidification, compared with controls; this may result in inadequate neutralization of acid, although that may be a secondary phenomenon caused by S cell damage by duodenitis. Somatostatin is an inhibitor of gastric acid and gastrin release. Somatostatin is less effective in inhibiting meal-stimulated acid and gastrin release in duodenal ulcer patients than in controls [30], and ulcer patients also have diminished concentrations of somatostatin in their antrums [17] and decreased concentrations of D cells in their duodenums [43]. Thus somatostatin deficiency may be important in duodenal ulcer disease.

Bombesin, a peptide capable of stimulating the release of gastric acid, may play a part in this condition. An increased concentration of bombesin cells has been found in the duodenums of patients with duodenal ulcer [36]. Recently it has been shown that duodenal ulcer patients have higher postprandial plasma insulin, GIP, and GI glucagon levels [29] than healthy persons, and it has been suggested that the resulting hypoglycemia may activate the vagus nerve, resulting in increased gastric acid secretion.

HYPERGASTRINEMIA

Raised levels of gastrin in the plasma may occur in a number of conditions.

Hypochlorhydria. Here there is a diminution or loss of the normal acid inhibitory effect on the G cells, with resultant hypergastrinemia. This occurs under physiological conditions with increasing age, and with severe atrophic gastritis. Both vagotomy and treatment with H_2-receptor antagonists give rise to hypergastrinemia. In pernicious anemia, the serum gastrin level may be markedly raised because of the profound hypochlorhydria.

Short bowel syndrome. After massive small intestinal resection or severe small intestinal inflammatory disease, gastric hypersecretion of acid with resultant peptide ulceration may occur as the result of hypergastrinemia [53]. The mechanism of the hypergastrinemia is obscure; because patients with jejunoileal bypass done for morbid obesity have serum gastrin levels less high than patients who have had an equivalent small intestinal resection, it has been postulated that the small intestine acts as an organ for the catabolism and removal of gastrin [6].

Renal failure. Peptic ulceration caused by hypergastrinemia and hypersecretion of acid may occur in advanced renal failure. Although this may be explained partly on the basis of failure of disposal of gastrin, the mechanism is probably more complex.

Retained gastric antrum. Rarely, after gastrectomy for peptic ulceration, residual antral mucosa left at the duodenal stump site may give rise to hypergastrinemia, hypersecretion of acid, and recurrent peptic ulceration.

Hyperparathyroidism. The chronic hypercalcemia seen in hyperparathyroidism may lead to hypergastrinemia, hypersecretion of acid, and peptic ulceration. It is now known that most such patients also have a gastrinoma, although this may only become evident many years later with the development of a full-blown Zollinger-Ellison syndrome. Such patients usually have the multiple endocrine adenopathy type 1 syndrome (MEA 1), and parathyroidectomy is often successful initially in controlling the hypergastrinemia.

Gastrinoma. Gastrinomas are apudomas, which is a term used to denote a proliferative lesion, either hyperplasia or neoplasia, of the APUD cells. These lesions most often involve the pancreas. Zollinger and Ellison in 1955 described a condition (Zollinger-Ellison syndrome), characterized by severe peptic ulceration (often recurrent after previous gastric operations), gross gastric hypersecretion, and a non-beta islet-cell tumor or tumors of the pancreas. These tumors were later shown to secrete gastrin and named *gastrinomas*. A number of other conditions form variants of the Zollinger-Ellison syndrome. Antral G-cell hyperplasia gives rise to hypersecretion of acid and hypergastrinemia, but no gastrinoma is found. The number of antral G cells is many times the normal mean, yet it may be that this condition is simply an extreme in the spectrum of patients with duodenal ulcer disease, rather than a separate entity [46]. Retained gastric antrum, after gastrectomy for duodenal ulcer, may mimic the Zollinger-Ellison syndrome. Hyperparathyroidism giving rise to hypergastrinemia is probably part of the MEA 1 syndrome, and has been discussed. The hypergastrinemia is usually caused by hypercalcemia, but parathyroid adenomas themselves may also secrete gastrin.

The single most useful investigation in instances of suspected gastrinoma is the serum gastrin estimation. Values for fasting gastrin level vary from one reference laboratory to another, but in general levels of less than 50 pmol/L are normal, while levels above 100 pmol/L represent hypergastrinemia. Any patient with recurrent duodenal ulceration after a previous ulcer operation, or with gastric hypersecretion (basal acid output $<$ 10 mmol/hr), should have a serum gastrin estimation. Two provocation tests have been described for instances in which there is doubt about the diagnosis. The secretin stimulation test [51] involves intravenous administration of 1 IU/kg of the gastric inhibitory hormone secretin. In patients with gastrinoma, there is a rise in serum gastrin level (greater than 50 percent of basal), while in patients with hypergastrinemia not caused by gastrinoma, the serum gastrin level falls. With the calcium provocation test [31], calcium gluconate is infused intravenously (5 mg/kg/hr), and a rise in gastrin level occurs in patients with gastrinoma but not in healthy persons. Both tests, however, may give rise to false positive and false negative results.

Once a gastrinoma is diagnosed, it is desirable to localize the lesion in the pancreas, although many of these tumors are small or multiple, making detection difficult. Endoscopic retrograde cholangiopancreatography and scanning by ultrasound, computerized tomography, and radioisotopes have had varying degrees of success. Better results at localization of pancreatic apudomas have been obtained with selective arteriography using subtraction techniques [20] and transhepatic selective venous sampling [25], which can also detect hepatic metastases secreting a particular peptide. All patients with a raised fasting gastrin level should have an endoscopic antral biopsy to exclude antral G-cell hyperplasia. The plasma calcium level should be estimated, and if hypercalcemia is present parathormone estimations become mandatory.

Before the advent of the H_2-receptor antagonist, treatment for gastrinoma usually involved total gastrectomy, and, if possible, the primary tumor was removed. Although many gastrinomas are malignant, and thus often not cured by removal of the primary lesion, they are slow-growing tumors, and good long-term results have often been obtained by total gastrectomy. The advent of cimetidine has altered traditional treatment. Gastric hypersecretion can be controlled for prolonged periods with this drug, obviating the need for total gastrectomy as initial treatment [12, 34, 35, 45, 60]. The dose for individual patients may range from 1.2 gm to 3.6 gm per day to suppress acid secretion below 10 mmol/hr between doses. Favorable long-term results have been obtained with this approach. Some patients may require increasing doses of cimetidine to suppress acid secretion, and in some instances "escape from" H_2-receptor blockade may occur, thus making total gastrectomy necessary.

Pirenzepine has been shown to enhance the effect of H_2-receptor blocking agents [32], and it will be of interest to see if this drug is of use in the treatment of gastrinoma. Although some success has been achieved with anticholinergic drugs, chemotherapeutic agents have little beneficial effect in this condition. Patients with hypergastrinemia and hyperparathyroidism should have parathyroidectomy first. Patients with antral G-cell hyperplasia are cured by antrectomy and do not require total gastrectomy.

Gastrointestinal Hormonal Changes After Gastric Operations

Gastric operations alter the profile of some of the GI tract hormones, often profoundly, and it has been suggested that these changes may play a part in the pathophysiology of some of the syndromes seen after both gastrectomy and vagotomy.

GASTRECTOMY

The main peptide to alter after gastrectomy is gastrin, which is not surprising considering that gastrin is found predominantly in the antrum and duodenal bulb. A fall in serum gastrin level, both basally and after a meal, is seen after gastrectomy. The basal gastrin release is only slightly reduced after Billroth I gastrectomy or antrectomy, but very much lower basal gastrin levels are seen after Billroth II gastrectomy [14, 52]. After Billroth I gastrectomy or antrectomy postprandial gastrin release is significantly reduced [8, 9, 52], while no gastrin is released postprandially after Billroth II gastrectomy [52]. The difference in release of gastrin seen in the two types of gastrectomy is probably caused by resection of the duodenal bulb in Billroth II gastrectomy [50], because when the duodenal bulb is additionally resected after antrectomy or Billroth I gastrectomy, basal serum gastrin concentrations decrease significantly.

Hypergastrinemia after gastrectomy is found in the condition of retained gastric antrum. When antral tissue is retained in the gastric remnant, there is a postprandial rise in serum gastrin level [3] with production of recurrent ulceration in the gastric remnant, which can be cured by resection of the residual antral mucosa. Retained antral mucosa at the duodenal stump may lead to massive hypergastrinemia and recurrent fulminating ulceration, with signs and symptoms similar to the Zollinger-Ellison syndrome [54], and the secretin and calcium provocation tests may be required to differentiate the two conditions.

Besides changes in gastrin following gastrectomy, there are also changes in glucose homeostasis [13] and in release of insulin [14], enteroglucagon [11], and GIP [49]. There is a significantly greater postprandial rise in serum insulin, glucose, enteroglucagon, and GIP levels in patients after gastrectomy compared with controls. These changes are greater after Billroth II than Billroth I gastrectomy and the levels can be returned to near normal by jejunal loop interposition; it is thus likely that the changes are caused by rapid gastric emptying after gastrectomy.

The dumping syndrome may occur after

gastrectomy, pyloroplasty, or gastroenterostomy. It has been attributed to the rapid passage of hyperosmolar nutriments into the upper small intestine, resulting in a shift of fluid from the vascular compartment into the intestine, with a resultant fall in plasma volume. The levels of a number of humoral agents such as serotonin [42], kinins [59], enteroglucagon [11], neurotensin [10], and, more recently, VIP [48] have been shown to rise postprandially in the dumping syndrome. The part played by these hormones in the pathogenesis of this condition is unclear. Some of these peptides have been shown to rise in the plasma to a greater extent in postgastrectomy patients with symptoms of dumping compared with postoperative patients who have no symptoms. Furthermore, many of these hormones are vasoactive, and it has been suggested that they may be involved in the production of dumping symptoms by contributing to the fall in plasma volume in a situation in which the circulation is already compromised by osmotic fluid shifts [48]. However, it may well be that these changes are simply epiphenomena [23].

VAGOTOMY

After vagotomy, there is an increase in basal and postprandial gastrin. This is caused mainly by a reduction in gastric acid secretion and thus a loss in pH-dependent inhibition of the antral G cells. It has also been shown that there is an increase in G cells in the antrum [5] and gastrin content of antral mucosa [7] after vagotomy. The vagus nerve contains inhibitory fibers for gastrin release, and this inhibition may act by a humoral factor (vagogastrone) probably released from the antrum and duodenal bulb. Truncal vagotomy abolishes this inhibitory effect. There is evidence that the extent of vagotomy affects serum gastrin levels. Thus the highest postprandial gastrin levels are found after truncal vagotomy, followed by selective vagotomy, and then proximal gastric vagotomy; this may be the result of preservation of the inhibitory vagal fibers in the more selective procedures.

Basal and postprandial insulin levels are unchanged after selective vagotomy and proximal gastric vagotomy [47]. After truncal vagotomy, some studies have shown postprandial insulin levels to be reduced [1, 24], while other studies show them to be unchanged [47]. An increase in the basal GIP occurs following proximal gastric vagotomy and truncal vagotomy [19], while postprandial GIP response to glucose is increased after truncal vagotomy and pyloroplasty [56]. While basal pancreatic glucagon levels are not altered after selective gastric vagotomy or truncal vagotomy, the concentration of this peptide does fall during hypoglycemia after truncal but not after selective gastric vagotomy [47]. All types of vagotomy reduce the pancreatic polypeptide response to a meal [2].

Trophic Effect of Gastrin on the Stomach and Duodenum

The trophic effect of gastrin has been reviewed by Johnson [27]. There seems little doubt that gastrin is trophic to the gastric mucosa (with the exception of the antrum) and the duodenum. Most work relating to this effect has been carried out in laboratory animals. However, some clinical evidence supports the experimental data. Thus the hypergastrinemia in the Zollinger-Ellison syndrome leads to marked gastric mucosal hyperplasia [39], while after antrectomy or partial gastrectomy resultant hypogastrinemia may be partly responsible for the atrophic gastritis and decrease in parietal cell mass [21].

Knowledge of the peptide hormones of the upper gastrointestinal tract has expanded rapidly over the last decade, and our understanding of various disease processes has improved concomitantly. For the surgeon, this advance is well exemplified in the changes in hormone profile brought about by various surgical procedures on the stomach and duodenum. The future holds exciting prospects in this field, in terms of both diagnostic and therapeutic aspects of gastrointestinal peptides, and we can anticipate that some of these hormones, or drugs that mimic them or block their action, will be used in the management of some gastrointestinal disorders.

References

1. Aagaard, P., Decker, T. and Fenger, H. J. Serum insulin after intravenous administration of glucose before and after total vagotomy. *Scand. J. Gastroenterol.* 8:699, 1973.
2. Adrian, T. J. C., Bloom, S. R., Besterman, H. S., et al. Mechanism of pancreatic polypeptide release in man. *Lancet* 1:161, 1977.
3. Amdrup, E., Brandborg, M., Brandsborg, O., and Lovgren, N. A. Interrelationship between serum gastrin concentration, gastric acid secretion, and gastric emptying rate in recurrent peptic ulcer. *World J. Surg.* 3:235, 1979.
4. Baron, J. H. The clinical use of gastric function tests. *Scand. J. Gastroenterol.* 5 (Suppl. 6):9, 1970.
5. Becker, H. D., Arnold R., Börger, H. W., et al. Influence of truncal vagotomy on serum and antral gastrin and G cells. *Gastroenterology* 72:811(A), 1977.
6. Becker, H. D., Reeder, D. D., and Thompson, J. C. Extraction of circulating endogenous gastrin by the small bowel. *Gastroenterology* 65:903, 1973.
7. Becker, H. D., Reeder, D. D., and Thompson, J. C. Influence of vagotomy on tissue gastrin levels in the stomach and pancreas in rats. *Surgery* 74:744, 1973.
8. Becker, H. D., Reeder, D. D., and Thompson, J. C. Direct measurement of vagal release of gastrin. *Surgery* 75:101, 1974.
9. Becker, H. D., Reeder, D. D., and Thompson, J. C. Direct measurement of gastrin release from duodenum and jejunum in dogs. *Am. J. Physiol.* 227:897, 1974.
10. Blackburn, A. M., Christofides, N. D., Ghatei, M. A., et al. Elevation of plasma neurotensin in the dumping syndrome. *Clin. Sci.* 59:237, 1980.
11. Bloom, S. R., Royston, C. M., and Thompson, J. P. Enteroglucagon release in the dumping syndrome. *Lancet* 2:789, 1972.
12. Bonfils, S., Mignon, M., Jian, R., and Kloeti, G. Biological Studies During Long-term Cimetidine. In *Proceedings of the 2nd International Symposium on Histamine H_2-Receptor Antagonists*. Amsterdam: Excerpta Medica, P. 311, 1977.
13. Breuer, R. J., Moses H., Hagen, T. C., and Zuckerman, L. Gastric operations and glucose homeostasis. *Gastroenterology* 62:1109, 1972.
14. Breuer, R. J., Zukerman, L., Hauch, T. W., et al. Gastric operations and glucose homeostasis. II. Glucagon and secretin. *Gastroenterology* 69:598, 1975.
15. Bryant, M. G., Bloom, S. R., Polak, J. M., et al. Possible dual role for vasoactive intestinal peptide as gastrointestinal hormone and neurotransmitter substance. *Lancet* 1:991, 1976.
16. Byrnes, D. J., Lam, S. K., and Sircus, W. The relation between functioning parietal cell and gastrin cell masses in two groups of duodenal ulcer patients. *Clin. Sci. 50:375, 1976.*
17. Chayvialle, J. A. P., Descos, S., Bernard, C., et al. Somatostatin in mucosa of stomach and duodenum in gastroduodenal disease. *Gastroenterology* 75:13, 1978.
18. Crean, G. P. Marshall, M. W., and Rumsey, R. D. E. Parietal cell hyperplasia. *Gastroenterology* 67:601, 1974.
19. Ebert, R., and Creutzfeldt, W. Aspects of GIP pathology. In S. R. Bloom (Ed.), *Gut Hormones*. Edinburgh: Churchill Livingstone, 1978, P. 453.
20. Fulton, R. E., Sheady, P. E., Mellrath D. C., and Feris, D. O. Preoperative angiographic localization of insulin-producing tumors of the pancreas. *Am. J. Radiol.* 123:367, 1975.
21. Gjeruldsen, S. T., Myren, J., and Fretheim, B. Alterations of gastric mucosa following a graded partial gastrectomy for duodenal ulcer. *Scand. J. Gastroenterol.* 3:465, 1968.
22. Guiss, C. W. and Stewart, F. W. Histologic basis of an acidity in gastric disease. *Arch. Surg.* 57:618, 1948.
23. Hobsley, M. Dumping and Diarrhoea. *Br. J. Surg.* 68:681, 1981.
24. Humphrey, C. S., Dykes, T. R, and Johnston, D. Effects of truncal, selective, and highly selective vagotomy on glucose tolerance and insulin secretion in patients with duodenal ulcer. *Br. Med. J.* 2:112, 1975.
25. Ingemensson, S., Holst, J., Larson, L., and Lunderquist, A. Localisation of glucagonomas by catheterisation of the pancreatic veins with glucagon assay. *Surg. Gynecol. Obstet.* 145:509, 1977.
26. Isenberg, J. I., Grossman, M. I., Maxwell, V., and Walsh, J. H. Increased sensitivity to stimulation of acid secretin by pentagastrin in duodenal ulcer. *J. Clin. Invest.* 55:330, 1975.
27. Johnson, L. R. The trophic action of gastrointestinal hormones. *Gastroenterology* 70:278, 1976.
28. Johnson, L. R., Lichtenberger, L. M., Copeland, E. M., et al. Action of gastrin on gastrointestinal structure and function. *Gastroenterology* 68:1184, 1975.
29. Knight, N. F., Zahedi-ASL, S., Sanders, D. J.,

et al. Gut-glucagon and GIP may cause sufficient hypoglycemia in duodenal ulcer patients to activate the vagus nerve. *Gut* 22:A426, 1981.
30. Konturek, S. J., Zwieczek, J., Kwiecien, N., et al. Effect of somatostatin on meal-induced gastric secretion in duodenal ulcer patients. *Gastroenterology* 72:818, 1977.
31. Lamers, C. B. H., and van Tongren, J. H. M. Comparative study of the value of calcium, secretin, and meal stimulated increase in serum gastrin in the diagnosis of the Zollinger-Ellison syndrome. *Gut* 18:128, 1977.
32. Longdon, W., Longdon, V., Ruthe, C., and Weizert, P. Complete inhibition of food stimulated gastric acid secretion by combined application of pirenzepine and ranitidine. *Gut* 22:542, 1981.
33. Mayston, P. D., Borrownan, J. A., and Dowling, R. H. Effect of pentagastrin on small bowel structure and function in the rat. *Digestion* 12:79, 1975.
34. McCarthy, D. M. Report on the clinical states experience with cimetidine in Zollinger-Ellison syndrome and other hypersecretory states. *Gastroenterology* 74:453, 1978.
35. McCarthy, D. M., Peckin, S. R., Lopatin, R. N., et al. H_2-Receptor Antagonists in Gastric Hypersecretory States. In W. Creutzfeldt (Ed.), *Cimetidine. Proceedings of an International Symposium on Histamine H_2-Receptor Antagonists*. Amsterdam: Excerpta Medica, 1978, P. 153.
36. McCrossan, M. V., Polak, J. M., Bloom, S. R., et al. Duodenal bombesin cell pathology. *Gut* 18:A410, 1977.
37. McGuigan, J. E., and Trudeau, W. L. Differences in rates of gastrin release in normal persons and patients with duodenal ulcer disease. *N. Engl. J. Med.* 288:64, 1973.
38. Morin, C. C., and Ling, V. Effect of pentagastrin on the rat small intestine after resection. *Gastroenterology* 75:224, 1978.
39. Neuburger, P., Lewin, M., and Bonfils, S. Parietal cell and chief cell populations in four cases of the Zollinger-Ellison syndrome. *Gastroenterology* 63:937, 1972.
40. Panson, D., Berard, A., Dechelette, M. A., and Lampert, R. Influence of secretin and pentagastrin on the rhythm of cell proliferation in the intestinal mucosa in rats. *Digestion* 11:266, 1974.
41. Pearse, A. G. E. The diffuse neuro-endocrine system and the APUD concept: Related "endocrine" peptides in brain, intestine, pituitary placenta, and anuran cutaneous glands. *Med. Biol.* 55:115, 1977.
42. Peskin, G. W., and Miller, C. C. The role of serotonin in the "dumping syndrome." *Arch. Surg.* 85:701, 1962.
43. Polak, J. M., Bloom, S. R., McCrossan, M. V., et al. Morphology of somatostatin in gastrointestinal health and disease. *Gut* 17:816, 1976.
44. Raptis, S., and Rosenthal, J. Somatostatin: Potential diagnosis and therapeutic value. *Acta Hepatogastroenterol.* (Stuttg.) 24:61, 1977.
45. Richardson, C. T., Peters, M. N., Feldman, M., et al. Treatment of Zollinger-Ellison syndrome with exploratory laparotomy, proximal gastric vagotomy, and H_2-receptor antagonists: A prospective study. *Gastroenterology* 89:357, 1985.
46. Royston, C. S., Polak, J. M., Bloom, S. R., et al. G cell population of the gastric antrum, plasma gastrin, and gastric acid secretion in patients with and without duodenal ulcer. *Gut* 19:689, 1978.
47. Russell, R. C. G., Thompson, J. P. S., and Bloom, S.R. The effect of truncal and selective vagotomy on the release of pancreatic glucagon, insulin, and enteroglucagon. *Br. J. Surg.* 61:821, 1974.
48. Sagor, G. R., Bryant, M. G., Ghatei, M. A., et al. Release of vasoactive intestinal peptide in the dumping syndrome. *Br. Med. J.* 282:5057, 1981.
49. Schafmayer, A., Börger, H. W., Colle, E. F., and Becker, H. D. Glucose-Homeostase bei resezlirenden und nicht resezieren den verfuhren am Magen. *Langenbecks Arch. Chir.* (Suppl.):115, 1979.
50. Sjxödin, L., and Nilsson, G. Role of the antrum and duodenum in the control of postprandial gastric secretion and plasma gastrin concentration in dogs. *Gastroenterology* 69:928, 1975.
51. Stage, J. G., Stachl, F., Rehfeld, J. F., et al. Secretin and the Zollinger-Ellison syndrome: Reliability of secretin tests and pathogenic role of secretin. *Scand. J. Gastroenterol.* 13:501, 1978.
52. Stern, D. H., and Walsh, J. H. Gastrin release in postoperative ulcer patients: Evidence for release of duodenal gastrin. *Gastroenterology* 64:363, 1973.
53. Strauss, E., Gerson, C. D., and Yalow, R. S. Hypersecretion of gastrin associated with the short bowel syndrome. *Gastroenterology* 66:175, 1974.
54. Strauss, E., and Yalow, R. S. Differential Diagnosis of Hypergastrinaemia. In J. C. Thomp-

son (Ed.), *Gastrointestinal Hormones*. Austin, Tex.: University of Texas Press, 1975, P. 99.
55. Tapia, F. J., Barbosa, A. J. A., Marangos, P. J. et al. Neuron-specific enolase is produced by neuroendocrine tumours. *Lancet* 1:808, 1981.
56. Thomford, N. R., Sirineck, K. R., Crockett, S. E., et al. Gastric inhibitory polypeptide: Response to oral glucose after vagotomy and pyloroplasty. *Arch. Surg*. 109:177, 1974.
57. Walsh, J. H., Richardson, C. T., and Fordtran, J. S. pH dependence of acid secretion and gastric release in normal and ulcer subjects. *J. Clin. Invest*. 55:462, 1975.
58. Walsh, J. H., Yalow, R. W., and Berson S. A. The effect of atropine on plasma gastrin response to feeding. *Gastroenterology* 60:16, 1971.
59. Zeitlin, I. J., and Smith, A. N. 5-Hydroxindoles and kinins in the carcinoid and dymping syndromes. *Lancet* 2:986, 1966.
60. Zollinger, R. M., Ellison, R. C., O'Dorsio, T. M., and Sparks, J. Thirty years' experience with gastrinoma. *World J. Surg*. 8:493, 1984.

Special Comment

THE GASTRIC MUCOSAL BARRIER

David C. Carter

In the last edition of this book, Professor Horace Davenport in his authoritative comment on the gastric mucosal barrier considered that "interest in the barrier will wane, as all scientific interests do, but there will be a residuum of useful knowledge." Research developments in the intervening years have caused interest to continue, and their addition to the residuum of useful knowledge has increased our understanding of the barrier in health and disease, offering exciting prospects for therapeutic advance.

Mucus and the Barrier

Hollander [6] proposed that the barrier had two components: a superficial "mucous barrier" and an underlying "mucosal barrier" formed by the surface layer of columnar epithelial cells. Until recently the importance of the mucous barrier was often denied. It was argued that H^+ ions diffused through it rapidly and that it had only a limited capacity to buffer and neutralize influxing acid. Reappraisal of the structure and properties of mucus now suggests that the mucous layer does delay H^+ transfer by acting as an unstirred layer and by immobilizing water in its interstices, a characteristic dependent on its viscosity [17]. The viscous and gel-forming properties of mucus depend on the polymeric structure of its undegraded glycoprotein [12], and glycoprotein secretion rates must be sufficient to exceed the threshold concentration for gel formation and maintain mucous gel depth.

Indirect evidence suggests that the surface epithelial cells of antral and oxyntic mucosa also secrete HCO_3^-, but secretory capacity is only 5 to 10 percent of maximal acid secretory capacity. Basal rates of HCO_3^- secretion can be demonstrated in antral mucosa and fundic mucosa when acid secretion is blocked by H_2-receptor antagonists. Agents known to stimulate HCO_3^- secretion included carbachol, calcium, and prostaglandin [7], although basal HCO_3^- secretion was not increased by prostaglandin in isolated amphibian gastric mucosa [14]. If gastric mucosa can secrete only one-tenth to one-twentieth of the amount of HCO_3^- needed to neutralize secreted acid, it appears at first that this alkali is unlikely to contribute significantly to mucosal protection. However, useful protection might be afforded if the relatively small amount of alkali were held where it would be of most value, namely, in the unstirred mucous gel covering the surface epithelium.

Elegant experiments involving measurement of pH at varying depths in the mucous layer support this concept, showing that pH values rise as the measuring electrode passes through the mucous layer from the lumen [1]. During periods of non–acid secretion, continuous basal HCO_3^- production might make good any losses and saturate the gel, while increased rates of acid production might invoke additional secretion of HCO_3^- and mucus by the epithelium.

Mucosal Function and Barrier Integrity

Healthy gastric mucosa has a great capacity to resist free ionic diffusion, a fact reflected in the small amounts of H^+ that normally enter the mucosa despite a lumen-to-blood concentration gradient on the order of three million to one. Increased ionic flux during barrier damage probably results from increased passive diffusion of ions down their concentration gradients once the impediment posed by the barrier has been removed. However, measurement of the absolute rate of disappearance of H^+ from the gastric lumen does not necessarily reflect mucosal injury, and given rates of acid back-diffusion cause erosion formation in animal models only when other factors such as decreased mucosal blood flow are also implicated [16].

Silen and his group have made a number of critical observations regarding the relationship between secretory status and mucosal susceptibility to damage. They have shown that in vitro preparations of amphibian mucosa are more susceptible to injury when acid secretion is blocked by H_2-receptor antagonists [11] and that exposure to 120 mM HCl consistently causes erosion of unstimulated rabbit gastric mucosa but not of mucosa stimulated by histamine [15]. In the same context, the carbonic anhydrase inhibitor, acetazolamide, causes ulceration of rabbit antral mucosa without affecting the rate of luminal H^+ loss or degree of mucosal acidification [9]. The hypothesis proposed is that a secreting gastric mucosa can contend with acid back-diffusion by virtue of the HCO_3^- generated within it as part of the alkaline tide, whereas a nonsecreting mucosa, denied this defense, may ulcerate more readily when exposed to similar amounts of influxing acid.

In addition to maintaining mucosal metabolic and secretory activity, the gastric mucosal microcirculation may additionally protect the mucosa by "sweeping away" excess influxing H^+ and preventing mucosal acidosis. Some support has been provided for this thesis by demonstrations that intravenous HCO_3^- infusion protects the mucosa against injury induced by bile salt and hemorrhagic shock in dogs [5]. The protection afforded is not the result of reduction in the amount of influxing acid, but presumably relates to enhanced ability of the mucosa to buffer H^+ ion.

Mucosal Cytoprotection

It has been recognized for some time that prostaglandins, including the most recently described member of this group of substances, prostacyclin, are synthesized by gastric mucosa. The compounds prevent gastric mucosal injury in a wide variety of animal models, and at first it was assumed that this was a function of their ability to inhibit gastric secretion [4]. However, prostaglandins were found to protect rats against intestinal ulceration induced by indomethacin, a model in which acid secretion cannot be implicated, and the term *cytoprotection* was introduced to describe this phenomenon. It is now apparent that the cytoprotective ability of prostaglandins extends to gastric mucosa, and Robert and colleagues [13] have demonstrated that they protect against injury induced by such varied agents as absolute ethanol, 0.6M HCl, 0.2M NaOH, hypertonic saline solution, and boiling water. Cytoprotection is unrelated to antisecretory activity in that it is observed in the presence of exogenous acid, with doses of prostaglandin that do not affect secretion, and with prostaglandins that have no antisecretory activity. While cytoprotection by prostaglandins is now generally accepted, it is still uncertain whether agents such as cimetidine and anticholinergic drugs have protective actions over and above their ability to inhibit secretion [3, 8].

The mechanism of cytoprotection by prostaglandins is unknown, but as mentioned earlier, increased mucous and HCO_3^- secretion might prevent mucosal injury by reducing the amount of luminal H^+ entering the mucosa. Although prostaglandins are vasoactive, cytoprotection does not depend on altered mucosal blood flow as it is observed in isolated amphibian gastric mucosa [2]. Additional elucidation of the manner in which agents such as prostaglandins protect the mucosa from injury may allow considerable therapeutic advance, not only with regard to promoting healing in disease but also in preventing damage by prostaglandin synthetase inhibitors such as aspirin and indomethacin, which diminish mucosal production of prostaglandin E_2 and prostacyclin [10].

References

1. Bahari, H. M. M., Ross, I. N., and Turnberg, L. A. The "mucus-bicarbonate barrier": Demonstration of a pH gradient within the mucus layer of human stomach. *Br. J. Surg.* 68:365, 1981.
2. Barzilai, A., Schiessel, R., Kivilaakso, E., et al. Effect of 16-16-dimethyl-prostaglandin E_2 on ulceration of isolated amphibian gastric mucosa. *Gastroenterology* 78:1512, 1980.
3. Carmichael, H. A., Nelson, L., and Russell, R. I. Cimetidine and prostaglandin: Evidence for different modes of action on the rat gastric mucosa. *Gastroenterology* 74:1229, 1978.
4. Carter, D. C., Karim, S. M. M., Bhana, D., and Ganesan, P. A. Inhibition of human gastric secretion by prostaglandin. *Br. J. Surg.* 60:828, 1973.
5. Cheung, L. Y., and Porterfield, G. Protection of gastric mucosa against acute ulceration by infusion of sodium bicarbonate. *Am. J. Surg.* 137:106, 1979.
6. Hollander, F. The two-component mucus barrier: Its activity in gastroduodenal mucosa against peptic ulceration. *Arch. Intern. Med.* 93:107, 1954.
7. Kauffman, G. L. Gastric bicarbonate secretion: An update. *Brain Res. Bull.* 5(Suppl. 1):15, 1980.
8. Kauffman, G. L., and Grossman, M. I. Prostaglandin and cimetidine inhibit the formation of ulcers produced by parenteral salicylates. *Gastroenterology* 75:1099, 1978.
9. Kilvilaakso, E., Barzilai, A., Schiessel, R., et al. Ulceration of isolated amphibian gastric mucosa. *Gastroenterology* 77:31, 1979.
10. Konturek, S. J., Piastucki, I., Brzozowski, T., et al. Role of prostaglandins in the formation of aspirin-induced gastric ulcers. *Gastroenterology* 80:4, 1981.
11. O'Brien, P. E., and Silen, W. Influence of acid secretory state on the gastric mucosal tolerance to back diffusion of H^+. *Gastroenterology* 71:760, 1976.
12. Pearson, J., Allen, A., and Venables, C. Gastric mucus: Isolation and polymeric structure of the undegraded glycoprotein: Its breakdown by pepsin. *Gastroenterology* 78:709, 1980.
13. Robert, A., Nezamis, J. E., Lancaster, C., and Hanchar, A. J. Cytoprotection by prostaglandins in rats: Prevention of gastric necrosis produced by alcohol, HCl, NaOH, hypertonic NaCl, and thermal injury. *Gastroenterology* 77:433, 1979.
14. Schiessel, R., Allison, J. G., Barzilai, A., et al. Failure of 16-16-dimethyl-prostaglandin E_2 to stimulate alkaline secretion in the isolated amphibian gastric mucosa. *Gastroenterology* 78:1513, 1980.
15. Smith, P., O'Brien, P. E., and Silen, W. Secretory state of gastric mucosa and resistance to injury by exogenous acid. *Am. J. Surg.* 133:81, 1977.
16. Whittle, B. J. R. Mechanisms underlying gastric mucosal damage by indomethacin and bile salts and the actions of prostaglandins. *Br. J. Pharmacol.* 60:455, 1977.
17. Williams, S. E., and Turnberg, L. A. Retardation of aid diffusion by pig gastric mucus: A potential role in mucosal protection. *Gastroenterology* 79:299, 1980.

II

Diagnostic Techniques

4

Gastric Secretion Tests

J. H. Baron

Surgeons use gastric secretion tests to try to answer various questions: Does this patient have an ulcer? Does this patient have a gastrin-secreting tumor? Should this patient be treated surgically? What type of operation should I perform? Is a recurrent ulcer likely to develop? Have I performed a complete vagotomy? Have I cured the ulcer?

Although secretion tests may help to answer some of these questions, the test results can provide direct answers to only three questions: (1) How many parietal (or chief) cells are there in the stomach? (2) Are some or all of these cells innervated by branches of the vagus nerves? (3) Are the parietal cells being stimulated by excess gastrin?

This chapter describes how to perform and interpret standard tests of gastric secretion and specifies the clinical situations in which these measurements may help the surgeon. Recent work is cited, and additional information may be found in my monograph [13] and in reviews [7–12, 36, 53].

Procedure

A standardized procedure for gastric secretion tests will improve the reliability of the results and their comparability both with tests performed elsewhere and with published standards. The current protocol in the Department of Surgery, Royal Postgraduate Medical School, London, has been described in detail [8, 9, 13, 14] and is summarized in the following sections.

BASAL SECRETION AND PENTAGASTRIN-STIMULATED ACID OUTPUT

Basal secretion is collected as four 15-minute aspirates followed by a maximum stimulus of 6 μg/kg of pentagastrin given intramuscularly (IM) and by an additional series of four 15-minute (or six 10-minute) aspirates. If pentagastrin is not available, tetragastrin, 20 μg/kg IM; gastrin, 2 μg/kg IM; betazole (Histalog), 1.5-2 mg/kg IM; or histamine acid phosphate, 40 μg/kg subcutaneously, preceded by an antihistamine injection, will also yield the highest acid output from the stomach not yet operated on. Thin patients may need higher doses such as 8 μg/kg pentagastrin [95] or 50–55 μg/kg histamine acid phosphate [34].

Volume, pH, and titratable acidity (pH 7–7.4) are measured. Volume × titratable acidity (mmol/L) = acid output (mmol). Acid output can be expressed as the whole hour after pentagastrin or as the sum of the two highest consecutive collection periods; this peak acid output (expressed for convenience as mmol/hr) is approximately the same as the plateau acid output after an intravenous infusion of pentagastrin, 6 μg/kg/hr, an alternative but less convenient method of measuring maximum secretion.

THE INSULIN TEST

After the basal secretion hour, 2 ml of venous blood is drawn for determination of blood glucose, 0.2 unit/kg regular insulin is injected intravenously, and eight more 15-minute aspirates are collected. Further blood samples are taken at 30 and 45 minutes. Medical supervision is essential, and 50% dextrose should be available for intravenous injection if necessary. In healthy persons and patients with duodenal ulcer, single intravenous injections of insulin over the range 0.01–0.4 unit/kg give peak acid outputs higher (generally 0.2 unit/kg) than after either smaller or greater doses. After apparently incomplete vagotomy, most patients also give their highest peak outputs after 0.2 unit/kg of insulin. Peak acid output is correlated with the lowest blood glucose level as well as with the extent and rate of fall of blood glucose level, so the acid response to insulin is not an all-or-none phenomenon. Hypoglycemia provides a quantitative glycopenic stimulus that produces a quantitative vagal secretory response. The optimum dose of insulin of 0.2 unit/kg in most persons lowers blood glucose level sufficiently to elicit a maximum vagal acid response without reducing blood glucose so much that secretion is depressed. In some healthy persons and in patients after vagotomy, the greatest fall in blood glucose level and the highest peak acid output may occur after 0.1 rather than 0.2 unit/kg of insulin.

After the basal secretion hour and the 2-hour collection period after insulin administration, it is both possible and practical to perform a pentagastrin test, making this a 4-hour basal-insulin-pentagastrin test.

Intravenous Infusion

An intravenous infusion of insulin, 0.04 unit/kg/hr for 2.5 hours, does not reduce blood glucose as severely as a standard insulin test and has milder side effects, yet it achieves comparable acidity and acid output both in patients who have undergone vagotomy and in patients who have not been operated on [24, 25, 45].

SHAM FEEDING

In this technique the patient chews and spits out a tasty meal, such as steak and salad or a toasted sandwich. A mouthful of food is well chewed and then spat out, and the mouth washed out with a small amount of water to ensure that no food particles are swallowed. The chew, spit, and rinse sequence is repeated for several cycles for a total of 10 minutes, during which gastric secretion is continually aspirated with additional aspiration for another five 10-minute periods. Peak, or maximum, acid output is calculated as for pentagastrin-stimulated acid.

ASPIRATION, NEUTRALIZATION, AND LOSS

The stomach secretes an acid parietal component from the parietal cells and alkaline nonparietal components. These secretions are partly diluted and neutralized by swallowed saliva, mucus, and duodenal reflux. This pyloric reflux of bile and pancreatic secretion by the duodenum is variable; can be minimized by separate duodenal intubation; is greater after pyloroplasty, gastroduodenostomy, and gastrojejunostomy [38]; and can be estimated from measurements of chloride [51] or sodium [52]. Some gastric contents are lost through the pylorus, but recovery has been estimated at about 90 percent by the use of markers. Pyloric loss is probably a constant rather than a fixed proportion of secretion, so the effect of this loss is perhaps lower at the high rates of secretion associated with duodenal ulcer.

Table 4-1. Mean (and range) of basal and peak acid output (mmol/hr) in healthy persons and in patients with peptic ulcer

	Normal		Duodenal ulcer		Gastric ulcer	
Sex of subject	Basal	Peak	Basal	Peak	Basal	Peak
Men	1 (0–5+)	22 (< 1–45)	4 (0–15+)	42 (15–100+)	1 (0–5+)	23 (3–40)
Women	1 (0–5+)	12 (< 1–30)	2 (0–5+)	32 (15–100+)	1 (0–2+)	10 (1–30)

Source: Data from Baron [6].

In most published series no correction has been made for pyloric loss or reflux.

OTHER TESTS

A gastric residue of more than 250 ml 4 hours after a meal indicates pyloric stenosis.

Tubeless tests such as the Diagnex Blue dye tests, radiotelemetry, and isotopic scans are not reliable measures of basal or maximum acid output. They may give false positives and false negatives in the assessment of anacidity and are therefore not recommended for routine clinical use. However, serum pepsinogen I promises to become the first reliable tubeless test of gastric secretory capacity suitable for routine use.

Principles of Tests

MAXIMUM SECRETION AND PARIETAL CELL MASS

The gastric juice of patients with duodenal ulcer is significantly higher than normal in volume and acidity, both in basal conditions and in responses to stimuli such as test meals, caffeine, submaximal and maximal histamine, betazole, and pentagastrin [59] (Table 4-1).

This hypersecretion is of profound pathophysiological importance, but the results of all clinical tests overlap the normal range, so the various tests differ in their diagnostic value. The diagnostic value of a secretion test depends on (1) the proportion of duodenal ulcer patients who in a particular test have values above the upper limit of normal and are thus in the hypersecretory range, indicating duodenal ulcer, and (2) the proportion of healthy persons who in a particular test have values below the lowest value of patients with duodenal ulcer and are thus in the hyposecretory range, excluding patients with duodenal ulcer.

Estimates of basal secretion can help to diagnose duodenal ulcer, since about one-fourth of patients have significantly high outputs; the higher the basal output, the more likely it is that there is an underlying gastrinoma (Fig. 4-1). The diagnostic advantages of a test of maximum secretion are twofold (Fig. 4-2). First, the proportion of patients with duodenal ulcer in the diagnostic hypersecretory range is about one-third to one-half; second, and in many ways more important, there appears to be a threshold of peak acid output below

Fig. 4-1. Diagnostic discrimination of measurements of basal acid output. ZE = Zollinger-Ellison syndrome; PA = pernicious anemia. (From Baron [8].)

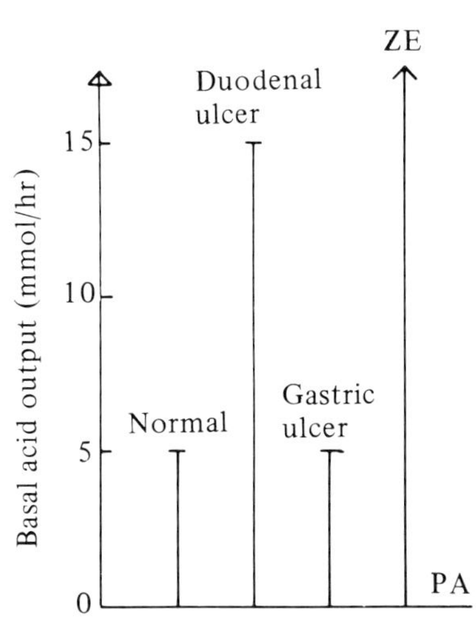

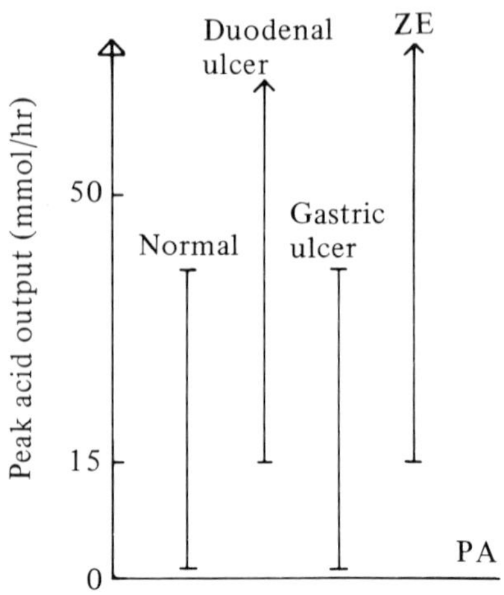

Fig. 4-2. Diagnostic discrimination of measurements of peak acid output. ZE = Zollinger-Ellison syndrome; PA = pernicious anemia. (From Baron [8].)

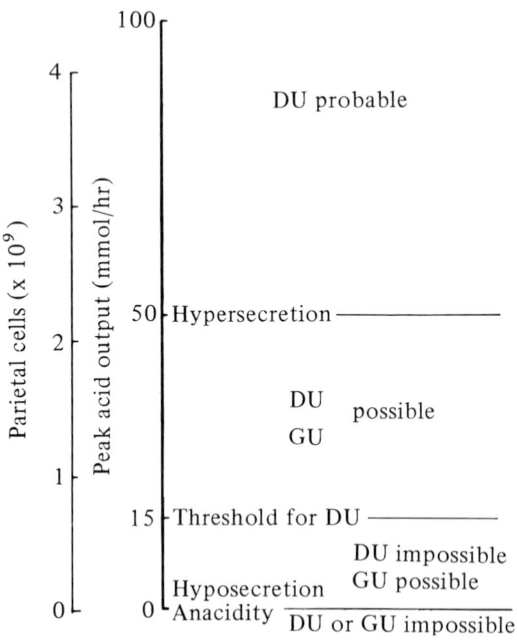

Fig. 4-3. Parietal cell mass and the secretory situation in peptic ulcer. DU = duodenal ulcer; GU = gastric ulcer. (From Baron [8].)

which patients with duodenal ulcer are seldom found [6]. This threshold is about 15 mmol/hr for peak acid output or 12 mmol/hr for maximum acid output, and it is similar in men and women. About one-fifth of controls have peak acid outputs below this threshold for duodenal ulcer. This diagnostic discrimination is of a similar order irrespective of the stimulant or its route of administration.

The difference in maximum acid output in different individuals has a morphological basis. The total number of parietal cells counted postmortem in the stomachs of patients with duodenal ulcer was double the number found in the stomachs of patients without ulcers, and there was a threshold parietal cell count of 10^9, below which duodenal ulcers were not seen, with about one-half of controls' stomachs having parietal cell counts below this number [32] (Fig. 4-3).

ASSESSMENT OF VAGAL INNERVATION

After vagotomy all phases of gastric secretion are markedly reduced. The reductions in basal and maximum acid output are similar for truncal, selective, and proximal gastric vagotomy, regardless of whether or not the vagotomy is accompanied by gastrojejunostomy or pyloroplasty. The "maximal" secretory response used in these calculations is the output following a conventional maximum dose of stimulus [2], even though it is known that higher doses of histamine or pentagastrin are needed after vagotomy to elicit the highest rate of acid secretion. A cholinergic stimulus can increase the "maximal" acid output after vagotomy, bringing it back to the preoperative level of acid output, indicating there probably has been no reduction in the number of parietal cells. The parietal cells of patients with duodenal ulcer may be abnormally sensitive to stimuli such as pentagastrin [60]. Although these cells are less sensitive to pentagastrin and histamine after vagotomy, it has not been possible to restore the preoperative output in humans. After proximal gastric vagotomy, both the sensitivity and maximal secretory capacity of the parietal (and chief) cells were reduced [96]. The Oslo group of Roland et al.

was able with carbacholine to restore the sensitivity of the parietal cells to prevagotomy levels, but in only two of nine patients.

Intraoperative Tests
Vagotomists in many countries are now reassessing tests that might indicate at the time of operation that there are still important uncut vagal fibers, especially if these tests can help them to locate and cut these residual nerves. The three most widely used are the electrical stimulation (Burge) test, the intragastric pH probe mapping (Grassi) test, and the Congo red test [35, 76]. Preliminary reports have suggested that these tests may lead to lower postoperative insulin-stimulated acid output and fewer recurrent ulcers, and adequate large scale follow-up data are eagerly awaited [2].

Postoperative Tests
Unfortunately, glycopenic stimulation of the hypothalamus produces both parasympathetic and sympathetic responses, and hypoglycemia may also affect the gastric parietal and antral G cells and the adrenal glands. The adrenal-sympathetic system may be a neural nonvagal pathway, but in the healthy individual, insulin-stimulated secretion is unaffected by α- and β-adrenergic receptor blockade [54]. However, β-adrenergic blocking agents reduce insulin-stimulated acidity and acid output after truncal vagotomy [46, 74, 94], possibly through release of gastrin by epinephrine [105], so some acid response after vagotomy may be caused by factors other than inadequate vagal section (Fig. 4-4).

Sham feeding by chew and spit [72, 112] evokes acid secretion from the stomach similar to that resulting from adequate sham feeding with an esophagostomy [64]. The sham feeding vagal stimulus is highly reproducible [39, 72] and produces comparable acid output to the insulin test, that is, about half the maximum. Sham feeding is probably preferable to the insulin test because it is simpler, safer, and less unpleasant for the patient. Moreover, it does not seem to have two other drawbacks of insulin: Insulin may stimulate nonvagal pathways, either those inhibiting gastric acid leading to a false negative result,

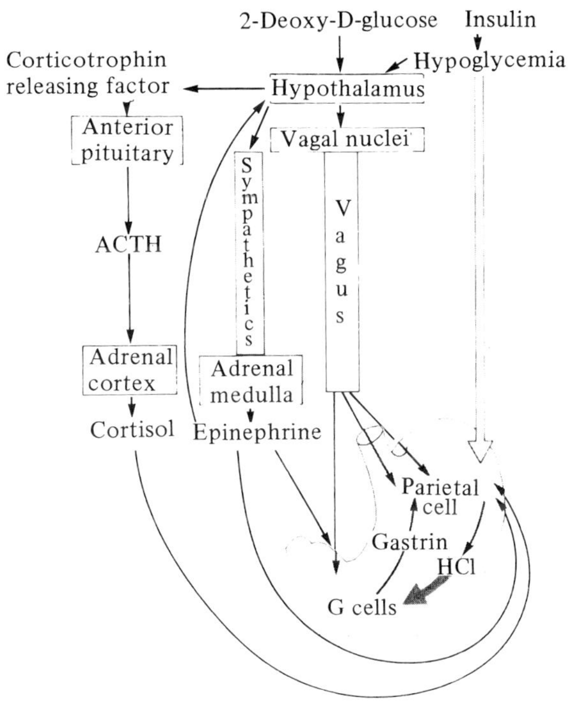

Fig. 4-4. Glycopenia and the stomach. ACTH = adrenocorticotropic hormone. (Modified from Hodge et al. [54].)

or those stimulating the adrenal-adrenaline-gastrin cells giving a false positive response.

Criteria of Vagal Activity
The insulin test is in general use for assessing vagal innervation, even if there has been no general agreement as to how to perform the test or how to interpret the results. The old statement that an insulin test was positive implied that vagal denervation is incomplete, and was arrived at by considering various qualitative (acid concentration) and quantitative (acid output) criteria.

QUALITATIVE CRITERIA. The Hollander positive criterion of an incomplete vagotomy (Δ [H] > 20 mmol/l, or > 10 mmol/l if [H] basal = 0) [55] was qualitative and arbitrary, as were the divisions into early positive (0 to 45 [97] or 60 minutes [62]) and late positive (after 45 or 60 to 120 minutes) and different criteria for men and women [103].

QUANTITATIVE CRITERIA. The quantitative approach uses basal and peak acid outputs after pentagastrin and sham feeding or insulin [3, 4, 5, 18, 37, 39, 57, 72, 109, 120]. Multiple criteria for assessing the completeness of vagotomy have been recommended by some researchers [5, 44] but were found unhelpful by others [33]. Some users of criteria assume that an insulin test yields a positive or negative answer and that vagal innervation is either present or absent. Today we no longer assume that a surgeon cuts either all or none of the vagal fibers to the stomach. No secretory value can be defined as an absolute dividing line between an incomplete and a complete vagotomy, and it is probable that the higher the peak acid output after sham feeding or insulin, the more parasympathetic fibers remain and the more likely is recurrent ulceration. Other approaches to peak acid output after sham feeding (PAO_{sh}) include subtracting basal acid output [72] and expressing PAO_{sh} as a proportion of peak acid output after pentagastrin (PAO_{pg}) [39]. This quantitative approach to vagally mediated gastric secretion is only presumptive in humans, but it has experimental support [89, 90, 110, 111].

Thus the task is to compare the various measurements after vagotomies with the incidence or absence of subsequent recurrent duodenopyloric or gastrojejunal ulcer rather than with the numbers of uncut vagal fibers, which are unknown. As well as using the many published criteria, Kronborg [71] followed, for six to eight years, 99 percent of 500 patients with duodenal ulcer treated by truncal vagotomy and pyloroplasty or gastrojejunostomy and used discriminative analysis to place the highest possible proportion of recurrences and nonrecurrences in relation to a critical level of secretion.

Kronborg's discriminative analysis was done for fasting, basal acid output (BAO), and peak acid outputs after insulin (PAO_I) and histamine (PAO_H) in 428 survivors by comparing the 27 patients with ulcer recurrence to both the 80 dyspeptic patients without ulcer recurrence and the 321 patients free of dyspepsia [68–71]. Unfortunately, these studies were done before duodenoscopy became available, so the criteria of ulcer recurrence were roentgenographic, and actual ulcer craters were found in only 16 of the 25 patients with ulcer recurrence who had reoperation [68]. The prognostic value of these calculated criteria was compared with the many older, arbitrary criteria, both for tests done before or 10 days after vagotomy, and for tests done three to four years after, since acid secretion may increase in the years after operation. Kronborg's results, which bear careful scrutiny, are presented in Table 4-2. Because the sensitivity and specificity of all tests are low, their predictive value and discriminatory ability are also poor [31, 68–71].

PEPSIN. A few patients after vagotomy may show a rise in pepsin concentration or output or both after insulin administration, without a rise in acidity or acid output [79]; therefore, Venables et al. [119] assessed residual vagal innervation as full, partial, or none by comparing the insulin-pentagastrin ratios of acid and pepsin.

GASTRIN. The serum gastrin response to hypoglycemia [49] is correlated, like the acid response, with the degree of hypoglycemia evoked by intravenous injection [29] or infusion [45] of insulin. The gastrin response may depend on intact vagal fibers [50], but there have been reports of rises in serum gastrin levels in patients after vagotomy with no rise in acidity or acid output [75, 104]. Gastrin measurements after intravenous infusion with insulin, as after single injections, do not give additional information of value in assessing vagotomy [45].

Serum pancreatic polypeptide (PP) levels normally rise after hypoglycemia. This rise is abolished by truncal vagotomy [99], but it is unlikely that PP is a valid index of vagal activity alone, and the procedure cannot be recommended as a tubeless test of vagal innervation.

INTERPRETATION OF TESTS OF VAGAL ACTIVITY. The Hollander criteria should be abandoned even though they are the oldest and most widely used, because they incorrectly imply an all-or-none vagal innervation and do

Table 4-2. Discriminative analysis of acid tests for ulcer recurrence

Discriminative test and result threshold	% recurrence in men 6–8 yr postop. in relation to test result threshold >	<
Preoperative PAO_H, 46 mmol/hr	21	5
PAO_H 10 days after operation, 21 mmol/hr	25	5
Reduction in PAO_H 10 days after operation to 68%	2	16
BAO 10 days after operation, 1.3 mmol/hr	22	6
PAO_I 10 days after operation, 1.5 mmol/hr	27	5
Hollander test 10 days after operation, + or −	26	7
Hollander test 3–4 years after operation, + or −	19	5

Note: PAO_H = peak acid output after histamine stimulation; BAO = basal acid output; PAO_I = peak acid output after insulin stimulation.
Source: Data from Kronborg [68–71].

not provide the best means of selecting those patients after vagotomy in whom recurrent ulcer has developed or in whom it is most likely to develop. It is more helpful to use quantitative statements of postvagotomy secretion, such as basal acid output and peak acid outputs after sham feeding or administration of insulin and pentagastrin.

THE ZOLLINGER-ELLISON SYNDROME

The Zollinger-Ellison syndrome of intractable peptic ulcer and gastric hypersecretion and a pancreatic tumor is usually caused by excess secretion of gastrin from a gastrinoma (see Chap. 18).

Acid Tests

Various criteria for the diagnosis of gastrinoma have been suggested, based on the acidity or acid output of unstimulated or stimulated gastric secretion and on various secretory ratios, such as the following:

1. Basal acid output more than 15 mmol/hr in a stomach that has not been operated on, or more than 5 mmol/hr in a stomach that has been operated on
2. 12-hour night acid more than 100 mmol
3. Basal acidity more than 100 mmol/l in a stomach that has not been operated on, or 70 mmol/l in a stomach that has been operated on
4. Basal acid output: maximum acid output ratio of more than 60 percent
5. Basal: peak acidity ratio of more than 60 percent
6. A disproportionate increase in gastric acidity compared with pepsin concentration.

Unfortunately, these criteria are not reliable and may lead to false positive or false negative diagnoses [7, 17, 19, 78]. A gastrinoma should be suspected if any of the criteria is positive or if the history arouses suspicion, even if some or all of these criteria are negative. A patient with a suspicious history should first have measurements of basal and maximum gastric secretion. Clinicians faced with suspicious clinical signs and symptoms or suspicious gastric hypersecretion (e.g., basal acid output more than 10 mmol/hr) should measure serum gastrin. Gastrin should always be measured in patients with recurrent ulceration after gastric operations.

Immunoassays for Gastrin

Immunoassay tests for gastrin are now available in special laboratories and provide a logical, definitive, sensitive, and nearly specific diagnostic test for gastrinoma [48, 82, 83, 91]. Just as in other endocrine disorders, blood levels of the hormone can be measured under basal conditions as well as after stimulation and suppression, and some laboratories can fractionate gastrin into its seven or more components [121, 122].

FASTING SERUM GASTRIN LEVELS. Fasting serum gastrin levels in patients with gastrinoma are usually well above the upper limit of normal for that laboratory (Fig. 4-5). Occasionally, the level may be in the normal range (Fig. 4-6). In patients with duodenal ulcer, the plasma gastrin level may treble within 30 minutes of a meal, but patients with duodenal ulcer may have fasting serum gastrin concentrations below normal because of the negative feedback control of the normal release of gastrin by antral pH (their basal interdigestive acid secretion keeps the antrum acid). A fasting serum gastrin level is thus of no value for distinguishing a patient with duodenal ulcer from a healthy person, but it is an almost complete discriminant for distinguishing a patient with duodenal ulcer from a patient with gastrinoma. The secretion of gastrin by gastrinomas is extragastric and autonomous and cannot be suppressed by antral acidification. Conversely, patients with anacidity, such as those with pernicious anemia, may have very high serum gastrin levels in the gastrinoma range, a situation that is analogous to the high plasma adrenocorticotropic hormone levels found in primary hypoadrenalism. In clinical practice, however, a patient with gastrinoma has basal acid hypersecretion and basal hypergastrinemia ("inappropriate hypergastrinemia") and could not be confused with a patient who had a false positive result because of pernicious anemia.

As with other endocrinopathies such as hyperinsulinism and hyperparathyroidism, patients with gastrinoma may not have continuous elevation of serum gastrin level. If the clinical situation is suspicious and a single serum gastrin value is normal, this measurement should be repeated; if the serum gastrin level is on the high side of normal, a stimulation test should be performed.

SECRETIN. Secretin, either as a single intravenous injection of 1-2 cu/kg or as an intravenous infusion of 1-3 cu/kg/hr, inhibits gastric acid secretion in healthy persons but may increase gastric acid (and serum calcium and gastrin) in some patients with gastrinoma [22, 23, 52, 66, 77, 84, 85, 98, 107, 115, 121]. This secretin provocation test was found reliable in patients with gastrinoma who had not been operated on, but after partial gastrectomy false positives and false negatives may occur [20].

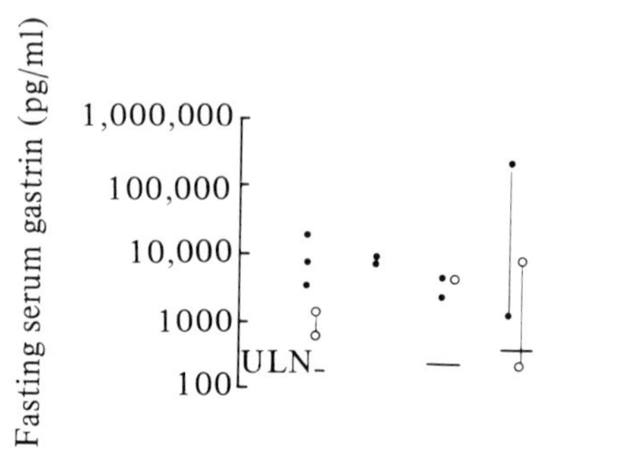

Fig. 4-5. Radioimmunoassay of serum gastrin in patients with Zollinger-Ellison syndrome (●) and with pernicious anemia (○). The upper limits of normal (ULN) are shown by horizontal lines. (From Baron [8]; based on data *(left to right)* from McGuigan and Trudeau [82, 83], Odell et al. [91], Hansky and Cain [48], and Yalow and Berson [124].)

CALCIUM INFUSION. Intravenous infusion of calcium (4 mg/kg/hr) for 3 hours can be given to patients with hypersecretion to raise the serum calcium level to 3–3.5 mmol/L (12–14 mg/100 ml) and to stimulate gastrin release [118]. In healthy persons and in patients with duodenal ulcer, calcium infusion produces modest increases in gastric acid (and serum gastrin), whereas in patients with gastrinoma, acid output usually doubles to more than 80 percent of the response to maximum stimulation, and serum gastrin doubles and rises to more than 500 pg/ml [15]. This test has now been simplified to a calcium challenge test with a single intravenous injection of 2 mg/kg of calcium [92]. If there is a very high basal hypergastrinemia, there may be little response to calcium, but the calcium test would have been supererogatory in this situation [121]. Calcium tests may be unreliable after total gastrectomy.

ANTRAL G-CELL HYPERPLASIA. Gastric hypersecretion and high levels of fasting gastrin may not be caused by a gastrinoma, but by hyperplasia of the G cells of the gastric antrum, as demonstrated by immunofluores-

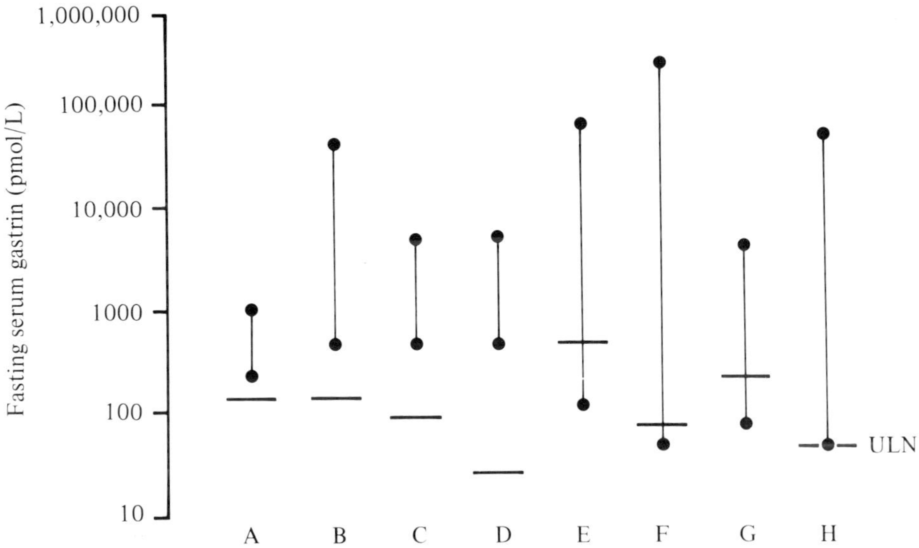

Fig. 4-6. Recent studies of fasting serum gastrin level in patients with gastrinoma. (From Baron [13]; based on data *(left to right)* of Korman et al. [65], Ganguli and Hunter [42], Lewin et al. [78], Moore and Wolfe [88], Stadil and Rehfeld [106], Walsh [121], Thompson et al. [116], and Straus and Yalow [113].)

cence studies of preoperative biopsies or of the whole antrum after antrectomy [30, 43, 93]. In this condition, as in gastrinomas, the hypergastrinemia is not inhibited by antral acidification. However, the hypergastrinemia of antral G-cell hyperplasia may increase further after a meal and decrease after secretin, whereas the hypergastrinemia of gastrinomas is unchanged by a meal and increased by secretin [41, 47].

A RETAINED GASTRIC ANTRUM. A retained gastric antrum after Billroth II partial gastrectomy (see Chap. 19) is a third possible cause of hypergastrinemia, gastric hypersecretion, and recurrent ulceration. This hypergastrinemia from an isolated antrum may be inhibited by secretin [66].

The plasma calcium level should always be measured if there is hypergastrinemia. Conversely, the serum gastrin level should be measured in every patient with hyperparathyroidism.

Use of Tests by Gastric Surgeons

ROLE OF PREOPERATIVE TESTING

Gastric Ulcer, Benign or Malignant

Patients with gastric ulcer have normal basal and peak acid outputs corresponding to the normal number of parietal cells in their stomachs (see Table 4-1). Tests of gastric secretion are therefore of little value in the diagnosis of gastric ulcer, because these patients fall within the normal range. A benign ulcer of the stomach can occur with extreme hyposecretion (minimum pH 6.1 for corpus ulcer, pH 3.7 for antral), and it is not possible to say that a particular patient does not have a benign gastric ulcer unless there is an absolute anacidity [40].

There have been many attempts, all unsuccessful, to distinguish benign from malignant lesions by various measurements of gastric secretion. It is true that more benign than malignant ulcers are associated with the following secretory states: (1) maximal acid outputs above 20 mmol/hr; (2) both an acidity of more than 80 mmol/l and a chloride concentration of more than 125 mmol/l; (3) an intrinsic factor output of more than 5000 ng B_{12}/hr; (4) protein concentration less than 400 mg/100 ml; or (5) β-glucuronidase activity less than 400 units. However, the overlap between the ranges of benign ulcer and carcinoma is too great for these measures to be of diagnostic help. The only definitive criterion is that absolute anacidity is found only in association with carcinomatous lesions, but it is found in only one-fifth of these [40].

Some doctors measure acid in these circumstances in the hope of being able to diagnose even 20 percent of the carcinomas. However, the carcinomas that could be picked out by the associated anacidity are likely to be large or infiltrating, are probably obvious by other diagnostic methods, and are likely to be incurable. This diagnostic yield seems too scant to justify routine gastric function tests in these patients, since the surgeon's time could be more fruitfully employed in gastroscopy, biopsy, and cytology.

X-Ray–Negative Ulcerlike Dyspepsia

Many patients with ulcerlike dyspepsia show no evidence of peptic ulcer on barium meal examination. Some of these patients are found on follow-up to have evidence of gastric or duodenal ulcer, or gallbladder or other alimentary tract disease; others probably have so-called nervous dyspepsia. A gastric secretion test cannot diagnose a gastric ulcer (discussed previously); gastroscopy can. Gastric hypersecretion may suggest the presence, and hyposecretion, the absence, of an underlying duodenal ulcer (see Figs. 4-1, 4-2, 4-3), but duodenoscopy is a more direct and useful procedure. Endoscopy, not gastric secretory tests, should be performed on patients with dyspepsia and normal barium meal studies because so few of them have diagnostic hypersecretion [86, 87].

Some patients with dyspepsia have radiological, gastroscopic, and histological evidence of hypertrophy of the gastric mucosa with hypersecretion of acid and pepsin and no excess protein loss in the gastric juice. *Hypertrophic, hypersecretory gastropathy* is perhaps the best term for this condition. It can be found in association with x-ray evidence of gastric ulcer, duodenal ulcer, or the Zollinger-Ellison syndrome; however, it may also be seen when there is no radiological evidence of ulcer, although duodenal ulceration may later be found at operation.

Relatively coarse hypertrophic gastric folds are also found in Menetrier's disease, but this is a hypertrophic exudative gastritis with edematous, inflamed mucosa. This exudative condition can easily be distinguished from hypertrophic, hypersecretory gastropathy by the results of secretion tests, which show excess protein but little or no acid in the gastric juice. Coarse mucosal folds may also be seen in the duodenum and have been correlated with histological duodenitis on biopsy as well as with duodenal acidity and gastric secretion. Less than half these patients have duodenal ulcers, but some develop an ulcer later. The acid output of patients with coarse duodenal folds has been found to be similar to that of duodenal ulcer patients as a whole, and very coarse duodenal folds indicate very marked gastric hypersecretion. The hypersecretion, histological duodenitis, and symptoms may improve after vagotomy [108].

These syndromes of radiological, hypersecretory, and histological changes in the folds of the stomach and duodenum are probably interrelated. The coarse gastric folds are probably caused by a large parietal cell mass with gastric hypersecretion that damages the duodenum, producing duodenitis, coarse duodenal folds, and eventually, duodenal ulcer [67].

Unoperated Duodenal Ulcer

In theory, tests could help in the diagnosis and prognosis of a duodenal ulcer. They could assist in deciding whether the patient should have an operation, and, if so, which operation should be performed.

DIAGNOSIS, ACTIVITY, AND COMPLICATIONS. The diagnosis of duodenal ulcer is normally made by radiologists and checked, if possible, with duodenoscopy. If the diagnosis is still in doubt, a test result of hypersecretion or hyposecretion can suggest the probable presence or absence of duodenal ulcer disease.

The activity of a duodenal ulcer is associated with higher levels of basal acid output, urine pepsinogen output, pepsin response to pentagastrin, and antral response to distention and broth than are found in patients with inactive ulcers. Such results are interesting, but they cannot help the clinician, who assesses activity from the history and, if possible, by duodenoscopy.

Complications are associated with higher acid outputs than are found in patients with uncomplicated ulcers. Peak acid output in patients whose symptoms recur at least once a year, necessitating hospitalization, was found to be significantly higher than in patients with intermittent histories and long intervals between symptoms [123]. In several series ulcers that have bled, perforated, or developed pyloric obstruction have been associated with higher peak acid output than those without complications [58, 114, 123]. These series were selected and retrospective, and the overlap between groups was complete. In the one prospective, consecutive series [21], there was no significant correlation between basal or peak acid output at the time of initial hospital admission and the severity of symptoms two to four years later.

INDICATIONS FOR OPERATION. In two series [26, 123] the patients selected for operation on clinical grounds, without consideration of secretory data, had significantly higher peak acid outputs than those chosen to continue medical treatment. Those patients who had high gastric acidity after an Ewald meal between 1936 and 1945 were significantly more likely, when followed up in 1963, to have had a poor clinical course and a higher frequency of gastric operations than those with low acidity [67]. However, the overlap between groups was complete, and two studies [1, 21] failed to show any such differences in the basal or peak acid outputs of patients chosen for clinical reasons to have medical or surgical treatments, nor was the acid secretion of patients who originally were selected for medical treatment but who were operated on during the follow-up period different from the acid secretion of those who continued with medical treatment.

SELECTIVE SURGERY FOR DUODENAL ULCER. Patients with chronic duodenal ulcer have a wide range of maximal acid outputs. If the hope of gastric surgery is to reduce gastric acid below a threshold level, and if acid-lowering operations tend to reduce gastric acid by a fixed amount or a fixed percentage, then patients with higher acid outputs should require an operation with more acid-lowering effect than is required by those with lower acid outputs [10]. Somervell and Orr [102] introduced the concept of selective operation for duodenal ulcer, advocating gastrojejunostomy for those patients without very marked hyperacidity and partial gastrectomy for those with excess hyperacidity. There have been at least 13 such schemes in which various increasingly radical operations with greater acid-lowering effect have been used for patients with higher acid outputs. A review of their results [8] suggested a paucity of convincing follow-up studies. The most careful data are from Edinburgh [101], where about a quarter of the patients who would formerly have been selected for Pólya gastrectomy are now treated by other operations; these operations, however, achieve only a slight reduction in mortality and in recurrent jejunal ulceration.

An adequate vagotomy is generally considered an appropriate operation for almost all patients with chronic duodenal ulcer if it is judged merely by the result that acid secretion of nearly all patients after this operation falls below the mean value of the normal population [117]. More radical surgical operations, such as partial gastrectomy, with or without vagotomy, reduce acid secretion more effectively than the less radical operations of vagotomy and/or drainage, but are they necessary and justifiable in view of the possible associated increased mortality and morbidity [10]?

Preoperative basal acid output and maximal acid output do not influence the postoperative incidence of recurrence or side effects after gastrojejunostomy, according to Clark and Kay [27], or after partial gastrectomy, according to Small et al. [101]. For truncal vagotomy and drainage operations, the data are conflicting. In three British series [16, 28, 31], recurrent ulcer was equally common in the lower and upper halves of the range of preoperative maximal acid outputs. These British series are small, and none of them can be compared with the 99 percent follow up study by Kronborg [71] of 500 patients studied six to eight years after truncal vagotomy and pyloroplasty (see Table 4-2). In these patients recurrent ulceration occurred at an unacceptably high rate of 21 percent among the one-third of men with duodenal ulcer who had had a preoperative maximal acid output of more than 46 mmol/hr.

If long-term follow-up studies in Copenhagen and other centers suggest that preoperative acid studies are of prognostic value, there will be a testable, formulated hypothesis of a rational scheme for selective acid-lowering operations for duodenal ulcer, as follows:

1. Higher acid outputs: an antrectomy and a vagotomy procedure
2. Lower acid outputs: a vagotomy procedure
3. Lowest acid output: gastrojejunostomy alone(?)

Policies of selective operation cannot be said to have proved their usefulness, nor have there been prospective, randomized trials of such policies. A vagotomy procedure may still be a suitable basic operation for all patients with duodenal ulcer (except those with gastrinoma or antral G-cell hyperplasia), whatever their acid status. It is possible that a more radical procedure should be selected as a first operation for a proportion of those patients with marked hypersecretion, but data to decide this point do not yet exist.

ROLE OF POSTOPERATIVE TESTING

Acid Tests After Partial Gastrectomy

Patients with dyspepsia after gastrectomy are difficult to assess clinically. Peptic ulcer may recur after gastrectomy, vagotomy, or drainage procedures in the gastric remnant, at the stoma, or in the duodenum or jejunum. Both radiology and endoscopy may fail to confirm or exclude such ulcers. Gastric secretory studies may provide diagnostic information [7, 14]. It is particularly important that the holes in the tip of the tube be positioned fluoroscopically in the gastric remnant. Technically, the test is less satisfactory than in the stomach not operated on because the stoma tends to increase loss of gastric juice as well as increase duodenal reflux. It is difficult to block the stoma with a balloon, but stomal loss can be measured with markers [38, 100].

EXCLUSION OF RECURRENT ULCERATION. As would be expected from the "no acid, no ulcer" postulate, anacidity after a maximum stimulus excludes a diagnosis of recurrent ulceration. There is no lower limit of basal acid output below which a recurrent ulcer can be excluded or even said to be unlikely. A recurrent ulcer is extremely rare if the patient's peak acid output is less than 1 mmol/hr, but there is no lower limit of peak acid output (except zero) below which a recurrent ulcer can be excluded.

ESTABLISHMENT OF A DIAGNOSIS OF RECURRENT ULCER. Basal acid outputs more than 5 mmol/hr are found only in the presence of recurrent ulcer, but such outputs occur in only about one-fifth of patients. Peak acid outputs more than 15 mmol/hr are unusual except in the presence of recurrent ulcer and are present in about half of such ulcers. Peak acid outputs more than 22 mmol/hr are found only in the presence of recurrent ulcer; however, only one-third of these recurrent ulcers are accompanied by such peak acid outputs.

Acid hypersecretion not only may indicate a recurrent ulcer but also may suggest a cause and a rational policy of revision operation. A high basal acid output that is little increased by maximum stimulation (i.e., a basal-peak acid output ratio of more than 60 percent) suggests an increased "basal drive" on the parietal cells, probably from excess gastrin. Such excess gastrin would suggest a search for a gastrinoma or a retained gastric antrum, as discussed previously. A low basal output and a very high peak acid output indicate a large parietal cell mass and suggest the need for a higher gastric resection or the addition of a vagotomy.

Acid Tests after Vagotomy

There are four possible reasons for performing some test of vagal innervation after a vagotomy operation [2]. The test may be done routinely after every vagotomy operation as a measure of the efficacy of the surgeon's technique and as a means of assessing the likelihood of recurrent ulceration in that patient.

The test may be done in patients with dyspepsia after vagotomy in the hope of determining whether the dyspepsia is caused by recurrent ulceration, and, if so, whether there is still substantial vagal innervation that needs exploration and division.

ASSESSING THE TECHNIQUE OF THE SURGEON. There have been two studies of the results of insulin tests after operations. Sheffield [63] found early positive responses in 13 of 54 patients whose vagotomies had been performed by surgeons in training, but there were no positive responses among 73 patients who had vagotomies performed by experienced surgeons. The first 24 vagotomy patients treated by one of Kay's surgical trainee showed the following pattern of early positive and negative responses:

1	2	3	4	5	6	7	8	9	10	11	12	13	14	15	16	17	18	19	20	21	22	23	24
+	+	−	−	+	+	−	−	−	−	+	−	−	−	−	+	−	−	−	−	−	−	−	−

However, in Leeds [61] the mean percentage of incomplete truncal vagotomies by nine consultant surgeons (18 percent) was higher than that obtained by 15 senior registrars and registrars (12 percent), even though the range was smaller among the consultants (8–45 percent) than among their assistants (0–52 percent). There were similar results after selective vagotomy, but there was a marked decrease over the years 1966–1970 in the incidence of positive Hollander tests after selective vagotomy.

Acid output tests are of even greater value to trainee and trained vagotomists in assessing the efficacy of their technique of denervation. In one center patients operated on by general surgeons produced more than twice as much acid in response to insulin than did patients operated on by gastric surgeons; these patients also showed more than 5 times the incidence of recurrent ulceration [56, 73].

PROGNOSIS OF THE PATIENT. Although the various tests described previously do indicate the relative risk of recurrent ulcer, there is overlap between the groups. Hobsley's group [37] assessed insulin-stimulated secretion after correcting juice volume (V_G) for pyloric loss and duodenal reflux. After vagotomy, of men with $V_G > 140$ ml/hr (that is, within the preoperative range), half had recurrent ulcers develop, and all of those with $V_G < 140$ ml/hr remained symptom-free (Fig. 4-7). The discriminant for conventional peak acid output was 8 mmol/hr (Fig. 4-8). Standardization for height improved discrimination slightly, retrospectively [80] and prospectively [81]. It is impossible to predict reliably in an individual patient whether recurrent ulceration will develop and whether any patient would therefore need more careful follow-up study. For this reason basal, pentagastrin, and sham feeding or insulin-stimulated acid secretion should be measured routinely after vagotomy as a quality control of the operative procedure rather than to predict which patients have a greater chance of recurrence. There are other reasons why patients should be followed regularly after vagotomy. Patients soon tell their doctors if their dyspepsia has returned, and those patients with recurrent symptoms can then have endoscopy.

DYSPEPSIA AFTER VAGOTOMY. Patients with dyspepsia after vagotomy are more likely to have recurrent ulcers, not only if they have positive Hollander tests or higher peak acid outputs after sham feeding or insulin administration, but also if they have higher basal or maximal pentagastrin-stimulated acid outputs.

Absolute anacidity excludes a diagnosis of recurrent ulceration. A low basal secretion with a low sham feeding or insulin-stimulated but a high pentagastrin-stimulated acid output suggests that the patient has a very large functional parietal cell mass, even if there is no obvious vagal or gastrin drive. High basal and high peak acid outputs after sham feeding or insulin, especially in relation to the pentagastrin-stimulated acid output, suggest not only that recurrent ulceration is likely, but also that it is associated with significant remaining vagal innervation.

Planning Revision Operation

A high basal secretion with a low peak acid output after sham feeding or insulin, especially in relation to the pentagastrin-stimulated acid output, suggests that any recurrent ulceration is unlikely to be caused by inadequate vagotomy; rather, it is probably caused

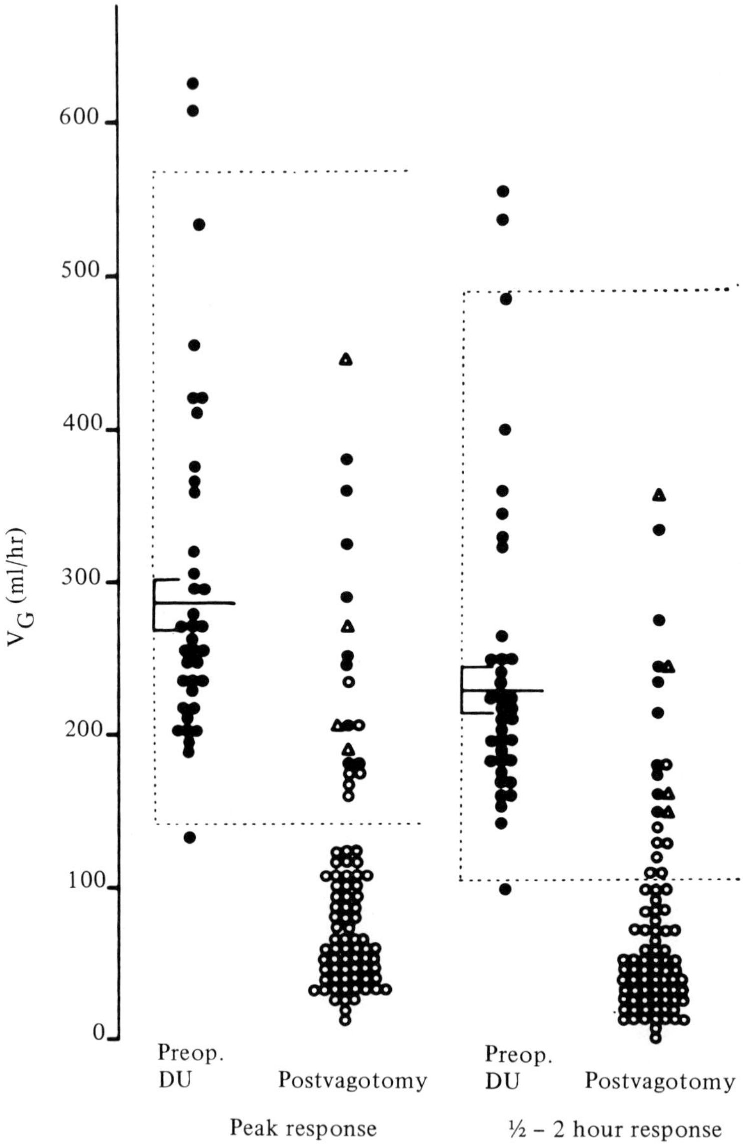

Fig. 4-7. Comparison of secretion, expressed as V_G, in duodenal ulcer patients not operated on and after vagotomy. Mean, standard error of mean, and 95 percent tolerance limits of the range of the unoperated group were calculated after logarithmic transformation. In the postvagotomy group: ○ = no symptoms; △ = recurrent symptoms; ● = recurrent ulcer. (From Faber et al. [37].)

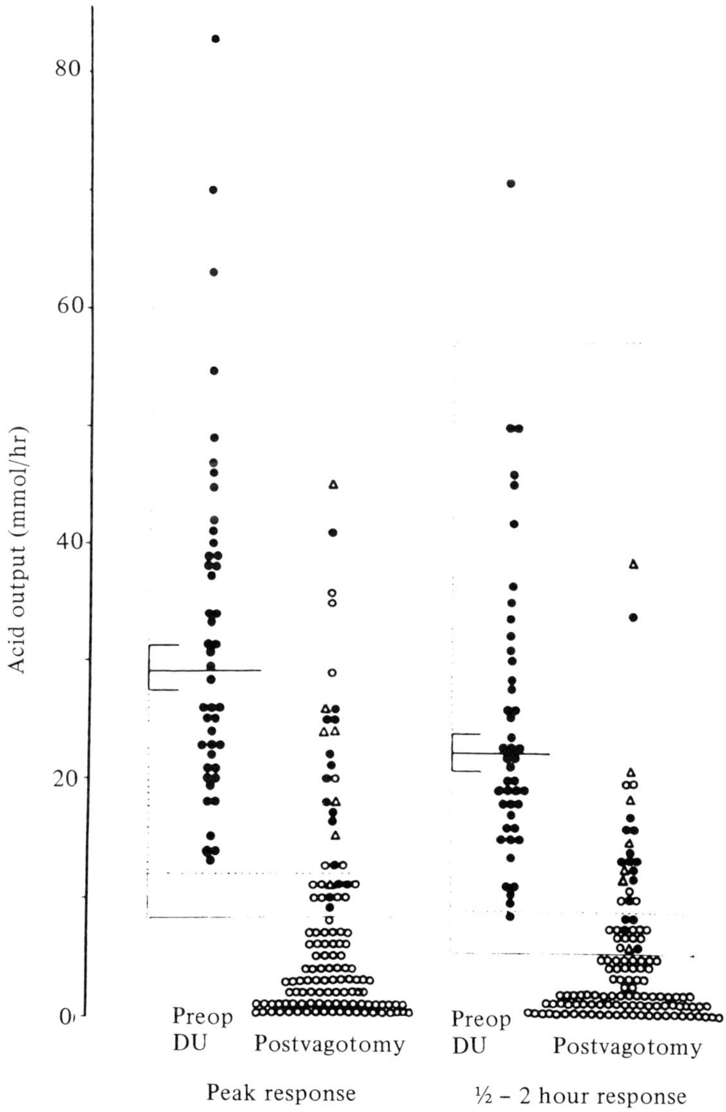

Fig. 4-8. Comparison of secretion, expressed as acid output in duodenal ulcer patients not operated on and after vagotomy. Symbols as in Figure 4-7. (From Faber et al. [37].)

by excess antral or extragastric gastrin secretion, which needs appropriate investigation (discussed previously). If, however, the primary surgical treatment for recurrent ulcers after vagotomy (except for gastrinoma) is antrectomy, then a repeat vagotomy is of secondary importance and the value of acid tests in assessing vagal innervation is also less important.

Thus after vagal denervation, routine basal, sham-feeding (or insulin), and pentagastrin-stimulated acid tests are probably useful as part of the systematic assessment of the vagotomy and of the surgeon, and in symptomatic patients these tests may be useful in the evaluation of residual innervation in planning a revision operation.

Acid tests are occasionally helpful in patients with x-ray-negative, endoscopy-indefinite, ulcerlike dyspepsia in that they may suggest that a particular patient probably has, or probably does not have, duodenal ulcer disease.

Basal secretion and pentagastrin-stimulated acid output should be measured in all patients before all operations for duodenal ulcer, in patients with dyspepsia after gastrectomy (serum gastrin should also be tested in these patients), and routinely together with sham-feeding (or insulin) in all patients after vagotomy as part of the assessment of the trainee surgeon rather than to predict the prognosis of the patient. These tests, and serum gastrin, should be done in patients with dyspepsia after vagotomy to seek a cause for recurrent ulceration and to help in planning revision operations.

References

1. Aagaard, P. Comparison of Gastric Acid Secretion in Patients with Duodenal Ulcer in a Surgical and a Medical series. In O. Gregor and O. Riedl (Eds.), *Modern Gastroenterology*. Stuttgart: Schattauer, 1969.
2. Baron, J. H., Alexander-Williams, J., Allgower, M., Muller, C., and Spencer, J. (Eds.), *Vagotomy in Modern Surgical Practices*. London: Butterworths, 1982.
3. Bachrach, W. H. Laboratory criteria for the completeness of vagotomy. *Am. J. Dig. Dis.* 7:1071, 1962.
4. Bachrach, W. H., and Bachrach, L. B. Re-evaluation of the Hollander test. *Ann.N.Y. Acad. Sci.* 140:915, 1967.
5. Bank, S., Marks, I. N., and Louw, J. H. Histamine-and insulin-stimulated gastric acid secretion after selective and truncal vagotomy. *Gut* 8:36, 1967.
6. Baron, J. H. An assessment of the augmented histamine test in the diagnosis of peptic ulcer. *Gut* 4:243, 1963.
7. Baron, J. H. The clinical use of gastric function tests. *Scand. J. Gastroenterol.* 5(Suppl.6):9, 1970.
8. Baron, J. H. Gastric Function Tests. In C. Wastell (Ed.), *Chronic Duodenal Ulcer.* London: Butterworths, 1972.
9. Baron, J. H. The clinical application of gastric secretion measurements. *Clin. Gastroenterol.* 2:293, 1973.
10. Baron, J. H. The Rationale of the Different Operations for Peptic Ulcer. In J. Alexander-Williams and A. G. Cox (Eds.), *Vagotomy on Trial*. London: Heinemann, 1973.
11. Baron, J. H. Acid secretion in duodenal ulcer disease before and after surgery. *Mt. Sinai J. Med.* 41:732, 1974.
12. Baron, J. H. Gastric Secretion in Duodenal Ulcer Disease. In J. E. Murphy (Ed.), *Aspects of Peptic Ulceration*. Cambridge Medical Publications, 1978. Pp 21–38.
13. Baron, J. H. *Clinical Tests of Gastric Secretion: History, Methodology, and Interpretation*. London, Macmillan; New York: Oxford University Press, 1978.
14. Baron, J. H., and Alexander-Williams, J. Gastric Secretion Tests in Clinical Surgery. In S. Taylor (Ed.), *Recent Advances in Surgery* (no. 8). Edinburgh: Churchill Livingstone, 1973.
15. Basso, N., and Passaro, E. Calcium stimulated gastric secretion in the Zollinger-Ellison syndrome. *Arch. Surg.* 101:399, 1970.
16. Bell, P. R. F., Checketts, R. G., Johnston, D., and Duthie, H. L. Augmented histamine response after incomplete vagotomy. *Lancet* 2:978, 1965.
17. Bernades, P., Mignon, M., Bensalem, R., Dubrasquet, M., Bader, J. P., and Bonfils, S. Discriminative interest of the study of basal acid secretion and pepsin acid correlation in Zollinger-Ellison syndrome and peptic ulcer. *Digestion* 9:1, 1973.

18. Bitsch, V., Christiansen, P. M., Faber, V., and Rødbro, P. Gastric Secretory pattens before and after vagotomy. *Lancet* 1:1288, 1966.
19. Bonfils, S., and Bernades, P. Zollinger-Ellison syndrome: Natural history and diagnosis. *Clin. Gastroenterol.* 3:539, 1974.
20. Bonfils, S. Mignon, M., and Accary, J. P. The secretin provocation test in the diagnosis of Zollinger-Ellison syndrome. *Gut.* 15:841, 1974.
21. Bonnevie, O., Kallehauge, H. E., Wulff, H. R., and Wulff, M. R. Prognostic value of the augmented histamine test in ulcer disease and x-ray negative dyspepsia. *Scand. J. Gastroenterol.* 6:727, 1971.
22. Bradley, E. L., and Galambos, J. T. Failure of a secretin feedback loop in the Zollinger-Ellison syndrome? The gastric factor revisited. *Am. J. Dig. Dis.* 17:939, 1972.
23. Bradley, E. L., Galambos, J. T., Lobley, C. R., and Chan, Y. K. Secretin-gastrin relationships in Zollinger-Ellison syndrome. *Surgery* 1:73:550, 1973.
24. Carter, D. C., Dozois, R. R., and Kirkpatrick, J. R. Insulin infusion test of gastric secretion. *Br. Med. J.* 2:202, 1972.
25. Carter, D. C., Dozois, R. R., and Kirkpatrick, J. R. Gastric secretory response to insulin infusion in vagotomised subjects. *Br. J. Surg.* 60:702, 1973.
26. Christiansen, P. M. Gastric Secretion in Relation to Duodenal and Gastric Ulcer. In L. S. Semb and J. Myren (Eds.), *The Physiology of Gastric Secretion.* Oslo: Universitetsforlaget, 1968.
27. Clark, D. H., and Kay, A. W. The results of partial gastrectomy and selected gastrojejunostomy in treatment of duodenal ulcer. *Scott. Med. J.* 4:158, 1959.
28. Clark, C. G., Murray, J. G. Slessor, I. M., and Wyllie, J. H. Complete vagotomy and its consequences: Follow-up of 146 patients. *Br. Med. J.* 2:900, 1964.
29. Cowley, D. J., Baron, J. H., Hansky, J., and Korman, M. G. The effect of insulin hypoglycaemia on serum gastrin and gastric acid in normal subjects and patients with duodenal ulcer. *Br. J. Surg.* 60:438, 1973.
30. Cowley, D. J. Dymock, I. W., Boyes, B. E., Wilson, R. G., Stagg, B. H., Lewin, M. R., Polak, J. M., and Pearse, A. G. E. Zollinger-Ellison syndrome type I: Clinical and pathological correlations in a case. *Gut* 14:25, 1973.
31. Cowley, D. J., Spencer, J., and Baron, J. H. Acid secretion in relation to recurrence of duodenal ulcer after vagotomy and drainage. *Br. J. Surg.* 60:517, 1973.
32. Cox, A. J. Stomach size and its relation to chronic peptic ulcer. *Arch. Pathol.* 54:407, 1952.
33. Decker, G. A. G. An assessment of vagotomy by means of the insulin test using different criteria of a positive response. *S. Afr. Med. J.* 43:867, 1969.
34. Desai, H. G., Anita, F. P., Gupte, U. V., and Potnis, P. R. Dose of histamine for maximal stimulation of gastric acid secretion. *Gastroenterology* 57:636, 1969.
35. Donahue, P. E., and Nyhus, L. M. The simplified endoscopic Congo red test. *Surg. Gynecol. Obstet.* In press, 1986.
36. Elder, J. B., Ganguli, P. C. Gastric Function. In S. S. Brown, E. L. Mitchell, and D. S. Young (Eds.), *Chemical Diagnosis of Disease.* Amsterdam: Elsevier, 1979. Pp. 663-88.
37. Faber, R. G., Russell, R. C. G., Parkin, J. V., Whitfield, P., and Hobsley, M. The predictive accuracy of the postvagotomy insulin test: A new interpretation. *Gut* 16:337, 1975.
38. Faber, R. G., Russell, R. C. G., Royston, C. M. S., Whitfield, P., and Hobsley, M. Duodenal reflux during insulin-stimulated secretion. *Gut* 15:880, 1974.
39. Feldman, M., Richardson, C. T., and Fordtran, J. S. Experience with sham feeding as a test for vagotomy. *Gastroenterology* 79:792, 1980.
40. Fischermann, K., and Køster, K. H. The augmented histamine test in the differential diagnosis between ulcer and cancer of the stomach. *Gut* 3:211, 1962.
41. Ganguli, P. C., Elder, J. B., Polak, J. M., and Pearse, A. G. E. Antral-gastrin cell hyperplasia in peptic-ulcer disease. *Lancet* 1:1288, 1974.
42. Ganguli, P. C. and Hunter, W. M. Radioimmunoassay of gastrin in human plasma. *J. Physiol.* 220:499, 1972.
43. Ganguli, P. C., Pearse, A. G. E., Polak, J. M., Elder, J. B., and Hegarty, M. Antral-gastrin-cell hyperplasia in peptic-ulcer disease. *Lancet* 1:583, 1974.
44. Gillespie, G., Gillespie, I. E., and Kay, A. W. An analysis of the insulin test after vagotomy using single and multiple criteria. *Gut* 9:470, 1968.
45. Girvan, D. P., Hansky, J. Spencer, J., and Baron, J. H. The response of gastric secretion and serum gastrin to an insulin infusion in pa-

tients with duodenal ulcer. *Am. J. Dig. Dis.* 19:977, 1974.
46. Hall, W. H., Durkin, M. G., and Read, R. C. Propranolol and serum gastrin in post-vagotomy insulin tests. *Digestion* 9:325, 1973.
47. Hansky, J. Antral-gastrin-cell hyperplasia in peptic ulcer disease, *Lancet* 1:1344, 1974.
48. Hansky, J., and Cain, M. D. Radioimmunoassay of gastrin in human serum. *Lancet* 2:1388, 1969.
49. Hansky, J., Korman, M. G., Cowley, D. J., and Baron, J. H. Serum gastrin in duodenal ulcer: II. Effect of insulin hypoglycaemia. *Gut* 12:959, 1971.
50. Hansky, J., Soveny, C., and Korman, M. G. Role of the vagus in insulin-mediated gastrin release. *Gastroenterology* 63:387, 1972.
51. Hassan, M. A., Gardham, J. R., and Hobsley, M. Evaluation of errors in gastric secretion studies, *Br. J. Surg.* 56:384, 1969.
52. Hobsley, M. Pyloric reflux: A modification of the two-component hypothesis of gastric secretion. *Clin. Sci. Mol. Med.* 47:131, 1974.
53. Hobsley, M. Tests of Gastric Secretory Function. In W. Sircus and A. N. Smith (Eds.), *Scientific Foundations of Gastroenterology*. London: Heinemann, 1980. Pp. 316–332.
54. Hodge, A. J., Masarei, J. R., and Catchpole, B. N. The role of the sympathetic nervous system in hypoglycaemia-stimulated gastric secretion. *Gut* 13:341, 1972.
55. Hollander, F. The insulin test for the presence of intact nerve fibres after vagal operations for peptic ulcer. *Gastroenterology* 7:607, 1946.
56. Holst-Christensen, J., Hansen, O. H., Pedersen, T., and Kronborg, O. Recurrent ulcer after proximal gastric vagotomy for duodenal and pre-pyloric ulcer. *Br. J. Surg.* 64:42, 1977.
57. Hubel, K. A. Insulin-induced gastric acid secretion in young men. *Gastroenterology* 50:24, 1966.
58. Hunt, J. N., and Kay, A. W. The nature of gastric hypersecretion of acid in patients with duodenal ulcer. *Br. Med. J.* 2:1444, 1954.
59. Isenberg, J. I., Walsh, J. H., Best, W. R., and Grossman, M. I. Effect of graded doses of pentagastrin on gastric acid secretion in duodenal ulcer and non-duodenal ulcer subjects. *Gastroenterology* 62:764, 1972.
60. Isenberg, J. I., Walsh, J. H., Passaro, E., Moore, E. W., and Grossman, M. I. Unusual effect of secretin on serum gastrin, serum calcium and gastric acid secretion in a patient with suspected Zollinger-Ellison syndrome. *Gastroenterology* 62:626, 1972.
61. Johnston, D., and Goligher, J. C. The influence of the individual surgeon and of the type of vagotomy upon the insulin test after vagotomy. *Gut* 12:963, 1971.
62. Johnston, D., Thomas, D. G., Checketts, R. G., and Duthie, H. L. An assessment of postoperative testing for completeness of vagotomy. *Br. J. Surg.* 54:831, 1967.
63. Kay, A. W. Introduction. In J. Alexander Williams and A. G. Cox (Eds.), *After Vagotomy*. London: Butterworth, 1969.
64. Knutson, U., and Olbe, L. Gastric acid response to sham feeding in the duodenal ulcer patient. *Scand. J. Gastroenterol.* 8:513, 1973.
65. Korman, M. G., Soveny, C., and Hansky, J. Serum gastrin in duodenal ulcer. I. Basal levels and effects of food and atropine. *Gut* 12:899, 1971.
66. Korman, M. G., Soveny, C., and Hansky, J. Paradoxical effect of secretin on serum immunoreactive gastrin in the Zollinger-Ellison syndrome. *Digestion* 8:407, 1973.
67. Krag, E. Enlarged gastric and duodenal rugae: The prognostic significance of the radiological finding of coarse mucosal folds in the stomach and duodenum. *Acta Med. Scand.* 179:343, 1966.
68. Kronborg, O. The value of the insulin test in predicting recurrence after vagotomy and drainage for duodenal ulcer. *Scand. J. Gastroenterol.* 6:471, 1971.
69. Kronborg, O. Influence of the number of parietal cells on risk of recurrence after truncal vagotomy and drainage for duodenal ulcer. *Scand. J. Gastroenterol.* 7:423, 1972.
70. Kronborg, O. The discriminatory ability of gastric acid secretion tests in the diagnosis of recurrence after truncal vagotomy and drainage operations for duodenal ulcer. *Scand. J. Gastroenterol.* 8:483, 1973.
71. Kronborg, O. Gastric acid secretion and risk of recurrence of duodenal ulcer within 6–8 years after truncal vagotomy and drainage. *Gut* 15:714, 1974.
72. Kronborg, O., and Andersen, D. Acid response to sham feeding as a test for completeness of vagotomy. *Scand. J. Gastroenterol.* 15:119, 1980.
73. Kronborg, O., Joergensen, P. M., Hart Hansen, O., Pedersen, T. Assessment of completeness of vagotomy and surgical experience 10 days and 3 months after proximal gastric vagotomy. *Acta Chir. Scand.* 144:495, 1978.

74. Kronborg, O., Pedersen, T., Stadil, F., and Rehfeld, J. F. The effect of beta-adrenergic blockade upon gastric acid secretion and gastrin secretion during hypoglycaemia before and after vagotomy. *Scand J. Gastroenterol.* 9:173, 1974.
75. Kronborg, O., Stadil, F., Rehfeld, J., and Christiansen, P. M. Relationship between serum gastrin concentrations and gastric acid secretion in duodenal ulcer patients before and after selective and highly selective vagotomy. *Scand. J. Gastroenterol.* 8:491, 1973.
76. Kusakari, K., Nyhus, L. M., Gillison, E. W., and Bombeck, C. T. An endoscopic test for completeness of vagotomy. *Arch. Surg.* 105:386, 1972.
77. Lamers, C. B. H., and Van Tongeren, J. H. M., Comparative study of the value of calcium, secretin, and meal-stimulated increase in serum gastrin to the diagnosis of the Zollinger-Ellison syndrome. *Gut* 18:128, 1977.
78. Lewin, M. R., Stagg, B. H., and Clark, C. G. Gastric acid secretion in the diagnosis of Zollinger-Ellison syndrome. *Br. Med. J.* 2:139, 1973.
79. Limbosch, J. M., Woussen-Colle, M. C., and deGraef, J. Acid and pepsin secretion in response to insulin after truncal vagotomy in man. *Digestion* 4:281, 1971.
80. Maybury, N. K., Faber, R. G., and Hobsley, M. Post-vagotomy insulin test: Improved predictability of ulcer recurrence after corrections for height and collection errors. *Gut* 18:449, 1977.
81. Maybury, N. K., Faber, R. G., and Hobsley, M. A new interpretation of the insulin test validated and the usefulness of the Burge test confirmed. *Gut* 18:A405, 1977.
82. McGuigan, J. E., and Trudeau, W. L. Immunochemical measurement of elevated levels of gastrin in the serum of patients with pancreatic tumors of the Zollinger-Ellison variety. *N. Engl. J. Med.* 278:1308, 1968.
83. McGuigan, J. E., and Trudeau, W. L. Studies with antibodies to gastrin: Radioimmunoassay in human serum and physiological studies. *Gastroenterology* 58:319, 1970.
84. Mignon, M., Accary, J. P., and Bonfils, S. Signification diagnostique du test à la sécrétine dans le syndrome de Zollinger-Ellison. Analyse statistique de la réponse gastrinique et acide dans une série de 21 tests positifs. *Gastroenterol. Clin. Biol.* 1:425, 1977.
85. Mihas, A. A., Hirschowitz, B. I., and Gibson, R. G. Calcium and secretin as provocative stimuli in the Zollinger-Ellison syndrome. *Digestion* 17:1, 1978.
86. Mollman, K. M., Bonnevie, O., Gudmand-Hoyer, E., and Wulff, H. R. A diagnostic study of patients with upper abdominal pain. *Scand. J. Gastroenterol.* 10:805, 1975.
87. Mollman, K. M., Bonnevie, O., Gudmand-Hoyer. E., and Wulff, H. R. Nosography of x-ray negative dyspepsia. *Scand. J. Gastroenterol.* 11:193, 1976.
88. Moore, J. G., and Wolfe, M. The relation of plasma gastrin to the circadian rhythm of gastric acid secretion in man. *Digestion* 9:97, 1973.
89. Nundy, S., and Baron, J. H. An evaluation of the Hollander test by graded vagotomy in the dog. *Gut* 14:665, 1973.
90. Nundy, S., and Baron, J. H. Graded vagotomy and gastric secretion. *Am. J. Dig. Dis.* 19:137, 1974.
91. Odell, W. D., Charters, A. C., Davidson, W. D., and Thompson, J. C. Radiommunoassay for human gastrin using unconjugated gastrin as an antigen. *J. Clin. Endocrinol.* 28:1840, 1968.
92. Passaro, E., Basso, N., and Walsh, J. H. Calcium challenge in the Zollinger-Ellison syndrome, *Surgery* 72:60, 1972.
93. Polak, J. M., Stagg, B., and Pearse, A. G. E. Two types of Zollinger-Ellison syndrome: Immunofluorescent, cytochemical and ultrastructural studies of the antral and pancreatic gastrin cells in different clinical states. *Gut* 13:501, 1972.
94. Read, R. C., Thompson, B. W., and Hall, W. H. Conversion of Hollander tests in man from positive to negative. *Arch. Surg.* 104:573, 1972.
95. Rocha-Afodu, J. T., and Adesola, A. O. Dose-response studies of gastric acid secretion in Nigerians using pentagastrin stimulation. *Niger. Med. J.* 4:225, 1974.
96. Roland, M., Berstad, A., and Liavag, T. Acid and pepsin secretion in duodenal ulcer patients in response to graded doses of pentagastrin and carbacholine before and after proximal gastric vagotomy. *Scand. J. Gastroenterol.* 9:511, 1974.
97. Ross, B., and Kay, A. W. The insulin test after vagotomy. *Gastroenterology* 46:379, 1964.
98. Schrumpf, E., Petersen, H., Berstad, A., Myren, J., and Rosenlund, B. The effects of secretin on plasma gastrin in the Zollinger-Elli-

son syndrome, *Scand. J. Gastroenterol.* 8:145, 1973.
99. Schwartz, T. W., Holst, J. J., Fahrenkrug, J., Lindkaer Jensen, S., Nielsen, O. V., Rehfeld, J. F., and Schaffalitzky de Muckadell, O. B. Vagal, cholinergic regulation of pancreatic polypeptide secretion. *J. Clin. Invest.* 61:781, 1978.
100. Scobie, B. A., and Rovelstad, R. A. Anastomotic ulcer: Significance of the augmented histamine test. *Gastroenterology* 48:318, 1965.
101. Small, W. P., Bruce, J., Falconer, C. W. A., Sircus, W., and Smith, A. N. The results of a policy of selective surgical treatment of duodenal ulcer. *Br. J. Surg.* 54:838, 1967.
102. Somervell, T. H., and Orr, I. M. Some contributions to the causation, pathology and treatment of duodenal ulcer and its complications. *Br. J. Surg.* 24:227, 1936.
103. Spencer, J., Burns, G. P., Cheng, F. C. Y., Cox, A. G., and Welbourn, R. B. Differences between males and females in a Hollander insulin test. *Gut* 10:307, 1969.
104. Stadil, F. Effect of vagotomy on gastrin release during insulin hypoglycaemia in ulcer patients. *Scand. J. Gastroenterol.* 7:225, 1972.
105. Stadil, F., and Rehfeld, J. F. Release of gastrin by epinephrine in man. *Gastroenterology* 65:210, 1973.
106. Stadil, F., and Rehfeld, J. F. Determination of gastrin in serum: An evaluation of the reliability of a radioimunoassay. *Scand. J. Gastroenterol.* 8:112, 1973.
107. Stage, J. G., Stadil, F., Rehfeld, J. F., Fahrenkrug, J., and Schaffalitzky de Muckadell, O. B. Secretin and the Zollinger-Ellison syndrome: Reliability of secretin tests and pathogenetic role of secretin. *Scand. J. Gastroenterol.* 13:501, 1978.
108. Stempien, S. J., Dagardi, A. E., Reingold I. M., Heiskell, C. L., Goodman, J. R. Bloom, A., and Weaver, D. S. Hypertrophic hypersecretory gastropathy: Analysis of 15 cases and a review of the pertinent literature. *Am. J. Dig. Dis.* 9:471, 1964.
109. Stempien, S. J., Lee, E. R., and Dagradi, A. E. Clinical appraisal of insulin gastric analysis. *Am. J. Dig. Dis.* 13:21, 1968.
110. Stening, G. F., and Grossman, M. I. Effect of partial vagotomy in the neck or lower thorax on insulin-stimulated acid secretion in dogs. *Gastroenterology* 59:376, 1970.
111. Stening, G. F., and Isenberg, J. I. Insulin-induced acid secretion after partial vagotomy in dogs and cats. *Am. J. Physiol.* 217:962, 1969.
112. Stenquist, B., Knutson, U., and Olbe, L. Gastric acid responses to adequate and modified sham feeding and to insulin hypoglycemia in duodenal ulcer patients. *Scand. J. Gastroenterol.* 13:357, 1978.
113. Straus, E., and Yalow, R. S. Differential Diagnosis of Hypergastrinaemia. In J. C. Thompson (Ed.), *Gastrointestinal Hormones: A Symposium.* Austin: University of Texas Press, 1975, 99–113.
114. Sun, D. C. H., Ryan, M. L., Chang, P. L., and Keogh, R. Augmented histamine test. *Ann. N.Y. Acad. Sci.* 140:875, 1967.
115. Thompson, J. C., Reeder, D. D., Bunchman, H. H. Becker, H. D., and Brandt, E. N. Effect of secretin on circulating gastrin. *Ann. Surg.* 176:384, 1972.
116. Thompson, J. C., Reeder, D. D., Villar, H. V., and Fender, H. R. Natural history and experience with diagnosis and treatment of the Zollinger-Ellison syndrome. *Surg. Gynecol. Obstet.* 140:721, 1975.
117. Tovey, F. I., Sevaniathan, M., Parker, K., and Daniell, A. Effect of vagotomy on the gastric secretion of acid chloride and pepsin in response to an antral stimulus and to insulin and maximal histamine stimulation. *Gut* 9:659, 1968.
118. Trudeau, W. L., and McGuigan, J. E. Effect of calcium on serum gastrin levels in the Zollinger-Ellison syndrome. *N. Engl. J. Med.* 281:862, 1969.
119. Venables, C. W., and Wheldon, E. J., and Johnston, I. D. A. The pentagastrin-insulin secretion test: Its value in diagnosis and surgical management of recurrent ulceration following previous vagotomy. *Gut* 16:830, 1975.
120. Waddell, W. R. The acid secretory response to histamine and insulin hypoglycemia after various operations on the stomach. *Surgery* 42:652, 1957.
121. Walsh, J. H. Use of radioimmunoassay in endocrine G.I. tumors. *Clin. Gastroenterol.* 3:643, 1974.
122. Walsh, J. H., and Grossman, M. I. Gastrin. *N. Engl. J. Med.* 292:1324, 1377, 1975.
123. Wormsley, K. G., and Grossman, M. I. Maximal histalog test in control subjects and patients with peptic ulcer. *Gut* 6:427, 1965.
124. Yalow, R. S., and Berson, S. A. Radioimmunoassay of gastrin. *Gastroenterology* 58:1, 1970.

EDITOR'S COMMENT

In the previous edition, Dr. Baron was introduced as the only internist who is a member of the Surgical Research Society in England; what was omitted was the fact that he also works, at least for part of his time, in the Department of Surgery at the Royal Postgraduate Medical School, Hammersmith Hospital. It remains true therefore that his contribution to a surgical textbook is appropriate. His work as a Research Fellow at the Mount Sinai Hospital in New York and subsequently at Hammersmith has been continued and extended, and the chapter that precedes this comment is particularly welcome.

In the past few years we have seen several important trends in the development of gastric secretion tests. First, there is the use of the sham feeding technique, in which the subject "chews and spits." Second, although various methods for testing the completeness of vagotomy during operation have been described previously, they have now been subjected to more detailed analysis and comparison with one another. Harold Burge was one of the first to tackle this problem with his rather cumbersome apparatus to test gastric motility after electrical stimulation of the nerve. The need to map the stomach accurately for proximal gastric vagotomy led to the development of the Congo red technique. Another method involves the placement of the pH probe directly on the surface of the mucosa. The third method we have used is to pass a small pH probe through the mouth and sample the mucosa by manipulation of the tip of the probe through the wall of the inflated stomach. All these perioperative tests are described but are rather cumbersome and time-consuming, and surgeons therefore tend to use their knowledge of the anatomy of the nerves. Third, Hobsley has repeatedly cautioned those who would measure gastric acid to remember the error occasioned by loss of gastric juice through the pylorus. Although methods to measure this loss have employed nonabsorbable markers, it would seem that an acceptable estimate can be made simply by measuring the sodium content of the aspirated gastric juice.

Should a surgical department go to the trouble and expense of setting up a gastric secretion laboratory? Dr. Baron's answer is unequivocally affirmative, since he believes that all patients should have their acid measured before vagotomy, and vagotomy in some form or another is the most common operation for chronic duodenal ulceration. He cites other examples of when gastric acid measurement is useful or essential. I wholeheartedly agree with his judgment and also agree that in the realm of gastric surgery "acid is important."

For the future what we really need is a simple, accurate, safe, and acceptable method for ensuring completeness of vagotomy during operation. This has yet to be devised, but when and if such a test is developed it would resolve the endless speculation that goes on as to the relationship between incomplete vagotomy and recurrent ulceration. (C. W.)

5

Diagnostic and Therapeutic Aspects of Upper Gastrointestinal Endoscopy

Robert L. Goodale
John F. O'Leary

Growth of Endoscopy, Guidelines, and Training of Endoscopists

The development of high-quality fiberoptic endoscopes, mainly in Japan in the 1960s, permitted the direct visualization of intestinal lesions and quickly showed the shortcomings of the conventional barium roentgenographic studies. Endoscopy has been responsible for a vast improvement in accuracy in the diagnosis of gastrointestinal (GI) disease, resulting in a revolution in and revitalization of gastroenterology, to which the large increase in the number of qualified endoscopists attests. The American Society of Gastrointestinal Endoscopy (ASGE) grew from a few members in the 1950s to more than 2300 by 1980. The fiberoptic revolution has enabled biopsies, directed brush cytology, and photographs to become a normal part of GI evaluations. The minimal discomfort and general safety of the procedure have resulted in good patient acceptance. In contrast, the less well tolerated rigid esophagoscope is used now only for the occasional extraction of foreign bodies, special biopsies, and sometimes, sclerotherapy.

To overcome the limitations of single-contrast roentgenography revealed by endoscopy, roentgenologists have adopted the technique of double-contrast roentgenography pioneered in the 1960s in Japan. As shown in Table 5-1, double-contrast techniques reduce the error rate of a normal upper GI series to about 6 percent. In fact, by using the double-contrast technique, it is possible to reveal superficial gastric and esophageal erosions with an accuracy nearly as high as that achieved by endoscopy, i.e., 95–97 percent.

In 1980 the American College of Surgeons recommended that fiberoptic endoscopic instruction be included in all surgical training programs so that residents might become familiar with, if not competent in, endoscopy. Unfortunately, only 59 percent of university programs currently offer formal training in endoscopy [67], and this is provided within the surgery department in only some. Endoscopy should be of particular interest to surgical res-

Support for this chapter came from NCI Grant No. 2 R26 CA20115

Table 5-1. Error rates of single contrast and double contrast roentgenograms following a normal barium meal in dyspeptic patients with clinically relevant endoscopic findings*

		Single contrast		Double contrast	
Author	Year	No. of patients	False negatives	No. of patients	False negatives
Schuman [100]	1972	843	160 (13%)		
Cotton [15]	1973	200	64 (32%)		
Cumberland [18]	1975	96	16 (17%)		
Laufer [59]	1975	62	20 (32%)	41	2 (5%)
Herlinger [44]	1977			16	5 (32%)
Salter [96]	1977			140	7 (5%)
Salter [97]	1978			88	4 (5%)
Total		1201	260 (22%)	285	18 (6%)

*Active bleeding excluded.

idents because it exposes them firsthand to lesions they must deal with at the operating table.

Because of the tremendous increase in the number of endoscopic procedures done in this country, the American Gastroenterological Association and the Society for Surgery of the Alimentary Tract have established guidelines including standards for endoscopic training and indications for endoscopic procedures to ensure quality medical care and to discourage misuse. Although the guidelines have not been substantiated by published data, studies to evaluate them are underway. These guidelines are presented with the caution that exceptional circumstances have to be taken into account.

The following supervised experiences are suggested as minimal requirements for trainees to achieve a level of competence in endoscopy to qualify them for membership in the ASGE: 50–100 upper GI endoscopies, 25 endoscopic retrograde cholangio(pancreato)grams (ERCPs), and 50–100 colonoscopies. Along with documentation of procedures done, the trainee should study the endoscopic literature and ASGE teaching files. Attendance at conferences on GI issues and periodic peer review of accuracy and morbidity is also recommended. Surgical residents do not have to be trained within their departments. A three-month rotation on an approved gastroenterology service is recommended by Starling and Morrissey [106].

Endoscopy training is greatly aided by use of several good monographs on endoscopy. These are listed at the end of the chapter. In addition, there are courses and workshops in endoscopy sponsored annually by the ASGE that update endoscopic techniques of particular interest to trainees.

Fiberoptic endoscopy has enhanced surgeons' capabilities. They can now plan operations with more information about the extent, resectability, and histology of the primary lesion. Furthermore, they become aware of other lesions that may affect the patient, because endoscopy is a procedure that requires routine inspection of the esophagus, stomach, and duodenum in every instance.

Because of the special problems presented to the endoscopist by bleeding lesions, we discuss bleeding and nonbleeding lesions separately.

Nonbleeding Lesions of Esophagus, Stomach, and Duodenum

ESOPHAGUS

Roentgenography remains the initial examination for most esophageal diseases, although accuracy of roentgenograms alone is quite variable, as shown in Table 5-2. Endoscopy usually follows barium esophagogram in patients with severe or progressive dysphagia, even if the barium study is normal. Endoscopy is also helpful for atypical symptoms or symptoms of uncertain cause. For example, it may demonstrate esophagitis in the patient with atypical anginal symptoms and a normal cardiac evaluation. The guidelines state that patients who have mild symptoms of heartburn, intermittent dyspepsia, or nonspecific chest pain do not generally require endoscopy. In these instances, an upper GI series with a normal barium esophagogram is usually sufficient to rule out serious disease. However, mild strictures and early cancers can be missed if there is too rigid an observance of the guidelines.

Esophagitis

Roentgenograms are less accurate than endoscopy in the diagnosis of esophagitis (Table 5-2). Esophagitis is detected endoscopically by the gross appearance of friability, exudates, a fine nodularity of the mucosa, erosion, ulceration, and stricture [43]. Stricture is a late finding. Congestion of the capillaries is a useful biopsy finding according to Geboes et al. [28], occurring in 83 percent of patients with symptomatic reflux, and in 10 percent of controls. Reddening of esophageal mucosa is not a reliable indicator of esophagitis. Neither symptoms nor histological findings on biopsy correlate well with reddening alone [121]. Rarely, the diagnosis of esophagitis is uncertain endoscopically and the Bernstein test or pH monitoring of the lower esophagus and tests of acid clearance by swallowing are required to confirm or exclude the diagnosis. These tests are not necessary in most patients.

Monilial and viral infections can cause severe esophagitis and should be suspected in diabetic and immunosuppressed patients and those undergoing long-term antibiotic therapy. Brushings or biopsies or both will confirm monilial esophagitis, according to Nash et al. [77]. A thick, creamy white exudate that when peeled off leaves a friable bleeding surface is seen in esophageal thrush.

Barrett's esophagus is now considered an acquired disorder of the distal esophagus in which columnar epithelium replaces the usual stratified squamous epithelium. Esophagoscopy with biopsy is the most widely used procedure to establish the diagnosis; a velvety red mucosa is seen in the distal esophagus. The pattern can be circumferential, extending up from the lower esophageal sphincter, or there can be tongues or islands of red mucosa in the distal esophagus. The condition is probably the result of chronic gastroesophageal reflux caused by a motility disorder. In one study by Naef et al [75], 11 percent of patients with reflux esophagitis were found to have Barrett's esophagus. The true incidence of Barrett's esophagus in patients with reflux is unknown. It may be present in patients with hiatal hernia as well. The columnar epithelium can undergo ulceration, strictures (typically in the mid-esophagus), and, eventually, malignant transformation. Adenocarcinoma was found in 8 percent of 140 patients followed for 12 years by Naef [75]. The association with cancer indicates the need for periodic endoscopic surveillance. Brush cytology alone may be positive. It is suggested that endoscopic examination be done every one or two years.

Sliding Hiatal Hernia

The appearance of gastric mucosal rugae above the diaphragmatic crura is typical in this condition. If the hernia is small, it may only be elicited by the Valsalva maneuver. By retroflexing the tip of the endoscope 180 degrees inside the stomach, the hernia can be viewed from below and a widened diaphragmatic hiatus seen. Peptic ulcerations of strictures may occur above the hernia at the so-called Z-line of the squamocolumnar junction. Endoscopic confirmation is not required if a small sliding hiatal hernia is demonstrated roentgenographically in a patient who is not experiencing symptoms. Patients with roentgenographic evidence of esophageal ulceration and stricture, those with moderate-to-marked symptoms of esophagitis, and any with a history of bleeding should undergo endoscopy for purposes of biopsy. If surgical correction of hiatal hernia is contemplated, endoscopy is indi-

Table 5-2. Sensitivity of barium roentgenogram, endoscopy, biopsy, and directed brushings

				Sensitivity				
Author	Year	No. of patients	Disease	Roentgenogram (%)	Gross endoscopic appearance (%)	Biopsy (%)	Cytology (%)	Biopsy and cytology combined (%)
LESIONS OF THE ESOPHAGUS								
Ward [121]	1970	83	Esophagitis	76	100	56		
Hiatt [45]	1977	52	Esophageal stricture	40	100			
Waldram [119]	1977	44	Varices	86	100			
Gifford [30]	1979	60	Benign lesion		92	98		
Anselm [2]	1979	109	Benign stricture	67	100			
Geboes [28]	1980	15	Reflux esophagitis		100	83		
Kobayashi [57]	1972	35	Cancer			91	91	100
Graham [39]	1978	14	Cancer		93	100	92.8	100
Gifford [30]	1979	40	Cancer		85	90		95
Hanson [41]	1980	85	Cancer	71	89	64.7	91	99
Batra [3]	1982	24	Cancer			92	67	100

LESIONS OF THE STOMACH[a] AND DUODENUM								
Laufer [59]	1975	25	Erosions	52[b]	100			
Graham [39]	1978	61	Gastritis		82	100	100	
			Benign ulcer					
Salter [97]	1978	25	Marginal ulcer	84[b]	100			
Gifford [30]	1979	220	Benign lesions		92	100		
Kobayashi [57]	1972	348	Early cancer		86	97	83[c]	
Morrissey [74]	1976	126	Early cancer	7	65	84	60	
Nelson [79]	1976	14	Benign-appearing cancer	0	0			79
Graham [39]	1978	7	Cancer		86	86	86	100
Sancho-Poch [98]	1978	7	Early cancer		57	71		
		174	Advanced cancer		90	94		
Gifford [30]	1979	94	Cancer		85	74		90
Ito [48]	1979	14	Early cancer		43	86	54	86
		150	Advanced cancer			81	81	92
Hanson [41]	1980	69	Cancer	72	99	91		
Batra [3]	1982	36	Cancer			78	61	92
Tatsuta [111]	1982	35	Early cancer		40 (86[d])			
Belber [4]	1971	59	Duodenal ulcer	71	93			

[a]Excludes active bleeding.
[b]Double contrast study.
[c]Washings only.
[d]After Congo red dyeing.

cated to determine the extent of esophagitis or stricture and to exclude the possibility of more distal lesions (Fig. 5-1A).

Benign Stricture
These strictures are usually caused by many years of chronic peptic acid reflux. They have symmetrical, round, smooth tapering edges. The squamous epithelium may look pale until the narrowest point is reached and then may appear inflamed. All strictures, even those presumed to be of peptic origin, should be examined endoscopically to perform a biopsy. The sensitivity of biopsy for esophageal cancer is more than 90 percent, and the specificity of esophageal biopsy for benign lesions is even higher. If the stricture is too tight to allow the endoscope to pass easily (force is never advised), biopsy forceps and direct brush cytology can be used successfully. Repeat endoscopy is recommended after dilation of benign strictures to resolve any uncertainty about the distal esophagus or stomach.

Esophageal Varices
The gross endoscopic appearance of varices is characteristic and is accepted as the sine qua non of this condition (Table 5-2). Roentgenographic demonstration of varices is somewhat less certain. Thus endoscopy is indicated to confirm the presence of suspected varices. They appear as tortuous folds in the lower esophagus, and as they extend upward they become smaller, disappearing in the upper third (Fig. 5-1B). They are distinguished from normal longitudinal folds by their accentuation by the Valsalva maneuver and their persistence during air distention. Varices vary from pale white to bluish red. The size and presence of thin red areas of the varices, called cherry spots, correlate with bleeding tendency.

Caustic Injury
Lye ingested in solid or liquid form is an important caustic affecting the esophagus. Strong acid may also cause esophageal injury. Even though the esophagus becomes friable, esophagogastroscopy should be done promptly. Mucosal slough or full-thickness necrosis of the esophagus or stomach may evolve within a week. Therefore, endoscopy should be repeated during the first week even if the patient is relatively free of symptoms. Stricturing may start to be noticeable after two weeks.

Mechanical Injury
A history of hematemesis following vomiting, coughing, or straining is an indication for prompt endoscopy. Endoscopy can detect Mallory-Weiss mucosal tears better than roentgenography and does not cause additional damage to any rent that is seen (Fig. 5-1C). If dysphagia follows the ingestion of a swallowed bone or foreign body, a roentgenogram should first be done to localize the object. Endoscopy is indicated if dysphagia is persistent despite a normal roentgenogram, since small bones may be radiolucent. In instances of suspected acute esophageal perforation after instrumentation, or in acute anastomotic breakdown, roentgenograms using a small amount of water-soluble contrast will locate the site of fistula. Endoscopic confirmation is not necessary.

Malignant Tumors of the Esophagus
Endoscopy is indicated when roentgenographic examination shows an irregularity of the esophageal contour. A carcinoma appears as an abrupt transition in color or texture of the mucosa (Fig. 5-D). It is often nodular and irregular, and tends to obstruct and ulcerate. If probing with the biopsy forceps reveals a stiff mucosa, this indicates infiltration. Stasis of food and necrotic tissue result in a fetid odor. Despite their friability, esophageal cancers can be safely subjected to biopsy without risk of perforation or much bleeding. If the clinical impression of carcinoma is strong but the stricture is tight and biopsy findings are normal, brush cytology, which has an accuracy of about 90 pecent, is advised [57]. In several series, brushing and biopsy together have a reported sensitivity of 100 percent. A strong case for brush cytology to detect early cancer of the esophagus can be made; cytologic results may be abnormal even when the gross endoscopic appearance does not suggest tu-

Fig. 5-1

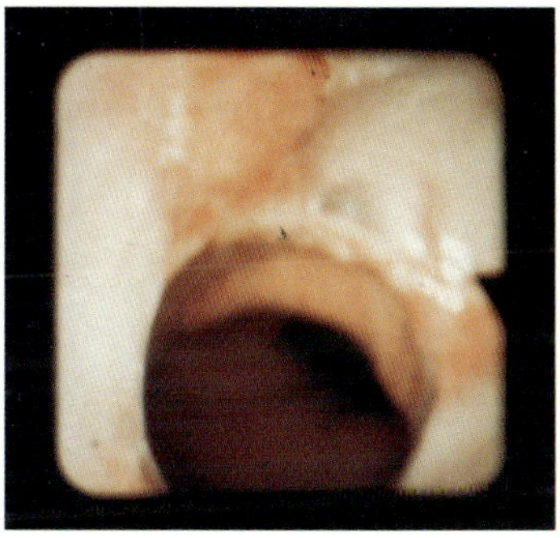

(A) Hiatal hernia and chronic esophagitis showing early stricture formation just above the hernia. Note the contrast between pink gastric mucosa and dark esophageal mucosa. Columnar epithelium extends above the stricture in two places.

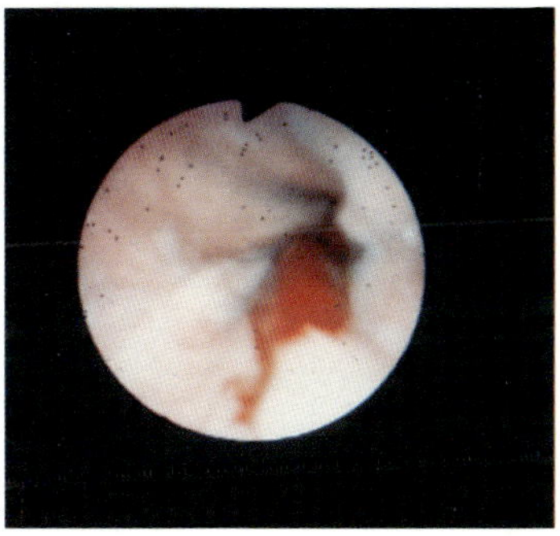

(B) Bleeding distal esophageal varix. The varices are often pale, as shown here. The patient was treated with sclerotherapy.

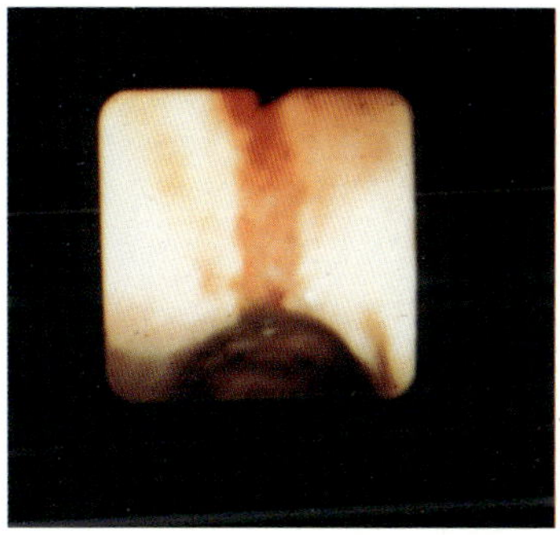

(C) A Mallory-Weiss esophageal laceration, which extends upward from the esophagogastric junction.

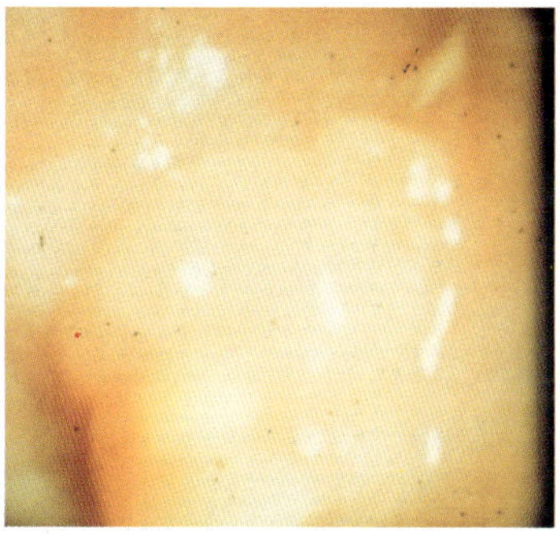

(D) An early squamous cell carcinoma of the esophagus showing pale irregular border of infiltrating tumor. It has not caused significant obstruction.

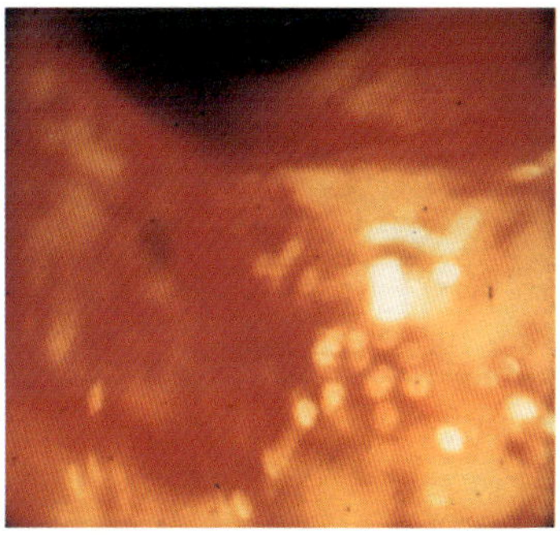

(E) Bleeding gastric erosion, which occurred one week after renal transplantation.

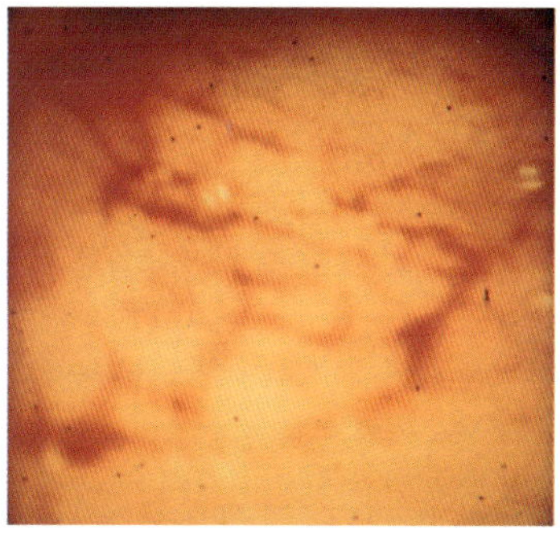

(F) Bleeding gastric erosions in a patient who had been taking aspirin.

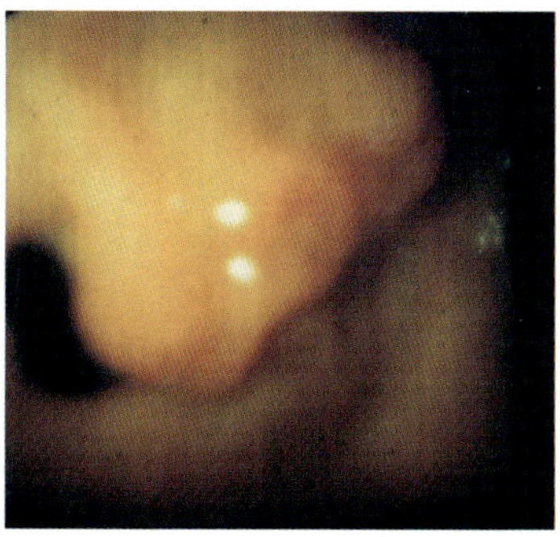

(G) A single hypertrophied rugal fold of antral mucosa. Although it gives a polypoid appearance, note the smooth borders and uniform appearance. Forceps biopsies showed normal antrum.

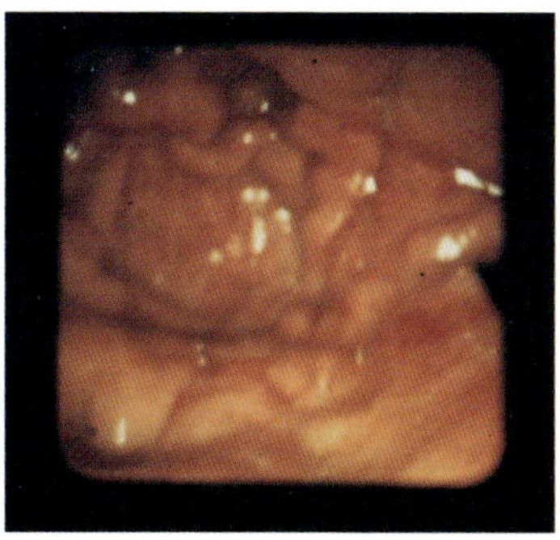

(H) Early linitis plastica in a 49-year-old patient. Large rugal folds have a bizarre pattern, not effaced by air insufflation. Patient was alive five years after total gastrectomy.

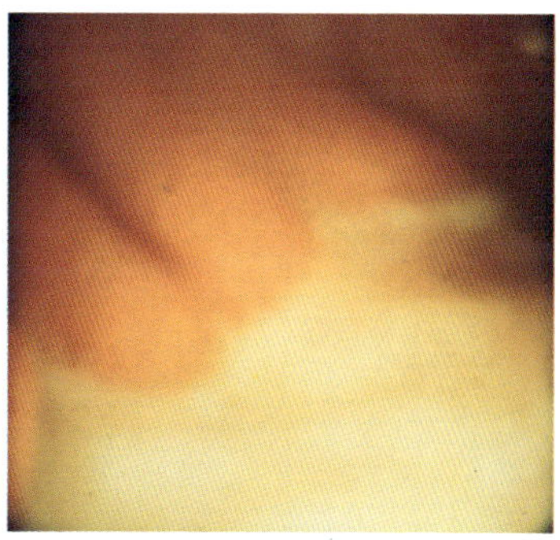

(I) Closeup of a benign ulcer margin showing typical smooth radiating rugal folds. Note the clean edge of the ulcer without overhanging mucosa.

Fig. 5-1. (continued)

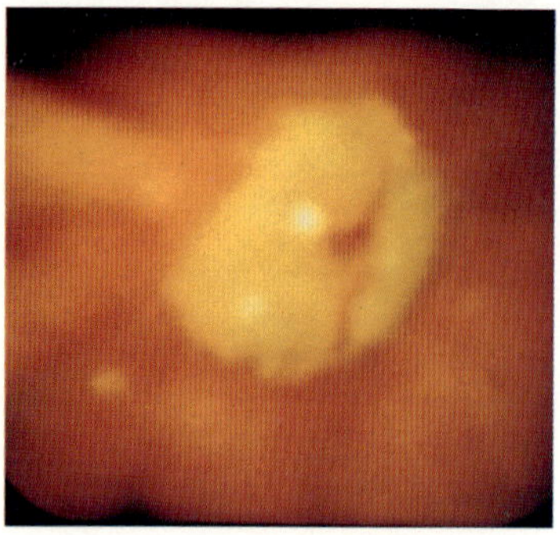

(J) A benign gastric ulcer in a patient who had taken Excedrin for many months. Note the radiating gastric folds and red stigma of an artery in the ulcer base.

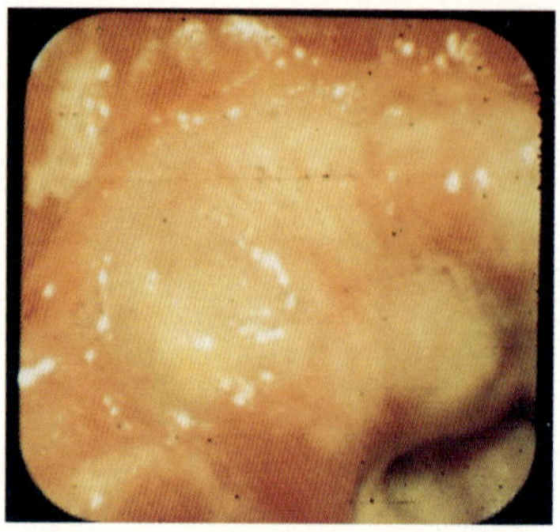

(K) Gastric lymphoma showing irregular edge of infiltrating ulcerating tumor and lack of normal surrounding rugal folds.

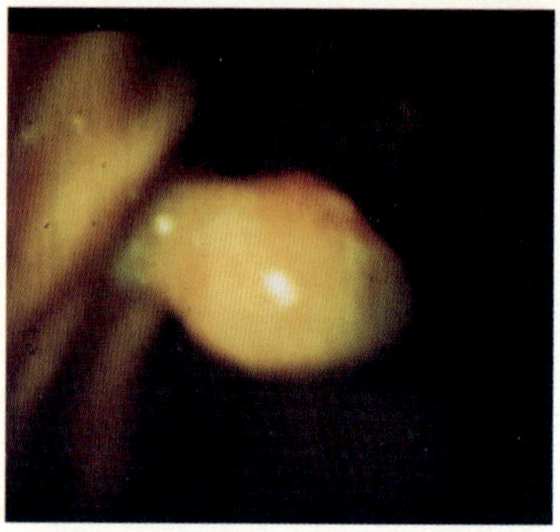

(L) Benign adenomatous polyp of the stomach. The best method for performing biopsy on pedunculated polyps such as this is electrocautery snare followed by aspiration.

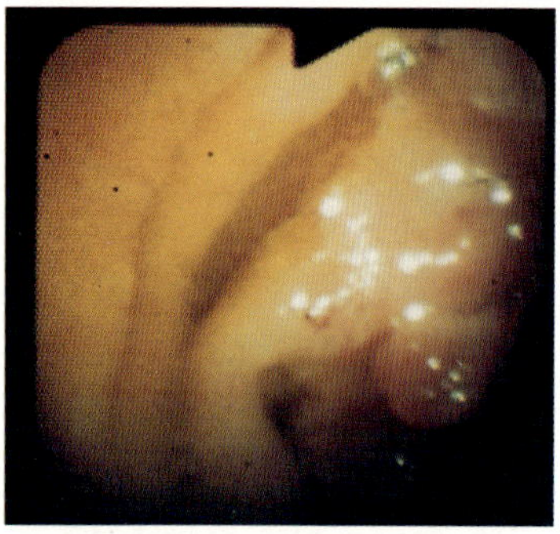

(M) Well-differentiated adenocarcinoma in the fourth portion of the duodenum caused chronic bleeding. Note the abrupt transition between the exophytic tumor and normal mucosa of small intestine.

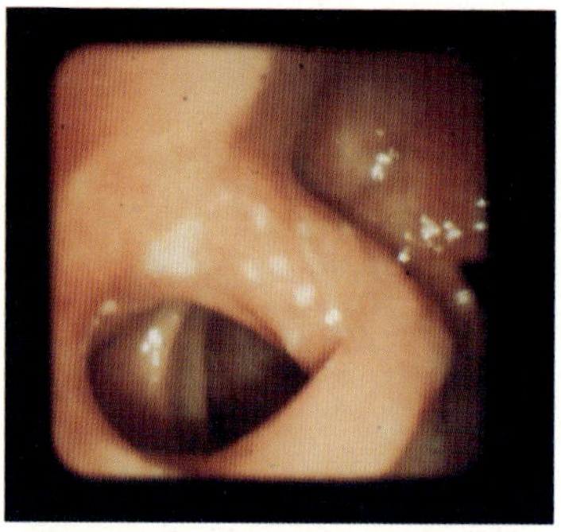

(N) Gastrointestinal bleeding occurred nine years after subtotal gastrectomy, vagotomy and Billroth II reconstruction. This photograph of gastric pouch shows a small white ulcer crater at the anastomotic line.

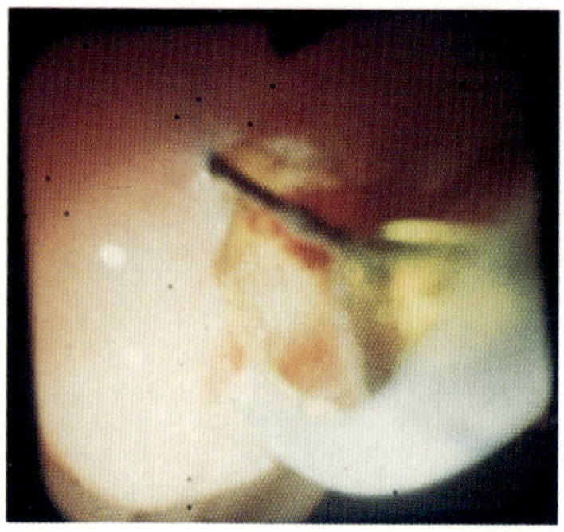

(O) Endoscopic sphincterotomy for treatment of retained biliary tract stones. The sphincterotome is introduced in the papilla of Vater; the cautery wire is pulled taut, cutting the distal 1 cm of the common bile duct.

mor [11]. Directed brushing is more accurate than washing for cytology. Tumors just below the esophagogastric junction may extend upward submucosally and appear as benign esophageal strictures. When viewed from the stomach, the correct diagnosis can be made.

Miscellaneous Conditions

Leiomyomas and lipomas are the most frequent mural tumors. They appear as smooth, round polypoid lesions with intact movable overlying mucosa. Biopsies often reveal only mucosa, although multiple or deep biopsies may provide a diagnosis. Schatzki rings are thin webs that appear briefly in the lower esophagus at the squamocolumnar junction and are seldom the cause of obstruction or symptoms. Achalasia is a condition that can be diagnosed by manometric studies of the esophagus along with roentgenographic studies. Endoscopy is indicated for two reasons. The ease with which the scope passes through the esophagogastric junction will reveal or rule out an underlying stricture and eliminate the possibility of a malignant obstruction. Cancer of the esophagus has been reported in up to 8 percent of these patients.

STOMACH

The stomach is more difficult to view in its entirety than the esophagus because of greater size and angulation. The stomach can usually be more fully seen using some of the following maneuvers. For ulcers seen tangentially or poorly by forward-viewing scopes, we substitute a side-viewing scope. For spasm in the antrum or pyloric channel, we administer glucagon intravenously to provide smooth-muscle relaxation. For secretions or blood obscuring the view, we shift the patient and clean the mucosa with a water jet through the hollow channel of the scope.

Gastritis

This is an important and frequent cause of epigastric pain and occult bleeding. Gastritis may be caused by stress, sepsis, shock, gastric stasis, bile reflux, or a growing list of drugs including indomethacin, steroids, aspirin, and alcohol (Fig. 5-1E, F). Edema and erythema of gastric rugae are present in mild gastritis and may be diffuse or localized. The fundus is more often affected by stress. Antral gastritis is more typical of chronic bile reflux. More severe forms show intense erythema, small punctate erosions, occult or frank bleeding, and friability. Duodenal erosions or ulcers frequently accompany gastritis. Esophagitis may also reflect the chronic vomiting or reflux of bile seen in gastritis. Biopsy is not indicated and does not add any more information than the gross appearance unless there are areas with bizarre mucosal folds suggesting a malignant tumor. Brushings should also be done.

Giant Rugal Gastritis

This condition is characterized by the finding of rugal folds that fail to become effaced with air distention and by a fold thickness of greater than 1 cm (Fig. 5-1G). Gastric lymphoma, pseudolymphoma, Ménétrier's disease, and linitis plastica all show large rugal folds (Fig. 5-1H). If the pattern of rugae is abnormal and localized, a special biopsy technique is recommended since the small fragments of tissue obtained from the 2 mm biopsy forceps are inadequate. A two-channel scope used with a snare technique as described by Martin et al. [66] and by Bjork et al. [7] is recommended. The lift and cut technique gets 10 mm specimens of tissue. In a small series of patients with giant rugal folds, Bjork found that the correct diagnosis was only made by snare, and was missed by standard biopsy forceps [7].

Gastric Ulcer and Erosions

Roentgenography is still the most useful initial procedure in patients with symptoms of gastric ulcer. Endoscopy is not indicated if a good double-contrast roentgenographic study is unequivocally normal. Almost all patients with roentgenographically suspected ulcers should undergo endoscopy *and* biopsy, with as many as eight biopsy specimens taken and four quadrants sampled. The benign gastric crater typically has a smooth round edge that appears "punched out," has no heaping-up mucosa at the edge, and has a uniform increase in vascular pattern at the edges. Gastritis usually surrounds an ulcer. Chronic ulcers show smooth, straight, radiating ridges, which represent contraction scars. These ridges converge at the ulcer edge (Fig. 5-1I). A frequent site of benign ulcer is the lesser curvature near the incisura, but they can occur anywhere. An ulcer base with a persistent clot or visible vessel is thought especially likely to rebleed, and the endoscopist should alert the physicians caring for the patient to this possibility (Fig. 5-1J). Ulcers should be followed after medical treatment. Most authors recommend repeat endoscopy after four to six weeks of intensive medical treatment even if roentgenography shows healing. The endoscopist should do a repeat biopsy on nonhealed or scarred areas that persist despite intensive medical treatment. Probably the only benign-appearing ulcers on roentgenography that do not require endoscopy are in patients younger than 40 years of age with a history of ulcerogenic drug use and with no history of bleeding.

Gastric Carcinoma and Polypoid Lesions

The sensitivity of gross endoscopic impression of gastric cancer varies from 80 percent to greater than 90 percent. The endoscopic features of cancer include an asymptomatic ulcer base with irregular, heaped-up, or granular tissue overhanging the edge (Fig. 5-1K). If there are converging mucosal folds (frequently there are not), they do not reach the ulcer margins or else are clubbed or show irregularity. Exophytic and ulcerated lesions may involve an entire region of the antrum, body, or fundus. About six or eight multiple forceps biopsies should be taken at the edges of ulceration, avoiding the necrotic areas of the ulcer bed. The sensitivity of biopsy alone varies from about 75 to 85 percent in most series. Malignant biopsy specimens are "chunky" and white in contrast to the soft pink mucosa surrounding a benign ulcer.

Sensitivity increases with the number of biopsies taken. The sensitivity of directed brush cytology is less than that of biopsy (about 55 to 80 percent), but it is additive to the overall accuracy and is recommended when the biopsy results are normal despite the visual appearance of a malignant tumor [41]. Indeed, directed brushings and biopsy together yield an accuracy over 90 percent for gastric cancer in many reported series.

Early Gastric Cancers

As many as 33 percent of all gastric cancers in Japan are "early," according to Kawai [53], but the incidence is only 2 to 8 percent in the United States. Early cancer in the Japanese classification system indicates that the lesion is confined to the mucosa and submucosa. Early gastric cancer may appear as a polypoid lesion in the mucosa (type I) or as a slight elevation or depression (type II). Early cancer may be associated with an ulcer and may involve only one quadrant of a benign ulcer. It is important to perform a biopsy on any erosion in the vicinity of an ulcer. Morrissey [74] found that only 2 percent of gastric cancers in this country could be classified as early in his study. Despite a low pickup rate by roentgenography (Table 5-2), the accuracy of gross appearance in early lesions was about 65 percent [74]. In the United States, mass screening with gastrocamera or upper GI series is impractical, but in a large-scale screening study using routine upper GI series and endoscopy of all patients with positive Hemoccult results, four of ten gastric cancers found were early [32]. The value of Hemoccult screening and of roentgenographic and endoscopic studies to detect early and potentially curable gastrointestinal cancer is under active study here and at other centers.

Polyps

Gastric polyps wider than 3 mm in diameter should undergo biopsy endoscopically and, if possible, should be retrieved by suction after snare and electrocautery of the base so that the whole polyp can be sectioned for histological examination. If multiple polyps are present, larger polyps and areas of pallor or irregularity should undergo biopsy or snaring. Most (79 percent according to Ming and Goldman [70], and Tomasulo [113]) are hyperplastic or regenerative. While hyperplastic polyps themselves do not undergo malignant degeneration, cancer may eventually develop in other areas of the stomach in up to 28 percent of patients [113].

The adenomatous polyp is the next most frequent type, and malignant degeneration occurs in up to 40 to 59 percent (Fig. 5-1L). Follow-up examination every one or two years is recommended after endoscopic removal. The incidence of cancer increases in polyps that exceed 2 cm, yet smaller adenomas can contain cancer. When carcinoma in situ is found, a partial gastrectomy is advised since recurrence at the base has been reported [95]. Sessile polyps of the stomach greater than 1 cm in diameter should not undergo biopsy and removal by snare electrofulguration since the stump may bleed heavily.

Multiple Polyps

Gastric polyposes are of several types. They have a definite malignant potential if adenomatous elements predominate. A form of polyposis recently described by Tatsuta et al. [110] is polypoid glandular hyperplasia. These multiple, small (< 5 mm) polyps that arise in the acid-secreting mucosa of the body or fundus may spontaneously regress. Because the chance of malignant degeneration is 10 percent, periodic follow-up study is advised. The rarer types of polyps caused by Peutz-Jeghers syndrome, Brunner's gland adenomas, pancreatic rests, and juvenile polyposis have no association with gastric cancer.

Recurrent and Postgastrectomy Cancer

Periodic follow-up examination is indicated to detect recurrence at the anastomotic line in patients who undergo resection for gastric cancer. A biopsy should be performed on any thickening or granularity.

According to many authors, there is an increased incidence of gastric stump cancer (as high as 9 percent) in patients after gastric resections for benign conditions. The average latent period was 26 years [20]. New symptoms should alert the physician to this possibility. Domellof et al. [19] state that the cancer arises at the stoma and extends in the deep submucosal plane with little mucosal distortion. Deep biopsies should be taken.

DUODENUM

Duodenal Ulcer

Roentgenographic contrast study is the first procedure in patients with suspected duodenal ulcer. If the symptomatic response to treatment is not rapid or the roentgenographic findings are equivocal, duodenoscopy is indicated and may detect very small ulcers or duodenitis. Duodenoscopy is not indicated if a duodenal ulcer is clearly seen roentgenographically and prompt healing is apparent. Many studies have confirmed that endoscopy is more accurate than single-contrast barium studies in detecting an ulcer. The difference between diverticula and ulcer is easily seen endoscopically but is sometimes confusing roentgenographically. A biopsy of a duodenal ulcer in the first portion of the duodenum is not needed, but an unusual appearance or location of ulcer in the second or third portions is an indication for biopsy. A duodenal ulcer in the vicinity of an abdominal aortic graft is an extremely hazardous lesion, and spontaneous exsanguinating hemorrhage has been reported; therefore, duodenoscopy is especially indicated in all persons with abdominal aortic grafts and suspected upper GI tract bleeding. Endoscopy has been reported to be more accurate than aortography [13].

Duodenitis

This can be associated with ulcer symptoms and bleeding and is recognized by the presence of mucosal erythema, friability, edema, and hypermotility but may not be apparent roentgenographically. Duodenitis is most marked around duodenal ulcers and is associated with gastritis, gastric ulcer, and pancreatitis.

Duodenal Tumors

Benign and malignant tumors occur with about equal frequency; however, malignant tumors of the first portion of the duodenum are quite rare. Large adenomatous polyps can give intermittent obstruction as they prolapse through the pylorus. Villous adenomas, Brunner's gland adenomas, and leiomyomas are the most common benign tumors. Benign tumors do not cause obstruction. Multiple biopsies should be taken of sessile or villous polyps. The most common malignant lesion of the duodenum is an adenocarcinoma, followed by leiomyosarcoma. Malignant duodenal tumors cause chronic obstruction, bleeding, and jaundice (Fig. 5-1M). Extramural tumors of the stomach, pancreas, colon, and kidney compress the duodenum only when they reach an advanced stage.

Papillae of Vater and Santorini
These structures often are not seen easily by the end-viewing scopes. When it is difficult to obtain a satisfactory view for good biopsy, a side-viewing scope should be used. Benign villous tumors of the papilla may cause partial obstruction of the pancreatic and common bile duct, and in such instances the forceps biopsy can be done safely. Carcinoma of the ampulla is often associated with ulceration and bleeding.

MISCELLANEOUS LESIONS
Fistulas
Endoscopic confirmation of the size and location of a fistula can help in the management of these difficult problems. Biopsy should be performed for chronic fistula tracts if a history of cancer is present. A flexible probe passed into a tiny fistula by the endoscopist at the operating table can guide the surgeon through adhesions. The presence of any distal intestinal obstructions are noted, which aids in management.

Marginal Ulcers
These often cause pain and bleeding. At best, 80 percent of marginal ulcers can be detected by double-contrast roentgenography. However, endoscopy is indicated in every suspected instance because biopsy may be required (Fig. 5-1N). If a marginal ulcer is on the jejunal or duodenal side of the gastric anastomosis, an inadequate ulcer operation may have been performed. If the ulcer involves the stomach, the same presumption may hold. In addition, however, gastric cancer must be ruled out by a biopsy. Ulcers may form around nonabsorbable sutures that project into the lumen, and these also may cause symptoms. Sutures can be cut endoscopically with special cutting forceps allowing the ulcer to heal.

Endoscopic Retrograde Cholangiopancreatography

A beneficial and important development has been the ability of the endoscopist to cannulate selectively the biliary and pancreatic ducts through the papilla of Vater. The cholangiograms and pancreatograms obtained endoscopically by retrograde cannulation (endoscopic retrograde cholangiopancreatography, or ERCP) reveal fine and accurate morphological detail. This is of great aid in patient management and frequently obviates the need for an exploratory laparotomy. In patients with abdominal pain of obscure origin or with suspected biliary or pancreatic disease, the recommended initial study is the abdominal echogram, which is inexpensive and fairly sensitive, or the computerized tomographic scan. If these studies demonstrate extrahepatic obstruction or pancreatic enlargement, or are equivocal, ERCP is indicated.

The success rate of cannulation of the desired duct ranges from 63 to 92 percent for cholangiograms (Table 5-3). The accuracy of a successful cholangiogram in the detection of stones or tumors of the biliary tree is very high, approaching 100 percent. The biliary tree is harder to cannulate because of its acute angulation with respect to the ampulla, so the rate of success is about 10 to 20 percent less than that of pancreatic duct cannulation (Table 5-3).

An analysis of the sensitivity of the pancreatogram is given in Table 5-4. Although patient numbers are small, it is apparent from these studies that ductal abnormalities are present in only about 50 percent of instances of acute relapsing pancreatitis. In patients with chronic pancreatitis, ductal abnormalities that were diagnostic were more frequent, found in up to 90 percent of attempted ERCPs. However, highly respected endoscopists have had lower success rates. About the same range of sensitivity pertains to the diagnosis of pancreatic cancer. Although some do not think ERCP

Table 5-3. Selective cannulation of clinically relevant ducts by endoscopic retrograde cholangiopancreatography

Author	Year	Instances papilla successfully cannulated out of total attempted procedures (percent)	Rate of success of cannulation (percent)		Complications				
			Pancreatic duct	Biliary duct	Drug-related	Pancreatitis	Cholangitis sepsis	Death	Overall complications
Cotton [16]	1972	/60	11/13 (84%)	29/47 (73%)	0	0	2	0	7%
Rohrman [94]	1974	265/300 (88%)	203/300 (68%)	[N/A]	---------- N/A ----------				
Zimmon [123]	1978	300/? (92%)			7	5	3	2	5%
Belohlavek [5]	1976	2336/2507 (93%)	1315/1604 (82%)	790/1254 (63%)		4		4	3.5%
Bilbao [6]	1976	10,435/?			5	119	72	15	3%
Gaisford [26]	1976	395/407 (97%)	[N/A]	145/157 (92%)	1	4	0	0	1%
Hatfield [42]	1976	/61	53/61 (87%)						
Liguory [63]	1976	93/130 (72%)	93/130 (72%)	[N/A]		5			
Silvis [102]	1976	3884/?		[N/A]	[N/A]	51	25	5	2.1%
Montori [72]	1978	978/1067 (92%)	[N/A]	[N/A]					
Geenen [29] (survey)	1981	[N/A]	[N/A]	[N/A]	0.01–6%	0.7–7%	0.6–.8%	0.001–0.08%	

Note: N/A = not applicable to study, or no information.

Table 5-4. Sensitivity of endoscopic retrograde cholangiopancreatography (ERCP) in acute pancreatitis, chronic pancreatitis, pseudocyst, and pancreatic cancer

		Acute relapsing pancreatitis (no. of patients)		Chronic pancreatitis (no. of patients)		Pseudocyst (no. of patients)		Pancreatic cancer (no. of patients)			
Author	Year	Attempted cannulations	Abnormal pancreatic duct	Attempted cannulations	Abnormal pancreatic duct (diagnostic study)	Attempted cannulations	Cyst filled	Attempted cannulations	Positive biliary duct or pancreatic duct sign	Cytology alone	Combined cytology and ERCP
Rohrman [94]	1974	21	5	15	(93%)	16	10	23	(90%)		
Endo [22]	1974							29	19 (66%)	23/29 (79%)	28/29 (96%)
Freeny [23]*	1976							11	11 (100%)		
Hatfield [42]	1976			9	6 (67%)	N/A		26	18 (69%)	(54%)	(92%)
Liguory [63]	1976	53	25	77	22	29	22	32	20 (62%)		
Ralls [89]*	1980			41	38 (93%)	Included in chronic panc.		8	6 (75%)		
Goodale [34]	1981			51	46 (90%)	Included in chronic panc.		26	19 (73%)	(54%)	(85%)
Frick [24]*	1982			41	33 (80%)	Included in chronic panc.		33	30 (91%)		
Gilmore [33]	1982							32	20 (62%)		

*Patients with successful ERCP only.
Note: N/A = not applicable to study.

should be done for pseudocyst, useful information can be obtained about the size, location, communication, and multiplicity of pseudocysts. The few studies available indicate that about 60 to 70 percent of attempted cannulations show a communication with the main pancreatic duct.

A feature of ERCP requiring additional study is aspiration cytology. The fluid can be aspirated by the cannula in the duct, and the sensitivity is much greater than that obtained by duodenal fluid analysis. Although aspiration cytology is positive in only 50 to 80 percent of instances, when it is combined with the impression of the ductogram, the combined accuracy of cancer diagnosis rises to nearly 90 percent.

Since pancreatic cancer usually presents with advanced signs and symptoms of spread, such as jaundice and abdominal pain denoting extension beyond surgical curability, ERCP has not changed the survival statistics of this disease. The value of ERCP in accurate preoperative diagnosis of cancer, however, is great.

With growing experience, totaling many thousands of instances, a definite procedure-related morbidity has been defined (Table 5-3). Although mortality is low (0.08 to 0.001 percent), there is a significant incidence of pancreatitis and/or cholangitis and sepsis. Infectious complications can be minimized to a degree by not overdistending the pancreatic duct with dye and by use of prophylactic antibiotics given systematically beforehand and within the contrast medium. More important, when a poorly draining pseudocyst or obstructed bile duct is to be cannulated, a standby surgical team must be prepared to drain the collections within 6 hours to prevent cholangitis or pancreatic abscess.

Endoscopy for Bleeding Lesions

ACCURACY OF DIAGNOSIS

No one today will contest the superiority of endoscopy over contrast radiography in the localization of upper GI bleeding. As summarized in Table 5-5, six fairly representative studies all indicated that the sensitivity of endoscopy was greater than that of contrast roentgenography. In no study was the opposite true. The overall sensitivity of endoscopy was 87 percent, versus 55 percent for contrast studies. There is a definite place for barium studies, as discussed in a subsequent section, but for acute bleeding, endoscopy takes precedence and is indicated in virtually every circumstance.

In a survey of the endoscopic experience in 2097 bleeding patients (Table 5-6), Gilbert et al. [31] found a high correlation between endoscopically identified bleeders and the final diagnosis at discharge or death. The correlations between endoscopy and final diagnosis were quite high for bleeding duodenal and gastric ulcers or Mallory-Weiss tears (about 90 to 95 percent) but were lower for the bleeding inflammatory and erosive conditions. This may reflect the transient nature (i.e., rapid healing) of inflammations that at time of discharge or death may no longer be detectable.

TIMING OF ENDOSCOPY

The severity of bleeding dictates the timing of endoscopy. Immediate endoscopy is needed in patients who require more than 4 units of blood per day, have unstable blood pressure, or have copious blood loss. In bleeding of a more moderate and self-limited nature with hemodynamic stability maintained, endoscopy should still be done as soon as possible.

Adequate gastric lavage is the secret of accurate endoscopic diagnosis in the face of active bleeding. It is hard to overstress the importance of lavage. A wide-bore clear plastic tube (No. 35F; Edlich) is passed orally into the stomach, and irrigation with 2 or more liters of cold saline solution or water is performed until the returns are clot-free. If there are clots on the tube when it is removed, the lavage is not adequate. The tube is cleaned and reinserted, and lavage is begun again. An hour of lavage may be required before a clot-free tube is removed. An end-viewing scope is then passed. A jet of water directed through the biopsy channel from a Water Pik device is useful for dislodging any clots in the stomach and exposing an underlying ulcer or rent. One

Table 5-5. Sensitivity of barium roentgenogram versus endoscopy in diagnosis of upper gastrointestinal bleeding

			Sensitivity (%)		False positives (%)		Combined accuracy (%)
Author	Year	No. of patients	Roentgenogram	Endoscopy	Roentgenogram	Endoscopy	
Allan and Dykes [1]	1974	100	86	94	2	2	89
McGinn [68]	1975	138	51	86	8	1	91
Morris [73]	1975	54	22	67	?	?	70
Keller [55]	1976	68	34	72	18	7	75
Graham [37]	1980	95	62	97	?	?	?
Cello [12]	1980	100	68*	96	9	1	96
Total		555					
Average			55%	87%	9%	2%	87%
No. Successes/No. Patients			254/459	454/519	32/364	9/370	400/460

*Double contrast.

must be sparing in the use of the suction channel because fresh clots will clog it and obscure the view. The patient should be positioned so that the area of interest is not dependent. The duodenum, stomach, and esophagus must be easily seen because lesions are frequently multiple. The freshest blood comes from the active bleeding site; clots that are expanding are lying on actively bleeding vessels.

Does early endoscopic diagnosis favorably affect the outcome of patients with upper GI hemorrhage? Table 5-7 addresses the problems typically encountered with prospective randomization studies of bleeding patients. First, although many patients may stop bleeding spontaneously, they still have a high mortality because of the often irreversible sequelae of prolonged hemorrhagic shock. In these instances the precise knowledge of the bleeding site as given by endoscopy makes no difference in outcome. Second, there is a temptation to remove patients from study protocols when massive bleeding requiring surgical intervention occurs. Furthermore, most physicians now are biased in favor of endoscopy and are reluctant to treat patients without the diagnostic information endoscopy provides. These factors inevitably interfere with the randomization of prospective controlled studies.

In a study by Allan and Dykes [1], 40 percent of patients who had routine endoscopy had a different or new diagnosis established. In 17 of the 50 controls, endoscopy was performed because bleeding did not stop or roentgenographic findings were equivocal and surgical intervention was under consideration. Again, endoscopy provided either an important new diagnosis or an exclusion of diagnosis. Endoscopy did not lower the mortality. However, the control group contained some patients who had endoscopy.

In a study by Graham [37], 49 patients and their physicians were told the immediate results of endoscopy and in 11, relevant new information was gleaned. In 46 patients, the result of endoscopy was not told to the clinicians for 48 hours. Protocol violations occurred in the control group, and again no difference in mortality was seen. Since physicians consistently balk at withholding endoscopy from patients who are bleeding heavily, it is unlikely that a truly well-controlled randomized prospective study of immediate endoscopy in upper GI hemorrhage will ever be performed.

Table 5-6. Agreement of endoscopic and final diagnosis in 2097 bleeding patients

Lesion	Identified at endoscopy	As final diagnosis (% agreement)
1. Duodenal ulcer	477	450 (94)
2. Gastric ulcer	459	421 (92)
3. Stomal ulcer	39	36 (92)
4. Mallory-Weiss syndrome	168	150 (89)
5. Gastric erosion	620	468 (75)
6. Esophageal varices	323	214 (66)
7. Esophagitis	269	130 (48)
8. Duodenitis	191	124 (65)
9. Neoplasm	78	49 (63)
10. Esophageal ulcer	46	33 (72)
11. Osler-Rendu-Weber disease	10	8 (80)

Source: Data from Gilbert et al. [31].

Upper Gastrointestinal Therapeutic Endoscopy

There has been exciting growth in the field of upper GI therapeutic endoscopy over the past ten years. Therapeutic procedures should be attempted only after the endoscopist has achieved a high degree of competency, since these procedures have a considerable inherent risk. Endoscopic complications may include serious perforations, bleeding, or sepsis, and a surgical team may be required on a standby basis.

ENDOSCOPIC ESOPHAGEAL DILATION

Benign stricture dilation is almost uniformly successful by endoscopic means, the mortal-

Table 5-7. Effect of routine early endoscopy in patients with active upper gastrointestinal bleeding (prospective randomized studies)

		Immediate endoscopy			Selective or delayed endoscopy		
Author	Year	No. of patients	Caused change in treatment	Hospital mortality	No. of patients	Caused change in treatment	Hosptial mortality
Sandlow [99]	1974	58 {42}	?	6 (10%)	70 {11}	?	6 (9%)
Allan and Dykes [1]	1974	50	20	4 (13%)	50 {17}	10	4 (8%)
Morris [73]	1975	32[a]	?	5 (16%)	28	?	0 (0%)
Keller [55]	1976	38	15	1 (3%)	38	10	1 (3%)
Graham [37]	1980	49	11	4 (8%)	46 {15[b]}	10	6 (13%)
Total		227	46/137 (34%)	20 (9%)	232	30/134 (22%)	17 (7%)

[a]Excludes massive bleeders.
[b]Protocol violations or crossover to endoscopy.
Note: { } = only patients who actually underwent endoscopy.

Table 5-8. Complications of esophageal dilations

Author	Year	No. of patients	Perforations No.	Perforations Rate (%)	Deaths
FIBEROPTIC CONTROL (PUESTOW-EDER DILATOR)					
Puestow [88]	1955	6	0		0
Price [87]	1974	28	1	3.5	0
Olsen [81]	1977	40	0		0
Silvis (survey) [102]	1976	9431*	33	0.6	0
RIGID ESOPHAGOSCOPY					
Raptis [90]	1972	100	4	4.0	1
Williamson [122]	1975	83	7	8.4	1

* = No. of procedures.

ity is nearly zero, and the perforation rate is only about 0.6 percent (Table 5-8). A great advance in dilation was achieved when Rockman et al., in 1970 [93], described a method of endoscopic placement of the guide wire through the stricture. There is no absolute contraindication to esophageal dilation. Peptic strictures can be dilated by the metal Puestow olives or by the mercury-filled rubber bougies. In tight firm strictures that cannot be dilated by rubber bougies, a guide wire is passed through the stricture under direct vision by the endoscope. The scope is withdrawn, and over the guide wire left in place several graduated sizes of metal olive dilators are advanced through the stenotic area. Ideally, the procedure is monitored by fluoroscopy both to keep the alignment of the guide wire with the advancing olive and push rod, and to be sure the stricture is passed. Factors determining the extent of dilatation accomplished at each setting are (1) the pressure required to dilate, (2) patient tolerance, and (3) the amount of scarring around the stricture. Dilation should be discontinued after blood is found on the metal olive. It may not be wise to attempt more than three or four progressive size changes. Additional dilation can be done every four to seven days. If concern exists about a perforation or laceration in the esophagus, one can rescope immediately. A small mucosal rent at the stricture after dilation is an acceptable finding. Unfortunately, as the stricture is dilated diminishing dysphagia may be accompanied by esophageal reflux and esophagitis. Once the stricture is opened up, additional maintenance of patency can be achieved by periodic bougienage; a mercury-filled rubber Hurst or Maloney dilator is used. Some patients can be instructed in self-dilation with the mercury dilators. In patients who are at low operative risk, an antireflux operation can be considered to provide long-term protection against reflux and restricture.

Lye Strictures

Strictures of the esophagus may develop up to six months after lye ingestion. Immediate use of steroids is advocated, though evidence that they prevent scarring is lacking. Repeated dilation should be done after the period of extreme friability has passed (two weeks) and may be required over one or two years. Adults may be taught self-dilation. This stricture is associated with a slight increased risk of esophageal cancer with a latent period of many years.

Achalasia

This condition is preferably handled by surgical myotomy unless the patient's extreme debility requires prolonged preoperative nutritional support. In that circumstance, a trial of pneumatic dilation is recommended. This procedure carries a risk of perforation between 1 and 5 percent. The issue of whether a trial of pneumatic dilation in low-risk patients is worthwhile is not resolved. In our experience, the effect is only temporary.

Some lesions are not suited to dilation, including the neck of a Zenker's diverticulum and cricopharyngeal spasm induced by stroke or brain stem disease. Here, dilation is of no help and can be hazardous.

GASTRIC ANASTOMOTIC DILATION

Anastomotic strictures at the gastric outlet can be dilated with endoscopically directed dilators. A set of metal olive dilators ranging in size from 20F to 38F can be preloaded onto the endoscope. In our experience, five of seven patients were successfully relieved of their gastric obstruction and reoperation was avoided. Several were in the early postoperative period, and the narrowing of the stoma may have been caused by soft adhesions. The stoma seems to pop open as the dilator is passed through. We do not advise anastomotic dilation earlier than two weeks postoperatively for fear of suture line breakdown. No postdilation bleeding has occurred. A hydrostatic balloon dilator as described by Grüntzig [40] can be passed through a 3-mm endoscopic channel and forcefully dilates up to a diameter of 10 mm [64].

ESOPHAGEAL ENDOPROSTHESIS INSERTION

Many patients with advanced unresectable malignant stricture of the esophagus reach the point at which they start to regurgitate even liquids. A tracheo-esophageal fistula is another unfortunate complication that occurs. Esophageal endoprosthesis insertion may improve the quality of life in either situation, while not actually increasing survival. Success rates in terms of improved swallowing vary from 50 to 100 percent. The hospital mortality ranges from 12 to 80 percent. Nevertheless, some patients accept the risks in order to be able to swallow liquids or avoid aspiration through the tracheo-esophageal fistula. The method of insertion of the Hering or Proctor and Celestin tubes endoscopically also entails a risk of hemorrhage, perforation and tube migration, as well as tube malfunction, i.e., plugging or kinking. In addition, failure or absence of a distal antireflux flap valve may result in severe regurgitation or aspiration.

An endoscope is preloaded with its outer sheath as a push rod, after which an endoprosthesis is slid over the scope. The stricture may have to be dilated first to accommodate the scope. The prosthesis is then pushed into the stricture using the scope as a guide, and seated with the flanged end resting on the proximal edge of the tumor, with the distal end extending below the tumor. The scope and push rod are then withdrawn, leaving the prosthesis in place. The position of the prosthesis is checked by barium swallow or by endoscope. Retention sutures placed before insertion can be used to pull the prosthesis back if necessary. The distal end of the prosthesis is secured in some instances by doing the procedure in the operating room and surgically placing a sleeve or flutter valve over the distal end within the stomach.

FOREIGN BODY REMOVAL

Bezoars

Phytobezoars can impede gastric emptying. They occur in patients who eat before good motility returns after gastric resection or who have gastric outlet stenosis or gastric stasis. A diet consisting largely of fiber and fruits may cause bezoars. A mass lesion in the stomach may be demonstrated roentgenographically. Bezoars usually pass in time with a liquid diet; however, endoscopy is sometimes indicated. They can be broken up by the endoscope with the snare or by irrigation, or enzymatic degradation by papain may be used. Trichobezoars (hairballs) cannot be dissolved safely by any substance; if massive, they have to be removed surgically.

Ingested Foreign Bodies

Although it has been reported that as many as 75 percent of ingested foreign bodies pass through the GI tract, these objects can still pose a serious problem [69]. Pills or meat may become impacted above esophageal strictures or by esophageal spasm. They can often be pushed through the stricture using a small nasogastric tube or pediatric scope. If the stricture is too tight, impacted material should be broken up by a biopsy forceps or by snare and then removed or pushed through. Although swallowed coins frequently lodge in the antrum, they usually pass. Sometimes they have to be dislodged first by the endoscope and their passage aided by a high fiber diet. Objects that are irregular in shape can be grasped by snare or special grasping forceps. Sharp, broken glass, straight pins, or nails should be grasped if possible and may be removed, without esophageal trauma, inside a protective sheath enclosing the endoscope. This technique is described by Sugawa and Schuman [107]. Razor blade fragments may be softened by the acid in the stomach. A high fiber diet may help coat other sharp objects and prevent injury during passage. Since sharp objects may become impacted and perforate the intestine, patients need periodic roentgenographic follow-up examinations. Surgical treatment should be withheld until obstruction or perforation occurs.

ENDOSCOPIC RETROGRADE SPHINCTEROTOMY

Endoscopic sphincterotomy is gaining acceptance as an alternative to operation. Endoscopic retrograde sphincterotomy is indicated in patients with previous cholecystectomy who have retained common duct stones. It can be considered preoperatively in high-risk patients as a temporizing measure to allow stabilization of their general medical status and permit an elective cholecystectomy. Its use in patients with so-called papillary stenosis has been advocated by some, but its value is unproved. A contraindication to the procedure is a disproportion in size between the stone and the terminal duct. Stones that approach 3 cm in diameter may not be extractable. A bleeding tendency is a relative contraindication. Too long a strictured segment of distal duct invites a perforation of the duodenum by the cutting wire. Active pancreatitis is also a contraindication. This procedure should only be attempted when an endoscopist has mastered the technique of ERCP (Fig. 5-1O). A surgical team should be alerted and ready to operate immediately should there be an endoscopic complication.

Table 5-9 outlines the history of the technique as it evolved both in Japan and Germany nearly simultaneously. Kawai, in 1973, performed transduodenal papillotomy in dogs and showed its feasibility and safety. This was followed by clinical reports of Kawai et al. [54] and also of Classen and Ossenberg [14] and Koch et al. [58] and Demling in Germany. The

Table 5-9. Experience with endoscopic retrograde sphincterotomy

				Complications				
Author	Year	No. of patients	Successful stone passage	Moderate–severe pancreatitis (operations)	Bleeding (operations)	Perforation (operations)	Cholangitis (operations)	Death
RESULTS OF ENDOSCOPIC PAPILLOTOMY								
Kawai [54]	1974	3	2	1				0
Koch [58]	1977	267	192/222 (86%)	9	7 (5)	2 (2)	2	2 (0.7%)
Montori [72]	1978	64	47/49 (96%)		2 (0)		2	0
Nakajima [76]	1979	80	65/75 (87%)	1	1 (0)			0
Sohma [105]	1979	70	57/66 (86%)		4		3	
Geenen [29] (U.S.A. review)	1981	1250		41 (3)	29 (5)	14 (6)	25 (9)	15 (1.2%)
RESULTS OF SURGICAL SPHINCTEROPLASTY								
Bohmig [9]	1969	268						3 (1.1%)
Jones [51]	1972	5750						244 (4.2%)

*Papillotomy also done for papillary stenosis and ampullary carcinoma.

overall success rate ranges from 86 to 96 percent in most large series. There is a 3 to 10 percent morbidity and a 0.4 to 1.2 percent mortality. This is somewhat lower than the mortality of surgical sphincteroplasty, which can be as high as 4 percent or greater. Bleeding is the most frequent complication of endoscopic sphincterotomy and can be caused by cutting too quickly or too far up the common duct. Unfortunately, there is no way to know in advance whether a branch of the gastroduodenal artery lies in the path of the papillotome. The safest technique is to apply 1- or 2-second bursts of cutting and cautery current at moderate settings. Mortality is related to perforation of the duodenum, cholangitis, and bleeding. The incidence of restenosis is 1 to 2 percent. An alternative method of extraction if patients have a retained T tube in the common duct is the so-called Burhenne technique. Stones are removed by a directed basket under fluoroscopic control. However, this technique requires a mature T-tube tract, i.e., one that has been present for four to six weeks.

Therapy for Bleeding

Endoscopy has taught us a great deal about upper GI bleeding. We now appreciate that multiple lesions are often present and that only by endoscopy can the bleeding sites be identified. Lesions suspected by history or shown by roentgenography may not be bleeding. Furthermore, endoscopy is often the only means to diagnose bleeding from superficial lesions such as Mallory-Weiss mucosal tears and hemorrhagic gastritis.

Although early endoscopic diagnosis of bleeding has not improved survival rates, a variety of schemes for endoscopic control of GI bleeding have been tried, and some of these have been well tested in randomized prospective trials. The results of the studies have begun to demonstrate the potential therapeutic effectiveness of some of these new modalities. Following are discussions of three of the most promising and widely used endoscopic techniques for control of bleeding.

ESOPHAGEAL INJECTION SCLEROTHERAPY FOR BLEEDING VARICES

Bleeding varices carry a formidable mortality in patients with poor hepatic reserve. Portal-systemic shunts became established in the 1940s as the definitive surgical method to control bleeding esophageal varices. Compared with all other procedures, shunts carry the lowest long-term risk of rebleeding. Serious questions about the morbidity and mortality of shunts arose after the randomized prospective studies by Jackson et al. [49], in 1965, and Resnick et al. [92], in 1969 and 1974. These large cooperative studies showed that the survival rate of patients with varices was approximately the same for medically treated patients as for those treated prophylactically with shunts. They also showed that the morbidity and mortality of shunt-related encephalopathy and accelerated liver failure counterbalanced the beneficial effects of decreased bleeding in these patients. The distal splenorenal shunt (the Warren shunt) carries the lowest risk of encephalopathy, but the procedure is technically difficult. Because of the pressures of mounting hospitalization and surgical costs (as high as $52,900 for hospitalization for portacaval shunt as calculated by O'Donnell et al. [80]), the cost-effectiveness of major surgical procedures is being questioned.

Crafoord and Frenckner, in 1939 [17], first conceived of the method of esophageal sclerotherapy and reported the successful treatment of a young woman with bleeding varices that were controlled and obliterated after a course of 15 injections. They used a rigid esophagoscope and a quinine-uretan solution as the sclerosant. This method never gained wide acceptance as long as general anesthesia and rigid esophagoscopes were used, though Moersch [71], Johnston and Rodgers [50], Paquet and Fleig [86], and Terblanche et al. [112] have reported good results (Table 5-10).

Sclerotherapy is being reevaluated because it now can be done with fiberoptic scopes, which are far easier to use and better tolerated, and the deficiencies of shunts have become apparent. Sclerotherapy is indicated for the high-risk patient with Child's class B or C

Table 5-10. Clinical experience with sclerotherapy for bleeding esophageal varices[a]

				Total control of bleeding			Complications					
Author	Year	Scope (rigid vs. flexible)	No. of patients	Immediate control of active bleeding	Instances of re-bleeding	Obliteration	Esophageal ulcer	Necrosis or perforation	Pleural effusion	Stenosis	Death (30 days)	All complications combined
Raschke [91]	1973	R	30	11/12	2 (?)[b]	?		1			10	
Terblanche [112]	1979	R	22				1	2		2	9	
Lewis [62]	1981	F	19	16/19	3 (0)	9/14	5		5	0	8	
Paquet [86]	1981	R	909	871	?	?	28	18	18	22	123	12%
Sivak [104]	1981	F	22	1/3	16	?	?	0		0	8	
MacDougall [65]	1982	F	51[c]	[N/A]	22	[N/A]	15	0		9	9	
Goodale [36]	1982	F	42	9/11	20 (7)	6/25	14	1	2	0	9	
Hughes [46]	1982	F	75	?/14	27	?	7	2	45	2	6	
Jorge [52]	1982	F	29	3/4	7	?					5	
Sivak (survey) [103]	1982	F	610	75%	39 (33%)	?	50	4 (3%)		4 (3%)	(3%)	19%

[a]Excludes prophylactic procedures.
[b]Parentheses indicate number treated surgically.
[c]All nonbleeding.
Note: N/A = not applicable to study.

hepatic functional reserve. The indications for its use in lower risk patients are debatable. Although the risk of sclerotherapy is low in this population, the risk of an operation is also acceptably low.

The best method of performing sclerotherapy is not yet well defined. Both rigid and flexible scopes have been used, with more groups favoring the latter since they avoid use of anesthesia, are well tolerated, and cause less trauma to the esophagus. The most common sclerosant is sodium morrhuate (cleared for use by the United States Food and Drug Administration), but ethanolamine oleate is favored by several European groups. Obliteration or substantial improvement has occurred in 30 to 60 percent of patients after multiple injection treatments. The incidence of recurrence of varices has not been established. Rebleeding occurs in roughly half the patients, especially after the first two or three treatments.

Esophageal ulceration was noted as a frequent complication. The ulcers preceded healing and obliteration of varices. In our own experience, sclerotherapy did not seem to jeopardize the outcome of surgical treatment since six of seven patients who underwent emergency portal-systemic shunting lived [36]. The presence of severe hepatic dysfunction, active bleeding at the time of sclerotherapy, the occurrence of rebleeding, and comorbid conditions all adversely affected survival. Other complications include fever, pleural effusion, esophageal necrosis, and mesenteric infarction. Mesenteric infarction is associated with prolonged vasopressin administration and a probable low flow state in the portal system. Our own results from a nonrandomized study can be compared with those of historic control patients with roughly comparable severity of hepatic impairment. At six months, 52 percent of our patients were alive after sclerotherapy; this compares favorably with survival rates in the series of Graham and Smith [38], whose patients underwent medical treatment, and also with survival figures in patients who underwent emergency shunt operations reported by Orloff et al. in 1980 [82].

Although comparison of sclerotherapy with conventional medical treatment and emergency shunt suggests that sclerotherapy provides a better survival rate, far better evidence for this is found in two prospective randomized trials (Table 5-11). The first, by MacDougall et al., in 1982 [65], reported a lower risk of rebleeding after sclerotherapy than in medically treated controls ($p < .01$). There was also a significantly better two-year survival rate in the sclerotherapy-treated group compared with medically treated controls ($p < .01$).

Paquet's study in 1982 [85] also shows a definite survival benefit of sclerotherapy compared to medical treatment. In his study, sclerotherapy was done as a prophylactic measure, and bleeding incidence was also reduced. The long-term results of sclerotherapy are uncertain. Whether esophageal varices will reform and require continued periodic treatments are questions awaiting answer. Meanwhile, many endoscopists, internists, and surgeons are turning to sclerotherapy for the short-term control of variceal bleeding for which it does appear to have definite merit.

LASER PHOTOCOAGULATION

Laser treatment of acute bleeding lesions of the GI tract has made a promising start, though conclusive proof is lacking that the survival rate is improved. Part of the difficulty lies in the choice of laser. We used the CO_2 continuous wave laser experimentally in 1970 for control of gastric bleeding induced in dogs [35]. Though we applied CO_2 laser radiation in two patients with bleeding erosive gastritis, the laser arm had to be aimed by hand and directed through an open incision to the mucosal surface. Hemostasis was achieved and the patients survived. The 10.2-mm infrared wavelength of the CO_2 laser was unsuitable for transmission in fiberoptic bundles.

The argon laser was successfully used in experimental animal trials by Nath et al. in 1973 [78], and later by Fruhmorgen et al. [25], Waitman et al. [118], Dwyer [21], and Silverstein et al. [101]. The argon laser beam has a wavelength of 0.44–0.52 mm and can be transmitted by quartz fibers as a blue light. It is feasible for use in fiberoptic scopes. One drawback

Table 5-11. Sclerotherapy compared to medical treatment for bleeding varices

		Sclerotherapy group				Control group (medical treatment)		
Author	Year	No. of patients	Instances of rebleeding	Obliteration of varices	Death	No. of patients	Instances of rebleeding	Death
Paquet[a] [85]	1982	32	2 (6%)		2 (6%)	33	22 (66%)	14 (42%)
MacDougall [65]	1982	51	22 (43%)	42	11 (22%)[b]	56	42 (75%) (2 surg)[c]	22 (39%)

[a]Prophylactic sclerotherapy for grade 3 and 4 varices.
[b]Two years.
[c]Two patients underwent surgical treatment.

with the argon laser is the complete absorption by a thin layer of blood. For the energy to penetrate to the underlying tissue, an air or CO_2 jet has to clear blood from the target.

The neodymium-YAG laser has an infrared wavelength and can also be transmitted by quartz fibers. It has a better tissue penetration than the argon laser and is not absorbed by hemoglobin. Table 5-12 summarizes some of the leading clinical trials of both argon and neodymium-YAG lasers.

Three randomized prospective trials have been done. For arterial pumping lesions there was an immediate hemostatic effect in about two-thirds of patients after laser therapy in the study of Vallon et al. [114], but the numbers are small. The mortality was not much different from that of the control group. For oozing ulcers, there may be a greater effect. The study of Van Trappen et al. [116] showed 100 percent immediate arrest with laser, versus 78 percent arrest in the control group ($p < .005$), with no difference in mortality. The effectiveness of laser on the nonbleeding ulcer with the visible vessel was assessed in studies of Vallon and Cotton [115] and Swain et al. [109]. The Vallon study showed no effect in prevention of rebleeding, but Swain found significant lowering of the rebleeding rate and a lower mortality. These studies all showed no immediate risk or complication from laser therapy, though the authors noted that a percentage of lesions could not be reached by the laser.

One can conclude that for the arterial pumping lesion, laser treatment can achieve perhaps better hemostasis than medical treatment alone but that mortality and the need for surgical treatment is probably not diminished. For oozing lesions, at present it seems that the laser is most effective as a hemostatic agent, again with no proven effect on mortality. For the nonbleeding ulcer with stigmata of recent hemorrhage, there are conflicting results that may be resolved by more trials.

ELECTROFULGURATION OF ULCERS

Within the last 10 years, endoscopic electrofulguration of bleeding ulcers has been used in a few centers in this country and abroad (Table 5-13). It is not an established method to control bleeding and to date there have been no randomized controlled studies of its effectiveness. The first experimental studies of monopolar electrocoagulation in dogs were carried out by Blackwood and Silvis [8]. The current of injury diffuses outward from the electrode to the grounding plate. The safety and reproducibility of effects were studied by Papp [84]. Bipolar electrofulguration was introduced to reduce the depth of injury seen with monopolar techniques. In the bipolar electrode, the current flows only a short distance between the two electrodes at the tip of the probe, confining the heat to a small area. A multipolar probe is now available with six longitudinal electrodes placed at the sides and tip. The heating current is even more localized to the tissue adjacent to the tip of the instrument. Present coagulator probes are hollow to

Table 5-12. Clinical experience with laser photocoagulation for control of upper gastrointestinal bleeding, including randomized prospective trials of laser photocoagulation vs. medical management

		Laser treatment					Controls (medical treatment)				
Author	Year	Type of laser	Total no. of patients	Type of lesion	Immediate control	Rebleeding (operations)	Deaths	Total no. of patients	Immediate control	Rebleeding (operations)	Deaths
Fruhmorgen [25]	1976	A	7		6		?				
Kiefhaber [56]	1977	Nd	116	Acute arterial bleeding	105	49 (32)	42 (36%)				
Dwyer [21]	1979	Nd	58	Active bleeding	56	?	?				
Lawrence [60]	1980	A	36	Arterial spurting	25	3 (10)	4				
Bown [10]	1981	A	19	Visible vessel	?	9		20	?	9	
Ihre [47]	1981	Nd	19		11	4	1	13	8	4 (9)	2
LeBodic [61]	1981	A	15		13	1 (0)	3	10	5	7 (0)	1
Vallon [114]	1981	A	15	Arterial spurting	10	7 (7)	2	13	4	11 (9)	3
		A	19	Ulcers with visible vessels		8(6)	3	16		8 (5)	3
		A	34	Ulcers with red spot		5 (2)	0	39		4 (4)	4
Van Trappen [116]	1981	Nd	18	Arterial spurting	16	8 (9)	2				
		Nd	51*	Active bleeding and stigmata	51	5 (1)	2	51*	36	15 (6)	5

*Assuming equal distribution of 102 patients total.
Note: A = argon; Nd = neodymium-YAG.

Table 5-13. Experience with electrofulguration for arrest of upper gastrointestinal bleeding

Author	Year	No. of patients	Lesion	Initial control	Rebleeding (operations)	Deaths
Sugawa [108]	1975	6	Mallory-Weiss syndrome Gastric ulcers	6	2 (2)	?
Gaisford [27]	1979	6	Mallory-Weiss syndrome	6	1 (1)	?
		12	Gastric ulcer	12	4 (0)	?
		13	Duodenal ulcer	13	0 (?)	?
Volpicelli [117]	1978	5	Gastric ulcer	5	1 (1)	1
		6	Duodenal ulcer	6	0 (?)	0
Wara [120]	1980	16	Spurting arterial bleeding	12	4 (4)	
		49	Oozing	42	7 (6)	5
		4	Overlying clot	2	2 (1)	
Papp [84]	1980	12	Active Mallory-Weiss syndrome	10	(2)	6
		69	Gastric and duodenal lesions	63	10 (11)	

permit a water jet to be played on the bleeding site. The jet washes away the blood, allowing the probe to gain contact with tissue and minimizes the coagulum of charred tissue adherent to the electrode. This lets the electrode pull cleanly away from the ulcer without disturbing the fragile eschar produced. The electrode is applied circumferentially around the bleeding vessel and not on the vessel per se. A perivascular zone of edema is thought to occlude the vessel.

Uncontrolled trials of this therapy are summarized in Table 5-13. Gaisford [27] has treated 29 patients with actively bleeding gastric ulcers and 13 with duodenal ulcers with electrocoagulation, and reports an immediate arrest of bleeding in 92 percent. In two small series, Sugawa et al. [108] and Volpicelli et al. [117] noted rebleeding in 33 percent and 8 percent, respectively. Wara et al. [120] reported an 81 percent success rate in achieving hemostasis.

The cause of rebleeding was investigated in one study by Papp [83], who found that four of five patients with a visible vessel in the ulcer rebled. In a subsequent prospective randomized study, 10 of 13 medically treated control patients rebled and required surgical treatment, compared with 1 of 13 in the group who underwent electrofulguration.

In three patients who had electrocoagulation for bleeding ulcers, we noted one with a visible vessel. This ulcer rebled 24 hours after electrocoagulation.

Papp [84] successfully electrocoagulated a Mallory-Weiss tear with arterial bleeding in 1973 and summarized his experience in 1980. Ten of 13 patients' active arterial bleeding stopped with a monopolar Cameron Miller hollow-tipped coagulation electrode. There were no deaths.

In summary, endoscopic electrocoagulation is currently undergoing evaluation as a method to treat active ulcer bleeding. Animal studies indicate that bipolar cautery and argon lasers cause the least thermal damage to tissue, and neodymium and monopolar cautery cause the greatest. In general the laser is easier to apply, but this is offset by its great expense. The cautery is relatively inexpensive, and warrants controlled clinical studies to demonstrate the degree of its effectiveness.

References

1. Allan, R., and Dykes, P. A comparison of routine and selective endoscopy in the management of acute gastrointestinal hemorrhage. *Gastrointest. Endosc.* 20:154, 1974.
2. Anselm, K. Comparison of endoscopy and barium swallow in the diagnosis of esophageal stricture. *Gastrointest. Endosc.* 25:95, 1979.

3. Batra, S. K., Kini, S. R., Schuman, B. M., and Smith, M. J. Evaluation of brush rinsings for the cytologic diagnosis of esophageal and gastric cancer. *Gastrointest. Endosc.* 28:23, 1982.
4. Belber, J. P. Endoscopic examination of the duodenal bulb: A comparison with x-ray. *Gastroenterology,* 61:55, 1971.
5. Belohlavek, D., Koch, H., Rosch, W., et al. Five years experience in endoscopic retrograde cholangiopancreatography (ERCP). *Endoscopy* 8:115, 1976.
6. Bilbao, M. K., Dotter, C. T., Lee, T. G., et al. Complications of endoscopic retrograde cholangiopancreatography. *Gastroenterology* 70:314, 1976.
7. Bjork, J. T., Geenen, J. E., Soergel, K. H., et al. Endoscopic evaluation of large gastric folds: A comparison of biopsy techniques. *Gastrointest. Endosc.* 24:22, 1977.
8. Blackwood, W. D., and Silvis, S. E. Gastroscopic electrosurgery. *Gastroenterology* 61:305, 1971.
9. Bohmig, H. J., Fritsch, A., Kax, M., et al. Indikationen und ergebniese der transduodenalen sphincterotomie langenbecks. *Arch. Klin. Chir.* 323:173, 1969.
10. Bown, S., Storey, D., Swain, P., et al. Controlled trial of argon laser photocoagulation for hemorrhage from peptic ulcers. *Gut* 22:A414, 1981.
11. Burke, E. L., Sturm, J., and Williamson, D. The diagnosis of microscopic carcinoma of the esophagus. *Am. J. Dig. Dis.* 23:148, 1978.
12. Cello, J. P., and Thoeni, R. I. Gastrointestinal hemorrhage: Comparative values of double contrast upper gastrointestinal radiography and endoscopy. *J.A.M.A.* 243:685, 1980.
13. Champion, M. C., Sullivan, S. N., Coles, J. C., et al. Aortoenteric fistula: Incidence, presentation, recognition, and management. *Ann. Surg.* 195:314, 1982.
14. Classen, M., and Ossenberg, F. W. Nonsurgical removal of common bile duct stones. *Gut* 18:760, 1977.
15. Cotton, P. B. Fiberoptic endoscopy and the barium meal. *Br. Med. J.* 2:161, 1973.
16. Cotton, P. B., Blumgart, L. H., Davies, G. T., et al. Cannulation of papilla of Vater via fiber duodenoscope. *Lancet* 53:58, 1972.
17. Crafoord, C., and Frenckner, P. New surgical treatment of varicose veins of the oesophagus. *Acta Otolaryngol.* 27:422, 1939.
18. Cumberland, D. C. Fiberoptic endoscopy and radiology in the investigation of the upper gastrointestinal tract. *Clin. Radiol.* 26:223, 1975.
19. Domellof, L., Ericksson, S., and Jannuger, K. G. Late occurrence of precancerous changes and carcinoma of the gastric stump after Billroth II resection. *Acta Chir. Scand.* 141:292, 1975.
20. Dougherty, S. H., Foster, C. A., and Eisenberg, M. M. Stomach cancer following gastric surgery. *Arch. Surg.* 117:294, 1982.
21. Dwyer, R. M. Safe and effective laser phototherapy in man using the Nd:YAG laser. *Gastroenterology* 76(abstract):1126, 1979.
22. Endo, Y., Morii, T., Tamura, H., and Okuda, S. Cytodiagnosis of pancreatic malignant tumors by aspiration under direct vision using a duodenal fiberscope. *Gastroenterology* 67:944, 1974.
23. Freeny, P. C., Bilbao, M. K., and Katon, R. M. "Blind" evaluation of ERCP in diagnosis of pancreatic carcinoma: The double duct and other signs. *Radiology* 119:271, 1976.
24. Frick, M. P., O'Leary, J. F., Walker, H. C., and Goodale, R. L. Accuracy of endoscopic retrograde cholangiopancreatography (ERCP) in differentiating benign and malignant pancreatic disease. *Gastrointest. Radiol.* 7:241, 1982.
25. Fruhmorgen, P., Bodem, F., Reidenbach, H. D., et al. Endoscopic laser coagulation of bleeding gastrointestinal lesions with report of the first therapeutic application in man. *Gastrointest. Endosc.* 23:73, 1976.
26. Gaisford, W. D. Endoscopic retrograde cholangiopancreatography in the diagnosis of jaundice. *Am. J. Surg.* 132:699, 1976.
27. Gaisford, W. D. Endoscopic electrohemostasis of active upper gastrointestinal bleeding. *Am. J. Surg.* 137:47, 1979.
28. Geboes, K., Desmet, V., Van Trappen, G., and Mebis, J. Vascular changes in the esophageal mucosa: An early sign of esophagitis. *Gastrointest. Endosc.* 26:29, 1980.
29. Geenen, J. E., Vennes, J. A., and Silvis, S. E. Resume of a seminar on endoscopic retrograde sphincterotomy (ERS).*Gastrointest. Endosc.* 27:31, 1981.
30. Gifford, R. M., Dressel, T. D., and Goodale, R. L. The importance of Gastroscopy to the Surgeon. In J. S. Najarian and J. P. Delaney (Eds.), *Gastrointestinal Surgery*. Miami: Symposia Specialists, 1979. Pp. 155–64.
31. Gilbert, D. A., Silverstein, F. E., Tedesco, F. J., et al. The national A.S.G.E. survey on

upper gastrointestinal bleeding. *Gastrointest. Endosc.* 27:94, 1981.
32. Gilbertson, V. A. Colon Cancer Control Study, University of Minnesota. Unpublished data, 1982.
33. Gilmore, I. T., Pemberton, J., and Thompson, R. P. H. Retrograde cholangiopancreatography in the diagnosis of cancer of the pancreas. *Gastrointest. Endosc.* 28:77, 1982.
34. Goodale, R. L., Gajl-Peczalska, K., Dressel, T. D., et al. Cytologic studies for the diagnosis of pancreatic cancer. *Cancer* 47:1552, 1981.
35. Goodale, R. L., Okada, A., and Gonzales, R. Rapid endoscopic control of bleeding gastric erosions by laser radiation. *Arch. Surg.* 101:211, 1970.
36. Goodale, R. L., Silvis, S. E., O'Leary, J. F., et al. Early survival after sclerotherapy for bleeding esophageal varices. *Surg. Gynecol. Obstet.* 155:523, 1982.
37. Graham, D. Limited value of early endoscopy in the management of upper gastrointestinal bleeding. *Am. J. Surg.* 140:284, 1980.
38. Graham, D. Y., and Smith, J. L. The course of patients after variceal hemorrhage. *Gastroenterology* 80:800, 1981.
39. Graham, D. Y., Spjut, H. J., and Estrada, R. E. Directed cytology of the esophagus and stomach: A comparison of three rapid collection methods. *Gastrointest. Endosc.* 24:277, 1978.
40. Grüntzig, A. R., Senning, A., and Siegenthaler, W. E. Nonoperative dilation of coronary stenosis. *N. Engl. J. Med.* 301:61, 1979.
41. Hanson, J. T., Thoreson, C., and Morrissey, J. F. Brush cytology in the diagnosis of upper G.I. malignancy. *Gastrointest. Endosc.* 26:33, 1980.
42. Hatfield, A. R. W., Smithies, A., et al. Assessment of endoscopic retrograde cholangiopancreatography (ERCP) and pure pancreatic juice cytology in patients with pancreatic disease. *Gut* 17:14, 1976.
43. Hatorri, I., Winans, C., Archer, F., et al. Endoscopic diagnosis of esophageal inflammation. *Gastrointest. Endosc.* 20:102, 1974.
44. Herlinger, H. An evaluation of the double contrast barium meal against endoscopy. *Clin. Radiol.* 28:307, 1977.
45. Hiatt, G. A. The roles of endoscopy vs. radiography in diagnosing benign peptic strictures. *Gastrointest. Endosc.* 23:194, 1977.
46. Hughes, R. W., Larson, D. E., Viggiano, T. R., et al. Endoscopic variceal sclerosis: A one-year experience. *Gastrointest. Endosc.* 28:62, 1982.
47. Ihre, I., Johansson, C., Seligson, U., and Torngren, S. Endoscopic YAG laser treatment in massive gastrointestinal bleeding. *Scand. J. Gastroenterol.* 16:633, 1981.
48. Ito, Y., Blackstone, M. O., Riddell, R. H., and Kirsner, J. B. The endoscopic diagnosis of early gastric cancer. *Gastrointest. Endosc.* 25:96, 1979.
49. Jackson, F. C., Perrin, E. B., DeGradi, A. E., et al. Clinical investigation of the portacaval shunt. I. Study design and preliminary survival analysis. *Arch. Surg.* 91:43, 1965.
50. Johnston, G. W., and Rodgers, H. W. A review of 15 years' experience in the use of sclerotherapy in the control of acute hemorrhage from oesophageal varices. *Br. J. Surg.* 60:797, 1973.
51. Jones, S. A., and Smith, L. L. A reappraisal of sphincteroplasty (not sphincterotomy). *Surgery* 71:565, 1972.
52. Jorge, A. D. Injection sclerotherapy of esophageal varices. *Endoscopy* 14:115, 1982.
53. Kawai, K. Diagnosis of early gastric cancer. *Endoscopy* 1:23, 1971.
54. Kawai, K., Nakajima, M., Kunoto, K., et al. Endoscopic sphincterotomy of the ampulla of Vater. *Gastrointest. Endosc.* 20:148, 1974.
55. Keller, R. T., and Logan, G. M. Comparison of emergent endoscopy and upper gastrointestinal series radiography in acute upper gastrointestinal hemorrhage. *Gut* 17:180, 1976.
56. Kiefhaber, P., Nath, G., and Moritz, K. Endoscopic control of massive gastrointestinal hemorrhage by irradiation with a high power neodymium-YAG laser. Prog. Surg. 15:140, 1977.
57. Kobayashi, S., Yoshii, Y., and Kasugai, T. Selective use of brushing cytology in gastrointestinal strictures. *Gastrointest. Endosc.* 19:77, 1972.
58. Koch, H., Rosch, W., Schaffner, O., and Demling, L. Endoscopic papillotomy. *Gastroenterology* 73:1393, 1977.
59. Laufer, I., Hamilton, J., and Mullens, J. E. Demonstration of superficial gastric erosions by double contrast radiography. *Gastroenterology* 68:387, 1975.
60. Lawrence, B. H., Vallon, A. G., and Cotton, P. B. Endoscopic laser photocoagulation for bleeding peptic ulcers. *Lancet* 1:124, 1980.
61. LeBodic, L., and Sudry, P. Cited in: P. B. Cotton and A. G. Vallon, European Clinical Ex-

perience in Laser Photocoagulation in Upper Gastrointestinal Tract. In J. P. Papp (Ed.), *Endoscopic Control of Gastrointestinal Hemorrhage*. Boca Raton, Fl: C.R.C. Press, 1981. Pp. 103–10.
62. Lewis, J., Chung, R. S., and Allison, J. G. Injection sclerotherapy for control of acute variceal hemorrhage. *Am. J. Surg*. 142:592, 1981.
63. Liguory, Cl., and Caletti, C. A. An evaluation of endoscopic retrograde pancreatography in chronic and relapsing acute pancreatitis. *Endoscopy* 8:59, 1976.
64. London, R. L. Trotman, B. W., DiMarino, A. J., et al. Dilation of severe esophageal strictures by an inflatable balloon catheter. *Gastroenterology* 80:173, 1981.
65. MacDougall, B. R. D., Theodossi, A., Westaby, D., et al. Increased long-term survival in variceal haemorrhage using injection sclerotherapy. *Lancet* 1:124, 1982.
66. Martin, T. R., Onstad, G. R., Silvis, S. E., and Vennes, J. A. Lift and cut biopsy technique for submucosal sampling. *Gastrointest. Endosc*. 23:29, 1976.
67. Max, M. H., and Polk, H. C. Perceived needs for gastrointestinal endoscopic training in surgical residencies. *Am. J. Surg*. 143:150, 1982.
68. McGinn, F. P., Guyer, P. B., Wilken, B. J., et al. A prospective comparative trial between early endoscopy and radiology in acute upper gastrointestinal haemorrhage. *Gut* 16:707, 1975.
69. McManus, J. E. Perforations of the intestine by ingested foreign bodies. *Am. J. Surg*. 53:393, 1941.
70. Ming, S. C., and Goldman, H. A histogenic classification and its relation to carcinoma. *Cancer* 18:721, 1965.
71. Moersch, H. J. Treatment of esophageal varices by injection of a sclerosing solution. *J. A. M. A*. 135:754, 1947.
72. Montori, A., Viaconte, G. W., and Pastorino, C. ERCP, endoscopic papillotomy, and gallstone removal by JFBs Olympus and PFSB 1200 Machida. *Endoscopy* 10:103, 1978.
73. Morris, D. W., Levine, G. M., Soloway, R. D., et al. Prospective randomized study of diagnosis and outcome in acute upper gastrointestinal bleeding: Endoscopy vs. conventional radiography. *Am. J. Dig. Dis*. 20:1103, 1975.
74. Morrissey, J. F. The diagnosis of early gastric cancer. *Gastrointest. Endosc*. 23:13, 1976.
75. Naef, A. P., Savary, M., and Ozzello, L. Columnar-lined lower esophagus: An acquired lesion with malignant predisposition. *J. Thorac. Cardiovasc. Surg*. 70:826, 1975.
76. Nakajima, M., Akasaka, Y., and Kawai, K. Endoscopic Sphincterotomy. In T. Takemoto and T. Kasugai (Eds.), In *Endoscopic Retrograde Cholangiopancreatography*. Tokyo; Igaku-Shoin, 1979.
77. Nash, G., and Ross, J. S. Herpetic esophagitis: A common cause of esophageal ulceration. *Hum. Pathol*. 5:339, 1974.
78. Nath, G., Gorisch, W., and Kiefhaber, P. First laser endoscopy via a fiberoptic transmission system. *Endoscopy* 5:208, 1973.
79. Nelson, R. S., Urrea, L. H., and Lanza, F. L. Evaluation of gastric ulcerations. *Am. J. Dig. Dis*. 21:389, 1976.
80. O'Donnell, T. F., Gembarowicz, R. M., Callow, A. D., et al. The economic impact of acute variceal bleeding: Cost-effectiveness implications for medical and surgical therapy. *Surgery* 88:693, 1980.
81. Olsen, H. W., Lawrence, W. A., Bottarini, G., et al. The fiberoptic approach to dilation of stenotic lesions of the esophagus. *Gastrointest. Endosc*., 23:201, 1977.
82. Orloff, M. J., Bell, R. H., Hyde, P. V., et al. Long-term results of emergency portacaval shunt for bleeding esophageal varices in unselected patients with alcohol cirrhosis. *Ann. Surg*. 192:325, 1980.
83. Papp, J. P. Endoscopic electrocoagulation of the nonbleeding visible ulcer vessel. *Gastrointest. Endosc*. 25(abstract):45, 1979.
84. Papp, J. P. Electrocoagulation of actively bleeding Mallory-Weiss tears. *Gastrointest. Endosc*. 26:128, 1980.
85. Paquet, K. J. Prophylactic endoscopic sclerosing treatment of esophageal wall in varices: A prospective controlled randomized trial. *Endoscopy* 14:4, 1982.
86. Paquet, K. J., and Fleig, W. E. Sclerotherapy of Esophageal Varices. In J. R. Papp, (Ed.), *Endoscopic Control of Gastrointestinal Hemorrhage*. Boca Raton, Fla.: C.R.C. Press, 1981. Pp. 43–71.
87. Price, J. O., Stancia, C., and Bennett, J. R. A safer method of dilating esophageal strictures. *Lancet* 1:1141, 1974.
88. Puestow, K. L. Conservative treatment of stenosing diseases of the esophagus. *Postgrad. Med*. 18:6, 1955.
89. Ralls, P. W., Halls, T., Renner, I., et al. Endoscopic retrograde cholangiopancreatogra-

phy (ERCP) in pancreatic disease. *Radiology* 134:347, 1980.
90. Raptis, S., and Milne, D. M. A review of the management of 100 cases of benign stricture of the esophagus. *Thorax* 27:599, 1972.
91. Raschke, E., and Paquet, K. J. Management of hemorrhage from esophageal varices using the esophagoscopic sclerosing method. *Ann. Surg.* 177:99, 1973.
92. Resnick, R. H., Chalmers, T. C., Ishihara, A. M., et al. A controlled study of the prophylactic portacaval shunt: A final report. *Ann. Intern. Med.* 70:675, 1969.
93. Rockman, S., Morrissey, J. F., and Koizumi, H. A simple approach to narrow esophageal strictures. *Gastrointest. Endosc.* 16:212, 1970.
94. Rohrman, C. A., Silvis, S. E., and Vennes, J. A. Evaluation of the endoscopic pancreatogram. *Radiology* 113:297, 1974.
95. Rosato, F. E., and Noto, J. A. Gastric polyps. *Am. J. Surg.* 111:647, 1966.
96. Salter, R. H. X-ray negative dysepsia. *Br. Med. J.* 21:235, 1977.
97. Salter, R. H., Girdwood, T. G., Scott-Harden, W. G., and Cole, T. P. Endoscopic and radiological assessment of recurrent ulceration after peptic ulcer surgery. *Br. J. Radiol.* 51:257, 1978.
98. Sancho-Poch, F. J., Balanzo, J., Ocana, J., et. al. An evaluation of gastric biopsy in the diagnosis of gastric cancer. *Gastrointest. Endosc.* 24:281, 1978.
99. Sandlow, L. J., Becker, G. H., Spellberg, M. H., et al. A prospective randomized study of the management of upper gastrointestinal hemorrhage. *Am. J. Gastroenterol.* 61:282, 1974.
100. Schuman, B. M. The gastroscopic yield from the negative upper G.I. series. *Gastrointest. Endosc.* 19:79, 1972.
101. Silverstein, F. E., Protell, R. L., Gilbert, D. A., et al. Argon vs. neodymium-YAG laser photocoagulation of experimental canine gastric ulcers. *Gastroenterology* 77:491, 1979.
102. Silvis, S. E., Nebel, O., Rogers, G., et al. Endoscopic complications: Results of the 1974 American Society for Gastrointestinal Endoscopy Survey. *J.A.M.A.* 235:928, 1976.
103. Sivak, M. V. Endoscopic injection sclerosis of esophageal varices (ASGE Survey). *Gastrointest. Endosc.* 28:41, 1982.
104. Sivak, M. V., Stout, D. J., and Skipper, G. Endoscopic injection sclerosis (EIS) of esophageal varices. *Gastrointest. Endosc.* 27:52, 1981.
105. Sohma, S., and Fiyita, R. Significance of Endoscopy Sphincteropapillotomy. In T. Takemoto and T. Kasugai (Eds.), *Endoscopic retrograde cholangiopancreatography.* Tokyo, Igaku-Shoin, 1979.
106. Starling, J. R., and Morrissey, J. F. One solution to the dilemma of endoscopic requirements for general surgical residents. *Surg. Gynecol. Obstet.* 155:65, 1982.
107. Sugawa, C., and Schuman, B. M. *Primer of Gastrointestinal Fiberoptic Endoscopy.* Boston: Little, Brown, 1981.
108. Sugawa, C., Shier, M., Lucas, C. E., and Walt, A. J. Electrocoagulation of bleeding in the upper part of the gastrointestinal tract. *Arch. Surg.* 110:975, 1975.
109. Swain, C. P., Brown, S. G., Storey, D. W., et al. Controlled trial of argon laser photocoagulation in bleeding peptic ulcers. *Lancet* 2:1313, 1981.
110. Tatsuta, M., Okuda, S., Tamura, H., and Taniguchi, H. Polyps in the acid-secreting area of the stomach. *Gastrointest. Endosc.* 27:145, 1981.
111. Tatsuta, M., Okuda, S., Tamura, H., et al. Endoscopic determination of the extent of early ulcerated gastric cancer. *Endoscopy* 14:41, 1982.
112. Terblanche, J., Northover, J. M. A., Bornman, P., et al. A prospective evaluation of injection sclerotherapy in the treatment of acute bleeding from esophageal varices. *Surgery* 85:239, 1979.
113. Tomasulo, J. Gastric polyps: Histologic types and their relationship to gastric carcinoma. *Cancer* 27:1346, 1971.
114. Vallon, A. G., Cotton, P. B., Laurence, B. H., et al. Randomized trial of endoscopic argon laser photocoagulation on bleeding peptic ulcers. *Gut* 22:228, 1981.
115. Vallon, A. G., and Cotton, P. B. Visible vessel in peptic ulcers (letter). *N. Engl. J. Med.* 306:872, 1982.
116. Vantrappen, G., Rutgeerts, P., Broeckaert, L., et al. Controlled trial of neodymium-YAG laser treatment for upper digestive haemorrhage. *Gastrointest. Endosc.* 27:139, 1981.
117. Volpicelli, N. A., McCarthy, J. D., Bartlett, J. D., et al. Endoscopic electrocoagulation: An alternative to operative therapy in bleeding peptic ulcer disease. *Arch. Surg.* 113:483, 1978.

118. Waitman, A. M., Spira, I., Chryssanthou, C. P., et al. Fiberoptic coupled argon laser in the control of experimentally produced gastric bleeding. *Gastrointest. Endosc.* 22:78, 1975.
119. Waldram, R., Nunnerley, H., Davis, M., et al. Detection and grading of oesophageal varices by fiberoptic endoscopy and barium swallow with and without buscopan. *Clin. Radiol.* 28:137, 1977.
120. Wara, P., Hojsgaard, A., and Amdrup, E. Endoscopic electrocoagulation: An alternative to operative hemostasis in active gastroduodenal bleeding? *Endoscopy* 12:237, 1980.
121. Ward, A. S., Wright, D., and Collis, L. J. The assessment of esophagitis in hiatus hernia patients. *Thorax* 25:568, 1970.
122. Williamson, R. C. N. The management of peptic oesophageal stricture. *Br. J. Surg.* 62:448, 1975.
123. Zimmon, D. S. Endoscopic management of biliary calculi. *Hosp. Pract.* 13:103, 1978.

Further Readings

Berci, G. (Ed.), *Endoscopy*. New York: Appleton-Century-Crofts, 1976.

Cotton, P. B., and Williams, C. B. (Eds.), *Practical Gastrointestinal Endoscopy*. Oxford: Blackwell, 1980.

Kawai, K. (Ed.), *Early Diagnosis of Pancreatic Cancer*. Tokyo, New York: Igaku-Shoin, 1980.

Papp, J. R. (Ed.), *Endoscopic Control of Gastrointestinal Hemorrhage*. Boca Raton, Fla.: C.R.C. Press, 1981.

Pearl, R. K. *Gastrointestinal Endoscopy for Surgeons*. Boston: Little, Brown, 1984.

Salman, P.R. (Ed.), *Fiberoptic Endoscopy*. New York: Grune & Stratton, 1974.

Schiller, K. F. R., and Salmon, P. R. (Eds.), *Modern Topics in Gastrointestinal Endoscopy*. Chicago: Year Book, 1976.

Silvis, S. E. (Ed.), *Therapeutic Gastrointestinal Endoscopy*. New York: Tgaku–Shoin, 1985.

Stewart, E. T., Vennes, J. A., and Geenen, J. E. (Eds.), *Atlas of Endoscopic Retrograde Cholangiopancreatography*. St. Louis: Mosby, 1977.

Sugawa, C., and Schuman, B. M. (Eds), *Primer of Gastrointestinal Fiberoptic Endoscopy*. Boston: Little, Brown, 1981.

SPECIAL COMMENT

Massive Upper Gastrointestinal Hemorrhage: What Role for Endoscopic Control?

Philip E. Donahue

Although the use of flexible fiberoptic endoscopes has increased diagnostic accuracy in patients with gastrointestinal hemorrhage, there is no definite evidence that the morbidity and mortality of bleeding episodes are lower in patients who have had the advantage of accurate endoscopic diagnosis. The first of several possible explanations for this situation is that medical treatment of bleeding lesions in the upper gastrointestinal tract is quite nonspecific; therefore, changes in morbidity indices may not be observed until specific and effective treatments become widely available. Second, if the patients in all treatment groups have serious associated illnesses, mortalities may still be high even though the patients do not die of hemorrhage per se. Last, since individuals without associated illnesses or of younger age have lower mortality risks in association with major hemorrhage than persons with associated illnesses or of advanced age, a relatively small survival advantage in one treatment group might escape detection in a series of fewer than 100 patients. The recent advent of transendoscopic techniques for stopping gastrointestinal hemorrhage is of extreme interest in this regard and may allow a more precise evaluation of the benefits of endoscopic devices as adjuncts in the management of patients with gastrointestinal hemorrhage than could previously be done.

Now that the endoscopist can use a coagulation or laser device to stop bleeding at the time of diagnosis, there is a possibility that patients whose evaluation and treatment include modern endoscopic devices will have fewer complications, fewer blood transfusions, and lower overall morbidity than previously. My associates and I have used the BICAP (American AMCI) bipolar probe for the control of nonvariceal upper gastrointestinal bleeding sites. Based on that experience we believe that endoscopic coagulation is not only an established means of controlling bleeding, but probably the most desirable one in light of overall cost, efficiency, and ease of use.

Believing that randomized controlled trials are not the only way to assess efficacy, and because it is doubtful that convincing randomized controlled studies can ever be performed to evaluate therapeutic devices for control of hemorrhage, we have adopted the approach that endoscopic coagulation be used only in patients with active bleeding, patients with serious episodes of hemorrhage, or victims of recent hemorrhage who have a bleeding site with a visible vessel. This stance avoids the application of therapy to all patients with hemorrhage, a group in which 80 percent will stop bleeding spontaneously; parenthetically, the last point has made the interpretation of laser data quite difficult at times.

Since any patient whose bleeding was not controlled by endoscopy would have been operated on, we did not have a separate control group. Patients served as their own controls, because until the time of the endoscopic examination they had received optimal conservative management.

During a one-year period, 279 patients were investigated for recent or continued bleeding. Twenty-eight (10 percent) of these patients had active bleeding sites, and another eight (3 percent) had visible vessels in the base of a chronic ulcer; these 36 patients (13 percent of the total) had endoscopic coagulation with the bipolar probe. The 28 with active bleeding had a mean transfusion requirement of seven units before attempts at control. Initial control was achieved in 23 of the 28 who bled from one of the following: duodenal or gastric ulcers (14), gastritis (11), Mallory-Weiss lesions (2), and gastric tumors (1).

Most of these patients did not have spurting arterial vessels; nonetheless, they had continuous, troublesome bleeding that was stopped at endoscopy. Five patients required additional transfusion therapy because of rebleeding, including three patients with lesions in which additional bleeding was inevitable.

No patient in the study died of hemorrhage, but the mortality was similar (20 percent) in those who required operation and those who were treated medically; two of nine patients treated by surgical means died, compared to four of the 19 patients treated nonoperatively. The 20 percent mortality was higher than expected in a population of bleeders but was not unexpected in this 10 percent subgroup of patients with the worst hemorrhage; almost all of these patients had serious associated illnesses and composed a group in whom high mortality was inevitable.

It is surprising that some physician- and surgeon-endoscopists have been slow to use coagulation devices for the endoscopic control of hemorrhage. The excellent results of several pioneers have been noted and were made possible by experimental definition of the safe ranges of current density that could be used. Consequently, there have been few adverse experiences reported in the literature. If concern about safety has restricted the use of endoscopic coagulation, however, the bipolar devices should become increasingly popular since they have an inherently safer mode of function and small risk of transmural injury.

Endoscopic devices for the control of nonvariceal upper gastrointestinal hemorrhage should be viewed as state-of-the-art technology that has had sufficient testing and that deserves wider application than it now has. Furthermore, when the laser and coagulation devices are compared, it seems that they are comparable in efficacy but differ greatly in cost and maintenance. Also, the lasers are stationary, whereas coagulation probes are portable. All of these considerations are valid in the assessment of endoscopic treatment methods, which may not affect overall mortality in patients at highest risk but can control acute bleeding in most instances.

EDITOR'S COMMENT

The surgeon-endoscopist is becoming recognized as a bona fide member of the patient care team (Donahue, Abcarian, Nyhus, *Surg. Gastroenterol.* 1:73, 1982).

Dr. Donahue and I detailed the role of the surgeon-endoscopist in the assessment of postoperative patients (*South. Med. J.* 75: 1570, 1982):

The sometimes extraordinary specificity of modern diagnostic techniques has made the practice of both medicine and surgery more scientific and enjoyable during the past 25 years. Much of this progress, with respect to gastrointestinal diseases, is a result of the impact of flexible fiberoptic endoscopes. These instruments have had an almost universal effect on the recognition and management of diseases and in several instances have altered our view of the natural history of particular digestive tract problems.

Because they have always had an interest in their patients' postoperative problems and because of their commitment to patients' long-term care, surgeons have become involved in many of the postoperative examinations, including endoscopy, that are sometimes required. As a direct result, surgeons have been able to make many observations that have had a direct effect on treatment recommendations; in several situations, the insights and experience of the surgeon-endoscopist have been of unique value.

It is important to stress the proficiency of modern-day gastrointestinal tract surgeons in the diagnosis and management of many gastrointestinal diseases; indeed, the process of learning who will or will not be a candidate for primary or remedial surgical procedures is the essence of surgical training.

Whenever an operation on a digestive structure is suggested, the operating surgeon bears the responsibility for ensuring that the diagnosis is sound and that the patient is adequately informed about the contemplated operation. The surgeon must decide among alternative operations, basing this decision on experimental as well as scientific data. That the surgeon must make such a decision is especially true in the treatment of patients who have had previous gastrointestinal operations. Sometimes these determinations involve the performance or interpretation of gastrointestinal endoscopic studies, with the information so obtained contributing to the pool of data that must be analyzed. The technical aspects of such an endoscopic examination are analogous to those of any other procedure on a patient: Endoscopy is a potentially harmful procedure that must be performed safely by a competent individual. In every instance, the well-being of the patient and the accuracy of observation are paramount.

Several anatomical areas and their endoscopic study have long been the purview of the surgeon. For example, direct laryngoscopy, bronchoscopy, esophagoscopy, choledochoscopy, laparoscopy, and proctoscopy have been practiced extensively, and sometimes exclusively, by surgeons. All reputable training programs have included in their curriculum the indications for several of these endoscopic examinations, as well as supervised experience in their application.

For these reasons, it is apparent that every surgeon who performs endoscopy is merely continuing the traditions of the profession, as opposed to expanding its scope. The imperative that surgeons perform postoperative follow-up studies on their patients and that they be aware of the consequences of their art finds additional expression when the surgeon obtains direct endoscopic views of the digestive tract.

In the postoperative clinic the manifestations of specific problems are often vague. There may not be pathognomonic signs and symptoms; there may only be suggestive patterns of complaints, which may be misinterpreted as neurosis. Individuals who evaluate these patients must be thoroughly familiar with and experienced in the interpretation of digestive tract complaints. There is no sequential and foolproof algorithm.

In terms of specific diagnostic tests, contrast studies of the upper gastrointestinal tract, endoscopic examinations, sonograms, gastric emptying studies, scintigraphic cholecystography, or laparotomy may be crucial, but the important catalyst in the process is experienced clinical judgment, which determines the sequence of investigation and interpretation.

Surgeons and physicians both have a role at times in the evaluation of patients who have had previous surgical procedures. A collaborative evaluation is in the patient's best interest.

(L. M. N.)

III

Gastritis and Gastric Ulcer

6

Gastritis and Duodenitis

Richard Whitehead

Chronic Gastritis

It is now usual to use the pathological term *chronic gastritis* in reference to the inflammatory lesion of the stomach that affects more or less of the gastric mucosa, that may or may not be associated with peptic ulcer or pernicious anemia, and that increases in frequency with age. Histologically, it is characterized by mucosal inflammation with or without destruction and architectural modification of the epithelial components. It emerged as an entity after the work of Faber [26] and Magnus and Ungley [57] which was primarily concerned with the lesion of pernicious anemia. With the examination of laparotomy biopsies and excised stomach specimens [55, 56, 72], it became clear that chronic gastritis occurred in association with a wide variety of disease states. However, the methods used in all these studies are open to criticism. Necropsy studies, even when performed with fixation immediately after death, are not ideal because of possible agonal changes and autolysis.

Gastrectomy specimens have two disadvantages. First, often only the distal segment of the stomach is available for examination, and second, operative maneuvers have been shown to cause inflammatory changes in the gastric mucosa [70, 73]. The advent of flexible-tube biopsy instruments [87, 98] was the beginning of a new era of investigation into mucosal lesions of the stomach. The association of chronic gastritis with the anemias, peptic ulceration, cancer, and autoimmune phenomena was studied in great detail, but the results showed a good deal of discrepancy. In part this was the result of the lack of good control studies in ostensibly normal populations, but to a greater extent it was caused by the inherent shortcomings of the biopsy instruments. It was possible to obtain a biopsy of only a limited area of stomach, never the highest part of the fundus and hardly ever the antrum. The normal site of biopsy was the greater curvature on the anterior or posterior wall, and it was never accurately sited.

The promise of rapid progress in the understanding of gastritis and its relationships to other diseases was thus understandably not fulfilled. With justification MacDonald and Rubin [54] wrote that the definition and classification of chronic gastritis remained unsatisfactory. Motteram [63], for example, subdivided chronic gastritis into superficial gastritis with minimal atrophy, atrophic gastritis with moderate or severe atrophy, and gastric atrophy. Wood and Taft [99] used the terms *superficial gastritis, atrophic gastritis,* and *gastric atrophy.* The superficial gastritis of Williams et al. [96] was classified by Davidson and Markson [18] as mild atrophic gastritis. These and other classifications were based on the appearances in body mucosa, whereas Schrager et al. [75] used an entirely different classification for antral mucosa.

The development of fiberoptic instruments permitting biopsy under direct vision meant that gastric mucosa free from serious artifact could now be obtained from all parts of the stomach and duodenum. Although the biopsy specimens are small, they usually include the muscularis mucosa; with careful handling, good, informative histological sections can be prepared. Interest in gastritis, particularly in relation to peptic ulceration and gastric cancer, is currently running at a high level.

TWO TYPES OF CHRONIC GASTRITIS

There is an overall similarity in the histological appearance of the chronic gastritis that occurs in association with a variety of disease states. Despite this, two broad groups can be recognized. These two groups are associated with different geographical distributions of gastritis within the stomach.

Strickland and MacKay [84] designate type A gastritis as that in which the serum contains parietal cell antibodies and there is a markedly reduced acid secretion. Impairment of vitamin B_{12} absorption will eventually develop in some but not all of these patients. It is this type of gastritis for which there appears to be familial or genetic predisposition [89]. The antrum is relatively spared, but there is a hyperplasia of gastrin-producing cells, which accounts for the high circulating serum levels. Antibodies to intrinsic factors are regularly found in the serum and gastric juice in patients in whom pernicious anemia develops. Type B gastritis is that formed in association with a negative parietal cell antibody test; there is a moderate or slight reduction in acid secretion, and only rarely is there an impairment of vitamin B_{12} absorption. In type B the gastritis is distal, always involving the pyloric region and extending backward to a variable extent along the lesser curvature. When severe, it fans out to involve the anterior and posterior walls of the body and sometimes the fundus, but usually only in a patchy manner.

As stated previously, the involved mucosa in both types of gastritis may not differ histologically. However, in a proportion of patients with pernicious anemia and type A gastritis the picture is better described as a gastric mucosal atrophy rather than atrophic gastritis, because at the time of examination active inflammatory destruction is absent. However, the gastritis not associated with pernicious anemia usually shows evidence of acute inflammatory epithelial destruction characterized not only by the presence of plasma cells and lymphocytes but also by the presence of polymorphonuclear leukocytes. This latter type of gastritis (type B) is that seen in association with duodenal and gastric ulcer, and it also occurs with increasing frequency as age advances. It is numerically the much more frequent of the two and is thus more important, since both types are associated with an increased risk of gastric cancer.

NEW CLASSIFICATION OF CHRONIC GASTRITIS

Based on experience with well over 4000 biopsy specimens from patients with a wide range of clinical conditions and from normal volunteer controls, Whitehead et al. [94] proposed a new classification of chronic gastritis applicable to all areas of the stomach.

In the normal stomach the pyloric mucosa occupies a triangular area in the lower third of the stomach. On the greater curvature it is found only in the immediate pyloric region for 1 or 2 cm proximal to the pyloric ring. On the lesser curvature the upper limit of the pyloric mucosa is usually in the region of the incisura angularis; but this is more variable, and the pyloric type of mucosa rarely extends to the esophagus. The cardiac glands are found distal to the cardioesophageal junction for a distance of about 1 cm, and all the remaining mucosa of the stomach is of the body type. The junction between the three areas may be abrupt, but it is often occupied by a transitional zone. At the pylorus-body junction in the lesser curvature region, the width of the transitional zone is variable, and sometimes the whole lesser curvature shows a transitional structure. When the mucosa of the various parts of the stomach is inflamed, differences in the appearances that are produced can best be classified by establishing four biopsy features:

1. The mucosal type
2. The grade of chronic gastritis
3. The activity of the gastritis
4. The presence and type of metaplasia

Mucosal Type

The recognition of the mucosal type is usually a simple matter, but when gastritis is severe and there is marked atrophy or metaplasia, it can be difficult or impossible. If all the tubules remaining are of the pyloric type, the mucosa could have originated in any part of the stomach, because gastritis in pyloric or cardiac mucosa is similar to gastritis with pseudopyloric metaplasia in the body or the junctional mucosa. However, if residual body glands remain, the mucosa must be of the body or junctional type. One of the great values of fiberoptic instruments is that the site of the biopsy specimen is fairly accurately located, except in stomachs altered by previous operations. In practice, difficulty arises only in biopsy specimens from the lesser curvature area, where the demarcation of one region from its neighbor is often poorly defined even in the normal stomach. A helpful point in the differentiation of normal pyloric glands from pseudopyloric glands is that, while the former may contain occasional parietal cells, the latter do not.

Grade of Chronic Gastritis

In common with most previous authors, I advocate two major subdivisions of chronic gastritis, i.e., superficial gastritis and atrophic gastritis. In the former the inflammatory and reactive changes affect only the superficial epithelium, gastric pit region, and related lamina propria. Deeper involvement with inflammation and destruction of gland tubules constitutes atrophic gastritis. Clearly, the difficult line of demarcation is between superficial gastritis and early atrophic gastritis; the later and more severe grades of atrophic gastritis are obvious. Deep extension of the inflammatory infiltrate around the tubules is usual in atrophic gastritis, but the best criterion for diagnosis is the recognition of atrophy of the tubules. In this respect the preparations stained for reticulin are most valuable, since loss of tubules, even in small numbers, is reflected by characteristic changes in reticulin pattern [94]. Atrophic gastritis could be classified more accurately by quantifying the number of glands that remain, but a convenient subdivision is into mild, moderate, and severe. If only one or two groups of tubules have disappeared, the mucosa is classified as showing mild atrophy; if all normal tubules are lost or only one or two groups remain, the designation is severe; all appearances between these two extremes are classed as moderate. It is important for this scheme that only normal glands be considered and that those showing metaplasia be discounted.

In severe atrophic gastritis with widespread metaplasia, a negligible inflammatory cell infiltrate is sometimes seen. Any lymphoid aggregates appear sparsely cellular and frequently show a fatty infiltration that may also appear in other areas of the lamina propria; these appearances are often referred to as gastric mucosal atrophy.

Activity of Gastritis

Some biopsy specimens exhibit an invasion of polymorphonuclear leukocytes into and severe degenerative changes of the epithelial elements of the gastric mucosa. Crypt abscess formation may also be present. If these features reflect an active stage of inflammatory epithelial destruction, as seems likely, it is clear that their presence should be brought into any scheme of classification. Epithelial degenerative changes associated with an infil-

Table 6-1. Proposed classifications of chronic gastritis

Mucosal type	Grade of gastritis				Metaplasia
Pyloric	Superficial	quiescent active	acute chronic		Pseudopyloric
Body	—				Intestinal
Cardiac	Atrophic	mild moderate severe	quiescent active	acute chronic	—
Junctional	—				—
Indeterminate	—				—

Source: Whitehead [91].

trate of the chronic type should be recorded as chronic activity.

In both types of chronic gastritis—superficial and atrophic—the activity can be graded simply on the basis of whether it is diffuse throughout the mucosa or is patchy in distribution. In mucosa with little or no epithelial degenerative changes and only a slight, insignificant chronic inflammatory infiltrate, the appearances should be classified as a quiescent or burned-out stage of the process. This quiescent phase is seen par excellence in mucosa with severe atrophy and metaplasia, i.e., in tissue showing so-called gastric mucosal atrophy.

Metaplasia

Intestinal metaplasia almost invariably occurs in a mucosa that is the site of atrophic gastritis. Occasionally it is present in the superficial epithelium and pits in superficial gastritis, and rarely isolated islands are seen in otherwise normal mucosa. Pseudopyloric metaplasia, on the other hand, occurs only in atrophic gastritis. There is some evidence that pseudopyloric metaplasia may be reversible [36]. Both types should be recorded separately, and the degree to which they are present can be graded. A full classification based on the principles outlined previously is shown in Table 6-1. From the point of view of investigation of the relationship of gastritis to other diseases or of exploring possible etiological factors, part or all of the classification may be employed, depending on the circumstances. Figures 6-1 through 6-15 show normal and gastric mucosa as seen in biopsy specimens. A detailed histological consideration of both is found in an article by Whitehead [91].

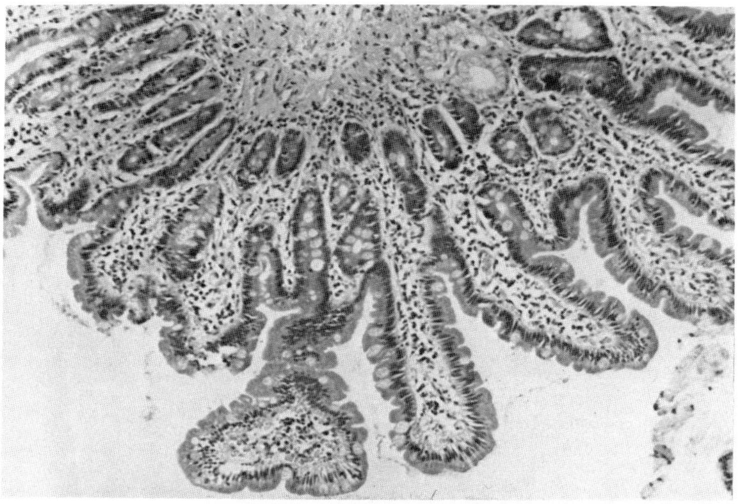

Fig. 6-1. Duodenal biopsy (grade 0). (H&E, ×100)

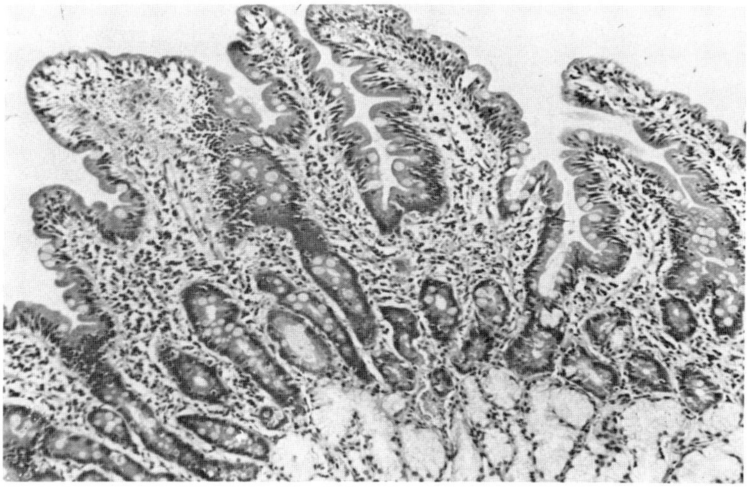

Fig. 6-2. Duodenal biopsy: Principal feature is increased cellularity of the lamina propria (grade 1). (H&E, ×100)

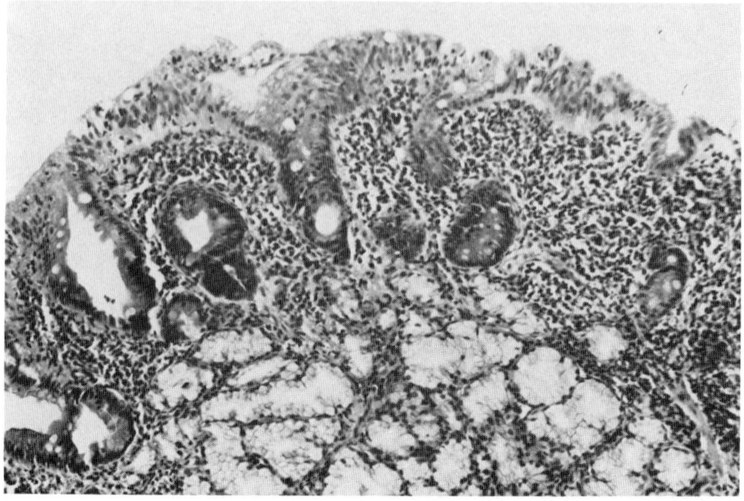

Fig. 6-3. Duodenal biopsy: Apart from cellularity of lamina propria, there is altered superficial epithelium (grade 2). Compare biopsies in Figures 6-2 and 6-3. (H&E, ×100)

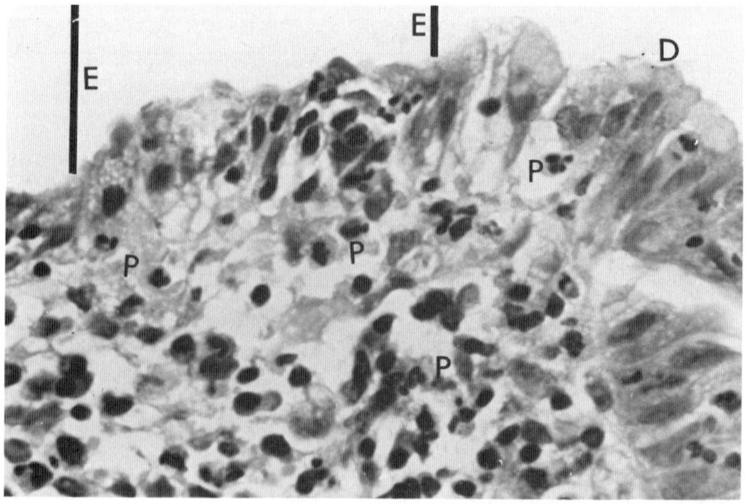

Fig. 6-4. Duodenal biopsy at a higher magnification. There is erosion of abnormal surface epithelium between the two lines marked E and residual degenerate epithelium marked D (grade 3). Note also the obvious polymorphs in the inflammatory infiltrate, some of which are marked P. (H&E, ×400)

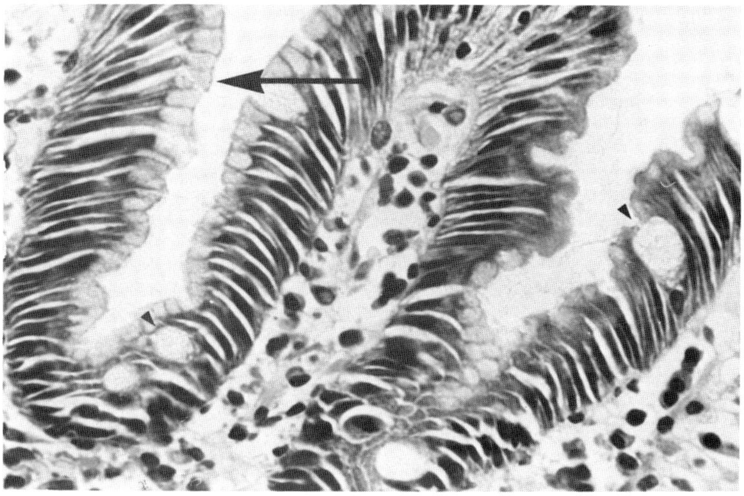

Fig. 6-5. Duodenal biopsy showing replacement of normal epithelium by gastric superficial epithelial cells *(arrow)*. Note residual goblet cells *(arrowheads)*. (H&E, ×300)

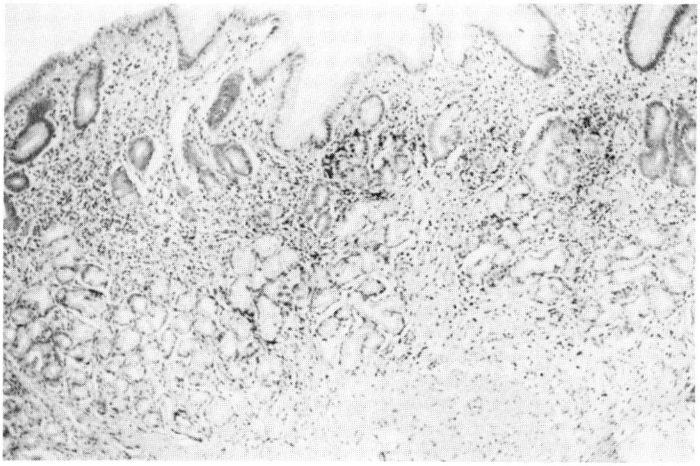

Fig. 6-6. Pyloric mucosa in mild atrophic gastritis. The infiltrate is more extensive, and some glands have disappeared.

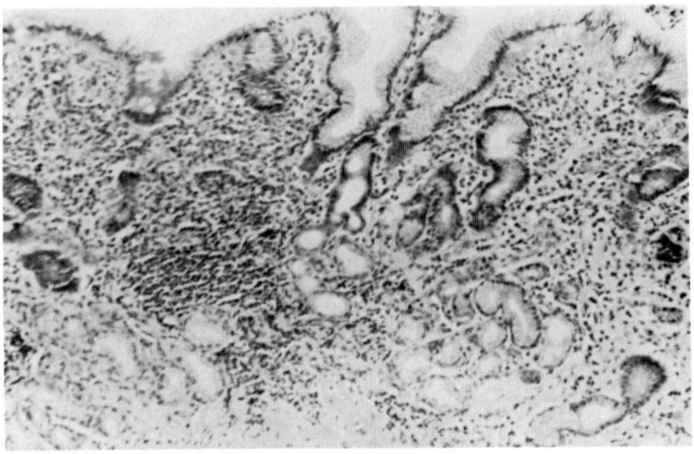

Fig. 6-7. Pyloric mucosa in moderate atrophic gastritis.

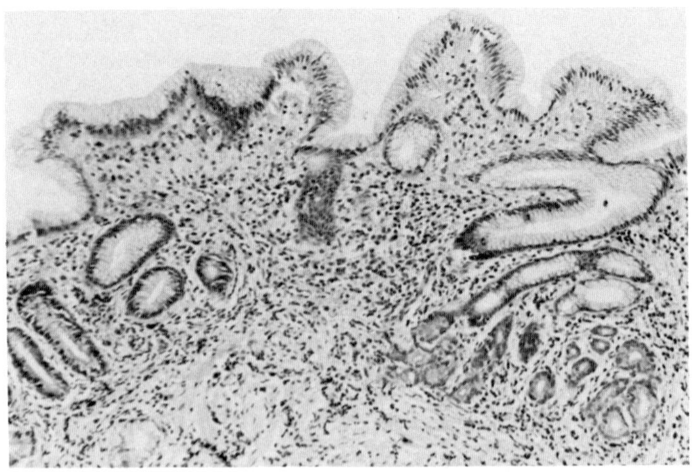

Fig. 6-8. Pyloric mucosa in severe atrophic gastritis. Occasional groups of glands are all that remain. As in Figure 6-7, a dense infiltrate still persists.

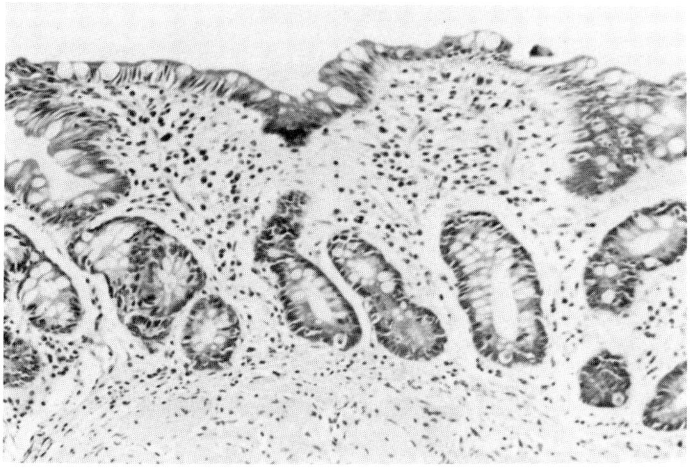

Fig. 6-9. Pyloric mucosa in severe atrophic gastritis with total replacement of residual mucosal elements by metaplastic small intestinal epithelium. Note that the infiltration has become minimal. These histological features are often diagnosed as representing gastric mucosal atrophy.

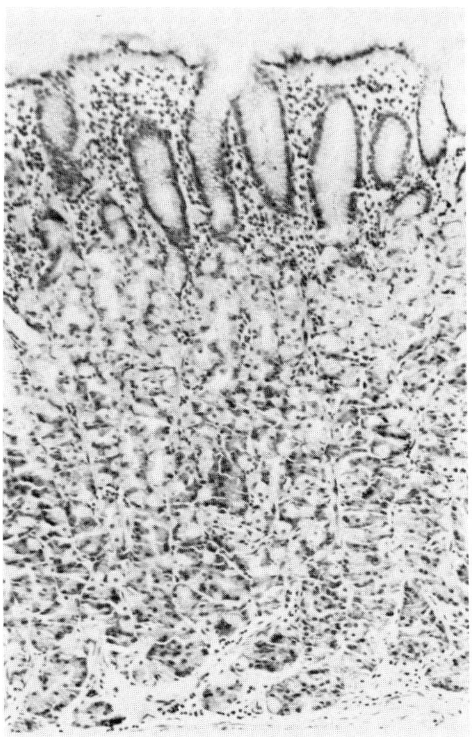

Fig. 6-10. Body mucosa in superficial gastritis.

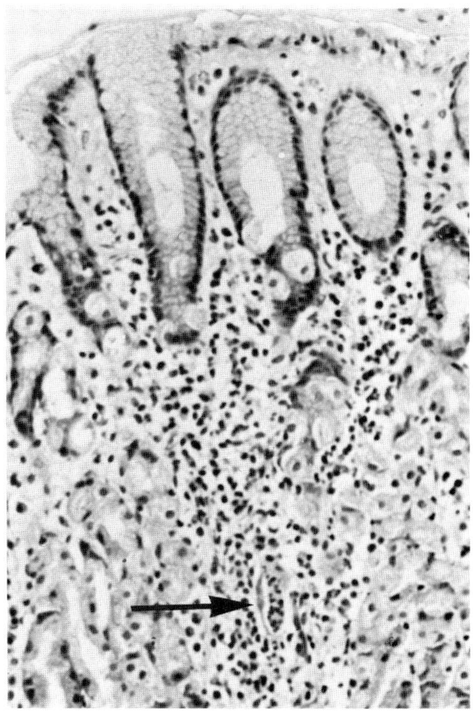

Fig. 6-11. Body mucosa in mild atrophic gastritis. An inflammatory infiltrate is beginning to extend into the gland layer. Note the tubule degeneration and associated luminal polymorphs *(arrow)*.

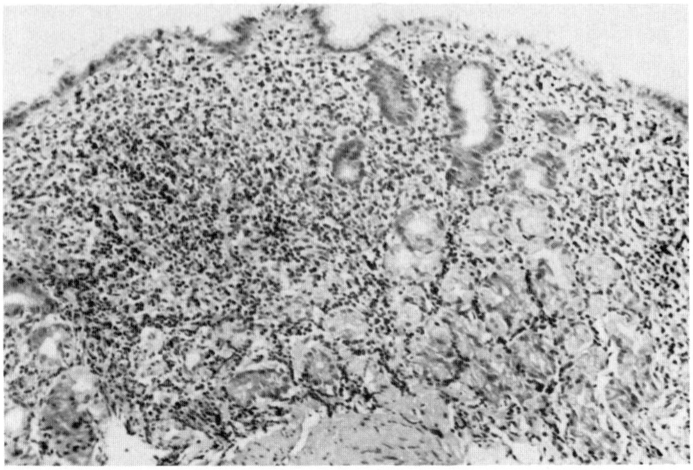

Fig. 6-12. The body mucosa in moderate atrophic gastritis. There is full-thickness inflammation with disappearance of several glands.

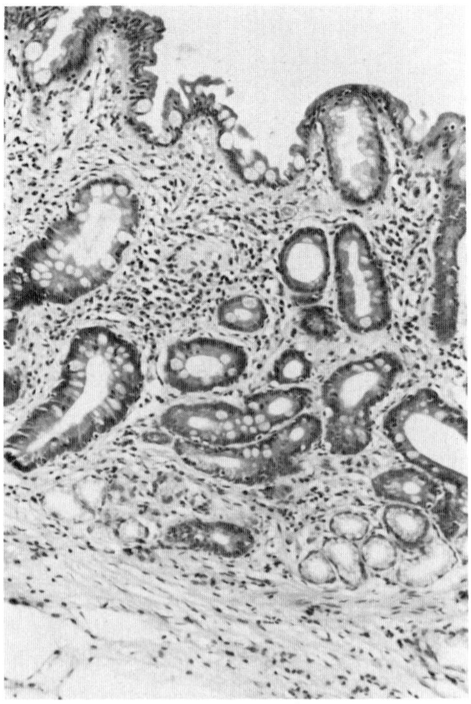

Fig. 6-13. Body mucosa in severe atrophic gastritis. There is widespread intestinal metaplasia, and the only glands remaining are of simple mucous type, i.e., there is pseudopyloric metaplasia. Note that there is still a fairly prominent inflammatory infiltrate, but it is not as marked as it is in Figure 6-12. Compare also with Figure 6-9.

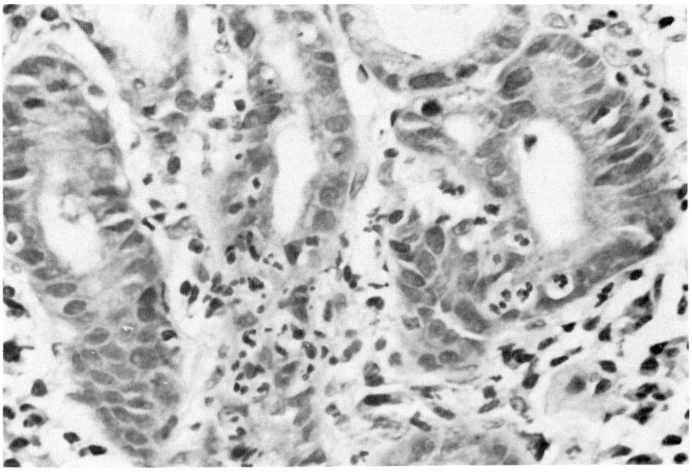

Fig. 6-14. Acute activity in gastritis. There is obvious polymorph infiltration and degeneration of the epithelial elements.

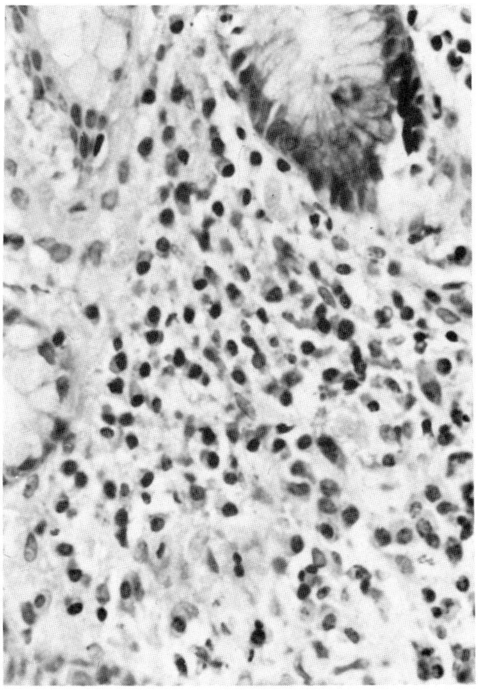

Fig. 6-15. Chronic activity in gastritis. The infiltrating cells are wholly lymphocytic or plasma cell in type. The epithelium shows less damage.

ETIOLOGY OF GASTRITIS

The etiology of chronic gastritis is poorly understood. There is some evidence that immune mechanisms are involved in the gastric mucosal lesion of pernicious anemia, but this is not so for the more common type B gastritis. Nevertheless autoantibodies reacting with the antral gastrin cells have been demonstrated in just less than 10 percent of patients with type B gastritis [88]. This would support the concept of an autoimmune variant. On the other hand, it is a characteristic of the often widespread gastritis in the postgastrectomy stomach to be unassociated with the presence of gastric autoantibodies [27]. Similarly, genetic factors that are strongly implicated in the causation of pernicious anemia play no apparent role in chronic gastritis (type B). What of its relationship to acute gastritis? The pathology of acute gastritis has not been adequately studied, and the term is often used incorrectly to refer to lesions of an acute erosive nature related to drug ingestion or other insults. Characteristic symptoms following bouts of acute alcohol intoxication, dietary indiscretions, or symptoms associated with certain viral infections or ingestion of drugs are commonly ascribed to acute inflammation of the gastric mucosa. There is little direct histological evidence for this. Palmer [66] reported acute superficial gastritis in all of 34 men on whom biopsies were performed within 6 hours of an episode of acute alcohol intoxication, but he did not illustrate his findings. In 9 of 11 men on whom biopsies were performed three weeks later, the mucosa was said to have returned to normal. The reported incidence of chronic gastritis in chronic alcoholics varies between 10 and 70 percent [20, 46, 95], but concrete evidence that excessive long-term alcohol usage causes chronic gastritis is still lacking. Indeed it is of interest that the incidence of chronic gastritis among patients with alcoholic cirrhosis was no higher than in a control series [7].

External X-ray Therapy

External x-ray therapy for peptic ulceration induces acute gastric mucosal damage within two weeks. There is a patchy but severe coagulative necrosis with subsequent secondary inflammatory infiltration [35]. This is usually followed by a reversion to normal after about four months. Intragastric irradiation, however, causes permanent tissue damage and it occasionally induces frank ulceration [30].

Foods, Condiments, Drugs, Age

Palmer [65] ascribed epithelial necrosis and intraluminal sloughing in the region of the gastric pits to acute staphylococcal food poisoning, but on critical appraisal the illustrations published show only a series of traumatic artifacts. Virtually nothing is known of the morphological changes induced by various foods, condiments, or drugs. Certainly the ingestion of pickles can produce acute surface epithelial cytological degeneration [92], and environmental circumstances related to diet probably determine the higher incidence of gastritis in some countries, such as Finland and Japan. The ingestion of aspirin [59] accelerates epithelial cell turnover [14] and is associated with the back-diffusion of acid [16, 77]. If exfoliation exceeds regeneration, this might explain the surface erosions and hemorrhage that may occur. After an episode of aspirin-induced acute gastrointestinal hemorrhage, erosions are commonly visualized gastroscopically, but good biopsy studies have not been reported. If the erosions and hemorrhage are diffuse, however, radical surgical treatment may be indicated. Histological examination of the excised specimen reveals loss of the superficial epithelium and upper pits with a diffuse hemorrhage into the upper layers of the mucosa. This constitutes acute hemorrhagic gastritis, which is also occasionally seen after major operations or trauma [28].

Numerous chemicals and drugs act as gastric irritants or corrosives, and these produce a variety of histological appearances ranging from hyperemia, surface erosion, and inflammation to more massive mucosal necrosis and sloughing.

Thus there is no direct evidence that the known causes of gastric mucosal injury or repeated attacks of acute gastritis lead to the development of chronic gastritis. There is, however, circumstantial evidence based on blind biopsy studies that links chronic gastritis of the body with the drinking of hot liquids [24]. Gastritis of the body is also said to increase in frequency with age. A recent fiberoptic biopsy study in Japan [48] seems to bear this out; in this study gastritis was found to spread backward from the pylorus as age advanced.

Long-term salicylate use and cigarette smoking seem to be contributory factors in chronic gastritis [23]. Jarvis and Whitehead [41] showed that the administration of nicotine to rats in their drinking water results in a decrease in the mucus-producing component of the gastric mucosa. Theoretically, this would tend to decrease its ability to withstand the effects of any other ingested agents with a propensity for gastric mucosal injury. It is perhaps significant that both age and cigarette smoking are also related to atherosclerosis. Peptic ulceration, which is always associated with chronic gastritis in some part of the stomach (see the section Two Types of Chronic Gastritis), is more common in patients with severe atherosclerosis, especially if aortic calcification and/or atheromatous aneurysms are present [25, 45]. The relationship of gastritis to duodenal reflux will be considered in the following section. Siurala and Salmi [78] produced evidence, using a blind biopsy method, that superficial gastritis eventually develops into the more severe lesion of atrophic gastritis, but there is no hard guarantee that sequential biopsies are even approximately from the same site. Gear et al. [32], however, showed a progression of the severity of chronic gastritis in patients with peptic ulcer when biopsies were accurately located to the same site in the stomach using a fiberoptic instrument. It seems likely, therefore, that the chronic gastritis lesion is a progressive one and that it has a multifactorial etiology involving exogenous and endogenous factors.

CHARACTERISTICS OF CHRONIC GASTRITIS AND ASSOCIATED PROBLEMS

The importance of chronic gastritis as a clinical entity is hard to assess. The ability to secrete acid, pepsinogen, and intrinsic factor is reduced as the body mucosa atrophies [34], but normally the ability to produce some intrinsic factor persists longer than the ability to secrete acid. This is interesting, because in humans both acid and intrinsic factor come from the parietal cell [37].

As atrophic gastritis progresses, the pattern of mucoprotein secretion alters, and albumin and globulin in high concentrations may be found in the gastric juice [33]. It has been postulated by Coghill [12] that otherwise obscure instances of hypoalbuminemia in the elderly may be caused by albumin loss from the stomach with diffuse atrophic gastritis, but this is an issue still to be settled.

Dyspepsia

Despite such disturbances of function, the evidence that chronic gastritis of the body mucosa is associated with dyspepsia is not convincing [11, 46, 76]; however, the studies that have been done were based on blind biopsy methods and were carried out at an early stage in the understanding of chronic gastritis. It seems that chronic gastritis of the body may be present in patients without symptoms, whereas patients with persistent non-ulcer dyspepsia may show no changes. It is obvious that there is need for further work in this field utilizing modern techniques.

Iron Deficiency

It has been shown repeatedly that patients with iron deficiency anemia have an incidence of body gastritis of between 30 and 60 percent [3, 13], and it is more common in those patients with no other known cause for iron deficiency. The view that iron deficiency causes gastritis is unfounded, and there are follow-up studies [39, 40] that show that gastritis persists after the anemia has been treated and that recurrent anemia is seen more frequently in those patients in whom the gastritis progresses in severity. This would indicate that the gastritis may be the cause of the anemia; in postgastrectomy patients blood loss from the atrophic gastric mucosa has been shown to be increased [38]. Loss of free iron is also increased in patients with atrophic gastritis [85] and is probably caused by the increase in cell turnover that occurs. There is some evidence that the presence of chronic gastritis makes the stomach mucosa more susceptible to damage by other agents such as aspirin or alcohol [97].

Peptic Ulcer

The relationship between gastritis and peptic ulcer of the stomach becomes less obscure if only type B gastritis is considered. The very early observations of Cruveilhier in 1862 [15] are still true: Ulcer and gastritis are invariably present in the same stomach. The gastritis always involves the antrum in prepyloric ulcers and extends proximally to involve a larger area in body ulcers [32]. Body ulcers are always situated in a pyloric type of mucosa either distal to or at its junction with body mucosa [64]; consequently, when the ulcer is high, the antrum appears to be enlarged. This could be the result of atrophic gastritis with pseudopyloric metaplasia, or it might mean that persons with an abnormally large antrum are prone to ulcer. There is increasing evidence that the former is the case, but clearly this also needs further study.

What is the extent to which the body and fundic mucosae are involved by atrophic gastritis in gastric ulcers? Gear et al. [32] have shown that gastritis does indeed occur in these areas, but frequently it is in a patchy distribution. Patients with gastric ulcer show duodenal reflux [21], and bile and pancreatic juice combined are potent producers of gastritis, as seen both in postgastrectomy patients and in experimental situations [10, 17]. Mucosa showing atrophic gastritis is very prone to ulceration [69], and Gear et al. have shown that the gastritis associated with ulcer persists or gets worse after the ulcer is healed. More recently, Aukee and Krohn [2] have confirmed this observation and established that it is a significant change. They found that after operation for peptic ulcer, not only does the gastritis progress in severity, as judged by biopsy examination, but also acid production falls. It would seem very probable, therefore, that it is the gastritis that precedes and predisposes to gastric ulcer, but whether all gastric ulcers can be explained in this way is as yet unsolved.

CANCER RISK

The importance of the phenomena discussed previously is plain because of the cancer risk in patients with atrophic gastritis. Morson [60] has shown that atrophic gastritis with intestinal metaplasia is seen in over 90 percent of patients with cancer of the stomach. After 25 years the incidence of cancer in patients who have had a gastric operation is 6 times the expected rate [81], and gastritis in these patients is the rule. Deaths from gastric cancer occur at 3 or 4 times the expected frequency in patients with pernicious anemia [6, 62]. In a follow-up study of atrophic gastritis unassociated with pernicious anemia, Siurala and Seppala [79] showed that about 10 percent develop cancer; and since this type of gastritis is much more frequent than pernicious anemia, it represents a more important precancerous condition.

By implication this finding poses an important clinical problem in the management of patients known to have widespread atrophic gastritis and intestinalization. There is recent evidence that carcinoma arising in chronic gastritis does so by evolution through progressive dysplasia involving the areas of intestinalization [61]. Furthermore, the tumor arising in such circumstances is often of the so-called intestinal type [51], and studies suggest that the intestinal mucosa from which it arises is colonic rather than small intestinal, based on the histochemical difference in their epithelial mucins [42]. It is this intestinal type of carcinoma that forms the excess of tumors in countries with a high incidence of gastric cancer.

Electron microscopy and immunological and histochemical studies have shown, however, that almost all gastric cancers show a proportion of cells with characteristics of intestinal epithelium [19, 71, 82, 86]. Cells with intestinal characteristics are also found in the base of the pits of normal gastric mucosa, which is the zone of cell proliferation. In atrophic gastritis there is a marked increase in cell turnover and a tendency for the intestinal type of cell to be produced. In such circumstances cancer might be expected to supervene in a proportion of instances. This also explains why intestinal metaplasia and cancer cells with intestinal characteristics are so commonly associated. After the examination of 64 gastrectomy specimens, Skinner et al. [80] showed that the gastritis and intestinal metaplasia associated with gastric ulcer of the body of the stomach has a similar distribution and severity to that of gastric cancer but is more localized in association with pyloric ulcer. In patients with recurrent stomal or pyloric ulcer after gastrojejunostomy for duodenal ulcer, however, the gastrectomy specimen showed a distribution and severity of gastritis that was also like that seen in cancer (Table 6-2). This similarity points to a higher cancer risk in the stomach with body ulcer and after gastrojejunostomy.

The practical implications of these facts are obvious. The choice of a surgical treatment of peptic ulcer that ensures cure must be influenced by the relative postoperative tendencies to accelerate the premalignant condition of chronic gastritis.

Duodenitis

The duodenum, like the rest of the small and large intestine, has a lamina propria that contains an easily discernible lymphocyte, plasma cell, histiocyte, and eosinophil polymorphonuclear leukocyte population. Together with the intraepithelial lymphocytes, solitary lymphoid follicles, and Peyer's patches, the lymphohistiocytic cells form the whole of the intestinal-associated lymphoid tissue. Changes in the density of these cell types will occur when that system is stimulated. This may occur in viral, bacterial, or parasitic infection or in other circumstances of antigenic stimulation such as gluten-sensitive enteropathy or protein intolerance, or when the duodenum is involved in a specific disease process such as Crohn's disease.

The duodenum may also exhibit changes in cellularity of the lamina propria as the result of involvement in a "field" change caused by lesions of neighboring organs, e.g., stomach, pancreas, or bile ducts. It is only by exclusion that one is able to define a form of duodenal inflammation that is a distinct and separate entity. Such a lesion—"duodenitis" or "nonspecific duodenitis"—has emerged over almost a century and a half; it was first described by Baudin in 1837 [4]. This discovery has not occurred without considerable debate. Konjetzny [49] recognized duodenitis in the mucosa immediately adjacent to a duodenal ulcer, and MacCarty [53] showed that identical appearances are sometimes seen in operative specimens from patients who have a typical duodenal ulcer history but no ulcer. Thus the lesion of duodenitis and its importance as a cause of non-ulcer dyspepsia and as a precursor of duodenal ulcer became a subject of great interest [47].

With the advent of flexible-tube biopsy procedures, interest in duodenitis was renewed and the study of the relationship between duodenitis and ulcer was intensified. The results proved conflicting. The findings of Fraser et al. [29], Beck et al. [5], Rhodes et al. [68] and Gear and Dobbins [31] supported the concept of a diathesis comprising hyperchlorhydria and duodenitis leading to duodenal ulcer. Rhodes et al. [68] also stressed the roentgenographic features of duodenitis and concluded that the presence of coarse duodenal folds was related to the duodenal inflammation, Brunner's gland hyperplasia, or both. Other workers [1, 22, 44], however, found no significant association between duodenitis and non-ulcer dyspepsia or between duodenitis and duodenal ulcer. Cheli [8] concluded that duodenitis in duodenal ulcer was simply a local phenomenon in the immediate vicinity of the ulcer with no pathogenetic importance.

The reasons for these discordant results become clear when it is realized that in all these studies patient selection was made on the ba-

Table 6-2. Atrophic gastritis, intestinal metaplasia, and superficial gastritis in 64 gastrectomy specimens

Ulcer type and number	Atrophic gastritis						Intestinal metaplasia						Superficial gastritis					
	P	LC	LGC	UGC	BA	BP	P	LC	LGC	UGC	BA	BP	P	LC	LGC	UGC	BA	BP
Before gastrojejunostomy																		
Body, 23	23	23	20	19	19	21	21	21	18	18	19	21	0	0	0	2	1	0
Pyloric, 14	5	4	3	2	0	0	3	3	3	2	0	0	8	1	1	0	0	0
After gastrojejunostomy																		
Pyloric, 3	3	3	3	3	2	1	3	3	3	3	2	1	0	0	0	0	1	0
Stomal, 3	3	3	3	3	3	3	3	3	3	2	3	2	0	0	0	0	0	0
Cancer, 21	19	19	19	20	20	18	19	19	18	18	18	17	0	0	0	0	0	0

Note: Sites indicated in the various groups studied: P = pyloric; LC = lesser curvature above the pyloric region; LGC = lower greater curvature; UGC = upper greater curvature; BA = anterior wall of body mucosa; BP = posterior wall of body mucosa.
Source: Skinner et al. [80].

sis of the roentgenographic appearance and that the biopsies assessed for the presence of duodenitis were taken from sites localized by fluoroscopy. Even the best roentgenologists miss duodenal ulceration, and the interpretation of the roentgenographic signs of an irritable duodenum or one with thickened mucosal folds is notoriously difficult. Furthermore, the fluoroscopic siting of the tip of the biopsy instrument in the normal duodenum, and especially in a deformed duodenum, is subject to inaccuracy. Another cause of difficulty is in the histological classification of what is a significant duodenitis. Clear descriptions of criteria for the diagnosis have been lacking.

It has proved possible for even small increases in cells of the lamina propria, as well as other changes in structure, to be accurately quantified. Whitehead et al. [93] have shown, however, that by noting the presence of easily identifiable histological features used as criteria, three grades of duodenitis can be recognized (Table 6-3). These results correlate well with the results from morphometric methods, which objectively measure lamina propria cell numbers and surface-to-volume ratios of mucosal biopsies.

In grade 1 or mild duodenitis the only important deviation from normal is an increase in the cellularity of the lamina propria. The villous pattern, although frequently showing abnormality in the form of shortening and blunting, is too inconsistent to be a useful criterion in classification. The epithelial cells in grade 1 are always normal in height and structure. It is this type of lesion that seems likely to be associated with abnormalities in neighboring structures, e.g., the pancreas or stomach. It probably corresponds to the interstitial duodenitis of Cheli [8], in which the patchy distribution of the increased cellularity is ascribable to the inclusion of reactive lymphoid aggregates.

In grade 2 or moderate duodenitis the same features as in grade 1 are seen, but with the addition of abnormality of the surface epithelial cells. The cells may appear flatter than normal or show nuclear hyperchromasia and increased cytoplasmic basophilia of the diminished cytoplasm. The brush border becomes less distinct and the cells may appear stratified with nuclei at different levels. Sometimes budlike syncytial masses project from the surface, the crypt zone shows hyperplasia, and there is a failure of differentiation such that primitive cells without the features of enterocytes or goblet cells come to occupy the surface. Once again the tendency is for villous effacement, and the cellular infiltrate of the lamina propria and the interepithelial compartment is increased.

The most severe grade, grade 3, is characterized by the critical features of erosion of the abnormal epithelial surface. It is usual for there to be severe or complete effacement of the villous pattern, and this grade is associated with the heaviest degree of cellular infiltration.

Table 6-3. Histological grading of duodenitis

Grade of duodenitis	Distinguishing histological features	General histological features	
0	Normal	↓ Increasing cellularity of lamina propria and loss of the villous pattern (applies to grades 0–3)	Neutrophil polymorph infiltration + or − ; Gastric superficial epithelial metaplasia + or −
1	Superficial epithelium and general morphology normal; increased cellularity of lamina propria		
2	Abnormality of the surface epithelium		
3	Erosion of the surface epithelium		

When the inflammatory infiltrate contains a neutrophil polymorphonuclear component, this should be noted separately. It is commonly associated with a separation of the epithelial elements, which is usually interpreted as tissue edema. Neutrophil polymorphs are usually seen in the grade 2 and 3 biopsies but not always, and their importance may lie as an indicator of activity or progression of the lesion.

The presence of gastric superficial epithelial metaplasia should also be recorded. It is important to realize that this is an entity distinct from gastric heterotopia of the duodenum, which occurs as slightly elevated isolated islands of gastric mucosa composed of superficial epithelium, crypts, and specialized glands, usually containing parietal cells, but occasionally chief cells also. Furthermore, it is not sufficiently well recognized that the pyloroduodenal junction is frequently not well demarcated. Biopsies from the transitional zone can easily be misinterpreted as duodenal mucosa showing gastric metaplasia, and vice versa. This probably accounts in part for the extremely high incidence of "gastric metaplasia" found in some published series of duodenal biopsy studies even in healthy persons [50]. Indeed if gastric surface epithelium is seen in the absence of considerable duodenal inflammation, the biopsy site is probably at the junction of the pylorus and duodenum or just beyond. True gastric superficial epithelial metaplasia, which can be induced in cats by stimulating hypersecretion of hydrochloric acid [67], is usually only seen in an extensive manner in grades 2 and 3 duodenitis. It is hardly ever seen in grade 1 duodenitis or when appearances are entirely normal, especially when biopsies are taken well into the bulb. The principal histological features referred to here are illustrated in Figures 6-1 through 6-5.

Duodenitis and Brunner's gland hyperplasia are thought to be associated [58], but there is a difficulty in assessing Brunner's gland mass in fiberoptic biopsies because of their superficial nature. Certainly they can be seen in some duodenal mucosal biopsies, especially those from the bulb and descending part. It is not usual in duodenitis for those parts of the Brunner's glands that extend below the muscularis mucosa to show periglandular inflammatory infiltrates, although naturally those lying above the muscularis mucosa will do so.

The blood vessel changes of congestion or dilatation, which are normally associated with inflammation in vivo, are notoriously difficult to assess in histological preparations. It is likely that they disappear during the biopsy procedure and the fixation and tissue processing with its associated shrinkage that occurs in slide preparation. As a consequence, there is a poor correlation between histological inflammation and mild or even severe erythema seen at endoscopy. Reddening with erosion and petechiae, however, correlate well with severe histological duodenitis.

For the pathologist, therefore, the histological variations from normality that occur in duodenal biopsies are readily recognized and have been verified in quantitative studies [9, 50, 52, 74, 93]. They have also been related to patients' symptoms in clinicopathological investigations [83, 90]. In the last few years these pathological changes have been seen increasingly in proper perspective. In patients with non-ulcer dyspepsia and no other demonstrable disease, a severe duodenitis with microerosions and a neutrophil polymorph infiltration may well be causally related. Alternatively, mild increases in chronic inflammatory cells in patients with pancreatitis may only be a secondary or field effect. There is already evidence to show that severe duodenitis is the lower end of the spectrum of duodenal ulcer disease [43]. There is no doubt that in the not too distant future, well-planned collaborative research will provide a better understanding of duodenitis. A better time for the treatment of duodenal ulcer disease is surely the preulcerative phase.

References

1. Aronson, A. R., and Norfleet, R. G. The duodenal mucosa in peptic ulcer disease: A clinical pathological correlation. *Am. J. Dig. Dis.* 7:506, 1962.
2. Aukee, S., and Krohn, K. Occurrence and pro-

gression of gastritis in patients operated on for peptic ulcer. *Scand. J. Gastroenterol.* 7:541, 1972.
3. Badenoch, J., Evans, J. R., and Richards, W. C. D. The stomach in hypochromic anemia. *Br. J. Haematol,* 3:175, 1957.
4. Baudin, J. B., M. D. thesis, University of Paris, 1837. Cited by Ostow, J. D., and Resnick, R. H. *Ann. Intern. Med.* 51:1303, 1959.
5. Beck, I. T., Kahn, D. S., Lacerte, M., et al. Chronic duodenitis: A clinical pathological entity. *Gut* 6:376, 1965.
6. Blackburn, E. K., Callendar, S. T., Dacie, J. V., et al. Possible association between pernicious anaemia and leukaemia: A prospective study of 1,625 patients with a note on the very high incidence of stomach cancer. *Int. J. Cancer* 3:163, 1968.
7. Brown, R. C., Hardy, G. J., Temperley, J. M., et al. Gastritis and cirrhosis: No association. *J. Clin Pathol.* 34:744, 1981.
8. Cheli, R. Duodenitis and duodenal ulcer. *Digestion* 1:175, 1968.
9. Cheli, R., and Giacosa, A. Inflammatory cell count and identification in chronic non-specific duodenitis. *Endoscopy* 9:91, 1977.
10. Cheng, J., Ritchie, W. P., Jr., and Delaney, J. Atrophic gastritis: An experimental model. *Fed. Proc.* 28:513, 1969.
11. Coghill, N. F. The significance of gastritis. *Postgrad. Med. J.* 36:733, 1960.
12. Coghill, N. F. Chronic Idiopathic Gastritis: Cause and Effect. In R. Williams (Ed.) *Fifth Symposium on Advanced Medicine.* Bath, England: Pitman, 1969. P. 14.
13. Coghill, N. F., and Williams, A. W. Gastric mucosa in hypochromic anaemia. *Proc. Soc. Med.* 51:464, 1958.
14. Croft, D. N. Aspirin and exfoliation of gastric epithelial cells: Cytological and biochemical observations. *Br. Med. J.* 2:897, 1963.
15. Cruveilhier, J. *Traité D'anatomie Pathologique Générale.* Paris: Ballière, 1862. P. 484.
16. Davenport, H. W. Salicylate damage to the gastric mucosal barrier. *N. Engl. J. Med.* 276:1307, 1967.
17. Davenport, H. W. Destruction of gastric mucosal barrier by detergents and urea. *Gastroenterology* 54:175, 1968.
18. Davidson, W. M. B., and Markson, J. L. The gastric mucosa in iron deficiency anaemia. *Lancet* 2:639, 1955.
19. De Boer, W. G. R. M., Forsyth, A. and Nairn, R. C. Gastric antigens in health and disease: Behaviour in early development, senescence, metaplasia and cancer. *Br. Med. J.* 3:93, 1969.
20. Debray, C., Hardouin, J. P., Laumonier, R., et al. La gastrite ethylique sous le contrôle de la gastrobiopsie. *Arch. Mal. App. Dig. Nutr.* 46:925, 1957.
21. Delaney, J. P., Cheng, J. W. B., Butler, B. A., and Ritchie, W. P. Gastric ulcer and regurgitation gastritis. *Gut* 11:715, 1970.
22. Doniach, I., and Shiner, M. Duodenal and jejunal biopsies. II. Histology. *Gastroenterology* 33:71, 1957.
23. Edwards, F. C., and Coghill, N. F. Aetiological factors in chronic atrophic gastritis. *Br. Med. J.* 2:1409, 1966.
24. Edwards, F. C., and Edwards, J. H. Tea drinking and gastritis. *Lancet* 2:543, 1956.
25. Elkeles, A. Gastric ulcer in the aged and calcified atherosclerosis. *Am. J. Roentgenol. Radium Ther. Nucl. Med.* 91:744, 1964.
26. Faber, K. *Gastritis and Its Consequences.* London: Oxford University Press, 1935.
27. Fisher, J. M., Mackay, I. R., Taylor, K. B., and Ungar, B. An immunological study of categories of gastritis. *Lancet* 1:176, 1967.
28. Flowers, R. S., Kyle, K., and Hoerr, S. O. Post-operative haemorrhage from stress ulceration of the stomach and duodenum. *Am.J. Surg.* 119:632, 1970.
29. Fraser, G. M., Pitman, R. G., Lawrie, J. H., et al. The significance of the radiological finding of coarse mucosal folds in the duodenum. *Lancet* 2:979, 1964.
30. Fruin, R. C., Littman, M. S., and Littman, A. Intragastric beta-irradiation with ruthenium-rhodium 106 in patients with peptic ulcer and gastric neoplasm. *Gastroenterology* 45:34, 1963.
31. Gear, E. V., and Dobbins, W. O. The histologic spectrum of proximal duodenal biopsy in adult males. *Am. J. Med. Sci.* 257:90, 1969.
32. Gear, M. W. L., Truelove, S. C., and Whitehead, R. Gastric ulcer and gastritis *Gut* 12:639, 1971.
33. Glass, G. B., and Ishimori, A. Passage of serum albumin into the stomach: Its detection by paper electrophoresis of gastric juice in protein-losing gastropathies and gastric cancer. *Am. J. Dig. Dis.* 6:103, 1961.
34. Glass, G. B., Speer, F. D., Neiburgs, H. E., et

al. Gastric atrophy, atrophic gastritis and gastric secretory failure: Correlative study by suction biopsy and exfoliative cytology of gastric mucosa, paper electrophoretic and secretory assays of gastric secretion and measurements of intestinal absorption and blood levels of vitamin B_{12}. *Gastroenterology* 39:429, 1960.
35. Goldgraber, M. B., Rubin, C. E., Palmer, W. L., et al. The early gastric response to irradiation: A serial biopsy study. *Gastroenterology* 27:1, 1954.
36. Harvey, B. C. H. A study of the structure of the gastric glands of dogs and the changes which they undergo after gastroenterostomy and occlusion of the pylorus. *Am. J. Anat.* 6:207, 1907.
37. Hoedemaeker, P. J., Abels, J. Wachters, J. J., et al. Investigations about the site of production of Castles' gastric intrinsic factor. *Lab. Invest.* 13:1394, 1964.
38. Holt, J. M., Gear, M. W. L., and Warner, G. T. The role of chronic blood loss in the pathogenesis of post gastrectomy iron deficiency anemia. *Gut* 11:847, 1970.
39. Ikkala, E., Salmi, H. J., and Siurala, M. Gastric mucosa in iron deficiency anaemia. Results of a follow-up examination. *Acta Haematol.* (Basel) 43:228, 1970.
40. Ikkala, E., and Siurala, M. Gastric lesion in iron deficiency anaemia. *Acta Haematol.* (Basel) 31:313, 1964.
41. Jarvis, L. R., and Whitehead, R. Effect of nicotine on the morphology of the rat gastric mucosa. *Gastroenterology* 78:1488, 1980.
42. Jass, J. R., and Filipe, M. I. Variants of intestinal metaplasia associated with gastric carcinoma: A histochemical study. *Histopathology* 3:191, 1979.
43. Joffe, S. N., Lee, F. D., and Blumgart, L. H. Duodenitis. *Clin. Gastroenterol.* 7:635, 1978.
during continuous or interrupted aspirin ingestion in humans. *Am. J. Dig. Dis.* 21:963, 1976.
60. Morson, B. C. Intestinal metaplasia of the gastric mucosa. *Br. J. Cancer* 9:365, 1955.
61. Morson, B. C., Sobin, L. H., Grundmann, E., et al. Precancerous conditions and epithelial dysplasia in the stomach. *J. Clin. Pathol.* 33:711, 1980.
62. Mosbech, J., and Videbaek, A. Mortality from and risk of gastric carcinoma among patients with pernicious anaemia. *Br. Med. J.* 2:390, 1950.
63. Motteram, R. A biopsy study of chronic gastritis and gastric atrophy. *J. Pathol. Bacteriol.* 63:389, 1951.
44. Johnston, D. H. Blind gastric and duodenal mucosal biopsies in patients with duodenal ulcer and those with an ulcer-like syndrome. *South. Med. J.* 57:79,1964.
45. Jones, A. W., Kirk, R. S., and Bloor, K. The association between aneurysms of the abdominal aorta and peptic ulceration. *Gut* 11:679, 1970.
46. Joske, R. A., Finckh, E. S., and Wood, I. J. Gastric biopsy: A study of 1,000 consecutive successful gastric biopsies. *Q. J. Med.* 24:269, 1955.
47. Judd, E. S., and Nagel, W. G. Duodenitis, *Ann. Surg.* 85:380, 1927.
48. Kimura, K. Chronological transition of the fundic-pyloric border determined by stepwise biopsy of the lesser and greater curvatures of the stomach. *Gastroenterology* 63:584, 1972.
49. Konjetzny, G. E. Zur Pathologie und chirurgischen Behandlung des Ulcus duodeni. *Dtsch. Z. Chir.* 184:85, 1924.
50. Kreuning, J., Bosman, F. T., Kuiper, G., et al. Gastritis and duodenal mucosa in "healthy" individuals: An endoscopic and histopathological study of 50 volunteers. *J. Clin. Pathol.* 31:69, 1978.
51. Lauren P. The two histological main types of gastric carcinoma: Diffuse and so-called intestinal type carcinoma. *Acta Pathol. Microbiol. Scand.* 64:31, 1965.
52. Lev, R., Thomas, E., Parl, F. F., and Pitchumoni, C. S. Pathological and histomorphometric study of the effects of alcohol on the human duodenum. *Digestion* 20:207, 1980.
53. MacCarty, W. C. Excised duodenal ulcers: A report of four hundred and twenty-five specimens. *J.A.M.A.* 83:1894, 1924.
54. MacDonald, W. C., and Rubin, C. E. Gastric biopsy: A critical evaluation. *Gastroenterology* 53:143, 1967.
55. Magnus, H. A. The pathology of simple gastritis. *J. Pathol. Bacteriol.* 58:431, 1946.
56. Magnus, H. A. Gastritis. In F. H. Jones (Ed.), *Modern Trends in Gastroenterology* (1st ser.). London: Butterworth, 1952. Pp. 323-51.
57. Magnus, H. A., and Ungley, C. C. The gastric lesion in pernicious anaemia. *Lancet* 1:420, 1938.
58. Maratka, Z., Kociánová, J., Kudrmann, J., Jirk, P., and Pirk, F. Hyperplasia of Brunner's glands: Radiology, endoscopy and biopsy. *Acta Hepatogastroenterol.* 26:64, 1979.

59. Metzger, W. H., McAdam, L., Bluestone, R., and Guth, P. H. Acute gastric mucosal injury
64. Oi, M., Oshida, K., and Sugimura, S. The location of gastric ulcer. *Gastroenterology* 36:45, 1959.
65. Palmer, E. D. The morphologic consequences of acute exogenous (staphylococcic) gastroenteritis on the gastric mucosa. *Gastroenterology* 19:462, 1951.
66. Palmer, E. D. Gastritis: A reevaluation. *Medicine* 33:199, 1954.
67. Rhodes, J. Experimental production of gastric epithelium in the duodenum. *Gut* 5:454, 1964.
68. Rhodes, J., Evans, K. T., Lawrie, J. H., and Forest, A. P. M. Coarse mucosal folds in the duodenum. *Q. J. Med.* 37:151, 1969.
69. Ritchie, W., Jr., and Delaney, J. Gastric ulcer: An experimental model. *Surg. Forum* 19:312, 1968.
70. Sanders, G. B., and McCray, P. M. Pseudogastritis of operative origin. *Ann. Surg.* 114:986, 1941.
71. Sasano, N., Nakamaru, K., Arai, M., and Akazaki, K. Ultrastructural cell patterns in human gastric carcinoma compared with non-neoplastic gastric mucosa: Histogenetic analysis of carcinoma by mucin histochemistry. *J. Natl. Cancer Inst.* 43:783, 1969.
72. Schindler, R. *Gastritis*. London: Heineman, 1947.
73. Schindler, R., Necheles, H., and Gold, R. L. Surgical gastritis: Study on genesis of gastritis found in resected stomachs with particular reference to so-called "antral gastritis" associated with ulcer. *Surg. Gynecol. Obstet.* 69:281, 1939.
74. Schmitz-Moorman, P., Schmidt-Sløordahl, R., Peter, J. H., and Massarrat, S. Morphometric studies of normal and inflamed duodenal mucosa. *Pathol. Res. Pract.* 167:313, 1980.
75. Schrager, J., Spink, R., and Mitra, S. The antrum in patients with duodenal and gastric ulcers. *Gut* 8:497, 1967.
76. Shiner, M., and Doniach, I. A study of x-ray negative dyspepsia with reference to histologic changes in the gastric mucosa. *Gastroenterology* 32:313, 1957.
77. Silen, W. New concepts of the gastric mucosal barrier. *Am. J. Surg.* 133:8, 1977.
78. Siurala, M., and Salmi, H. J. Long-term follow-up of subjects with superficial gastritis or a normal gastric mucosa. *Scand. J. Gastroenterol.* 6:459, 1971.
79. Siurala, M., and Seppala, K. Atrophic gastritis as a possible precursor of gastric carcinoma and pernicious anaemia. Results of follow-up examinations. *Acta. Med. Scand.* 166:455, 1960.
80. Skinner, J. M., Heenan, P. J., and Whitehead, R. Atrophic gastritis in gastrectomy specimens. *Br. J. Surg.* 62:23, 1975.
81. Stalsberg, H., and Taksdal, S. Stomach cancer following gastric surgery for benign conditions. *Lancet* 2:1175, 1971.
82. Stemmerman, G. N. Comparative sudy of histochemical patterns in non-neoplastic and neoplastic gastric epithelium. A study of Japanese in Hawaii. *J. Natl. Cancer Inst.* 39:375, 1967.
83. Stephen, J. G., Lesna, M., and Venables, C. W. Endoscopic appearances and histological changes in ulcer-associated duodenitis. *Br. J. Surg.* 65:438, 1978.
84. Strickland, R. G., and MacKay, I. R. A reappraisal of the nature and significance of chronic atrophic gastritis. *Am. J. Dig. Dis.* 18:426, 1973.
85. Sutton, D. R., Baird, I. M., Stewart, J. S. and Coghill, N. F. "Free" iron loss in atrophic gastritis, post-gastrectomy states, and adult coeliac disease. *Lancet* 2:387, 1970.
86. Tarpila, S., Telkkä, A., and Siurala, M. Ultrastructure of various metaplasias of the stomach. *Acta pathol. Microbiol. Scand.* 77:187, 1969.
87. Tomenius, J. An instrument for gastrobiopsies. *Gastroenterology* 15:498, 1950.
88. Vandelli, C., Bottazzo G. F., Doniach, D., and Franceschi, F. Autoantibodies to gastrin-producing cells in antral (type B) chronic gastritis. *N. Engl. J. Med.* 300:1406, 1979.
89. Varis, K. Family behaviour of chronic gastritis. *Ann. Clin. Res.* 13:123, 1981.
90. Venables, C. W., Stephen, J. G., and Lesna, M. Duodenitis. *Scand. J. Gastroenterol.* 15(Suppl. 63):45, 1980.
91. Whitehead, R. Mucosal Biopsy of the Gastrointestinal Tract. In *Major Problems in Pathology*, Vol. 3. Philadelphia:Saunders, 1973.
92. Whitehead, R. *Mucosal Biopsy of the Gastrointestinal Tract* (2nd ed.). Philadelphia: Saunders, 1979. Volume 3 in the series *Major Problems in Pathology*.
93. Whitehead, R., Roca, M., Meikle, D. D., et al. The histological classification of duodenitis in fibreoptic biopsy specimens. *Digestion* 13:129, 1975.
94. Whitehead, R., Truelove, S. C., and Gear, M. W. L. The histological diagnosis of chronic gastritis in fibreoptic gastroscope biopsy specimens. *J. Clin. Pathol.* 25:1, 1972.

95. Williams, A. W. The effects of alcohol on gastric mucosa. *Br. Med. J.* 1:256, 1956.
96. Williams, A. W., Edwards, R., Lewis, T. H., and Coghill, N. F. Investigation of non-ulcer dyspepsia by gastric biopsy. *Br. Med. J.* 1:372, 1957.
97. Winawer, S. J., Bejar, J., McCray, R. S., and Zamcheck, N. Haemorrhagic gastritis: Importance of associated chronic gastritis. *Arch. Intern. Med.* 127:129, 1971.
98. Wood, I. J., Doig, R. K., Motteram, R., and Hughes, A. Gastric biopsy: Report on 55 biopsies using new flexible gastric biopsy tubes. *Lancet* 1:18, 1949.
99. Wood, I. J., and Taft, L. I. *Diffuse Lesions of the Stomach*. London: Arnold, 1958. P 86.

EDITOR'S COMMENT

Although gastritis has been a recognized entity for years, it has become much more prominent since the advent of the flexible endoscope. There is little question that gastritis is the prominent abnormality found during endoscopy of the stomach after an operation. In a study of 400 patients who had operations, Bowden and colleagues (*Ann. Surg.* 197:637, 1984) found various degrees of gastritis in 127 (37 percent) of the patients after the operation. More specifically, bile gastritis was found in 53 patients.

The problem with clinical observations is the inability to be more specific in terms of the variations in pathology described by Whitehead. It is obvious that the term *gastritis* by itself is almost meaningless unless carefully defined in each instance. What does the term *bile gastritis* mean? The gastrointestinal endoscopist must expect a total analysis of the biopsy material as outlined. Only then will we be able to sort out fact from fiction in each patient complaining of symptoms after a gastric operation. Too often the endoscopic appearance of the mucosa, the presence of bile, the pathological diagnosis of *gastritis*, and the patient's symptoms are interpreted to mean alkaline reflux gastritis (see Chap. 7). The answer is not that simple. Svenson again confirmed that in patients with and those without a history of heartburn, bile vomiting, and postprandial pain after a gastric operation, the gastritis was of the same severity and was not related to the degree of bile reflux (*Scand. J. Gastroenterol.* 18:729, 1983).

The answer to this dilemma can be found only with additional basic studies within the realm of the pathologist, biochemist, or neurophysiologist. I find it exciting that evasive gastritis has been linked with the release of pancreatic polypeptide and the autonomic centers in the midbrain (Larson, et al. *Am. J. Surg.* 147:97, 1984).

(L.M.N.)

Duodenal Reflux Syndrome

Richard G. Fiddian-Green
William E. Strodel

A distinct postgastrectomy syndrome exists, characterized by the symptom of epigastric pain in the absence of recurrent ulceration. This pain can be reproduced by the intragastric infusion of autologous duodenal juice. The pathogenesis of the syndrome can be attributed to effects on the gastric mucosa produced by contact with duodenal juice and to an abnormal gastric motor response to the presence of duodenal juice in the stomach. The syndrome is best termed the *duodenal reflux syndrome*. It has also been called *alkaline reflux gastritis* or *bile gastritis*, but these terms are misleading. The symptoms of the syndrome cannot be attributed to the presence of gastritis or to the appearance of bile alone in the stomach. In addition, duodenal juice is not truly alkaline.

Historical Background

Bile vomiting was recognized as a distinct postgastrectomy syndrome by Wolfer in 1881 [95] and later by Billroth in 1885 [5]. The symptom was initially attributed to the intermittent or partial obstruction of the afferent limb of a gastrojejunostomy or Billroth II (BII) gastrectomy [91]. Thus bile vomiting was first treated by a side-to-side enteroenterostomy between the afferent and efferent limbs and later by the conversion of a BII anastomosis to a Billroth I (BI) anastomosis. These operations were not found to be very successful in the treatment of bile vomiting. It was subsequently observed that bile vomiting could also occur after vagotomy and pylorplasty even though an afferent limb had not been created. Afferent loop obstruction is now recognized as a definite but rare cause of bile vomiting. The syndrome of bile vomiting is more likely caused by an abnormal gastric motor response to the presence of duodenal juice in the stomach [91].

The possibility that alkaline reflux gastritis might be a distinct postgastrectomy syndrome that could be treated by a Roux-en-Y diversion was first suggested by du Plessis in 1965 [21]. This syndrome became popular in the United States after van Heerden's report in 1975 [92].

Although bile vomiting was described as a feature of this new syndrome, epigastric pain was the dominant symptom [7]. Du Plessis [21] attributed the pain to the presence of gastritis and the gastritis to the regurgitation of duodenal contents into the stomach. It had been appreciated for some time that chronic peristomal gastritis developed after partial gastrectomy or gastrojejunostomy. Since the gastritis changes could be reversed by a Roux-en-Y diversion, du Plessis and others assumed that the gastritis was caused by exposure of the gastric mucosa to regurgitated duodenal contents [9, 20, 39, 68, 76, 85]. This assumption was later confirmed in animal experiments performed by du Plessis' associate, Lawson [65, 66, 67]. High concentrations of bile conjugates were subsequently found to be present in fasting gastric juice of patients believed to have the alkaline reflux gastritis syndrome [21, 80]. This observation has since been confirmed by other investigators [16, 82]. The possibility that peristomal gastritis and the syndrome were caused by the regurgitation of bile into the gastric remnant was additionally supported by the demonstration that bile broke the "gastric mucosal barrier" [13, 37, 38, 50, 51, 52, 53, 83]. These observations led to the suggestion that the regurgitation of bile was responsible for the gastritis *and* for the syndrome. Hence the terms alkaline reflux gastritis and bile gastritis were coined.

Despite du Plessis' recognition of the alkaline reflux syndrome as a specific postgastrectomy syndrome and his recognition that both the pain and the bile vomiting could be relieved by a Roux-en-Y diversion, he also acknowledged many unresolved problems with his concept, as the following quotation indicates [22]:

> Why do only some people develop symptoms of reflux gastritis after operations which remove or bypass the pylorus? Some degree of reflux gastritis is seen around the artificial stoma in every case, but it is symptomatic in only some cases. Is there, in fact, an "active" type of gastritis which is symptomatic and progressive, with a marked cellular reaction on histologic examination, as opposed to an "inactive" variety which is asymptomatic, not progressive, and without a cellular infiltration? If so, what is the basic difference in pathogenesis between these two types? Is it merely a matter of degree, or does the improvement reported in some cases about six months postoperatively [39] indicate that another factor is involved?

It is these questions raised by du Plessis that perplex those who do not accept alkaline reflux gastritis as a specific postgastrectomy syndrome [1].

Cause of Reflux

Small amounts of duodenal juice are found in gastric juice in healthy persons [83]. Larger amounts are found in gastric juice in patients with peptic ulcers [8, 17, 21, 23, 24, 29, 79–81, 84] and in patients with biliary disease [58, 80, 93]. Even larger amounts are found in patients who have a gastroenterostomy.

In persons with normal anatomy, duodenal juice regurgitates into the stomach whenever the rate of fluid entering the duodenum exceeds the rate at which it exits to the more distal gastrointestinal tract. Thus duodenal juice appears in large amounts in the stomach in patients with intestinal obstruction and in patients whose duodenal motility is impaired by atropine [34]. Regurgitation of duodenal juice into the stomach under these circumstances may be impaired by pyloric sphincteric contraction [28]. When saline solution, which does not induce pyloric sphincteric contraction, is infused into the duodenum at a high rate, duodenal juice regurgitates into the stomach. But when acid, which does induce pyloric sphincteric contraction, is infused into the duodenum at the same rate, regurgitation is either abolished or markedly reduced. When acid is infused into the duodenum of gastric and duodenal ulcer patients, however, the pyloric sphincter does not contract, and the regurgitation of duodenal juice into the stomach occurs unabated [29, 96].

In healthy persons, any duodenal juice that regurgitates into the stomach is returned very rapidly into the duodenum. On the other hand, duodenal juice that regurgitates into the stomach in patients with duodenal or gastric ulcers persists in the stomach for a long time [96]. The importance of gastric emptying to an abnormal accumulation of duodenal juice in the stomach is additionally emphasized by the reduction in the amount of duodenal juice present in the stomach after the administration of metoclopramide hydrochloride, an agent that stimulates gastric emptying [14, 55]. It appears, therefore, that a combination of abnormalities may contribute, independently of a gastric operation, to the abnormal presence of duodenal juice in the stomach in patients with peptic ulcer disease and biliary disease.

The abnormal presence of duodenal juice in the stomach is most marked in patients who have had gastric operations. It is seen more frequently in patients who have a gastrojejunostomy than in patients who have had a pyloroplasty, and least frequently in patients who have had a highly selective vagotomy with preservation of the pylorus [45, 46, 49]. In patients who have had only a gastrojejunostomy, regurgitation of duodenal juice into the stomach may be reduced by taking down the gastrojejunostomy [32]. Normal anatomy cannot be restored in patients who have had an antrectomy; however, the regurgitation of duodenal juice into the stomach may be markedly reduced by the interposition of an isoperistaltic segment of jejunum between the stomach and the duodenum [43, 86], or it may be eliminated by the construction of a Roux-en-Y limb [87].

Effect of Reflux on Gastric Mucosa

The appearance of duodenal juice in the stomach is responsible for the development of gastritis. Gastritis is present before operation in patients with gastric ulcers and, to a more limited degree, in patients with duodenal ulcers [69]. The extent of the gastritis is increased by destruction or bypass of the pylorus [9, 21, 46, 59, 76, 85]. The abnormal presence of duodenal juice in the stomach is associated with the endoscopic evidence of mucosal hyperemia and histological features of gastritis [45]. The presence of gastritis is directly related to the concentration of duodenal juice and of bile acids in the stomach [26, 82]. The association is stronger for bile acids measured in the supine position than for bile acids measured in the erect position or after a meal. The gastritic changes may be reversed by the diversion of duodenal juice from the stomach [67, 82].

Several factors in duodenal juice appear to be responsible for the gastritic changes seen in the stomach after gastrojejunostomy. Bile has a cytolytic action of its own [31]. The action of bile may be enhanced by the addition of acid [13]. Because the effect of duodenal juice is much more marked than the effect of bile alone, some other agent in duodenal juice must also contribute to the presence of the gastritis [65, 66].

Acid may be a cause of the gastritis. Acid has been shown to be an important factor in the genesis of acute gastric mucosal injury and, of course, is important in the genesis of peptic ulceration [13]. The noxious effect of luminal acid appears in part to be a function of the rate at which acid can enter gastric mucosa [62, 63]. The rate at which luminal acid diffuses into the stomach can be calculated from the product of the hydrogen ion concentration (in mEq/L) in gastric juice, and the permeability of gastric mucosa to H^+ (0.048 mEq/hr/mEq of gradient) [25]. The rate at which luminal acid must diffuse into gastric mucosa to induce damage in a normally perfused stomach appears to be approximately 12.5 mEq/hr. This rate may be achieved by exposing the stomach to bile, which increases gastric mucosal permeability, and to acid in a concentration of 160 mEq/L. Because the concentration of acid in the stomach of patients with the duodenal reflux syndrome is seldom greater than 10 mEq/L and usually less than 1 mEq/L, the back-diffusion of acid in the form of H^+ is unlikely to be a factor contributing to gastric mucosal damage. The buffering of acid by bicarbonate in the stomach, however, is accompanied by a large rise in the pCO_2 of gastric juice. The CO_2 formed may appear transiently in a much higher gradient than H^+ and is able to diffuse through gastric mucosa much more rapidly than H^+ [25]. In this manner the buffering of acid by bicarbonate in the stomach may increase the rate at which acid enters the gastric mucosa. Thus the back-diffusion of acid may be important in the production of gastric mucosal injury in the duodenal reflux syndrome even though the hydrogen ion concentration is usually less than 1 mEq/L. An analysis of the possible effects of regurgitated duodenal juice on the back-diffusion of acid, based on the Henderson-Hasselbalch equation, suggests that the back-diffusion of acid will occur at a maximum rate when the pH of gastric juice is between 2 and 5 and at a minimum rate when the pH is above 6.1, the pKa of carbonic acid (Fig. 7-1).

In animals and humans the appearance of acute gastric mucosal injury is associated with a fall in pH in gastric mucosa below normal levels [22, 62, 63]. The pH in gastric mucosa falls below normal levels when the rate of acid, diffusing from the lumen into gastric mucosa or being generated in the mucosal cells, exceeds the rate at which acid can be buffered by the mucosa and removed by the blood. The magnitude of the fall in the intramucosal pH is directly related to the rate at which acid diffuses into the mucosa. The fall in pH may be markedly increased by the gastric buffering of acid by bicarbonate, which converts acid present at a low gradient and in a relatively impermeable form (H^+) to acid present at a higher gradient and in a more permeable form (CO_2). A fall in intramucosal pH may also be enhanced by an impaired ability to dispose of acid entering the gastric mucosa. This disposal occurs in part through the microcirculation, which can be compromised by decreased perfusion as seen in hypotension and perhaps occlusive arteriosclerotic lesions [62].

In conclusion, there is an abundance of evidence incriminating duodenal juice as a causative factor in gastritis. A *multitude* of factors (bile [13], proteolytic enzymes [65, 66], lysolecithin [54, 61], and bicarbonate [22]) in duodenal juice and possibly mucosal ischemia have been implicated as possible causative factors. The mechanism by which these factors induce mucosal damage is uncertain but may be related to the induction of a fall in intramucosal pH below critical levels.

Cause of Symptoms

Histological evidence of gastritis correlates poorly with symptoms in patients with the duodenal reflux syndrome and persists long after the symptoms have been relieved by a diversionary procedure [45]. Endoscopic evidence of severe hyperemia correlates better with symptoms [59], and both the symptoms and hyperemia can be reversed by procedures [67, 82]. However, 50 percent of patients experiencing symptoms do not have any endoscopic evidence of hyperemia, and endoscopic evidence of hyperemia may be present in patients without symptoms. Thus the symptoms of the duodenal reflux syndrome cannot be attributed with any certainty to the presence of either gastritis or severe hyperemia.

The intragastric infusion of bile alone in concentrations and composition found in the duodenal juice of patients with symptoms does not reproduce the symptoms [73]. Thus it is difficult to ascribe the symptoms of the duodenal reflux syndrome to the presence of bile in the stomach alone.

The intragastric infusion of autogenous duodenal juice obtained from patients with symptoms *does* reproduce the symptoms in these patients. It seems, therefore, that the appearance of some constituent, other than bile, of duodenal juice in the stomach of patients with symptoms is responsible for the epigastric pain in the duodenal reflux syndrome.

The symptoms may also be induced by the exogenous agent NaOH. The importance of this observation is the suggestion that the symptoms of the syndrome may be induced by other exogenous agents [94]. Therefore, any procedure that only diverts endogenous stimuli such as duodenal juice will not be successful in relieving the symptoms in all patients with the duodenal reflux syndrome.

The mechanism by which the intragastric infusion of autogenous duodenal juice induces symptoms in patients is not known. Circum-

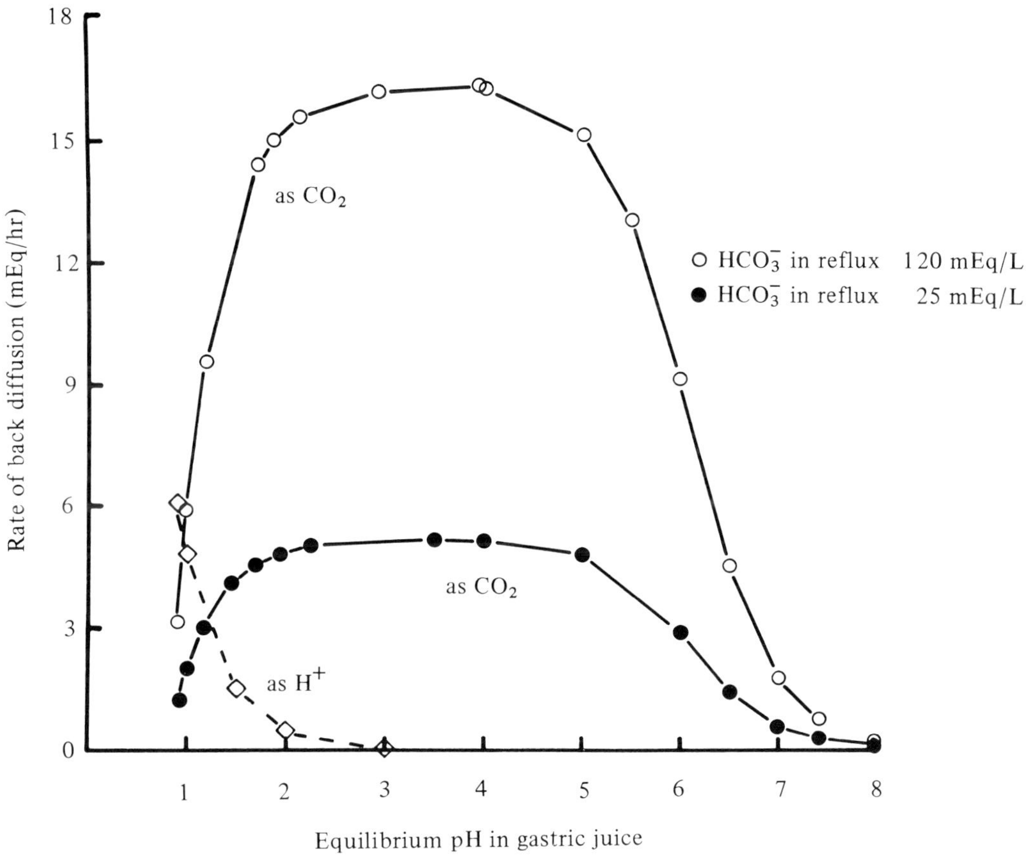

Fig. 7-1. Rate of back-diffusion of acid (calculated from data obtained from experiments in dogs [25]), which occurs as either H^+ or CO_2 at different equilibrium pH values in gastric juice. The rate of back-diffusion of CO_2 varies with the varying concentration (25–120 mEq/hr) of bicarbonate present in regurgitated duodenal juice.

stantial evidence suggests that the pain might occur as a result of a fall in tissue pH in gastric mucosa [22]. The appearance in the stomach of bicarbonate in duodenal secretions may induce a precipitous fall in tissue pH in the gastric mucosa. The magnitude of the fall induced will depend on the amount of bicarbonate regurgitating into the stomach proportionate to the amount of gastric acid, and on the equilibrium pH in gastric juice. The effect will approach maximum levels when the equilibrium pH of gastric juice is between 2 and 5 and is insignificant above pH 6.1, the pKa of carbonic acid (Fig. 7-1). The relationship of the fall in tissue pH to the occurrence of pain is suggested by the following patient history.

A patient was admitted to the University of Michigan Medical Center complaining of epigastric pain precipitated by drinking large volumes of water and by eating food. This patient had a basal acid output (BAO) of 0.7 mEq/hr and a maximal acid output (MAO) of 3 mEq/hr. He had endoscopic evidence of gastric hyperemia but no evidence of peptic ulceration. Biliary and pancreatic disease were also eliminated from the differential diagnosis. Angiography showed complete occlusion of the celiac axis and of the left gastric artery. The blood supply to the stomach appeared to come from the splenic artery in a retrograde manner through collaterals from the superior mesenteric artery. The tissue pH in the gastric mucosa was measured in this patient in the manner previously described [25] and was found to be consistently below the lower limit of normal in the stomach (pH 7.3). Under fasting conditions, while the patient was not experiencing symptoms, the tissue pH was 7.27 on one day and 7.21, 7.15, and 7.29 on a separate day. Drinking a large volume of water and eating food reproduced the symptoms and induced a fall in tissue pH to 6.87 and 7.03, respectively. The intriguing possibility that a fall in tissue pH might cause the pain in patients with the duodenal reflux syndrome requires additional evaluation.

The roentgenographic studies of Toye and Alexander-Williams [91] indicate that the occurrence of bile vomiting after gastric operation for ulcer disease is part of an abnormal motor response initiated by the appearance of endogenous duodenal juice in the stomach [91]. This motor response is characterized by gastric atony, gastroesophageal reflux, and bile vomiting. Patients with duodenal and gastric ulcers have also been observed to have an impaired ability to empty the stomach of regurgitated duodenal juice before gastric operations [96]. This raises the possibility that the abnormality responsible for the duodenal reflux syndrome may be present in these patients preoperatively and may be accentuated by the performance of procedures that increase the reflux of duodenal juice into the stomach. Metoclopramide hydrochloride increases gastric emptying of regurgitated duodenal juice and decreases the symptoms of regurgitation in some patients with the duodenal reflux syndrome [14]. These findings suggest that the symptoms of the duodenal reflux syndrome may be related, in part, to an abnormal gastric motor response to the presence of regurgitated duodenal juice in the stomachs of patients with previous ulcer disease but not in healthy persons.

Clinical Presentation

Van Heerden et al. [92] initially defined a group of patients who satisfied the following criteria: (1) previous gastroduodenal operation, (2) presence of upper abdominal symptoms, (3) decreased or absent gastric acid secretion, (4) exclusion of the diagnosis of recurrent peptic ulcer, and (5) endoscopic (histological) evidence of gastritis. Almost 80 percent of their patients experienced constant midepigastric pain that had a boring quality and was *unrelated* to food or antacid ingestion. Only 35 percent of patients reported bilious vomiting as a major symptom. Anemia, dumping, and hemorrhage were present in 24 percent, 12 percent, and 2 percent of instances, respectively. Several authors have subsequently expanded and modified the clinical criteria to include weight loss and nausea (Table 7-1). Others used bilious vomiting as the major criterion for patient selection and excluded gastric analysis for acid secretion. The syndrome has been observed after all types of gastroduodenal operations performed for peptic ulcer disease (Table 7-2). Warshaw [93] suggested that the symptoms of bile gastritis can also occur in patients who have not had a previous gastroduodenal operation. All 10 patients in Warshaw's series, however, had undergone previous cholecystectomy. Basal achlorhydria was noted in 8 of 10 patients. Maximal acid stimulatory studies were normal in only 3 patients; the rest had values below normal. Similarly, Scudmore et al. [88], van Heerden et al. [92], and Johnson et al. [56] noted the occurrence of some of the symptoms attributed to "alkaline reflux" in patients who did *not* undergo gastric operations.

Diagnosis

The clinical hallmarks of the syndrome are nonspecific and variable. They cannot be used to establish conclusively the diagnosis of the duodenal reflux syndrome. More objective criteria are needed to confirm the diagnosis in patients with symptoms suggestive of the syndrome [7, 44].

The preliminary goal when evaluating patients with symptoms who have undergone operations for peptic ulcer disease is to eliminate recurrent or marginal ulceration as a cause for their symptoms. Other causes such as biliary disease, pancreatitis, and gastric, pancreatic,

Table 7-1. Presenting symptoms in patients from collected series of "alkaline reflux gastritis" or "bile gastritis"

Author	Year	Pain	Bile vomited	Anemia	Weight loss	Dumping	GI bleeding
Joseph [57]	1973	11	11	11	11		
Herrington [43]	1974	48	48	19	31		6
Drapanas [19]	1974	24	19	—	19	—	9
van Heerden [92]	1975	38	17	12	—	6	—
Zimmerman [97]	1976	10	11	5	9	—	3
Hoare [45]	1977	18	31	—	—	—	—
Berardi [4]	1976	5	1	—	4	—	—
Ritchie [82]	1980	11	9	5	8	5	—

Table 7-2. Types of peptic ulcer operations performed on patients before the diagnosis of "alkaline reflux gastritis" or "bile gastritis"

Author	Year	No. of patients	Previous operations						
			V&P	V&BI	GR	V&BII	GJ	BII	PCV
Conyers [10]	1960	46							
Joseph [57]	1973	11	3	4	—	4	—	—	—
Pyrtek [77]	1973	10	—	1	—	7	—	—	—
Coppinger [12]	1973	26	2	3	—	17	2	—	—
Herrington [43]	1974	44	5	10	—	17	3	11	—
Griffiths [33]	1974	91	26	—	58	—	7	—	—
Drapanas [19]	1974	24	2	5	—	8	2	7	—
Davidson [14]	1975	22	1	5	—	16	—	—	—
van Heerden [92]	1975	51	4	4	—	10	9	25	—
Berardi [4]	1976	40	4	—	—	33	3	—	—
Zimmerman [97]	1976	11	1	1	—	3	—	6	—
Hoare [45]	1977	84	22	20	—	32	—	—	10
Ludwig [68]	1979	13	—	13	—	—	—	—	—
Meshkinpour [73]	1980	11	3	5	—	3	—	—	—
Boren [6]	1980	39	9	6	—	11	6	7	—
Ritchie [82]	1980	21	—	1	—	13	—	6	—

Note: V&P = vagotomy and pyloroplasty; V&BI = vagotomy and Billroth I partial gastrectomy; GR = gastric resection; V&BII = vagotomy and Billroth II partial gastrectomy; GJ = gastrojejunostomy; BII = Billroth II partial gastrectomy without vagotomy; PCV = parietal cell vagotomy.

or right colonic neoplasms must also be eliminated.

ENDOSCOPY

Since the introduction of the fiberoptic gastroscope, a variety of endoscopic findings in patients with the alkaline reflux gastritis syndrome have been described, including bile staining, hyperemia, friability, and granularity of the mucosa. Bile reflux is common among all patients who have had any of the operations usually performed for peptic ulcer disease (except highly selective vagotomy). Hoare [45] evaluated 84 patients who had different operations for peptic ulcer disease. Endoscopy and gastric biopsy were performed on all patients, half of whom were experiencing symptoms. Antral and stomal gastritis were observed in most instances (89 percent), regardless of symptoms. Hyperemia, bile staining, bile reflux, contact bleeding, edema, and erosions were seen with equal frequency in patients with and those without symptoms, and the extent of hyperemia was the same. A granular mucosa was observed only in patients with symptoms. The presence of the endoscope itself probably alters the movement of duodenal contents across the pylorus. In addition, there is no objective method for visually quantifying bile flow. In several other studies, the subjective assessment of bile reflux had no correlation with symptoms or the presence of gastritis. Histological assessment of endoscopically obtained biopsy specimens demonstrates superficial gastritis in many of the patients who have undergone ulcer operations. These findings do *not* correlate with symptoms or with the gross endoscopic appearance of gastritis.

EVALUATION OF REFLUX

Quantitative and qualitative evaluation of bile reflux and assessment of gastric emptying may be of benefit in establishing the diagnosis in patients with symptoms.

Hoare [47] sampled gastric fluid in patients who had operations for peptic ulcer disease. Aspirates were obtained by a nasogastric tube after fasting, postcibally, after pentagastrin stimulation, and overnight. The significant discriminant between patients with and those without symptoms was the amount of bile reflux per half hour from the fasting stomach. Of 22 patients with symptoms, 17 had reflux of more than 120 mol/hr. Patients with less than this amount did not experience symptoms.

Ritchie [82] demonstrated that a subset of patients with symptoms, those experiencing epigastric pain, nausea, and vomiting, had significantly decreased recumbent and postcibal bile acid concentration compared with controls and with other patients with symptoms. The net bile acid reflux per hour was also significantly increased. The data also suggest that intragastric bile acid concentration and net bile reflux per hour may differentiate among postgastrectomy patients with symptoms and identify those with the alkaline reflux syndrome. These patients had more severe gastritis by histological criteria and also complained of bilious vomiting more frequently than did controls and patients who had symptoms but who did not have increased bile acid reflux.

Gadacz [30] also evaluated patients who had undergone procedures for peptic ulcer disease. Fasting gastric aspirates were obtained at the time of endoscopy. In contrast to Ritchie, he noted no significant difference in the total amount of bile acid in patients with and those without symptoms. Patients who had symptoms, however, did have a significantly increased proportion of secondary bile acids present in the samples, particularly deoxycholic acid.

Meshkinpour [74] noted, in patients with symptoms, colonization of the upper gastrointestinal tract with stains of enteric gram-negative bacteria and Pseudomonas. The presence of free bile acids was correlated with heavier bacterial colonization. Patients who did not have symptoms were not colonized. Antibiotic treatment did not alter symptoms, and no specific species emerged in the bacterial flora after treatment. Gastric motility and pH values of gastric secretions did not correlate with the type or numbers of the microflora.

Tolin [90] studied enterogastric reflux using radioisotopic techniques (^{99m}Tc and ^{111}In) in healthy persons and postgastrectomy patients. Activities were recorded over the liver, gallbladder, and stomach, and an enterogastric reflux index was determined. The index was significantly lower (indicating increased reflux) in postoperative patients without symptoms than in healthy controls. In addition, postoperative patients with symptoms had significantly greater indices than postoperative patients without symptoms. Others have corroborated these findings [36, 49].

Attention has also been given to gastric stasis. Davidson [15] evaluated 22 patients with duodenal reflux syndrome who underwent diversionary procedures. Patients with poor clinical responses had altered gastric emptying, manifested in atony and stasis, both preoperatively and postoperatively. Administration of metoclopramide hydrochloride improved gastric emptying and alleviated symptoms in most patients. Hocking et al. [48] generated data in the canine model that corroborated the high incidence of delayed gastric emptying observed clinically after a Roux-en-Y diversion. The delays in gastric emptying were observed mainly with solids and to a lesser degree with liquids. Ludwig [68] noted a tendency for patients with slow emptying to have increased bile acid output. Differences between patients with symptoms and those without symptoms, however, were not statistically significant. In addition, high bile acid output was not a good indicator of symptoms.

PROVOCATIVE TESTS

Meshkinpour [73] evaluated 11 patients with the "alkaline reflux syndrome" (postcibal epigastric pain, bilious vomiting, and nausea) and 10 postgastrectomy patients without symptoms. Concentrations of bile acids were determined. Autologous upper gastrointestinal contents, normal saline solution, and artificial bile acid solutions (similar in composition and concentration to the upper intestinal contents of both patients with symptoms and those without symptoms) were infused in a random, double-blind manner into the stomachs of the patients (Table 7-3). Of 11 patients with symptoms, 10 had their symptoms reproduced by infusion of autologous intestinal contents.

Table 7-3. Provocative test using the infusion of autologous duodenal juice

1. Patient fasts overnight.
2. Rehfuss tube inserted through the nose into the duodenum under fluoroscopic control.
3. Cholecystokinin (4 ng/kg IV) administered.
4. 75 ml of duodenal contents collected.
5. Duodenal tube withdrawn into the stomach (recheck position with fluoroscopy).
6. 60 ml of intestinal contents and 60 ml of 154 mmol NaCl solution infused through the tube at 4 ml/min for 15 minutes in a random sequence.
7. Test infusions separated by 15-minute intervals.
8. Solution containers covered. A laboratory technician switches solutions without the patient's or investigator's knowledge.
9. Symptoms monitored every 5 minutes.

Source: After Meshkinpour [73].

Only 2 of 10 patients without symptoms had symptoms develop with the autologous solution. Both patients also responded to saline solution. Patients with symptoms had a significantly greater concentration of bile acids compared to the group without symptoms. No difference in bile acid composition was noted between groups. Administration of the artificial bile acid solution did not produce symptoms in either group of patients. None of the patients in this study underwent diversion of duodenal juice from the stomach; therefore the predictive value for success of diversionary procedures is unknown.

Warshaw [94] described a provocative test that uses hydrochloric acid, saline solution, sodium hydroxide (NaOH), and the patient's own gastric contents. A positive test is interpreted as reproduction of the patient's pains with NaOH or gastric contents but not with HCl or saline solution. Seventy-one percent of patients with the clinical diagnosis of alkaline reflux gastritis had a positive test, while only 6 percent of healthy controls had a positive test. Only 5 of the 15 patients who had positive tests had responses to both NaOH and gastric contents. The remainder responded to NaOH alone. Fifteen of the 21 patients diagnosed as having bile gastritis were treated with a Roux-en-Y diversion. Nine of 10 patients with a positive response had relief of symptoms after the operation. None of the five patients with a negative test was relieved of pain after an operation. While this study reproduced symptoms, it did not provide information regarding the role of endogenous secretions in the production of the syndrome. Patients were not used as their own controls, so it is not clear whether this response is acquired after gastrectomy or whether it indicates a native characteristic of the individual's stomach. No studies have been conducted on patients who subsequently underwent a Roux-en-Y diversion to assess their response to NaOH.

GASTRIC ANALYSIS

Patients reported to have the syndrome of alkaline reflux either have achlorhydria or hypochlorhydria. Histamine administration to the patient does not evoke an acid secretory response. If the back-diffusion of CO_2, generated by the buffering of acid by bicarbonate, is active in this syndrome, the appearance of symptoms should be associated with a pH of gastric juice between 2 and 5 (Fig. 7-1).

Treatment

MEDICAL

A variety of medical treatments have been proposed, including antiulcer regimens, cholestyramine, parenteral nutrition, and metoclopramide. None of these measures has been shown conclusively to be of any therapeutic value.

Antacids have been widely used, but their effect and role remain questionable. The acidic secretions that bathe the stomach in patients with the alkaline reflux syndrome are already neutralized. It has been suggested that aluminum hydroxide may bind bile salts and thus decrease their concentration in the stomach [3, 70, 88], but no consistent relief has been afforded by this agent. Anticholinergic agents, especially, are of dubious benefit since gastric atony and stasis may be contributing factors to the syndrome.

Cholestyramine directly binds bile salts in the gastrointestinal tract. Meshkinpour [72] compared cholestyramine with placebo and antacid treatment in a randomized, double-blind, crossover study. No differences in the frequency of symptoms were observed among the various regimens. Most other reports concur with these results.

Parenteral nutrition and stomach "rest" have been advocated by some, but no studies have shown this to be an effective treatment except in the overall preparation of the malnourished patient for a major abdominal operation.

The beneficial effects reported for metoclopramide hydrochloride have been mentioned previously. Preliminary data suggest that this agent may be useful not only in patients who have duodenal reflux but also in those with gastric stasis who do not obtain pain relief after diversionary operations [14, 55].

SURGICAL

The primary goal of surgical treatment is to provide total diversion of pancreatobiliary and duodenal secretions from the stomach. Originally, this was accomplished by the performance of a side-to-side enteroenterostomy (Braun's loop) between the afferent and efferent limbs of the gastrojejunostomy [91]. Experience with this technique showed incomplete diversion of duodenal juice from the stomach.

Subsequently, three other operations were developed: the Roux-en-Y gastrojejunostomy [2, 18, 21], the Tanner 19 [89], and the Henley loop (interposed isoperistaltic jejunal segment) [40, 41, 42] (Fig. 7-2). With each of these procedures truncal vagotomy is also performed, if it has not been done already, to prevent stomal ulceration. If vagotomy has been performed, some assessment of its completeness must be made before one of the diversionary procedures is performed, since they are potentially ulcerogenic preparations. In addition, in instances in which a gastrojejunostomy alone has been performed for the

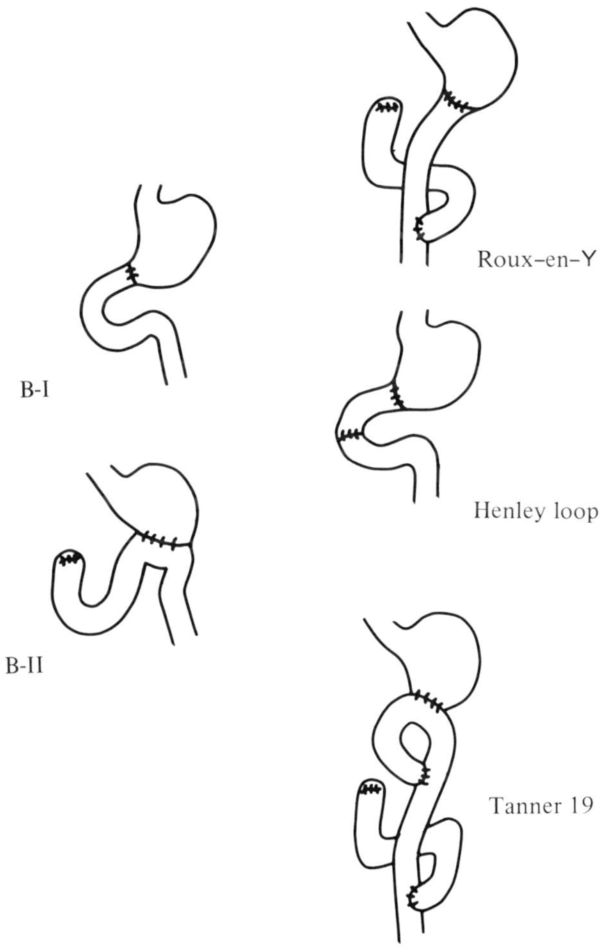

Fig. 7-2. Both Billroth I (B-I) and Billroth II (B-II) gastric reconstructions may be converted by the procedures depicted on the right to provide diversion of duodenal juice from the stomach. In addition, complete vagotomy is performed.

treatment of peptic ulcer disease, the anastomosis can be dismantled and the original anatomy restored provided there is no obstruction to the gastric outlet.

Roux-en-Y Operation

Conversion to a Roux-en-Y gastrojejunostomy has been the most common operation performed.

BI CONVERSION. When the abdomen is entered, the gastroduodenostomy is mobilized and the old anastomosis transected. The end of the duodenum is freshened and then closed in at least two layers. Attention is directed to the proximal jejunum, which is transected just distal to the ligament of Treitz. The distal cut end is based on the second and third jejunal vessels. The distal end is oversewn and an end-to-side gastrojejunostomy is performed. Intestinal continuity is reestablished by anastomosing the proximal cut end of the jejunum to the side of the jejunum at least 50 cm distal to the gastrojejunostomy [2, 18, 27, 87]. The Roux limb may be placed in either an antecolic or retrocolic position.

BII CONVERSION. The afferent limb is transected immediately at the stomal inlet and the distal cut end oversewn. The proximal cut end is anastomosed to the side of the jejunum 50 cm distal to the gastrojejunostomy.

Good or excellent results have been variably reported in 50 to 100 percent of instances [4, 6, 10, 11, 12, 15, 19, 28, 35, 48, 53, 57, 71, 75, 78, 92, 97]. Most series report nearly a 75 percent success rate with the Roux-en-Y procedure. In addition to pain relief, most patients also experience weight gain. Bilious vomiting is also relieved if present preoperatively (Table 7-4). In Ritchie's series [82] patients were studied 6–22 months after revision. Bile acid reflux was completely abolished, the MAO increased, the hematocrit reading rose, and gastritis (by histological assessment) improved.

Gastroscopy performed several months after the remedial operation usually shows gross improvement in the severity of hyperemia present [67]. Overall operative mortality for the Roux-en-Y conversion procedure has been approximately 1 percent.

Tanner 19 Operation

The Tanner procedure is a modification of the Roux-en-Y operation, used when exposure and dissection around the gastrojejunostomy stoma is difficult [89].

BI CONVERSION. After mobilization and division of the gastroduodenostomy, the duodenal end is closed in at least two layers. As in the Roux-en-Y procedure, a 5-cm-long defunctionalized limb of jejunum is created. The end of this limb is looped and anastomosed to the side of the limb 10 cm distal to the gastrojejunostomy. An end-to-side gastrojejunostomy is created at the midpoint of the segment between the segments of the end-to-side enteroenterostomy.

BII CONVERSION. The afferent limb is transected 10–12 cm proximal to the gastrojejunostomy. The distal cut end is anastomosed to the side of the jejunum distal to the gastrojejunostomy. The proximal cut end is anastomosed to the side of the jejunum 50 cm distal to the gastrojejunostomy.

Clinical response, morbidity, and mortality with this operation have been similar to those reported with the Roux-en-Y conversion (Table 7-4).

Henley Jejunal Interposition Operation

The Henley loop has been infrequently used to treat alkaline reflux syndrome [38, 86].

BI CONVERSION. The abdominal cavity is approached through a midline incision, and the gastroduodenal anastomosis is mobilized. The ligament of Treitz is identified, and a segment of jejunum is selected as near as possible to this point. A graft of 10–20 cm in length is optimum; if the graft is longer, gastric stasis may result. In the selection of the graft, the blood supply to the segment must be adequate, with as little interruption of the vascular arcade as is compatible with the mobility of the segment. The segment is isolated between clamps or by using the surgical stapler. The continuity of the jejunum is restored with a two-layer anastomosis, and a hole is made in the transverse mesocolon on either side of the middle colic artery. The jejunal segmental graft is passed through this hole and the distal end of the graft is anastomosed (end-to-end) to the duodenum in two layers after division of the gastroduodenostomy. The proximal position of the graft is anastomosed to the stomach in an end-to-end or side-to-side manner. The hole in the transverse mesocolon is closed and attached to the jejunal mesentery.

BII CONVERSION. This operation can be converted into a jejunal graft by resection of the afferent limb immediately at the stomal inlet and the efferent limb 10 cm distal to the stomal outlet. The mesentery to this segment is isolated from the rest of the small intestinal mesentery. The afferent end is oversewn, and the efferent limb is anastomosed end-to-side to the duodenum just distal to the end of the duodenal stump. The two free ends of jejunum are anastomosed in two layers to restore GI continuity.

Herrington et al. [43] treated 20 patients with Henley loops and obtained excellent results in 14 patients and good results in 4 patients. However, because the procedure requires more dissection, additional anastomoses, and longer operating time, it has no advantage over the more commonly used Roux-en-Y operation (Table 7-4).

Some authors have suggested the routine use of primary Roux-en-Y gastrojejunal recon-

Table 7-4. Type of operative procedure performed and results of operation in patients with "alkaline reflux gastritis" or "bile gastritis"

Author	Year	No. of patients	Roux	Tanner	Henley	Pain relief	Weight gain	No bile vomited
Conyers [10]	1960	46	46	—	—	42	21	35
Joseph [57]	1973	11	11	—	—	11	11	—
Coppinger [12]	1973	26	26	—	—	20	11	—
Herrington [43]	1974	48	27	—	20	17R, 18H	17	—
Griffiths [33]	1974	91	22	—	6	—	—	—
Drapanas [19]	1974	24	15	5	3	13R, 5T, 3H	—	—
Davidson [14]	1975	22	21	1	1	—	—	—
van Heerden [92]	1975	51	31	—	12	26R, 6H	—	—
Zimmerman [97]	1976	11	10	—	1	—	—	11
Kennedy [60]	1978	36	36	—	—	25	—	—
Hoare [47]	1978	18	18	—	—	9	—	—
Malagelada [70]	1979	13	13	—	—	12	—	—
Berardi [4]	1976	5	5	—	—	4	—	—
Boren [6]	1980	52	52	—	—	—	—	—
Menguy [71]	1980	—	21	—	2	18R, 1H	—	—
Davidson [15]	1980	59	51	4	1	—	—	—
Warshaw [94]	1981	16	16	—	—	9	—	—

Note: R = Roux-en-Y conversion; T = Tanner 19 conversion; H = Henley loop construction.

struction after partial gastrectomy to preclude the development of alkaline reflux [64]. This is unwise for two reasons. First, diversion of alkaline secretions from the gastric outlet increases the incidence of marginal ulceration (Mann-Williamson preparation). The occurrence of stomal ulceration can be minimized but not completely avoided by the performance of a truncal vagotomy. Second, it appears that the incidence of the duodenal reflux syndrome is quite low. Thus many patients would be placed at risk of marginal ulceration to prevent development of a syndrome that occurs in only a few instances.

University of Michigan Experience

The University of Michigan experience with the duodenal reflux syndrome has been similar to that of other institutions. Only 23 patients have been treated over the past 15 years, 15 men and 8 women. Their mean age was 49 years. All patients were originally diagnosed with peptic ulcer disease and underwent surgical treatment.

The initial surgical procedure performed in these patients was vagotomy and pyloroplasty in eight patients, Billroth I gastrectomy in six patients, and Billroth II gastrectomy in nine patients. Eight patients subsequently underwent a second operation for either marginal ulceration, outlet obstruction, or afferent loop syndrome. Three patients had a Billroth II converted to a Billroth I reconstruction. Five patients, who had had a vagotomy and pyloroplasty, underwent antrectomy and Billroth II reconstruction. Four patients were operated on a third time: two underwent Billroth II to Billroth I conversion and two others had the vagotomy redone (Table 7-5). Other operations performed on the patients in this group included cholecystectomy (seven patients) and hiatal hernia repair (six patients).

The average interval between operation and the onset of symptoms consistent with duodenal reflux was 43.6 months. Epigastric pain was present in all patients and occurred post-

Table 7-5. Types of peptic ulcer operations performed on patients before diagnosis of the duodenal reflux syndrome—University of Michigan experience

Operation	No. of patients
Initial	
Vagotomy and pyloroplasty	8
Vagotomy and Billroth I partial gastrectomy	6
Vagotomy and Billroth II partial gastrectomy	9
Second	
Billroth II converted to Billroth I	3
Vagotomy and pyloroplasty converted to Billroth II	5
Third	
Billroth II converted to Billroth I	2
Vagotomy (redone)	2

Table 7-6. Presenting symptoms in patients with the diagnosis of the duodenal reflux syndrome—University of Michigan experience

Symptoms	No. of patients
Pain	23
Postcibal	8
Vomiting	18
Bilious	5
Weight loss	8
Anemia	6
Diarrhea	3

prandially in eight patients. Fourteen patients characterized the pain as sharp and nonradiating, while nine patients described it as a burning sensation. Antacids were tried by all patients, but only five patients reported any consistent relief. Vomiting was a predominant feature in 18 patients and in five patients, the emesis was bilious. Relief of epigastric pain with vomiting was noted in six patients. Weight loss, diarrhea, and anemia were observed in eight, six, and three patients, respectively (Table 7-6).

All patients underwent gastric analysis and were found to have either achlorhydria or hypochlorhydria. A fasting serum gastrin level was determined in eight patients and the mean level was 78.2 pg/dl. Upper GI contrast studies were nondiagnostic in 21 patients and showed delayed gastric emptying in 2 patients. Flexible fiberoptic gastroscopy was performed in all patients. Mild, moderate, and severe hyperemia was observed in 6, 13, and 14 patients, respectively. In instances in which moderate or severe hyperemia was noted, the entire gastric remnant was inflamed. In addition, eight patients had endoscopic evidence of distal esophagitis. Gastric biopsies were performed on six patients and all specimens showed histological characteristics of superficial gastritis.

Twenty patients eventually underwent a Roux-en-Y conversion. Three patients had the Tanner 19 procedure (Table 7-7). No operative deaths occurred. Wound infection was noted in one patient and prolonged ileus in three patients.

Overall, 18 patients indicated that their symptoms (pain and vomiting) were improved by the operation. The remaining five patients noted no change in their symptoms (Table 7-7). Eight patients resumed a regular diet, while 15 patients required dietary restrictions (usually smaller feedings). Repeat endoscopy was performed in seven patients (two months after operation), and improvement in the gross appearance of the gastritis was seen in six patients. Repeat biopsies were not obtained.

Summary

There is a postgastrectomy syndrome characterized by epigastric pain, duodenogastric reflux, weight loss, anemia, and hypochlorhydria or achlorhydria. The syndrome cannot be attributed to the histological presence of gastritis. Thus the term *gastritis* is best deleted from the name of the syndrome. The symptoms have also been associated with the abnormal presence of bile in the stomach but

Table 7-7. Types of remedial operations and results of operation in patients with the duodenal reflux syndrome—University of Michigan experience

Operation	No. of patients	Pain relief	No vomiting
Roux-en-Y	20	16	14
Tanner 19	3	2	2

cannot be ascribed solely to the intragastric presence of bile. The term *bile* is therefore also best deleted from the name of the syndrome. Because the pH of duodenal secretions is usually below 7.0, the fluid that regurgitates into the stomach in patients with this syndrome is not truly alkaline. The term *duodenal reflux syndrome* is perhaps most appropriate, and the syndrome is best defined as epigastric pain reproduced by intragastric instillation of autologous duodenal juice.

The fact that the symptoms may be induced by the intragastric administration of an exogenous agent in addition to autologous duodenal juice raises the possibility that multiple factors may be capable of initiating the symptoms in these patients. Only patients whose symptoms are reproduced by the intragastric instillation of autologous duodenal juice can be expected to be relieved by treatments that reduce duodenogastric reflux, such as diversionary operative procedures, or possibly, metoclopramide. Since bile alone does not cause symptoms, agents that bind bile salts cannot be expected to produce an improvement in symptoms. The use of a provocative test may reduce the number of patients who fail to attain relief of their symptoms after diversionary procedures.

References

1. Alexander-Williams, J. Alkaline reflux gastritis: A myth or a disease? *Am. J. Surg.* 143:17, 1982.
2. Bartlett, M. K., and Burrington, J. D. Bilious vomiting after gastric surgery: Experience with a modified Roux-Y loop for relief. *Arch. Surg.* 97:34, 1968.
3. Begemann, F., Schumpelick, V., and Bandomer, G. Adsorption of bile acids and lysolecithin by antacids. *Scand. J. Gastroenterol* 16(Suppl.67):191, 1981.
4. Berardi, R. S., Siroospour, D., Ruiz, R., et al. Alkaline reflux gastritis: A study in forty postoperative duodenal ulcer patients. *Am. J. Surg.* 132:552, 1976.
5. Billroth, T. *Clinical Surgery.* Translated by C. Dent. London:New Sydenham Soc., 1885.
6. Boren, C. H., and Way, L. W. Alkaline reflux gastritis: A reevaluation. *Am. J. Surg.* 140:40, 1980.
7. Bushkin, F. L., Wickbom, G., Deford, J. W., et al. Postoperative alkaline reflux gastritis. *Surg. Gynecol. Obstet.* 138:933, 1974.
8. Capper, W. M. Factors in the pathogenesis of gastric ulcer. *Ann. R. Coll. Surg. Engl.* 40:21, 1967.
9. Capper, W. M., Butler, T. J., and Buckler, K. G. Alkaline areas in gastric mucosa after gastric surgery. *Gut* 7:220, 1966.
10. Conyers, J. H., Hall, R. A., and Laing, D., et al. The use and risks of the Roux-en-Y anastomosis in the relief of post-gastrectomy symptoms. *Br. J. Surg.* 47:533, 1960.
11. Cooperman, A. M. Postoperative alkaline reflux gastritis. *Surg. Clin. North Am.* 56:1445, 1976.
12. Coppinger, W. R., Job, H., DeLamo, J. E., et al. Surgical treatment of reflux gastritis and esophagitis. *Arch. Surg.* 106:463, 1973.
13. Davenport, H. W. Gastric mucosal injury by fatty and acetylsalicylic acids. *Gastroenterology* 46:245, 1964.
14. Davidson, E. D., and Hersh, T. Bile reflux gastritis: Contribution of inadequate gastric emptying. *Am. J. Surg.* 130:514, 1975.
15. Davidson, E. D., and Hersh, T. The surgical treatment of bile reflux gastritis: A study of 59 patients. *Ann. Surg.* 192:175, 1980.
16. Delaney, J. P., Broadie, T. A., and Robbins, P. L. Pyloric reflux gastritis: The offending agent. *Surgery* 77:764, 1975.
17. Delaney, J. P., Cheng, J. W. B., Butler, B. A., et al. Gastric ulcer and regurgitation gastritis. *Gut* 11:715, 1970.
18. Dragstedt, L. R., Woodward, E. R., Seito, T., et al. Question of bile regurgitation as cause of gastric ulcer. *Ann. Surg.* 174:548, 1971.
19. Drapanas, T., and Bethea, M. Reflux gastritis following gastric surgery. *Ann. Surg.* 179:618, 1974.
20. du Plessis, D. J. Gastric mucosal changes after

operations on the stomach. *S. Afr. Med. J.* 36:471, 1962.

21. du Plessis, D. J. Pathogenesis of gastric ulceration. *Lancet* 1:974, 1965.
22. duPlessis, D. J. Alkaline Reflux Gastritis. In H. N. Harkins and L. M. Nyhus (Eds.), *Surgery of the Stomach and Duodenum.* London: Churchill Livingstone, 1969.
23. du Plessis, D. J., Myburgh, J. A., Lawson, H. H., et al. Experiences with the treatment of duodenal ulceration in Johannesburg Hospital. *S. Afr. Med. J.* 39:918, 1965.
24. Fiddian-Green, R. G., and Hobsley, M. Hypoacidity in gastric juice in chronic gastric ulceration caused by neutralization. *S. Afr. Med. J.* II:580–582, 1976.
25. Fiddian-Green, R. G., Pittenger, G., and Whitehouse, W. M. Back-diffusion of CO_2 and its influence on the intramural pH in gastric mucosa. *J. Surg. Res.,* 33:39, 1982.
26. Fiddian-Green, R. G., et al. The quantification in human gastric juice of duodenogastric reflux by sodium output . . . *Klin. Wochenschr.* 57:815, 1979.
27. Fielding, J. W. L., Bradby, H., Tulley, N. J., et al. Inadequate methods for bile diversion after total gastrectomy. *Surg. Res. Soc. Abstr.* 67:830, 1980.
28. Fisher, R., and Cohen, S. Physiological characteristics of the human pyloric sphincter. *Gastroenterology* 64:67, 1973.
29. Fisher, R., and Cohen, S. Pyloric dysfunction in patients with gastric ulcer. *N. Engl. J. Med.* 288:273, 1973.
30. Gadacz, T. R., and Zuidema, G. D. Bile acid composition in patients with and without symptoms of postoperative reflux gastritis. *Am. J. Surg.* 135:48, 1978.
31. Grant, R., Grossman, M. I., Wang, K. J., et al. The cytolytic action of some gastrointestinal secretions and enzymes on the epithelial cells of the gastric and duodenal mucosa. *J. Cell. Comp. Physiol.* 37:137, 1951.
32. Green, R., Spencer, E. A., and Kennedy, T. Closure of gastrojejunostomy for post-vagotomy symptoms. *Br. J. Surg.* 65:161, 1978.
33. Griffiths, J. M. T., Smith, A. N., Small, W. P., et al. The results of reoperation for bile vomiting following surgery for peptic ulcer. *Br. J. Surg.* 61:838, 1974.
34. Gustke, R. F., Varma, R. R., and Soergel, K H. Gastric reflux during perfusion of the proximal small bowel. *Gastroenterology* 59:890, 1970.
35. Halpern, N. B., Hirschowitz, B. L., and Moody, F. G. Failure to achieve success with remedial gastric surgery. *Am. J. Surg.* 125:108, 1973.
36. Halter, F. Therapeutic implications of duodenogastric reflux. *Scand. J. Gastroenterol.* 16(Suppl. 67):257, 1981.
37. Harmon, J. W., Doong, T., and Gadacz, T. R. Bile acids are not equally damaging to the gastric mucosa. *Surgery* 84:79, 1978.
38. Harmon, J. W., Lewis, C. D., and Gadacz, T. Bile salt composition and concentration as determinants of canine gastric mucosal injury. *Surgery* 89:348, 1981.
39. Harvey, B. C. A study of the structure of the gastric glands of the dog and the changes they undergo after gastro-enterostomy and occlusion of the pylorus. *Am. J. Anat.* 6:207, 1906.
40. Hedenstedt, S. Gastrectomy with jejunal replacement. *Acta Chir. Scand.* 117:295, 1959.
41. Henley, F. A. Gastrectomy with replacement. A preliminary communication. *Br. J. Surg.* 40:118, 1952.
42. Henley, F. A. Gastrectomy with replacement. *Ann. R. Coll. Surg. Engl.* 13:141, 1953.
43. Herrington, J. L., Sawyers, J. L., and Whitehead, W. A. Surgical Management of reflux gastritis. *Ann. Surg.* 180:526, 1974.
44. Himal, H. S. Alkaline gastritis and alkaline esophagitis: A review. *Can. J. Surg.* 20:403, 1977.
45. Hoare, A. M., Jones, E. L., Alexander-Williams, J., et al. Symptomatic significance of gastric mucosal changes after surgery for peptic ulcer. *Gut* 18:295, 1977.
46. Hoare, A. M., Keighley, M. R. B., Starkey, B., et al: Measurement of bile acids in fasting gastric aspirates: An objective test for bile reflux after gastric surgery. *Gut* 19:166, 1978.
47. Hoare, A. M., McLeish, A., Thompson, H., et al. Selection of patients for bile diversion surgery: Use of bile acid measurement in fasting gastric aspirates. *Gut* 19:163, 1978.
48. Hocking, M. P., Vogel, S. B., Falasca, C. A., et al. Delayed gastric emptying of liquids and solids following Roux-en-Y biliary diversion. *Ann. Surg.* 194:494, 1981.
49. Hollinger, A., Ammann, R., Sialer, G., et al. Quantitative assessment of duodenogastric reflux after vagotomy with or without pyloroplasty: A clinical investigation. *Scand. J. Gastroenterol.* 16(Suppl. 67):55, 1981.
50. Ivey, K. Acute haemorrhagic gastritis: Modern concepts based on pathogenesis. *Gut* 12:750, 1971.

51. Ivey, K. Gastric mucosal barrier. *Gastroenterology* 61:247, 1971.
52. Ivey, K. J., DenBesten, L., and Clifton, J. A. Effect of bile salts on the ionic movement across the human gastric mucosa. *Gastroenterology* 59:683, 1970.
53. Janowitz, H. D. Bile in the stomach. *Gastroenterology* 57:356, 1969.
54. Johnson, A. G. The action of metoclopramide on human gastroduodenal motility. *Gut* 12:421, 1971.
55. Johnson, A. G. Pyloric function and gall-stone dyspepsia. *Br. J. Surg.* 59:449, 1972.
56. Johnson, A. G., and McDermott, S. J. Lysolecithin: A factor in the pathogenesis of gastric ulceration. *Gut* 15:710, 1974.
57. Joseph, W. L., Rivera, R. A., O'Kieffe, D.A., et al. Management of postoperative alkaline reflux gastritis. *Ann. Surg.* 177:655, 1973.
58. Kalima, T., and Sjoberg, J. Bile reflux after cholecystectomy. *Scand. J. Gastroenterol.* 16(Suppl. 67):153, 1981.
59. Keighley, M. R. B., Asquita, P., and Alexander-Williams, J. Duodenogastric reflux: A cause of gastric mucosal hyperaemia and symptoms after operations for peptic ulceration. *Gut* 16:28, 1975.
60. Kennedy, T., and Green, R. Roux diversion for bile reflux following gastric surgery. *Br. J. Surg.* 65:323, 1978.
61. Kivilaakso, E., Ehnholm, C., Kalima, T. V., et al. Duodenogastric reflux of lysolecithin in the pathogenesis of experimental porcine stress ulceration. *Surgery* 79:65, 1976.
62. Kivilaakso, E., Fromm, D., and Silen, W. Relationship between ulceration and intramural pH of gastric mucosa during hemorrhagic shock. *Surgery* 84:70, 1978.
63. Kivilaakso, E., and Silen, W. Pathogenesis of experimental gastric mucosal injury. *N. Eng. J. Med.* 301:364, 1979.
64. Langhans, P., Schonleben, K., and Bunte, H. The routine use of Roux-en-Y anastomosis in gastric surgery. *Scand. J. Gastroenterol.* 16(Suppl. 67):241, 1981.
65. Lawson, H. H. Effect of duodenal contents on the gastric mucosa under experimental conditions. *Lancet* 1:469, 1964.
66. Lawson, H. H. The effect of the duodenal contents on the gastric mucosa. *S. Afr. J. Surg.* 3:79, 1965.
67. Lawson, H. H. The reversibility of postgastrectomy alkaline reflux gastritis by a Roux-en-Y loop. *Br. J. Surg.* 59:13, 1972.
68. Ludwig, S., and Ippoliti, A. Objective evaluation of symptomatic bile reflux after antrectomy. *Gastroenterology* 76:1189, 1979.
69. Magnus, H.A. *Gastritis.* In F. Avery Jones (Ed.), *Modern Trends in Gastroenterology.* London: Butterworth, 1952.
70. Malagelada, J. R., Phillips, S. F., Higgins, J. A., et al. A prospective evaluation of alkaline reflux gastritis: Bile acid finding agents and Roux-Y diversion. *Gastroenterology* 76:1192, 1979.
71. Menguy, R., and Chey, W. Experience with the treatment of alkaline reflux gastritis. *Surgery* 88:482, 1980.
72. Meshkinpour, H., Elashoff, J., Stewart, H., et al. Effect of cholestytramine on the symptoms of reflux gastritis. *Gastroenterology* 73:441, 1977.
73. Meshkinpour, H., Marks, J. W., Schoenfield, L. J., et al. Reflux gastritis syndrome: Mechanism of symptoms. *Gastroenterology* 79:1283, 1980.
74. Meshkinpour, H., Thrupp, L. D., Shiffer, P., et al. Reflux gastritis syndrome: Role of upper gastrointestinal microflora. *Arch. Surg.* 116:1148, 1981.
75. Mosimann, R., Loup, P., Fontolliet, C., et al. Post-operative reflux gastritis: Results of surgical treatment. *Scand. J. Gastroenterol.* 16(Suppl. 67):237, 1981.
76. Palmer, E. D. Gastritis: A reevaluation. *Medicine* 33:199, 1954.
77. Pyrtek, L. J., and Bartus, S. A. Reflux bile gastritis. *Am. J. Surg.* 125:408, 1973.
78. Reber, H. A., and Way, L. W. Surgical treatment of late postgastrectomy syndromes. *Am. J. Surg.* 129:71, 1975.
79. Rhodes, J., Apsimon, H. T., and Lawrie, J. H. pH of the contents of the duodenal bulb in relation to duodenal ulcer. *Gut* 7:502, 1966.
80. Rhodes, J., Bernardo, D. E., Phillips, S. E., et al. Increased reflux of bile into the stomach in patients with gastric ulcer. *Gastroenterology* 57:241, 1969.
81. Rhodes, J., and Prestwich, C. J. Acidity at different sites in the proximal duodenum of normal subjects and patients with duodenal ulcer. *Gut* 7:509, 1966.
82. Ritchie, W. P. Alkaline reflux gastritis: An objective assessment of its diagnosis and treatment. *Ann. Surg.* 192:288, 1980.
83. Ritchie, W. P., and Felger, T. S. Differing ulcerogenic potential of dihydroxy and trihy-

mimics complete gastric outlet obstruction. Endoscopy is mandatory and most often demonstrates a widely patent anastomosis. Most patients respond to "tincture of time," parenteral or oral bethanechol therapy, or no specific treatment at all, and leave the hospital after a prolonged postoperative stay.

The late Roux syndrome is quite subtle, and the patients are often not referred back to the primary surgeon. In our experience, the symptoms are always the same: intermittent vomiting, epigastric fullness with or without pain, and a history of numerous and normal endoscopic and upper gastrointestinal barium examinations. Retrospective studies in these patients almost always demonstrate delayed emptying after either radionuclide or "barium burger" examination. In this rather homogeneous group, oral bethanechol has been moderately effective when used before each meal and at bedtime. Metoclopramide has had no effect on this delayed emptying syndrome.

Does a preexisting motility disorder predispose to more severe postoperative symptoms of delayed gastric emptying? This review cannot evaluate this question adequately since most patients did not undergo more sophisticated gastric emptying studies before Roux-Y diversion. It is interesting, however, that among 34 patients who had unequivocal preoperative symptoms of gastric retention there appeared to be an increased incidence of post-Roux-Y delayed emptying symptoms and a higher number of Visick 4 failures. The hypothesis suggested by Davidson and Hersh, that a preexisting motility problem predisposes to a more severe postoperative course, is probably correct. The question remains whether all post-Roux-Y failures result from a preexisting condition or whether the syndrome of alkaline gastritis itself is caused, in part, by a postvagotomy or postgastrectomy motility disorder.

Does Roux-Y biliary diversion alter upper gastrointestinal emptying? Using a canine model to evaluate standard dog chow and liquid emptying, my group documented considerably more gastric retention in dogs who had undergone truncal vagotomy and Roux-Y gastrectomy compared with dogs who underwent vagotomy and Billroth II gastrectomy [5]. These initial studies tended to support the overall clinical impression. Since most if not all patients evaluated for alkaline gastritis have undergone previous vagotomy, it was important to evaluate the role of vagal denervation in delayed upper gastrointestinal emptying. Recent canine experiments using a technetium 99 radionuclide emptying technique demonstrated rapid gastric emptying in dogs after antrectomy and Roux gastroenterostomy without vagotomy. The subsequent addition of a truncal vagotomy dramatically alters gastrointestinal emptying. Significant radionuclide retention was observed in the stomach only, in both the stomach and the Roux limb, and, in some experiments, in the Roux limb only with intermittent flow of the radionuclide between the Roux limb, stomach, and back to the Roux limb [8].

Although authors have traditionally discussed and evaluated gastric emptying per se, it has become clear to my group that in the patient or experimental animal who has undergone vagotomy the problem may indeed reside in both the stomach and the Roux limb. During recent clinical evaluations, and in reviewing post-Roux-Y radionuclide and "barium burger" upper GI examinations, I have corroborated my experimental data and observed prolonged retention of solid food in the Roux limb as well as the stomach in many patients. No data are available evaluating selective or highly selective vagotomy with Roux antrectomy. It has become evident that these findings may play an important role in the early and late delayed emptying syndrome, and furthermore, may explain the successful use of a Roux limb in treating postgastrectomy dumping. Additionally, the success and minimal side effects of total gastrectomy with Roux-Y esophagojejunostomy may certainly be caused by the delayed emptying in the vagotomized Roux limb. Although I am uncertain of the cause of this phenomenon, a combination of factors in the presence of complete vagal denervation may contribute to altered gastrointestinal emptying, namely, transection of the jejunum with alteration of electrical activity, complete diversion of duodenal contents,

51. Ivey, K. Gastric mucosal barrier. *Gastroenterology* 61:247, 1971.
52. Ivey, K. J., DenBesten, L., and Clifton, J. A. Effect of bile salts on the ionic movement across the human gastric mucosa. *Gastroenterology* 59:683, 1970.
53. Janowitz, H. D. Bile in the stomach. *Gastroenterology* 57:356, 1969.
54. Johnson, A. G. The action of metoclopramide on human gastroduodenal motility. *Gut* 12:421, 1971.
55. Johnson, A. G. Pyloric function and gall-stone dyspepsia. *Br. J. Surg.* 59:449, 1972.
56. Johnson, A. G., and McDermott, S. J. Lysolecithin: A factor in the pathogenesis of gastric ulceration. *Gut* 15:710, 1974.
57. Joseph, W. L., Rivera, R. A., O'Kieffe, D.A., et al. Management of postoperative alkaline reflux gastritis. *Ann. Surg.* 177:655, 1973.
58. Kalima, T., and Sjoberg, J. Bile reflux after cholecystectomy. *Scand. J. Gastroenterol.* 16(Suppl. 67):153, 1981.
59. Keighley, M. R. B., Asquita, P., and Alexander-Williams, J. Duodenogastric reflux: A cause of gastric mucosal hyperaemia and symptoms after operations for peptic ulceration. *Gut* 16:28, 1975.
60. Kennedy, T., and Green, R. Roux diversion for bile reflux following gastric surgery. *Br. J. Surg.* 65:323, 1978.
61. Kivilaakso, E., Ehnholm, C., Kalima, T. V., et al. Duodenogastric reflux of lysolecithin in the pathogenesis of experimental porcine stress ulceration. *Surgery* 79:65, 1976.
62. Kivilaakso, E., Fromm, D., and Silen, W. Relationship between ulceration and intramural pH of gastric mucosa during hemorrhagic shock. *Surgery* 84:70, 1978.
63. Kivilaakso, E., and Silen, W. Pathogenesis of experimental gastric mucosal injury. *N. Eng. J. Med.* 301:364, 1979.
64. Langhans, P., Schonleben, K., and Bunte, H. The routine use of Roux-en-Y anastomosis in gastric surgery. *Scand. J. Gastroenterol.* 16(Suppl. 67):241, 1981.
65. Lawson, H. H. Effect of duodenal contents on the gastric mucosa under experimental conditions. *Lancet* 1:469, 1964.
66. Lawson, H. H. The effect of the duodenal contents on the gastric mucosa. *S. Afr. J. Surg.* 3:79, 1965.
67. Lawson, H. H. The reversibility of postgastrectomy alkaline reflux gastritis by a Roux-en-Y loop. *Br. J. Surg.* 59:13, 1972.
68. Ludwig, S., and Ippoliti, A. Objective evaluation of symptomatic bile reflux after antrectomy. *Gastroenterology* 76:1189, 1979.
69. Magnus, H.A. *Gastritis.* In F. Avery Jones (Ed.), *Modern Trends in Gastroenterology.* London: Butterworth, 1952.
70. Malagelada, J. R., Phillips, S. F., Higgins, J. A., et al. A prospective evaluation of alkaline reflux gastritis: Bile acid finding agents and Roux-Y diversion. *Gastroenterology* 76:1192, 1979.
71. Menguy, R., and Chey, W. Experience with the treatment of alkaline reflux gastritis. *Surgery* 88:482, 1980.
72. Meshkinpour, H., Elashoff, J., Stewart, H., et al. Effect of cholestytramine on the symptoms of reflux gastritis. *Gastroenterology* 73:441, 1977.
73. Meshkinpour, H., Marks, J. W., Schoenfield, L. J., et al. Reflux gastritis syndrome: Mechanism of symptoms. *Gastroenterology* 79:1283, 1980.
74. Meshkinpour, H., Thrupp, L. D., Shiffer, P., et al. Reflux gastritis syndrome: Role of upper gastrointestinal microflora. *Arch. Surg.* 116:1148, 1981.
75. Mosimann, R., Loup, P., Fontolliet, C., et al. Post-operative reflux gastritis: Results of surgical treatment. *Scand. J. Gastroenterol.* 16(Suppl. 67):237, 1981.
76. Palmer, E. D. Gastritis: A reevaluation. *Medicine* 33:199, 1954.
77. Pyrtek, L. J., and Bartus, S. A. Reflux bile gastritis. *Am. J. Surg.* 125:408, 1973.
78. Reber, H. A., and Way, L. W. Surgical treatment of late postgastrectomy syndromes. *Am. J. Surg.* 129:71, 1975.
79. Rhodes, J., Apsimon, H. T., and Lawrie, J. H. pH of the contents of the duodenal bulb in relation to duodenal ulcer. *Gut* 7:502, 1966.
80. Rhodes, J., Bernardo, D. E., Phillips, S. E., et al. Increased reflux of bile into the stomach in patients with gastric ulcer. *Gastroenterology* 57:241, 1969.
81. Rhodes, J., and Prestwich, C. J. Acidity at different sites in the proximal duodenum of normal subjects and patients with duodenal ulcer. *Gut* 7:509, 1966.
82. Ritchie, W. P. Alkaline reflux gastritis: An objective assessment of its diagnosis and treatment. *Ann. Surg.* 192:288, 1980.
83. Ritchie, W. P., and Felger, T. S. Differing ulcerogenic potential of dihydroxy and trihy-

droxy bile acids in canine gastric mucosa. *Surgery* 89:342, 1981.
84. Russell, R. C. G., Fiddian-Green, R. G., Hassan, M. A., et al. The relationship between pyloric reflux and gastric ulcer. *Br. J. Surg.* 59:905, 1972.
85. Schindler, R. *Gastritis*. New York: Grune & Stratton, 1947.
86. Schumpelick, V., Schwoy, M., Begemann, F., et al. Clinical results of jejunal transposition. *Scand. J. Gastroenterol.* 16(Suppl. 67):241, 1981.
87. Scott, H. W., and Weidner, M. G. Total gastrectomy with Roux-en-Y esophagojejunostomy in treatment of gastric cancer. *Ann. Surg.* 143:682, 1956.
88. Scudmore, H. H., Eckstam, E. E., Fencil, W. J., et al. Bile reflux gastritis: Diagnosis, medical and surgical therapy. *Am. J. Gastroenterol.* 60:9, 1973.
89. Tanner, N. C. The surgical treatment of peptic ulcers. *Br. J. Surg.* 51:5, 1964.
90. Tolin, R. D., Malmud, L. S., Stelzer, F., et al. Enterogastric reflux in normal subjects and patients with Billroth II gastroenterostomy. *Gastroenterology* 77:1027, 1979.
91. Toye, D. K. M., and Alexander-Williams, J. Post-gastrectomy bile vomiting. *Lancet* 2:524, 1965.
92. van Heerden, J. A., Phillips, S. F., Adson, M. A., et al. Postoperative reflux gastritis. *Am. J. Surg.* 129:82, 1975.
93. Warshaw, A. L. Bile gastritis without prior gastric surgery: Contributing role of cholecystectomy. *Am. J. Surg.* 137:527, 1979.
94. Warshaw, A. L. Intragastric alkali infusion. *Ann. Surg.* 194:297, 1981.
95. Wolfer, A. Gastroenterostomie. *Zentralbl. Chir.* 8:705, 1881.
96. Wormsley, K. G. Aspects of duodeno-gastric reflux in man. *Gut* 13:243, 1972.
97. Zimmerman, G. J., Westbrook, K. D., and Thompson, B. W. The surgical management of reflux gastritis. *Am. J. Surg.* 132:787, 1976.

SPECIAL COMMENT
Alkaline Reflux Gastritis

Stephen B. Vogel

During the past 15 years, clinicians have observed a dramatic increase in both the diagnosis and treatment of alkaline or bile reflux gastritis. The appearance of this "new clinical entity" seems to be in part coincident with the increasing and now widespread use of perioperative flexible endoscopy. Postoperative endoscopy has revealed the presence of copious amounts of refluxed bile and gastritis in patients with essentially asymptomatic disease. This finding, however, does not appear to negate the described syndrome, as most reviews refer only to symptomatic disease with bile vomiting and burning abdominal pain that is resistant to medical therapy and shows histological or endoscopic evidence of severe gastritis. In describing the results of Roux-Y biliary diversion for alkaline gastritis, most investigators have reported from 80 to 95 percent successful results. Recent reviews, however, have documented a less successful outcome. Several investigators have questioned whether "alkaline reflux gastritis" exists as a separate disease entity, whether the criteria used for patient selection are adequate, whether a preexisting motility disorder is present, and perhaps most important, whether or not biliary diversion is an entirely safe procedure.

Does the syndrome of alkaline gastritis exist and, if so, which patients benefit from remedial surgical treatment? These intriguing questions have been discussed in excellent reviews by Ritchie, Alexander-Williams, Warshaw [1, 6, 7, 9], and others. In an effort to evaluate this elusive "syndrome" more adequately these authors have advocated the use of additional diagnostic criteria including measurements of intragastric bile acid concentration, radionuclide enterogastric reflux testing, and a provocative intragastric alkaline infusion test. In response to the decreasing success rate following biliary diversion, they have provided more accurate means of selecting patients to undergo remedial operations and suggest that the more stringent the diagnostic criteria, the better the postoperative results. This approach is reasonable, appropriate, and perhaps should be mandatory in evaluating patients with symptomatic bile gastritis. It is somewhat perplexing, however, to observe that most patients evaluated in other series have benefited from remedial operations without this critical approach. Additionally, it has become apparent that the increasing failure rate of biliary diversion is caused by the undesirable symptoms of severe gastric retention—not recurrence of abdominal pain [2].

Roux-Y biliary diversion has been assumed to be a relatively safe procedure with minimal morbidity. When reviewing the British and American literaure since 1965, one notes sporadic reports of prolonged postoperative hospitalization, and occasional suggestions of delayed gastric emptying. More recent reviews have documented an incidence of up to 60 percent of severe gastric emptying problems after Roux-Y duodenal diversion. Davidson and Hersh [3, 4] in 1975 suggested that symptoms of alkaline gastritis may be indistinguishable from those of delayed gastric emptying and more recently reported that patients with preexisting gastric emptying problems had not benefited from Roux-Y diversion. Is delayed gastric emptying unique to the formation of a Roux-Y gastroenterostomy or simply the result of operating upon a select group of patients with a preexisting motility disorder? Although I had observed post-Roux-Y emptying problems before and had even reported the beneficial effect of Roux-Y diversion for postgastrectomy dumping, these observations prompted me to evaluate my experience with biliary diversion.

Patients and Procedures

From 1970 to 1980, 97 patients underwent Roux-Y biliary diversion for bile gastritis at the Shands Teaching Hospital. Follow-up periods lasted two to twelve years. Most of the patients were referred to us after their primary or secondary gastric procedure. The indication for the primary operation was usually duodenal or gastric ulcer, although a small but significant number underwent ulcer operations, prophylactically or combined with hiatal hernia repair, for "ulcer diathesis" when no ulcer was present. For the most part, as was common then, the diagnosis of bile gastritis was made by history, exclusion of other diseases, resistance to extensive medical therapy at numerous institutions, gastric secretory studies, and numerous endoscopic procedures. The initial results of Roux-Y diversion were quite similar to most of the reported series. Complete relief from the pain of bile gastritis was observed in nearly all the patients early and in about 95 percent of patients at three months.

Results

The long-term results were somewhat different from the early successful outcome. During the follow-up period, 50 of 97 patients were considered to have moderate-to-severe symptoms of delayed gastric emptying. The group's entire clinical course was evaluated by Visick grading. The results were as follows: excellent, 29 percent; good, 30 percent; fair, 18 percent; and poor or failure, 23 percent. It is intriguing, however, and quite pertinent to the entire issue of alkaline gastritis, that nearly all the patients in the fair and poor groups readily discriminated between resolution of their preoperative pain and the more subtle postoperative symptoms of delayed gastric emptying. Essentially all of the Visick 4 patients had results considered failures only because of the severe and debilitating effects of gastric retention. Almost all of the Visick 3 patients (18 percent) were extremely satisfied with the results of Roux-Y diversion. These patients' results were downgraded to fair because of moderate symptoms of delayed emptying, frequent visits to their local physicians, or numerous hospitalizations.

Discussion

The "Roux syndrome," as I have taken the liberty of calling this condition, can occur either early in the postoperative period or late, from months to years after Roux-Y diversion. The early syndrome (19 of 97 patients) is characterized by prolonged hospitalization and persistent vomiting of either liquids or solids. Gastrografin or barium swallow occasionally mimics complete gastric outlet obstruction. Endoscopy is mandatory and most often demonstrates a widely patent anastomosis. Most patients respond to "tincture of time," parenteral or oral bethanechol therapy, or no specific treatment at all, and leave the hospital after a prolonged postoperative stay.

The late Roux syndrome is quite subtle, and the patients are often not referred back to the primary surgeon. In our experience, the symptoms are always the same: intermittent vomiting, epigastric fullness with or without pain, and a history of numerous and normal endoscopic and upper gastrointestinal barium examinations. Retrospective studies in these patients almost always demonstrate delayed emptying after either radionuclide or "barium burger" examination. In this rather homogeneous group, oral bethanechol has been moderately effective when used before each meal and at bedtime. Metoclopramide has had no effect on this delayed emptying syndrome.

Does a preexisting motility disorder predispose to more severe postoperative symptoms of delayed gastric emptying? This review cannot evaluate this question adequately since most patients did not undergo more sophisticated gastric emptying studies before Roux-Y diversion. It is interesting, however, that among 34 patients who had unequivocal preoperative symptoms of gastric retention there appeared to be an increased incidence of post-Roux-Y delayed emptying symptoms and a higher number of Visick 4 failures. The hypothesis suggested by Davidson and Hersh, that a preexisting motility problem predisposes to a more severe postoperative course, is probably correct. The question remains whether all post-Roux-Y failures result from a preexisting condition or whether the syndrome of alkaline gastritis itself is caused, in part, by a postvagotomy or postgastrectomy motility disorder.

Does Roux-Y biliary diversion alter upper gastrointestinal emptying? Using a canine model to evaluate standard dog chow and liquid emptying, my group documented considerably more gastric retention in dogs who had undergone truncal vagotomy and Roux-Y gastrectomy compared with dogs who underwent vagotomy and Billroth II gastrectomy [5]. These initial studies tended to support the overall clinical impression. Since most if not all patients evaluated for alkaline gastritis have undergone previous vagotomy, it was important to evaluate the role of vagal denervation in delayed upper gastrointestinal emptying. Recent canine experiments using a technetium 99 radionuclide emptying technique demonstrated rapid gastric emptying in dogs after antrectomy and Roux gastroenterostomy without vagotomy. The subsequent addition of a truncal vagotomy dramatically alters gastrointestinal emptying. Significant radionuclide retention was observed in the stomach only, in both the stomach and the Roux limb, and, in some experiments, in the Roux limb only with intermittent flow of the radionuclide between the Roux limb, stomach, and back to the Roux limb [8].

Although authors have traditionally discussed and evaluated gastric emptying per se, it has become clear to my group that in the patient or experimental animal who has undergone vagotomy the problem may indeed reside in both the stomach and the Roux limb. During recent clinical evaluations, and in reviewing post-Roux-Y radionuclide and "barium burger" upper GI examinations, I have corroborated my experimental data and observed prolonged retention of solid food in the Roux limb as well as the stomach in many patients. No data are available evaluating selective or highly selective vagotomy with Roux antrectomy. It has become evident that these findings may play an important role in the early and late delayed emptying syndrome, and furthermore, may explain the successful use of a Roux limb in treating postgastrectomy dumping. Additionally, the success and minimal side effects of total gastrectomy with Roux-Y esophagojejunostomy may certainly be caused by the delayed emptying in the vagotomized Roux limb. Although I am uncertain of the cause of this phenomenon, a combination of factors in the presence of complete vagal denervation may contribute to altered gastrointestinal emptying, namely, transection of the jejunum with alteration of electrical activity, complete diversion of duodenal contents, and bypass of the duodenal pacemaker. Post-Roux-Y delayed gastrointestinal emptying is a real syndrome that occurs both clinically and experimentally and can be documented objectively even in patients without symptoms.

The syndrome of bile reflux gastritis and its treatment by Roux-Y biliary diversion presents an intriguing dilemma. Even though Roux diversion caused altered upper gastrointestinal emptying with severe effects in some patients, almost 80 percent of the patients believed the diversion successful in eliminating their preoperative symptoms. A small but significant number of patients from this group, as well as other patients, have undergone additional remedial operations in an attempt to alleviate their post-Roux-Y retention symptoms. The results following either extensive (90–95 percent) gastrectomy with Roux reconstruction (17 patients) or total gastrectomy (6 patients) have for the most part been gratifying.

I remain cautious in evaluating patients with alkaline gastritis, especially in the presence of preoperative symptoms of gastric retention. All patients now undergo evaluation of gastric emptying using the described methods both pre- and postoperatively. Even in the absence of such symptoms or objective documentation, I agree that more critical diagnostic criteria need to be applied when evaluating post-gastrectomy abdominal pain and bile gastritis. Although I am still enthusiastic about Roux-Y diversion, I hope future pharmacological advances will not only alleviate preoperative symptoms but also resolve postvagotomy-gastrectomy and Roux-Y motility disorders.

Comment References

1. Alexander-Williams, J. Alkaline reflux gastritis: A myth or a disease? *Am. J. Surg.* 143:17, 1982.
2. Boren, C. H., and Way, L. W. Alkaline reflux gastritis: A re-evaluation. *Am. J. Surg.* 140:40, 1980.
3. Davidson, E. D., and Hersh, T. Bile reflux gastritis. *Am. J. Surg.* 130:514, 1975.
4. Davidson, E. D., and Hersh, T. The surgical treatment of bile reflux gastritis: A study of 59 patients. *Ann. Surg.* 192:175, 1980.
5. Hocking, M. P., Vogel, S. B., Falasco, C. A., and Woodward, E. R. Delayed gastric emptying of liquids and solids folloing Roux-en-Y biliary diversion. *Ann. Surg.* 194:494, 1981.
6. Ritchie, W. P., Jr. Alkaline reflux gastritis: An objective assessment of its diagnosis and treatment. *Ann. Surg.* 192:288, 1980.
7. Ritchie, W. P. Jr. Alkaline reflux gastritis: A diagnosis in search of a disease? *J. Clin. Surg.* 1:414, 1982.
8. Vogel, S. B., Vair, B., and Woodward, E. R. Alterations in gastrointestinal emptying of 99m-technetium labeled solids following sequential antrectomy, truncal vagotomy, and Roux-Y gastroenterostomy. *Ann. Surg.* 198:506, 1983.
9. Warshaw, A. L. Intragastric alkali infusion: A simple, accurate, provocative test for diagnosis of symptomatic alkaline reflux gastritis. *Ann. Surg.* 194:297, 1981.

8

Gastric Ulcer

Jack Rudick

Although the surgical procedures for treatment of gastric ulceration have not changed dramatically since the last edition of this book, we have gained clearer insight into the pathogenesis and natural history of this disease. The advent of flexible fiberoptic endoscopy has changed the way in which gastric ulcers are investigated and managed by permitting more accurate distinction between benign and malignant ulceration.

Incidence

The incidence of gastric ulceration varies with the type of population examined, the age of the population, and the type of study conducted (antemortem versus postmortem). It has been estimated that 3,500,000 persons in the United States were affected annually by duodenal and gastric ulceration during the period 1963–1965 [6]. If the usual ratio for duodenal ulcer to gastric ulcer of 4 : 1 is correct [60], then approximately 700,000 persons per year in the United States, or 0.4 percent of the total population, would have had a gastric ulcer during that time period. Autopsy studies demonstrate a somewhat higher incidence of gastric ulceration.

AGE AND SEX DISTRIBUTION

Gastric and duodenal ulcers are usually more common in men than in women [31], but the relative frequency varies with the type of ulcer, the age of the patient, the mode of presentation, and the geographic distribution. Although ulcers are not universally gastric in the elderly, gastric ulcer tends to occur with increased frequency in this age group; in elderly patients 30 to 50 percent of peptic ulcers are gastric.

RATIO OF GASTRIC TO DUODENAL ULCER

The ratio of gastric to duodenal ulcer is 1 : 4 [60], but it may range from 1 : 12 to 1 : 17. A reversal of this ratio has been noted in the high Peruvian Andes [44], where gastric ulcers are 20 times more prevalent than duodenal ulcers.

CHRONOLOGICAL CHANGE IN INCIDENCE

The pattern of peptic ulceration has changed from a disease predominant in young women in the nineteenth century to one that is more common in men and in the elderly.

OCCUPATION AND SOCIOECONOMIC STATUS

Gastric ulceration is 2 to 5 times more common in poor men than in men of the upper socioeconomic classes. The reportedly higher mortality from gastric ulcers in patients with low socioeconomic status may simply reflect a poorer standard of available medical care, while the higher rate of perforation in the rural population may be due to a possible reluctance to seek early medical advice.

DIETARY FACTORS

On the basis of broad epidemiological comparisons, it has been suggested that a high protein diet with a low refined carbohydrate content is associated with a low ulcer frequency [17]. In contrast, a high carbohydrate diet has been suggested as less likely than protein to stimulate acid output by the stomach. It has also been hypothesized that overrefinement of staple (carbohydrate) foods may predispose to ulcer by removing the fiber content. However, none of these hypotheses has been proved. The consumption of hot curries and spices as a cause of peptic ulceration has been disproved, since there is no clear geographical association between ulcer frequency in India and the consumption of spices [29]. Indeed, the prevalent semisolid, nonfibrous diet in southern India, where ulcer is common, bears a superficial resemblance to the often recommended Western ulcer diet.

GEOGRAPHICAL DISTRIBUTION

The pattern of gastric ulceration varies with different countries and also from area to area within a given country. Japan is one of the few places where gastric ulcer may be more common than duodenal ulcer [101]. The ratio of males to females for peptic ulcer has been found to be 3.1 : 1.0; for duodenal ulcer, 3.5 : 1.0; and for gastric ulcer, 2.7 : 1.0. Regional differences have also been noted. In fishing communities in northern Norway [87] the ratio of gastric to duodenal ulcers was 2.7 : 1.0. In the high Peruvian Andes, 96 percent of peptic ulcers were gastric in location, whereas at sea level in Peru the usual ratio prevailed.

ULCER MORTALITY

Gastric and duodenal ulceration ranks thirteenth among causes of death in white American men. The higher mortality in men reflects the overall frequency of the disease pattern [70] (Table 8-1), while the high mortality from gastric ulceration is probably due to the tendency of gastric ulcer to afflict the elderly.

Etiology

ALCOHOL

Alcohol clearly damages the gastric mucosal barrier. Davenport [22] demonstrated the threshold for damage to be between 8 and 14 percent ethanol (w/v). Solutions of 8 percent or less did not damage the mucosal barrier; however, ethanol solutions of 14 percent (the equivalent of a cocktail sherry) and 27 percent (the equivalent of a martini made of 4 parts gin and 1 part vermouth) broke the barrier, allowing insorption of H^+ and exsorption of Na^+ and K^+. These are acute changes; the role of ethanol in the production of chronic gastric lesions in experimental animals remains inconclusive. Clinical studies indicate that acute transient gastritis is frequent after the excessive intake of alcohol. Endoscopic evidence of chronic superficial or atrophic gastritis is found in from 30 to 70 percent of chronic alcoholics [83], yet there is no sound evidence to show that mild-to-moderate alcohol consumption increases the likelihood of development of chronic gastric or duodenal ulceration [5].

INDOMETHACIN

Therapy with this synthetic nonsteroidal antiinflammatory agent carries a high incidence of gastrointestinal side effects. Lack of prospective studies of indomethacin ingestion

Table 8-1. Age-adjusted death rates per 100,000 population from gastric and duodenal ulcer in the United States in 1965

Population	Gastric ulcer	Duodenal ulcer
White males	3.3	3.5
White females	1.3	0.9
Nonwhite males	4.0	2.8
Nonwhite females	1.5	0.9

Source: Data from A. I. Mendeloff and J. P. Dunn. *Digestive Diseases.* (Vital and Health Statistics Monographs.) Cambridge, Mass.: American Public Health Association, Harvard University Press, 1971.

with matched controls makes it impossible to decide whether or not it is ulcerogenic. Available evidence indicates an ulcer incidence of 5.5 percent with its use [56], a figure no greater than that given for the frequency in the general population. Nevertheless, indomethacin should not be used in patients with active peptic ulcer disease, and it should be used with caution if there is a history of previous ulcer disease.

SALICYLATES

Although aspirin is well documented as a cause of occult bleeding and acute gastric erosions, there is little evidence to suggest that it causes gastric ulceration. Aspirin alters the mucosal barrier of the stomach, making it abnormally permeable to water-soluble compounds and ions; it disrupts the lipid-protein layer on the surface of cells, causing desquamation by breaking the tight junctions between cells. Back-diffusion of acid then occurs, resulting in damage to the mucosa [20, 22]. This damage to the mucosal barrier may produce bleeding, and this can be demonstrated by ^{51}Cr-labeled red cell loss in the feces [52]. For most persons the bleeding produced by aspirin is trivial: The blood loss after taking two 300-mg tablets is usually only about 0.5–2.0 ml. Given daily for three days, 2 gm unbuffered aspirin will increase the fecal blood loss to about 3–5 ml per day. Some susceptible people, however, may lose several hundred milliliters of blood. Thus the effects of salicylates in producing bleeding can be highly variable in different people or at different times.

The ability of salicylates to diffuse through the mucosal barrier at varying rates can be explained on the basis of the pK of aspirin. Salicylate solubility in fat depends on the acidity of the medium in which it is dissolved. In a neutral solution aspirin becomes ionized, the hydrogen being removed from its carboxyl group (COOH) so that the group is left with a negative charge (COO^-); in that state the molecule is relatively insoluble in fat and does not penetrate the lipid barrier of the mucosa readily. On the other hand, in an acid solution the carboxyl group remains un-ionized; aspirin is then soluble in fat and diffuses rapidly through the mucosal barrier. Once in the mucosa, the salicylate is immediately ionized and prevented from crossing the barrier in the opposite direction. A steep gradient for diffusion of the salicylate into the mucosa builds up, and salicylate enters the gastric mucosa at a rate dependent on the acid content of the stomach.

Despite these experimental observations, prospective clinical studies do not allow a firm conclusion and only suggest that aspirin is ulcerogenic. Nevertheless, they do imply that smoking and aspirin ingestion together are strongly associated with the development of gastric ulcers.

PHENYLBUTAZONE

In the experimental animal, phenylbutazone is ulcerogenic orally or parenterally, but a certain concentration in the gastric mucosa is necessary for the ulcerogenic action to become apparent. Epigastric pain, nausea, vomiting, acute ulcer, activation of preexisting peptic ulcer disease, development of gastric or duodenal ulcer, hematemesis, melena, and perforation have been reported after oral or intramuscular administration in humans [98]. The precise incidence of phenylbutazone ulceration (probably 2–4 percent) is not clear, but apparently de novo ulceration is more commonly gastric in location. Susceptibility to phenylbutazone ulceration is increased in the elderly and in patients with rheumatoid arthritis or with a family history of peptic ulcer disease. Perhaps the gastric mucosa in these groups of patients is more vulnerable. The incidence of ulceration increases with larger doses (more than 400 mg per day) and with prolonged continuous therapy (more than two weeks).

CORTICOSTEROIDS

Despite experimental demonstration of delayed healing, the preponderance of gastric over duodenal ulceration, and the high incidence of free perforation, the relationship of adrenocorticotropic hormone and the adrenocorticosteroids to gastroduodenal ulcer is controversial. "Steroid ulcers" are claimed to be relatively painless ("silent"), develop rapidly, and often present with complications such as perforation. Such ulcers have been described as being shallow, often multiple, and usually located in the pyloric antrum, as well as being pliable and having little fibrous reaction.

Garb et al. [43] have questioned the basis for the steroid ulcer entity. Of 1084 patients who underwent gastrectomy for gastric ulcer, 57 (5.6 percent) had received adrenal corticosteroids; in only 23 of these 57 (40 percent), the ulcer was thought to be directly attributable to the corticosteroids. Twenty-three patients who had undergone gastric resection for benign gastric ulcer, but who had not received corticosteroids, were selected as controls and were matched as far as possible for sex, age, location of the ulcer, and use of salicylates. Neither specific roentgenographical differences between the two groups nor correlation with duration or dosage of corticosteroids was found. Multiple ulcers occurred equally in both groups, and differences in size were not found. Finally, the steroid ulcers were similar histologically to those in the control group. It appears that the steroid ulcer in humans is identical to the nonsteroid ulcer.

The question of whether corticosteroids interfere with the healing of chronic peptic ulcers has not been investigated. There is adequate evidence that corticosteroids do interfere with the healing of experimental ulcers, and it would seem reasonable that they may have the same effect in humans.

SMOKING

The association between smoking and peptic ulceration has been studied by several investigators; the proportion of smokers is higher in gastric ulcer patients of both sexes. Smoking appears to be a factor delaying the healing of a gastric ulcer [32] and is associated with an increase in deaths of gastric ulcer. By interfering with the healing of a gastric ulcer, smoking probably maintains the chronicity, but it is probably not a direct causal agent. When considered in relation to data concerning aspirin ingestion [45], smoking plus the frequent use of aspirin may be more ulcerogenic than either alone.

Pathophysiology of Gastric Ulcer

LOCATION OF THE ULCER

Most gastric ulcers occur on or near the lesser curvature. Fifteen to twenty percent are distal to the incisura angularis, 60 percent are at or a little above the incisura, and 15 to 20 percent are high on the lesser curvature. A minority of ulcers occur well away from the lesser curvature and may frequently be malignant. Although large gastric ulcers are more likely to be malignant than are small gastric ulcers, most large gastric ulcers are benign.

Peptic ulcer nearly always develops in junctional epithelium [67, 75]. Thus esophageal ulcers occur just above the junction of fundic and esophageal mucosa, gastric ulcers just below the junction of fundic and antral mucosa, and duodenal ulcers just below the junction of pyloric and duodenal mucosa. Less than 3 percent occur in areas other than mucosal junctions. Peptic ulcer almost never occurs in acid-secreting mucosa; when this does occur, the ulcer is usually located in aberrant antral mucosa [74] rather than in parietal mucosa. Chronic gastric ulcers are predominantly found in the antrum of the stomach. Portis and Jaffe [79] found 59.1 percent within 6 cm of the pyloric ring, while Niwayama and Terplan [73] found 64.4 percent of gastric ulcers in the same area. Oi et al. [75] found that 96.4 percent of all gastric ulcers occurred within 2 cm of the border zone, which they defined as the zone between the body and antrum that contains both fundic and pyloric glands. The width of this border zone was 2.0 cm or less in all their patients. Gastric ulcers appear at different distances from the pyloric sphincter because the antrum extends a variable distance from the pylorus, especially along the lesser curvature. The junction between the acid-bearing and pyloric gland areas on the lesser curvature varies from 2 to 16 cm from the pyloric ring [75]. This striking localization of peptic ulcer to the junctional epithelium suggests that these areas are more sensitive to acid and pepsin than are other parts of the gastrointestinal mucosa; they may also be exposed to higher concentrations of acid and pepsin.

The alkaline area of the stomach has been found by Capper et al. [11] to be very small in patients with duodenal ulcer, whereas in gastric ulcer patients the alkaline area is extensive. The alkaline area was lined by true antral mucosa and not degenerated fundic mucosa. These findings suggest that gastric ulcer develops in patients who have a large antrum, whereas duodenal ulcer occurs in patients with a small antrum. The inverse relationship between the size of the antrum and the extent of the parietal cell mass may be of great importance [11]. Nevertheless, the G-cell population in the pyloric gland area of gastric ulcer patients was found to be less than half that in duodenal ulcer patients [92]. The difference was due to a higher incidence of intestinal metaplasia and a decrease in the thickness of the antral mucosa in patients with gastric ulcers.

Oi [74] also stated that peptic ulcer tends to occur in relation to certain muscular bands in the stomach, especially where these muscular bands coincide with junctional epithelium. The effective focus of this dual mechanism (junctional epithelium and muscle anatomy) producing gastric ulcers is located at or near the incisura angularis, which agrees with the clinical observations that gastric ulcers tend to occur in this location.

THE GASTRIC MUCOSAL BARRIER TO ACID

Numerous investigators have studied the relationship between the gastric mucosal barrier and gastric ulcers. Although the barrier is usually referred to as a mucosal barrier to ion diffusion, this is incorrect. *It is a mucosal barrier to hydrogen (acid).* Davenport [24] defined the gastric mucosal barrier as "that property of the gastric mucosa which impedes diffusion of acid from the lumen into the mucosa, and impedes diffusion of sodium ions from mucosal interstitial space into the lumen." The barrier is one of the means by which the stomach protects itself against damage by its own secretion. This property enables the stomach to contain an acid solution against a high concentration gradient, preventing insorption of hydrogen ions from the lumen into the interstitial tissues. If the pH of the interstitial tissues is 7.4 and the pH of gastric juice is 1.0, then the concentration gradient for hydrogen from the lumen to interstitial tissues is more than 3,000,000 : 1.

Elements Composing the Barrier

The mucosal barrier is a composite of several elements. The apical plasma membrane of the surface epithelial cells is composed of a lipid bilayer with a protein core and is penetrated by water-filled channels. Adjacent cells are linked by tight junctions at their superolateral surface. Water, electrolytes, and water-soluble substances such as glucose and urea can enter the intact mucosal surface through the channels; hydrogen cannot. Ionized materials are poorly absorbed, but un-ionized lipid-soluble substances are absorbed.

There is a gradient of permeability to the insorption of hydrogen [39, 50, 82]. Hydrogen is lost across the normal fundic mucosa only at very slow rates (5 to 10 percent per hour); in the antrum, hydrogen loss is 14 times greater per unit surface area than in the corpus [39]; and the duodenum is 30 to 50 times more permeable to hydrogen than the corpus [50]. This gradient of permeability may account for the relative vulnerability of antral and duodenal mucosa to acid-pepsin ulceration [39].

Agents Damaging to the Barrier

A variety of agents can damage the mucosal barrier. Cytotoxic agents, because of their lipid solubility, can penetrate the barrier and destroy it. Topical application of salicylates [18, 20, 22], fatty acid [18], ethanol [22], lysolecithin [23], and bile salts [21] to the gastric mucosa disrupts the normal barrier. Hydrogen diffuses rapidly from the lumen into the mucosa, and sodium ions diffuse from the mucosa into the lumen. The sodium ion movement is bidirectional, the net flux being into the lumen [25]; potassium ion movement is also bidirectional, with an increase in potassium movement into the lumen. This intraluminal potassium is derived from exfoliation of living cells and from extracellular fluid [19]. Although bile disrupts the barrier, pancreatic juice does not [85]. When the gastric mucosa is actively secreting in response to, for example, histamine or gastrin, it becomes less permeable to acid and is more able to contain an acid load [84].

The Disrupted Barrier

Once the barrier is disrupted, hydrogen is insorbed. In addition to cellular destruction, vasodilatation and increased capillary permeability occur because of the release of histamine within the damaged mucosa. The histamine further stimulates acid secretion, which in turn stimulates pepsin secretion. Histamine also dilates the precapillary sphincters and mucosal capillaries, increasing capillary blood pressure and blood flow. The vessels become more permeable, and there is extravasation of plasma proteins and fluid into the interstitial fluid, producing mucosal edema. Acid insorption also stimulates gastric motility, probably by arousing reflexes within the intrinsic plexuses of the stomach; this may at least partially account for the pain of gastric ulceration.

In addition to the mucosal barrier to hydrogen, there is a second safeguard to the damage produced by insorbed acid. The mature cells of the gastric mucosa continuously desquamate and are replaced by new cells. The human stomach sheds about 500,000 cells per minute, enabling the surface mucosa of the stomach to be renewed every three days. Even severe damage can be repaired in a matter of hours or days.

Exogenous acid instillation into the human stomach is more rapidly insorbed in patients with gastric ulcer than in healthy persons, suggesting increased permeability in the gastric ulcer patients [12]. During stimulation with intravenous pentagastrin, the insorbed acid can be trapped by the instillation of glycine buffer [13]. Although the stomach of the gastric ulcer patient is more permeable to acid than normal, it remains more permeable even after the ulcer has undergone complete healing according to roentgenographical and endoscopic criteria [13]. The increased acid insorption thus is a function of gastric mucosal permeability rather than hydrogen loss through the ulcer.

Antral Inflammatory Changes

There is general agreement that gastric ulcer is almost always accompanied by antral inflammatory changes. Du Plessis [34], in a histological study of resected stomachs in patients with gastric ulcer, found inflammatory and atrophic changes in the antrum in all patients, and in 61 of 75 he observed severe chronic gastritis in the pyloric gland area. Chronic gastritis was thought to be the predisposing factor in these patients. Increased bile reflux has been demonstrated in gastric ulcer patients. Capper [9] suggested that gastric ulcer may be caused by the regurgitation of duodenal contents into the stomach, causing gastric atrophy with disappearance of parietal cells. The pyloric regurgitation test of Capper et al. [10] using an injection of 20 ml of barium mixture into the duodenal cap through a duodenal tube showed pyloric incompetence and regurgitation in 20 of the 29 patients with active gastric ulceration. Pyloric reflux was much more common in gastric ulcer patients than in duodenal ulcer patients or healthy persons. By labeling the bile salt pool with ^{14}C, Rhodes and co-workers [81] found a mean postprandial bile salt concentration of 5.3 mmol as compared with 0.13 mmol in controls. With healing of the ulcer, the levels of bile salts returned to normal. Decreased pyloric pressure may account for increased duodenogastric reflux in patients with gastric ulcer [96]. It is of interest that reflux of duodenal contents into the stomach can be produced by smoking [97].

THE DRAGSTEDT THEORY (ANTRAL STASIS)

Drawing from a large experimental and clinical experience, Dragstedt [33] postulated that gastric ulcers develop primarily as a result of antral stasis with concomitant hypersecretion of gastric juice of humoral origin. This antral stasis may be secondary to pyloric obstruction following duodenal ulcer disease. In patients with gastric ulcer independent of pyloric obstruction, Dragstedt suggests that the antral stasis is dependent on hypofunction of the motor fibers in the vagi. A major weakness in this theory is that most of these patients do not have delayed gastric emptying. Mangold [66] noted delayed emptying by roentgenogram in only 19 percent of 157 patients, and Capper et al. [10] found stasis in only 7 of 83 patients with combined ulcer disease. The ultimate proof of the hypothesis will be to see whether patients with both duodenal and gastric ulcers have higher gastrin levels than patients with ulcer in only a single location. This experiment has not been reported. Vagotomy (truncal or selective) without a drainage procedure impairs gastric emptying and leads to gastric ulceration [16].

GASTRIC MUCUS

Mucus has been implicated in the defense against injury of the gastrointestinal mucosa. Hollander [51] emphasized this role of mucus in his two-component mucosal barrier theory. The layer of mucous secretion constitutes the first line of defense of the gastric wall and comprises one component. It functions by its tenacious adherence to the underlying tissue, through its general impermeability to destructive chemical agents made possible by its cohesiveness because of a specific impermeability to pepsin, and through its adsorptive properties and its buffering action. Normally this viscous surface is continually being removed and replaced. If the rate of removal exceeds the rate of secretion, the mucous layer will be broken and the second line of defense, the layer of columnar and cuboidal cells of the surface and crypts of the mucosa, will be exposed. It is the normal function of this cell layer to supply mucus to replace that being removed from the surface. These cells have an amazing rate of reconstitution. Ulceration, according to Hollander's concept, occurs in an area of defensive defect that is subjected to autodigestion by acid and pepsin.

It must be pointed out, however, that the principal function of the layer of mucus is lubrication; it has only weak neutralization capacity, and acid diffuses quickly through it to reach the surface border of the epithelial cells. Moreover, acid diffuses through mucus as rapidly from lumen to mucosa as it does from mucosa to lumen. Thus the protective function of the mucous layer is not thought to be as important as it once was.

ISCHEMIA

Local ischemic factors have again been implicated in the causation of chronic gastric ulceration [77]. However, the stomach has an excellent blood supply. Even when the entire main arterial supply has been ligated, the submucosal vascular anastomosis ensures the viability of the stomach. The lesser curvature is not as well vascularized and is supplied by end-arteries; this has been the reason given for the lesser curvature being the most common site for chronic ulceration. There is little concrete evidence that chronic gastric ulcer in humans is related to ischemia.

SUMMARY

Currently damage to the gastric mucosal barrier seems to be the most plausible mechanism in the genesis of gastric ulceration. The sequence of events would be as follows: pyloric sphincter incompetence → reflux of bile and duodenal contents into stomach → alteration of mucosal barrier to hydrogen → if acid is present, acid insorption → mucosal injury. Nevertheless, one must be cautious in accepting this theory uncritically, for it still has to be explained why gastric mucosal permeability remains increased even after an ulcer has healed.

An altered mucosal barrier by itself is insufficient to cause a gastric ulcer. It also requires the presence of acid. This may explain why surgical procedures that do not improve mucosal permeability may, by the reduction of acidity, heal the ulcer.

Acid Secretion in Gastric Ulcer

The rate of acid secretion (basal or maximal acid output [MAO]) varies with the location of the ulcer in the stomach. Ulcers of the body of the stomach are associated with lower than normal rates of secretion. Patients with prepyloric gastric ulcers (GU) as well as those with concomitant gastric and duodenal ulcers (DU) tend to be hypersecretors of gastric acid. Since gastric ulcers usually occur marginally and caudally to the area of parietal cells, Baron [3] has confirmed a theoretical gradient for MAO:

DU > prepyloric GU >
incisura angularis GU > body (corpus) GU

The hypoacidity of patients with ulcers in the corpus may not be a true hypoacidity but an apparent one [12, 13]. Measured acid output not only measures the secretory capacity of the parietal cell mass, it also is affected by the flux rate from lumen to mucosa. Under normal circumstances the latter is negligible, but in patients with corpus ulcers the back-diffusion of H^+ may be considerable. Exogenous acid instilled into the stomach is more rapidly insorbed in patients with gastric ulcer (16.9 mEq/hr) than in controls (8.8 mEq/hr), which suggests that there is abnormal permeability in gastric ulcer patients [12, 13]. The instillation of glycine buffer to trap H^+ during maximal pentagastrin secretion results in an increased recovery of acid, the increase being identical to the insorption during acid instillation [13]. If the insorbed H^+ is added to the maximal acid output, the true secretory rate falls within the range of normal secretion rather than hyposecretion. In Chapman's study [13] the increased H^+ insorption was still present even after healing of the ulcer, suggesting that the increased acid insorption is not a local phenomenon related to the ulcer but rather is a generalized alteration in gastric mucosal permeability, which does not return to normal after healing.

Serum Gastrin Levels

Using radioimmunoassay, Trudeau and McGuigan [95] correlated the rate of acid secretion with the fasting serum gastrin levels in patients with gastric and duodenal ulcers and in a control group (Table 8-2). They demonstrated an inverse relation between the rate of basal acid secretion and the serum gastrin concentration. Gastrin values averaged approximately twice the normal level in patients with gastric ulcer; this increase correlated with the tendency for reduced acid secretion in this disease. The elevated gastrin levels might be due to decreased inhibition of antral gastrin release because of higher antral pH; they might also be related to antral stasis or to antral gastritis.

The Natural History of Gastric Ulcers

Patients with gastric ulceration managed medically show a high incidence of recurrence. Natvig et al. [71] reported a recurrence of 56 percent after 3 years, Smith and Jordan [89] found a 46.8 percent recurrence rate at 5 years, while Flood and Hennig [42] reported one or more recurrent ulcers in 99 of 101 patients followed for an average of 5.6 years. In the Veterans Administration (VA) cooperative study [49] on gastric ulcer there were 377 patients whose initial ulcer healed completely and who were followed for 2 years. Of this group, 41.9 percent had one or more recurrent ulcers: 30.2 percent had one documented recurrence during the follow-up period, while 11.6 percent had two episodes of recurrent ulceration. In Copenhagen [14, 72] 329 patients with gastric ulcer were treated medically and followed for 5 to 15 years; 61 percent had recurrent ulceration, 5 percent had gastric carcinoma, and 11 percent died of the ulcer.

Table 8-2. Correlation of fasting serum gastrin concentration and gastric acid secretion rate

Study group	Basal secretion (mEq/hr)	Peak secretion (mEq/hr)	Serum gastrin (pg/ml)
Controls	2.0	17.4	85
Duodenal ulcer	4.6	26.2	78
Duodenal ulcer with high basal secretion	> 8.0	—	52
Gastric ulcer	1.5	16.4	159

Source: Data from W. L. Trudeau and J. E. McGuigan, *N. Engl. J. Med.* 284:408, 1971.

FACTORS ASSOCIATED WITH RECURRENCE

Several factors have been claimed to affect the incidence of gastric ulcer recurrence, but recent data cast doubt on a number of these factors:

1. Although it has been stated that men have a poorer prognosis than women, neither age [49] nor sex [42] has any effect on the rate of recurrence.
2. The incidence of recurrence is slightly lower when the patients have had symptoms of ulcer disease for less than one year when first treated [42], but the difference is not statistically significant.
3. It has been suggested that a slower rate of healing means a slightly poorer than average clinical course [42], but the VA study showed that the question of whether or not the time required for initial healing affected the recurrence rate was still unsettled [49].
4. The location or size of the initial ulcer does not affect the likelihood of recurrent ulceration [9].
5. No definite correlation has been shown between gastric acid output and prognosis [4].
6. Hemorrhage occurs at some time during the course of the ulcer in 37 percent of patients [42]. The recurrence rate in this group does not differ from that in patients with no history of bleeding.

LOCATION AND SIZE OF RECURRENT ULCERS

In the VA study [62] the recurrent ulcer often occurred at a different site from the original ulcer; however, the percentage of ulcers in the various anatomical segments and curvatures of the stomach was almost the same for the original and recurrent ulcers. For example, 88 percent of initial ulcers and 94 percent of recurrent ulcers were on the lesser curvature. Three recurrent ulcers were located on the greater curvature; in each instance, the original ulcer had been located on the greater curvature. With regard to distance from the pylorus, the recurrent ulcer group on the average closely resembled the initial ulcer group, with the exception that there were no recurrent ulcers located more than 12 cm from the pylorus, whereas 26 of the initial ulcers were located in that area.

Many of the recurrent ulcers were small in comparison with the original ulcer. The median product size for the initial ulcer was 97 sq mm; for the first recurrence, 35 sq mm; and for the second recurrence, 20 sq mm. The difference in size between the initial ulcer and the first recurrence was statistically significant, whereas the difference in size between the first and second recurrences was not significant. The most likely explanation for the difference in the size of the initial ulcer and the recurrences is that the recurrences were detected at an earlier stage of development than was the initial ulcer.

BEHAVIOR OF RECURRENT ULCERS

Benign recurrent gastric ulceration probably heals as readily as does an initial ulcer. The ulcers of 73 of the 84 patients with recurrent ulceration in the VA study [62] healed within the allotted 12-week period. This figure certainly compares favorably with and actually surpasses the 75.9 percent healing rate of initial ulcers that healed within the protocol time period. It must be remembered, however, that any recurrent ulcer group may be a select group in that the patients with a tendency for slow healing have already been labeled as "refractory" on the basis of their initial ulcer and have been referred for surgical treatment.

COEXISTENCE OF GASTRIC AND DUODENAL ULCERATION

Wilkie in 1926 [100] reported that 42 of 79 patients with a gastric ulcer also had a concomitant duodenal ulcer. A VA study [86] demonstrated an overall incidence of 41.6 percent of patients with a gastric ulcer having coexisting deformity of the duodenal bulb, a duodenal ulcer, or both. There was a higher incidence of duodenal ulceration when the gastric ulcer was located below (± 50 percent) than above (± 35 percent) the incisura angularis. The size of the gastric ulcer was not related to the incidence of concomitant duodenal ulcers. Associated duodenal ulcer or duodenal bulb deformity has been found to have no effect on the healing rate of gastric ulcers [78], but it does result in an increased incidence of recurrent gastric ulceration [69].

Coexistent duodenal ulcer or duodenal bulb deformity lessens the chances of an apparently benign gastric ulcer actually being malignant. In the VA study [86] gastric carcinoma occurred in 6.0 percent of the gastric ulcer patients without coexistent duodenal ulceration but in only 1.2 percent of the gastric ulcer patients with coexistent duodenal ulceration; 12 percent of the patients with malignant ulcers had coexistent duodenal ulceration, whereas 42.7 percent of the patients with benign ulcers had evidence indicating a diseased duodenum. Thus a benign-appearing gastric ulcer is more likely to be benign if associated duodenal ulcer disease is present, but in an individual patient a deformed duodenal bulb does not rule out a malignant tumor of the stomach.

MALIGNANT CHANGE IN BENIGN GASTRIC ULCERS

Finsterer [41] stated that malignant degeneration of a benign ulcer was so frequent an occurrence that resection of a gastric ulcer might be regarded as an early operation for carcinoma of the stomach. Although earlier studies claimed evidence of carcinoma originating in chronic benign gastric ulcers, more recent investigators [65, 68] did not find sufficient evidence to warrant a conclusion that gastric ulcers present a high potential origin for a malignant tumor.

Gastric ulcers that appear to be benign roentgenologically may turn out to be malignant; 5 to 10 percent may in fact be ulcerating carcinomas [35]. The prognosis of these small carcinomas is excellent. A cure rate of up to 80 percent may be achieved by radical surgical resection [28].

Surgical Approach to Gastric Ulcer

Pyloric channel ulcers, prepyloric ulcers, and gastric ulcers that occur concomitantly with duodenal ulceration or pyloric stenosis behave pathophysiologically as duodenal ulcers and should be treated surgically as duodenal ulcers. The standard operative approach to benign gastric ulcer is antrectomy (distal gastrectomy)—resection of 50–60 percent of the stomach—with excision of the ulcer [1]. Since the duodenum is usually normal and mobile, a gastroduodenal (Billroth I) anastomosis is advocated. Postgastrectomy symptoms are much milder after antrectomy for gastric ulcer than after subtotal gastrectomy for duodenal ulcer because a considerably smaller amount of stomach is removed. Mortality for gastric ulcer treated by gastrectomy has been reported as low as 2.7 percent [99], 1.0 percent [26, 80], and 0.3 percent [76]. Surgeons experienced in gastric surgery should be able to achieve a mortality figure for elective gastrectomy of the Billroth I type of about 1.0 percent. The incidence of recurrent ulcer after gastrectomy for gastric ulcer is low; Tanner [93] reported a series of more than 1000 before encountering a recurrent ulcer.

A Billroth II anastomosis is favored by some surgeons, especially if the ulcer is high on the lesser curvature. Patients with a Billroth II anastomosis are less likely to have gastric stasis, and this procedure should certainly be used if a Billroth I anastomosis would produce tension on the suture line.

Clearly an operation with such low mortality and recurrence rates is difficult to give up in favor of alternative procedures. Nevertheless, advocates for vagotomy and pyloroplasty (usually with wedge resection or four-quadrant biopsy) claim that however low the operative mortality from antrectomy for gastric ulcer, it will be even lower with vagotomy [8, 36, 40]. Recurrence rates after vagotomy and pyloroplasty, however, range from 7 to 38 percent [102]. Admittedly in elderly, high-risk patients, ulcer recurrence is not as critical as the low mortality that is gained by vagotomy and pyloroplasty; also, recurrence may not develop before such older patients die of other causes.

The Maki pylorus-preserving partial gastrectomy [64] is comparable to a Billroth I gastrectomy except that the distal 1.5 cm of antrum is retained and anastomosed to the proximal stomach. Although Maki claims that the remaining antrum and pylorus allow better regulation of gastric emptying and prevent stasis [88], Teigan et al. [94] found an unacceptable rate of gastric stasis and recurrent ulceration in long-term follow-up studies.

Based on a prospective, randomized, controlled trial in gastric ulcer patients, Duthie and Kwong [38] reported that 14 percent of patients undergoing vagotomy and pyloroplasty required subsequent gastrectomy. In sharp contrast, none of the patients who underwent Billroth I antrectomy required reoperation. Comparable results were obtained in a similar study by Madsen et al. [63]. It should also be remembered that there is a small but definite risk of missing a curable carcinoma when vagotomy and drainage are used.

Johnston [54] has advocated proximal gastric vagotomy for the surgical management of gastric ulcer; he has had excellent results with the procedure. A randomized trial of the operation combined with excision of the ulcer, however, showed that the rate of ulcer recurrence was more than double that of the Billroth I antrectomy [37]. When only patients with prepyloric ulceration are considered, the recurrent ulcer rate becomes 22 percent after proximal gastric vagotomy [2]. Lawson [61] developed an interesting scenario of gastritis *and* hypersecretion in patients with these unusually placed gastric ulcers. The subject of alternative surgical management approaches is reviewed by Greenhall and Lehnert [46].

Other alternatives to antrectomy have been suggested based on the postulate that gastric retention is one of the prime mechanisms for the development of gastric ulcer. Wedge resection with pyloroplasty or gastrojejunostomy has been reported. The high incidence of recurrent ulceration makes wedge resection unacceptable for the elective treatment of gastric ulcer unless a situation of extreme urgency should arise during the operation that prohibits other procedures. There is no evidence, therefore, to support the abandonment of the Billroth I antrectomy as the operation of choice for most patients with gastric ulcer.

The rationale for the surgical management of duodenal ulceration is well understood, but it is not so clear for gastric ulceration. Elevated fasting serum gastrin levels in gastric ulcer patients are probably caused by decreased inhibition of antral gastrin release because of higher antral pH. Moreover, apart from the gastric ulcers associated with duodenal deformity or pyloric stenosis, few patients with gastric ulcer have delayed emptying. It is my opinion that the reasons for the efficacy of these procedures can best be explained when the gastric mucosal barrier to hydrogen is understood. Gastric ulcers probably arise as a result of an incompetent mucosal barrier, perhaps mediated by bile reflux. When a strongly acid solution is present on the mucosal surface of a stomach with an impaired barrier, back-diffusion of hydrogen ions occurs; this damages the mucosa, and an ulcer ensues. When a neutral solution or very weak acid is present on the mucosal surface of an incompetent barrier, very little or no back-diffusion of hydrogen occurs, and no ulcer is produced. In other words, two factors are necessary for the production of an ulcer: (1) an impaired barrier from whatever cause, and (2) the presence of hydrogen ions, although not necessarily in large amounts. Although research is being directed at improving the impaired barrier, we do not yet have an effective method to achieve this. We therefore direct our efforts at elimination or reduction of the second factor, the presence of hydrogen ions. It thus becomes evident that any satisfactory acid-reducing operation will result in a high cure rate; the degree of reduction of acidity need not be as great as that required for duodenal ulceration.

Moreover, when the operative procedure, e.g., a Billroth I antrectomy, is not associated with a significant amount of bile reflux, a superior result can be anticipated.

GASTRIC ULCER PERFORATION

Although the mortality for perforated peptic ulcers in general has fallen (especially if operated on), the mortality in patients over 60 years of age remains high. Gastric ulcers are much more common in older persons, and there is an increasing percentage of perforations in the sixth, seventh, and eighth decades of life. Similar criteria have generally been used to select the operation of choice for perforated gastric ulcer as for perforated duodenal ulcer. However, a more aggressive approach should be directed toward the surgical management of perforated gastric ulcer for the reasons stated in the following discussion.

Most perforated gastric ulcers are found on the anterior or anterosuperior surface of the lesser curvature. Although large ulcers usually perforate anteriorly, perforation may occur into the lesser sac or even between the layers of the gastrohepatic omentum. The higher the perforation, the greater the mortality; perforations of the upper stomach carry a mortality of 80 percent [59]. Furthermore, the larger the perforation and the older the patient, the higher are the morbidity and mortality; gastric perforations are usually larger than duodenal perforations and occur more commonly in elderly patients.

An abnormally high percentage of perforated gastric ulcers that are diagnosed as simple gastric ulcers at operation prove to be malignant; the rates are as high as 12 percent [27, 30]. In a prospective study of 72 patients with perforated gastric ulcer treated by gastrectomy, 9 of the ulcers proved to be carcinoma in situ [27]; all these patients survived, free of malignant disease, for 1 to 8 years.

After the occurrence of a perforation, chemical peritonitis ensues, which develops into bacterial peritonitis. Independent investigators [47, 58] have demonstrated that the spillage is really sterile; cultures taken at operations performed even after 24 hours were more often negative and less often grew pathogens than cultures taken at earlier operations. The magnitude of the spillage, especially when preoperative antibiotics were administered, did not influence the development of peritonitis; only in the grossly neglected case or in the debilitated patient with poor resistance to infection did frank bacterial peritonitis supervene.

Because gastric ulcer perforations are usually anterior, the operation is technically easy. There is no problem with mobilization and transection of the duodenum. A very large ulcer may make resection easier than simple closure of the ulcer; placing sutures in a friable, edematous stomach may cut through tissues and enlarge the hole, making resection the only feasible procedure. For all these reasons, as well as the high risk of malignancy, an antrectomy with removal of the ulcer should be advocated in low-risk patients.

EMERGENCY OPERATION FOR BLEEDING GASTRIC ULCER

It has been repeatedly demonstrated that the prognosis is worse for hemorrhage from a gastric ulcer than from a duodenal ulcer. The mortality for hemorrhage from gastric ulcers is more than double that for duodenal ulcers [55, 90], even allowing for the greater proportion of elderly patients in the former group. Because of the greater tendency for hemorrhage from gastric ulcers to be both severe and persistent, we have practiced immediate operation (after initial resuscitation) on all patients diagnosed or known to have a gastric ulcer as the source of hemorrhage [57].

Gastric resection including the bleeding ulcer is the procedure of choice. Simple suture ligation of the vessel in the ulcer base is fraught with an unacceptable risk of recurrent hemorrhage. Vagotomy plus pyloroplasty with suture ligation of the bleeding vessel is certainly superior to ligation alone; however, clinical experience with this method remains meager, and the technique should be used sparingly. Whereas the feeding vessels may be readily identified in the patient with bleeding duodenal ulcer, this is not the case in the patient with bleeding gastric ulcer. Circumferential suturing may be necessary and even then may inadequately control the vessels and dispose the area to recurrent hemorrhage. In my personal experience, suture ligation of bleeding gastric ulcers, even though accompanied by vagotomy and drainage, has yielded results inferior to antrectomy with excision of the ulcer. Hampson et al. [48] demonstrated what can be accomplished by gastric resection. They operated on 50 patients with massively bleeding gastric ulcer, with only 1 death; 46 of these patients were treated by resection, and 4 had vagotomy and pyloroplasty. Early gastrectomy should be advocated in patients with bleeding gastric ulcer. In contrast to most surgeons, Johnston [53] advocates a policy of underrunning the bleeding point followed by vagotomy.

THE HIGH BENIGN GASTRIC LESION

Most gastric ulcers are found in the middle or distal stomach, but about 5 percent occur high on the lesser curvature, near or at the esophagogastric junction [7]. How gastric ulcers may occur here can be readily understood when one remembers that the antrum extends like a tongue for a greater distance along the lesser curvature than along the greater curvature. Like other gastric ulcers, the high lesser curvature ulcer occurs at the junction of parietal and alkaline areas of the stomach [75]. This junction is very variable in humans, particularly along the lesser curvature. Whereas the antrum-corpus ratio is small in the duodenal ulcer patient, it becomes larger in patients with gastric ulcers [9, 75]. The variability of the junction explains the variable location of gastric ulcers. The larger the alkaline area of the stomach, the higher the ulcer will be.

If malignancy can be excluded with certainty at endoscopy, a distal gastrectomy of the Billroth I type, leaving the ulcer in situ (Kelling-Madlener procedure), should be the procedure of choice. This avoids a suture line in inflamed, edematous tissue near the esophagus, thus avoiding suture line leakage, and it achieves excellent healing of the ulcer. However, because of the fear of cancer, most surgeons still prefer gastrectomy with inclusion of the ulcer in the specimen. Either the Pauchet or the Schoemaker operation (antrectomy plus excision of a tongue of proximal lesser curvature) may be performed when the high gastric ulcer is not too large, not surrounded by too much inflammatory reaction, and not too near the esophagogastric junction. The rotation gastrectomy of Tanner [93] is an eminently suitable alternative. Vagotomy and pyloroplasty, with or without wedge excision of the ulcer, may also be used; although recurrence rates may be higher than with resection, morbidity and mortality are low. Both proximal gastrectomy and total gastrectomy yield an unacceptably high mortality (10 percent in some series) because of leakage of the esophagogastric anastomosis.

THE RECURRENT GASTRIC ULCER

The gastric ulcer recurrence rate after antrectomy is very low, but it is appreciable after vagotomy and drainage [102]. If there is recurrence after antrectomy, a gastrinoma should be excluded, and, if found, it should be treated by total gastrectomy. Retained antrum within the duodenal stump may create problems after a Billroth II but not after a Billroth I resection. Unlike the gastrinoma, the elevated gastrin levels will only be modestly elevated by a calcium or magnesium challenge and will be inhibited by secretin or glucagon injections. If retained antrum is present, its removal suffices. It should be remembered that antrectomy for gastric ulceration is usually accompanied by a gastroduodenal anastomosis, where, if a retained antrum is present, the retained antrum will be subjected to normal acid inhibition of gastrin release. If gastric ulcers recur after a simple antrectomy, it should be suspected that they are part of a duodenal ulcer diathesis and that antrectomy alone was inadequate as the primary procedure. Recurrences after antrectomy should be treated by vagotomy and a moderate resection of the stomach. Recurrences after vagotomy and drainage (as in the case of duodenal ulcers) may be related to incomplete vagotomy, inadequate drainage procedure (wherein drainage is retarded rather than facilitated), or inadequacy of the procedure for the control of the ulcer diathesis. If vagotomy and drainage have been performed and the gastric ulcer recurs, an antrectomy should be carried out; this is effective in controlling the peptic ulcer diathesis and in preventing further recurrence.

GASTRIC ULCER IN OLD AGE

Gastric ulcers in the elderly pose a special problem. There is an increased risk of bleeding from the ulcer (47 percent), with a mortality of 33 percent [15]. Complicating diseases are common (47 percent) and render the prognosis even more unfavorable (mortality, 64 percent). Moreover, the incidence of healing is less frequent. These factors should be borne in mind when treating gastric ulcers in patients older than 70 years of age.

UNSUSPECTED MALIGNANT CHANGE

From time to time, gastric resection is performed for a benign gastric ulcer that is subsequently found to be malignant. Desmond et al. [28] found the five-year survival rate in such instances to be 23 percent. However, when a revisional operation was undertaken six to eight weeks later, the five-year survival rate was 56 percent. If the surgeon is confronted with a malignant ulcer after nonradical gastric resection for a supposedly benign ulcer, a revisional operation should be undertaken if the age and general condition of the patient permit. The lymphatic drainage should be cleared, and a second resection (even total gastrectomy) should be performed if the line of gastric resection is too close to the ulcer edge. It should be emphasized, however, that this situation is now rare, since routine endoscopy virtually prevents this misdiagnosis.

References

1. Adkins, R. B., DeLozier, J. B., III, Scott, H. W., Jr., and Sawyers, J. L. The management of gastric ulcers: A current review. *Ann. Surg.* 201:741, 1985.
2. Andersen, D., Høstrup, H., and Amdrup, E. The Aarhus County vagotomy trial. II. An interim report on reduction in acid secretion and ulcer recurrence rate following parietal cell vagotomy and selective gastric vagotomy. *World J. Surg.* 2:91, 1978.
3. Baron, J. H. On assessment of the augmented histamine test in the diagnosis of peptic ulcer. *Gut* 4:243, 1963.
4. Barsby, B. Prognosis of healed gastric ulcers. *Lancet* 2:59, 1951.
5. Bingham, J. R. Precipitating factors in peptic ulcer. *Can. Med. Assoc. J.* 83:205, 1960.
6. Blumenthal, I. S. Digestive disease as a national problem. *Gastroenterology* 54:86, 1968.
7. Braasch, J. W., Cain, J. C., and Priestley, J. T. Juxtaesophageal gastric ulcer. *Surg. Gynecol. Obstet.* 101:280, 1955.
8. Burge, H. W., Gill, A. M., and Lewis, R. H. The pyloric-channel syndrome and gastric ulceration. *Lancet* 1:73, 1963.
9. Capper, W. M. Factors in the pathogenesis of gastric ulcer. *Ann. R. Coll. Surg. Engl.* 40:21, 1967.
10. Capper, W. M., Airth, G. R., and Kilby, J. O. A test for pyloric regurgitation. *Lancet* 2:621, 1966.
11. Capper, W. M., Laidlaw, C. D. A., Buckler, K., and Richards, D. The pH fields of the gastric mucosa. *Lancet* 2:1200, 1962.
12. Chapman, M. L., Werther, J. L., and Janowitz, H. D. Response of the normal and pathological human gastric mucosa to an instilled acid load. *Gastroenterology* 55:344, 1968.
13. Chapman, M. L., Werther, J. L., Rudick, J., and Janowitz, H. D. Pentagastrin infusion–glycine instillation as a measure of acid absorption in the human stomach: Comparison to an instilled acid load. *Gastroenterology* 63:962, 1972.
14. Christiansen, P., Amdrup, E., Fenger, C., et al. Gastric ulcer. III. Non-surgical treatment. *Acta Chir. Scand.* 139:466, 1973.
15. Christiansen, P., Jensen, H.-E., Amdrup, E., et al. Gastric ulcer in old age. *Acta Chir. Scand.* 144:491, 1978.
16. Clarke, R. J., and Alexander-Williams, J. The effect of preserving antral innervation and of a pyloroplasty on gastric emptying after vagotomy in man. *Gut* 14:300, 1973.
17. Cleave, T. L., Campbell, G. D., and Painter, N. S. *Peptic Ulcer in Diabetes, Coronary Thrombosis and the Saccharine Disease* (2d ed.). Bristol: Wright, 1967. P. 87.
18. Davenport, H. W. Gastric mucosa injury by fatty and acetylsalicylic acids. *Gastroenterology* 46:245, 1964.
19. Davenport, H. W. Potassium fluxes across the resting and stimulated mucosa: Injury by salicylic and acetic acid. *Gastroenterology* 49:238, 1965.

20. Davenport, H. W. Salicylate damage to gastric mucosal barrier. *N. Engl. J. Med.* 276:1307, 1967.
21. Davenport, H. W. Destruction of gastric mucosal barrier by detergents and urea. *Gastroenterology* 54:175, 1968.
22. Davenport, H. W. Gastric mucosal hemorrhage in dogs: Effects of acid, aspirin and alcohol. *Gastroenterology* 56:439, 1969.
23. Davenport, H. W. Effect of lysolecithin, digitonin and phospholipase upon the dog's gastric mucosal barrier. *Gastroenterology* 59:505, 1970.
24. Davenport, H. W. The gastric mucosal barrier. *Digestion* 5:162, 1972.
25. Davenport, H. W., Warner, H. A., and Code, C. F. Functional significance of gastric mucosal barrier to sodium. *Gastroenterology* 47:142, 1964.
26. Davis, Z., Verheyden, C. N., van Heerden, J. A., and Judd, E. S. The surgically treated chronic gastric ulcer: An extended followup. *Ann. Surg.* 185:205, 1977.
27. Desmond, A. M. Acute Perforated Peptic Ulcers. In R. Maingot (Ed.), *Abdominal Operations* (5th ed.). New York: Appleton-Century-Crofts, 1969. P. 347.
28. Desmond, A. M., Nicholls, J., and Brown, C. Further surgical management of gastric ulcer with unsuspected malignant change. *Ann. R. Coll. Surg. Engl.* 57:101, 1975.
29. Dogra, J. R. Studies on peptic ulcer in South India. IV. Incidence of peptic ulcer in India with particular reference to South India. *Indian J. Med. Res.* 29:665, 1941.
30. Doll, R. Perforated carcinoma of the stomach simulating perforated gastric ulcer. *Br. Med. J.* 1:215, 1950.
31. Doll, R. Epidemiology of Peptic Ulcer. In F. A. Jones (Ed.), *Modern Trends in Gastroenterology*. New York: Hoeber, 1952.
32. Doll, R., Jones, F. A., and Pygott, F. Effect of smoking on the production and maintenance of gastric and duodenal ulcers. *Lancet* 1:657, 1958.
33. Dragstedt, L. R. A concept of the etiology of gastric and duodenal ulcers. *Gastroenterology* 30:208, 1956.
34. du Plessis, D. J. Pathogenesis of gastric ulcer. *Lancet* 1:974, 1965.
35. Duthie, H. L. Vagotomy for gastric ulcer. *Gut* 11:540, 1970.
36. Duthie, H. L. Surgery for gastric ulcer. *World J. Surg.* 1:29, 1977.
37. Duthie, H. L., and Branson, C. J. Highly selective vagotomy with excision of the ulcer compared with gastrectomy for gastric ulcer in a randomized trial. *Br. J. Surg.* 66:43, 1979.
38. Duthie, H. L., and Kwong, N. K. Vagotomy or gastrectomy for gastric ulcer. *Br. Med. J.* 4:79, 1973.
39. Dyck, W. P., Werther, J. L., Rudick, J., and Janowitz, H. D. Electrolyte movement across canine antral and fundic gastric mucosa. *Gastroenterology* 56:488, 1969.
40. Farris, J. M., and Smith, G. K. Treatment of gastric ulcer (in situ) by vagotomy and pyloroplasty: A clinical study. *Ann. Surg.* 158:461, 1963.
41. Finsterer, H. Ulcer-cancer of the stomach. *Arch. Klin. Chir.* 131:71, 1924.
42. Flood, C. A., and Hennig, G. C. Recurrence in gastric ulcer under medical management. *Gastroenterology* 61:57, 1950.
43. Garb, A. E., Soule, E. H., Bartholomew, L. G., and Cain, J. C. Steroid-induced gastric ulcer. *Arch. Intern. Med.* 116:899, 1965.
44. Garrido-Klinge, G., and Pena, L. The Gastroduodenal Ulcer in High Altitudes (Peruvian Andes). In *Proceedings of the World Congress of Gastroenterology,* Vol 1. Baltimore: Williams & Wilkins, 1959. Pp. 68–78.
45. Gillies, M., and Skyring, A. Gastric and duodenal ulcer: The association between aspirin ingestion, smoking and family history of ulcer. *Med. J. Aust.* 2:280, 1969.
46. Greenhall, M. J., and Lehnert, T. Vagotomy or gastrectomy for elective treatment of benign gastric ulceration? *Dig. Dis. Sci.* 30:353, 1985.
47. Hamilton, J. E., and Harbrecht, P. J. Growing indications for vagotomy in perforated peptic ulcer. *Surg. Gynecol. Obstet.* 124:61, 1967.
48. Hampson, L. G., Mulder, D. S., Elias, G. L., and Palmer, J. D. The emergency surgical treatment of massively bleeding peptic ulcer. *Arch. Surg.* 97:450, 1968.
49. Hanscom, D. H., and Buchman, E. The follow-up period. *Gastroenterology* 61:585, 1971.
50. Himal, H. S., Young, S. B., Rudick, J., et al. Ionic flux across the duodenal mucosa. *Gastroenterology* 58:959, 1970.
51. Hollander, F. The two-component mucous barrier: Its activity in protecting the gastroduodenal mucosa against peptic ulceration. *Arch. Intern. Med.* 93:107, 1954.
52. Holt, P. R. Measurement of gastrointestinal blood loss in patients taking aspirin. *J. Lab. Clin. Med.* 56:717, 1960.

53. Johnston, D. Division and repair of the sphincteric mechanism at the gastric outlet in emergency operations for bleeding peptic ulcer. *Ann. Surg.* 186:723, 1977.
54. Johnston, D. Chronic Gastric and Duodenal Ulcer. In R. Maingot (Ed.), *Abdominal Operations* (7th ed.). New York: Appleton-Century-Crofts, 1980. P. 211.
55. Jones, F. A. Haematemesis and melaena with special reference to causation and to the factors influencing the mortality from bleeding peptic ulcers. *Gastroenterology* 30:166, 1956.
56. Katz, A. M., Pearson, C. M., and Kennedy, J. M. A clinical trial of indomethacin in rheumatoid arthritis. *Clin. Pharmacol. Ther.* 6:25, 1965.
57. Kim, U., Dreiling, D. A., Kark, A. E., and Rudick, J. Factors influencing mortality in surgical treatment for massive gastroduodenal hemorrhage. *Am. J. Gastroenterol.* 62:24, 1974.
58. Kincannon, W. M., McLenathen, C. W., and Weinberg, J. A. Vagotomy and pyloroplasty for acute perforated duodenal ulcer. *Am. Surg.* 29:692, 1963.
59. Kozoll, D. D., and Meyer, K. A. Laboratory findings in acute perforated gastroduodenal ulcers: A review of 1,904 cases. *Arch. Surg.* 84:646, 1962.
60. Kukral, J. C. Gastric ulcer: An appraisal. *Surgery* 63:1024, 1968.
61. Lawson, H. H. Prepyloric ulceration. *Surg. Annu.* 16:229, 1984.
62. Littman, A., and Hanscom, D. H. The course of recurrent ulcer. *Gastroenterology* 61:592, 1971.
63. Madsen, P., Kronborg, O., Hart Hansen, O., and Pedersen, T. Billroth I gastric resection versus truncal vagotomy and pyloroplasty in the treatment of gastric ulcer. *Acta. Chir. Scand.* 142:151, 1976.
64. Maki, T., Shirator, T., Hatakufu, T., and Sugawara, K. Pylorus-preserving gastrectomy as an improved operation for gastric ulcer. *Surgery* 61:838, 1967.
65. Mallory, T. B. Carcinoma in situ of stomach and its bearing on histogenesis of malignant ulcers. *Arch. Pathol.* 30:348, 1940.
66. Mangold, R. Combined gastric and duodenal ulceration: Survey of 157 cases. *Br. Med. J.* 2:1193, 1958.
67. Marks, I. N., and Shay, H. Observations on the pathogenesis of gastric ulcer. *Lancet* 1:1107, 1959.
68. Marshall, S. F. The relation of gastric ulcer to carcinoma of the stomach. *Ann. Surg.* 137:891, 1953.
69. McCray, B. S., Ferris, E. J., Herskovic, T., et al. Clinical differences between gastric ulcers with and without duodenal deformity. *Ann. Surg.* 168:821, 1968.
70. Mendeloff, A. I., and Dunn, J. P. Digestive Diseases. In *Vital and Health Statistics Monographs*. Cambridge, Mass.: American Public Health Association, Harvard University Press, 1971.
71. Natvig, P., Römcke, O., and Swaar-Seljesaeter, O. Results of medical treatment of gastric and duodenal ulcer. *Acta Med. Scand.* 113:444, 1943.
72. Nielsen, J., Amdrup, E., Christiansen, P., et al. Gastric ulcer. II. Surgical treatment. *Acta Chir. Scand.* 139:460, 1973.
73. Niwayama, G., and Terplan, K. A study of peptic ulcer based on necropsy records. *Gastroenterology* 36:409, 1959.
74. Oi, M., Ito, Y., Kumagai, F., Yoshida, K., et al. A possible dual control mechanism in the origin of peptic ulcer: A study on ulcer location as affected by mucosa and musculature. *Gastroenterology* 57:280, 1969.
75. Oi, M., Oshida, K., and Sugimura, S. The location of gastric ulcer. *Gastroenterology* 36:45, 1959.
76. Pearce, C. W., Jordan, G. L., and DeBakey, M. E. Intra-abdominal complications following distal subtotal gastrectomy for benign gastroduodenal ulceration. *Surgery* 42:447, 1957.
77. Piasecki, C. Role of ischaemia in the initiation of peptic ulcer. *Ann. R. Coll. Surg. Engl.* 59:476, 1977.
78. Pollard, H. M., Bachrach, W. H., and Block, M. The rate of healing of gastric ulcers. *Gastroenterology* 8:435, 1947.
79. Portis, S. A., and Jaffe, R. H. Study of peptic ulcer based on necropsy records. *J.A.M.A.* 110:6, 1938.
80. Priestley, J. T., Walters, W., Gray, H. K., et al. Annual report on surgery of stomach and duodenum for 1954. *Proc. Staff Meet. Mayo Clin.* 31:62, 1956.
81. Rhodes, J., Barnardo, D., Phillips, S. F., et al. Increased reflux of bile into the stomach in patients with gastric ulcer. *Gastroenterology* 57:241, 1969.

82. Ritchie, W. P., Jr. Pathogenesis of acute gastric mucosal injury. *Viewpoints Dig. Dis.* 15:17, 1983.
83. Roberts, D. M. Chronic gastritis, alcohol, and non-ulcer dyspepsia. *Gut* 13:768, 1972.
84. Rudick, J., Chapman, M. L., Werther, J. L., and Janowitz, H. D. Ionic fluxes across canine antral mucosa: Effects of pentagastrin and histamine. *Clin. Res.* 28:388, 1970.
85. Rudick, J., Werther, J. L., Chapman, M. L., et al. Hydrogen permeability of canine gastric antral and fundic mucosa following exposure to pancreatic juice. *J. Surg. Res.* 13:72, 1972.
86. Rumball, J. M. Coexistent duodenal ulcer. *Gastroenterology* 61:622, 1971.
87. Schanke, K. Behavior of ulcer in fishing district in north of Norway: Studies on frequency and localization. *Acta Chir. Scand.* 94(Suppl. 115):1, 1946.
88. Sekine, T., Sato, T., Maki, T., and Shiratori, T. Pylorus-preserving gastrectomy for gastric ulcer: One- to nine-year follow-up study. *Surgery* 77:92, 1975.
89. Smith, F. H., and Jordan, S. M. Gastric ulcer: A study of 600 cases. *Gastroenterology* 11:575, 1948.
90. Strange, S. L. Giant innocent gastric ulcer: Its behaviour and treatment. *Br. Med. J.* 1:476, 1959.
91. Sun, D. C. H., and Stempien, S. J. Site and size as determinants of outcome. *Gastroenterology* 61:576, 1971.
92. Takahashi, T., Shimazu, H., Yamagishi, T., and Tani, M. G-cell populations in resected stomachs from gastric and duodenal ulcer patients. *Gastroenterology* 78:498, 1980.
93. Tanner, N. C. Non-malignant affections of the upper stomach. *Ann. R. Coll. Surg. Engl.* 10:45, 1952.
94. Teigan, T., Liarag, J., and Roland, M. Pylorus-preserving gastric resection for gastric ulcer. *Acta Chir. Scand.* 144:249, 1978.
95. Trudeau, W. L., and McGuigan, J. E. Relations between serum gastrin levels and rates of gastric hydrochloric acid secretion. *N. Engl. J. Med.* 284:408, 1971.
96. Valenzuela, J., and Defilippi, C. Pyloric sphincter studies in peptic-ulcer patients. *Am. J. Dig. Dis.* 21:229, 1976.
97. Valenzuela, J., Defilippi, C., and Csendes, A. Manometric studies on the human pyloric sphincter. *Gastroenterology* 70:481, 1976.
98. Varro, V., and Csernay, L. Experimental Studies on the Ulcerogenic Effect of Phenylbutazone. In S. C. Skoryna (Ed.), *Pathophysiology of Peptic Ulcer.* Montreal: McGill University Press, 1963. P. 291.
99. Walters, W., and ReMine, W. H. Appraisal of the various operations for peptic ulcer. *Surgery* 55:585, 1964.
100. Wilkie, D. P. D. Coincident duodenal and gastric ulcer. *Br. Med. J.* 2:469, 1926.
101. Yamagata, S. Epidemiology of Ulcer in Japan. In *Proceedings Second World Congress of Gastroenterology,* Vol. II. Basel: S. Karger, 1963. P. 285.
102. Zahn, R. L., Stemmer, E. A., Hom, L. W., and Connolly, J. E. Delayed recurrence of gastric ulcer following vagotomy and drainage procedures. *Am. Surg.* 34:757, 1968.

EDITORS' COMMENT

Dr. Rudick provides an elegant description of the pathophysiology, natural history, and surgical treatment of chronic benign gastric ulceration.

As far as treatment of chronic gastric ulcer is concerned, a new challenge to the conventional Billroth I gastrectomy has just been mounted. This is proximal gastric vagotomy (PGV) with excision of the ulcer. Reid and associates have reported on a series of 56 patients treated either by this new method or by the conventional Billroth I gastrectomy with an average follow-up time of eight years (*Br. J. Surg.* 69:605, 1982). One of the interesting aspects of this series of patients is that from a symptomatic point of view, ulcer excision and PGV fare better than Billroth I gastrectomy. One of the implications of this series is that patients who have had Billroth I gastrectomy may have more symptoms than has been supposed. A similar study by Emmås and Hammarberg (*Am. J. Surg.* 146:631, 1983) concluded that because of long-term adverse results following partial gastrectomy, further trials of proximal gastric vagotomy with ulcer

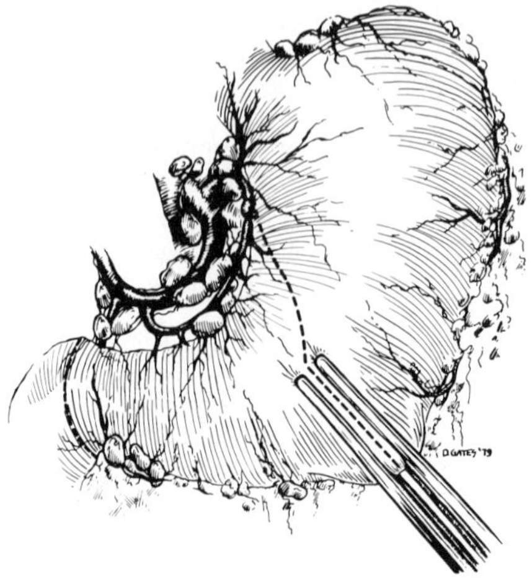

Fig. 8-1. A Payr clamp has been placed perpendicular to the greater curvature of the stomach and extends toward the angulus for 4.5–5.0 cm. Division of the duodenum just distal to the pylorus precedes this step. The dashed line shows a proposed resection, which would terminate just above the ulcer. The antrum and the ulcer will be removed with greater amounts of anterior or posterior gastric wall (respectively) included, depending on the location of the ulcer. (From P. E. Donahue and L. M. Nyhus, Surgical excision of gastric ulcers near the gastroesophageal junction. *Surg. Gynecol. Obstet.* 155:85, 1982. By permission of *Surgery, Gynecology & Obstetrics.*)

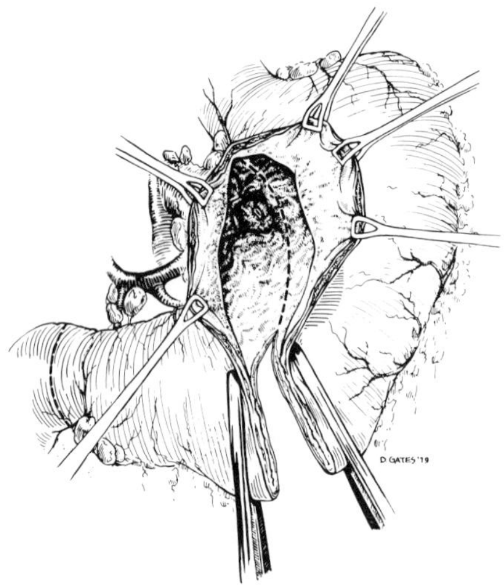

Fig. 8-2. A freehand completion of the excision proceeds rapidly, and bleeding is temporarily stopped with Babcock clamps. The posterior location of the ulcer accounts for the narrow amount of anterior resection and the generous amount of posterior wall in the planned resection. A suture should be placed just after the apex of the incision has been created to take advantage of the remaining stomach as a traction device and to avoid retraction of the proximal part of the stomach. (From P. E. Donahue and L. M. Nyhus, Surgical excision of gastric ulcers near the gastroesophageal junction. *Surg. Gynecol. Obstet.* 155:85, 1982. By permission of *Surgery, Gynecology & Obstetrics.*)

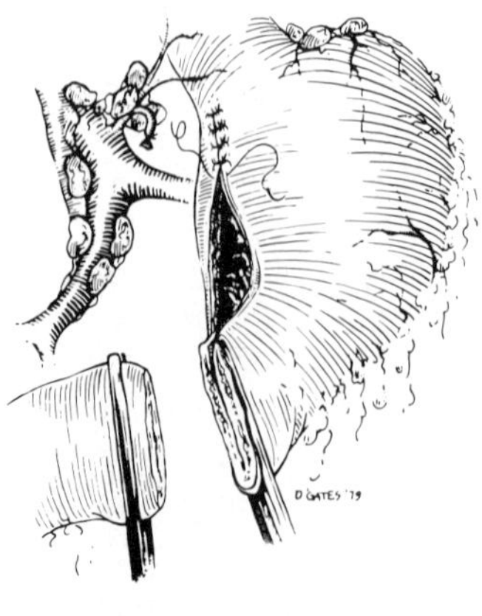

Fig. 8-3. A two-layer anastomosis is always advisable. We prefer an inner layer of running lock sutures of 00 chromic catgut. A larger needle will facilitate rapid placement of this hemostatic stitch, and interrupted nonabsorbable sutures complete the tubularization of the remaining part of the stomach. (From P. E. Donahue and L. M. Nyhus, Surgical excision of gastric ulcers near the gastroesophageal junction. *Surg. Gynecol. Obstet.* 155:85, 1982. By permission of *Surgery, Gynecology & Obstetrics.*)

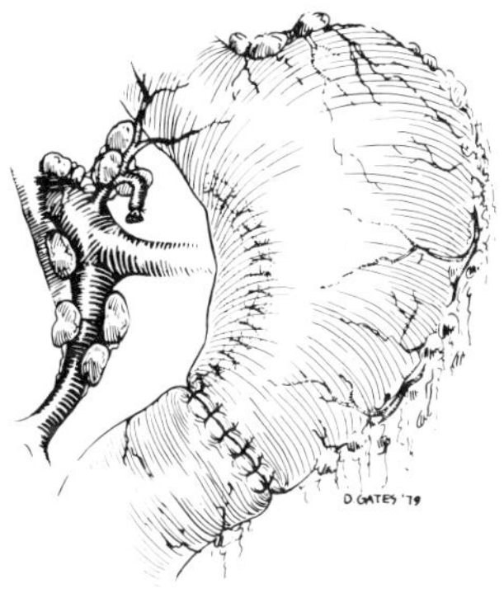

Fig. 8-4. The suture line has seemingly rotated posteriorly, a fact explained by the posterior location of the ulcer and the consequent resection of more of the posterior than the anterior lesser curvature. If the ulcer had been situated more anteriorly, the suture line would appear to have rotated anteriorly. (From P. E. Donahue and L. M. Nyhus, Surgical excision of gastric ulcers near the gastroesophageal junction. *Surg. Gynecol. Obstet.* 155:85, 1982. By permission of *Surgery, Gynecology and Obstetrics.*)

excision are justified for the treatment of corporeal gastric ulcer.

Donahue and Nyhus (*Surg. Gynecol. Obstet.* 155:85, 1982) renewed interest in the Pauchet or Tanner rotation gastrectomy for high-lying lesser curvature gastric ulcers. Although most gastric ulcers can be excised by conventional techniques, the principle of freehand excision of the ulcer, as illustrated in Figures 8-1 to 8-4, can be extremely useful in ulcers near the gastroesophageal junction.

C.W. and L.M.N.

9

Billroth I Gastrectomy

J. R. Siewert
A. H. Hölscher

Definition

Partial gastrectomy is the surgical removal of a part of the stomach. The partial gastrectomies connected with the name Theodor Billroth are resections of the distal stomach. According to the type of disease (ulcer or carcinoma) and the location of the basic disease (duodenal ulcer, gastric ulcer, high-situated gastric ulcer, cardial ulcer), they are performed as antral, two-thirds, four-fifths, or subtotal gastrectomies. Distal partial gastrectomy is named according to the type of anastomosis between the small intestine and the gastric remnant regardless of the extent of gastrectomy.

The Billroth I operation is a gastroduodenostomy that can be performed both end-to-end and end-to-side. A decisive difference between this method of operation and the Billroth II procedure is that the duodenal passage remains intact. Because of anastomotic requirements, the Billroth I operation as a rule is performed as either an antral or a two-thirds gastrectomy. Extended gastrectomies can only be reconstructed with difficulty, as in a gastroduodenostomy. Direct anastomoses of this kind between gastric fundus and duodenum are often followed by postoperative diseases.

History and Classification

After failures by Péan (1879) and Rydygier (1880)—both patients died after the operation—Theodor Billroth, on January 29, 1881, performed the first successful partial gastrectomy on a 43-year-old woman with an antral carcinoma [9]. He reconstructed the gastrointestinal passage with an end-to-end gastroduodenostomy (duodenum to lesser curvature) (Fig. 9-1).

After his third resection Billroth changed his operative technique to a gastroduodenostomy (duodenum to greater curvature) because of a better outflow (Fig. 9-2). In the course of time, the reconstruction of the gastroduodenal passage in the Billroth I procedure underwent numerous modifications (Fig. 9-2 and Table 9-1).

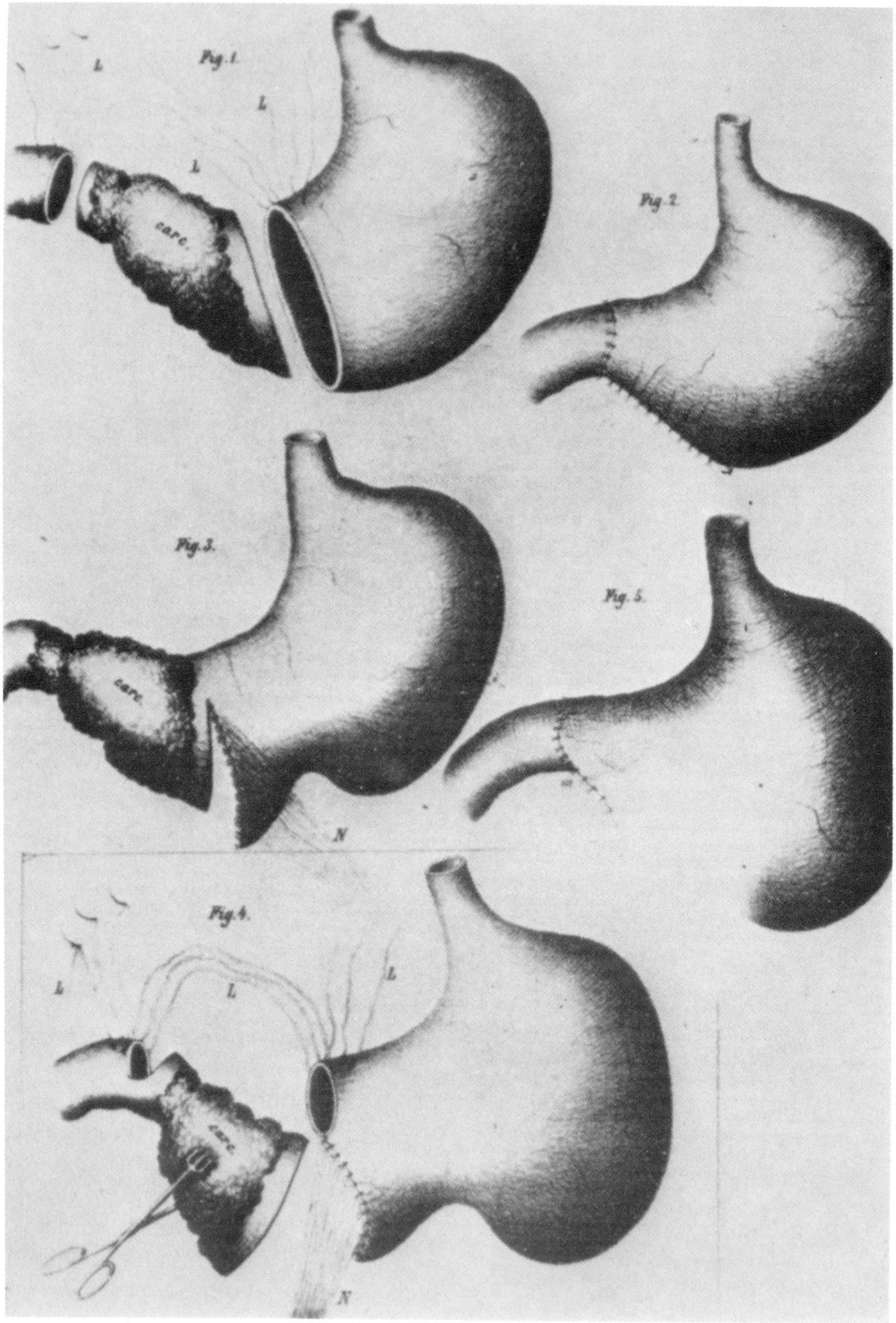

Fig. 9-1. Reproduction from Wölfler's original article on gastric resections from Billroth's clinic in 1881. (From Rutledge [64].)

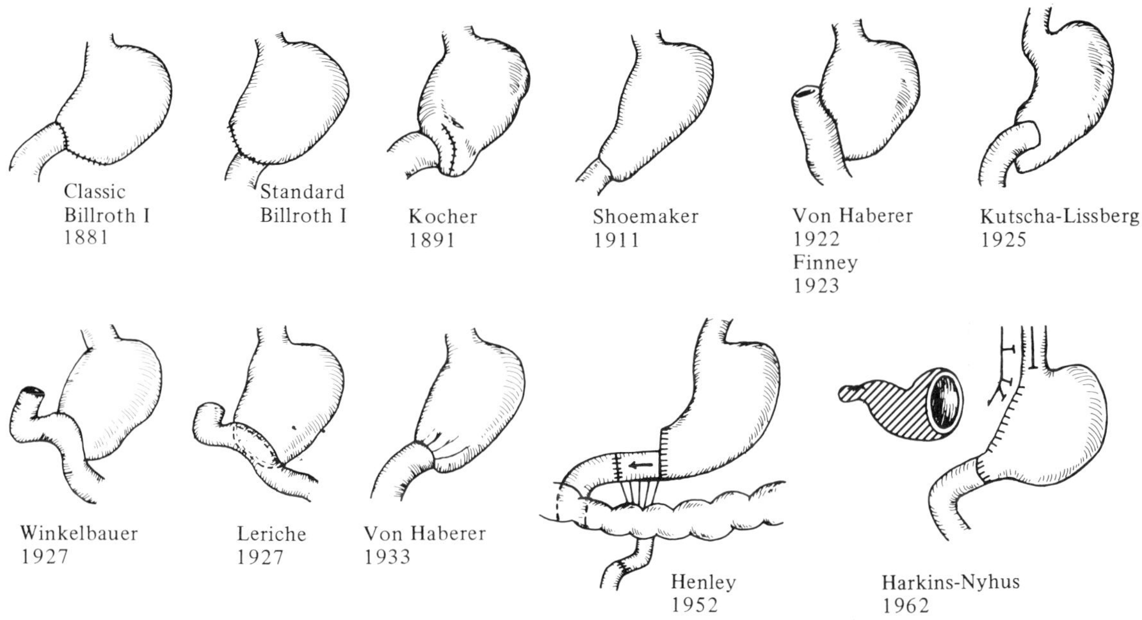

Fig. 9-2. Technical variations of the Billroth I gastrectomy.

The most frequently recommended technique is a combination of the second method applied by Billroth and the modification by Schoemaker with partial closure of the stomach remnant on the lesser curvature and an end-to-end gastroduodenostomy with the duodenum attached to the greater curvature side of the stomach.

Surgical Technique

RECOMMENDED METHOD: END-TO-END GASTRODUODENOSTOMY

The midline epigastric incision is the most frequently recommended access (Fig. 9-3). Alternatively, a transverse epigastric rectus muscle–splitting incision or an upper vertical muscle-splitting incision to the right can be chosen.

The dissection of the stomach begins in the middle level of the greater curvature with cutting of the gastrocolic omentum (Fig. 9-4A). Thus the omental bursa is opened. The dissection for gastric ulcer can take place between the gastroepiploic vessels and the gastric wall. In carcinoma the greater omentum corresponding to the extent of the resection in the greater curvature must be removed at the same time. When the omental bursa has been opened, the flimsy part of the gastrohepatic omentum can be pushed by the finger and a soft rubber Penrose drain placed around the stomach. The dissection is then continued step by step along the greater curvature toward the duodenum. Near the pylorus the greater omentum becomes thicker and divides into a front and a back layer. It is recommended to proceed in the loose intermediate tissue further in the direction of the duodenum and then to sever individually the layers of tissue carrying the vessels.

The preparation of the duodenum demands careful technique (Fig. 9-4B). It begins above or somewhat below the second portion of the duodenum from a lateral direction (so-called Kocher maneuver). The peritoneal duplication is sharply cut along the lateral duodenal wall between the second portion of the duodenum and the beginning of the hepatoduodenal ligament. When the second portion of the duodenum is stretched medially the retroperito-

Table 9-1. History of the Billroth I Operation

Author	Year	Procedure
Billroth	1881	GDST ter. or. part. cran.
Billroth	1881	Following resection GDST ter.-ter. or. part. caud.
Kocher	1891	GDST lat.-ter. or. post. to circumvent the "Jammer Ecke"
Schoemaker	1911	Resection of lesser curvature including GDST ter.-ter. or. tot.
von Haberer	1920	GDST ter.-ter. tot. with gathering sutures
Schmieden	1921	Modification of Schoemaker's procedure
von Haberer	1922	GDST ter.-lat. or. tot. part. contrapapillaris
Kirschner	1922	GDST ter.-ter. including rotating stomach dorsally
Mayo	1923	Modification of Schoemaker's procedure
Finney	1923	Modification of von Haberer's procedure
Goepel	1923	GDST with telescope-like invagination of duodenum into stomach
Kutscha-Lissberg	1925	GDST lat.-ter. or. anterior
Finsterer	1925	Modification of von Haberer's procedure
Horsley	1926	GDST ter.-ter. or. part. cran. with duodenoplasty
Horsley	1926	Modification of Goepel's procedure
Winkelbauer	1927	GDST ter.-lat. or. tot. caud. part. infrapapillaris
Leriche	1927	GDST lat.-lat. infrapapillaris ant.
Leriche	1928	GDST ter.-lat. infrapapillaris
Oliani	1929	GDST lat.-lat. contrapapillaris ant.
von Haberer	1933	GDST ter.-ter. or. tot.
Steinberg	1936	Modification of von Haberer's procedure; excision of triangular antral patch from anterior wall
Flechtenmacher	1942	GDST ter.-ter. or. tot. caud. part. contrapapillaris
Blagett	1948	Modification of Flechtenmacher 1942
Oloni	1951	GDST ter.-ter. with interposition of an isoperistaltic jejunal loop
Henley	1952	GDST ter.-ter. part. inferior with interposition of isoperistaltic loop
Nagel/Belcher	1953	GDST with resection of greater curvature and tubular repair
Johnson	1956	Modification of Nagel/Belcher (1953)
McQueen	1956	GDST with resection of lesser curvature and tubular repair
Schoemaker	1957	GDST with Z-plasty of lesser curvature and tubular repair
Viezian	1957	GDST with plastic coverage of lesser curvature
Corriero Bayer	1957	GDST ter.-lat. with tubular repair of stomach
Harkins-Nyhus	1960	Steplike hemigastrectomy with selective gastric vagotomy "combined operation"

GDST = gastroduodenostomy; ter. = terminalis (end); lat. = lateralis (side); or. = oralis (cephalad); part. = partialis (partial); tot. = totalis (total); cran. = cranialis (cephalad); caud. = caudalis (caudad); ant. = anterior; post. = posterior. For example: GDST posterior = anastomosis to posterior gastric wall; GDST anterior = anastomosis to anterior gastric wall; GDST termino-terminalis oralis totalis = end-to-end anastomosis of duodenum to entire end of cut stomach; GDST termino-lateralis contrapapillaris oralis totalis = end-to-side anastomosis of duodenum (opposite ampulla of Vater) to entire cut end of stomach; GDST oralis partialis inferior = end-to-end anastomosis with partial closure of lesser curvature of stomach.
Source: V. Schumpelick, and H. W. Schreiber: *Med. Welt* 27:2442, 1976.

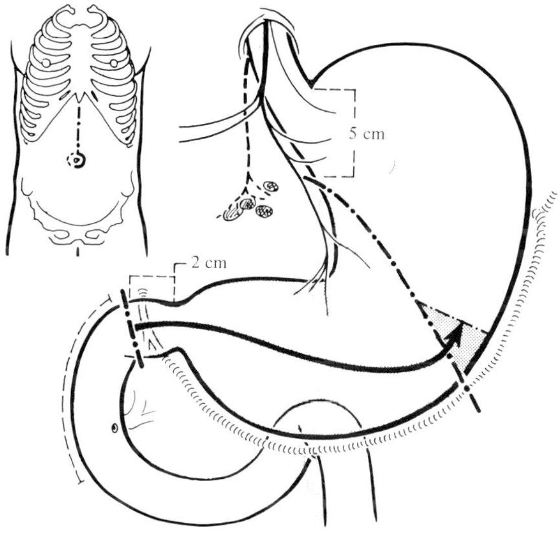

Fig. 9-3. The Billroth I gastrectomy: access (midline epigastric incision) and extension of the gastric resection.

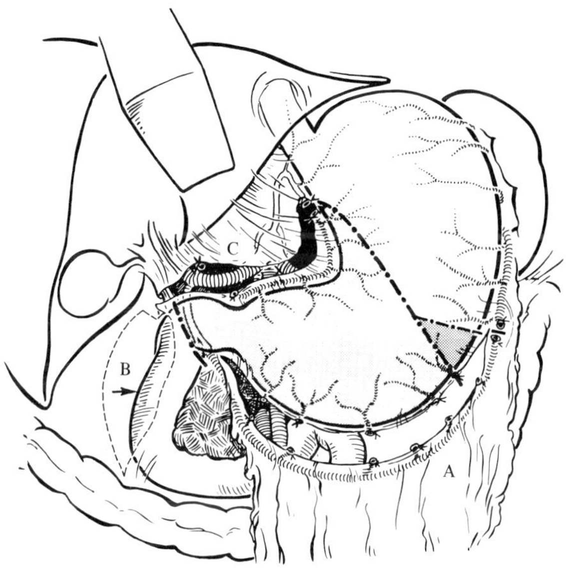

Fig. 9-4. Dissection of the stomach; cutting of the gastrocolic omentum (A); mobilization of the duodenum (B) and preparation of the lesser curvature (C).

neal tissue is loosened, partly bluntly, partly sharply, until the duodenum is mobilized. In this way a good general view can be achieved, which later is important for the gastroduodenostomy. The preparation of the free, first part of the duodenum is then continued.

With stretching of the stomach, the dissection proceeds along the greater curvature toward the left medial duodenal wall, then toward the back wall, and finally toward the lateral duodenal wall as far as the beginning of the hepatoduodenal ligament. In this way, from 3 to 5 cm of the duodenal back wall can be made free—in stomach ulcer or carcinoma usually without technical difficulty. The transition from the first free part of the duodenum to the part fixed dorsally on the pancreas can be recognized from the course of the gastroduodenal artery. At this point the serosa goes from the duodenum to the head of the pancreas. Here the preparation must be especially careful, as the artery is important for the blood supply to the duodenum.

After mobilization of the duodenum, the preparation is continued along the lesser curvature of the stomach (Fig. 9-4C). Here difficulties can arise as a result of perforation of a gastric ulcer. Frequently a perforating gastric ulcer can be pinched off by fingers. It is advisable to coagulate the base of the ulcer and to oversew the hole in the stomach. The dissection must always be continued so far orally that a sufficiently large area of intact stomach wall has been prepared. According to the findings, the preparation of the stomach on the lesser curvature can be continued directly into the area of the cardia. The layers of the gastrohepatic omentum sit at variously wide intervals on the front or back wall of the stomach. They encircle a tissue rich in fat with the branches of the left gastric artery. The preparation proceeds in the clearest possible way by bluntly forcing the intermediate tissue apart and severing individually the front and back layer of the gastrohepatic omentum. As long as the ascending trunk of the left gastric artery is not directly included, it will remain intact during the ulcer resection.

The resection starts with the cutting of the duodenum. For this purpose a soft intestinal clamp is fitted 1 to 2 cm behind the pylorus. The duodenum is cut orally to the clamp. This incision can also proceed in an open way between holding sutures. The duodenum is then temporarily closed with a swab. After this, the borders of the resection in the stomach are determined. The stomach is best removed with a suturing device (e.g., TA 90 stapler). The incision follows at an angle of 45 degrees to the lesser curvature. The line can, but need not, be oversewn. After removal of the distal stomach, a clamp is fitted at right angles to the greater curvature. The clamp is thus pushed so far orally until the removal level corresponds to the duodenal lumen. The remaining aboral end is cut off (Fig. 9-5). We recommend Von Haberer submucous sutures in the front and back wall to achieve hemostasis. The anastomosis can be performed freely, i.e., with clamps or without clamps.

The anastomosis is applied as a gastroduodenostomy (duodenum to greater curvature). For this purpose the two cut surfaces are placed on each other and the back wall is joined by seromuscular interrupted sutures (000 silk or polyglycolic acid [PGA]) (Fig. 9-6A); the suture of the mucosa (absorbent suture material, e.g., PGA 4-0 continuous) then forms a second row (Fig. 9-6B). The front wall is best covered with one row of all-layer interrupted sutures (nonabsorbent suture material of 000 PGA [Fig. 9-6C]). Special attention must be paid to the so-called Jammer Ecke (complaint corner) on the lesser curvature. Here it is advisable to use a triple seromuscular suture, which includes the duodenal wall as well as the front and back walls of the stomach (Fig. 9-6D).

Finally, a finger is used to check the anastomosis to be sure it is open, and the stomach tube is checked orad to the anastomosis to be sure it is in a good position. The surgical site is drained thoroughly by a soft rubber Penrose drain (Fig. 9-7).

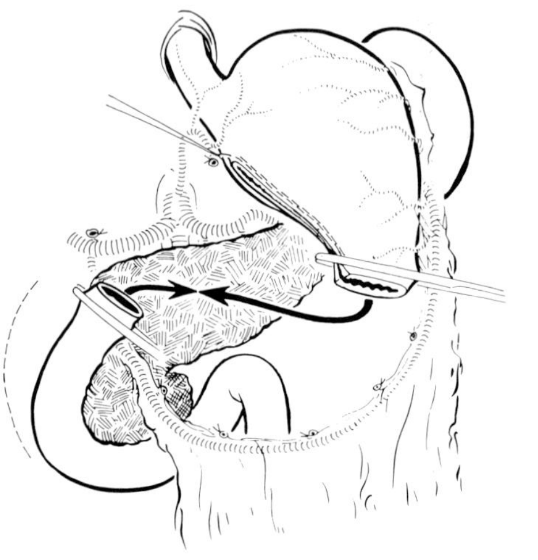

Fig. 9-5. Distal gastric resection: after removal of the distal stomach and the distal end of the greater curvature, the two cut surfaces are placed on each other.

ALTERNATIVE METHOD: END-TO-SIDE GASTRODUODENOSTOMY

In difficult-to-treat duodenal ulcers (duodenal ulcer or scars in the duodenal bulb), it can be impossible to preserve enough duodenal wall to be able to cut the duodenum without clamps and close the duodenal stump in the usual manner. The reconstruction of the intestinal passage can proceed by end-to-side anastomosis (end-to-side gastroduodenostomy). For this purpose the stomach is removed in the same way; the dissected gastric lumen, however, is anastomosed onto the front wall of the duodenum. Usually an oblique incision should be made on the front wall of the duodenum so that the incision level starts from oral-medial and goes to aboral-lateral (Fig. 9-8A). The suture technique is the same as for the end-to-end anastomosis. Here too, the back wall is sutured in two rows (Fig. 9-8A) and the front wall with all-layer interrupted sutures (Fig. 9-8B). In technically difficult duodenal stump closures, this practice is suitable for additional covering of the stump with the back wall of the stomach (Fig. 9-8C).

Anastomosis by Stapler Technique

The preparation of the stomach and duodenum proceeds as previously described. After the duodenum is severed, an EEA stapler is introduced transpylorically into the

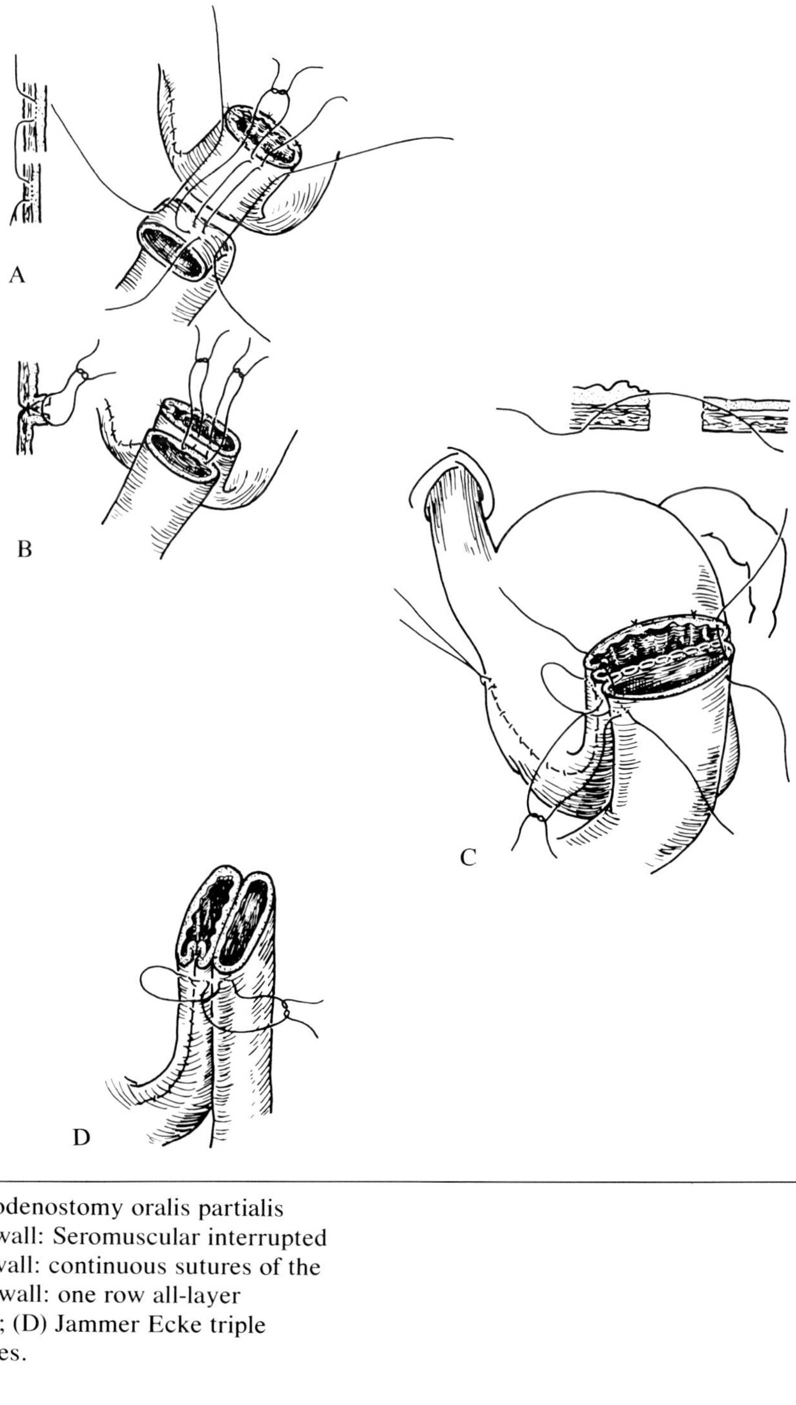

Fig. 9-6. Gastroduodenostomy oralis partialis inferior: (A) Back wall: Seromuscular interrupted sutures; (B) Back wall: continuous sutures of the mucosa; (C) Front wall: one row all-layer interrupted sutures; (D) Jammer Ecke triple seromuscular sutures.

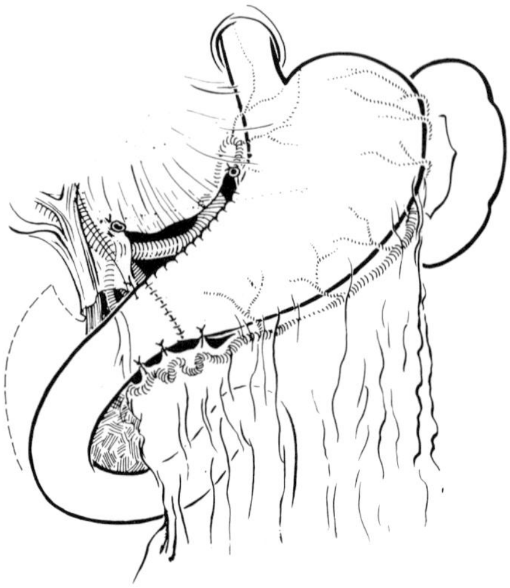

Fig. 9-7. Final aspect of Billroth I distal gastric resection.

stomach. A small incision is made through a pursestring suture at the point on the back wall of the stomach selected for the anastomosis. The head of the EEA stapler is brought through the incision (Fig. 9-9). The pursestring suture is tied above the stapler cartridge. The anvil of the stapler is then led into the duodenum after a pursestring suture has been made there as near to the end as possible. After these pursestring sutures are tied, the EEA stapler can be closed and the anastomosis performed.

After the anastomosis has been positioned between the duodenum and the back wall of the stomach, the stapler is removed and the stomach resection performed aborally to the anastomosis after closure of the proximal stomach with the TA 90 stapler (Fig. 9-10). The cut surface of the stomach can, but need not, be oversewn (Fig. 9-11).

Fig. 9-8. Gastroduodenostomy terminolateralis: After removal of the distal stomach, the stomach lumen is anastomosed onto the front wall of the duodenum (A). The suture technique is the same as described in Fig. 9-6 (A,B). The duodenal stump is covered with the posterior gastric wall (C).

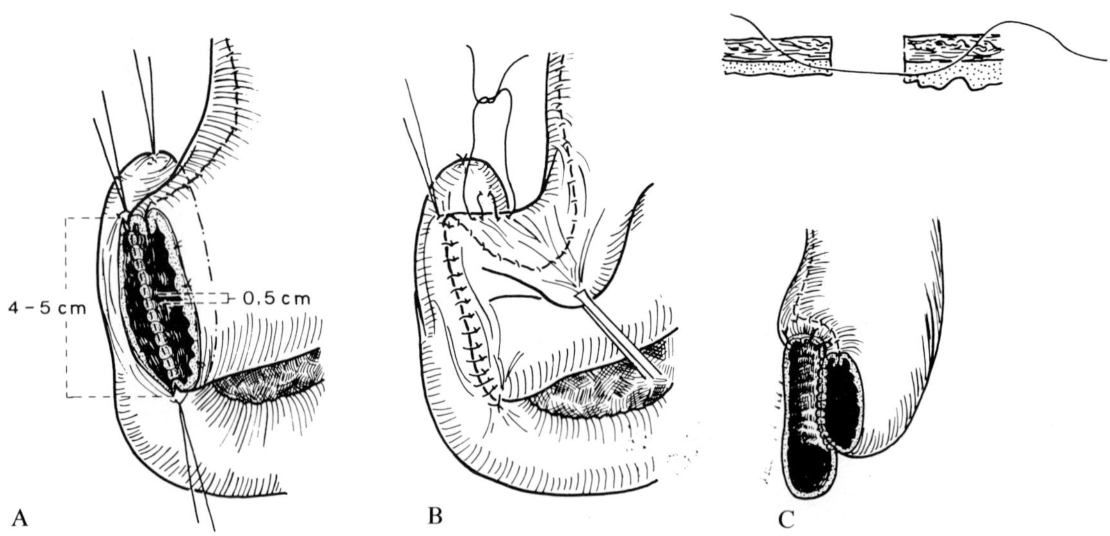

Early Complications

After a Billroth I gastrectomy, the following intra-abdominal complications may appear [78, 83]: suture insufficiency in the region of the anastomosis (3–4 percent; disorders of passage (2–5 percent); postoperative bleeding (2 percent); and postoperative pancreatitis (0.9 percent) (Fig. 9-12, Table 9-2).

An *early insufficiency* in the area of the gastroduodenostomy within the first three to four

Fig. 9-9. Billroth I stapler technique. The EEA stapler is introduced transpylorically and brought through a purse string suture on the back wall of the stomach.

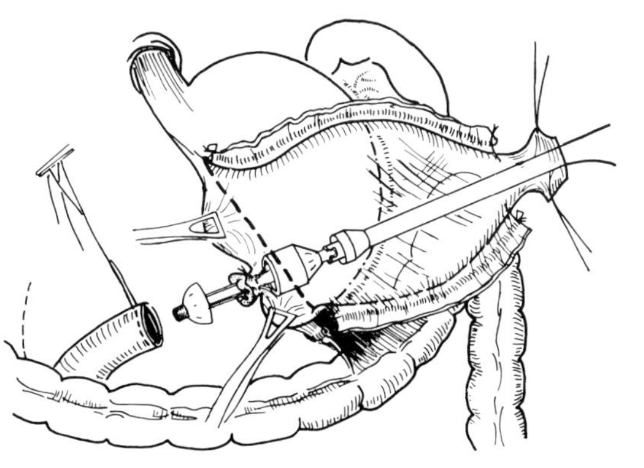

Fig. 9-10. The stomach resection is performed aborally from the anastomosis after closure of the proximal stomach with the TA 90 stapler.

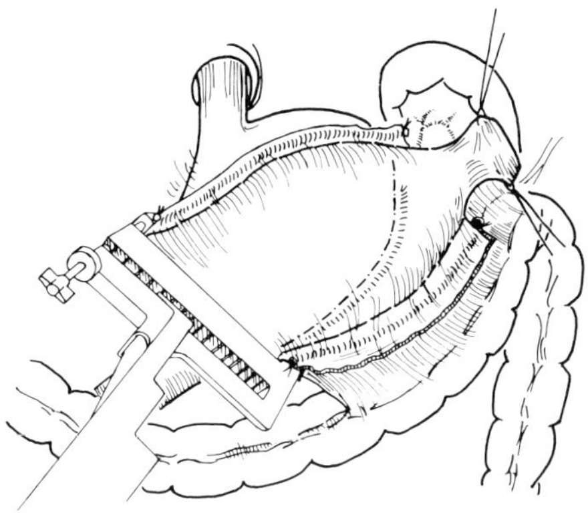

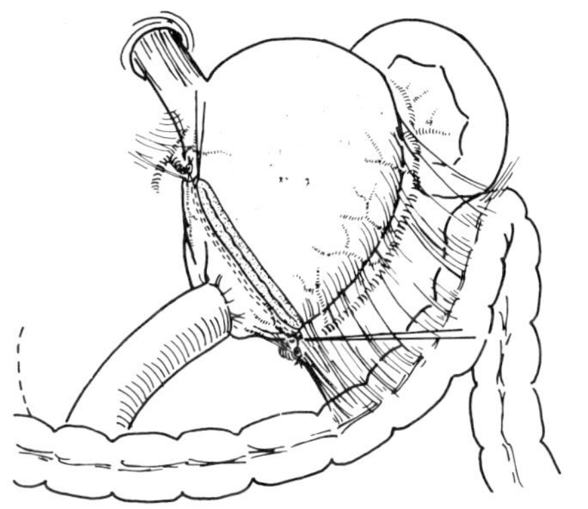

Fig. 9-11. After removal of the distal stomach, the cut surface can, but need not, be oversewn.

Fig. 9-12. Possible early complications after B I gastrectomy: 1) suture insufficiency in area of gastroduodenostomy (GD), 2) secondary hemorrhaging from GD into intra- or extraluminal space, 3) impairment of passage by obstruction of anastomosis, 4) postoperative pancreatitis, 5) secondary stenosis of cystic duct, 6) mechanical ileus, and 7) peritonitis.

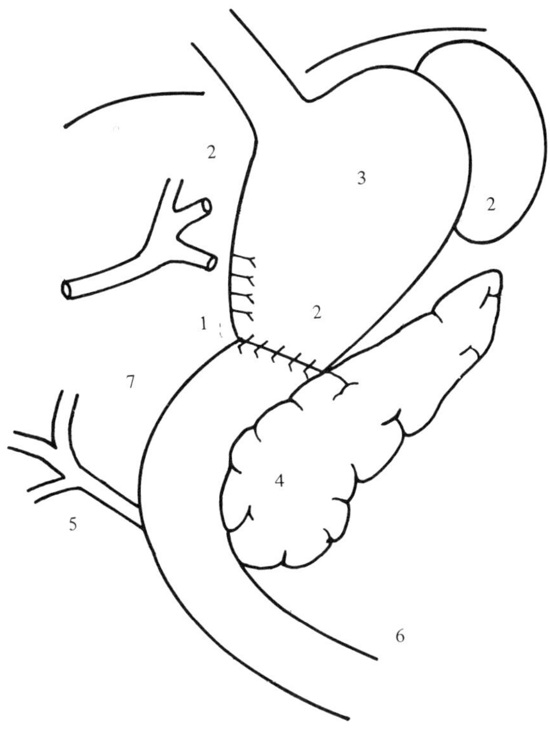

Table 9-2. Incidence of early postoperative complications following Billroth I gastrectomy for gastric or duodenal ulcer

Author	Year	No. of patients	Atony/ stenosis (%)	Suture insufficiency/ peritonitis (%)	Secondary hemorrhage (%)	Pancreatitis (%)
Horsburgh [35]	1965	113	—	0	0	—
Semb [74]	1973	130	3.8	0	0	—
Nielsen [53]	1973	97	5.1	2.1	4.1	—
Duthie [15]	1973	50	6	6	4	—
Madsen [48]	1976	22	4.5	—	—	—
Winkler [94]	1977	302	6.3	7.3	2.3	0.7
Kraft-Kinz [43]	1977	1023	0	1	0	—
Hollender [33]	1978	228	1.3	1.3	—	0.9
Hollender [33] Literature compilation	1978	2303	—	1.7	—	—
Baehrlehner [5] Single-row anastomosis	1979	155	0	3.9	0.6	—
Baehrlehner [5] Double-row anastomosis	1979	157	2.5	8.3	3.8	—
Range			0–6.3	0–8.3	0–4.1	0.7–0.9

postoperative days usually leads to diffuse peritonitis with an unfavorable prognosis. If the leakage appears later, the resulting local peritonitis most often can be kept under control if the insufficiency is drained properly. With good internal drainage by gastric tube, external drainage, and supplementary application of cimetidine—preferably somatostatin (for ischesis) and parenteral alimentation, also—drying of the anastomosis almost always occurs, and healing of the fistula must be awaited. Necrosis of the stomach remnant is a rare but fatal complication and frequently coincides with severe peritonitis.

Postoperative *disorders of passage* in the area of the gastroduodenostomy should not appear when good surgical technique is applied. If this problem develops, it is most often attributed to anastomotic edema, hematoma, or atony of the stomach, and will dissolve under sufficient internal drainage within the following 10 to 14 days. Revisions are necessary only in exceptional instances.

Intragastric or intraperitoneal *secondary bleeding* is rare. The indications for revision depend on the extent of bleeding. A revision should be performed when more than 6 units of blood per day are needed to make up the blood loss. With hemorrhage from the anastomotic site or the stomach remnant, a reopening of the stomach is performed through a transverse incision 3–5 cm above the anastomosis. From this location a close inspection of the anastomosis as well as the remaining stomach can be achieved, and furthermore, a ligature of hemorrhagic sites can easily be conducted. Closing of the incision again is achieved in a transverse direction. Extraluminal sources of hemorrhaging are treated in a typical manner. If the spleen is found to be the source of bleeding, a splenectomy is performed.

Postoperative pancreatitis is usually the edematous type with a rather good prognosis. In hemorrhagic necrotizing pancreatitis, a high mortality has to be expected. Postoperative pancreatitis of this kind should always raise the suspicion of mechanical deviation of the pancreas. A *sclerosing inflammation of the omentum* can be regarded as a rare postoperative complication. It almost always results from hypocirculation or infection. This so-called liposclerosis of the omentum can be the cause of unexplained rises in temperature. In rare instances it is directly responsible for partial or complete obstruction of the anastomosis. Rather frequently, however, we observe a benign intermittent *postoperative jaundice*. When this rise in bilirubin level cannot be explained by hemolysis or preexistent damage to the liver, frequently a so-called bilirubinostatic jaundice in combination with blood transfusions is responsible.

Postoperative disorders appear more often when local ulcer complications, such as bleeding or perforation, are present. In a series of 61 Billroth I resections done for acute hemorrhaging from an ulcer, all types of complications appeared at least twice as often as they did with elective Billroth I gastrectomy [94]. Stenosing or penetrating ulcers, however, showed no increased rate of complications in this group of patients.

According to published reports, the risks involved with a gastroduodenostomy are higher than those of a gastrojejunostomy. The overall risk, as expressed by mortality, is reported to amount to 0–6 percent for Billroth I gastrectomy (Table 9-3), whereas percentages ranging from 1.2 to 4.7 are associated with Billroth II anastomosis [50, 53, 60]. The mortality following gastrectomy is mainly caused by postoperative hemorrhage and anastomotic insufficiency, which accordingly is seen more often with Billroth I than with Billroth II operations. The higher rate of insufficiency of the gastroduodenostomy is mainly caused by the type of operative approach, especially in high gastrectomies in which only a tension-free anastomosis can be performed, usually with difficulty. It is not, however, the anastomosis alone that is more dangerous with a Billroth I procedure; the consequences of insufficiency are far more dangerous. Compared with gastrojejunostomy, which is almost dry, a leakage of a gastroduodenostomy leads to an effusion of duodenal contents with all its effects. The Billroth II resection, on the other hand, encompasses the risk of a duodenal stump insufficiency, which appears more rarely. By using improved suture techniques, especially the single row suture [5], the insufficiency rate after Billroth I resections could be lowered markedly, resulting in mortalities not higher than those of Billroth II resections, according to new statistics [5, 33, 43, 86].

Table 9-3. Mortality following Billroth I gastrectomy for gastric or duodenal ulcer

Author	Year	No. of patients (N = 4123)	Operative mortality* (%)
Horsburgh [35]	1965	113	2.7
Salzer [78]	1967	631	4.2
McKeown [50]	1970	124	0.6
Duthie [16]	1970	47	0.0
Duthie [16] (review)	1970	1252	1.8
Nielsen [53]	1973	97	6.0
Semb [74]	1973	130	0.8
Madsen [48]	1976	22	0.0
Kraft-Kinz [43]	1977	1023	1.0
Hollender [33]	1978	228	3.0
Baehrlehner [5]	1979		
Single-row anastomosis		155	1.3
Double-row anastomosis		157	4.5
Thomas [85]	1982	144	0.7
Emas [18]	1983	14	0.0

*Average = 2.1%; range = 0.0–6.0%.

Pathophysiological Considerations of Duodenal Passage

The question of whether a gastroduodenostomy or a gastrojejunostomy should be attempted after a distal gastric resection simultaneously poses the question of the sense of maintaining duodenal passage. Under physiological conditions, the duodenum serves four purposes in the course of digestion:

1. *Neutralization of acid.* The chyme emptied from the duodenum is neutral under physiological conditions. The act of neutralization is carried out with the help of three regulating mechanisms: (1) Emptying of the

stomach is regulated in such a way that the amount of acid reaching the duodenum from the stomach usually does not exceed the amount that can be compensated for in the duodenal bulb and the first few centimeters of the duodenum. (2) The release of secretin and cholecystokinin (CCK) from the duodenal mucosa accomplishes a stimulation of the pancreas and thereby effects an increased excretion of secretions containing bicarbonate. (3) A small amount of acid is absorbed by the duodenal mucosa or is neutralized by bicarbonate secreted directly from the duodenal mucosa.

2. The osmotic pressure of duodenal contents is balanced to *isotonicity*. During the complete duodenal passage, the chyme remains isotonic. Depending on the kind of food ingested, the contents emptied from the stomach usually are either hyper- or hypotonic. The adjustment of osmotic balance itself is affected by control of the stomach emptying as well as by secretion of fluids from the duodenal mucosa.
3. In part, *digestion* begins in the duodenum. After the excretion of CCK, stimulation of the pancreas and contraction of the gallbladder ensue. This leads to a decomposition of food by pancreatic enzymes and bile acid already in the duodenum. The fast, pendular peristalsis characteristic of the duodenum thereby accomplishes good mixture (segmentation).
4. *Resorption* of some processed food fractions starts in the duodenum. Monosaccharides, amino acids, smaller polypeptides, as well as free fatty acids are resorbed. Furthermore, the duodenum is the main location of iron and calcium resorption.

The essential condition for the timely performance of these sequential functions in the area of the duodenum is the control of *stomach-emptying* by the duodenum itself. This is performed by neural regulatory mechanisms and hormones.

Proximal parts of the stomach participate in the emptying of liquids from the stomach; even if only the antrum and pylorus are left intact, a controlled emptying of liquids is still possible. The decisive role in emptying solid food particles is performed by the antrum and pylorus. These two structures clearly are able to substitute for one another, and as long as one of the two is left intact, sufficient control of emptying of solid substances is provided. If both structures are absent, the emptying of solid food particles is seriously disturbed, causing a pathological condition [80]. In distal stomach resection, the total emptying mechanism of the stomach is removed. The B-II anastomosis excludes duodenal receptors from the food flow, whereas with the B-I resection these receptors are preserved. The size of the anastomosis influences the emptying process only to the extent that a too tight stoma leads to retention. The emptying process proceeds in almost the same way with a normal-sized or especially wide stoma. Proximal to the anastomosis, only the fundus and part of the corpus remain. The motility of these stomach segments causes emptying of fluids. The muscular prevention of emptying, the hindrance of reflux, the pacesetter, and the receptors are no longer present. The following consequences may be encountered:

1. Too rapid emptying of fluids and solid substances
2. Too rapid evacuation of fluids with simultaneous retention of solid substances
3. Too tight stoma retention of both solid and liquid substances

Quite clearly, the emptying process following distal resection of the stomach with gastroduodenal anastomosis (B-I) is not as rapid as it is with a gastrojejunal anastomosis (B-II).

It can be demonstrated roentgenologically that the duodenum slows liquid emptying of the stomach [80].

Gastroduodenostomy, as opposed to gastrojejunostomy, offers a synchronized interaction of digestive enzymes and food. This provides some advantages:

1. By adding secretions containing bicarbonate (pancreatic fluids, bile, duodenal mucosal secretions), with resorption of acids

through the duodenal mucosa and with distribution of acids by segmentation, a certain neutralization of acids is accomplished.
2. Osmotic pressure can still be regulated by secretion of fluids through the duodenal mucosa and by peristaltic distribution (segmentation) of duodenal contents.
3. It seems to be of prime importance, however, that the preserved early decomposition of food by pancreatic enzymes and bile acids as well as the maintained resorption of primary food particles, as iron and calcium, take place.

The better synchronization of digestion results in a diminished excretion of fat after a Billroth I as opposed to a Billroth II operation (pancreatocibal synchrony) [75].

DUODENAL PASSAGE AND FUNCTION OF THE PANCREAS

According to the available studies, it can be established that unencumbered *exocrine function* of the pancreas is possible after a Billroth I as well as after a Billroth II operation.

Measurements of pancreatic bicarbonate level and enzyme output in patients who had a Billroth II operation and in healthy controls revealed no difference in those measurements between the two groups [88]. In another study performed under liquid test meal conditions, it was found that patients with Billroth I as well as those with Billroth II operations secreted as much trypsin and bile acids within normal limits as controls did [49]. The low intraluminal enzyme concentrations that were measured in these experiments resulted from dilution caused by too rapid stomach emptying. Our own studies conducted with dogs [44] showed no discrepancy in exocrine pancreatic secretion after Billroth I or Billroth II gastrectomy.

Other studies, however, imply a reduction in *endocrine pancreatic* function. Distinct differences could be demonstrated in patients who had received total gastrectomy with and without duodenal passage.

After glucose loading, patients lacking duodenal passage as compared with a group with duodenal passage showed a significantly stronger rise of glucose concentration after 60 minutes (304 mg% versus 241 mg%), whereas the serum concentrations of insulin and gastric inhibitory peptide (GIP) were lower [40, 66, 81] (Fig. 9-13). The GIP levels found in duodenal biopsy specimens of patients with duodenal passage were significantly higher than those of the biopsy specimens taken from the jejunums of patients without duodenal passage.

The results confirm the role of the duodenum as the main source of the glucose-induced GIP release. Increased GIP secretion of patients with duodenal passage effects a pronounced release of insulin (insulinotrope activity) and thereby an improved glucose tolerance.

In the same study, patients with Billroth I and Billroth II gastric resections were examined. Similar results were obtained concerning duodenal passage, although with reduced distinctness [66]. In the same way, a study dealing with glucose homeostasis following total gastrectomy [10] showed that exclusion of the duodenum from the food passage leads to a significant deterioration of oral glucose tolerance (Fig. 9-14). Moreover, the capacity for insulin secretion in patients without duodenal passage was diminished by 50 percent (Fig. 9-15).

Oral fat loading leads to GIP release as well. It is higher in patients who have had gastrectomy without duodenal passage than in patients with preserved duodenal passage. This indicates that fat-induced GIP release takes place predominantly in the jejunum and not in the duodenum (Fig. 9-16).

DUODENAL PASSAGE AND FUNCTION OF THE LOWER ESOPHAGEAL SPHINCTER

Regulation of the function of the lower esophageal sphincter (LES) is accomplished through neural, myogenic, and hormonal pathways. It is possible that a distal gastrectomy might interfere with these regulatory mechanisms. Possibilities of impediments of this kind were once discussed in the context of mechanical changes (e.g., changes of the angle of His, lack of stomach weight) or as a result of

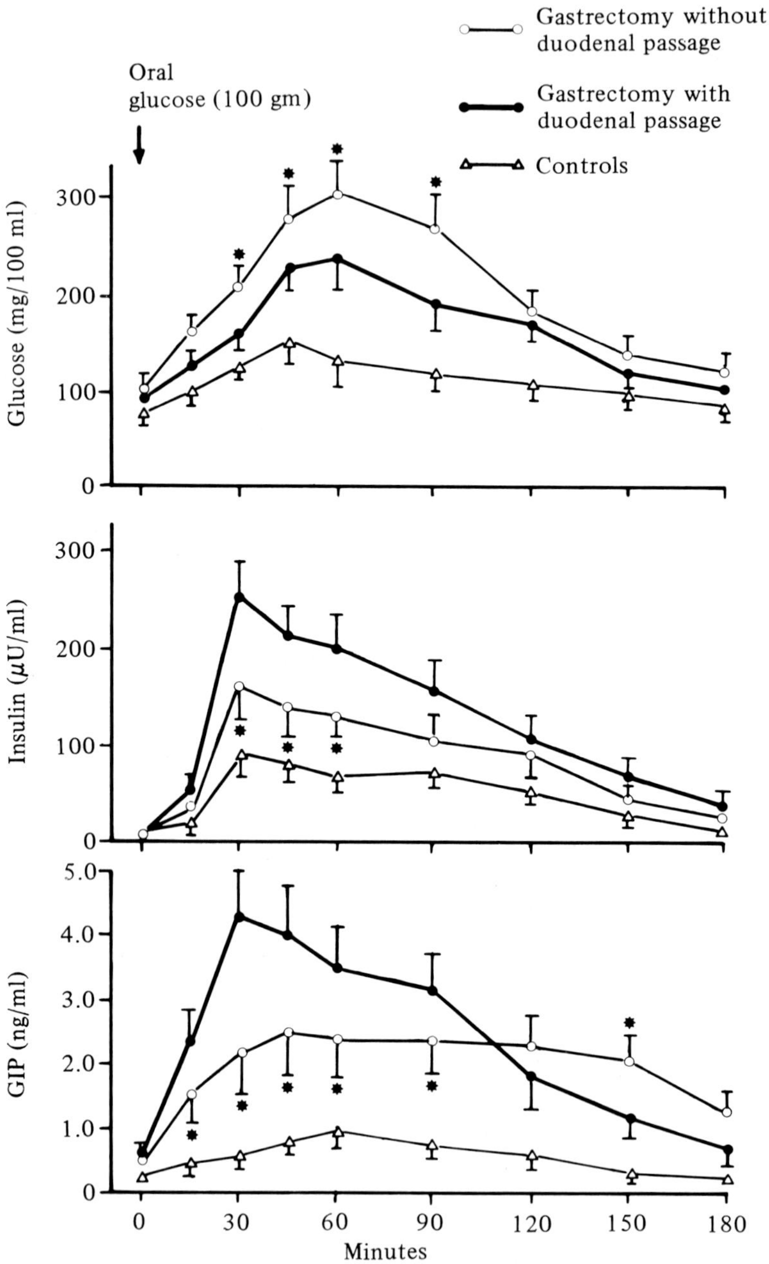

Fig. 9-13. Glucose, insulin, and gastric inhibitory peptide GIP levels after administration of 100 gm glucose in healthy probands (n = 18), gastrectomized patients with duodenal passage (n = 7), and gastrectomized patients without duodenal passage (n = 7). Error bars shown are average ± SEM. Asterisks indicate significant differences between the gastrectomy groups ($p < .005$).

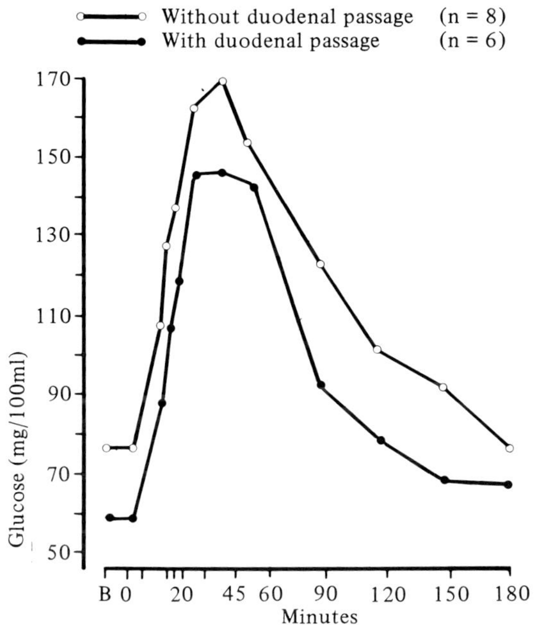

Fig. 9-14. Blood glucose concentration before (*point B*) and after oral glucose loading in gastrectomized patients without duodenal passage (n = 8) and in gastrectomized patients with duodenal passage (n = 6). (From Bittner [10].)

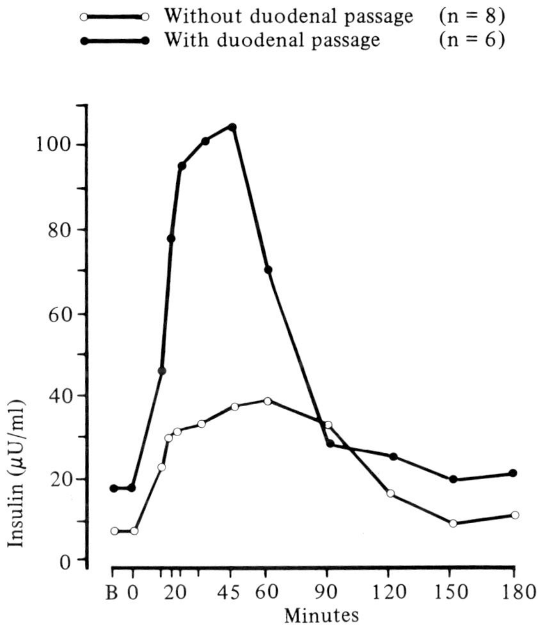

Fig. 9-15. Plasma insulin levels before (*point B*) and after oral glucose loading in gastrectomized patients without duodenal passage (n = 8) and in gastrectomized patients with duodenal passage (n = 6). (From Bittner [10].)

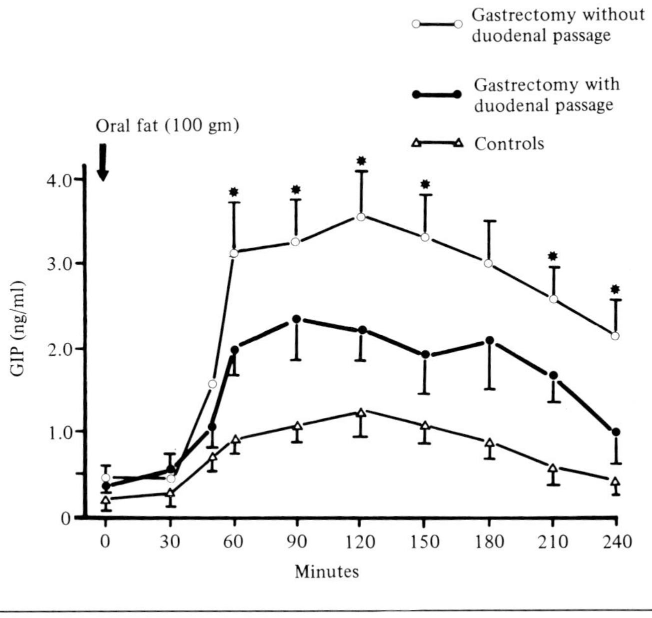

Fig. 9-16. Gastric inhibitory peptide (GIP) levels after administration of 100 gm of fat in healthy probands (n = 18), gastrectomized patients with duodenal passage (n = 7) and gastrectomized patients without duodenal passage (n = 7). Error bars shown are average ± SEM. Asterisks indicate significant differences between the gastrectomy groups ($p < .005$).

hypogastrinemia following antrectomy. Studies performed with unselected patient groups with distal gastrectomy have not demonstrated an increased rate of disturbances in LES function. Our own investigations showed 23 percent of an unselected patient group with Billroth II operations to have disorders of LES function, compared with 15 percent of healthy probands of a control group [82]. Of more interest are the more pathophysiologically oriented studies of LES regulatory mechanisms conducted on patients with Billroth I and Billroth II procedures [45]. Herein it was demonstrated that the LES reacted in the same way to a test meal as it had done before the antrectomy (Fig. 9-17). After a gastrojejunostomy, however, the typical postprandial pressure increase is absent even in clinically complaint-free patients (Fig. 9-18), the LES pressure is diminished, and reflux, which is especially demonstrable in patients suffering from a postgastrectomy syndrome, occurs. These disorders cannot be corrected, even with a remedial operation such as reconstruction of duodenal passage. Thomas and Earlam [85] published similar findings. In nine patients who had undergone a "Pólya partial gastrectomy," they discovered a shortening of the high pressure zone in combination with a significant decline in resting pressure. No direct correlation to clinical symptoms could be revealed, however. Endo et al. [19], on the other hand, found a marked shortening of the high pressure zone and a distinct increase in LES pressure in patients who underwent Billroth I resection (subtotal or two-thirds), although no increased clinical symptoms were associated with these findings.

In general, it must be said that the mentioned disorders in LES function following Billroth I and Billroth II gastric resection rarely assume clinical importance.

Therapeutic Effectiveness

ACID REDUCTION

One measurement of the therapeutic effectiveness of distal gastrectomy is the rate of acid reduction. According to Baron [6] basal acid secretion (BAO) is reduced by 87 percent, and maximal secretion (MAO) induced by pentagastrin stimulation is reduced by 86 percent. No differences regarding acid production of Billroth I and Billroth II stomachs are discernible if the extent of resection is the same [44]. A proximal gastric vagotomy (PGV) leads to a reduced acid production of 79 percent at BAO and 48 percent at MAO [79].

RECURRENCE RATES

In discussing rate of recurrence, patients with duodenal ulcers have to be distinguished from those with gastric ulcers. Follow-up studies have shown that patients who had undergone surgical treatment of a duodenal ulcer had recurrence more often after gastroduodenostomy than after gastrojejunostomy (Table 9-4). Certain aspects of operative technique, as mentioned in the section on early complications, may be responsible for this difference. To obtain a tension-free anastomosis, often a stomach resection set lower is preferred, resulting in an insufficient reduction in the number of parietal cells.

For *gastric ulcers* only two older studies [11, 65] report serious discrepancies concerning recurrence rates after Billroth I and Billroth II gastrectomies (Table 9-5). It has to be taken into consideration, however, that a clear classification of gastric ulcers was not always made in the older studies. Once ulcers of Johnson type II and III [37] are classified as gastric ulcers (with consideration to their pathogenesis, which resembles that of duodenal ulcers), a relatively higher rate of recurrence must be expected. On the other hand, when a statistic is limited entirely to type I gastric ulcers, as was done in the studies by Duthie, Madsen, and Becker [8, 16, 48], the problem of recurrence can be estimated to be lower. In studies of this kind, the Billroth I operation returned distinctly better results than PGV with ulcer excision (Table 9-5).

The pylorus-preserving Billroth I resection (see Chap. 12), as propagated by Maki, has been abandoned because of its high recurrence rate of more than 10 percent and the frequent appearance of postoperative stomach retention [84].

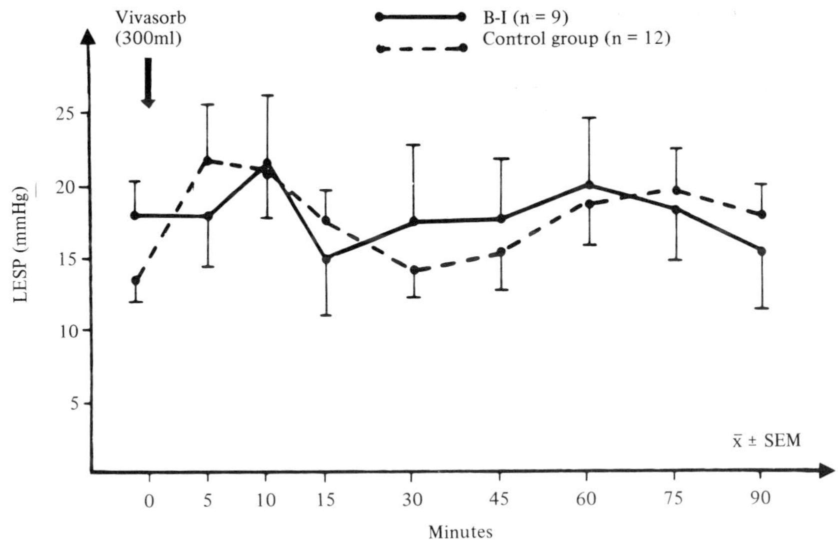

Fig. 9-17. LES pressure changes in 9 patients who underwent B-I resection after test meal stimulation compared with controls.

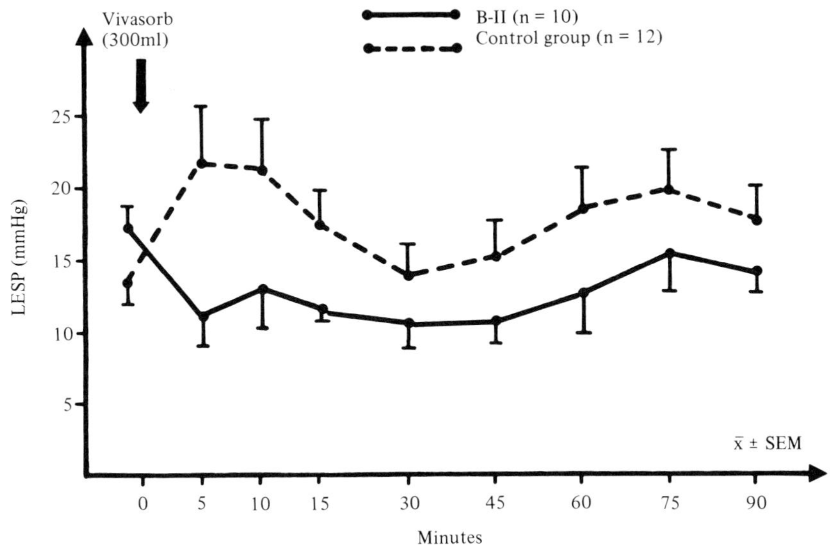

Fig. 9-18. LES pressure changes in 10 clinically symptom-free patients who underwent B-II resection compared with the results of controls.

Table 9-4. Percentage of ulcer recurrence after Billroth I gastrectomy, Billroth II gastrectomy, or proximal gastric vagotomy (PGV) for duodenal ulcer

Author	Year	B-I (%)	B-II (%)	PGV (%)
von Haberer [26]	1952	0.7	0.5	—
Wallensteen [90]	1953	4.0	—	—
Wallensteen [89]	1954	12.6	1.0	—
Moloney [52]	1954	0.0	2.8	—
Schuemann [68]	1953	1.5	—	—
von Redwitz [62]	1957	0.7	0.9	—
Ordahl [56]	1955	28.6	6.2	—
Goligher [24]	1956	17.5	—	—
Walters [91]	1956	21.9	—	—
Hickinbotham [30]	1956	10.0	—	—
Walters [92]	1957	7.4	3.6	—
Fisher [20]	1958	13.1	3.7	—
Localio [46]	1959	10.6	—	—
Hutchinson [36]	1960	10.0	—	—
Nyhus [55]	1962	3.7	7.5	—
Postlethwait [60]	1973	13.7	4.4	—
Borg [11]	1969	17.6	3.6	—
Goligher [22]	1970	13.7	1.1	—
Johnston [38]	1975	—	—	1.0
Hallenbeck [27]	1976	—	—	12.5
Holst-Christensen [34]	1977	—	—	12.0
Goligher [23]	1978	—	—	8.0
Junginger [39]	1979	—	—	10.9
Nilsell [54]	1979	—	—	19.2
Andersen [4]	1980	—	—	15.0
Madsen [47]	1980	—	—	26.0
Holle [32]	1980	—	—	2.7
Adami [1]	1980	—	—	12.7
Müller [7]	1981	—	—	5.6
Liavåg [7]	1981	—	—	13.0
Donahue [13]	1984	—	—	20.0
Emas [17]	1985	—	—	10.0
Range		0–28.6	0.5–7.5	1–26

Table 9-5. Percentage of ulcer recurrence after Billroth I gastrectomy, Billroth II gastrectomy, or proximal gastric vagotomy (PGV) for gastric ulcer

Author	Year	B-I (%)	B-II (%)	PGV (%)
Walters [91]	1956	5.0	—	—
Welch [78]	1958	—	1.0	—
Tanner [73]	1958	0.2	—	—
Harvey [78]	1961	—	1.5	—
Salzer [78]	1967	2.0	—	—
Borg [11]	1969	11.1	0.0	—
Harkins [28]	1969	0.7	—	—
McKeown [50]	1970	1.3	1.3	—
Duthie [16]	1970	2.4	—	14.3
Semb [74]	1973	1.5	—	—
Duthie [15]	1973	4.0	—	—
Sapala [65]	1973	16.1	—	—
Nielsen [53]	1973	5.0	5.0	—
Kraus [80]	1976	—	6.0	—
Madsen [48]	1976	0.0	—	13.0
Hollender [33]	1978	0.0	—	—
Duthie [14]	1979	7.0	—	15.0
Liedberg [79]	1979	0.0	—	21.1
German Study [79]	1980	—	—	14.3
Liavåg [7]	1981	6.0	—	20.0
Pichlmayr [7]	1981	5.0	—	25.5
Thomas [86]	1982	3.5	—	—
Becker [8]	1982	0.0	—	14.3
Range		0–16.1	0–6.0	14.3–25.5

VISICK GRADING

The Visick grading of Billroth I gastrectomies showed good results (Visick I and II) in 84 to 95.2 percent of patients (Table 9-6). These results were slightly better than those of the PGV, in which, extracted from a compilation of publications, Visick grades I and II were achieved in a mean of 86 percent of instances [79].

Table 9-6. Visick grading after Billroth I gastrectomy for gastric ulcer

Author	Year	Good (grade I + II) (%)	Poor (grade III + IV) (%)
Semb [74]	1973	88.0	12.0
Duthie [73]	1976	92.0	8.0
Madsen [48]	1976	95.2	4.8
Hollender [33]	1978	88.7	11.3
Thomas [86]	1982	84.0	16.0
Range		84–95.2	4.8–16

Sequelae of Billroth I Gastrectomies

Aside from ulcer recurrence rates, secondary diseases are important for an evaluation of late follow-up results of stomach resection.

STOMACH INCONTINENCE (DUMPING SYNDROME)

Dumping complaints in the form of early dumping phenomena are markedly more frequent after gastrojejunostomies than after gastroduodenostomies. In this context, the figures given for the Billroth I procedure range from 7 to 29 percent, whereas values between 17 and 39 percent are reported for Billroth II gastrectomy; thus the average dumping rates are approximately 10 percent higher for the Billroth II procedure (Table 9-7). Dumping complaints occur more rarely with PGV without pyloroplasty—about 8.1 percent (zero to 17 percent) according to a compilation of publications [79].

Table 9-7. Frequency of dumping syndrome after Billroth I gastrectomy and Billroth II gastrectomy for gastric or duodenal ulcer

Author	Year	B-I (%)	B-II (%)
Meurling [78]	1953	29.9	39.6
Wallensteen [89]	1954	19.9	29.4
Herrington [78]	1958	23.0	37.0
Horsburg [35]	1965	22.6	38.4
Amdrup [3]	1970	17.6	33.0
Borg [11]	1969	18.0	22.9
Nielsen [53]	1973	17.0	19.0
Sekine [72]	1975	7.4	17.3
Range		7.4–29.9	17.3–39.6

REFLUX ESOPHAGITIS

Postoperative reflux disease acquired wide attention only recently. As described earlier, it can be identified indirectly by manometry more often with Billroth II than with Billroth I resections. Pathophysiological considerations dictate the Billroth I operation, although their clinical relevance still remains unclear. In the context of postgastrectomy complaints, reflux esophagitis usually poses as nothing more than a partial aspect of various syndromes. A suggested conservative treatment is use of an H_2-receptor antagonist; bile acid binding substances such as cholestyramine or antacids are seldom effective. Roux-en-Y anastomosis is a surgical procedure that has proved its reliability with therapy-resistant reflux diseases following distal stomach resection.

ATROPHIC GASTRITIS

Five to ten years after stomach resection, atrophic gastritis of various grades is found in the gastric stump of 80 to 90 percent of patients operated on. So far there is no sufficient proof that the atrophic changes of the mucosa are of a lesser extent with Billroth I than Billroth II resections.

Compared with atrophic gastritis of a stomach that has been operated on, the atrophic gastritis that affects the gastric stump does not necessarily assume a manifest disease status. Most patients who have undergone gastrectomy do not complain of symptoms despite widespread histological abnormalities. Only 10 percent complain about symptoms that necessitate therapy, such as epigastric burning sensations, feelings of fullness and vomiting bile. It is characteristic that upper abdominal complaints resolve after bile vomiting and amplify after stimulation of bile or pancreatic secretion.

The cause of the described complaints evidently is not the atrophic gastritis of the stump, but rather the enterogastric reflux, which in most instances coincides with the endoscopic sign of hyperemia of the gastric mucosa (gastric erythema). Furthermore, the bacterial flora of the stomach may be regarded as a predisposing factor. Corresponding studies show a correlation between the degree of severity of the gastritis and the extent of the duodenogastric reflux [69, 93]. The studies of Schumpelick et al. [69] registered a maximum reflux with the retrocolic type of anastomosis, whereas smaller, but nevertheless pathological, values were obtained from the Billroth II resection with Braun's anastomosis and from the Billroth I stomach. An increase in the bacterial flora and elevated incidence of atrophic gastritis simultaneous with a rising intragastric pH were proved [70].

In another study, a causal connection was shown between therapeutically induced low production of hydrochloric acid by the gastric mucosa and the development of atrophic gas-

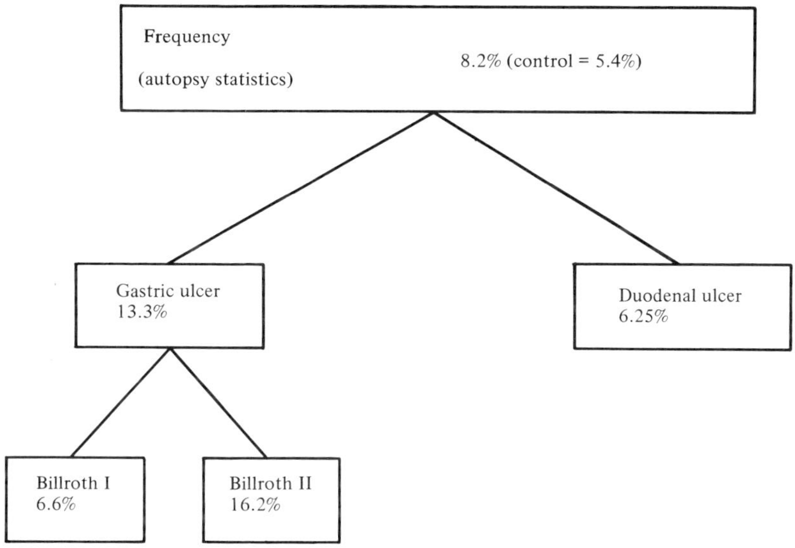

Fig. 9-19. Incidence of gastric stump cancer.

tritis [2]. According to the studies of Werner et al. [93], there is a lower frequency of atrophic gastritis with Billroth I than with Billroth II stomachs (Billroth I, 35.8 percent; Billroth II, 45.2 percent; controls 25 percent). In other studies, however, no discrepancy was found in the incidence of gastritis, which for both operative approaches ranged from 50 to 58.5 percent [61, 69]. In an endoscopic study, Kliems et al. [41] described the time factor in the development of atrophic gastritis; he reported an annual increase of atrophy of 3 percent after Billroth I resection.

CANCER OF THE GASTRIC STUMP

An especially important possible sequela of stomach resection is the development of cancer of the gastric stump emerging from atrophic gastritis. Chronic atrophic gastritis of the stump in combination with intestinal metaplasia is regarded as *optional precancerosis*. The number of observed gastric stump cancers has increased drastically in recent years [12, 25, 58]. This circumstance definitely can be attributed to the large number of gastrectomies performed 20 to 30 years ago, and furthermore, to the present-day widespread use of endoscopy.

From the wealth of studies dealing with this theme, two are of interest because they review Billroth I resection separately from Billroth II resection [25, 31]. The incidence of gastric stump cancer when all gastric resections were considered was 8.2 percent, as compared with 5.4 percent for a group of controls taken from autopsy statistics. The incidence increased to 13.3 percent when only the resections performed for gastric ulcers were considered. When the types of stomach resections were differentiated, an incidence of 6.6 percent was derived for the Billroth I and 16.2 percent for the Billroth II resection (Fig. 9-19).

Other statistical studies did not reproduce a discrepancy of this extent [59, 67]. The question of whether or not gastric stump carcinoma actually appears more infrequently with the Billroth I than with the Billroth II resection therefore has to remain unanswered for the moment.

GENERAL POSTGASTRECTOMY PROBLEMS

Malnutrition

Loss of weight after a stomach resection is considered a result of insufficient intake as well as inadequate digestion of food caused by impaired intestinal resorption. There are nu-

Table 9-8. Changes in body weight following Billroth I and Billroth II gastrectomy

Author	Year	B-I (%)	B-II (%)	Variable
French [21]	1960	24.0	43.0	Percentage of patients with postoperative weight loss
Borg [11]	1969	57.2	71.2	
Hedenstedt [29]	1974	28.0	36.0	
Paakonen [57]	1982	−1.2	—	Mean percentage of postoperative weight loss compared with preoperative weight
Thomas [86]	1982	+2.8	—	
Mellström [51]	1982			Percentage of postoperative weight loss in patients correlated to that of healthy probands of same age
70 years		−2.5	−4.5	
75 years		−2.9	−8.4	

merous causes of malnutrition and malabsorption. Most of these disorders are usually minor and rarely gain clinical importance.

Malnutrition necessitating therapeutic intervention predominantly develops after Billroth II resections [21, 29]. In a study dealing with long-term effects of gastrectomy, Mellström and Rundgren [51] described the body weight of 70-year-old patients who underwent Billroth II resections as being a mean of 6 kg lighter and that of 75-year-old patients who underwent Billroth II resections as being a mean of 11 kg lighter than healthy probands of the same age [51]. In contrast to older studies, newer studies could not demonstrate any significant loss of weight on comparing preoperative initial weight to that after Billroth I resections; at times an increase in weight was even witnessed in these patients [51, 57, 86] (Table 9-8).

Anemia

In estimating reasonably it may be projected that approximately half the patients who undergo gastrectomies will suffer anemia after 20 years.

The anemia seems more frequent and distinct after Billroth II than after Billroth I resections and is more frequent in patients who have been operated on for gastric rather than duodenal ulcers [29, 51, 87]. With declining incidence, anemia is caused by low iron supply, lack of vitamin B_{12}, or deficient folic acid levels, leading to frequent discovery of combined anemia types [63]. Hypoferremia is the result of various factors. On the one hand, patients who have had a gastrectomy often do not include enough iron in their diet; on the other hand, impaired iron resorption caused by reduced acid concentration, absent duodenal passage (with the main location for iron resorption being the proximal duodenum), and accelerated intestinal food passage additionally aggravates the problem. Postgastrectomy anemia can be treated by oral or intravenous administration of iron and regular replacement of vitamin B_{12}.

Osseous Changes after Gastrectomy

Several factors have been held responsible for the appearance of osteomalacia and osteoporosis after gastrectomy. These are a diminished resorption of vitamin D in combination with malabsorption of fat, the formation of saponified Ca^{++} in the event of steatorrhea, and exclusion of the duodenum, which is considered to be the main location of calcium resorption. Osseous changes following gastrectomy are described in up to 42 percent of all patients. Although many of these alterations are of a discrete nature, it can be demonstrated clearly that patients with partial stomach resections experience fractures far more often than do probands [51]. Following the same mode of pathogenesis as described earlier, indications are presented in published articles that suggest heavier osseous changes after Billroth II than after Billroth I resections. Patients who have undergone Billroth II rather than Billroth I resections show a significant increase in concentration of vitamin D and disorders of calcium metabolism [51, 76]. In contrast to this, no loss of minerals in bones and no diminished calcium absorption could be demonstrated in patients with Billroth I resections four years postoperatively [57].

Conclusions

ARGUMENTS IN FAVOR OF BILLROTH I GASTRECTOMY

Raising the question concerning the advantages and disadvantages of the two resections—Billroth I and Billroth II—simultaneously poses the question of the purpose of maintaining duodenal passage. On reviewing statements in the literature on this topic, it may be assessed that the Billroth I resection on the average combines slightly higher operative risk with somewhat superior long-term results. The sequelae of distal stomach resections may be basically the same for both procedures; they are, however, of a lesser degree with the Billroth I operation.

From this information it can be concluded that the difference between the Billroth I and Billroth II operations is not of a fundamental or qualitative nature but rather is of a quantitative nature. Under these circumstances, the argument of a possibly reduced risk of cancer of the gastric stump gains special weight. For the patient it is equally important to have the advantages of preserved synchrony of digestion that are obtainable with gastroduodenostomies, which find pronounced expression in fewer instances of dumping and improved body mass postoperatively. To this extent statements in the literature conform, yet the final evidence in favor of Billroth I gastrectomy needs to be gathered by a randomized study on a homogeneous patient group.

The studies presented still differ with respect to the pathophysiological importance of a duodenal passage maintained after antrectomy. There was no discrepancy worth mentioning with regard to stomach emptying and exocrine pancreatic function. Favorable consequences, however, seem to be produced by duodenal passage in endocrine pancreatic function and function of the cardia (Table 9-9).

INDICATIONS

Gastric Ulcers

The main indication for a Billroth I resection is a gastric ulcer that displays a high rate of recurrence after proximal gastric vagotomy in combination with ulcer excision. The following arguments advocating the Billroth I resection for gastric ulcers prevail:

1. A gastric ulcer can be removed completely transmurally and can be studied histologically for exclusion of malignant growths.
2. The point of least resistance situated at the border between antrum and corpus on the lesser curvature is eliminated.
3. The number of parietal cells is reduced by removing parts of the corpus and fundus.
4. The antrum, the main producer of gastrin, is removed.
5. In skeletonizing the lesser curvature beyond the resection line, the remaining stomach receives a partial vagotomy.

Prepyloric Ulcers

Prepyloric ulcers also are a good indication for Billroth I resections. Because of their secreting characteristics and because of their surgical and therapeutic consequences, these ulcers were labeled as duodenal and as a rule were treated accordingly by vagotomy. A five-year follow-up study of patients who received this form of therapy disclosed rather high recurrence rates; it may be concluded that prepyloric ulcers should, for the purposes of choosing a surgical procedure, be classified as gastric ulcers and be considered indications for resection [8].

Recurrent Ulcers in the Stomach and Duodenum after Vagotomy

Here the distal gastrectomy of the Billroth I normally is part of a combined operation. In view of the simultaneously performed secondary vagotomy (selective gastric vagotomy or truncal), the distal resection can be restricted to an antrectomy. A gastrectomy after vagotomy, however, especially PGV, most often turns out to be a technically difficult procedure.

In the event that a recurrent duodenal ulcer

Table 9-9. Sequelae after Billroth I gastrectomy, Billroth II gastrectomy, and proximal gastric vagotomy

Sequela	B-I	B-II	PGV
Secretion	Strongly reduced	Strongly reduced	Reduced
Recurrent ulcers			
Gastric ulcers	Rare	Rare	Very frequent
Duodenal ulcers	Frequent	Rare	Often
Reflux of bile (vomiting of bile)	Frequent	Dorsal gastroenterostomy necessary; with Braun's anastomosis as B-I	Rare
Atrophic gastritis	Frequent	Frequent	More infrequent
Gastric stump cancer	More rare (?)	More frequent (?)	So far not seen
Dumping	More rare	More frequent	Very rare, more often after pyloroplasty
Stomach emptying			
Solids	Rarely delayed	Rare, delayed	Intermittently delayed
Liquids	Slightly accelerated	Heavily accelerated	Accelerated
Pancreatic function			
Endocrine (release of insulin)	Slightly reduced	More heavily reduced	Unchanged
Exocrine	Unchanged	Unchanged (pancreaticocibal asynchrony?)	Unchanged
Cardiac function	Unimpaired (?)	Unimpaired (?)	Unchanged (definitely after 1 year)
Anemia	Slight	Stronger	None
Weight change	Unchanged	Reduced	Unchanged
Osseous changes	Slight	Stronger	None
Loop syndrome	None	Possible	None

has been identified or that a pyloroplasty has been performed in a previous operation, dissection of the duodenum may be extremely difficult, necessitating an end-to-side anastomosis instead.

Early Gastric Cancer

Cancer of the stomach itself presents an unfavorable indication for a Billroth I operation because it has not been proved that as radical an operation as may be necessary can be performed. An exception to this rule is an early cancer of the distal stomach. In that situation, even a Billroth I resection can be sufficiently radical.

References

1. Adami, H. O., Enander, L. K., Ingvar, C., and Rydberg, B. Clinical results of 229 patients with duodenal ulcer 1–6 years after highly selective vagotomy. *Br. J. Surg.* 67:29, 1980.
2. Alexander-Williams, J., and Hoare, A. M. Partial Gastric Resection. In A. L. Blum and J. R. Siewert (Eds.), *Postsurgical Syndromes, Clinics in Gastroenterology,* Vol. 8. London, Philadelphia, Toronto: Saunders, 1979. Pp. 321–54.
3. Amdrup, E., Nielsen, J., and Jensen, H. E. Treatment of benign gastric ulcer by segmental gastric resection with and without pyloroplasty. *Surgery* 68:759, 1970.
4. Andersen, D., Amdrup, E., Høostrup, H., and Søorensen, F. H. Aarhus County vagotomy

trial: Five year recurrence rate after PGV and SGV. *Acta Hepatogastroenterol.* (Stuttg.) 27(Suppl.):344, 1980.

5. Baehrlehner, E., Lenschel, D., Fischer, R., et al. Die einreihige extramuköse Adaptationsnaht ("Naht auf Stoss") bei der Magenresektion nach Billroth I. *Dtsch. Gesundh. Wesen* 31:1466, 1979.
6. Baron, J. H. The Rationale of the Different Operations for Peptic Ulcer. In A. G. Cox and J. Alexander-Williams (Eds.), *Vagotomy on Trial.* London: Heinemann, 1973.
7. Baron, J. H., Alexander-Williams, J., Allgöwer, M., et al. (Eds.) *Vagotomy in Modern Surgical Practice.* London: Butterworth, 1982.
8. Becker, H. D., Lehmann, L., Löhlein, D., et al. Selektiv-proximale Vagotomie mit Ulcusexzision oder Billroth-I-Resektion beim chronischen Ulcus ventriculi. *Chirurg* 53:773, 1982.
9. Billroth, T. Offenes Schreiben an Herrn Wittelshöfer. *Wien. Med. Wochenschr.* 31:161, 1881.
10. Bittner, R., Bittner, B., and Beger, H. G. Glukosehomöostase und Magenresektion. Die Bedeutung der Nahrungspassage durch das Duodenum. *Z. Gastroenterol.* 19:698, 1981.
11. Borg, J., and Bergström, S. Spätergebnisse der Resektionsbehandlung nach Billroth I und Billroth II in der Ulcuschirurgie. *Bruns Beitr. Klin. Chir.* 217:481, 1969.
12. Clemençon, G., Baumgartner, R., Leuthold, H., et al. Das Carcinom des operierten Magens. *Dtsch. Med. Wochenschr.* 101:1015, 1976.
13. Donahue, P. E., Bombeck, C. T., Condon, R. E., and Nyhus, L. M. Proximal gastric vagotomy versus selective vagotomy with antrectomy: Results of a prospective, randomized clinical trial after four to twelve years. *Surgery* 96:585, 1984.
14. Duthie, H. L., and Branson, C. J. Highly selective vagotomy with excision of the ulcer compared with gastrectomy for gastric ulcer in a randomized trial. *Br. J. Surg.* 66:43, 1979.
15. Duthie, H. L., and Kwong, N. K. Vagotomy or gastrectomy for gastric ulcer. *Br. Med. J.* 4:79, 1973.
16. Duthie, H. L., Moore, K. T. H., Bardsley, D., and Clark, R. G. Surgical treatment of gastric ulcers: Controlled comparison of Billroth I gastrectomy and vagotomy and pyloroplasty. *Br. J. Surg.* 57:784, 1970.
17. Emas, S., and Fernstrom, M. Prospective, randomized trial of selective vagotomy with pyloroplasty and selective proximal vagotomy with and without pyloroplasty in the treatment of duodenal, pyloric and prepyloric ulcers. *Am. J. Surg.* 149:236, 1985.
18. Emas, S., and Hammarburg, C. Prospective, randomized trial of selective proximal vagotomy with ulcer excision and partial gastrectomy with gastroduodenostomy in the treatment of corporeal gastric ulcer. *Am. J. Surg.* 146:631, 1983.
19. Endo, A., Okamura, S., Kono, N., and Katsumi, M. Esophageal reflux after gastrectomy: A hazard after Billroth I subtotal gastrectomy. *Int. Surg.* 63:53, 1978.
20. Fisher, P. B., and Jordan, G. L., Jr. Billroth I gastrectomy for the treatment of duodenal ulcer. *Am. Surg.* 24:922, 1958.
21. French, A. B., Pallard, H. M., and Ratner, J. T. Incidence of postgastrectomy malabsorption. *Gastroenterology* 38:964, 1960.
22. Goligher, J. C. The comparative results of different operations in the elective treatment of duodenal ulcer. *Br. J. Surg.* 57:780, 1970.
23. Goligher, J. C., Hill, G. L., Kenny, T. E., and Nutter, E. Proximal gastric vagotomy without drainage for duodenal ulcer: Results after 5–8 years. *Br. J. Surg.* 65:145, 1978.
24. Goligher, J. C., Moir, P. J., and Wrigley, J. H. The Billroth I and Polya operations for duodenal ulcer. *Lancet* 1:220, 1956.
25. Grieser, G., and Schmidt, H. Statistische Erhebungen über die Häufigkeit des Carcinoms nach Magenoperation wegen eines Geschwürleidens. *Med. Welt* 15:1836, 1964.
26. Haberer, H. V. Ulcus jejuni postoperativum nach Resektion Billroth II. *Chirurg* 23:164, 1952.
27. Hallenbeck, G., Gleysteen, J. C., and Aldrete, J. S. Proximal gastric vagotomy: Effects of two operative techniques on clinical and gastric secretory results. *Ann. Surg.* 184:435, 1976.
28. Harkins, H. N. Gastric Resection: Billroth I. In H. N. Harkins and L. M. Nyhus (Eds.), *Surgery of the Stomach and Duodenum* (2d ed.). Boston: Little, Brown, 1969. P. 491.
29. Hedenstedt, S., and Moberg, S. Gastric ulcer treated with selective proximal vagotomy (SPV): A preliminary report. *Acta Chir. Scand.* 140:309, 1974.
30. Hickinbotham, P. The Billroth I gastrectomy. *Br. J. Surg.* 44:206, 1956.
31. Hilbe, G., Salzer, G. M., Hussl, H., and Kutschera, H. Die Carcinomgefährdung des Resektionsmagens. *Langenbecks Arch. Klin.*

Chir. 323:142, 1968.
32. Holle, F., Holle, G. E. (Eds.). *Vagotomy and Pyloroplasty.* Berlin, Heidelberg, New York: Springer, 1980.
33. Hollender, L. F., Bur, F., van Peteghem, R. P., Alexion, D., and Starlinger, M. Hat die Resektion nach Billroth I beim Magengeschwür an Bedeutung verloren? *Zentralbl. Chir.* 103:329, 1978.
34. Holst-Christensen, J., Hart-Hensen, O., and Pedersen, T. Recurrent ulcer after proximal gastric vagotomy for duodenal and prepyloric ulcer. *Br. J. Surg.* 62:42, 1977.
35. Horsburgh, A. G., and Cox, R. A comparison of Polya and Billroth gastrectomies. *Gastroenterology* 49:381, 1965.
36. Hutchinson, W. B., and Kiriluk, L. B. Billroth I gastric resection for chronic duodenal ulcer. *Am. J. Surg.* 100:251, 1960.
37. Johnson, H. D., Love, A. H. G., Rogers, N. C., and Wyatt, A. B. Gastric ulcer blood groups and acid secretion. *Gut* 5:402, 1964.
38. Johnston, D. Highly selective vagotomy. *Prog. Surg.* 14:1, 1975.
39. Junginger, T., and Pichlmaier, H. Ergebnisse nach proximaler selektiver Vagotomie wegen Gastroduodenalulcus. *Dtsch. Med. Wochenschr.* 104:127, 1979.
40. Klapdor, R. Release of gastric inhibitory polypeptide (GIP) and gastrin after a test meal with low glucose load in patients after B-II resection, proximal duodenopancreatectomy (PDP) and jejunal bypass. *Res. Exp. Med.* (Berl.) 181:11, 1982.
41. Kliems, G., Paquet, K. J., Lindstaedt, H., and Miederer, S. Atrophic gastritis after Billroth I gastrectomy. *Endoscopy* 2:127, 1979.
42. Koelz, N. R., Lepsien, G., Blum, A. L., and Siewert, J. R. The duodenum regulates the lower esophageal sphincter. *Gastroenterology* 75:283, 1978.
43. Kraft-Kinz, J., and Kronberger, L. Operationsbedingte Mißerfolge bei der Magenresektion nach Billroth I. *Zentralbl. Chir.* 102:1194, 1977.
44. Lankisch, P. G., Siewert, J. R., and Jennewein, H. M. Trophischer Einfluß des Gastrins auf Magen- und Pankreassekretion beim Hund. *Verh. Dtsch. Ges. Verdauungs Stoffwechselkr.* 31:25, 1976.
45. Lepsien, G., Weiser, H. F., and Siewert, J. R. Die Rolle des Duodenums in der Regulation des unteren Oesophagussphinkters (UOS). *Langenbecks Arch. Chir.* (Suppl. 77):231, 1977.
46. Localio, S. A., and Dwyer, W. The results of adequate gastrectomy with gastroduodenostomy. *Surg. Gynecol. Obstet.* 108:207, 1959.
47. Madsen, P., and Kronberg, O. Recurrent ulcer 5 ½–8 years after highly selective vagotomy without drainage and selective vagotomy with pyloroplasty. *Scand. J. Gastroenterol.* 15:193, 1980.
48. Madsen, P., Kronberg, O., Hart-Hansen, O., and Pedersen, T. Billroth I gastric resection versus truncal vagotomy and pyloroplasty in the treatment of gastric ulcer. *Acta Chir. Scand.* 142:151, 1976.
49. McGregor, I. L., Deveney, C., Way, L. W., and Meyer, J. H. The effect of acute hyperglycemia on meal-stimulated gastric, biliary and pancreatic secretion, and serum gastrin. *Gastroenterology* 70:197, 1976.
50. McKeown, K. D. A study of peptic ulcer. *Br. J. Surg.* 57:131, 1970.
51. Mellström, D., and Rundgren, Å. Long-term effects after partial gastrectomy in elderly men. *Scand. J. Gastroenterol.* 17, 433, 1982.
52. Moloney, G. E. Back to Billroth I: A comparison of results of Billroth I and II operations. *Br. Med. J.* 1:1186, 1954.
53. Nielsen, J., Amdrup, E., Christiansen, P., et al. Gastric ulcer. II. Surgical treatment. *Acta Chir. Scand.* 139:460, 1973.
54. Nilsell, K. Five to nine years' results of selective proximal vagotomy with and without pyloroplasty for duodenal ulcer. *Acta Chir. Scand.* 145:251, 1979.
55. Nyhus, L. M. Evaluation of the Billroth I gastric resection. *Am. J. Dig. Dis.* 7:224, 1962.
56. Ordahl, N. B., Ross. F. P., and Baker, D. V., Jr. The failure of partial gastrectomy with gastroduodenostomy in the treatment of duodenal ulcer. *Surgery* 38:158, 1955.
57. Paakonen, M., Alhava, E. M., and Karjalainen, P. Bone mineral and intestinal calcium absorption after partial gastrectomy. *Scand. J. Gastroenterol.* 17:369, 1982.
58. Peitsch, W., and Becker, H. D. Was ist gesichert in der Pathogenese und Häufigkeit des primären Carcinoms im operierten Magen? *Chirurg* 50:33, 1979.
59. Peitsch, W., and Burkhardt, K. Zur Pathogenese und Klinik des Magenstumpfcarcinoms. *Langenbecks Arch. Klin. Chir.* 341:195, 1976.
60. Postlethwait, R. W. Five year follow-up results of operations for duodenal ulcer. *Surg. Gynecol. Obstet.* 137, 387, 1973.
61. Pulimood, B. M., Knudsen, A., and Coghill, N. F. Gastric mucosa after partial gastrectomy.

Gut 17, 463, 1976.
62. Redwitz, E. v. Cited in A. Kiczián. Modifizierte Billroth-I-Resektion. *Chirurg* 28:363, 1957.
63. Rothmund, M. Therapeutisches Prinzip: Resektion. In A. L. Blum and J. R. Siewert (Eds.), *Ulcus-Therapie*. Berlin, Heidelberg, New York: Springer, 1982. Pp. 418–49.
64. Rutledge, R. W. In commemoration of Theodor Billroth on the 150th anniversary of this birth. *Surgery* 86:672, 1979.
65. Sapala, J. A., and Ponka, J. Operative treatment of benign gastric ulcers. *Am. J. Surg.* 125:19, 1973.
66. Schattenmann, G., Ebert, R., Greutzfeld, W., and Siewert, J. R. Die Bedeutung des Duodenums und Jejunums für die nahrungsinduzierte GIP-Freisetzung. *Langenbecks Arch. Chir.* 28:141, 1981.
67. Schmid, E., Adlung, J., Belohlavek, D., et al. Anastomosenulcera als Spätkomplikationen des Billroth-I- und Billroth-II-Magens. *Z. Gastroenterol.* 15:626, 1977.
68. Schuemann, V. Zur Behandlung des perforierten Magen-Zwölffingerdarmgeschwüres. *Zentralbl. Chir.* 78:1945, 1953.
69. Schumpelick, V., Begemann, F., Peterhoff, G., and Flashoff, D. Reflux und Refluxkrankheit im Resektionsmagen. *Langenbecks Arch. Chir.* 348:61, 1979.
70. Schumpelick, V., and Schassan, H. H. Bakteriologie des operierten Magens. *Langenbecks Arch. Chir.* 350:271, 1980.
71. Schumpelick, V., and Schreiber, H. W. Chirurgie des Magens. *Med. Welt* 27:2442, 1976.
72. Sekine, T., Sato, T., Maki, T., and Shiratori, T. Pylorus-preserving gastrectomy for gastric ulcer. *Surgery* 77:92, 1975.
73. Semb, L. S. Billroth I Gastrectomy. In L. M. Nyhus and C. Wastell (Eds.), *Surgery of the Stomach and Duodenum* (3d ed.). Boston: Little, Brown, 1978.
74. Semb, L. S., Monclair, T., and Brunsgaard, C. Partial gastrectomy with gastroduodenal anastomosis with or without truncal vagotomy in the treatment of peptic ulcer. *Acta Hepatogastroenterol.* 20:178, 1973.
75. Shingelton, W. W., Floyd, I. K., and Sonders, A. P. Studies on postgastrectomy steatorrhea using radioactive triolein and oleic acid. *Surgery* 42:12, 1957.
76. Siebert, H., Werner, E., Schmidt-Gayk, K., and Pannike, A. *Calcif. Tissue Res.* (Suppl.)27:43, 1979.
77. Siewert, J. R. Chirurgische Verfahrenswahl: Billroth I oder Billroth II. In H. D. Becker and H. J. Peiper (Eds.), *Ulcus Ventriculi*. Stuttgart: Thieme, 1977.
78. Siewert, J. R. Operative Therapie des unkomplizierten Ulcus ventriculi. In M. Allgoewer, F. Harder, L. F. Hollender, H.-J. Peiper, and J. R. Siewert (Eds.), *Chirurgische Gastroenterologie*. Berlin, Heidelberg, New York: Springer, 1981. Pp. 436–50.
79. Siewert, J. R., and Bauer, H. Therapeutisches Prinzip: Vagotomie. In A. L. Blum, and J. R. Siewert (Eds.), *Ulcus-Therapie*. Berlin, Heidelberg, New York: Springer, 1982. Pp. 355–97.
80. Siewert, J. R., and Hinder, R. A. Der operierte Magen. In L. Demling (Ed.), *Klinische Gastroenterologie*. Stuttgart: Thieme, 1984. Pp. 429–40.
81. Siewert, J. R., Schattenmann, G., and Ebert, R. Importance of the Duodenal Passage Following Gastrectomy. In C. Herfarth and P. Schlag (Eds.), *Gastric Cancer*. Berlin, Heidelberg, New York: Springer, 1979.
82. Siewert, J. R., Stuhler, T., Koch, A., and Wallat, H. Cardiafunktion und gastrooesophagealer Reflux nach distaler Magenresektion. *Z. Gastroenterol.* 12:583, 1974.
83. Stuecker, F. J., Larena, A., Hoffmann, K., and Zumtobel, V. Frühe und späte Reinterventionen nach Resektion wegen Gastro-Duodenalulcus. *Chirurg* 44:7, 1973.
84. Teigan, T., Liavåg, J., and Roland, M. Pylorus preserving gastric resection for gastric ulcer. *Acta Chir. Scand.* 144:249, 1978.
85. Thomas, P. A., and Earlam, R. J. The gastroesophageal junction before and after operations for duodenal ulcer. *Br. J. Surg.* 60:717, 1973.
86. Thomas, W. E. G., Thompson, M. H., and Williamson, R. C. N. The long-term outcome of Billroth I partial gastrectomy for benign gastric ulcer. *Ann. Surg.* 195:189, 1982.
87. Tovey, F. I., and Clark, C. G. Anemia after partial gastrectomy: A neglected curable condition. *Lancet* 1:956, 1980.
88. Tymper, F., Roesch, W., Domschke, W., and Demling, L. The functions of the exocrine pancreas after exogenous and endogenous stimulation in Billroth II patients. *Acta Hepatogastroenterol.* 23:444, 1976.
89. Wallensteen, S. Results of the surgical treatment of peptic ulcer by partial gastrectomy, according to Billroth I and Billroth II methods: A clinical study based on 1256 operated cases. *Acta Chir. Scand.* (Suppl. 191):1, 1954.

90. Wallensteen, S., and Goethmann, L. An evaluation of the Billroth I operation for peptic ulcer. *Surgery* 33:1, 1953.
91. Walters, W., and Lynn, T. E. Results of 237 Billroth I gastric resections for peptic ulcer: A 6- to 15-year follow-up. *Ann. Surg.* 144:464, 1956.
92. Walters, W., and Lynn, T. E. The B-I and B-II operation: Comparison of results six to ten years after operation for gastric, duodenal and gastrojejunal ulcers. *Arch. Surg.* 74:680, 1957.
93. Werner, B., Leppin, A., and Seiler, J. Duodenaler Reflux und Gastritis im Billroth-I-Magen. *Dtsch. Med. Wochenschr.* 100:2385, 1975.
94. Winkler, R., Farthmann, E., and Eichfuss, H. P. Die B-I-Resektion in der Ulcuschirurgie. *Langenbecks Arch. Chir.* 343:123, 1977.

SPECIAL COMMENT
Billroth I Gastrectomy

Herbert L. Duthie

In my practice Billroth I gastrectomy is used mainly for the treatment of simple gastric ulcer unassociated with duodenal ulcer; my colleagues and I have been comparing its outcome with that of more conservative operations during the past 15 years. The pressure to change arose from the general trend to avoid resection in the primary surgical treatment of peptic ulceration, combined with initially encouraging reports of the use of vagotomy and drainage for gastric ulcer. Two prospective, randomized, controlled trials have been undertaken. In the first, standard Billroth I gastrectomy was compared with vagotomy and pyloroplasty [2]; in the second, Billroth I gastrectomy was compared with proximal gastric vagotomy (highly selective vagotomy). In these trials prepyloric ulcers were excluded, as were gastric ulcers combined with duodenal ulcers.

As might be expected, significantly less morbidity was found after the more conservative operations. There were no deaths. Specimens for histological examination of the ulcer in the vagotomy groups were obtained by excising the edge of the ulcer in the first trial and by excising the whole ulcer in the second trial. Initially all patients obtained symptomatic relief, and the impression was that results after Billroth I gastrectomy were more likely to be excellent than after vagotomy and pyloroplasty (Table 9-10). In fact, up to three years postoperatively there was statistical support for this concept. However, this distinction was blurred with the passage of time, and at five years no significant difference was found between the groups in percentage of functional results. The disturbing feature of the conservative surgical treatment was the frequent need for another operation. Seven of the 50 patients after vagotomy and pyloroplasty had a later gastrectomy—1 for bleeding, 4 for recurrent ulcer, and 2 for gastric cancer. At this stage it appeared that Billroth I gastrectomy had maintained its place against the more conservative operation, which still could be useful when resection would be technically difficult, for example, for an ulcer high on the lesser curvature.

Table 9-10. Gastric ulcer trial I: percentage of functional results

Operation	Follow-up period (yr)	Functional results (%) Good	Fair	Poor
Billroth I gastrectomy	1	92	8	0
	3	88	7	5
	5	78	14	8
Truncal vagotomy and pyloroplasty	1	78	13	9
	3	60	20	20
	5	68	12	20

It might seem rather obstinate at this stage to proceed with another comparison involving a vagotomy procedure. However, my group was of the opinion that the results could be improved by using proximal gastric vagotomy (highly selective vagotomy) without pyloroplasty. This procedure was expected to prevent an increase in biliary reflux after operation, and since reflux of duodenal content is held to be one of the main causative factors in gastric ulcer, it seemed reasonable to assume that there would be less recurrent ulceration. Another potential benefit in the avoidance of a pyloroplasty would be the reduction in postoperative symptoms connected with altered gastric emptying, such as dumping and diarrhea. However, it must be stated that the latter symptoms had not been a cause of failure of vagotomy and pyloroplasty in the first series. The other change in technique in the second series was to excise the full thickness of the stomach wall in an area 1 cm around the ulcer. Full histological examination could then be done and the possibility of overlooking a cancer could be eliminated.

The length of the follow-up period in the second series is now an average of eight years, and both procedures show a high recurrent ulcer rate—23 percent after proximal gastric vagotomy with excision of the ulcer and 17 percent after Billroth I gastrectomy. The functional results have shown no significant differences up to four years [1], but the figures at eight years show a difference in favor of proximal gastric vagotomy [5] (Table 9-11); the poor results after Billroth I gastrectomy were divided almost equally between recurrent ulcer and postprandial symptoms, whereas nearly all those after proximal gastric vagotomy were attributed to recurrences.

Because one of the objectives of these studies was to assess the general applicability of the more conservative methods, all grades of surgeons were involved in the trial, not only those with extensive experience of the newer forms of vagotomy. However, most of the operations were performed by consultants who had used proximal gastric vagotomy in the management of duodenal ulcer for at least one year before taking part in the study. The main disappointment has been the high rate of recurrent ulcer in both groups [3]. Certainly much better results have been achieved by surgeons treating consecutive series of patients. For example, Johnston in Leeds [4] has a personal series of 30 instances after proximal gastric vagotomy and ulcer excision with only one recurrence on a 5- to 12-year follow-up study; of a total of 70 patients treated in his unit, only 4 (6 percent) have recurrent ulcers.

Table 9-11. Gastric ulcer trial II: percentage of functional results

Operation	Follow-up period (yr)	Functional results (%)		
		Good	Fair	Poor
Billroth I gastrectomy	1	76	12	12
	3	76	20	4
	4	74	15	11
	8	52	12	36
Proximal gastric vagotomy and ulcer excision	1	81	19	0
	3	88	8	4
	4	78	0	22
	8	71	0	29

The overall symptomatic result was good in 84 percent of the patients. In addition, a series of Billroth I gastrectomy patients followed for 9.4 years showed a good result in 84 percent, with 3.5 percent having recurrent ulcers [6].

One of the main indications for a conservative operation is to avoid the technical difficulty of a gastrectomy for lesser curvature ulcers near the cardia. The so-called conservative procedure has now been so complicated by including excision of the ulcer that the advantage is seriously diminished, if not lost. This fact is underlined by the exclusion from the trial at operation of eight patients, either because of a strong suspicion of malignant tumor when they had a gastrectomy (six patients) or because of technical difficulty with proximal gastric vagotomy and excision of the ulcer when they had a truncal vagotomy and pyloroplasty (two patients). In a patient with such an ulcer near the cardia, it would probably be sensible to do an open biopsy at operation and to submit it for immediate histological examination. If it is benign, the ulcer can then be left in situ and either gastrectomy or vagotomy can be used.

In summary, my associates and I have compared Billroth I gastrectomy with two types of vagotomy in more than 170 patients with simple gastric ulcer over 15 years. The potential advantage of the more conservative procedures in avoiding mortality did not materialize, since no patient died within one month of the operation. Recurrent ulcers have been more frequent than in many other series, but the long-term follow-up study shows a shift to favor proximal gastric vagotomy with ulcer excision.

Comment References

1. Duthie, H. L., and Bransom, C. J. Highly selective vagotomy with excision of the ulcer compared with gastrectomy for gastric ulcer in a randomised trial. *Br. J. Surg.* 66:43, 1979.
2. Duthie, H. L., and Kwong, N. K. Vagotomy or gastrectomy for gastric ulcer. *Br. Med. J.* 4:79, 1973.
3. Greenall, M. J., and Lehnert, T. Vagotomy or gastrectomy for elective treatment of benign gastric ulceration? *Dig. Dis. Sci.* 301:353, 1985.
4. Johnston, D. Highly selective vagotomy for gastric ulcer 1982 (personal communication).
5. Reid, D. A., Duthie, H. L., Bransom, C. J., and Johnson, A. G. Late follow-up of highly selective vagotomy with excision of ulcer compared with Billroth I gastrectomy for treatment of benign gastric ulcer. *Br. J. Surg.* 69:605, 1982.
6. Thomas, W. E. G., Thompson, M. H., and Williamson, R. C. N. Long term outcome of Billroth I partial gastrectomy for benign gastric ulcer. *Ann. Surg.* 195:189, 1982.

EDITOR'S COMMENT

The Billroth I gastrectomy has an important place in the history of gastric surgery, but it is used now only for benign gastric ulcer, and when combined with vagotomy, for chronic duodenal ulcer. It is a most elegant technique, demonstrating a perfect harmony between anatomical surgery and the physiological result that is achieved. Thus the strip of mucosa along the lesser curvature of the stomach in which a gastric ulcer is most likely to occur is removed, and at the same time the antrum with its contained G cells is also excised.

One of the problems never adequately dealt with when considering the use of Billroth I gastrectomy with vagotomy for chronic duodenal ulcer is the difficulty of the dissection and anastomosis of a distorted and inflamed duodenum. Accounts of series of patients treated by this method sometimes seem to suggest that the very much lower recurrence rate is obtained at no cost. Billroth I gastrectomy in a patient with a severe, active duodenal ulcer can be an extremely difficult and therefore dangerous operation. Unfortunately it is probably in this very situation, with a severe duodenal ulcer diathesis, that this type of procedure is indicated. Duodenal closure is easier than anastomosis; therefore, why not perform the operation of vagotomy with a Billroth II procedure? There are theoretical, practical, and metabolic reasons why the Billroth I operation is preferred. The crux of the problem lies in our inability to identify patients (excluding those with the Zollinger-Ellison syndrome) who will have recurrent ulcers after lesser procedures such as proximal gastric vagotomy. If we could identify such patients, the extra time and risks involved in performing the combined operation of vagotomy and Billroth I resection would be acceptable.

The Jammer Ecke, or angle of sorrow, is mentioned several times by Dr. Siewert. This is the point at which the Schoemaker closure of the lesser curvature meets the duodenum. Early in the experience with this technique, an anastomotic leak was frequent. Finsterer suggested a buttressing suture at the corner, and placing this suture has removed the danger of breakdown. A single suture with two bites to the stomach and one bite to the duodenum will suffice to infold the corner.

The concern for carcinoma developing in the retained gastric pouch years after resection is probably overstated. At least in the United States, this serious complication failed to materialize in a careful study of the problem at the Mayo Clinic (*N. Engl. J. Med.* 309:1210, 1983).

C. W.

IV

Duodenal Ulcer

10

Chronic Duodenal Ulcer

Christopher Wastell

Duodenal ulcer is distinct from all the other ulcers of the gastrointestinal tract that occur in contact with luminal acid and pepsin. Papers are still being written that include the results of a particular form of treatment for duodenal, prepyloric, and even gastric ulcer as if there were no distinction among these conditions. Duodenal ulcer and gastric ulcer are two distinct diseases with different frequencies, pathophysiologies, and treatments. Other "peptic" ulcers, such as those in the lower esophagus, Meckel's diverticulum, and gastrojejunal junction after operation, are clearly separate.

Diagnosis of Duodenal Ulcer

The answer to the question, "Is a duodenal ulcer present?" at first seems to be simple. The question asks whether there is an ulcer in which the surface mucosa is breached and in which the base extends down to the muscularis mucosa. The problem in answering it is related, first, to the difficulty of inspecting in vivo the whole of the duodenal mucosa; second, to the fact that the disease is remittent; and third, to the unreliability of the symptomatology [15]. Thus an ulcer may be present one week and may have healed the next, with or without indigestion.

The problem of diagnosis amounts really to a problem of definition, particularly when the question of recurrent ulceration after operation is being considered (see Chap. 13). Since the appearance of the third edition of this book, articles [119] have appeared that define the term *recurrence;* we have attempted our own definition, also in Chapter 13. The follow-up assessment after surgical treatment of duodenal ulcer is notoriously difficult [32]. Patients attending follow-up clinics may complain of indigestion. If endoscopy reveals only an "inflamed" duodenal mucosa, perhaps with an inadequate examination of the whole of the first part of the duodenum, and if a barium meal examination shows distortion of the duodenum because of the previous documented ulceration, at what point does the diagnosis of recurrent ulcer truly apply? If on later review the symptoms have abated, it is difficult to record the patient as having an active ulcer.

SYMPTOMS OF DUODENAL ULCER

The pain of duodenal ulcer, which may be extremely severe, is usually epigastric, although it may extend through to the back if the ulcer is posterior. Initially the pain is relieved by either food or alkalis, but as time passes the relief that these agents give is much less certain and of a shorter duration. The pain commonly wakes the patient at night, often at about 2 A.M. Typically a patient loses little time from work. When the patient is admitted to the hospital, the symptoms usually disappear within hours. When symptoms first occur they usually are troublesome for several hours each day for a period of one or two weeks. This experience is followed by a remission period, often extending for several months. The cylce is then repeated, with the difference that the episodes of pain become longer and the periods of remission shorter.

It bears emphasis that the principal symptom of chronic duodenal ulcer is pain. All other abdominal symptoms, such as nausea and a feeling of being bloated, the variable site of the pain, and symptoms occuring in other areas and systems tend to detract from the diagnosis. The pain probably originates from the ulcer and its margins, as was demonstrated by Dragstedt [47] when he instilled hydrochloric acid down a tube sited in the duodenum and found that the symptoms could be "switched" on and off by altering the pH of the contents of the duodenum. It has been claimed that the pain arises from the lower esophagus [53], but others besides Dragstedt have found this not to be so [40]. Heartburn occurs in a number of patients, but it usually follows closely the development of the abdominal pain.

Many patients consult the doctor for the first time after several years of self-medication at home. Chronicity is thus an important feature; there are few other diseases associated with such prolonged, severe symptoms in a patient who is otherwise quite well.

OBJECTIVE METHODS OF DIAGNOSIS

The mainstays of objective diagnosis are the barium meal examination and endoscopy (see Chap. 5). Together these two procedures provide considerable accuracy, whether in the elective situation [10] or when there is hemorrhage [50, 76, 80, 152]. However, as Whitehead points out in Chapter 6, an actual mucosal lesion in the duodenum is merely one event in a process of progressive inflammatory change, and the situation is made more complicated by the fact that the small mucosal lesions undoubtedly heal. The duodenal ulcer diathesis exists when the food-related epigastric pain is caused by inflammatory duodenal changes; a duodenal ulcer exists when these changes progress to the point of mucosal breakdown. In the latter situation the diagnosis can be made with absolute certainty only by endoscopy or direct inspection.

Pathology

ETIOLOGY OF CHRONIC DUODENAL ULCER

Acid Secretion

It has been abundantly recorded that persons with chronic duodenal ulcers secrete on the average more acid at night, while fasting, and in response to food and stimulants than do those without such ulcers [11, 59, 71, 92, 100, 101, 124, 141]. As Wormsley [171] points out in his review, however, except for measurements over a few hours in any one individual, little is known about the actual quantity of acid present in the duodenal bulb because of the technical difficulties in measuring it.

The reason for the secretion of larger volumes of gastric juice containing normal concentrations of acid is still controversial. In postmortem studies, Cox [38] demonstrated that the stomachs of those who had duodenal ulcers were larger, thicker, and more densely populated with parietal cells than normal. Why the number of parietal cells should be increased, at least in some patients with duodenal ulcer, is not known. It has been suggested that there is a form of work hyperplasia, as the hypersecretion has been related to the duration of symptoms [141]. Alternatively, the large numbers of parietal cells may depend on genetic inheritance, which is suggested by the fact that for any individual there is a 30 percent increased risk if a parent or sibling has a duodenal ulcer [43, 45, 64, 156].

It has also been suggested that the gastric hypersecretion is a response to maximal stimulation and that therefore the parietal cell hyperplasia presumably follows and may be dependent on the development of the duodenal ulcer [77]. The Zollinger-Ellison syndrome is associated with hyperplasia of the gastric mucosa [130], and gastrin produces parietal cell hyperplasia in rats [143]; however, the relationship between gastrin and parietal cell hyperplasia has not yet been defined in human beings.

The quantity of gastrin in the antrum in patients with duodenal ulcer is currently a source of disagreement [36]. Fasting blood gastrin levels as measured by radioimmunoassay in patients with duodenal ulcer are reported to be high [30, 74], low [96], or within the normal range [7, 154]. However, there is agreement that levels of serum gastrin are higher after food stimulation in those with duodenal ulcer than in those without [19, 30]. Histochemical and immunofluorescence studies have shown that there is an increase in the number of antral and possibly duodenal gastrin-secreting cells (G cells) [131]. This finding is supported by the observation that if the antral pH is maintained at a constant level by continuous aspiration of acid, vagal stimulation by hypoglycemia induced by intravenous insulin results in elevation of serum gastrin level in duodenal ulcer patients to levels at least twice those in healthy individuals. Another possible factor in sustained gastric secretion is gastrin release from duodenal G cells [145]. Hypersecretion of both gastrin and glucagon has been demonstrated in severely burned patients, who are liable to develop duodenal ulcer [125].

At the present time, therefore, the evidence suggests that in most patients the role of gastrin in the pathophysiology of duodenal ulcer has not been elucidated.

Inhibition of Gastric Secretion

It has been demonstrated that a low antral pH inhibits the release of gastrin from the G cell that is under the influence of stimulation [17, 70]. When placed in the duodenum, acid, fat, and hyperosmotic solutions inhibit gastric acid secretion [22]. This effect must be mediated in part at least by humoral mechanisms, as it persists in spite of extrinsic duodenal denervation. It has been shown that acid secretion has been inhibited by such hormones as secretin [20], cholecystokinin [24], glucagon [34], gastric inhibitory peptide (GIP) [26, 27], and vasoactive intestinal peptide (VIP) [28]. The physiological roles of GIP and VIP have not been established. The quantity of secretin and cholecystokinin required to produce significant inhibition of acid secretion suggests that these hormones do not play an important physiological role in this respect, although failure of secretin release has been shown in duodenal ulcer patients [21]. Much more information is required about the interrelationships of the intestinal hormones before it can be stated that they do or do not have a part to play in the pathophysiology of duodenal ulcer. One abnormality of inhibition has been demonstrated in humans so far: It was found that if the antrum is maintained at a pH of 2.5, the degree of inhibition of gastrin release is significantly less in duodenal ulcer patients than in healthy individuals [160].

Blood Groups

A person with group O blood is more likely to have a duodenal ulcer than one having group A, B, or AB blood in a ratio of 133 : 100 [2]. Furthermore, those who do not secrete the mucopolysaccharide blood group substances in their saliva and other body fluids have an increased tendency toward development of duodenal ulcer when compared with secretors, in a ratio of 150 : 100. In group O patients who are nonsecretors, the chance of duodenal ulceration is more than double that of patients with group A, B, or AB blood who are secretors [14, 110]. Some have found that patients with group O blood without a duodenal ulcer have a higher acid output in response to the augmented histamine test [90], just as group O duodenal ulcer patients who are nonsecretors have a higher acid output than group A, B, or AB duodenal ulcer secretors. But others have found that in those with a duodenal ulcer, maximum acid output does not vary with either the blood group or the secretor status [25, 155].

Apart from the effect on gastric secretion of a particular blood group, it was not found that patients with group O blood underwent operation more frequently than those with other blood groups, but nonsecretors did [99]. In addition, patients with a duodenal ulcer and group O blood more commonly bled and had perforation than those with other blood groups [56].

Smoking
Although smoking cannot be directly incriminated as an important factor in the cause of duodenal ulcer, there is considerable evidence linking smoking with duodenal ulcer. The frequency of smoking was higher in those with duodenal ulcer than in a control population [42, 64], and although the duodenal ulcer patients did not smoke more cigarettes than those in the control group, a greater proportion inhaled. Among doctors with duodenal ulcer, those who smoked had a higher death rate than those who did not smoke [44]. Perhaps one of the main reasons for this is the association between duodenal ulcer and chronic bronchitis, in which smoking may be the causal link [65]. Sputum retention leading to bronchopneumonia is the most common cause of death following vagotomy and pyloroplasty.

Diet
The studies that relate diet and duodenal ulcer are largely unsatisfactory. The high incidence of "peptic" (largely duodenal) ulcers in southern India compared with the incidence in northern India has been ascribed to the difference in diet [105], the effect of diet on saliva production [108], and the effect of saliva production on gastric function [106]. Patients with duodenal ulcer swallow more frequently than do controls [61].

Emotional Factors
It is a belief deeply held by many, including clinicians, that there is a basic personality defect in patients who suffer from chronic duodenal ulcer. It is therefore strange that so little work has been carried out to examine this part of the problem. Baron [13] has reviewed the evidence that any particular personality trait is associated with duodenal ulcer and concludes only that "patients with duodenal ulcers are abnormally anxious but do not show specific personality patterns." When more accurate methods of psychometric testing are developed, this will no doubt be a fruitful area of investigation, as will the entire subject of abdominal pain.

Cirrhosis
It is likely that duodenal ulcer is more common in patients with cirrhosis of the liver, and it is certainly more common after portacaval anastomosis [109].

Atheroma
There may be an association between atheroma and peptic, particularly duodenal, ulcer in that patients with coronary disease were shown to have a higher incidence of duodenal ulcer than would be expected [165]. In addition, patients with abdominal aortic aneurysms have a greater than expected incidence of duodenal ulcer [88]. It has been suggested that the reason for the association is dietary, since ulcer patients drink large quantities of milk, which contains a high fat content.

Renal Transplantation
Dudoenal ulceration is common in patients who have undergone renal transplantation [170].

Incidence of Duodenal Ulcer

There is debate as to whether or not duodenal ulcer is a disease of this century. In his Harveian oration, Hunt [79] considered that the condition existed in the distant past but was largely unrecognized. Albertus [3] (quoted by Jennings [83]) referred to it in 1725 as a rare cause of sudden death, thus emphasizing that it was recognized as a clinical entity. Other reports occurred during the nineteenth century [1, 63, 139, 153], but the impression is that duodenal ulcer was quite rare before 1900.

Moynihan [118] in 1907 was perhaps one of the first to record duodenal ulcer as a separate clinical entity. The steeply rising incidence was recorded in 1929 in Sweden by Bager [9], who analyzed all instances of perforated duodenal ulcer in 50 hospitals between 1911 and 1925. Whereas the incidence in women was constant at between 12 and 25 cases per year, that in men rose from 25 cases in 1911, to over 50 per year in 1914, and then to 125 cases per year by 1925. Watkinson [166] reported the prevalence of duodenal ulcer in Leeds, England, between 1930 and 1949 to be 4.6 percent for men and 1.3 percent for women, the data being obtained from analyses of 13,000 autopsies. This sort of survey is always open to the criticism that the population sample is not representative, but the prevalence nevertheless is similar to that observed by others, e.g., Doll et al. [41], who found it to be 3.1 percent for men over the age of 14.

From mortality statistics it has been found that new duodenal ulcers now tend to develop later in life than previously. Analysis revealed an increasing mortality beginning with those born in the middle of the nineteenth century, with a recent decline [147]. However, in Great Britain the decline in mortality for duodenal ulcer has occurred in association with the decline in the incidence in the male population, for example, in York from 0.3 percent from 1952 to 1954 to 0.15 percent from 1961 to 1963 [134].

The problem of diagnosis of a condition that does not frequently cause death or even require hospital admission was to some extent overcome by two studies of duodenal ulcer in persons medically qualified to diagnose their own ulcers. In the first of these, the incidence of duodenal ulcer in the age range 35–64 fell from 0.21 percent in 1947–1950 to 0.1 percent in 1961–1965 [112]. In the second study the incidence in male physicians in Massachusetts was between 0.25 percent and 0.4 percent in all age groups over 25, and this had been declining for between 10 and 20 years [114].

If perforated duodenal ulcer is considered—and it has been claimed that this constitutes a relatively fixed proportion of all ulcers [140]—there appears to have been a rise in its incidence in Scotland from 1924 to the mid-1950s that was followed by a decline [82, 167]; however, the incidence has now stabilized [111]. The number of perforations in the Oxford area has also declined during the years 1957–1963 [140].

AGE INCIDENCE

In the United Kingdom the peak age incidence seems to be changing; duodenal ulcers are developing at a later age. They are rare in people below the age of 15, and their incidence reaches a peak between ages 35 and 44 in both men and women (Table 10-1). The age incidence is probably the same in much of Europe and North America [98].

To summarize, it would appear that there has been a wave of duodenal ulcers with an increased incidence in men starting in approximately 1920, reaching a peak in 1950–1955, thereafter declining, and now probably stabilizing. This phenomenon has occurred in England, North America, and other parts of Europe. In women the incidence seems to have been stable for approximately two decades.

SEX RATIO

In 1938 the male-female ratio was 4.5 : 1, and the ratio has progressively decreased year by year until currently it is approximately 2 : 1 (Table 10-2) [114, 134]. These figures are mixed in that they are from various locations within the United Kingdom and the United States; in spite of this, they suggest a decreased incidence, in men at least, since the mortality for women has not risen. If the sex ratio for perforation is examined in the same way, it is seen that in 1928 it was 19 : 1 and fell to 5 : 1 by 1967 (Table 10-3). Once again the figures are not precisely comparable because they are not from repeated samples of the same population, but the differences are so

Table 10-1. Distribution by age ranges of patients with new ulcers in the United Kingdom in 1968

Age	Men	Women
15–19	680	221
20–24	2,026	665
25–34	3,713	1,197
35–44	4,274	1,411
45–54	3,985	1,396
55–64	3,095	1,147
Total	17,773	6,037

Source: Data from the *Registrar General's Statistical Review, England and Wales for the year 1968* [137]; the *Annual Report of the Registrar General for Scotland*, 1967 [136]; and C. Wastell [162].

Table 10-2. The male-female ratio for the prevalence of uncomplicated duodenal ulcer since 1938

Author	Year	Male-female ratio
Jennison (U.S.A.) [84]	1938	4.5 : 1
Jones and Pollack (U.K.) [87]	1945	4.7 : 1
Doll et al. (U.K.) [41]	1950	3.0 : 1
Watkinson (U.K.) [166]	1958	3.5 : 1
Pulvertaft (U.K.) [134]	1968	2.8 : 1
Monson and MacMahon (U.S.A.) [114]	1969	1.9 : 1

Table 10-3. The male-female ratio for the incidence of perforated duodenal ulcer since 1928

Author	Ratio year	Male-female ratio
MacKay (1966) [102]	1928	19 : 1
MacKay (1966) [102]	1938	18 : 1
MacKay (1966) [102]	1948	12 : 1
Weir (1960) [163]	1951	9.4 : 1
MacKay (1966) [102]	1958	6 : 1
Sanders (1967) [140]	1967	5 : 1
Donovan (1979) [46]	1979	7.6 : 1

marked as to suggest that a true change is occurring. According to these figures, men seem to be at least twice as likely to have perforated duodenal ulcers as are women, at least in Scotland.

GEOGRAPHICAL AND SOCIOECONOMIC FACTORS

As with variations in incidence within one country, comparison between countries is difficult because of the differences in diagnostic and population sampling techniques. Added to these problems is the well-recognized variation in incidence within one country. For example, in the United Kingdom the incidence of duodenal ulcers is higher in Scotland and lower in southern England; in Nigeria it is higher in the south and lower in the north; it is higher in southern India and lower in northern India; and it varies between different ethnic groups within Uganda, Malaysia, and Indonesia [98]. It is probably true, however, that the differences in incidence within the United Kingdom are reflected in similar differences in Europe as a whole [98].

The World Health Organization in 1956 [117] published comparative mortality statistics for different countries (Table 10-4). Although the rates depend heavily on the conditions of certification of the cause of death and on the type of health care available, it is likely that the standard of care in the countries listed is comparable. Thus the figures quoted probably represent real differences in incidence and prevalence of the disease.

Apart from mortality, duodenal ulcer in India appears to be much more common in younger, poor men and more likely to be complicated by stenosis [103]. In Israel the peak age of incidence is higher and the social class is higher for those affected [172], but the overall incidence seems similar to that in Europe and the United States [113].

OCCUPATIONAL AND SOCIAL FACTORS

In 1950 in England it was reported by Doll and co-workers [41] that there were four groups of occupations in which the incidence of duodenal ulcer was apparently higher than the average. Doctors, unskilled laborers, and work-

Table 10-4. Relative mortality from duodenal ulcer per 100,000 population in men and women for all ages

	Mortality	
Country	Men	Women
England and Wales	9.9	1.9
Sweden	6.1	1.3
Australia	4.8	1.0
United States	4.5	0.9
Italy	4.4	0.6
Canada	3.8	0.7
Netherlands	3.4	0.7
Japan	2.3	0.9
France	0.6	0.1

Source: Data from *Chronicle W.H.O.* [117]

ers in responsible jobs seemed to have a high incidence, while agricultural workers had a significantly lower incidence than expected. However, the diagnosis in doctors often depended on informed observation, and barium meal examinations were undertaken at an earlier stage than is common in the population as a whole. It was therefore concluded that, contrary to previous reports [8, 138], doctors were not more prone to duodenal ulcer than the general population. This observation is strengthened by the fact that mortality statistics in England [135] and the United States [51] do not show an unusually high death rate from peptic ulcers in doctors.

Unskilled laborers appear to have a high incidence, which in the study by Doll et al. was based on bias in selection, since these workers seemed to be employed in this capacity because they had ulcers. However, there have been changes in the mortality from both gastric and duodenal ulcer in the last 50 years: The standardized mortality for men is now higher in the poorer social classes [98].

Business executives and foremen, considered together, underwent operation more frequently than the population as a whole [52]. However, this finding may merely reflect the fact that executives and foremen are more likely to make use of medical services than poorer patients, and the findings may have little bearing on the actual numbers of ulcers within the populations studied. Agricultural workers appear to have had a lower incidence than the general population [41], but this difference was shown to have disappeared, at least in York, by 1963 [134].

When all the changes in incidence in this disease are considered, there are no gross differences between social classes, but there is a significantly higher mortality in the poor. There is a possibility that countries with populations emerging from a largely agricultural, land-based existence to a more highly organized industrial society have a higher incidence of duodenal ulcer that affects younger men. This statement is not based on population surveys but on impressions gained while traveling to such areas as Ecuador, South Africa, the Middle East, and Malaysia, and it is in accord with the observations of Susser and Stein [147]. Why these changes occur is entirely unknown.

Natural History of Duodenal Ulcer

Because up to half the deaths of duodenal ulcer occur as a result of hemorrhage [133], it is important to know which patients are liable to bleed. In 1968 Pulvertaft [134] assessed the risk of hemorrhage according to age, sex, and manner of presentation (Table 10-5). From the data it can be seen that the main risk of bleeding is carried by men and women who have already presented with a previous episode of bleeding. For men there is a 64–75 percent and for women a 30–52 percent chance of rebleeding within a 10-year period, depending on age. (For a detailed description of this complication, see Chap. 15.)

The risks of perforation are less; Pulvertaft [133] presents data in a form similar to that for hemorrhage (Table 10-6). It has been stated [140] that perforation occurs as a constant fraction—11 percent of all duodenal ulcers—but this is at variance with both Pulvertaft's data and that of others. In India, for example, both perforation and hemorrhage seemed to be common complications of the disease [107],

Table 10-5. Risk of hemorrhage from duodenal ulcer (percentages within a 10-year period)

	Percent risk within 10 years			
Presentation	Men under 50	Men over 50	Women under 50	Women over 50
Symptoms	11	24	13	24
Previous hemorrhage	75	64	30	52
Perforation	13	15	—	—

Source: Data from Pulvertaft [134].

Table 10-6. Risk of perforation from duodenal ulcer (percentages within a 10-year period)

	Percent risk within 10 years			
Presentation	Men under 50	Men over 50	Women under 50	Women over 50
Symptoms	4	9	3	7
Hemorrhage	7	3	—	—
Previous perforation	15	13	—	—

Source: Data from Pulvertaft [134].

although admittedly selection may be a factor here (see Chap. 16). Apart from perforation and hemorrhage, chronic duodenal ulcer may result in stenosis of the first part of the duodenum (see Chap. 17).

Continued use of cimetidine over a long period would seem to control the ulcer diathesis at least for as long as five years and presumably longer [68], but this represents suppression rather than an alteration of the natural history. Surgery remains the only way in which the natural history can be premanently changed.

Location of Duodenal Ulcer

Most duodenal ulcers occur in the first part of the duodenum, but ulcers occurring in different locations must be considered also, in particular those occurring just proximal to the pyloric sphincter, those in the pyloric canal, and those distal to the bulb and in the descending and other portions of the duodenum. The classic work of Oi et al. [121, 122] provides some explanations regarding why ulcers may occur in these other areas (see Special Comment). Oi extended the original work of Berger [18] by counting the parietal cells in a series of 20 to 40 biopsies taken from stomachs removed at either operation or autopsy. From this work developed the concept that ulcers, whether esophageal, gastric, or duodenal, occur at mucosal junctions. Gastric ulcers, for example, were found in the pyloric gland area just distal to the fundopyloric mucosal boundary. Some 86 bulbar duodenal ulcers in 71 resected stomachs all conformed to this "mucosal rule"; all were found just distal to the pyloroduodenal boundary. Oi's studies were extended to consider the effect on the mucosa of the underlying gastroduodenal musculature. By gross observation it was concluded that there were two zones particularly liable to kinetic strain: an upper strain zone and a lower strain zone, which corresponded with the usual location of gastric ulcers and duodenal ulcers, respectively. All the duodenal ulcers of patients in Oi's study corresponded not only with the mucosal boundary rule but also with the muscular rule. Oi's theory is interesting, and it probably largely explains the localization but not the cause of some duodenal ulcers.

Another important consequence of Oi's work was the finding that the pyloroduodenal mucosal boundary was sharp and distinct and might extend for approximately 2 cm on either side of the apex of the pyloric muscular ring [123]. This provides an anatomical explanation for the prepyloric ulcer that has all the characteristics of a duodenal ulcer: The ulcer is located in duodenal mucosa.

POSTERIOR PENETRATING DUODENAL ULCER

Kirk [95] found that exactly as many duodenal ulcers were anterior as were posterior. The particular danger of the posterior variety is that if they penetrate, they may erode the gastroduodenal artery with consequent severe hemorrhage. Also, their proximity and fixity to the head of the pancreas, the common bile duct, and the accessory duct of Santorini makes damage to these structures a possibility during gastrectomy. Because fewer gastrectomies are performed, however, the problem of the posterior penetrating ulcer has become less now than it was formerly. Nevertheless, it is still occasionally necessary to carry out gastrectomy for either recurrent ulcer or when gastric and duodenal ulcers coexist (for technical details of operative management, see Chap. 14).

POSTBULBAR ULCER

The first postbulbar ulcer diagnosed by roentgenogram was reported by Parturier and Aimard [127]. Five percent of 158 duodenal ulcers in 9000 routine autopsies carried out by Portis and Jaffe [132] in Chicago were more than 5 cm distal to the pyloric ring. Postbulbar ulcers are more prone to bleed [148], cause stenosis [92, 128], require surgical treatment [39], and perforate [129], than other duodenal ulcers, and if they do perforate they may form a retroperitoneal (or, in the patient reported by Britt and Wolf [23], a retrocecal) abscess.

The important point about postbulbar ulcer is that it must not be missed at operation. The point, of course, is that the duodenum at first may look entirely normal and it is only when the second part is carefully inspected or palpated from the inside that the ulcer is found. It is even more vital to make the diagnosis before operation if proximal gastric vagotomy is to be carried out, because the duodenum is neither mobilized nor opened.

PYLORIC ULCER

Pyloric ulcers are in reality ulcers of duodenal mucosa [123]. Such an ulcer may result in gastric retention, which has been termed the *pyloric channel syndrome*. The condition, which may lead to secondary gastric ulceration, has been treated with vagotomy and drainage with good results [29, 55, 120].

Association of Gastric and Duodenal Ulcer

As mentioned at the beginning of this chapter, gastric ulcer is a different disease from duodenal ulcer; nevertheless, they do occur together [85]. In 175 patients with combined ulcers, Welsh and colleagues [169] found a 4 : 1 preponderance of men in whom there was a poor response to medical treatment, and they therefore advocated surgical intervention. Others [164] found that the peak acid output to pentagastrin stimulation in 16 patients with combined ulcers was similar to that in patients with duodenal ulcer alone. These patients were treated by truncal vagotomy and pyloroplasty in 15 instances and gastrojejunostomy in 1 instance, and it was found that at follow-up one to four years later, 14 of the patients were symptom-free.

Duodenal Ulcer and Esophagitis

There is clinical evidence that associates gastroduodenal ulceration with peptic esophagitis [31]. If an ulcer is present, it is frequently proximal to the esophagogastric mucosal boundary and may cause stricture. Esophagitis often occurs in association with gastroesophageal reflux due to incompetence of the sphincter mechanism of the lower esophagus, and in the past it has not resolved satisfactorily when patients were treated by means of acid-reducing operations. Thus this problem is approached by developing a new lower esophageal sphincter by various fundoplications (see Chap. 22).

Indications for an Operation

There are situations in which a decision to operate presents little difficulty. The first of these is pyloric stenosis (see Chap. 17), and the second is perforation (see Chap. 16). Acute, severe hemorrhage requires operation under certain circumstances (see Chap. 15). Very few instances of Zollinger-Ellison syndrome associated with a gastrinoma occur; but those that do may require some form of surgical treatment (see Chap. 18). However, most patients who are considered for an operation have severe, intractable symptoms. These symptoms and the previous history are evaluated, but the decision to operate finally rests on the assessment by the surgeon of the effect of the symptoms on the quality of life of the patient and the relief afforded by medical treatment [104]. Christiansen and colleagues in 1973 [33] found that truncal vagotomy and drainage for ulcerlike dyspepsia in the absence of an actual ulcer did not produce good results. Three of their 24 patients were actually worse after operation, and 15 remained unchanged. By contrast, patients with severe and active ulcers seemed to achieve a more satisfactory result.

What then are the indications of activity? Moore and colleagues [115] suggest that previous perforation, previous hemorrhage requiring transfusion, or progressive pain over two years are primary indications of virulence, and that onset of symptoms under the age of 20 or over 65 or failure of medical treatment were secondary criteria of virulence. If patients had two criteria, at least one of which was primary, they were considered to have virulent, progressive disease. The use of peak acid output is not by itself a good indicator of the subsequent course of events, although a peak acid output above 50 mmol/hr makes an ulcer likely [12] (see Chap. 4). The use of surgery remains a matter of opinion in this group of patients with symptoms only and tends to be decided by consensus between surgeon and patient.

Surgical Treatment

The surgical procedures currently used for uncomplicated chronic duodenal ulcer are as follows: truncal or selective vagotomy with pyloroplasty, gastrojejunostomy, or antrectomy of either the Billroth I or Billroth II type; subtotal gastrectomy of the Billroth II type; or proximal gastric vagotomy. More recently "lesser curve superficial seromyotomy" [149], experimental [151] or modified [159] with posterior truncal vagotomy [150], has been described. Since most of these procedures are discussed in detail later in this book, it would be repetitious to consider here which operation is appropriate to which situation; however, some general comments are appropriate.

Table 10-7 lists the chronology of the development of duodenal ulcer surgery. If this table is examined, it is apparent that during this century the trend has been in the direction of conservatism, from gastrectomy, to vagotomy, to selective vagotomy, to proximal gastric vagotomy, and now to lesser curve superficial seromyotomy. There is thus a spectrum of treatments ranging from those with greater certainty of cure but carrying the penalty of symptoms related to the operation, to those that bring the possibility of recurrent ulcers but with lesser postoperative sequelae.

The crux of the problem in using gastrectomy and vagotomy with drainage for the surgical treatment of duodenal ulcer is the extraordinary difficulty and intractability of the postoperative symptoms of dumping, diarrhea, and bilious vomiting, to mention the most important. To operate on this diathesis with the goal of achieving a nil recurrence rate is to condemn a considerable number of patients to incapacitating symptoms caused by the operation. Unfortunately, vagotomy has come under increasing attack because of its recurrent ulceration rate [97, 144]; most series quote a recurrent ulceration rate of between 5 and 7 percent. At the same time, in excellent trials of gastrectomy versus vagotomy with drainage, the latter has not been shown to be of any advantage with respect to expected postoperative symptoms [66, 67, 93]. Other trials of vagotomy with drainage against antrectomy and vagotomy also have not shown any advantage in the lesser procedure [89]. Perhaps vagotomy with drainage has not had a fair trial because of the tendency for truncal vagotomy to be included in trials when the clear advantage of selective vagotomy has been demonstrated [94, 97]. Following their monograph *After Vagotomy* in 1969 [4], Alexander-Williams and Cox wrote another one entitled *Vagotomy on Trial* in 1973 [37]—another indication that all was not well with

Table 10-7. The development of operations for chronic duodenal ulcer

Year	Type of operation
1884	Gastrojejunostomy (Rydygier, 1884 [139])
1915	Partial gastric resection (von Haberer, 1915, 1933 [157,158]; Strauss et al., 1930 [146])
1943	Vagotomy (Dragstedt and Owens, 1943 [48])
1945	Vagotomy plus gastrojejunostomy (Dragstedt and Schafer, 1945 [49])
1948	Selective vagotomy (Jackson, 1948 [81]; Franksson, 1948 [60])
1947–1952	Vagotomy plus antrectomy (Colp, 1952 [35]; Edwards and Herrington, 1953 [54]; Farmer and Smithwick, 1952 [57]; Smithwick et al., 1961 [142]; Harkins et al., 1953 [72]; Herrington et al., 1959 [75])
1956	Vagotomy plus pyloroplasty (Weinberg, 1956 [167])
1957–1967	Selective vagotomy plus drainage or antrectomy (Griffith, 1960 [69]; Harkins et al., 1967 [73])
1961	Proximal gastric vagotomy plus pyloroplasty (Holle, 1968 [78])
1969	Proximal gastric vagotomy without drainage (Johnston and Wilkinson, 1969 [86]; Amdrup and Jensen, 1970 [5])
1979	Lesser curve superficial seromyotomy (Taylor, 1979 [149])

vagotomy, be it truncal or selective, associated with gastric drainage. Now a third monograph *Vagotomy in Modern Surgical Practice* has been produced by multiple authors in an attempt to collate information on this subject up to 1982. [16].

Into these "troubled waters" has been thrown the new procedure of proximal gastric vagotomy. (Superficial lesser curve seromyotomy is essentially similar to proximal gastric vagotomy when carried out alone, although perhaps not when combined with posterior truncal vagotomy [126], but it is a procedure in its infancy.) Holle [78] carried out the operation first in 1969, but he always combined it with pyloroplasty, a combination that we [163] have found to be a potent cause of dumping. Proximal gastric vagotomy without drainage was then carried out both by Johnston, working in Leeds, and by Amdrup, then in Copenhagen; these two have been powerful advocates of the procedure ever since [6, 86]. It seems clear that serious side effects attributable to the operation itself are unusual. Dumping, diarrhea, and bilious vomiting are rare, and when they do occur, they are mild [163]. Recurrent ulceration whether accompanied by symptoms or not is the problem with proximal gastric vagotomy, leading to the question: When does a recurrent ulcer rate become unacceptable?

OPINION

Recurrence is not the only factor to be considered after operative mortality. Some persistent or recurrent ulcers can be treated, provided there is virtual certainty that the other postgastrectomy symptoms will not occur to a significant degree. As a clinical problem, a recurrent duodenal ulcer is easier to tackle than severe postvagotomy diarrhea or severe dumping.

In both the series from the Leeds/York trial [66] and the study from Glasgow [37] on vagotomy and gastrojejunostomy, consideration of one aspect of the postgastrectomy and postvagotomy with drainage problem was conspicuous by its absence: the metabolic effects of these operations some years later. A proportion of these patients have iron deficiency anemia [161], vitamin B_{12} deficiency, and metabolic bone disease [116]. All these are insidious conditions easily missed on follow-up, but they are of great importance nevertheless. Another, sinister problem is beginning to be recognized after gastrectomy: the development of epithelial dysplasia years after operation. Endoscopic review of 71 patients more than 15 years after a gastric operation [58] revealed 11 with epithelial dysplasia. Three of the lesions were severe and judged to be carcinomas in situ, 1 actually was a carcinoma, and in another patient carcinoma developed 18 months later. These changes were positively related to the degree of acid lowering that would be expected, i.e., greater in Billroth II than Billroth I gastrectomy. Although there can be no certainty, it seems likely that proximal gastric vagotomy will not be followed by this set of complications.

With the current state of knowledge, all procedures that involve interference with the pyloric sphincter carry with them some risk of undesirable sequelae. The development of proximal gastric vagotomy continues and to date is certainly the procedure of choice for most patients.

References

1. Abercrombie, J. *Diseases of the Stomach*. London: Murray, 1830.
2. Aird, I., Bentall, H. H., Mehigan, J. A., and Roberts, J. A. F. The blood groups in relation to peptic ulceration and carcinoma of the colon, rectum, breast, and bronchus: An association between the ABO groups and peptic ulceration. *Br. Med. J.* 2:315, 1954.
3. Albertus, M. *Systema Jurisprudenti Medicae*. Haloe, 1725. Cited in D. Jennings, Perforated peptic ulcer: Changes in age, incidence and sex distribution in the last 150 years. *Lancet* 1:395, 444, 1940.
4. Alexander-Williams, J., and Cox, A. G. *After Vagotomy*. London: Butterworth, 1969.
5. Amdrup, E., and Jensen, H. E. Selective vagotomy of the parietal cell preserving innervation of the undrained antrum. *Gastroenterology* 59:522, 1970.
6. Amdrup, E., Jensen, H. E., Johnston, D., et al. Clinical results of parietal cell vagotomy (highly selective vagotomy) two to four years after operation. *Ann. Surg.* 180:279, 1974.
7. Ardill, J., Buchanan, K. D., and Kennedy, T. L. Fasting plasma gastrin levels in man. *Gut* 12:860, 1971.
8. Avery, H. *Gastric and Duodenal Ulcers*. London: John, Bales & Staples, 1940. P. 30.
9. Bager, B. Beitrag zur Kenntnis über Vorkommen, Klinik und Behandlung von perforierten Magen und Duodenalgeschwuren nebst einer Undersuchung über die Spatresultatie nach verschiedenen Operations methoden. *Acta Chir. Scand.* 64(Suppl.):11, 1929.
10. Barnes, R. J., Gear, M. W. L., Nicola, A., and Dew, A. B. Study of dyspepsia in a general practice as assessed by endoscopy and radiology. *Br. Med. J.* 4:214, 1974.
11. Baron, J. H. The relationship between basal and maximum acid output in normal subjects and patients with duodenal ulcer. *Clin. Sci.* 24:35, 1963.
12. Baron, J. H. An assessment of the augmented histamine test in the diagnosis of peptic ulcer. *Gut* 4:243, 1963.
13. Baron, J. H. Aetiology of Chronic Duodenal Ulcer. In C. Wastell (Ed.), *Westminster Hospital Symposium on Chronic Duodenal Ulcer.* London: Butterworth, 1974. Pp. 19–52.
14. Baron, J. H. Gastric Function Tests. In C. Wastell (Ed.), *Westminster Hospital Symposium on Chronic Duodenal Ulcer.* London: Butterworth, 1974. Pp. 82–114.
15. Baron, J. H. Ulcers and Symptoms. In J. H. Baron, J. Alexander-Williams, M. Allgöwer, et al. (Eds.), *Vagotomy in Modern Surgical Practice*. London: Butterworth, 1982. Pp. 115–18.
16. Baron, J. H., Alexander-Williams J., Allgöwer, M., et al. (Eds.), *Vagotomy in Modern Surgical Practice*. London: Butterworth, 1982.
17. Becker, H. D., Reeder, D. D., and Thompson, J. C. The effect of changes in antral pH on the basal release of gastrin. *Proc. Soc. Exp. Biol. Med.* 143:238, 1973.
18. Berger, E. H. The distribution of parietal cells in the stomach: Histotopographic study. *Am. J. Anat.* 54:87, 1934.
19. Berson, S. A., Walsh, J. H., and Yalow, R. S. Radioimmunoassay of Gastrin in Human Plasma and Regulation of Gastrin Secretion. In S. Andersson (Ed.), *Frontiers in Gastrointestinal Hormone Research,* Nobel Symposium 16. Stockholm: Almqvist & Wiksell, 1973.
20. Berstad, A., and Peterson, H. Dose-response relationship of the effects of secretin on acid and pepsin secretion in man. *Scand. J. Gastroenterol.* 5:647, 1970.
21. Bloom, S. R., and Ward, A. S. Failure of secretin release in patients with duodenal ulcer. *Br. Med. J.* 1:126, 1975.
22. Bochenek, W., Rodgers, J. B., and Baling, J. A. Inhibition of pentagastrin stimulated gastric secretion by duodenal acidification or administration of fat in normal subjects and in patients with duodenal ulcer. *Am. J. Dig. Dis.* 16:865, 1971.

23. Britt, L. G., and Wolf, R. Y. Postbulbar ulcer with retrocecal abscess: A case report. *Arch. Surg.* 92:98, 1966.
24. Brooks, A. M., and Grossman, M. I. Effect of secretin and cholecystokinin on pentagastrin-stimulated gastric secretion in man. *Gastroenterology* 59:114, 1970.
25. Brown, D. A. P., Melrose, A. G., and Wallace, J. The blood groups in peptic ulceration. *Br. Med. J.* 2:135, 1956.
26. Brown, J. C. A gastric inhibitor polypeptide. I. The amino-acid composition and the tryptic peptides. *Can. J. Biochem.* 49:255, 1971.
27. Brown, J. C., and Dryburgh, J. R. A gastric inhibitory polypeptide. II. The complete amino-acid sequence. *Can. J. Biochem.* 49:867, 1971.
28. Bryant, M. G., Polak, J. M., Modlin, I., et al. Possible dual role for vasoactive intestinal peptide as a gastrointestinal hormone and neurotransmitter substance. *Lancet* 1:991, 1976.
29. Burge, H. W. The aetiology of benign lesser curve gastric ulcer: Vagotomy and pyloroplasty in its treatment. *Ann. R. Coll. Surg. Engl.* 38:349, 1966.
30. Byrnes, D. J., Young, J. D., Chisholm, D. J., and Lazarus, L. Serum gastrin in patients with peptic ulceration. *Br. Med. J.* 2:626, 1970.
31. Casten, D. F., Bernhang, A., Nach, R. J., and Spinzia, J. A physiological basis for the surgical treatment of sliding oesophageal hiatal hernia. *Surg. Gynecol. Obstet.* 117:87, 1963.
32. Cay, E. L., Philip, A. E., Small, W. P., et al. Patient's assessment of the result of surgery for peptic ulcer. *Lancet* 1:29, 1975.
33. Christiansen, J., Aagaard, P., and Kougahl, G. Truncal vagotomy in treatment of ulcer-like dyspepsia without ulcer. *Acta Chir. Scand.* 139:173, 1973.
34. Christiansen, J., and Hendel, L. The effect of glucagon on pentagastrin-induced gastric acid secretion and serum calcium concentration in man. *Scand. J. Gastroenterol.* 8:81, 1973.
35. Colp, R. Recent developments in the surgery of peptic ulcer. *Bull. N. Y. Acad. Med.* 28:785, 1952.
36. Cowley, D. J., and Baron, J. H. The G-Cell Mass in Duodenal Ulcer. In C. Wastell (Ed.), *Westminster Hospital Symposium on Chronic Duodenal Ulcer.* London: Butterworth, 1974. Pp. 99–106.
37. Cox, A. G., and Alexander-Williams, J. *Vagotomy on Trial.* London: Butterworth, 1973.
38. Cox, A. J. Stomach size and its relation to chronic peptic ulcer. *Arch. Pathol.* 54:407, 1952.
39. Cunningham, W. L., del Junco, T., and Wilk, S. P. Postbulbar duodenal ulcer. *West. J. Surg.* 69:26, 1961.
40. Dilwari, J. B., Blendix, L. M., and Edwards, D. A. W. Epigastric pain in duodenal ulcer. *Br. Med. J.* 1:254, 1975.
41. Doll, R., Avery Jones, F., and Buckatzsch, M. M. *Occupational Factors in the Aetiology of Gastric and Duodenal Ulcers with an Estimate of Their Incidence in the General Population* (Med. Res. Counc. Spec. Rep. Ser. No. 276). London: His Majesty's Stationery Office, 1951.
42. Doll, R., Avery Jones, F., and Pygott, F. Effect of smoking on the production and maintenance of gastric and duodenal ulcer. *Lancet* 1:657, 1958.
43. Doll, R., and Buch, J. Hereditary factors in peptic ulcers. *Ann. Eugen.* 15:135, 1950.
44. Doll, R., and Hill, A. B. Mortality in relation to smoking: 10 years observation of British doctors. *Br. Med. J.* 1:1399, 1460, 1964.
45. Doll, R., and Kellock, T. D. The separate inheritance of gastric and duodenal ulcers. *Ann. Eugen.* 16:231, 1951.
46. Donovan, A. J., Vinson, T. L., Maulsby, G. O., and Gewin, J. R. Selective treatment of duodenal ulcer with perforation. *Ann. Surg.* 189:627, 1979.
47. Dragstedt, L. R. Personal communication, 1971.
48. Dragstedt, L. R., and Owens, F. M. Supra-diaphragmatic section of the vagus nerve in the treatment of duodenal ulcer. *Proc. Soc. Exp. Biol. Med.* 53:152, 1943.
49. Dragstedt, L. R., and Schafer, P. W. Removal of the vagus innervation of the stomach in gastroduodenal ulcer. *Surgery* 17:742, 1945.
50. Dronfield, M. W., Langman, M. J. J., Atkinson, M., et al. Outcome of endoscopy and barium radiography for acute upper gastrointestinal bleeding: Controlled trial in 1037 patients. *Br. Med. J.* 284:545, 1982.
51. Dublin, L. I., Spiegelman, M., and Leland, R. G. Longevity and mortality of physicians. *Postgrad. Med. J.* 2:188, 1947.
52. Dunn, J. P., and Cobb, S. Frequency of peptic ulcer among executives, craftsmen and foremen. *J. Occup. Med.* 4:343, 1962.
53. Earlam, R. J. Further experience with epigastric pain reproduction test in duodenal ulceration. *Br. Med. J.* 2:683, 1972.

54. Edwards, L. W., and Herrington, J. L. Vagotomy and antral resection in the treatment of duodenal ulcer. *J. Tenn. Med. Assoc.* 46:8, 1953.
55. Ellis, H., Starer, F., Venables, C., and Ware, C. Clinical and radiological study of vagotomy and gastric drainage in the treatment of pyloric stenosis due to duodenal ulceration. *Gut* 7:671, 1966.
56. Evans, D. A. P., Horwich, L., McConnell, R. B., and Bullen, M. F. Influence of the ABO blood groups and secretor-status on bleeding and on perforation of duodenal ulcer. *Gut* 9:319, 1968.
57. Farmer, D. A., and Smithwick, R. H. Hemigastrectomy combined with section of the vagus nerve. *N. Engl. J. Med.* 247:1097, 1952.
58. Farrands, P. A., Blake, J. R. S., Ansell, I. D., et al. Endoscopic review of patients who have had gastric surgery. *Br. Med. J.* 286:755, 1983.
59. Fordtran, S. S., and Walsh, J. H. Gastric acid secretion rate and buffer content of the stomach after eating. *J. Clin. Invest.* 52:645, 1973.
60. Franksson, C. Selective abdominal vagotomy. *Acta Chir. Scand.* 96:409, 1948.
61. Galloway, S. P., Fonagy, P., and Pounder, R. F. Frequency of swallowing in duodenal ulceration and hiatus hernia. *Br. Med. J.* 285:23, 1982.
62. Gear, M. W. L. Proximal gastric vagotomy versus long-term maintenance treatment with cimetidine for chronic duodenal ulcer: A prospective randomised trial. *Br. Med. J.* 286:98, 1983.
63. Gerard, A. Des Perforations spontanees de l'Estomac. Paris: 1803. Cited in D. Jennings, Perforated peptic ulcer: Changes in age, incidence and sex distribution in the last 150 years. *Lancet* 1:395, 444, 1940.
64. Gillies, M. A., and Skyring A. Gastric and duodenal ulcer: The association between aspirin ingestion, smoking and family history of ulcer. *Med. J. Aust.* 2:280, 1969.
65. Glick, D. L., and Kern, F. Peptic ulcer and chronic obstructive bronchopulmonary disease: A prospective clinical study of prevalence. *Gastroenterology* 47:153, 1964.
66. Goligher, J. C., de Dombal, F. T., Conyers, J. H., et al. Five- to eight-year results of Leeds/York controlled trial of elective surgery for duodenal ulcer. *Br. Med. J.* 2:781, 1968.
67. Goligher, J. C., Pulvertaft, C. H., Irvin, T. T., et al. Five- to eight-year results of truncal vagotomy and pyloroplasty for duodenal ulcer. *Br. Med. J.* 1:7, 1972.
68. Gray, G. R., McWhinnie, D., and Smith, I. S. Five-year study of cimetidine or surgery for severe duodenal ulcer dyspepsia. *Lancet* 1:787, 1982.
69. Griffith, C. A. Gastric vagotomy vs. total vagotomy. *Arch. Surg.* 81:781, 1960.
70. Grossman, M. I. Antral Gastric Inhibitory Mechanisms. In L. S. Semb and J. Myren (Eds.), *The Physiology of Gastric Secretion* (NATO Advanced Study Institute). Oslo: Universitetsforlaget; Baltimore: Williams & Wilkins, 1968. Pp. 352–55.
71. Grossman, M. I., Kirsner, J. B., and Gillespie, I. E. Basal and histalog stimulated gastric secretion in control subjects and in patients with peptic ulcer or gastric cancer. *Gastroenterology* 45:14, 1963.
72. Harkins, H. N., Schmitz, E. J., Harper, H. P., et al. A combined physiologic operation for peptic ulcer (partial distal gastrectomy, vagotomy and gastroduodenostomy): A preliminary report. *West. J. Surg.* 61:316, 1953.
73. Harkins, H. N., Stavney, L. S., Griffith, C. A., et al. Selective gastric vagotomy. *Ann. Surg.* 33:546, 1967.
74. Herring, D. W., and Blair, E. L. Gastrin activity in the plasma of normal subjects and patients with duodenal ulceration. *Br. J. Surg.* 56:707, 1969.
75. Herrington, J. L., Edwards, L. W., Classen, K. L., et al. Vagotomy and antral resection in the treatment of duodenal ulcer: Results in 514 patients. *Ann. Surg.* 150:449, 1959.
76. Hoare, A. M. Comparative study between endoscopy and radiology in acute upper gastrointestinal haemorrhage. *Br. Med. J.* 1:27, 1975.
77. Hobsley, M., Whitefield, P. F., Faber, R. G., and Parkin, J. V. Hypersecretion and length of history in duodenal ulceration. *Lancet* 2:101, 1975.
78. Holle, F. Spezielle Magenchirurgie. Berlin: Springer, 1968. P. 508.
79. Hunt, T. Digestive disease: The changing scene. *Br. Med. J.* 2:689, 1972.
80. Iglesias, M. C., Dourdourekas, D., Adomavicius, J., et al. Prompt endoscopic diagnosis of upper gastrointestinal hemorrhage: Its value for specific diagnosis and management. *Ann. Surg.* 189:90, 1979.
81. Jackson, R. G. Anatomic study of the vagus nerves with a technique of transabdominal se-

lective gastric vagus resection. *Arch. Surg.* 57:333, 1948.
82. Jamieson, R. A. Acute perforated peptic ulcer: Freqency and incidence in the west of Scotland. *Br. Med. J.* 2:222, 1955.
83. Jennings, D. Perforated peptic ulcer: Changes in age, incidence and sex distribution in the last 150 years. *Lancet* 1:395, 444, 1940.
84. Jennison, J. Observations made on a group of employees with duodenal ulcer. *Am. J. Med. Sci.* 196:654, 1938.
85. Johnson, H. D. Associated gastric and duodenal ulcers. *Surg. Gynecol. Obstet.* 102:287, 1956.
86. Johnston, D., and Wilkinson, A. R. Selective vagotomy with innervated antrum without drainage procedure for duodenal ulcer. *Br. J. Surg.* 59:602, 1969.
87. Jones, A. F., and Pollack, H. Civilian dyspepsia. *Br. Med. J.* 1:797, 1945.
88. Jones, A. W., Kirk, R., and Bloor, K. The association between aneurysm of the abdominal aorta and peptic ulceration. *Gut* 11:679, 1970.
89. Jordan, P. H., Jr., and Condon, R. E. Prospective evaluations of vagotomy-pyloroplasty and vagotomy-antrectomy for treatment of duodenal ulcer. *Ann. Surg.* 172:547, 1970.
90. Jori, G. P., Mazzacca, G., Balestreieri, C., et al. Influence of blood group and secretory status on gastric activity. *Am. J. Dig. Dis.* 14:380, 1969.
91. Kaufman, S. A., and Levene, G. Postbulbar duodenal ulcer. *Radiology* 69:848, 1957.
92. Kay, A. W. Effect of large doses of histamine on gastric secretion of HCL. *Br. Med. J.* 2:77, 1953.
93. Kennedy, F., MacKay, C., Bedi, B. S., and Kay, A. W. Truncal vagotomy and drainage for chronic duodenal ulcer disease: A controlled trial. *Br. Med. J.* 2:72, 1973.
94. Kennedy, T. Selective Vagotomy. In C. Wastell (Ed.), *Westminster Hospital Symposium on Chronic Duodenal Ulcer.* London: Butterworth, 1974. P. 213.
95. Kirk, R. M. Site and localization of duodenal ulcers: A study at operation. *Gut* 9:414, 1968.
96. Korman, M. G., Soveny, C., and Hansky, J. Serum gastrin in duodenal ulcer. I. Basal levels and effect of food and atropine. *Gut* 12:899, 1971.
97. Kronborg, O., Malmström, J., and Christiansen, P. M. Comparison between results of truncal and selective vagotomy in patients with duodenal ulcer. *Scand. J. Gastroenterol.* 5:519, 1970.
98. Langman, M. The Changing Nature of the Duodenal Ulcer Diathesis. In C. Wastell (Ed.), *Westminster Hospital Symposium on Chronic Duodenal Ulcer.* London: Butterworth, 1974, Pp. 3–12.
99. Langman, M. J., and Doll, R. ABO blood group and secretor status in relation to clinical characteristics of peptic ulcers. *Gut* 6:270, 1965.
100. Levin, E., Kirsner, J. B., and Palmer, W. L. A simple measure of gastric secretion in man: Comparison of one hour basal secretion, histamine-secretion and 12-hour nocturnal secretion. *Gastroenterology* 19:88, 1951.
101. Littman, A. Basal gastric secretion in patients with duodenal ulcer: A long term study of variations in relation to ulcer activity. *Gastroenterology* 43:166, 1962.
102. MacKay, C. Perforated peptic ulcer in the west of Scotland. A survey of 5,343 cases during 1954–63. *Br. Med. J.* 1:701, 1966.
103. Madanagopalan, N., Subramaniam, R., and Krishnan, M. N. Comparative study of operated cases of peptic ulcer in Madras in the 1940s and 1960s. *Gut* 9:69, 1968.
104. Malagelada, J. R. Medical versus surgical therapy for duodenal ulcer: Making the right choice. *Mayo Clin. Proc.* 55:25, 1980.
105. Malhotra, S. L. Peptic ulcer in India and its aetiology. *Gut* 5:412, 1964.
106. Malhotra, S. L. Protective action of saliva in peptic ulceration. *Scand. J. Gastroenterol.* 2:95, 1967.
107. Malhotra, S. L., Majumdar, C. T., and Bardoloi, P. C. Peptic ulcer in Assam. *Gut* 5:355, 1964.
108. Malhotra, S. L., Saigal, O. N., and Moody, G. O. Role of saliva in the aetiology of peptic ulcer. *Br. Med. J.* 1:1220, 1965.
109. Martini, G. A., and Schmidt, H. A. Gastric Secretion in Chronic Liver Disease. In L. S. Semb and J. Myren (Eds.), *Physiology of Gastric Secretion.* Oslo: Universitetsforlaget, 1968. Pp. 646–56.
110. McConnell, R. B. *The Genetics of Gastrointestinal Disorders.* London: Oxford University Press, 1966.
111. McKay, A. J., and McArdle, C. S. Cimetidine and perforated peptic ulcer. *Br. J. Surg.* 69:319, 1982.
112. Meade, T. W., Arie, T. H. D., Brewis, M., et

al. Recent history of ischaemic heart disease and duodenal ulcer in doctors. *Br. Med. J.* 3:701, 1968.
113. Medalie, J. H., Birnbaum, D., Goldbourt, U., et al. Peptic ulcer history among 10,000 adult males. I. Prevalence and incidence. *Isr. J. Med. Sci.* 8:1673, 1972.
114. Monson, R. R., and MacMahon, B. Peptic ulcer in Massachusetts physicians. *N. Engl. J. Med.* 281:11, 1969.
115. Moore, F. D., Peete, W. P. J., Richardson, J. E., et al. The effect of definitive surgery on duodenal ulcer disease: A comparative study of surgical and non-surgical management in 997 cases. *Ann. Surg.* 132:652, 1950.
116. Morgan, D. B.,and Pulvertaft, C. N. Effects of Vagotomy on Bone Metabolism. In J. Alexander-Williams and A. G. Cox (Eds.), *After Vagotomy*. London: Butterworth, 1969. P. 161.
117. Mortality from ulcers of the stomach and duodenum. *Chronicle W.H.O.* 10:20, 1956.
118. Moynihan, B. G. A. Report on 334 cases of operation for nonmalignant disease of the stomach. *Medchir. Trans.* 90:393, 1907.
119. Mühe, E., Muller, C., Martinoli, S., et al. Five-Years' Results of a Prospective Multicentre Trial of Proximal Gastric Vagotomy. In J. H. Baron, J. Alexander-Williams, M. Allgöwer, C. Muller, and J. Spencer (Eds.), *Vagotomy in Modern Surgical Practice*. London: Butterworth, 1982. Pp. 176–86.
120. Murray, G. F., Ballinger, W. F., and Stafford, E. S. Ulcers of the pyloric channel. *Am. J. Surg.* 113:199, 1967.
121. Oi, M., Hoshiko, S., and Fumatsu, S. A study of the distribution of parietal cells in the human stomach. *Jikei Med. J.* 5:10, 1958.
122. Oi, M., Oshida, K., and Sugimura, S. The location of gastric ulcer. *Gastroenterology* 36:45, 1959.
123. Oi, M., and Sakurai, Y. The location of duodenal ulcer. *Gastroenterology* 36:60, 1959.
124. Orr, I. M. Selective surgery for peptic ulcer: A review. *Gut* 3:97, 1962.
125. Orton, C. I., Segal, A. W., Bloom, S. R., and Clarke, J. Hypersecretion of glucagon and gastrin in severely burned patients. *Br. Med. J.* 2:170, 1975.
126. Oostvogel, H. J. M., and van Vroonhoven, J. M. V. Anterior seromyotomy and posterior truncal vagotomy: Technique and early results of a randomized trial. *Netherlands J. Surg.* 37:69, 1985.
127. Parturier, G., and Aimard, J. Ulcus de la deuxième portion due duodénum: Contribution à la séméiologie objective clinique et radiologique basée sur dix-huit cas. *Bull. Soc. Med. Hôp.* (Paris) 44:1666, 1920.
128. Paterson, D. E., and Hancock, D. M. Duodenal stenosis due to postbulbar ulcer: A comparison of radiological and surgical findings. *Br. J. Radiol.* 31:660, 1958.
129. Pattison, A. C., and Stellar, C. A. Surgical management of postbulbar duodenal ulcers. *Am. J. Surg.* 111:313, 1966.
130. Polacek, M. A., and Ellison, E. H. Parietal cell mass and gastric acid secretion in the Zollinger-Ellison syndrome. *Surgery* 60:606, 1966.
131. Polak, J. M. Endocrine Cells of the Gut. In C. Wastell (Ed.), *Westminster Hospital Symposium on Chronic Duodenal Ulcer*. London: Butterworth, 1974. Pp. 27–52.
132. Portis, S., and Jaffe, R. Study of peptic ulcer based on necropsy records. *J.A.M.A.* 110:6, 1938.
133. Powis, S. J. A., Price, J. J., and Morrissey, D. M. Mortality after vagotomy and pyloroplasty for duodenal ulcer. *Br. Med. J.* 1:142, 1972.
134. Pulvertaft, C. N. Comments on the incidence and natural history of gastric and duodenal ulcer. *Postgrad. Med. J.* 44:507, 1968.
135. Registrar General. *Registrar General's Decennial Supplement, England and Wales*. London: His Majesty's Stationery Office, 1936.
136. Registrar General. *Annual Report of the Registrar General for Scotland* (No. 113). Edinburgh: Her Majesty's Stationery Office, 1967.
137. Registrar General. *Registrar General's Statistical Review, England and Wales for the year 1968* (Part 1). London: Her Majesty's Stationery Office, 1968.
138. Rivers, A. B. Clinical considerations of the etiology of peptic ulcer. *Arch. Intern. Med.* 53:97, 1934.
139. Rydygier, L. Pierwszy Przypade gastroenterostomii w obec zhezenia dwunastnicy pao wrzodzie; wyzdrowienie [gastro-enterostomy in stenosis of duodenum from ulceration, recovery]. *Przegl. Lek.* (Krakow) 23:249, 1884.
140. Sanders, R. Incidence of perforated duodenal and gastric ulcer in Oxford. *Gut* 8:58, 1967.
141. Sircus, W. The Aetiology of Peptic Ulcer. In C. Wells and J. Kyle (Eds.), *Peptic Ulceration*. Edinburgh: Livingstone, 1960. Pp. 11–36.
142. Smithwick, R. H., Harrower, H. W., and Farmer, D. A. Hemigastrectomy and vagot-

omy in the treatment of duodenal ulcer. *Am. J. Surg.* 101:325, 1961.
143. Stanley, M. D., Coalson, R. E., Grossman, M. I., and Johnson, L. R. Influence of secretin and pentagastrin on acid secretion and parietal cell number in rats. *Gastroenterology* 63:264, 1972.
144. Stempien, S. J., Dagradi, A. E., Lee, E. R., and Simonton, J. H. Status of duodenal ulcer patients 10 years or more after vagotomy-pyloroplasty. *Am. J. Gastroenterol.* 56:99, 1971.
145. Stern, D. H., and Walsh, J. H. Gastrin release in postoperative ulcer patients: Evidence for release of duodenal gastrin. *Gastroenterology* 64:363, 1973.
146. Strauss, A. A., Bloch, L., Friedman, J. C., et al. Subtotal gastrectomy for duodenal ulcer: Ten years' experience and clinical end results. *J.A.M.A.* 95:1883, 1930.
147. Susser, M., and Stein, Z. Civilization and peptic ulcer. *Lancet* 1:115, 1962.
148. Swarts, J. M., and Rice, M. L. Postbulbar duodenal ulcer with particular reference to its haemorrhagic tendency. *Gastroenterology* 26:251, 1954.
149. Taylor, T. V. Lesser curve superficial seromyotomy: An operation for chronic duodenal ulcer. *Br. J. Surg.* 66:733, 1979.
150. Taylor, T. V., Gunn, A. A., MacLeod, D. A. D., and MacLennan, I. Anterior lesser curve seromyotomy and posterior truncal vagotomy in the treatment of chronic duodenal ulcer. *Lancet* 2:846, 1982.
151. Taylor, T. V., Holt, S., Andrews, P. L. R., and Heading R. C. Vagotomy by chemoneurolysis: An experimental study in the rat. *Gut* 24:158, 1983.
152. Thoeni, R. F., and Cello, J. P. A critical look at the accuracy of endoscopy and double contrast radiography of the upper gastrointestinal (UGI) tract in patients with substantial UGI haemorrhage. *Radiology* 135:305, 1980.
153. Travers, B. *Medchir. Trans.* 8:231, 1816. Cited in D. Jennings, Perforated peptic ulcer: Changes in age, incidence and sex distribution in the last 150 years. *Lancet* 1:395, 444, 1940.
154. Trudeau, W. T., and McGuigan, J. E. Serum gastrin in patients with peptic ulcer disease. *Gastroenterology* 59:6, 1970.
155. Ventzke, L. E., and Grossman, M. I. Response of patients with duodenal ulcer to augmented histamine test as related to blood groups and to secretor status. *Gastroenterology* 42:292, 1962.
156. Vesely, K. T., Kubickova, A., Dvorakova, M., and Volankova, K. Z. Clinical data and characteristics differentiating types of peptic ulcer. *Gut* 9:57, 1968.
157. von Haberer, H. Meine Erfahrungen mit 183 Magenresektionen. *Arch. Klin. Chir.* 106:533, 1915.
158. von Haberer, H. Meine Technik der Magenresektion. *Munch. Med. Wochenschr.* 80:915, 1933.
159. Walker, W. J., and Taylor, T. V. A modification to the technique of lesser-curve vagotomy. *Ann. R. Coll. Surg. Engl.* 64:123, 1982.
160. Walsh, J. H., Richardson, C. T., and Fordtran, J. S. pH dependence of acid secretion and gastrin release in normal and ulcer subjects. *J. Clin. Invest.* 55:462, 1975.
161. Wastell, C. Long-term clinical and metabolic effects of vagotomy with either gastrojejunostomy or pyloroplasty. *Ann. R. Coll. Surg. Engl.* 45:193, 1969.
162. Wastell, C. Incidence, Appearances and Complications. In C. Wastell (Ed.), *Westminster Hospital Symposium on Ulcer.* London: Butterworth, 1974. Pp. 3–18.
163. Wastell, C., Wilson, T., and Pigott, H. Proximal gastric vagotomy. *Proc. R. Soc. Med.* 67:1183, 1974.
164. Wasunna, A. E. O., Kennedy, F., Gillespie, I. E., and Kay, A. W. Combined gastric and duodenal ulcers managed by vagotomy and drainage. *Lancet* 1:722, 1971.
165. Watkinson, G. Relation of chronic peptic ulcer to coronary sclerosis. *Gastroenterology* 89:292, 1958.
166. Watkinson, G. The autopsy incidence of chronic peptic ulceration, a national and regional survey of 20,000 examinations performed in Leeds, England, between 1930 and 1949 and in nine towns in England and Scotland. *Schweiz. Z. Pathol. Bakteriol.* 21:495, 1958.
167. Weinberg, J. A., Stempien, S. J., Movius, H. J., and Dagradi, A. E. Vagotomy and pyloroplasty in the treatment of duodenal ulcer. *Am. J. Surg.* 92:202, 1956.
168. Weir, R. D. Perforated peptic ulcer in northeast Scotland. *Scott. Med. J.* 5:257, 1960.
169. Welsh, J. S., Floyd, C. E., McKeon, J. A., et al. Combined gastric and duodenal ulcer: Comparison of medical and surgical treatment. *Am. Surg.* 31:590, 1965.
170. Williams, G., and Castro, J. E. Cimetidine in the treatment of peptic ulceration following

renal transplantation. *Br. J. Surg.* 66:510, 1979.

171. Wormsley, K. G. The pathophysiology of duodenal ulceration. *Gut* 15:59, 1974.
172. Yodfat, Y. A population study of peptic ulcer: Its relation to various ethnic and socio-economic factors. *Isr. J. Med. Sci.* 8:1680, 1972.

SPECIAL COMMENT

Duodenal Ulceration: Significance of the Relationship Between Gastric Mucosal Blood Flow and Acid Secretion

L. P. Fielding

The etiology of duodenal ulceration continues to interest clinicians and laboratory researchers, despite the availability of empirical treatments ranging from dietary manipulation and psychotherapy for mild disease to partial gastrectomy for patients having particularly aggressive disease or complications.

Because hydrochloric acid is easily aspirated from the stomach and can be measured under basal, stimulated, or restrained conditions, it has been the central focus of investigatory interest for half a century. This has been true despite the fundamental observation that the population of patients with duodenal ulcer diathesis cannot be differentiated from the normal population (irrespective of any statistical manipulation of the data) based on the measurement of acid secretion alone.

We all accept that the duodenal mucosa has great powers of spontaneous regeneration and repair, and this knowledge has led to the intuitive postulate that the expression of the ulcer diathesis in the form of a duodenal lesion is the resultant breakdown in the normal equilibrium of mucosal erosive factors to those of mucosal resistance. If this is a true statement, it follows that we might be able to identify the duodenal ulcer population by the simultaneous measurement of physiological markers of such "erosion and resistance" factors. It seems that hydrochloric acid is likely to be a principal player in the cast of characters on the "damaging" side of the equation [10, 15a]. By contrast, the agents involved with mucosal protection and repair have been more difficult to investigate. On general grounds, the secretion of mucus has been protective. However, in the laboratory one of the few moieties to influence the damaging effect of hydrochloric acid is the availability of adequate amounts of bicarbonate ions on the submucosal side of the lipid membrane that is the mucosal barrier [18]. This so called alkaline tide is a highly attractive concept supported by considerable evidence. Furthermore, a possible limiting factor to the delivery of such buffering ions at the potential site of damage is the rate of mucosal blood flow.

The thought that blood flow, or the lack of it, is part of the genesis of at least some duodenal ulcers is not new. Virchow [19] stated that mucosal necrosis occurs when the capacity of the mucosa to protect itself against acid fails because of insufficient local blood flow. Moody [14] confirmed this view when he discussed the role of mucosal blood flow in the pathogenesis of peptic ulcer.

Furthermore, the unique work of Piasecki [15] has demonstrated an anatomical area in the duodenum that is relatively oligemic, which coincides with the clinical observation that duodenal ulcer occurs at sites in the first part of the duodenum.

What then is known about the blood flow to the stomach and duodenum and its relation to acid secretion?

Methods of Measuring Gastric Blood Flow

Direct methods to measure gastric blood flow, such as collection of gastric venous drainage [6], radioactive microspheres [1], and indicator fractionation [16], are not applicable to humans, particularly if continuous repeated measurements in a conscious person are required. Indirect methods are therefore necessary. The most widely used indirect method was suggested by the finding that the stomach concentrates various organic bases given intravenously [17]. The authors [17] set out a pH partition theory to explain their findings: Lipid membranes are freely permeable to the undissociated lipid soluble form of the weak base, which is able to diffuse from blood at pH 7.4 into the gastric lumen. At pH 1.0 the weak base gains a proton and cannot diffuse back into the circulation.

This theory was used by Jacobson and coworkers [8] to develop a practical method to measure gastric mucosal blood flow. They showed in dogs that the diffusion of the weak base, amidopyrine, was limited only by blood flow. Therefore, clearance of amidopyrine by gastric juice reflected gastric mucosal blood flow. Later Curwain and Holton [7] used aniline as the clearance marker. Both these markers are too toxic for use in humans, and study of gastric mucosal blood flow in humans remained impossible until a new marker, neutral red, was introduced by Aures and associates [4]. The clearance of this substance, a cationic dye with physicochemical properties similar to those of amidopyrine and aniline, showed good correlation with the clearance of both amidopyrine [4] and aniline [5] when neutral red and an established marker were given together. In humans, however, when neutral red was used alone it failed to give adequate clearance measurements because a metabolite interfered with its estimation [3]; therefore, the marker was abandoned by its originators.

My colleagues and I, however, continued to investigate the use of neutral red because of the strong theoretical possibility that it is an effective marker of gastric mucosal blood flow. We found that when the extraction procedure was changed the problems with metabolite interference were resolved.

The important modification was the substitution of the nonpolar solvent diethylether for the semipolar solvent n-butanol [11]. This simplified method allowed extraction of only that part of the neutral red that was diffusible across the lipid mucosal membrane. Furthermore, we used whole blood because neutral red is distributed in red cells as well as in plasma. When these modified methods were used, clearance values for neutral red, given alone to dogs, correlated well with aniline clearance under similar conditions.

Encouraged by these results in dogs, my associates and I applied the method to humans, first in a small group of healthy volunteers [12] and then in a larger group. We compared these results with those for patients with symptomatic duodenal ulcers. Some of the volunteers and patients were studied again during cimetidine treatment, and 12 of the duodenal ulcer patients were investigated after highly selective vagotomy.

The details of the methods have been described previously for dogs [11], for healthy persons [12], and for patients with duodenal ulcers [13]. In short, the method consists in extraction of neutral red from blood (3 ml) and gastric juice (1 ml) with diethylether at pH 10. Neutral red is then reextracted from ether into O.IM HCl and the concentration measured with a spectrophotometer (Pye Unicam SP1800) at 540 nm. The clearance of neutral red from blood to gastric juice in milliliters per minute was calculated from the following formula:

$$\text{Clearance} = \frac{GV}{Bt}$$

where V = volume of gastric aspirate, G = concentration of neutral red in gastric juice, B = concentration of neutral red in blood, and t = time (15 minutes). Pooled data points were analyzed for skewness and kurtosis and found to be normally distributed. Acid secretion and neutral red clearance, including reproducibility of the method, were analyzed using (1) analysis of variance for population differences and for tests of significance of a single regression line within each group and (2) analysis of covariance for differences in slope and elevation between regression lines for each group [2].

Results

There were 23 volunteers (mean age 36, range 23–59) and 49 patients (mean age 37, range 31–70) in these studies, which were divided into three series. Acid secretion and neutral red clearance were measured simultaneously in each subject.

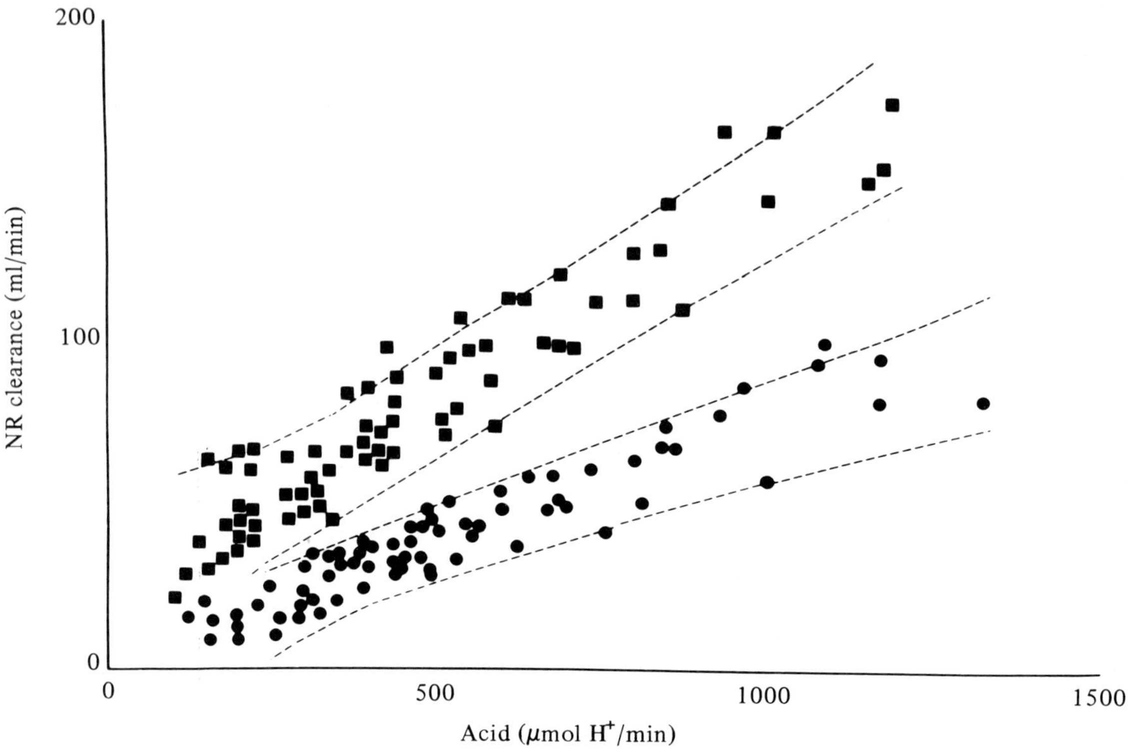

Fig. 10-1. Regression plot of the relationship between acid output and neutral red (NR) clearance for volunteers (*solid squares*) and duodenal ulcer patients (*solid circles*). Each data point represents simultaneous values for acid output and gastric mucosal blood flow at 15-minute intervals during the experiments. The 95 percent confidence limits are shown by the dashed lines for each group. (From McIsaac [13]. By permission of Churchill Livingstone.)

SERIES 1

Twenty-one volunteers and 25 patients received pentagastrin infusion alone for 1.5 hours. There was a linear relationship between clearance and acid output in both groups, but the slope of the regression line was significantly higher for normal volunteers than for patients (Fig. 10-1 and Table 10-8), there being no overlap of the 95% confidence limits during the period of pentagastrin stimulation.

SERIES 2

Twelve volunteers and 12 patients received pentagastrin and cimetidine infusions. Pentagastrin was infused for 2 hours. During the last hour cimetidine was added to the infusate. Acid output in the normal group was reduced by 72 percent and in the duodenal ulcer group by 74 percent; in contrast, neutral red clearance was reduced by 62 percent in the normal group but by only 40 percent in the patient group.

Figures 10-2 and 10-3 show the regression lines in these two groups before and after cimetidine infusion. Thus the relationship between acid secretion and neutral red clearance was different between the two groups. Statistical analysis showed that, in the volunteer group, the slope did not change significantly after cimetidine, although as stated above there was a reduction in both acid and neutral red clearance; the slope ± 95% confidence limits were .154 ± .061 before and .191 ± .071 after cimetidine ($p < .05$). The patient group showed an increase in the

Table 10-8. Regression equation for within-group variance[1]

Group	Correlation coefficient	Slope y = bx + a	95% confidence limits for slope
Volunteers	.80[2]	y = .158x + 21.5	.101–.215
Duodenal ulcer patients	.72[2]	y = .084x + 12.0	.042–.126

[1]Slopes are given with 95% confidence limits.
[2]$P < .001$ different from zero
By covariate analysis for difference between slopes:
$F_{1,82} = 30.4$ $P < .001$
and elevations:
$F_{1,83} = 121.9$ $P < .001$
Source: McIsaac [13]. By permission of Churchill Livingstone.

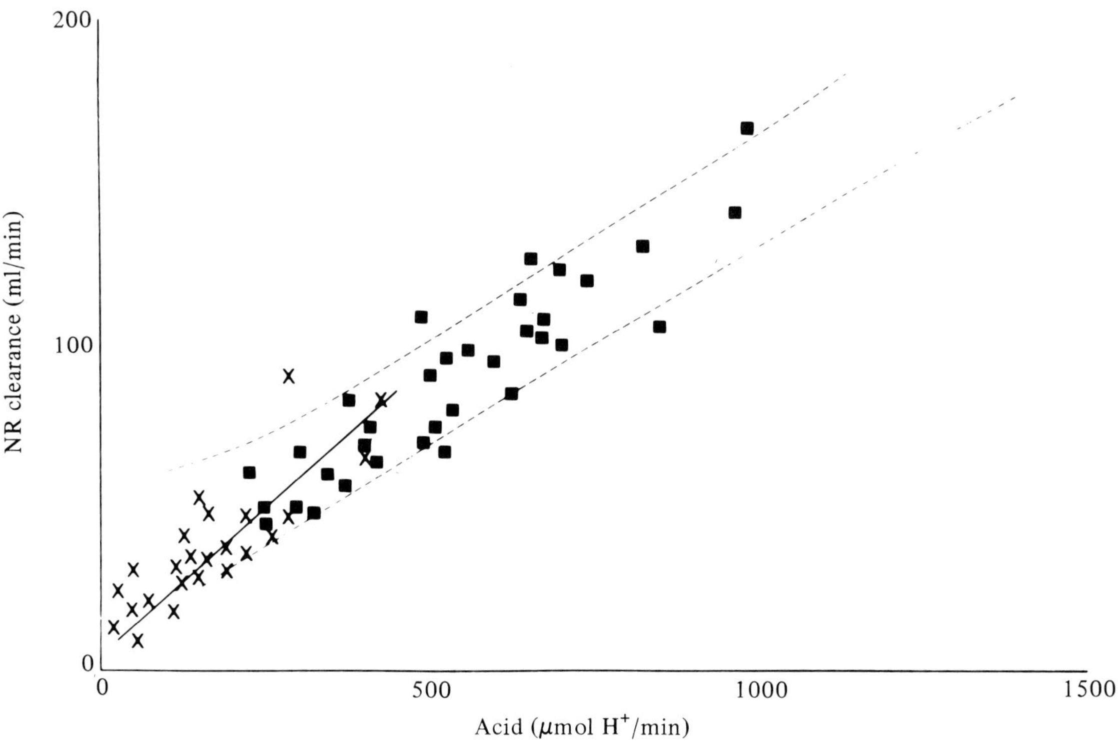

Fig. 10-2. Acid secretion and neutral red (NR) clearance in volunteers before (*solid squares*) and after cimetidine (*crosses*). The 95 percent confidence limits are shown by the dashed lines. (From McIsaac [13]. By permission of Churchill Livingstone.)

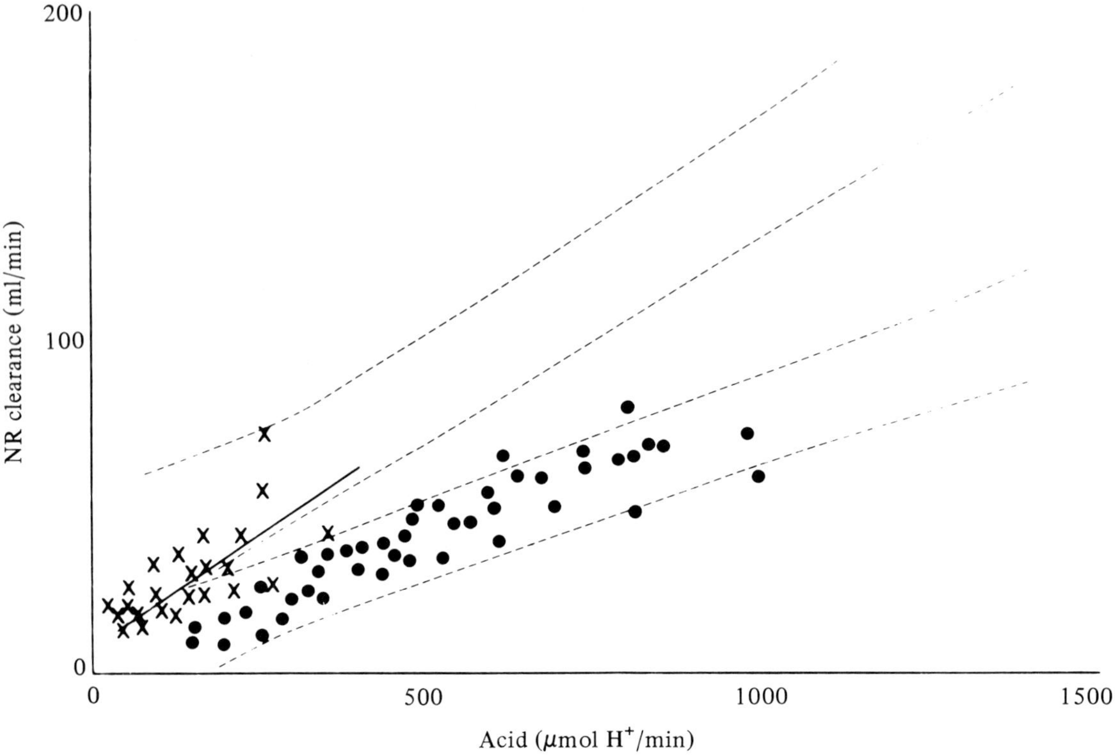

Fig. 10-3. Acid secretion and neutral red (NR) clearance in patients before (*solid circles*) and after cimetidine (*crosses*). The 95 percent confidence limits for the volunteers and the duodenal ulcer groups are shown. (From McIsaac [13]. By permission of Churchill Livingstone.)

regression slope after cimetidine infusion (.084 ± .046 to .210 ± .103, $p < .01$).

SERIES 3

Twelve patients with duodenal ulceration were studied in this series both before and 10–14 days after highly selective vagotomy; the completeness of vagotomy perioperatively was established by mapping of the acid-secreting area with a pH probe after stimulation with pentagastrin. Acid secretion was reduced by half, but neutral red clearance *increased* by one-fifth (Table 10-9). An analysis of variance comparing results before and after surgical treatment showed that changes in both acid output and blood flow were statistically significant. The slope of the regression line increased after the operation from .09 ± .042 to .191 ± .030 (Fig. 10-4), and this postoperative value came to lie in the range of the normal volunteers.

Summary of Experiment

In a series of studies, neutral red clearance was used to estimate gastric mucosal blood flow in humans. Measurement of neutral red clearance and acid secretion together showed a linear relationship between these two variables in healthy persons and patients with duodenal ulcers, but the slope of the regression line for patients was less than the slope for volunteers. After surgical treatment the relation between neutral red clearance and acid in patients increased into the normal range. Stimulation of the parietal cell after vagal section still produced a secretory response to

Table 10-9. Effect of cimetidine on acid output and NRC in normal volunteers and duodenal ulcer patients (mean ± SD)

Measure		Normals	Duodenal ulcer patients
Acid output, μmol min^{-1}	Before	540 ± 207.4	590 ± 195.7
	After	150 ± 113.8	122 ± 105
Neutral red clearance, ml min^{-1}	Before	77 ± 24.3	53 ± 18.5
	After	28 ± 12.6	32 ± 10.7

Source: McIsaac [13]. By permission of Churchill Livingstone.

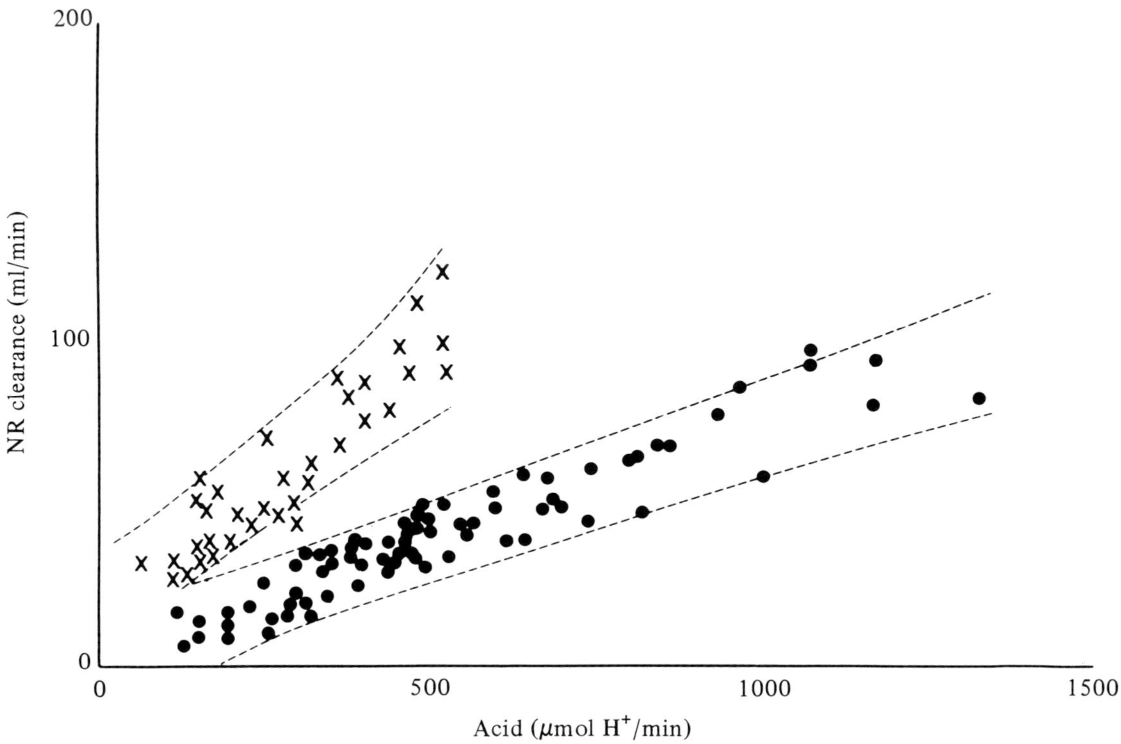

Fig. 10-4. Acid secretion and neutral red (NR) clearance for duodenal ulcer patients after highly selective vagotomy (*crosses*) compared with all duodenal ulcer patients before vagal section (*solid circles*). The 95 percent confidence limits for both groups are shown. (From McIsaac [13]. By permission of Churchill Livingstone.)

pentagastrin, but maximal acid output was reduced by 60 percent; by contrast, blood flow rose into the range for volunteers.

Discussion

The results of this work suggest that duodenal ulcer patients have a unique capacity to secrete acid under pentagastrin stimulation at a relatively low blood flow. Because pentagastrin-stimulated acid production is thought to be mediated by histamine [9], my co-workers and I suggest that the parietal cell is tuned to an increased sensitivity to histamine in duodenal ulcers patients. The ratio of blood flow to acid returns to normal after highly selective vagotomy and points to the vagus nerve as the tuning mechanism. The dissimilar effect of cimetidine to that of vagotomy is less easily understood. Perhaps it will be necessary in the future to look at the parietal cell and microvasculature as an integrated unit, capable of a joint response to stimulation and blockage. Unlike vagotomy, cimetidine diminishes the activity of the whole unit, but the detailed pathways and relative importance of histamine H_1 and H_2 effects must be a subject for further study.

We studied blood flow in the stomachs of patients with duodenal ulcers and cannot, therefore, comment precisely on the possibility, first suggested by Virchow, that reduced blood flow in the duodenum itself may be an important process in the initiation or perpetuation of an ulcer.

From the therapeutic viewpoint, a number of comments and conclusions follow from the data:

1. Vagotomy has been shown empirically to cure patients with symptomatic duodenal ulcer disease in all but a small minority of instances. These data seem to provide a more rational basis for its efficacy: It not only reduces acid output but increases local blood flow, bringing the ratio of these two measurements into the range previously found in normal volunteers.
2. Cimetidine seems to act differently from vagotomy, reducing the sensitivity of the whole system and diminishing both acid secretion and blood flow.
3. In patients who may have other reasons for systemic hypotension or relatively low blood flow to the gastrointestinal tract, the addition of cimetidine to protect the mucosa may be inappropriate because it may further reduce mucosal blood flow, leading to frank ischemia. Thus neutralization with antacids may be more appropriate; this concept coincides with the observation that patients in an intensive care setting are better protected from stress ulceration by the maintenance of gastric pH above 3 with the instillation of alkali than by the use of H_2 blocking agents.
4. Patients who have systemic acidemia (i.e., a reduced acid buffering capacity) will be at greater risk for duodenal ulceration, and every effort should be made to correct the metabolic and respiratory causes of this lowered pH.

The simultaneous measurement of gastric mucosal blood flow and acid secretion seems to confirm, on the basis of laboratory data, the concept of a deranged balance between mucosal damage and protection in patients with duodenal ulceration. Furthermore, the physiological significance of these biological mechanisms seems a fruitful area for additional study; we should assume that these processes are not unique to the stomach and duodenum but are part of many secretory clearance systems in other organs.

This work helps to highlight the need to treat systemic hypotension vigorously to protect against decreases in gastrointestinal blood flow. It is important to ensure that blood flowing to the gastrointestinal tract has a normal pH. Thus adequate buffering will occur and will mitigate the damaging effect of hydrogen ion back-diffusion, with resultant stress ulceration.

Comment References

1. Archibald, L. H., Moody, F. G., and Simons, M. Comparison of gastric mucosal blood flow

as determined by aminopyrine clearance and R-labeled microspheres. *Gastroenterology* 69:630, 1975.

2. Armitage, P. *Statistical Methods in Medical Research*. Oxford, England: Blackwell, 1973.
3. Aures, D., Bauman, H., Guth, P. H., and Grossman, M. I. A metabolite of neutral red that interferes with its use in measuring gastric mucosal blood flow in man. *Gastroenterology* 70:965, 1976.
4. Aures, D., Guth, P. H., and Grossman, M. I. The use of neutral red to measure gastric mucosal blood flow. *Gastroenterology* 68:175, 1975.
5. Chahal, P., and King, J. A. Comparison of neutral red and other markers used for the stimulation of gastric mucosal blood flow. *J. Physiol.* 256:29, 1976.
6. Cummings, J. D., Haigh, A. L., Harries, E. H. L., and Nutt, M. E. A study of gastric secretion and blood flow in the anesthetized dog. *J. Physiol.* 168:219, 1963.
7. Curwain, B. P., and Holton, P. The measurement of dog gastric mucosal blood flow by radioactive aniline clearance compared with amidopyrine clearance. *J. Physiol.* 229:115, 1973.
8. Jacobson, E., Linford, R. H., and Grossman, M. I. Gastric secretion in relation to mucosal blood flow studied by a clearance technique. *J. Clin. Invest.* 45:1, 1966.
9. Kahlson, G., Rosengren, E., and Svensson, S. E. Histamine and Gastric Secretion with Special Reference to the Rat. In P. Holton, (Ed.), *International Encyclopedia of Pharmacology and Therapeutics,* Section 39(a) Oxford, England: Pergamon, 1973. Pp. 41–102.
10. Kivilaakso, E., Fromm, D., and Silen, W. Relationship between intramural pH of gastric mucosa during hemorrhagic shock. *Surgery* 84:70, 1978.
11. Knight, S. E., and McIsaac, R. L. Neutral red as an estimate of gastric mucosal blood flow in dogs. *J. Physiol.* 267:45, 1977.
12. Knight, S. E., and McIsaac, R. L. Neutral red clearance as an estimate of gastric mucosal blood flow in man. *J. Physiol.* 272:62, 1977.
13. McIsaac, R. L., Fielding, L. P., and Knight, S. E. Studies of gastric mucosal blood flow in man: Cimetidine. *The Westminster Hospital Symposium* 20:220, 1979.
14. Moody, F. G. Role of Mucosal Blood Flow in the Pathogenesis of Gastric Ulcers. In P. Holton (Ed.), *International Encyclopedia of Pharmacology and Therapeutics,* Section 39(a) Oxford, England: Pergamon, 1973. Pp. 339–360.
15. Piasecki, C. The role of ischemia in the initiation of peptic ulcer. *Ann. R. Coll. Surg. Engl.* 59:476, 1977.

15a. Ritchie, W. P., Jr. Pathogenesis of acute gastric mucosal injury. Viewpoints on digestive diseases. 15:17, 1983.

16. Saperstein, L. A. Fractionation of the cardiac output of rats with isotopic potassium. *Circ. Res.* 4:689, 1956.
17. Shore, P. A., Brodie, B. B., and Hogben, C. A. M. The gastric secretion of drugs: A pH partition hypothesis. *J. Pharmacol. Exp. Ther.* 119:361, 1975.
18. Simpson, J. N. L., Merhav, A., and Silen, W. Alkaline r-secretion by amphibian duodenum. I. General characteristics. *Am. J. Physiol.* 240:G401, 1981.
19. Virchow, R. Historisches, kritisches, und positives zur lehre der unterleibsaffektionen. *Virchows Arch. (Pathol. Anat.)* 5:262, 1853.

SPECIAL COMMENT
Reappraisal of Subtotal Gastrectomy for Peptic Ulcer

Minoru Oi

My studies regarding the distribution of parietal cells and the location of chronic peptic ulcer on the gastric mucosal layer and the muscular coat were introduced in the previous editions (first to third) of this volume. The material used in these studies consisted mainly of stomachs removed in subtotal gastrectomies for peptic ulcer performed at the Department of Surgery, Jikei University School of Medicine, Tokyo, from 1947 to 1969. The large number of those stomachs, 1750, may indicate the breadth of my experience with subtotal gastrectomy. The period of time over which this experience occurred was concurrent with the prevalence of vagotomy as advocated by Dragstedt in 1943. Vagotomy, however, had never had a pervasive influence on us. Thus subtotal gastrectomy maintained its position as the procedure of choice in dealing with chronic peptic ulcer.

The subtotal gastrectomy my associates and I performed is illustrated in Figure 10-5. It

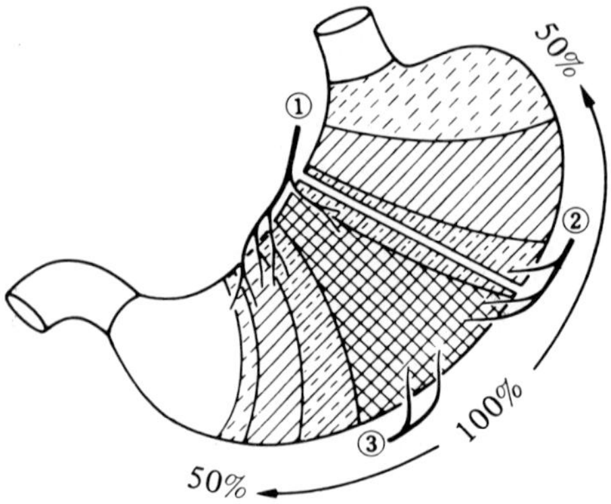

① Left gastric artery
② Left gastroepiploic artery
③ Right gastroepiploic artery
50% ← 100% → 50%
gradient in density of parietal cell distribution

Fig. 10-5. The extent of resection in subtotal gastrectomy as performed at Oi's hospital in Tokyo is shown. There is a gradient in the density of parietal cell distribution: its peak is the portion marked 100% at the middle of the gastric body, and it gradually declines to half (50%) toward both the cardia and the antrum. The resection line is placed on the lesser curvature just proximal to the group of preterminal (not terminal) branches of the left gastric artery and equally, on the greater curvature, just proximal to the preterminal (not terminal) branch of the left gastroepiploic artery. Thus the portion with 100% parietal cell density and the lower portion with 50% density are removed. This distal line (not depicted here) is placed 1–2 cm below the pyloric sphincter. (From Oi, M. *Peptic Ulcer: Gastric, Duodenal and Esophageal.* Tokyo: Nankodo, 1957.)

shows the gross extent of resection and the particular part of the stomach that we aim to include in the removal. The resection line basically considers the topography of parietal cell distribution that was revealed by our own histological studies. In the operative field this is conveniently placed in relation to the vascular insertions as the landmarks on the greater and lesser curvatures. The resection line is high enough and is in the proper direction for the "100 percent" portion to be included in the removal. In this way optimal reduction of the parietal cell mass can be obtained. It is presumed that an additional elevation of this line (greater resection) would add little to the extent of parietal cell mass reduction. No change in the technique of the procedure was attempted or was necessary depending on the site of ulcer (gastric or duodenal), type of anastomosis (Billroth I or Billroth II), or any difference in the relevant adjoining procedures, but it was always a rule to remove the ulcer. Of the 1750 subtotal gastrectomies mentioned before, 999 were for gastric ulcer, 566 for duodenal ulcer, and 185 for combined ulcer; 1126 were done as Billroth I and 624 as Billroth II anastomoses.

Here, note should be taken of the relation between the resection line and the gastric axis. In my design these two cross each other at a right angle, thus ensuring greater removal of the greater curvature portion and greater acid reduction. In the conventional design, in which the resection line is parallel to the body axis, considerably less of the parietal cell mass is removed. In patients with recurrent ulcer after gastrectomy (mostly referred from other surgeons), it was a common finding on reoperation that the greater curvature portion of the retained stomach was of substantial length. Additional resection of this greater curvature portion along a new line set perpendicular to the gastric axis successfully led to healing.

Here, however, readers should be reminded that no rule fits invariably. The anatomical arrangement of the stomach, like any other organ, varies from one individual to another; thus the location of the boundary between the fundic mucosa and antral mucosa varies. During our study it was generally observed that the aforementioned mucosal boundary was located lower in patients with duodenal ulcer than in those with gastric ulcer. This observation was thought to enhance the adequacy of subtotal gastrectomy in patients with duodenal ulcer and encouraged me to continue to use this procedure; therefore, my experience with subtotal gastrectomy became extensive. If the anatomical individuality of the patient were to be considered in other peptic ulcer operations, vagotomy in its many varieties would be no less a victim of these anatomical variations. Differences in anatomy seem to present a problem that cannot be overcome. We must continue to evaluate every aspect of these procedures so that an optimum experience can be obtained. Incidentally, the subtotal gastrectomy introduced here seems to have become the basic pattern of this kind of procedure in Japan. During the past 15 years I have been especially interested in seeing the surgical method of therapy for peptic ulcer (especially, duodenal ulcer) change. I see more than 10 variants "in confusion," and the basis for selection seems to be personal preference.

In Japan subtotal gastrectomy carries a distinctly lower recurrent ulcer rate than any other procedure. The operative mortality has no marked difference from that of other procedures, refuting criticism in this respect. Because Japan has a high incidence of gastric cancer, surgeons of the gastrointestinal tract are given frequent opportunities to accustom themselves to performing gastrectomy; this is believed to provide a firm background favoring subtotal gastrectomy as the procedure of choice when facing peptic ulcer too. Even surgeons who usually do other procedures are said to prefer gastrectomy in an emergency. The practicality of a procedure seems to provide an important base for its acceptability—an essential quality of a good operation. The final and seemingly largest shortcoming of subtotal gastrectomy is the remnant "small stomach." This criticism should be directed against, or the procedure looked at in comparison with, gastrectomy for cancer, in which an even "smaller stomach" is created. But here in Japan, by and large, this is a complaint of no consequence.

11

Truncal Vagotomy

Alan G. Johnson

In 1943 Dragstedt introduced gastric vagotomy, by a transthoracic approach, for the treatment of duodenal ulcer (DU). The technique was based on his assumption that the hypersecretion of acid in DU was of nervous origin, and on his desire to find an operation that could be performed by general surgeons without the high mortality of partial gastrectomy [9, 24, 44]. At the beginning, no drainage procedure was included and, to Dragstedt's disappointment, a number of patients had to have a drain added to relieve the symptoms of gastric stasis. Later Dragstedt advocated the transabdominal, perhiatal approach to the vagal trunks, followed by a pyloroplasty or gastroenterostomy. Since 1943 vagotomy of some type has become a standard operation for DU and, in some centers, for gastric ulcer (GU) also; more selective vagotomies have been introduced over the years. The purpose of this chapter is to review the present status of truncal vagotomy (TV) and to highlight its advantages and disadvantages compared with other operations.

Physiological Basis of Vagotomy

While vagotomy undoubtedly blocks the cephalic phase of gastric secretion, it also reduces the sensitivity of the parietal cells to circulating gastrin, reducing the acid response to pentagastrin or histamine by 65–70 percent [6]. To make matters more complicated, there is evidence that the vagus nerve not only provides a cholinergic stimulus to gastrin release but also may contain fibers that inhibit gastrin release [3]! Vagotomy, like atropine, completely abolishes the acid response to modified sham feeding in humans, while having no effect on gastrin release in either normal or DU patients [22]. The rise in fasting serum gastrin level seen after vagotomy is caused by lack of acid providing negative feedback in the antrum, and the rise seen with insulin stimulation may be through adrenaline release and independent of the vagus. The effect on symptoms of dividing the 90 percent of vagal fibers that are afferent is not clear.

In addition to acid secretion, the vagus

nerve influences receptive relaxation of the stomach and antral motility as well as function of the liver, pancreas, and small intestine. It is surprising that truncal vagotomy has so *few* side effects and how well the other control mechanisms can compensate.

Indications for Operation for Duodenal Ulcer

Since the introduction of H_2-receptor antagonists, claims have been made that peptic ulcer operations are a thing of the past. These claims have failed to recognize the differences between "healing" and "curing" an ulcer. The drugs merely suppress acid secretion while they are being taken, whereas vagotomy reduces the secretion permanently. The main indications for surgical treatment now are recurrent ulceration after each of several courses of drugs or relapse while on a maintenance dose, and the initial response to the drugs is a good indication that vagotomy will be successful. But the use of drugs has altered surgical treatment in two ways:

1. Usually the patient's symptoms can be controlled so that the timing of an operation can be planned.
2. Because only the more severe ulcers are being referred for surgical treatment, it is even more important that the operation succeed and that the incidence of recurrent ulcer be as low as possible.

There is, however, another group of patients who have "failed medical treatment"—those who have failed to respond at all to H_2-receptor blockade and might therefore be expected *not* to respond to vagotomy. Early indications are that symptoms do respond, but it is not yet clear whether the recurrence rate will be higher in these patients.

Indications for Truncal Vagotomy

There is still a wide variation among different countries and different surgeons in the practice of surgery for peptic ulcer. Some suggest that proximal gastric vagotomy (PGV) has relegated all other operations to the history book, whereas others still consider partial gastrectomy the best operation. Truncal vagotomy represents the middle ground between these two extremes and is probably the most common operation performed today for DU. But even for the surgeon who performs PGV there are still important indications for truncal vagotomy. These are as follows:

1. Some uncomplicated DUs
2. Emergencies—bleeding and perforation
3. Pyloric stenosis, in which a drainage operation is required
4. Recurrent ulcer after gastrectomy or PGV
5. Gastric ulcer
6. Gastric erosions

Even without controlled clinical trials, it is likely from first principles that truncal vagotomy will be safer than Pólya partial gastrectomy and quicker than either a partial gastrectomy or PGV. In the following sections I discuss the different indications in turn and review the published evidence.

CHRONIC UNCOMPLICATED DUODENAL ULCER

Once TV became established for DU, surgeons had the impression that the mortality and side effects were lower but the recurrence rate higher than after partial gastrectomy. The move toward vagotomy and antrectomy, particularly in the United States, confused the situation even more, and it became clear that the only way to answer the question, "Which is the best operation for DU?" was to design a controlled trial. Goligher and colleagues [14] did this in 1960, and their trial has become the prototype for assessing operations for peptic ulcer. They compared vagotomy and gastroenterostomy (V & GE), vagotomy and antrectomy (V & A), and subtotal gastrectomy. They subsequently compared patients who had these operations with an equivalent group of patients having vagotomy and pyloroplasty [13]. At 10–16 years after operation, the con-

Table 11-1. Recurrent ulcer rate 10–16 years after operation

	Proved (%)	Total recent ulcer symptoms (%)
Vagotomy and gastroenterostomy (94 instances)	4.2	10.6
Vagotomy and antrectomy (101 instances)	0	1.0
Subtotal gastrectomy (70 instances)	1.4	2.8
Vagotomy and pyloroplasty (134 instances)	10.4	15.7

clusions are that the resection operations gave a significantly lower recurrent ulcer rate (Table 11-1). The differences in Visick scores were not significant except for V & A being better than vagotomy and pyloroplasty (V & P). The questions raised regarding all such trials are whether the loss of 20 percent of patients to follow-up study affects the results and what the significance is of those who were excluded at the beginning because surgeons did not think they could perform each of the operations equally well. The authors, in their comments on the trial, draw attention to the inherently higher mortality of the resection operations. Further long-term follow-up studies [37] and multicenter controlled trials [6] confirm the impression that recurrence rates after TV are up to 10 percent but are considerably reduced by adding an antrectomy [19]. The side effects, although in different proportions, are about the same overall, but resection causes an inherently higher mortality. Trials against PGV [8, 21], which will be discussed in greater detail in Chapter 13, show more or similar [39] recurrences after PGV but a significant reduction in side effects. When assessing the Visick grading after all these operations, it is important to realize that the results are similar after hernia repair [35]!

Special Considerations

DIET. In some developing countries it is important not to resect the stomach because the staple diet is high in residue but low in protein and caloric value, and patients cannot eat a large enough volume of food to maintain their weight and nutritional status. On the other hand, in obese patients both resection and PGV are technically difficult.

SEX. In the Leeds-York trial the authors found that women fared worse than men after all the operations, confirming the surgical folklore that "women don't do well after gastrectomy." This, however, does not apply to PGV [26].

AGE. In an interesting study of patient age at the time of operation [37], it was found after a 10-year follow-up period that the recurrence rate in patients younger than 40 years of age was 9.5 percent but in those older than 40 only 0.5 percent. This may reflect the inherently lower acid secretion in the older patient and is another factor to consider.

ACID SECRETION. In the years following a variety of operations became available, and surgeons have tried to "tailor the operation to the patient" based on preoperative acid secretion. Kronberg [23], in a study of patients 6–8 years after TV and drainage, found that if the preoperative peak acid output (PAO) was above 46.1 mEq/hr (in humans), the recurrence rate was 21 percent, whereas if it was less than this, the recurrence rate was only 5 percent. In women the corresponding figures were 28 percent recurrence if above 41.5 mEq/hr, and 1 percent below this level. Whether this is because of antral "dominance" is still debated, but there is probably a small group of patients who need more than a truncal vagotomy. It is possible that measurement of pepsin will be more helpful than measurement of acid secretion.

When all the factors of recurrent ulcer, side effects, safety, simplicity and speed are taken together, truncal vagotomy with drainage compares favorably with all other operations for elective DU. It is likely to be used for many years to come and has, to a large extent, fulfilled Dragstedt's wish for a simple operation that can be safely performed by general surgeons [32, 34].

EMERGENCY SURGICAL INTERACTION

Modern drugs may have reduced the need for elective operations, but they have not reduced the prevalence of perforation and hemorrhage.

Perforation

There is still discussion about whether it is best simply to close the perforation at the first operation and reoperate later on the 50 percent who have recurrent ulcer symptoms, or to do a definitive operation on the first occasion. This is not the place to prolong this argument; however, if the patient has a long ulcer history and the surgeon decides to do a vagotomy, it is appropriate to do a truncal vagotomy with either a pyloroplasty through the perforation or closure of the defect and a gastroenterostomy. There is no evidence that opening the hiatus in the presence of a (chemical) peritonitis leads to problems.

Bleeding

The aims of an operation on a patient with a bleeding DU are first, to stop the bleeding, and second, to prevent its recurrence: It is a life-saving operation. The duodenum must be widely opened to undersew the bleeding artery (*both* sides of the bleeding point), and this usually means a pyloroplasty. A truncal vagotomy is the logical procedure and is quick to perform in such an emergency. Alternatively, the duodenostomy may be closed without a pyloroplasty and a gastroenterostomy added. The rebleeding rate after vagotomy is greater than after a Pólya partial gastrectomy, but the mortality is significantly less. McGregor et al. [28] report a remarkable 100 percent follow-up rate of 73 patients with massive hemorrhage, 68 percent older than 60 years of age. The mortality was only 8 percent and proven recurrences only 3 percent. This was not a controlled trial, but the results do show that an adequate vagotomy can be performed safely under emergency conditions.

PYLORIC STENOSIS

The main purpose of PGV is to avoid a pyloroplasty with its attendant side effects; there seems, therefore, little point in doing it if a drainage procedure is already required, although Holle [17] and Grassi [15] both recommended a PGV, rather than a TV, with a drainage procedure. Truncal vagotomy with either pyloroplasty or, preferably, gastroenterostomy, is the treatment of choice. A PGV with pyloric dilatation has been considered an alternative [10] based on the assumption that much of the "stenosis" is really edema that will subside when the ulcer heals. Recent results shed some doubts on the effectiveness of this technique [2]. If the stenosis is well distal to the pylorus a duodenoplasty may be done, thereby preserving the pylorus. On balance, however, TV with gastroenterostomy is the simplest and safest procedure, and there is good clinical evidence that the dilated stomach returns to normal size afterward. Although the new drugs have not made much difference in perforation or hemorrhage rates, they should decrease the incidence of pyloric stenosis by controlling the disease earlier in its course.

RECURRENT ULCERATION AFTER PARTIAL GASTRECTOMY OR PROXIMAL GASTRIC VAGOTOMY

Recurrent ulceration is discussed in more detail elsewhere. A truncal vagotomy is relatively easy after a previous Pólya gastrectomy because the hiatal area is undisturbed. It is more difficult after a previous PGV, and some surgeons still recommend the transthoracic approach in this instance. However, many would not try to complete the vagotomy and settle for an antrectomy [42]. Revagotomy is an unsatisfactory procedure without an intraoperative test, unless undivided trunks are easily found.

VAGOTOMY FOR GASTRIC ULCER

Gastric ulcer is commonly treated by Billroth I partial gastrectomy. A vagotomy *with excision of the ulcer,* however, seemed to give sufficiently good results to justify a controlled trial [11] (see Special Comment by Duthie, Chap. 9). Excision of the ulcer is important to confirm that the ulcer is benign, and every large series has a few unsuspected malignant tumors. Truncal vagotomy is particularly useful in the high, lesser curvature GU, which would otherwise entail an extensive resection. Good results over a mean follow-up time of 7.5 years were reported by Cade and Allan [5] with only 2 recurrences (one a DU) in 58 patients.

The reason vagotomy is effective in GU is difficult to explain on the basis of either the "bile reflux" or the "delayed emptying" hypothesis. Probably it reduces the already low acid secretion so much that no further mucosal damage occurs.

DIFFUSE GASTRIC EROSIONS (HEMORRHAGIC GASTRITIS)

The surgical treatment of bleeding gastric erosions is difficult, especially when they are diffuse and so cannot be resected except by a total gastrectomy. It was hoped that a vagotomy would reduce the acid and shunt blood from the mucosa sufficiently to heal the erosions, but this has not proved true in practice, and experimental evidence suggests that any change in mucosal blood flow is only temporary [25]. In uncontrolled studies [7], 25 percent of patients rebled after both vagotomy with pyloroplasty and vagotomy with resection, but the cause and distribution of the erosions also affected the outcome. If there is a strong suggestion that bile reflux is playing a part, a vagotomy and Roux-en-Y diversion may be appropriate.

Drainage Procedures

IS DRAINAGE REQUIRED AFTER TV?

Since Dragstedt's original experience, it has been assumed that a drainage procedure is necessary after truncal vagotomy. We know little about the degree of scarring in Dragstedt's patients, however, and not all needed to have a drainage procedure added at a later date. Therefore, if we are now operating on patients, most of whom have little scarring, it may be appropriate to question again the need for drainage. In a series of 74 patients with TV alone, Slaney et al. [36] reported no instances of serious gastric stasis. Glenn [12] found that stasis passed in 6 to 10 weeks, while Tanner's [40] patients commonly complained of foul eructations. Now the degree of preoperative scarring can be well assessed by fiberoptic endoscopy and patients can be selected for a "no drainage procedure." But a word of warning is required: Scarring takes place as the ulcer heals, so the preoperative assessment may not always be a safe guide, although much of the early stasis may be caused by edema.

Pyloric dilatation is being used instead of drainage after both TV [27] and PGV [10]. With truncal vagotomy it gives the same incidence of side effects as pyloroplasty, which is no advantage except that it avoids a suture line that may occasionally leak. We await results of trials of TV alone versus TV and dilatation in selected patients without severe preoperative scarring.

WHICH DRAINAGE PROCEDURE?

There are many drainage procedures, all of which can be classified as some form of pyloroplasty or some form of gastroenterostomy. They are shown in Figure 11-1. The individual side effects are discussed in detail in Chapter 20, but overall there is little difference among the various operations. Bilious vomiting is more common after gastroenterostomy [14], but ulcer recurrence is delayed with this procedure [42]. Diarrhea is more common after pyloroplasty, but dumping is the same for both [14]. The rationale for Tanner's juxtapyloric anterior gastroenterostomy [40] is sound, as the anastomosis is on alkaline mucosa, but it must be close to the pylorus to function properly. When dealing with a bleeding duodenal ulcer, the surgeon needs to open the duodenum widely to have a good view to undersew the bleeding point. It can be closed to exclude the ulcer from the duodenum if the ulcer is not large [20].

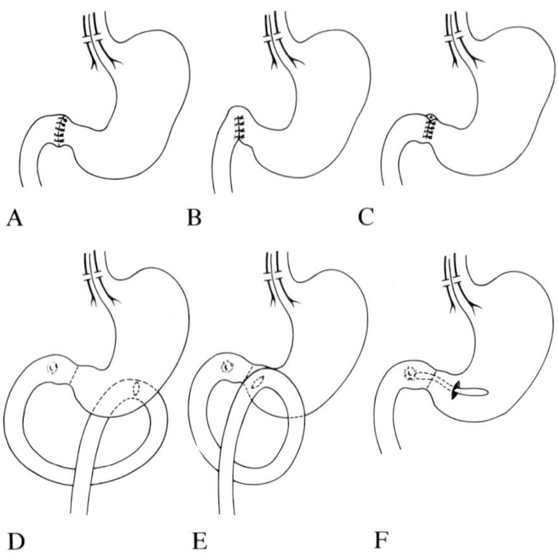

Fig. 11-1. Various drainage procedures. (A) Heineke-Mikulicz pyloroplasty. (B) Finney pyloroplasty. (C) Exclusion pyloroplasty. (D) Posterior gastroenterostomy. (E) Anterior juxtapyloric gastroenterostomy. (F) Pyloric dilatation by gastrotomy.

Selected Side Effects

ALCOHOL ABSORPTION

After TV and drainage, absorption of alcohol is more rapid than normal, leading to high peak levels soon after drinking. This fact has medicolegal importance, and patients should be warned, preferably in writing, to be especially careful with alcohol after the operation. (This change in absorption does not seem to occur after PGV [29]).

CHANGES IN MYOELECTRICAL ACTIVITY

After truncal vagotomy and pyloroplasty (TV & P) there is no difference in mean frequency of electrical activity, but the wave becomes more sinusoidal, with reduction of amplitude. These changes are permanent [38]. However, the duration of regular electrical activity is less than 50 percent immediately after the operation, increasing with time to 90 percent some years postoperatively. Occasionally marked arrhythmias are seen up to two years later, but the importance of these is not yet clear. Although TV produces profound permanent changes in the control mechanisms of gastric contractions, some of these changes progressively improve with time.

GALLSTONES

The question of whether or not TV increases the risk of gallstones developing has been debated for many years. However, vagotomy produces changes that would be expected to favor gallstone formation: There is reduced bile flow, an increase in gallbladder volume, a delay in emptying, and a reduced response to cholecystokinin [43]. Until recently, no controlled study had been done in which the state of the biliary tree was assessed before operation and the completeness of vagotomy checked postoperatively, and no study had a control group of medically treated duodenal ulcer patients. Ihasz and Griffith [18] compared TV & P patients in Hungary with selective vagotomy and pyloroplasty (SV & P) patients in the United States in whom the hepatic and celiac vagi had been carefully preserved. Two of 53 patients with SV had gallstones develop within seven years. In half the TV patients, gallbladder function did not change and gallstones developed in one, whereas in the other half the gallbladder became grossly dilated and contraction was impaired. Gallstones developed in nine patients. These findings are puzzling but strongly suggest that there is a group of patients who have an increased risk of gallstones after TV. They are not definable preoperatively, however.

When gallstones and peptic ulcer coexist, which is not uncommon, there is a high incidence of postvagotomy diarrhea (48 percent) 2–3 months postoperatively if TV & P and cholecystectomy are performed together or if either operation follows the other [41]. There is also a high incidence of bile reflux gastritis. A PGV is therefore recommended after, or at the same time as, cholecystectomy, even though the diarrhea improves with time.

DYSPHAGIA

Transient dysphagia is not uncommon if there has been enthusiastic dissection around the lower esophagus. It is caused by edema and perhaps a little hematoma in the wall, and passes off in a few weeks.

Techniques

We will describe here the key points of the standard abdominal approach. The transthoracic approach may be used occasionally for revagotomy if a drainage procedure has been done at the first operation.

EXPOSURE

A midline incision is satisfactory, extending up alongside the xiphisternum. To expose the hiatus and dissect under direct vision rather than high out of reach, a sternocostal retractor is invaluable. The Rochard is a good model; it is hooked to a strong frame attached to the operating table (Fig. 11-2). The left triangular ligament of the liver may be divided to give better access and the ligamentum teres and falciform ligament divided to avoid having the subcostal retractor tear the liver.

DISSECTION

The aim is to open the hiatus and divide the vagal trunks as proximal as possible before they branch. The peritoneal covering is incised to expose the white edge of the phrenoesophageal ligament (Fig. 11-3). This is lifted and the esophagus freed beneath it and on either side within the crura (Fig. 11-4). The anterior vagus is identified adherent to the anterior wall of the esophagus and divided high in the hiatus. The posterior vagus is then felt to the right and well away from the esophagus by the fingers encircling behind (Fig. 11-5); it is divided, together with the surrounding connective tissue, which often contains blood vessels. The esophagus is then rotated in both directions and all small branches divided, with careful clearance of the angle of His. There is little point in the traditional habit of sending a piece of vagal trunk for histological study, as this does not confirm that *all* vagal fibers have been divided. At the end the surgeon should be able to put three fingers around and behind the esophagus. Some surgeons recommend repair of the hiatus, but there is no evidence that this is necessary.

ERRORS

The most common technical error is to miss the posterior trunk completely [42] by dissecting too close to the esophagus. (Nyhus and colleagues [31] have pointed out important details of technique, including common anatomical variations.) Overenthusiastic dissection on the esophageal wall or not clearing the esophagus before encircling it can lead to a perforation, which *must* be recognized at the time and sutured; the stomach must be drained with a nasogastric tube for several days and a drain must be placed transperitoneally. Finally, care must be taken of the spleen and short gastric vessels, a task made easier by good exposure. Diathermy should be used only with caution on the esophageal wall.

INTRAOPERATIVE TESTING

Postoperative gastric secretory criteria for the completeness of vagotomy are discussed elsewhere, but there is an understandable desire to have a test that will tell the surgeon that the vagotomy is incomplete during the operation, when faults can be corrected. It is of little comfort to discover the incompleteness 10 days to 3 months postoperatively. Two groups of tests have been devised, one based on motility and the other on acid secretion. They can be used for all types of vagotomy (see Special Comment, Chap. 12).

In the Burge test [4] the rise in intragastric pressure is measured, using a nasogastric tube, in response to stimulation around the vagal trunks with an electrical current. If there are no residual vagal fibers supplying the stomach, there will be no rise in pressure. (With PGV, the antrum is intentionally left innervated and so a soft clamp has to be placed at an arbitrary point between the antral-body junction, which makes it impossible to know how far distal the denervation should be continued.) This test has been modified using small strain gauges on the surface of the stomach. A multicentric assessment of the Burge test showed a significantly reduced recurrence rate when the test was negative [30].

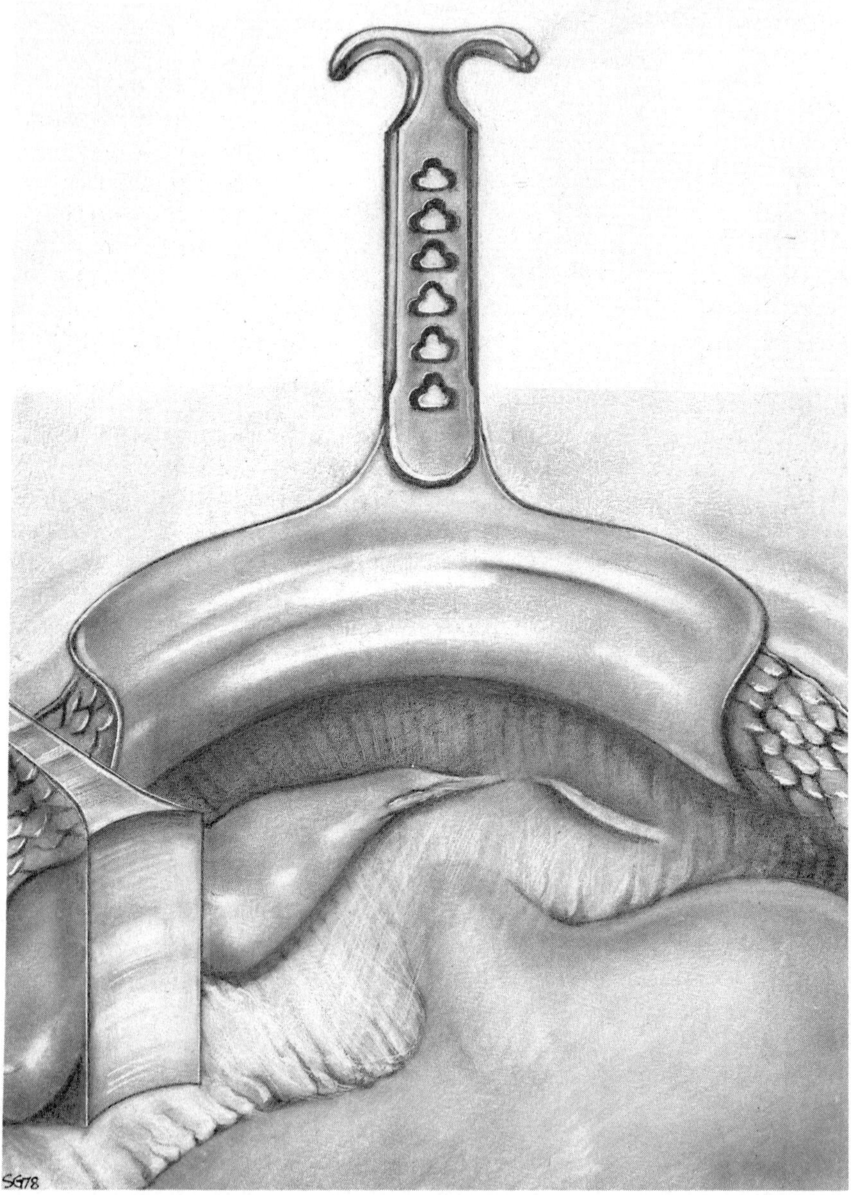

Fig. 11-2. Exposure of hiatus showing subcostal (Rochard) retractor. (From A. G. Johnson and K. W. Reynolds, *Techniques of Vagotomy*. London: Edward Arnold, 1979.)

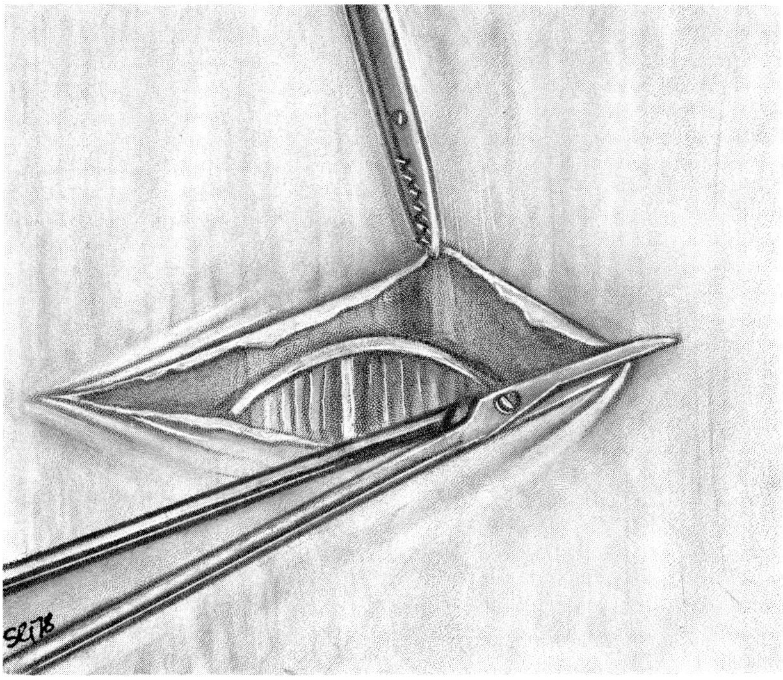

Fig. 11-3. Exposure of phrenoesophageal ligament after peritoneum is incised. (From A. G. Johnson and K. W. Reynolds, *Techniques of Vagotomy*. London: Edward Arnold, 1979.)

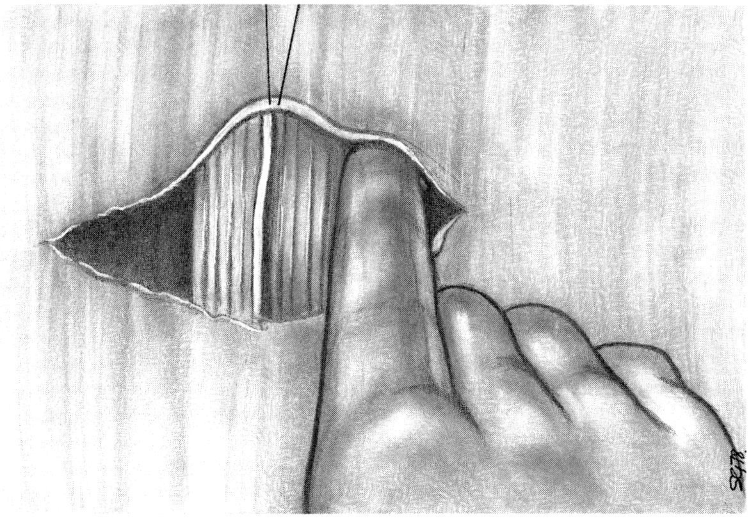

Fig. 11-4. Mobilization of lower esophagus. (From A. G. Johnson and K. W. Reynolds, *Techniques of Vagotomy*. London: Edward Arnold, 1979.)

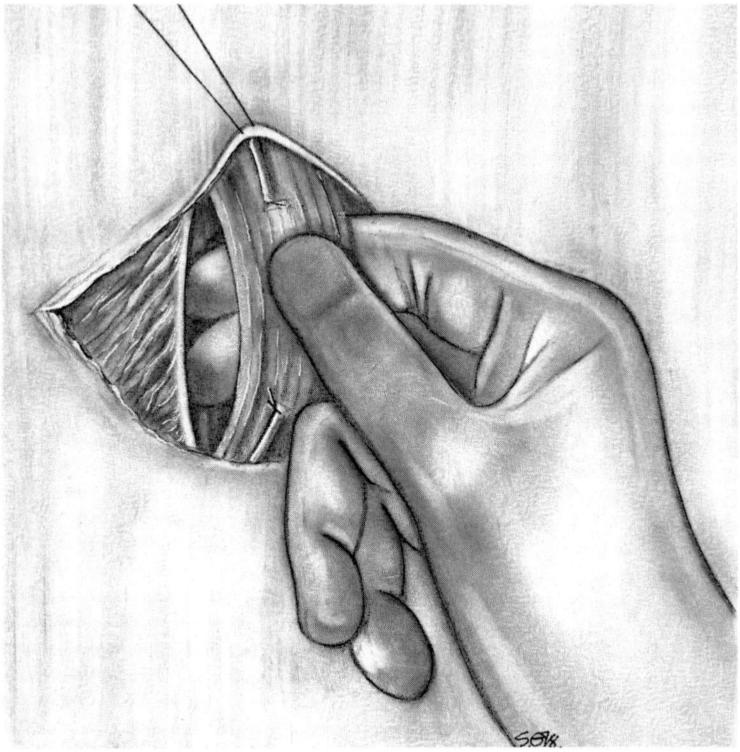

Fig. 11-5. Location of posterior vagus. (From A. G. Johnson and K. W. Reynolds, *Techniques of Vagotomy*. London: Edward Arnold, 1979.)

The Grassi, or pH, test [15] is based on the fact that denervated parietal cells are less sensitive to circulating (penta)gastrin than innervated cells. The stomach is washed out through a small gastrotomy, and a probe maps out the mucosal pH during an intravenous infusion of pentagastrin (6 μg/kg/hr). A pH below 5.0 shows residual innervation. This test has also been found to be effective in reducing acid secretion and has the advantage that the exact area of residual innervation can be detected, as can the distal extent of the parietal cell mass. A recent comparison of the two marginally favored the Grassi test for these reasons [33].

The tests have also shown the high proportion of patients with residual innervation after the first dissection [1], but this is considerably less with truncal vagotomy than with PGV.

Neither test is foolproof, and both have still to be evaluated in routine use in general surgical units; however, they may be of special use in the training of surgeons and during revagotomy.

POSTOPERATIVE PRECAUTIONS

There is commonly some delayed emptying of the stomach postoperatively, and therefore a nasogastric tube is a wise precaution for 48 hours, even though this may not be necessary after PGV. Acute dilatation of the stomach is a rare but dangerous complication. The patient is advised to avoid any foods that consistently cause indigestion, but there is no need for strict gastric regimens.

Anterior PGV and Posterior TV

Hill and Barker [16] have suggested this compromise operation for speed and simplicity, arguing that only one antral nerve need be preserved to ensure adequate emptying without a drainage procedure. Their example has not yet been followed.

Bilateral truncal vagotomy, at present with drainage, is not ideal but gives an acceptable incidence of side effects, particularly mortality, with an acceptable recurrent ulcer rate, in the hands of the average surgeon. Other operations have more recurrences with less side effects, and vice versa. If many surgeons cannot or are not prepared to take the extra time and trouble to do an adequate PGV, a return to TV is likely, especially if a drainage procedure can be avoided in selected patients.

References

1. Baxter, H., and Johnson, A. G. Where is your vagotomy incomplete? *Br. J. Surg.* 64:583, 1977.
2. Blackett, R. L., Axon, A. T. R., Barker, M. C., et al. HSV with pyloric dilatation for pyloric stenosis due to peptic ulcer. *Br. J. Surg.* 69:289, 1982.
3. Blair, E., Grund, E. R., Lund Kay, P., et al. Gastrin Release. In S. R. Bloom (Ed.), *Gut Hormones*. Edinburgh, London, New York: Churchill Livingstone, 1978. Pp. 151–55.
4. Burge, H., and Frohn, M. J. N. The technique of bilateral selective vagotomy with the electrical stimulation test. *Br. J. Surg.* 56:452, 1969.
5. Cade, D., and Allan, D. Long term follow-up of patients with gastric ulcers treated by vagotomy, pyloroplasty and ulcerectomy. *Br. J. Surg.* 66:46, 1979.
6. Christiansen, J., Jensen, H. E., Ejby-Poulsen, P., et al. Prospective controlled vagotomy trial for duodenal ulcer: Primary results, sequelae, acid secretion, and recurrence rates two to five years after operation. *Ann. Surg.* 193:49, 1981.
7. Cody, H. S., III, and Wichern, W. A., Jr. Choice of operation for acute gastric mucosal hemorrhage: Report of 36 cases and review of literature. *Am. J. Surg.* 134:322, 1977.
8. Donahue, P. E., Bombeck, C. T., Condon, R. E., and Nyhus, L. M. Proximal gastric vagotomy versus selective vagotomy with antrectomy: Results of a prospective, randomized clinical trial after four to twelve years. *Surgery* 96:585, 1984.
9. Dragstedt, L. R. Gastric vagotomy in the treatment of duodenal ulcer. In L. Nyhus and C. Wastell (Eds.), *Surgery of the Stomach and Duodenum* (3d ed.). Boston: Little, Brown, 1977.
10. Dunn, D. C., Thomas, W. E., and Hunter, J. O. Highly selective vagotomy and pyloric dilatation for duodenal ulcer with stenosis. *Br. J. Surg.* 68:194, 1981.
11. Duthie, H. L., and Kwong, N. K. Vagotomy or gastrectomy for gastric ulcer. *Br. Med. J.* 4:79, 1973.
12. Glenn, F. Present status of surgical treatment of peptic ulcer. *J.A.M.A.* 145:790, 1951.
13. Goligher, J. C., Feather, D. B., Hall, R., et al. Several standard elective operations for duodenal ulcer: Ten to 16 year clinical results. *Ann. Surg.* 189:18, 1979.
14. Goligher, J. C., Pulvertaft, C. N., and Watkinson, G. Controlled trial of vagotomy and antrectomy and subtotal gastrectomy in elective treatment of duodenal ulcer. *Br. Med. J.* 1:455, 1964.
15. Grassi, G. Highly selective vagotomy with intra-operative acid secretive test of completeness of vagal section. *Surg. Gynecol. Obstet.* 140:259, 1975.
16. Hill, G. L., and Barker, M. C. Anterior highly selective vagotomy with posterior truncal vagotomy: A simple technique for denervating the parietal cell mass. *Br. J. Surg.* 65:702, 1978.
17. Holle, F., and Hart, N. Nene Wege der Chirurgie des Gastroduodenalulkus. *Med. Klin.* 62:441, 1967.
18. Ihasz, M., and Griffith, C. A. Gallstones after vagotomy. *Am. J. Surg.* 141:48, 1981.
19. Jackson, D. S., Smith, E. E. J., Spencer, J., et al. Proximal gastric vagotomy or truncal vagotomy and antrectomy for chronic duodenal ulcer: Five to seven year results of a prospective randomised multicentre trial. *Br. J. Surg.* 69:282, 1982.
20. Kay, P. H., Johnson, A. G. The exclusion pyloroplasty. *Ann. R. Coll. Surg. Engl.* 63:277, 1981.
21. Koffman, C. G., Elder, J. B., Gillespie, I. E., et al. A prospective randomized trial of vagotomy in chronic duodenal ulceration. *Br. J. Surg.* 66:145, 1979.
22. Konturek, S. J., Dwiecien, N., Obtulowicz, W., et al. Cephalic phase of gastric secretion in healthy subjects and duodenal ulcer patients: Role of vagal innervation. *Gut* 20:875, 1979.
23. Kronborg, O. Gastric acid secretion and risk of

recurrences of duodenal ulcer within six to eight years after truncal vagotomy and drainage. *Gut* 15:714, 1974.
24. Landor, J. H. Lester Reynold Dragstedt: Physiologist–surgeon. *Gastroenterology* 80:846, 1981.
25. Levine, B. A., Gaskill, H. V., III, and Sirinek, K. R. Lack of sustained vagal control of gastric mucosal blood flow: Why vagotomy is not effective in preventing recurrent hemorrhage from stress ulcer. *Surgery* 90:631, 1981.
26. Linhardt, G., and Johnson, A. G. Do women do worse after proximal gastric vagotomy? *Br. J. Surg.* 69:321, 1982.
27. Longrigg, N., and Pringle, R. A new method of gastric drainage following truncal vagotomy. *Ann. Surg.* 113:905, 1978.
28. McGregor, D. B., Savage, L. E., and McVay, C. B. Massive gastrointestinal hemorrhage: A twenty-five year experience with vagotomy and drainage. *Surgery* 80:530, 1976.
29. Moodie, A. F., Royston, C. M., and Spencer, J. Alcohol tolerance after proximal gastric vagotomy. *Gut* 16:966, 1975.
30. Muller, C., Martinoli, S., and Allgöwer, M. The vagotomotor electrotest (modified Burge test) for completeness of vagotomy. In J. H. Baron, et al. (Eds.), *Vagotomy in Modern Surgical Practice*. London: Butterworth, 1982.
31. Nyhus, L. M., Donahue, P. E., Krystosek, R. J., et al. Complete vagotomy: The evolution of an effective technique. *Arch. Surg.* 115:264, 1980.
32. O'Leary, J. P., Woodward, E. R., Hollenbeck, H. I., and Dragstedt, L. R. Vagotomy and drainage procedure for duodenal ulcer: The results of seventeen years' experience. *Ann. Surg.* 183:613, 1976.
33. Pendower, J. A comparison of the Burge and Grassi intraoperative tests for completeness of nerve section in parietal cell vagotomy. *Br. J. Surg.* 68:83, 1981.
34. Saik, R. P., Greenburg, A. G., and Peskin, G. W. Pros and cons of parietal cell versus truncal vagotomy. *Am. J. Surg.* 148:93, 1984.
35. Salaman, J. R., Harvey, J., and Duthie, H. L. Importance of symptoms after highly selective vagotomy. *Br. Med. J.* 283:281, 1981.
36. Slaney, G., Bevan, P. G., and Brook, B. N. Vagotomy for chronic peptic ulcer. *Lancet* 2:221, 1956.
37. Smith, G., and Irving, A. D. Age at operation and the results of truncal vagotomy and gastroenterostomy for chronic duodenal ulcer. *Surg. Gynecol. Obstet.* 152:153, 1981.
38. Stoddard, C. J., Smallwood, R., Brown, B. H., and Duthie, H. L. The immediate and delayed effects of different types of vagotomy on human gastric myoelectrical activity. *Gut* 16:165, 1975.
39. Stoddard, C. J., Johnson, A. G., and Duthie, H. L. The four to eight year results of the Sheffield trial of elective duodenal ulcer surgery: Highly selective or truncal vagotomy? *Br. J. Surg.* 71:779, 1984.
40. Tanner, N. C. Drainage operations for vagotomy. *Proc. R. Soc. Med.* 60:221, 1967.
41. Taylor, T. V., Lambert, M. E., and Torrance, H. B. Value of bile-acid binding agents in post-vagotomy diarrhoea. *Lancet* 1:635, 1978.
42. Taylor, T. V., Pearson, K. W., and Torrance, B. Revagotomy for recurrent peptic ulceration. *Br. J. Surg.* 64:477, 1977.
43. Torrealba, V. Truncal vagotomy and cholelithiasis: Plea for a controlled study. *Br. Med. J.* 1:1160, 1977.
44. Woodward, E. R. Dr. Dragstedt's first vagotomy. *World J. Surg.* 7:554, 1983.

EDITOR'S COMMENT

Truncal vagotomy remains the method of vagal denervation used by most surgeons in the United States. This type of vagotomy is combined with pyloroplasty or antrectomy equally often. Surgeons in North America never aspired to the technique of selective vagotomy. A similar procrastination in the acceptance of proximal gastric vagotomy is occurring today, although there definitely is considerable interest in that procedure. It is my premise that the doomsayers of truncal vagotomy cannot overlook the vast population of surgeons and their patients who continue to be satisfied with the end results of truncal vagotomy in the treatment of duodenal ulcer disease. The surgical community of North America is not ultraconservative, yet after 40 years of experience, these surgeons dedicated to the welfare of their patients continue to practice the original technique.

Contrariwise, I maintain the nonvagotomy stance for patients with benign gastric ulcer: Billroth I antrectomy with excision of the ulcer. As time passes, this position may be less acceptable because the number of reported successes following truncal vagotomy, pyloroplasty, and ulcer excision is increasing (Madsen and Schousen, *Br. J. Surg.* 69:651, 1982; Madsen, et al., *Acta Chir. Scand.* 142:151, 1976).

We all have been perplexed as to the cause of postvagotomy diarrhea. Interesting changes in mucosal function of the ileum in patients with diarrhea after vagotomy and pyloroplasty have been reported (Sparsø et al. *Scand. J. Gastroenterol.* 18:669, 1983). Perfusion studies of the terminal ileum were performed in patients who had previously had vagotomy and pyloroplasty performed for peptic ulcer disease and who at follow-up study had diarrhea. The aim was to elucidate possible pathophysiological factors contributing to the sequelae. In patients with diarrhea the perfusion disclosed a large spontaneous ileal secretion that was not influenced by chenodeoxycholic acid. The secretion was caused mainly by a reduced mucosa-to-serosa flux of sodium and chloride and, to a lesser extent, by an increased serosa-to-mucosa flux. The patients with diarrhea showed an increased xylose absorption rate, suggesting an increased interepithelial leakiness. The authors suggested that the ileal epithelium of patients who have undergone vagotomy and suffered from diarrhea secretes spontaneously, possibly stimulated by an unidentified agent. All other studies have failed to help us understand the basic etiological mechanism of postvagotomy diarrhea. Investigations such as that of Sparsø et al. will ultimately give the answer.

L.M.N.

12

Selective Vagotomy Plus Suprapyloric Antrectomy: An Alternative Antidumping Operation

Charles A. Griffith

Terminology

For reasons described in the section in Chapter 2, Surgical Applications, Terminology, I prefer the words *total, selective,* and *parietal* to describe the three types of vagotomy. In *total abdominal* or *total vagotomy,* the surgeon cuts all abdominal vagi and denervates the stomach and midgut. In *selective gastric* or *selective vagotomy,* we cut all gastric vagi and confine denervation to the stomach by sparing the hepatic and celiac vagi. In *parietal cell* or *parietal vagotomy,* we cut the gastric vagi to the parietal mucosa and spare those to the gross antrum (and also the hepatic and celiac vagi).

Background

In the early 1950s, while working in the laboratory of H. N. Harkins (the senior editor of the first two editions of this book), my primary interest was to eliminate the side effects of the hepatic and celiac components of total vagotomy and also the dumping syndrome. The former entailed preservation of the hepatic and celiac vagi. The latter required preservation of both the valvular function of the pylorus and the reservoir function of the stomach. If the pylorus is saved but the segmental resection is too extensive, the gastric remnant is too small to serve as a reservoir and permits dumping through the intact pylorus [30, 31, 50].[1]

Unaware of the previous works of Latarjet

[1]In 1920 E. Wyllis Andrews [12] of Chicago coined the word *dumping* to describe rapid gastric emptying of a barium meal through a simple gastrojejunostomy.

> The striking thing was the abrupt disappearance of the barium into the bowel. It apparently did not lodge in the stomach at all, but passed instantly from the stomach into the intestine. . . . [H]is stomach no longer acted as a food reservoir, a digestive chamber, but immediately dumped its contents into the lesser bowel. . . . Hence I have applied the term "dumping stomach."

In subsequent years Andrews' terminology was discarded in favor of the term *dumping syndrome*. With the further passage of time, and despite the fact that Andrews relieved his patient of so-called gastric crippling by dismantling the gastrojejunostomy, the cause and effect relationship between the dumping stomach and the dumping syndrome was largely ignored. The relationship is now clear, and we may use the word *dumping* to mean either or both rapid gastric emptying and the syndrome that ensues.

[85] and Wertheimer [125] in the 1920s, and of Franksson [35] and Jackson [68] in the 1940s, I began studies of selective vagotomy alone in dogs. Although insulin tests were negative, gastric stasis was as severe after total vagotomy. The results of stasis indicated that effective antral motility is not preserved by the fibers descending from the hepatic vagal division to the pylorus (see Fig. 2-1). To preserve antral motility, parietal vagotomy was done. The results were no gastric stasis as determined by a barium meal, and negative or weakly positive insulin tests (the small and delayed adequate response in Fig. 2-16C). Before publication of these experiments [53], the results were sent to Drs. Dragstedt and Hollander for their review. Both rejected the concepts of parietal and selective vagotomy because they predicted that incomplete gastric vagotomy was inevitable. Their prediction was based on their belief that vagotomy obeyed the all-or-none law, which held that any single intact fiber after an incomplete vagotomy can innervate the entire stomach [26, 60]. In view of this rejection by the founders of vagotomy and the insulin test, and because we had not yet disproved the all-or-none law as described in Chapter 2, Dr. Harkins did not accept either parietal or selective vagotomy for clinical study at the University of Washington. Nor did my seniors in private practice accept it. Consequently, in private patients, I adopted hemigastrectomy (see Figs. 2-3 and 2-17) plus selective vagotomy and reported initial results in 1960 [44]. In the same year, Burge [18] independently reported on selective vagotomy plus pyloroplasty.[2]

[2]Because the insulin tests after parietal vagotomy in our dogs were negative or barely positive, I did not accept Dragstedt's and Hollander's rejection based on the law of all or none. Accordingly, in 1956 I did three parietal vagotomies in one of Seattle's private hospitals. The senior surgeons in this hospital quickly put the quietus on this surgical nonsense of a *purposely incomplete* vagotomy by a "dog surgeon from Harkins' lab" just starting his practice. They also objected to the *purposely incomplete* selective vagotomy, but tolerated it because of the complementary hemigastrectomy. I use the word *incomplete* to emphasize that all attention was then focused on cutting every vagal fiber that emerged through the esophageal hiatus. (This footnote is written in response to many queries asking why I did not begin evaluation of parietal vagotomy in the 1950s. The three patients with parietal vagotomy did quite well, without either dumping or recurrence.)

After these independent reports, the pros and cons of selective and total vagotomy became a frequent subject of debate during the 1960s. In the United States selective vagotomy has never been fully accepted because most surgeons have doubted the need for preserving the hepatic and celiac vagi. Of equal if not more importance, the idea of increased rates of incomplete vagotomy plus increased morbidity and mortality from the more difficult selective technique deterred general evaluation. With the advent of parietal vagotomy in the 1970s, interest in the selective versus total vagotomy debate was replaced by concern for the pros and cons of parietal and total vagotomy. In light of these controversial issues, I shall summarize my views concerning all three types of vagotomy.

Significant Sequelae of Hepatic and Celiac Vagotomy

Surgeons who favor total vagotomy argue that any sequelae from transecting the hepatic and celiac vagi do not occur frequently enough and are not significant enough to warrant the extra time and trouble necessary to preserve them. Contrary to this view, I believe that the hepatic and celiac vagi have definite functions that cannot be sacrificed with impunity in all patients. The main concerns are gallstones and diarrhea.

GALLSTONES

Total vagotomy has been found to result in rates of gallstone formation that range from 16 to 24 percent [20, 63, 95, 97, 98, 113, 124]. These rates are 4 to 6 times greater than the 4.5 percent control rate in the 10-year Framingham study of the general population [37]. In contrast, the rate of stone formation is not increased after selective vagotomy [63, 108]. Despite this evidence, many American surgeons either deny or ignore the existence of cholelithiasis as a sequela of total vagotomy, and most remain skeptical.

Essentially four considerations account for this skepticism. First, remarkably few valid studies *(long term with preoperative and post-*

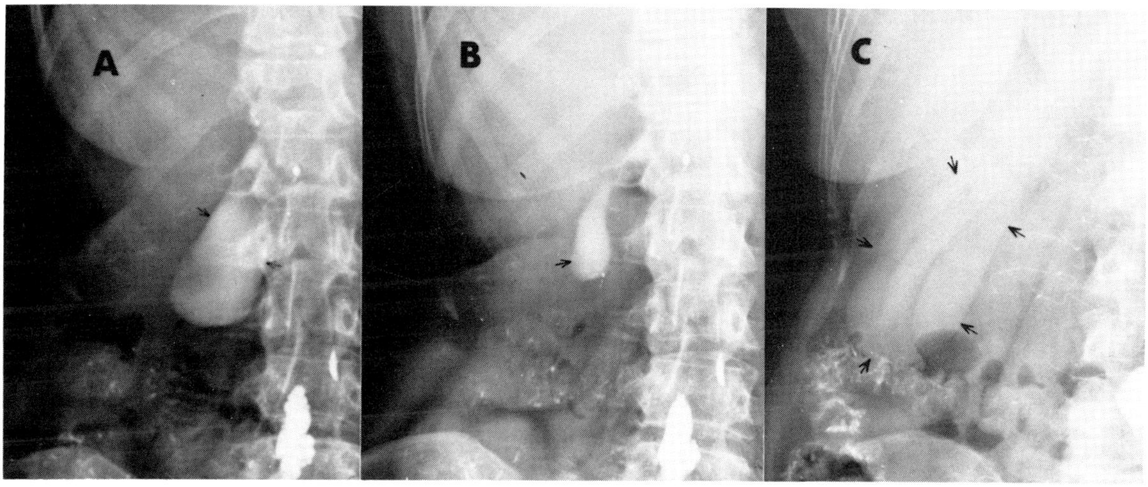

Fig. 12-1. Effects of complete hepatic vagotomy. The patient underwent transabdominal repair of a hiatal hernia, during which all of the hepatic vagi were transected in order to gain adequate exposure of the diaphragmatic crura; the gastric and celiac vagi were preserved. Cholecystograms before the operation demonstrate normal functions of concentration (A) and contraction in response to a fatty meal (B). Four years after the operation the patient suffered an attack of typical biliary colic that subsided spontaneously. Subsequent cholecystograms failed to visualize the gallbladder on two successive days, but on the third day a faint concentration of dye was demonstrated in a dilated gallbladder (C, *arrows*). No contraction occurred after a fatty meal. During the following year the patient had repeated attacks of biliary colic that necessitated cholcystectomy. At the operation the gallbladder was found to be unusually large and filled with inspissated bile and sludge. (The patient had undergone myelography several years before.)

operative cholecystograms) have been done in the past three decades since Johnson and Boyden [71] first observed a striking dilatation of the gallbladder and the development of gallstones in the long term after total vagotomy. Second, the interval between the vagotomy and the formation of gallstones is so long that, by the time the stones appear the past history of vagotomy is forgotten and the cause and effect relationship is overlooked, particularly when a preoperative cholecystogram is not available for comparison with the present cholecystogram. The third reason is the misconception that cholecystokinin is the only stimulus that causes the gallbladder to contract. My colleagues and I showed that electrical stimulation of the hepatic vagi also elicits contraction of the gallbladder. This finding demonstrates another of the many important neurohumoral mechanisms throughout the gastrointestinal tract [99, 100]. From this neurohumoral concept, it follows that the hepatic vagi maintain the muscular tonus of the gallbladder and keep its muscle primed in readiness for the humoral contraction. When this tonus is lost, as it is when the hepatic component of total vagotomy is complete, the gallbladder gradually dilates. With progressive dilatation for about three years or more, it becomes noncontractile. At this late stage, and not before, gallstones begin to form (Fig. 12-1).

The fourth and final reason for skepticism concerns the fact that most patients do not have these sequelae after total vagotomy. This lack of sequelae raises certain known and unknown considerations. For example, we know that motility of the gallbladder is preserved after parietal and selective vagotomy [63–65, 103, 111, 116] and also after total vagotomy in patients with positive insulin tests [71, 111]. In these patients both the gastric and hepatic vagotomies are presumably incomplete, but in any series of total vagotomy we do not know who has a complete hepatic vagotomy and who does not. Nor do we know whether complete hepatic vagotomy results in the same degree of hypotonia of the gallbladder in all patients. Our ignorance is due directly to the lack of any test for the completeness of hepatic vagotomy, and until such a test is available controversy from ignorance will continue.

In my study with Ihasz comparing selective and total vagotomy [63], increased stone formation occurred only in patients with advanced hypotonic changes of the gallbladder after total vagotomy. No increase occurred after selective vagotomy or after total vagotomy in patients without hypotonic gallbladders. Nor did stones form in *all* patients with hypotonia. This last finding suggests that stasis of bile is not the only factor. Numerous studies of bile flow and intrabiliary pressure [7, 13, 29, 38, 104, 115, 127] and studies of lithogenic substances in bile [15, 22, 25, 34, 90, 124, 126] are inconclusive. Nevertheless, the findings of Barnett and Hilbun [15] that total vagotomy retarded the rate of gallstone dissolution and that selective vagotomy did not, require some explanation other than biliary stasis in a hypotonic gallbladder (Fig. 12-2).

It is concluded that total vagotomy causes gallstones in some but not all patients over the long term, and that this sequela is prevented by preserving the hepatic vagi with parietal or selective vagotomy. In addition to the factors of age, sex, race, coexistence of peptic ulcer and gallstones, and the incidence of gallstones in the general population, any further comparative study must take into account the lack of any test for completeness of hepatic vagotomy. This lack means that surgeons familiar with the hepatic (and celiac) vagi should perform the operations and state in their operative reports whether these vagi are preserved or transected. This last criterion has never been met in a series of allegedly complete total vagotomies.

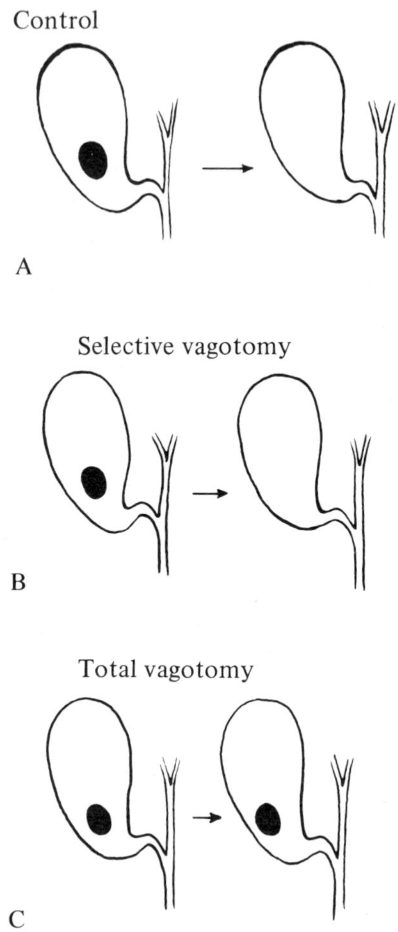

Fig. 12-2. Human cholesterol gallstones dissolve rapidly when placed in gallbladders of control dogs (A) and in dogs with selective vagotomy (B). In dogs with total vagotomy (C) this dissolution is delayed. The time factor is crucial in this type of experiment because, with continued observation, the stones in dogs with total vagotomy eventually dissolve and the difference between selective and total vagotomy is missed. (From Griffith [52].)

ILEUS

In the early days of total vagotomy the occurrence of postoperative ileus was a grave complication [36]. Now, with improved methods of treatment, it is much less serious but still results in prolonged hospitalization. The ileus involves the entire midgut consequent to the

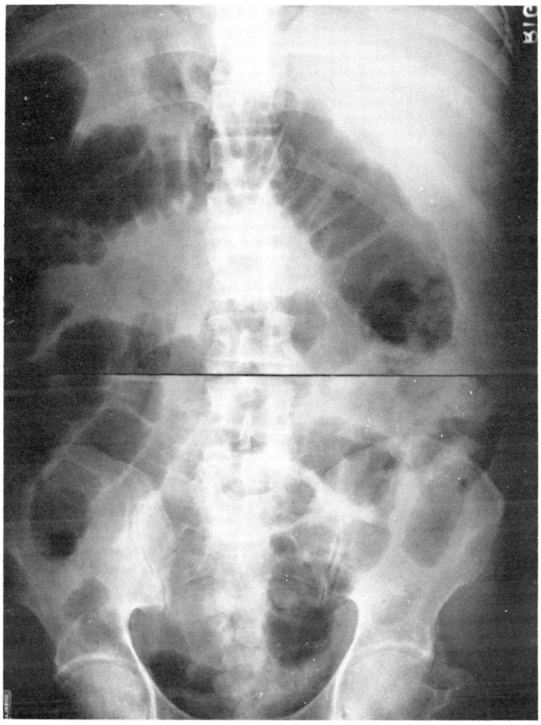

A

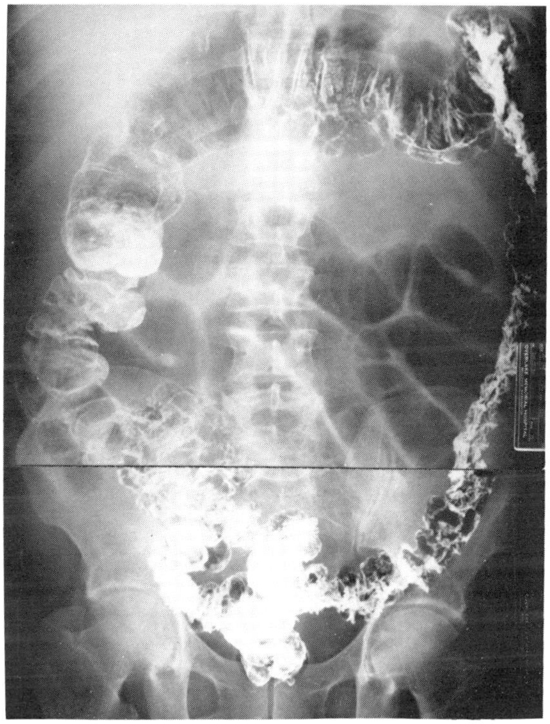

B

Fig. 12-3. Effects of complete celiac vagotomy. This patient underwent anterior selective–posterior total vagotomy plus antrectomy. Postvagotomy ileus resulted and was demonstrated on a flat roentgenogram (A) eight days postoperatively. Barium enema (B) showed dilated loops of small intestine and dilatation of the colon to the splenic flexure (the midgut is innervated by the celiac vagi). The descending colon and rectum were collapsed (the hindgut is innervated by the sacral parasympathetic nerves). Spontaneous expulsion of flatus did not occur until the twelfth postoperative day, but a flat roentgenogram (C) still showed intestinal dilatation and retention of barium in the cecum and proximal ascending colon.

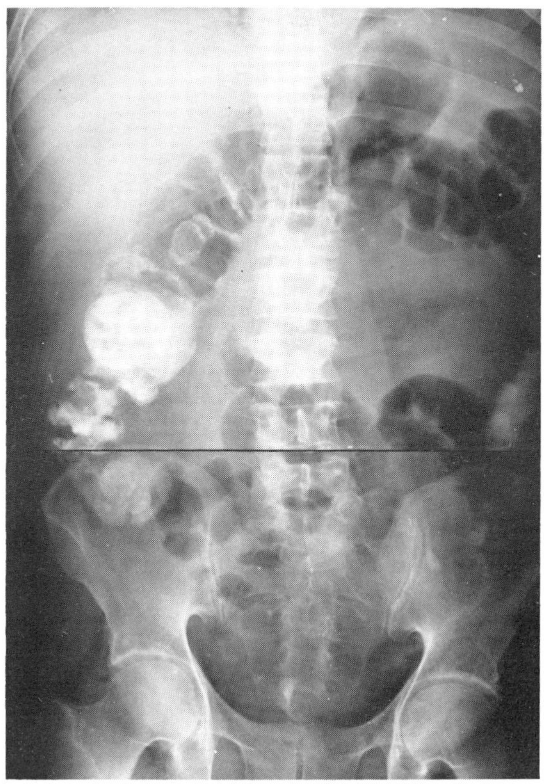

C

celiac component of total vagotomy (Fig. 12-3).

DIARRHEA

The first consideration in discussing postvagotomy diarrhea is its differentiation from the diarrhea associated with dumping, and also from diarrhea of bacterial origin in the blind jejunal loop after simple gastrojejunostomy or the Billroth II resection. Rapid gastric emptying from the "dumping stomach" [11] and consequent intestinal hurry often culminate in explosive diarrhea. In contrast to this postcibal diarrhea of dumping, true postvagotomy diarrhea occurs without rhyme or reason. It may be continuous or episodic with relapses and remissions lasting several days. Postvagotomy diarrhea severe enough to be disabling is rare—less than 5 percent—but diarrhea troublesome enough to constitute a complaint is more common. The infrequency of severe diarrhea explains why the surgeon who does an occasional total vagotomy may rarely if ever see an instance, but in large centers where total vagotomy is a common operation, disabling or troublesome postvagotomy diarrhea is a definite problem.

Celiac Vagotomy

Long-term if not permanent motile dysfunction of the midgut may occur after total vagotomy [14, 66]. Roentgenographic examinations with barium show intestinal dilatation, segmentation and puddling of content, stasis, and delayed transit time (Fig. 12-3). These sprue-like signs are a common denominator for many syndromes manifested by diarrhea. The patient whose roentgenograms are shown in Figure 12-3 underwent anterior-selective posterior-total vagotomy (preservation of only the hepatic vagi) and suffered the most severe nondumping postvagotomy diarrhea that I have ever encountered.

Hepatic Vagotomy

Another cause of diarrhea is an excessive excretion of dihydroxy bile acids [2] apparently caused by the hepatic component of total vagotomy. Large amounts of dihydroxy bile acids cause diarrhea by stimulating secretion of water and electrolytes. Binding the bile acids with cholestyramine has proved effective in relieving this type of postvagotomy diarrhea [3, 122]. Still unproved, however, are the suggestions that cholecystectomy exerts either a beneficial or a detrimental influence on the concentration of bile acids and on diarrhea [21]. Evaluation of the latter consideration must take into account the fact that a dilated and flaccid gallbladder cannot contract normally after *complete* total vagotomy (in contrast to its normal motility before vagotomy).

Comment

I have had minimal experience with the medical and surgical treatment of postvagotomy diarrhea. The only thing I can state with certainty is that it does not occur after vagotomy with preservation of the hepatic and celiac vagi [51, 64, 77].

LOSS OF GASTRIC ACID INHIBITION

The hepatic and celiac vagi regulate the release of a gastrone from the midgut. When the release of this gastrone is eliminated by total vagotomy, the loss of gastric acid inhibition is striking (Fig. 12-4).

Although most of the evidence for this acid inhibition is derived from Heidenhain pouch dogs [23, 27, 75, 79, 84, 94, 99, 100, 117, 121], the same mechanism occurs in humans [81]. In the previous edition of this book, I proposed that loss of the midgut gastrone was an important factor in explaining the lower rates of recurrence after selective vagotomy than after total vagotomy in patients with simple drainage. My proposal must now be modified because McVay's group [93] has since reported a recurrence rate with total vagotomy as low as ours with selective vagotomy [50].

Whether significant or not, the effect of acid inhibition by the hepatic and celiac vagi is not apparent with parietal vagotomy because it is overwhelmed by the antral vagal release of gastrin. With regard to the inhibitory influence of the antral vagi, we have not found any evi-

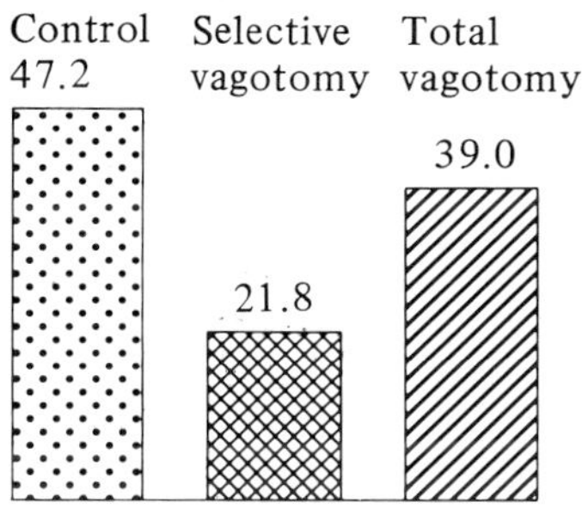

Fig. 12-4. Heidenhain pouch secretion expressed as mean mEq of total titrated acid (pH 7) in consecutive 24-hour collections for 30 days before and after each operative stage in dogs with pyloroplasty. (*Total vagotomy* is synonymous with *truncal vagotomy*.)

dence that this inhibition may be considered clinically significant.[3]

Completeness of Gastric Vagotomy

In the early 1960s we answered two basic questions in response to the criticism and skepticism concerning the completeness of gastric vagotomy by the selective technique.

DO THE HEPATIC AND CELIAC VAGI INNERVATE THE STOMACH?

This question implied that sparing the hepatic and celiac vagi would not permit complete vagotomy of the stomach. The following evidence showed that neither the hepatic nor the celiac vagus supplies efferent fibers to the stomach for motility or secretion.

Gastric Motility

Selective vagotomy eliminates the contractile response of the stomach to electrical vagal stimulation in animals [120] and humans [19].

[3]Consideration of the hepatic and celiac gastrone and other inhibitors [17, 24, 55, 67, 112] leads to the complex field of neurohumoral mechanisms. This field is beyond the scope of my knowledge, and I therefore defer to the senior editor (L. M. N.) of this book, referring the reader to an erudite resume of his studies [99, 100].

Gastric Secretion

Selective vagotomy eliminates the secretory response to insulin in animals [53, 106] and humans [46].

Vagal Release of Gastrin

Electrical stimulation of the gastric vagi to the isolated antrum elicits secretion of circulating neutral red dye from the parietal cell mass by the vagal release of gastrin [105]. Stimulation of the hepatic and celiac vagi does not [88].

WILL THE MORE COMPLICATED SELECTIVE TECHNIQUE INCREASE THE RATE OF INCOMPLETE VAGOTOMY?

During my initial experiments with parietal and selective vagotomy in his laboratory, Dr. Harkins repeatedly expressed curiosity about the completeness of gastric vagotomy. His curiosity increased when I started a clinical trial (see footnote 2), and he was not satisfied until he saw me do a selective vagotomy in 1960. Thereafter he became an enthusiastic convert from total to selective vagotomy—not because he was convinced of the rationale of sparing the hepatic and celiac vagi, but because he was convinced that the anatomical accuracy of the selective technique was the key to attaining consistently successful results of complete gastric vagotomy. His enthusiasm soon led to co-authorship with my group in the early 1960s [54, 56, 57] and extended to others (including Nyhus), who also reported a definite decrease in the incidence of incomplete vagotomy [77, 114].

The advantage of the anatomical accuracy of the selective technique is detailed in Chapter 2. Although this advantage has not led to general acceptance, it has resulted in consistently negative insulin tests [46] and no recurrent ulcers caused by incomplete vagotomy after a 12- to 17-year follow-up study [51].

Technique

The following technique [49] evolved through personal trial and error and observation of the techniques of others [1, 10, 19, 33, 43, 82,

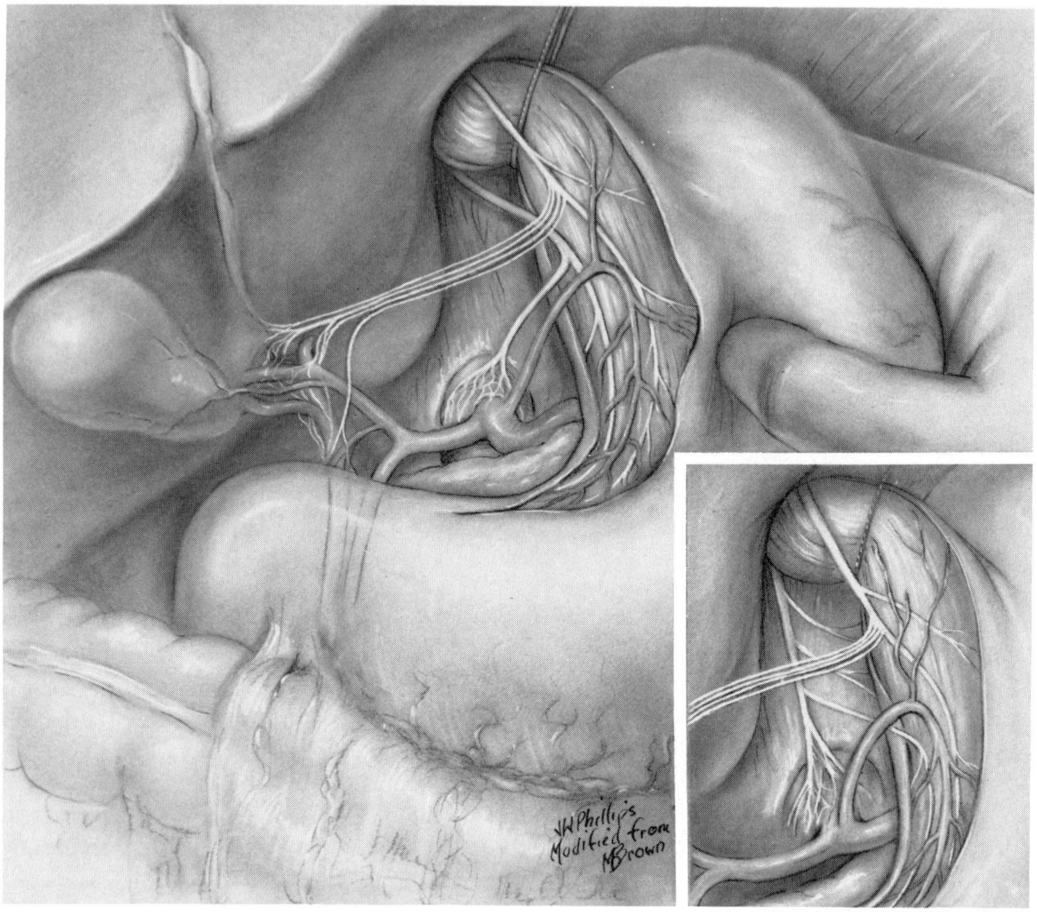

Fig. 12-5. The abdominal vagi. All vagal fibers shown in this illustration are readily identified by gross anatomical dissection. The hepatic vagal division (usually consisting of multiple fibers) from the anterior trunk courses within the lesser omentum to the porta hepatis. The celiac vagal division from the posterior trunk goes to the celiac autonomic plexus, usually in close association with the left gastric artery but occasionally with the right diaphragmatic crus (*inset*). The anterior and posterior gastric divisions from the anterior and posterior trunks run within the lesser omentum adjacent to the lesser curvature, sending off terminal branches to the anterior and posterior walls of the stomach from the cardia to the antrum.

123]. The illustration in Figure 12-5 provides overall orientation.

INCISIONS

The incision varies according to both the patient's body habitus and the hospital setting. The hospital setting may vary from a private hospital with one assistant to a university hospital with several assistants. The availability of the various self-retaining retractors is another important consideration for optimal exposure.

In patients with a narrow costal arch, a vertical midline incision is preferred. In patients with a wide costal arch, a conventional transverse or saber-slash incision [82] is preferred. In large, deep-chested, obese, and muscular men (who seem to present urgent indications

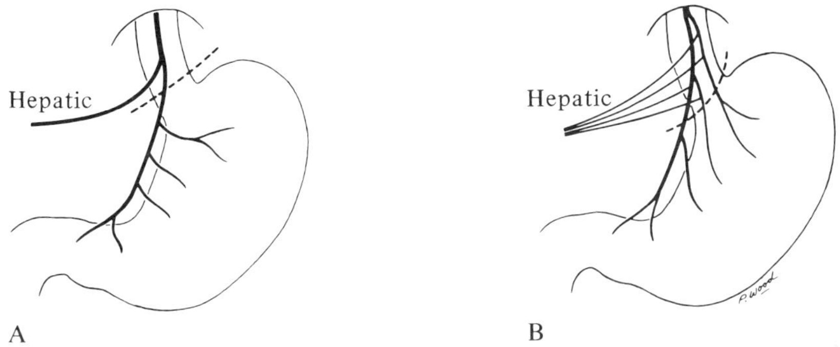

Fig. 12-6. Variations of the hepatic and anterior gastric vagi. (A) One anterior gastric truncal division at the cardia. (B) Multiple terminal gastric rami and low-lying hepatic vagi at the cardia.

for operation more often than not in the middle of the night, when minimal help is available), the Ross incision is most advantageous [110].

AVOIDING SPLENIC AND HEPATIC INJURY

Once the abdomen is entered, the first step is gentle retraction of the stomach and greater omentum to look for any omental attachments to the spleen. If any are present, it is often good judgment to divide them to prevent tearing the splenic capsule or pulp by retraction of the stomach and omentum during the subsequent operation. The next step is exposure of the hepatic vagi to ascertain the presence or absence of an aberrent left hepatic artery from the left gastric artery (the hepatogastric gastric artery). Both of these anomalies are described in Chapter 2.

VARIATIONS OF THE HEPATIC AND CELIAC VAGI

Although the course of the hepatic vagal division across the lesser omentum is constant, its origin varies. A selective vagotomy is quicker and easier when the patient has the anatomical pattern diagramed in Figure 12-6A than the pattern in Figure 12-6B.

The position of the posterior trunk–celiac division varies in the pancreatoduodenal fold (Fig. 12-7). This variability determines the ease or difficulty in identifying the division by palpation when the gastric vagi are first encircled.

THE VAGOTOMY

The technique for encircling all gastric vagi is illustrated in Figures 12-8 through 12-11. The anatomically positive inclusion of all gastric vagi within the surgical field is the sine qua non for accomplishing any complete vagotomy of the stomach.

Figures 12-12 through 12-15 illustrate selective vagotomy. Repair of a coexistent hiatal hernia plus posterior gastropexy is shown in Figure 12-16.

Variable Effects of Complete Gastric Vagotomy on Gastric Secretion

After initial experience with selective vagotomy complemented by distal resection, simple drainage by the Finney pyloroplasty [32] was evaluated. As determined by negative insulin tests [46, 51], this series with pyloroplasty provided material for study of the effect of complete vagotomy of the stomach alone on acid secretion. Among a total of 103 patients, preoperative and postoperative basal secretions were obtained from 90 patients. Results were expressed in terms of milliequivalents of free acid per hour. Using the levels of 1.5–2 mEq as the upper limit of normal secre-

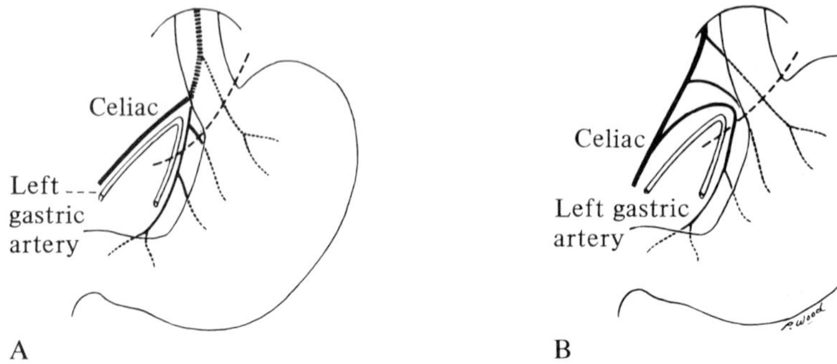

Fig. 12-7. Variations of the celiac and posterior gastric vagi. (A) The celiac division usually accompanies the main ascending left gastric artery, and the posterior gastric division follows the descending branch of the left gastric artery. (B) The celiac division of the posterior trunk lies close to the aorta and well away from the esophagus and gastric cardia. The posterior gastric vagi reach the stomach either independently (proximally) or in company with the left gastric artery (distally).

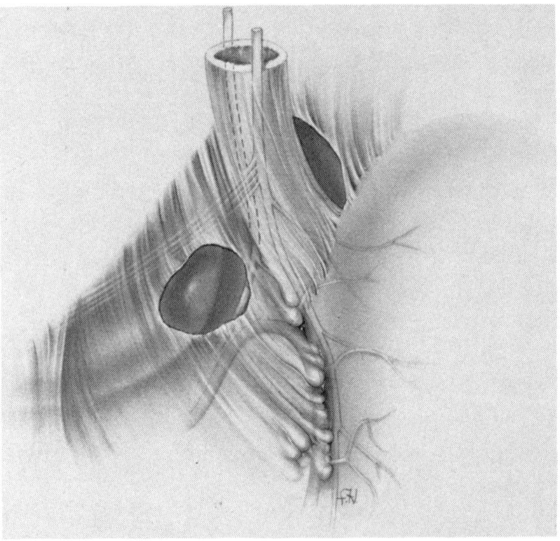

Fig. 12-8. For initial definition of the surgical field, the esophageal hiatus and vagal trunks purposely are not exposed. Instead, the hepatic vagi are identified. These vagi can always be seen in the avascular lesser omentum contrasted against the dark background of the caudate lobe of the liver. The lesser omentum is incised below the hepatic vagi well to the patient's right of the gastric cardia. No gastric vagi lie to the right of this incision in the lesser omentum. Next the peritoneum overlying the cardioesophageal angle of His is incised, and this opening is enlarged with the finger. No gastric vagi lie to the patient's left of this opening at the angle of His. Thus, between these two incisions in the lesser omentum and angle of His are included all anterior gastric vagi. None has been excluded. (From Griffith [49].)

tion, the 90 patients were divided into three groups.[4]

Group 1 (83 patients). Preoperative hypersecretion was not found in 12 patients. Hypersecretion in the other 71 patients ranged from 2.6 to 15.4 mEq. Vagotomy resulted in no free acid in 52 patients, and free acid less than 1.5 mEq in 31 patients. (Some patients with the highest levels of hypersecretion had no free acid after vagotomy. Conversely, some patients with the lowest levels of hypersecretion did have free acid after vagotomy.)

Group 2 (4 patients). Preoperative hypersecretion ranging from 4.2 to 7.8 mEq was reduced to high-normal levels of 1.7–1.9 mEq.

Group 3 (3 patients). Preoperative hypersecretion of 2.7, 3.2, and 8.9 mEq was not reduced. Each of these 3 patients had two insulin tests, and all tests were negative. This incidence of 3 of 90 patients with persistent

[4]This study was done *after* most American surgeons had adopted the method of basal acid output per hour in preference to Dragstedt's traditional method of output per 12 hours, but *before* we adopted the British refinement of maximal acid output. Although the latter is more accurate and reproducible, basal output still has some meaning.

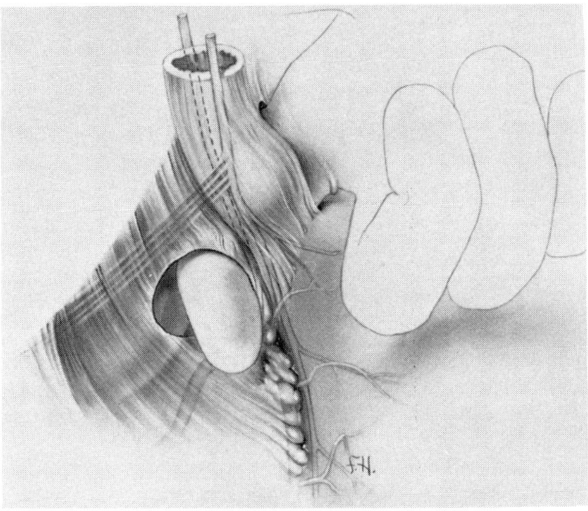

Fig. 12-9. The method of encircling all posterior gastric vagi cannot really be illustrated because it cannot be seen. It is done by finger dissection. The finger is worked into the angle of His, *not* with the aim of encircling the esophagus, but with the aim of palpating the posterior trunk–celiac division posterior to the esophagus. Once the posterior trunk–celiac division has been positively identified by palpating its course to the celiac plexus, the finger is dissected through the areolar tissue in the pancreatogastric fold behind the posterior trunk–celiac division. Encircling the posterior trunk–celiac division isolates all posterior gastric vagi since none lie behind the division. Next the fingertip encounters the peritoneum covering the patient's right surface of the gastropancreatic fold in the lesser peritoneal space. At this point the fingertip may be seen, or at least palpated with a finger of the other hand, through the incision in the lesser omentum initially made below the hepatic vagal division. The fingertip is then worked into the lesser peritoneal space through the peritoneum covering the gastropancreatic fold to emerge through the incision in the lesser omentum below the hepatic vagal division, as illustrated. The encirclement of *all* gastric vagi with the most distal part of the esophagus is thereby accomplished with anatomical certainty. (From Griffith [49].)

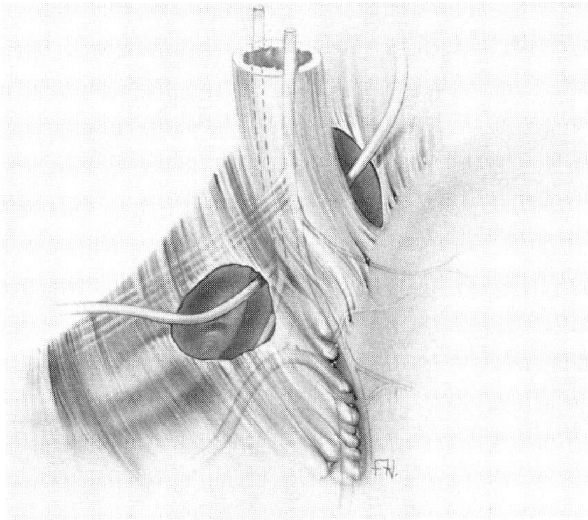

Fig. 12-10. The encircling finger in Figure 12-9 is replaced by a soft rubber urethral catheter to maintain the encirclement and exposure. (From Griffith [49].)

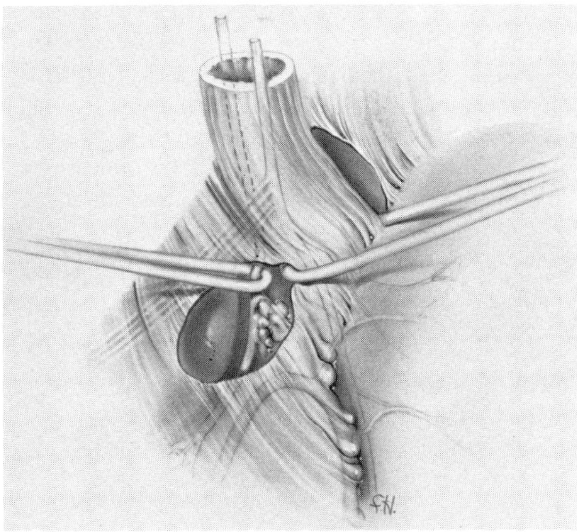

Fig. 12-11. By finger dissection the posterior trunk–celiac division is mobilized from its bed in the gastropancreatic fold and is encircled with another rubber urethral catheter so that it may be gently retracted to the patient's right. The original catheter in Figure 12-10 is then repositioned as shown to encircle all anterior gastric vagi with the most distal part of the abdominal esophagus, which then may be retracted to the patient's left.

At this stage two points should be noted: neither the esophageal hiatus nor the vagal trunks have been exposed or dissected, and either selective or total vagotomy may now be performed. (From Griffith [49].)

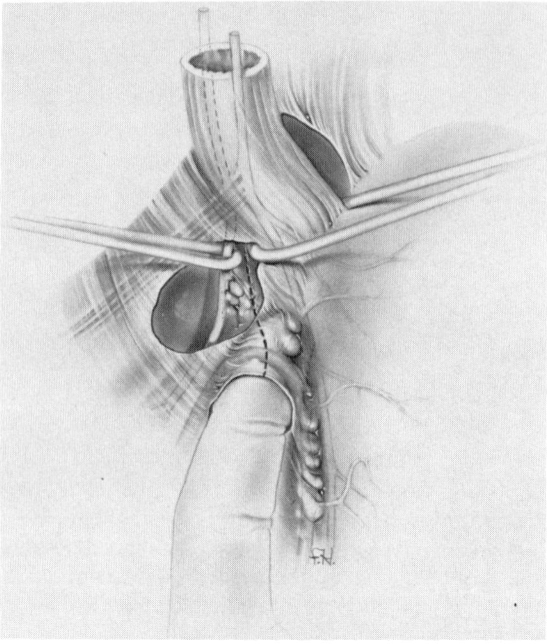

Fig. 12-12. Attention is now directed to the loop of the left gastric artery where it approaches the lesser curvature of the stomach and bifurcates into the descending gastric and ascending esophageal branches. I prefer finger dissection to isolate the descending left gastric artery in order to be able to transect any posterior gastric vagi that may accompany that vessel to the stomach. Then as indicated by the dashed line, the lesser curvature is freed entirely from the gastric cardia with successive transections between clamps and ligation up to the encircling catheters in order to transect any other posterior gastric vagi. Clearly this dissection is the step that makes selective vagotomy more difficult than total vagotomy. It may be even more complicated if an aberrant left hepatic artery from the left gastric artery is encountered (not illustrated, but present in approximately 10 percent of patients.) (From Griffith [49].)

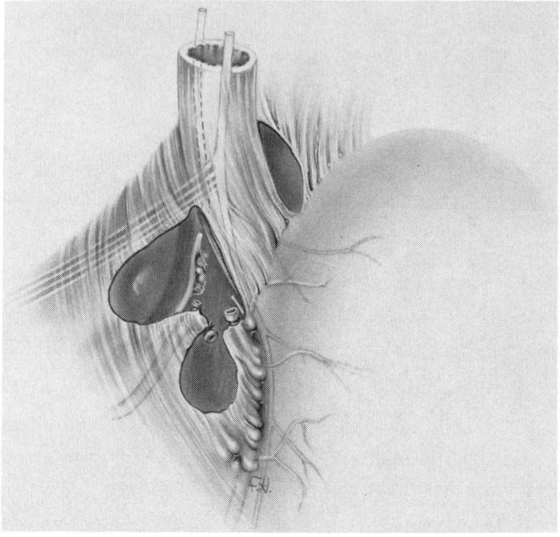

Fig. 12-13. The completed dissection described in Figure 12-12. By transecting all lesser omental attachments to the gastric cardia, thereby totally separating the posterior trunk–celiac division from the distal esophagus and gastric cardia, all posterior gastric vagi are severed. (From Griffith [49].)

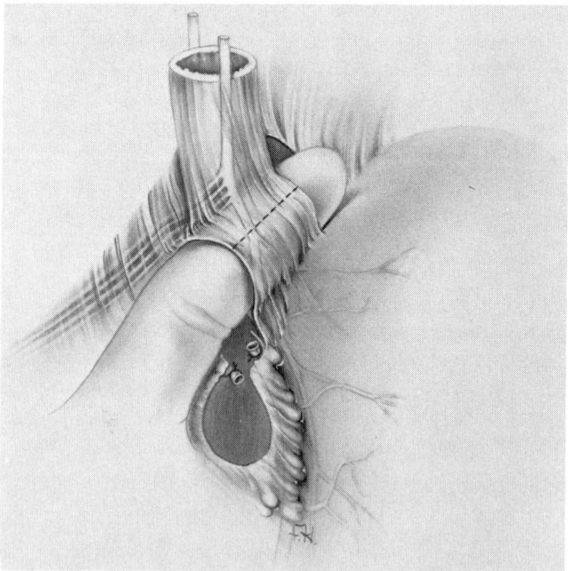

Fig. 12-14. All remaining tissue anterior to the esophagus—i.e., all tissue between the original incisions in the lesser omentum and angle of His—is dissected from the esophagus with the finger before division between right-angle clamps and ligation. This tissue contains all anterior gastric vagi and some esophageal vessels. (From Griffith [49].)

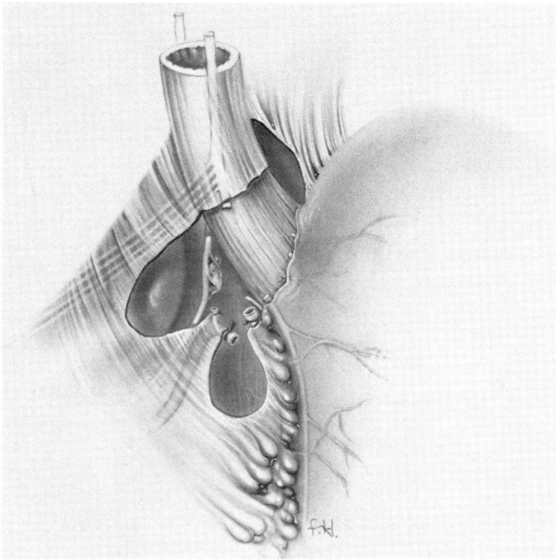

Fig. 12-15. The distal esophagus and gastric cardia are now completely separated from their attachments to all other tissue, including the vagal trunks. The only gastric vagi that can possibly remain are small twigs that may have arisen from the trunks or esophageal plexus above the surgical field. The usual careful search for these small twigs is therefore carefully conducted within and beneath the esophageal fascia propria. The esophageal muscle is thereby bared in its circumference. The esophageal muscle is not violated, for any nerves found within the muscle innervate the esophagus, not the stomach. Note that the completed dissection is identical to that currently emphasized for parietal vagotomy. At least two encircling fingers are used to feel for any intact fibers around the esophagus mobilized 5–7 cm. (From Griffith [49].)

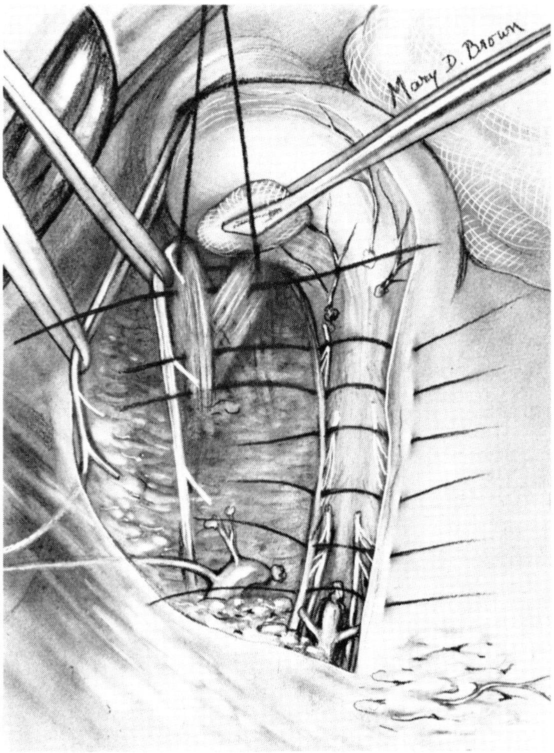

Fig. 12-16. Hiatal repair and posterior gastropexy. The two uppermost sutures approximate the diaphragmatic crura. The next two sutures anchor the gastric cardia to the right crus. (After observing this technique Lucius Hill refined it by incorporating the arcuate ligament for the so-called Hill repair.) In my early experience the lowest sutures imbricating the lesser curvature were placed when, as discussed in Chapter 2, vagal reinnervation and necrotic perforation were feared. (From Griffith [45].)

hypersecretion despite complete vagotomy compares with Dragstedt's finding of 3 similar patients in his first 70 vagotomies [128]. This type of hypersecretion has also been noted by others [40, 41]. It has never been observed after antrectomy, and therefore has been attributed to some type of antral hyperfunction [41] that is not associated with G-cell hyperplasia [39] or ulcerogenic endocrinopathy.

LACK OF CORRELATION BETWEEN SECRETION AND RECURRENCE

After follow-up periods of 12 to 17 years, one ulcer recurred, and that in the patient with the lowest level of persistent hypersecretion (2.7 mEq) among the three group-3 persistent hypersecretors. Inexplicably, the other two persistent hypersecretors have not had recurrences, nor have the four patients in group 2 with secretion on the border between high normal and low hypersecretion. The exact role of pyloroplasty in these patients is conjectural. Also, in four group-1 patients with satisfactory reductions of secretion, biliary reflux resulted in one gastric ulcer and two instances of hemorrhagic gastritis; the fourth patient had a gastric ulcer associated with stasis. The overall rate of actual recurrence plus the development of new gastric complications approximated 5 percent. No ulcer recurred because of incomplete vagotomy. It is to be noted that these results are from operations for duodenal ulcer. Our experience with vagotomy plus pyloroplasty for gastric ulcer has been poor [53].

COMMENT
In addition to the unsatisfactory reduction of acid in the few patients with pyloroplasty, dumping was as frequent and severe as after distal resection. These disadvantages prompted further experiments that led to the use of suprapyloric antrectomy for better control of both acid secretion and dumping [48].

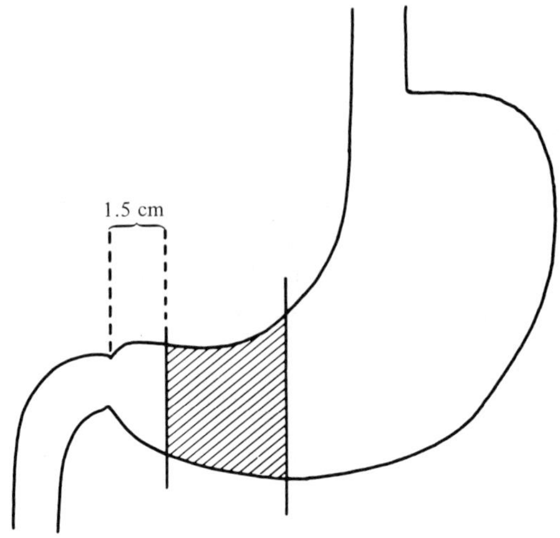

Fig. 12-17. Suprapyloric antrectomy. The distal line of transection is at a measured 1.5–2.0 cm from the middle of the pyloric ring. The proximal gastric remnant is anastomosed to the distal antral cuff. (From Griffith [47].)

Suprapyloric Antrectomy

For the treatment of gastric (and not duodenal) ulcer, Maki's group [91] reported their pylorus-preserving gastrectomy designed to prevent dumping. Shiratori of Maki's department demonstrated this operation when he visited us in Seattle in 1967. The extent of resection was quite limited and approximated an antrectomy rather than a subtotal gastrectomy. We therefore called it a *suprapyloric antrectomy* (Fig. 12-17).

Postoperative cineroentgenograms of gastric emptying were impressive. The meal was stored in an adequate gastric reservoir and was emptied of small amounts in a rhythmic manner as the pylorus opened and closed. Shiratori emphasized that the limited resection was adequate for gastric ulcer but inadequate for duodenal ulcer, and that a more extensive resection for duodenal ulcer would remove too much of the reservoir and permit dumping. Therefore, for duodenal ulcer he suggested that we combine suprapyloric antrectomy with selective vagotomy. When we raised the question of gastric stasis, he answered our question with another cineroentgenographic study of gastric emptying after vagotomy without drainage.

THE ANTIPERISTALTIC ANTRAL PUMP AFTER VAGOTOMY
Cineroentgenography showed quite clearly that the meal in the antrum was propelled by antiperistalsis proximally into the corpus with the net result of stasis. Subsequent studies in our laboratory were confirmatory [78]. This finding meant that hypotonia and pyloric tonus are not the only causes of gastric stasis.

We therefore studied selective vagotomy plus suprapyloric antrectomy in Heidenhain pouch dogs. Results were a marked decrease in pouch secretion and partial preservation of normally rhythmic gastric emptying as determined by cineroentgenography, and no stasis after test meals of solid food. Thus removal of the antiperistaltic antral pump did indeed prevent gastric stasis consequent to complete gastric vagotomy [28].

THE 1.5- TO 2-CM ANTRAL CUFF
The measured length of the antral cuff proved critical from the standpoints of both motility and secretion. Shorter cuffs evaluated by Maki's group destroyed pyloric function and permitted dumping. Longer cuffs in our dogs resulted in antiperistaltic dysfunction that caused both stasis and increased Heidenhain pouch secretion [4, 28]. Also, conversion of the selective vagotomy to total vagotomy resulted in a further increase in pouch secretion [79]. This finding added to the evidence for hepatic and celiac vagal inhibition of gastric secretion.

CLINICAL TRIAL
Of the first 20 patients with selective vagotomy plus suprapyloric antrectomy, 16 had excellent results without stasis or dumping in response to provocative meals. The remaining 4 patients had definite signs and symptoms of moderate gastric stasis. Why this stasis occurred in only a few patients (and, conversely, why stasis does *not* occur in a few patients after both selective and total vagotomy without drainage) is unknown. Whatever the reasons, removal of only the antiperistaltic antral pump is insufficient for preventing gastric stasis in all patients. Gastric hypomotility and pyloric tonus must still be considered.[5]

Pylorotomy (Not Pyloroplasty)
With the idea of only decreasing pyloric tonus and not destroying pyloric function completely by pyloroplasty, pylorotomy was added. In contrast to a pyloromyotomy, pylorotomy entails a full-thickness transection to eliminate any mucosal or submucosal stenosis that may be present. The longitudinal transection of the anterior pyloric ring (and only the ring) is closed transversely with interrupted sutures. In patients with a short and thick pylorus, the length of the pylorotomy approximates 1 cm or less. In patients with longer and thinner pyloric rings, a complete pylorotomy would require a significantly longer incision, and its transverse closure would seriously impair valvular function. Therefore, in these patients an *incomplete* pylorotomy is done. The length of the incision is determined by a finger passed through the antral cuff to determine the size of the new pyloric outlet. The finished pylorotomy provides a more patulous outlet that still imparts the sensation of a valvular ring when palpated from within. Endoscopy has shown that this ring still opens and closes, albeit partially in many patients.

Results
The addition of pylorotomy prevents gastric stasis and does not cause dumping in most patients. In the few patients with dumping, the frequency and severity are considerably less than previously observed with complete antrectomy or pyloroplasty. In no patient has dumping been disabling, and in no patient has intestinal hurry been fast enough to cause diarrhea. The cardiovascular symptoms have also been mild and, in most patients, manifest only with provocative meals containing raw sugar. Gastric secretion has been consistently decreased to normal or lower than normal levels. These results support our experimental findings that the gastrin from the entire antrum is for the most part removed by suprapyloric antrectomy [6, 28, 79] and that therefore the antral cuff kept in the acid stream is an unimportant source of gastrin. No ulcer has recurred to date. Furthermore, no signs or symptoms of reflux gastritis have appeared. Thus the pyloric valve serves to prevent both dumping and duodenal reflux [48].

[5]Gastric outlet obstruction was not the cause of stasis. The more one inspects and palpates the outlet at operation, the less is the surprise at finding moderate-to-severe stenosis in patients with no preoperative symptoms or roentgenographic signs of stasis. In a few patients the stenosis is caused by a mucosal and submucosal diaphragm without evidence of ulcer [109]. In the latter situation, and also in some instances of obvious ulcer, the stenosis cannot be seen or felt by palpation between thumb and finger. The open antral cuff during suprapyloric antrectomy provides ready access to determine the adequacy of the pyloric outlet. In contrast, parietal vagotomy requires either a gastrotomy or calibrators passed orally for an equally accurate assessment of the gastric outlet.

A Comparison

Since adopting selective vagotomy plus suprapyloric antrectomy rather than parietal vagotomy, I have been a keen observer of the many clinical trials of the latter operation. As far as I know, no other group has evaluated the former. This fact prompts a comparison of the two operations.

MAGNITUDE OF OPERATION

Parietal vagotomy is clearly a less extensive operation than selective vagotomy plus suprapyloric antrectomy, and, by not entering the stomach, eliminates wound contamination from gastric content. These advantages are partially outweighed by a meticulous and time-consuming dissection and more than outweighed in patients requiring a second operation for recurrence. Suprapyloric antrectomy with pylorotomy is obviously more extensive than pyloroplasty but, because it does not require dissection of the so-called difficult duodenum, it is definitely less extensive than complete antrectomy (see the section in Chap. 2, Necrotic Perforation of Lesser Curvature).

DUMPING

Parietal vagotomy has virtually eliminated dumping, and in this respect is definitely superior. Pylorotomy with suprapyloric antrectomy, however, does not cause complete loss of the valvular function of the pylorus. As previously noted, the completed pylorotomy still imparts the sensation of a valvular ring to the palpating finger, and the pyloric outlet still opens and closes when viewed through the endoscope in most but not all patients. This preservation of pyloric function, or at least partial preservation, explains why dumping is considerably less than after complete antrectomy or pyloroplasty.

RECURRENCE

In contrast to the recurrence rate to date—zero—after selective vagotomy plus suprapyloric antrectomy, the high rate of recurrence after parietal vagotomy is now recognized as the real problem that deters more general acceptance. This problem includes not only proven recurrent ulcers but recurrent symptoms without ulcer as well. The latter, as pointed out by Goligher [42], is "disturbingly frequent in Leeds." Fear of recurrence was the primary factor that dissuaded me from adopting parietal vagotomy after our final experiments in the late 1960s.[6]

In the United States the problem of recurrence has been approached primarily with emphasis on a thorough esophageal dissection—the same dissection illustrated in Figure 12-14. Although a complete vagotomy proximally results, recurrence has continued. It is therefore important to recognize other causes of recurrence and equally important to recognize these causes as a source of inevitable recurrence in some patients.

Incomplete Vagotomy Distally

Considerable variation exists in the location of the antral-parietal mucosal border (see Fig. 2-4) and also in the length of the nerve of Latarjet (see Fig. 2-7). The occurrence of a small extent of antral mucosa makes the accomplishment of a complete parietal vagotomy an-

[6]When devising parietal vagotomy in the mid-1950s, I was unaware of the occurrence of both persistent hypersecretion from antral hyperfunction and distal incomplete vagotomy from a small antrum. These entities were not discovered until the mid-1960s—the former by studying secretions of patients with selective vagotomy plus pyloroplasty, and the latter by delineating the antral-parietal mucosal border with Congo red in a few patients with Kirk's mucosal antrectomy [80] and, subsequently, in the pilot patients with suprapyloric antrectomy. During this period, as detailed in Chapter 2, experiments were continued that eventually disproved the law of all or none and proved that gastric vagal innervation is segmental [105, 107]. This finding was the breakthrough that provided an anatomical basis for the variable adequacy of vagotomy and its permanence [72–74, 86, 87, 89] (see Figs. 2-14 through 2-16) and also the anatomical basis for permanent parietal vagotomy. Accordingly, further study was done (in association with Bente and Erik Amdrup) that revealed a twofold increase in 24-hour Heidenhain pouch secretion [5] that was abolished by suprapyloric antrectomy and suprapyloric mucosal antrectomy [6]. These findings, plus the occurrence of antral hyperfunction and distal incomplete vagotomy, persuaded me to continue a clinical trial already started of selective vagotomy with suprapyloric antrectomy. Our final experiments showed that the increased pouch secretion was not so apparent in the fasting state [8, 9]. On the basis of these experiments Erik Amdrup started his clinical trial of parietal vagotomy on his return from Seattle to Copenhagen in 1969. His latest communication from Aarhus in 1982 reports a recurrence rate of about 10 percent, which he believes is primarily due to the retained antrum. He now believes that parietal vagotomy should not be done when the pH electrode defines a small antrum.

atomically impossible in about 20 percent of patients [96]. These incomplete results are usually harmless adequate vagotomies (see Figs. 2-14 through 2-16). But in patients with extremely small areas of antral mucosa that extend only 1–3 cm proximally from the pylorus [102] plus extremely short nerves of Latarjet that end 8 cm or more from the pylorus [11, 96, 118, 119], the results are inadequate vagotomies that pose the *potential* for a recurrence rate of about 5 percent. The *actual* rate is unknown because the antral-parietal mucosa is usually not determined when antrectomy is done for recurrence, and in most centers a parietal cell count is not done on the resected antrum. When a parietal cell count has been done, large concentrations of parietal cells have been found in some specimens [4].

Antral Hyperfunction

The incidence of persistent hypersecretion with or without G-cell hyperplasia poses the *potential* for recurrence in an additional 5 percent of patients. Here again the *actual* recurrence rate has not been established, particularly in centers where secretory studies have been abandoned in favor of gastrin determinations. Gastrin determinations per se cannot establish the diagnosis of persistent hypersecretion from antral hyperfunction.

Gastric Stasis

In his vast experience, Holle [61] has noted more epigastric fullness and dyspepsia from delayed emptying in patients with parietal vagotomy alone than in patients with parietal vagotomy plus his mucosal pyloroplasty. Others do not confirm the occurrence of clinically significant stasis after parietal vagotomy, but the fact that the innervated antrum has considerably more secretory potential than the denervated antrum [5, 117] raises two considerations. First, occult stasis can be detected in some patients without symptoms when the test meal is solid food [62]. Second, markedly increased and prolonged levels of gastrin are present when the allegedly empty stomach contains residue of stasis [16]. Although this combination of occult stasis plus excessive gastrin raises suspicion, it has not been proved or disproved as a cause of recurrence—even when the so-called recurrence is actually a new prepyloric gastric ulcer rather than a true recurrent duodenal ulcer.[7]

Reinnervation

The previously mentioned high rate of incomplete but adequate vagotomy results in the frequent observation of negative insulin tests in the early postoperative period converting to positive tests within a few weeks. This conversion is caused by so-called recovery and not reinnervation. Some reinnervation undoubtedly occurs, however—not by restoration of divided nerve ends but by sprouting. The latter type of reinnervation may take place in three areas. First, by virtue of the fact that parietal vagotomy cuts the intramural route of innervation to the antral mucosa and preserves the extramural route (see Fig. 2-10), vagotomy of the antral mucosa is incomplete. Sprouting from the residually innervated areas of mucosa reinnervates the denervated areas, but exactly how many G cells are initially denervated and exactly how many are eventually reinnervated is unknown. Second, sprouting from the residually innervated antral mucosa may reinnervate small areas of the adjacent parietal mucosa (see Fig. 2-15, bottom). Third, any residually innervated areas of adequate vagotomy within the parietal mucosa may enlarge slightly by sprouting (see Fig. 2-15, top).

Although reinnervation by sprouting may

[7]In his early experience Dragstedt became increasingly suspicious of stasis as a cause of gastric ulcer after total vagotomy without drainage or with a high-lying gastrojejunostomy. But his roentgenologists, using liquid barium, could not confirm stasis in all patients. Accordingly, Dragstedt supervised his own roentgenologic studies, using "a new test meal, consisting of meat, eggs, milk, toast, and cereal, mixed with barium sulfate" [101]. This new meal established the diagnosis of stasis that liquid barium could not and provided the basis for Dragstedt's diagnosis of the so-called stasis gastric ulcer. Consequently, he insisted that the antrum be drained by a low-lying gastrojejunostomy close to the pylorus and, later, by the Weinberg pyloroplasty. Although crude in this atomic age of nuclear methods of gastric emptying, Dragstedt's test meal still has some merit (to the amusement and then amazement of young roentgenologists who have never heard of it). Now, some 30 years after Dragstedt's work, more and more attention is being paid to solid rather than liquid test meals.

explain some or all of the gradual increase in secretion frequently noted after parietal vagotomy in the long term (in contrast to any increase by recovery in the short term), it has not been proved to be a cause of recurrence. It also has not been disproved. The microscopic studies revealing definite reinnervation by Joffe [69] and his group [70] are impressive, and the cause is probably sprouting rather than restoration of neural continuity.

Surgical Treatment of Recurrence

Although medical therapy has proved highly effective for recurrent symptoms without proved ulcer and also for proved ulcer in many patients, some patients require an operation. Antrectomy enjoys universal success because it removes both distal incomplete vagotomy and hypersecretion from antral hyperfunction; however, it also permits dumping. If the pylorus can be saved and if the prevention of dumping is still a goal, I recommend suprapyloric antrectomy. Furthermore, by the time a second operation becomes necessary, gastric motility has recovered enough to obviate the need for pylorotomy. This last consideration is in keeping with the success in closing a gastrojejunostomy (and occasionally in restoring the pylorus after pyloroplasty) for the relief of dumping after vagotomy plus drainage [76, 92].

Selection of Patients

In view of the various causes of recurrence, it is my conviction that parietal vagotomy should not be done routinely in all patients. Better results may be obtained by better patient selection.

WHERE IS THE ULCER?

Parietal vagotomy was devised for duodenal ulcer. In the case of gastric ulcer, and contrary to many reports, our results with vagotomy alone have been poor. Recurrence after parietal vagotomy for pyloric ulcer is also notorious. Channel ulcers may be either duodenal or gastric, because the location of the antral-duodenal mucosal border varies; it may lie proximal to, within, or distal to the pyloric ring.

WILL THE PATIENT EXPERIENCE DUMPING?

Hinshaw's group [59] injected concentrated glucose through an intrajejunal tube into preoperative patients and recorded the presence or absence of dumping. After gastric resection, this test was repeated with oral glucose. The postoperative results correlated exactly with the preoperative results, including the various degrees of severity of dumping. Hinshaw [58] writes that his test continues to be a reliable method for predicting who will and who will not have dumping.

With Hinshaw's test for dumping, the rationale of doing parietal vagotomy in patients innately immune to the dumping syndrome is open to serious question. So-called nondumpers are perhaps better served with the more definitive combination of vagotomy and antrectomy, preferably selective and suprapyloric—the former to prevent midgut dysfunction and the latter to avoid a difficult duodenum and to minimize postoperative reflux. For the dumpers, two other questions are posed before proceeding with parietal vagotomy.

WILL PARIETAL VAGOTOMY BE COMPLETE?

In centers where endoscopic examination has become a routine diagnostic study, application of the K test [83] would bring to light the presence of an extremely small antrum. This finding may well contraindicate parietal vagotomy and indicate suprapyloric antrectomy with pylorotomy plus selective vagotomy. (Routine antral biopsy is not generally considered worthwhile because the yield of G-cell hyperplasia is so low.)

IS ANTRECTOMY NEEDED?

Several surgeons, particularly the British (including one of the editors of this book, C. W.), have reduced the recurrence rate of parietal vagotomy by not doing it in patients whose maximal acid output is above a certain preset level and doing instead a vagotomy and antrectomy. Our data from selective vagotomy plus pyloroplasty support the validity of this method in most but not all patients. For example, some patients with very high levels of hypersecretion are rendered achlorhydric by complete vagotomy. Therefore, the predicted need for antrectomy in these patients results in needless antrectomies. Conversely, some patients with relatively low levels of hypersecretion maintain these low levels after complete vagotomy, but the levels are high enough to cause recurrence after any type of vagotomy. In these patients the needed antrectomy is not predicted. Thus the question to ask is, "Is antrectomy needed?" not, "Who will and who will not have a recurrence after parietal vagotomy?" Secretory testing can provide an answer to the first question for some patients. In any event, if antrectomy seems indicated, I again recommend suprapyloric antrectomy.

COMMENT

When selective vagotomy plus suprapyloric antrectomy was done as a routine procedure, the foregoing tests were unnecessary. With parietal vagotomy, however, this method of patient selection to contraindicate its use becomes mandatory if recurrence is to be eliminated or at least minimized. Selective vagotomy plus suprapyloric antrectomy is recommended for all nondumpers and dumpers with either or both high levels of hypersecretion and small antra. Parietal vagotomy is recommended for dumpers with low levels of hypersecretion and antra large enough to permit complete or adequate vagotomy.

The traditional school of surgical thought has emphasized lack of recurrence with definitive operations that cause dumping. Conversely, the new school of parietal vagotomy emphasizes no dumping and accepts recurrence. Some of the conflict between the old and the new may be resolved by recognizing selective vagotomy plus suprapyloric antrectomy as a procedure that meets the old requirement of no recurrence and the new requirement of no dumping, albeit not as effectively as parietal vagotomy. Ideally both operations have a place, and each may be used as indicated by the proposed methods of patient selection. Although these selection methods require more than the usual time and effort given to diagnostic study and may seem somewhat esoteric, the goal of no dumping and no recurrence requires proper patient selection and the use of both antidumping procedures.

Acknowledgment

For her patience and understanding during preparation of this chapter and Chapter 2, I want to thank my wife, Dolores (nee Meisner), whose gastrointestinal submucosal plexus is derived from the same genes as its namesake, Georg Meissner. Her great grandfather dropped one *s* from Meissner after immigrating to the United States in order to simplify the spelling and become "more American." It may be of some interest for British readers to note that another George, my paternal grandfather, sailed with the Royal Navy from Bristol, jumped ship in Boston, and homesteaded on the midwestern prairie a few miles north of the homestead that spawned Frank and Jesse James, whom he and others in the countryside befriended during the earliest forays against the hated railroad that disrupted the land with track.

References

1. Alexiu, O. Place de la vagotomie sélective avec antrectomie dans la chirugie de l'ulcère duodénal. *Acta Gastroenterol. Belg.* 28:154, 1965.
2. Allan, J. G., Gerskowitch, V. P., and Russell, R. I. The role of bile acids in the pathogenesis of postvagotomy diarrhoea. *Br. J. Surg.* 61:516, 1974.
3. Allan, J. G., and Russell, R. J. Double-blind controlled trial of cholestyramine in the treatment of post-vagotomy diarrhea. *Gut* 16:830, 1975.
4. Allgöwer, M. Personal visit, 1980.
5. Amdrup, B. M., and Griffith, C. A. Selective vagotomy of the parietal cell mass. I. With preservation of the innervated antrum and pylorus. *Ann. Surg.* 170:207, 1969.
6. Amdrup, B. M., and Griffith, C. A. Selective vagotomy of the parietal cell mass. II. With suprapyloric mucosal antrectomy and suprapyloric antral resection. *Ann. Surg.* 170:215, 1969.

7. Amdrup, B. M., and Griffith, C. A. The effects of vagotomy upon biliary function in dogs. *J. Surg. Res.* 10:209, 1970.
8. Amdrup, B. M., and Griffith, C. A. The effect of insulin upon the response to feeding in dogs with selective vagotomy of the parietal cell mass. *Scand. J. Gastroenterol.* 5:655, 1970.
9. Amdrup, B. M., and Griffith, C. A. The effect of a ganglion-blocking agent (hexamethonium bromide) upon the response to feeding in dogs with selective vagotomy of the parietal cell mass. *Scand. J. Gastroenterol.* 5:667, 1970.
10. Amdrup, E., Clemmesen, T., and Andreassen, J. Selective gastric vagotomy technic and primary results. *Am. J. Dig. Dis.* 12:351, 1967.
11. Andersen, D. Personal communication, 1982.
12. Andrews, E. W., Andrews, E., and Mix, C. L. "Dumping stomach" and other results of gastrojejunostomy: Operative cure by disconnecting old stoma. *Surg. Clin. Chicago* 4:879, 1920.
13. Baldwin, J. N., Heer, F. W., Albo, R., Pelso, O., Ruby, L., and Silen, W. Effect of vagus nerve stimulation on hepatic secretion of bile in human subjects. *Am. J. Surg.* 111:66, 1966.
14. Ballinger, W. F., II. The extragastric effects of vagotomy. *Surg. Clin. North Am.* 46:455, 1966.
15. Barnett, W. O., and Hilbun, G. R. Dissolution of human gallstone in the dog's gallbladder after various degrees of vagotomy. *Surgery* 60:840, 1966.
16. Bone, J., Host, V., Brandsborg, M., et al. An experimental study of parietal cell vagotomy with further graduated denervation of the antrum. *World J. Surg.* 2:249, 1978.
17. Brown, C. B. Gastric inhibitory polypeptide (GIP). *Gastroenterology* 67:733, 1974.
18. Burge, H. W. Vagal nerve section in chronic duodenal ulceration. *Ann. R. Coll. Surg. Engl.* 26:231, 1960.
19. Burge, H. W., and Frohn, M. J. N. The technique of bilateral selective vagotomy with the electrical stimulation test. *Br. J. Surg.* 56:452, 1969.
20. Clave, R. A., and Gaspar, M. R. Incidence of gall bladder disease after vagotomy. *Am. J. Surg.* 118:169, 1969.
21. Condon, J. R., Robinson, V., and Suleman, M. J. The cause and treatment of post-vagotomy diarrhoea. *Br. J. Surg.* 62:309, 1975.
22. Cowie, A., and Clark, C. G. The lithogenic effect of vagotomy. *Bull. Soc. Int. Chir.* 31:7, 1972.
23. Davis, J. L., Franklin, R. H., and Scott, H. W., Jr. Effects of selective gastric vagotomy and total abdominal vagotomy on Heidenhain pouch secretion in dogs with pyloroplasty. *Am. Surg.* 38:667, 1972.
24. Debas, H. T. Proximal gastric vagotomy interferes with a fundic inhibitory mechanism: A hypothesis for the high recurrence rate of peptic ulceration. *Am. J. Surg.* 146:51, 1983.
25. Deveny, C. W., Gardiner, B. N., and Way, L. W. Effect of truncal vagotomy on bile kinetics in rhesus monkeys. *Surg. Forum* 25:402, 1974.
26. Dragstedt, L. R. Personal communication, 1956.
27. Everett, M. T., and Griffith, C. A. Selective and total vagotomy plus pyloroplasty: A comparative study of gastric secretion and motility in dogs. *Ann. Surg.* 171:31, 1970.
28. Everett, M. T., and Griffith, C. A. The effects of selective vagotomy plus suprapyloric antrectomy upon gastric motility and Heidenhain pouch secretion. *Ann. Surg.* 171:36, 1970.
29. Fagerberg, S., Grevsten, S., Johansson, H., and Krause, U. Vagotomy and gallbladder function. *Gut* 11:789, 1970.
30. Ferguson, D. J., Billinger, H., Swensen, D., and Hoover, G. Segmental gastrectomy with innervated antrum for duodenal ulcer. *Surgery* 47:548, 1960.
31. Fielding, L. P., and Hittinger, R. The pylorus preserving gastrectomy: A prospective clinical trial in the treatment of duodenal ulceration. *Chir. Gastroenterol.* 10:251, 1976.
32. Finney, J. M. T. A new method of pyloroplasty. *Trans. Am. Surg. Assoc.* 20:165, 1902.
33. Fivoli, E. Accorgimenti tecnici nella Esecuzione della Deconnessione vagogastrica secondo Grassi. *Chir. Gastroenterol.* 1:89, 1967.
34. Fletcher, D. M., and Clark, C. G. Changes in canine bile-flow and composition after vagotomy. *Br. J. Surg.* 56:103, 1969.
35. Franksson, C. Selective abdominal vagotomy. *Acta Chir. Scand.* 96:409, 1948.
36. French, S. W., III. Morbidity of complete vagotomy. *Am. Surg.* 33:171, 1967.
37. Friedman, G. D., Kannel, W. B., and Dawber, T. R. The epidemiology of gallbladder disease: Observations of the Framingham study. *J. Chronic Dis.* 19:273, 1966.
38. Fritz, M. E., and Brooks, F. P. Control of bile flow in the cholecystectomized dog. *Am. J. Physiol.* 204:825, 1963.
39. Ganguli, P. C., Polak, J. M., Pearse, A. G. E.,

et al. Antral-gastrin-cell hyperplasia in peptic ulcer disease. *Lancet* 1:583, 1974.
40. Gelb, M., Baronofsky, I. D., and Janowitz, H. D. The effect of vagotomy on the maximal acid response to histamine. *Gut* 2:240, 1961.
41. Gillespie, I. E., and Kay, A. W. Effect of medical and surgical vagotomy on the augmented histamine test in man. *Br. Med. J.* 1:1557, 1961.
42. Goligher, J. C. Personal communication, 1979.
43. Grassi, G. La gastrovagotomia seletiva. *Minerva Chir.* 21:544, 1966.
44. Griffith, C. A. Gastric vagotomy vs. total abdominal vagotomy. *Arch. Surg.* 81:781, 1960.
45. Griffith, C. A. Selective gastric vagotomy. *West. J. Surg. Obstet. Gynecol.* 70:107 (part I), 195(part II), 1962.
46. Griffith, C. A. Completeness of gastric vagotomy by the selective technic. *Am. J. Dig. Dis.* 12:333, 1967.
47. Griffith, C. A. Significant functions of the hepatic and celiac vagi. *Am. J. Surg.* 118:251, 1969.
48. Griffith, C. A. Selective vagotomy plus suprapyloric antrectomy with and without pylorotomy for duodenal ulcer. *Ann. Surg.* 179:516, 1974.
49. Griffith, C. A. Selective Gastric Vagotomy. In R. A. Malt (Ed.), *Surgical Techniques Illustrated*. Philadelphia: Saunders, 1985.
50. Griffith, C. A. Editorial comment. *Curr. Surg.* 35:92, 1978.
51. Griffith, C. A. Long-term results of selective vagotomy plus pyloroplasty: 12 to 17 year follow-up. *Am. J. Surg.* 139:608, 1980.
52. Griffith, C. A. Types of Vagotomy. In R. Maingot (Ed.), *Abdominal Operations* (7th ed.). New York: Appleton-Century-Crofts, 1980.
53. Griffith, C. A., and Harkins, H. N. Partial gastric vagotomy: An experimental study. *Gastroenterology* 32:96, 1957.
54. Griffith, C. A., Stavney, L. S., Kato, T., and Harkins, H. N. Selective gastric vagotomy. *Am. J. Surg.* 105:13, 1963.
55. Grossman, M. E., et al. Candidate hormones of the gut. *Gastroenterology* 67:730, 1974.
56. Harkins, H. N., Griffith, C. A., and Nyhus, L. M. The revised combined operation with selective gastric vagotomy. *Am. Surg.* 33:510, 1967.
57. Harkins, H. N., Stavney, L. S., Griffith, C. A., Savage, M. A., Kato, T., and Nyhus, L. M. Selective gastric vagotomy. *Ann. Surg.* 158:448, 1963.
58. Hinshaw, D. V. Personal communication, 1982.
59. Hinshaw, D. V., Jorgensen, E. S., and Stafford, C. E. Postoperative dumping studies in peptic ulcer patients. *Arch. Surg.* 80:738, 1960.
60. Hollander, F. Personal communication, 1956.
61. Holle, F. Invited commentary. *World J. Surg.* 1:26, 1977.
62. Horton, J. W., McClelland, R. N., and Weger, R. V. Effect of parietal cell vagotomy on gastric emptying in duodenal ulcer disease. *Am. J. Surg.* 143:86, 1982.
63. Ihasz, M., and Griffith, C. A. Gallstones after vagotomy. *Am. J. Surg.* 141:48, 1981.
64. Inberg, M. V. Clinical experience with selective gastric and total abdominal vagotomy. *Ann. Chir. Gynaecol. Fenn.* 58(Suppl.):165, 1969.
65. Inberg, M. V., and Vuorio, M. Human gallbladder function after selective gastric and total abdominal vagotomy. *Acta Chir. Scand.* 135:625, 1969.
66. Isaac, F., Ottoman, R. E., and Weinberg, J. A. Roentgen studies of the upper gastrointestinal tract in vagotomy. *Am. J. Roentgenol. Radium Ther. Nucl. Med.* 63:66, 1950.
67. Isaza, J., Sugawara, K., Curt, J., and Woodward, E. R. The influence of mesenteric denervation on the inhibition of gastric secretion by fat in the intestine. *Gut* 12:34, 1971.
68. Jackson, R. G. Anatomic study of the vagus nerves, with a technique of transabdominal selective gastric vagus resection. *Arch. Surg.* 57:333, 1948.
69. Joffe, S. N. Personal communication, 1982.
70. Joffe, S. N., Crochet, A., and Doyle, D. Morphologic and functional evidence of reinnervation of the gastric parietal cell mass after parietal cell vagotomy. *Am. J. Surg.* 143:80, 1982.
71. Johnson, R. D., and Boyden, E. A. The effect of double vagotomy on the motor activity of the human gall bladder. *Surgery* 32:591, 1952.
72. Jones, W. M., and Griffith, C. A. On the question of vagal reinnervation of the stomach. I. The permanence of the amount of the residually innervated gastric mucosa. *Ann. Surg.* 171:365, 1970.
73. Jones, W. M., and Griffith, C. A. On the question of vagal reinnervation of the stomach. II. The unchanging secretory and ulcerogenic potential. *Ann. Surg.* 171:369, 1970.

74. Jones, W. M., and Griffith, C. A. A correlation of gastric motile and secretory responses after adequate incomplete vagotomy. Unpublished data, 1970.
75. Kelly, K. A., Nyhus, L. M., and Harkins, H. N. The vagal nerve and the intestinal phase of gastric secretion. *Gastroenterology* 46:163, 1964.
76. Kennedy, T. Personal visit, 1979.
77. Kennedy, T., and Connell, A. M. Selective or truncal vagotomy? *Lancet* 1:899, 1969.
78. Kilby, J. O., and Griffith, C. A. The relationships of gastric transection and vagotomy to gastric emptying. *Surgery* 69:633, 1971.
79. Kilby, J. O., and Griffith, C. A. Selective and total vagotomy with suprapyloric antrectomy: A comparative study of gastric secretion and emptying in dogs. *Surgery* 69:702, 1971.
80. Kirk, R. M. Mucosal antrectomy with vagotomy in the treatment of duodenal ulcer. *Br. J. Surg.* 52:604, 1965.
81. Korman, M. G., Hansky, J., Coupland, G. A. E., and Cumberland, V. H. Serum gastrin in duodenal ulcer. IV. Effect of selective gastric vagotomy. *Gut* 13:163, 1972.
82. Kraft, R. O., and Fry, W. J. Operative technic of selective gastric vagotomy. *Am. J. Surg.* 105:423, 1963.
83. Kusakari, K., Nyhus, L. M., Gillison, E. W., and Bombeck, C. T. An endoscopic test for completeness of vagotomy. *Arch. Surg.* 105:386, 1972.
84. Landor, J. H. The effect of extragastric vagotomy on Heidenhain pouch secretion in dogs. *Am. J. Dig.* 9:256, 1964.
85. Latarjet, A. Résection des nerfs de l'estomac. *Bull. Acad. Natl. Med.* (Paris) 87:681, 1922.
86. Legros, G., and Griffith, C. A. The anatomic basis for the variable adequacy of incomplete vagotomy. I. The various secretory and ulcerogenic potentials of various anatomic types of incomplete vagotomy in Shay rats. *Ann. Surg.* 168:1030, 1968.
87. Legros, G., and Griffith, C. A. The anatomic basis for the variable adequacy of incomplete vagotomy. II. The various responses to insulin of various anatomic types of incomplete vagotomy in dogs. *Ann. Surg.* 168:1035, 1968.
88. Legros, G., and Griffith, C. A. The anatomic pathways of the vagal fibers to the antral mucosa. *Surgery* 66:751, 1969.
89. Legros, G., and Griffith, C. A. The permanence of adequate incomplete vagotomy. *Surgery* 67:654, 1970.
90. Loeb, M., and Nicoloff, D. M. Gallbladder function in the dog following subtotal resection or vagotomy and pyloroplasty. *Surgery* 63:806, 1968.
91. Maki, T., Shiratori, T., Hatafuku, T., and Sugawara, K. Pylorus-preserving gastrectomy as an improved operation for gastric ulcer. *Surgery* 61:838, 1967.
92. Martin, C. J., and Kennedy, T. Reconstruction of the pylorus. *World J. Surg.* 6:221, 1982.
93. McGregor, D. B., Savage, L. E., and McVay, C. B. Vagotomy and drainage for elective treatment of peptic ulcers. *Surg. Gynecol. Obstet.* 146:349, 1978.
94. Middleton, M. D., Kelly, K. A., Nyhus, L. M., and Harkins, H. N. Selective vagal effects on the intestinal phase of gastric secretion. *Gut* 6:296, 1965.
95. Miller, M. C. Cholelithiasis developing after vagotomy. *Can. Med. Assoc. J.* 98:350, 1968.
96. Nielsen, H. O., Kronberg, M. O., and Andersen, D. The antrum in duodenal ulcer patients: Relationship between antrum size, nerve of Latarjet, gastrin cell quantity, and gastric acid secretion. *Scand. J. Gastroenterol.* 16:491, 1981.
97. Nielsen, J. R. Development of cholelithiasis following vagotomy. *Surgery* 56:909, 1964.
98. Nobles, E. R., Jr. Vagotomy and gastroenterostomy: 15-Year-follow-up of 175 patients. *Ann. Surg.* 32:177, 1966.
99. Nyhus, L. M. Two decades of gastrointestinal research: A perspective. *Am. J. Surg.* 131:1, 1976.
100. Nyhus, L. M. Neurohormonal observations and the gastrointestinal tract. *Am. J. Surg.* 143:6, 1982.
101. Oberhelman, H. A., and Dragstedt, L. R. New physiologic concepts related to the surgical treatment of duodenal ulcer by vagotomy and gastroenterostomy. *Surg. Gynecol. Obstet.* 101:194, 1955.
102. Oi, M., Oshida, K., and Sugimura, S. The location of gastric ulcer. *Gastroenterology* 36:45, 1959.
103. Parkin, G. J. S., Smith, R. B., and Johnston, D. Gallbladder volume and contractility after truncal, selective and highly selective (parietal-cell) vagotomy in man. *Ann. Surg.* 178:581, 1973.
104. Pitt, H. A., Doty, J. E., and DenBesten, L. Increased intragallbladder pressure response to cholecystokinin-octapeptide following va-

gotomy and pyloroplasty. *J. Surg. Res.* 35:325, 1983.
105. Pritchard, G. R., Griffith, C. A., and Harkins, H. N. A visual demonstration of the vagal release of gastrin. *Am. J. Surg.* 115:191, 1968.
106. Pritchard, G. R., Griffith, C. A., and Harkins, H. N. The insulin response of vagally innervated gastric pouches following selective gastric vagotomy. *J. Surg. Res.* 8:68, 1968.
107. Pritchard, G. R., Griffith, C. A., and Harkins, H. N. A physiologic demonstration of the anatomic distribution of the vagal system to the stomach. *Surg. Gynecol. Obstet.* 126:791, 1968.
108. Rehnberg, O., and Haglund, U. Gallstone disease following antrectomy and gastroduodenostomy with or without vagotomy. *Ann. Surg.* 201:315, 1985.
109. Rhind, J. A. Mucosal stenosis of the pylorus. *Br. J. Surg.* 46:534, 1959.
110. Ross, D. A. A new upper abdominal incision. *Am. J. Surg.* 79:841, 1950.
111. Rudick, J., and Hutchinson, J. S. F. Evaluation of vagotomy and biliary function by combined oral cholecystography and intravenous cholangiography. *Ann. Surg.* 162:234, 1965.
112. Said, S. I. Vasoactive intestinal peptide (VIP). *Gastroenterology* 67:735, 1974.
113. Sapala, M. A., Sapala, J. A., Resto Soto, A. D., and Bouwman, D. L. Cholelithiasis following subtotal gastric resection with truncal vagotomy. *Surg. Gynecol. Obstet.* 148:36, 1979.
114. Sawyers, J. L., Scott, H. W., Jr., Edwards, W. H., et al. Comparative studies of the clinical effects of truncal and selective gastric vagotomy. *Am. J. Surg.* 115:165, 1968.
115. Schein, C. J., Rosen, R. G., Warren, A., and Gliedman, M. L. A vagal factor in cholecystitis. *Surgery* 66:345, 1969.
116. Scheinin, T. M., and Inberg, M. V. Clinical experiences with selective vagotomy. *Acta Chir. Scand.* 133:533, 1967.
117. Shiina, E., and Griffith, C. A. Selective and total vagotomy without drainage: A comparative study of gastric secretion and motility in dogs. *Ann. Surg.* 169:326, 1969.
118. Skandalakis, J. E. Personal communication, 1982.
119. Skandalakis, J. E., Gray, S. W., Sorio, R. E., Sorg, J. L., and Rowe, J. S., Jr. Distribution of the vagus nerve in the stomach. *Am. Surg.* 46:130, 1980.
120. Stavney, L. S., Kato, T., Griffith, C. A., et al. A physiologic study of motility changes following selective gastric vagotomy. *J. Surg. Res.* 3:390, 1963.
121. Stening, G. F., and Grossman, M. I. Gastric acid response to pentagastrin and histamine after extragastric vagotomy in dogs. *Gastroenterology* 59:364, 1970.
122. Strauss, R., and Wise, L. New concepts in the prevention, causes, and treatment of postvagotomy diarrhea. *Curr. Surg.* 35:77, 1978.
123. Tanner, N. C. A technique of selective vagotomy. *Br. J. Surg.* 53:185, 1966.
124. Tompkins, R. K., Kraft, A. R., Zimmerman, E., et al. Clinical and biochemical evidence of increased gallstone formation after complete vagotomy. *Surgery* 71:196, 1972.
125. Wertheimer, P. *L'innervation et l'Énervation Gastriques: Etude Anatomique, Expérimentale et Clinique*. Lyon: Imprimérie-Express, 1922.
126. White, T. T., Tournut, R. A., Scharplatz, D., et al. The effect of vagotomy on biliary secretions and bile salt pools in dogs. *Ann. Surg.* 179:406, 1974.
127. Williams, R. D., and Huang, T. T. The effect of vagotomy on biliary pressure. *Surgery* 66:353, 1969.
128. Woodward, E. R., Harper, P. V., Jr., Tovee, E. B., and Dragstedt, L. R. Effect of vagotomy on gastric secretion in man and experimental animals. *Arch. Surg.* 59:1191, 1949.

SPECIAL COMMENT

Assessing the Completeness of Vagotomy

A. Gerson Greenburg
Richard P. Saik

With the increased sophistication concerning the use of various forms of vagotomy in surgical therapy for duodenal ulcer disease, it becomes necessary to establish methods for evaluating the completeness of vagotomy. Assessment of completeness is required in two situations—at operation and in postoperative clinical evaluation. The recurrence of symptoms after surgical treatment of duodenal ulcer disease is usually attributed to one of three factors. There is the possibility that some other disease is responsible for the symptoms;

fortunately, this situation is not common. More likely, the symptoms are related to either an incomplete vagotomy or inadequate drainage. It is now generally held that incomplete vagotomy represents the major contributing factor to recurrent ulcer disease.

Given this argument, there is excellent reason to consider the use of intraoperative adjuncts to assess the completeness of vagotomy and to have a reliable test that is useful in the postoperative period as well. The ideal intraoperative test should be performed easily, rapidly, and with a minimum of manipulation or instrumentation. If, additionally, a gastrotomy could be avoided so that the test could be used in proximal gastric vagotomy without drainage, universal applicability could be achieved.

Markers of Parietal Cell Mass

Although there has been interest in the use of azine dyes as in vivo markers of the parietal cell mass since 1908 [7], the first clinical application of an endoscopic technique with marker dye was reported in 1942 [10]. The use of intravenous neutral red supplemented with some form of vagal stimulation (electrical, insulin, or 2-deoxyglucose) has been advocated by various authors [3, 5, 12] but is generally assumed not to be applicable intraoperatively because of the physiological oscillations induced. Indeed, many of these tests have been used or documented only experimentally. Grassi and Orecchia [8, 9] reviewed these approaches. Other intraoperative techniques dependent on gastric motility changes rely on electrical stimulation of the vagus nerve or remnant fibers, require expensive, sophisticated instrumentation in the operating room, and cannot be used postoperatively [1].

Kusakari's Endoscopic Test

The endoscopic test (K test) for completeness of vagotomy described by Kusakari et al. in 1972 [10] meets the criterion of acceptability for use intraoperatively and postoperatively and, indeed, was designed for that purpose. Since early 1973 we have routinely used this test to assess the completeness of vagotomy intraoperatively as well as postoperatively [13, 14].

The K test is predicated on the well-documented existence in humans of a resting mucosal pH of less than 3.0 for intact vagally innervated areas of the gastric fundus [4]. Innervated mucosa can be distinguished from denervated areas or non-parietal-cell-containing areas, which have a mucosal pH greater than 3.0. Congo red, the azine dye used topically in this test, changes color at pH 3.0. When the pH is 3.0 or less it is black, and when the pH is 4.0 or greater the marker stays red. One can assess the extent of vagal innervation by observing, through a gastroscope or gastrotomy, the conversion from red to black and the extent of the area converted on a previously alkalinized parietal cell mucosa [6, 11, 15].

In our longitudinal, randomized prospective study of truncal and proximal gastric vagotomy and Jaboulay drainage for the treatment of duodenal ulcer disease, we have used this test intraoperatively and postoperatively to assess objectively the completeness of vagotomy and to correlate this finding with postoperative history, symptoms, and clinical course. Some minor modifications have been developed that enable us to make more effective use of the test in the operating room, particularly because anesthetic agents seem to depress basal gastric secretion [2, 13–16].

Procedure

Almost all patients are routinely given atropine as part of the preoperative medication. This agent's ability to block vagal innervation is well documented, and its administration could invalidate the test. Therefore all patients undergoing elective vagotomy as part of the protocol do not receive atropine or H_2 antagonists in their preoperative medication. We have omitted the use of a drying agent after consultation with our anesthesiologists.

After induction of general anesthesia just prior to endotracheal intubation, an end-viewing gastroscope is passed into the stomach. We have found this to be the easiest and safest time to accomplish this task, because we do not have to deflate the endotracheal cuff later in the operation, when secretions could be aspirated. Additionally, suction is available to clear any gastric contents or air insufflated during intubation. At the time of the incision, pentagastrin (0.5 μg/kg) is given IM to offset the vagolytic effects of general anesthesia.

It is exceedingly important that a positive test be ensured before vagotomy. A negative test before vagotomy invalidates any results, and testing is abandoned since either the depth of anesthesia or pharmacological manipulation may have inhibited acid secretion. After completion of the vagotomy, another test is performed: Normal saline solution, 250 ml, is used to irrigate the stomach and discarded. The saline irrigation is followed by irrigation with 150–200 ml of 5% sodium bicarbonate, which is also completely aspirated. At this time, 50 ml of a sterile solution of Congo red (1%) is sprayed over the gastric mucosa in a slightly insufflated stomach through the accessory port of the gastroscope using a polyethylene catheter and syringe. Viewing through the gastroscope or through transillumination in a darkened room for a period of 5–10 minutes, one searches for areas of incomplete vagotomy, which are evidenced as black patches. Inspection through a gastrotomy or through the open Jaboulay pyloroplasty eliminates the need for passage of a gastroscope. It has been our experience that when innervation is present, positive staining areas appear within 120 seconds of instilling the Congo red. Should an area of innervation appear in this time, the remaining vagal fibers are sought and divided, and the test is repeated. We have found that 1% Congo red solution is quite adequate to detect the rate and extent of innervation when endoscopic viewing is employed, but it is too dilute a solution to be adequate when transillumination is used. For the latter we prefer to use a 3% solution of Congo red. When using transillumination, it may not be necessary to use a gastroscope, since any fiberoptic light source passed into the gastric lumen perorally or through a gastrotomy may be sufficient. We have frequently used the light-source fiberoptic bundle from the bronchoscope when it is available.

K-Test Effectiveness

In conjunction with our gastroenterologists, we have studied more than 100 patients postoperatively to determine completeness of vagotomy in a prospective manner. Of interest are 11 patients in whom a positive test occurred. These patients were followed for recurrent ulcers and some were retested periodically. In those retested, positive testing could be reconfirmed after more than one year. In those whose tests were negative initially, only half (50 patients) were retested, and 6 patients had either small (1–2 cm^2) or questionable areas of positive results, which indicated remnant innervation, and in 4 of them an adequate reduction in postoperative maximal betazone (Histalog)-stimulated acid output was achieved. All 5 did well clinically. In 2 patients, both with large areas of positive staining, recurrent ulcers developed, in one despite a significant reduction in acid output. One other patient in a high risk category remained well. Neither parietal cell nor truncal vagotomy seems to be better than the other.

An additional 31 patients referred to us with postoperative symptoms of pain were similarly evaluated. Twenty-two had a vagotomy and drainage with all but 2 having a documented recurrent ulcer. One had no evidence of a recurrence after a complete vagotomy, and no cause for his symptoms was uncovered. The other patient without ulceration had gastritis only, but he also had an incomplete vagotomy and was treated medically. In 19 of the 20 patients with recurrent ulceration, evidence of incomplete vagotomy with positive Congo red staining and remnant innervation was uncovered. Fourteen of these patients had transthoracic vagotomy, which allowed the surgeon to avoid the previous operative site. Conversion to negative testing was achieved in all 14 patients whose ulcers healed, and they continued to be free of symptoms. Four patients were treated medically by their physician and one, by preference of the surgeon, underwent an antrectomy. Only one patient with an ulcer had a negative test. An antrectomy was performed because it was thought that the patient had had a complete vagotomy. Of interest were 4 of 6 patients who had recurrent ulcers after vagotomy and antrectomy. All but one of the 4 patients had an incomplete vagotomy discernible on Congo red testing despite the removal of the gastrin-containing area of the stomach. One patient declined a second vagotomy and the fourth patient with evidence of a complete vagotomy was treated with cimetidine in lieu of an extensive re-resection.

Thus far we have studied 42 patients intraoperatively with Congo red. Five patients were not included in the study because they never tested positively before vagotomy, even with pentagastrin stimulation. Failure to achieve a baseline positive result is considered to invalidate the test. Postoperative follow-up study of our 42 patients is thus far incomplete. In 4 instances, however, the surgeon was alerted to an incomplete vagotomy after performing what was thought to be an adequate operation. In 3 instances a second vagotomy resulted in a negative test, and the area of remnant innervation was identified by the area of the fundus staining black. In one instance, positive testing still occurred despite a second vagotomy, and an antrectomy was performed. This patient still had a positive test after operation. Until now, despite intraoperative testing with open mucosal inspection, tests appeared to be positive in small areas in 4 patients after their operation, but 2 of the 4 had received atropine before operation; thus their intraoperative tests were invalidated. All patients studied with transillumination were inspected with the endoscope as well. One patient had a questionably positive test, and no remnant vagal branches were uncovered. This patient has not been retested, but one patient with parietal cell vagotomy and recurrent ulcer had a positive test postoperatively that was apparently negative during operation. Thus there were 2 patients who had evidence of remnant innervation despite valid negative intraoperative testing by our technique.

The use of an intraoperative test for completeness of vagotomy becomes mandatory as we become more sophisticated in the types of vagotomy performed with omission of the drainage procedure. The modified endoscopic test described by Kusakari offers a safe and simple tool to acquire that information. That its use can be extended to the postoperative evaluation as well lends consistency and thus realistic interpretation. We have found it an invaluable adjunct and suggest that others consider its use in their practice.

Comment References

1. Allgöwer, M., and Perren, S. Comment concerning intraoperative electrotest for completeness of vagotomy. *Prog. Surg.* 8:69, 1970.
2. Bernard, R. A., and Kodekaro, M. The effect of anesthetics on the gastric secretory response to 2-deoxy-D-glucose. *Physiologist* 15:85, 1972.
3. Burge, H., and Vane, J. R. Method of testing for complete nerve section during vagotomy. *Br. Med. J.* 1:615, 1958.
4. Capper, W., Laidlaw, C., Buckler, K., and Richards, D. The pH fields of the gastric mucosa. *Lancet* 2:1200, 1962.
5. Cole, R. E. An intra-operative test for completeness of vagotomy. *Am. J. Surg.* 123:543, 1972.
6. Donahue, P. E., and Nyhus, L. M. The simplified endoscopic Congo red test for completeness of vagotomy. *Surg. Gynecol. Obstet.* in press.
7. Fuld, F. M. Briefkasten. *Munch. Med. Wochenschr.* 55:2264, 1908.
8. Grassi, G. Highly selective vagotomy with intra-operative acid secretive test of completeness of vagal section. *Surg. Gynecol. Obstet.* 140:259, 1975.
9. Grassi, G., and Orecchia, C. A comparison of intra-operative tests of completeness of vagal section. *Surgery* 75:155, 1974.
10. Kusakari, K., Nyhus, L. M., Gillison, E. W., and Bombeck, C. T. An endoscopic test for completeness of vagotomy. *Arch. Surg.* 105:386, 1972.
11. Lerner, H. H., Asher, L., and Andrew, K. The excretion of neutral red by the gastric mucosa as visualized gastroscopically. *Am. J. Dig. Dis.* 9:109, 1942.

12. Moe, R. E., and Klopper, P. J. Demonstration of the functional anatomy of the canine gastric antrum. II. Operative techniques not requiring gastrotomy. *Am. J. Surg.* 111:80, 1966.
13. Saik, R. P., Greenburg, A. G., Farris, J. M., and Peskin, G. W. The practicality of the Congo red test, or is your vagotomy complete? *Am. J. Surg.* 132:144, 1976.
14. Saik, R. P., Greenburg, A. G., and Peskin, G. W. The Congo red test to determine completeness of vagotomy: Clinical application. *Am. J. Surg.* 144:518, 1982.
15. Saik, R. P., Greenburg, A. G., and Peskin, G. W. Pros and cons of parietal cell versus truncal vagotomy. *Am. J. Surg.* 148:93, 1984.
16. Skyring, A. P., Milton, G. W., and Maxwell, G. A. Effect of sodium pentobarbital on histamine stimulated gastric secretion. *Am. J. Physiol.* 201:574, 1972.

EDITOR'S COMMENT

In the third edition of this monograph, Griffith's presentation highlighted the technique of selective vagotomy only. The addition of suprapyloric antrectomy to the presentation may surprise some readers. Two techniques infrequently used today by surgeons throughout the world are now combined into an operation for the treatment of the duodenal ulcer diathesis. Only after careful reading of this chapter, with appropriate reflection on all the anatomical, physiological, and clinical nuances presented, will the skeptic gain a better understanding of and thus perhaps a modicum of acceptance for the concept. The virtual absence of both recurrent ulceration *and* the dumping syndrome following selective vagotomy with antrectomy plus pylorotomy is an outstanding accomplishment. A controlled, comparative patient study is indicated.

The student of the history of vagotomy will find a wealth of material to whet the appetite. I was fortunate to have had the pleasure of friendly propinquity to many of the events described in this chapter and thus can vouch for the accuracy of the presentation. Skandalakis et al. have presented other historical perspectives (*Surg. Gynecol. Obstet.* 162:75, 1986).

L.M.N.

13

Proximal Gastric Vagotomy

Christopher Wastell

Proximal gastric vagotomy[1] is a logical step in the direction of conservatism in the surgical treatment of chronic duodenal ulcer, but the development of yet another operation can only be justified if there are serious objections to more established procedures. If the debate between gastrectomy and vagotomy has moved in favor of vagotomy—and the fact that truncal vagotomy with drainage is the procedure preferred by most [3] suggests that this is so—we need to consider the defects of truncal and selective vagotomy. Both of these procedures must be combined with either pyloroplasty or gastrojejunostomy. As a result of the vagotomy (whether truncal or selective) or the drainage, or a combination of the two, a significant proportion of patients will suffer from one or more of the following four major postoperative complications: (1) diarrhea [9, 12, 13, 25, 27, 28, 31, 67, 80, 84, 87, 90, 96]; (2) dumping syndrome [12, 21, 27, 28, 34, 44, 54, 58, 63, 80, 82, 87, 90, 94]; (3) bilious vomiting [57, 90]; or (4) recurrent or persistent ulceration [64, 86]. This is not to suggest that other symptoms such as postprandial fullness, flatulence, or difficulty in swallowing do not occur as well, but failure is usually laid at the door of one of these four major complications. It is true that severe diarrhea is seen much less often after selective than after truncal vagotomy [6, 58, 64], and there is some evidence to suggest that an inadequate vagotomy occurs less frequently after the selective procedure [36].

Nevertheless, the most ardent advocates of either truncal or selective vagotomy have to admit that neither of these procedures is absolutely reliable. It is pursuit of this utopian quality that has stimulated the research into

[1]We pointed out in the previous edition of this book the confusion [8] surrounding the term to be applied to this type of vagotomy. Unfortunately, confusion still exists, although the term *proximal gastric vagotomy* [91] is probably more widely used now than before. Historically, of course, *selective proximal vagotomy* (SPV), *highly selective vagotomy* (HSV), and *parietal cell vagotomy* (PCV) were the names coined by the three originators of the procedure. The fact that there are *three* names creates a problem, multiplied several times over by the use of other phrases to describe essentially similar procedures. For this reason we have elected to continue to use the term *proximal gastric vagotomy*.

and the development of an improved procedure—proximal gastric vagotomy (PGV).

Implicit in surgical teaching, especially in teaching of recent years, is the concept of preservation of both morphological and physiological integrity consistent with the attainment of the primary objective of the operation. This approach is clearly important in nonmalignant conditions such as duodenal ulcer. When the object of surgical treatment of this condition is to reduce acid secretion, the destruction of the coordinated, if ill-understood, antral-pyloric-duodenal mechanism is an undesirable side effect of both gastrectomy and gastric drainage. Recognition of this can be seen in the various attempts that have been made to preserve the pylorus. Thus in 1957 Griffith and Harkins [35] described experiments in which "partial gastric vagotomy" was carried out in 10 dogs. The procedure they described was in all ways similar to the modern operation of PGV, and they concluded that clinical application seemed feasible.

In 1960 Ferguson et al. [29] treated a series of patients with duodenal ulcer, apparently successfully, by means of PGV with a segmental gastric resection. A similar line of investigation was pursued by others [30, 61], who developed a "pylorus-preserving gastrectomy" in dogs. In this work the pyloric ring itself was retained, but the vagal nerve supply to it was not. After much debate as to how much of the prepyloric antrum should be left to enable the pylorus to function normally, Maki et al. in 1967 [69] described the use of a pylorus-preserving gastrectomy in patients with gastric ulcers. The fact that such an operation could be followed by normal gastric emptying in the long term was shown experimentally in dogs [32]. Recent results however, suggest that the pylorus-preserving gastrectomy, which leaves the denervated pylorus in situ, is unable to produce good long-term results in patients. The vagal nerve supply to the pylorus seems to be crucial for its normal function. The contrary view is given in Chapter 12.

Proximal gastric vagotomy, defined as vagal denervation of only that part of the stomach that is lined by mucosa that secretes acid and pepsin, was first performed on patients by Holle in 1961 [41], but he has always combined it with pyloroplasty. Working independently and at approximately the same time, Johnston in Leeds and Amdrup in Copenhagen began to carry out PGV without pyloroplasty in patients with duodenal ulcer; their first results were published in 1969 [51] and 1970 [5], respectively. This work has been followed by various other series of patients operated on in other centers in a variety of countries, and the task of assessment has begun. The technique of PGV used in our clinic is seen in Figures 13-1 through 13-7.

Results of Proximal Gastric Vagotomy

OPERATIVE MORTALITY

According to information collected by Johnston [48], the operative mortality in more than 5000 operations was 0.3 percent. Some of the deaths were caused by necrosis of the lesser curvature of the stomach with perforation [48, 74]. One possible cause of this complication is coincidental damage to the short gastric arteries necessitating splenectomy. Another possible cause is the use of diathermy to coagulate small vessels close to the gastric wall, which is already partially devascularized. Another

Fig. 13-1. Proximal gastric vagotomy technique. The front of the stomach, showing the usual arrangement of the anterior nerve of Latarjet. The dashed line represents the line of dissection. Note that the last major branch of the nerve of Latarjet is left intact and that the dissection starts 5–6 cm from the pylorus. At a point on the lesser curvature well below the separation of the nerve of Latarjet from the hepatic and fundic branches of the anterior vagus, the line of the section passes toward the angle of His across the front of the fundus of the stomach.

Fig. 13-2. Proximal gastric vagotomy technique, continued: The stomach has been turned up and to the right so as to reveal its posterior surface, the greater omentum having been omitted for clarity. The arrangement of the posterior nerve of Latarjet is shown, and again the dashed line indicates the line of the dissection. Not all of this dissection is carried out from within the lesser sac.

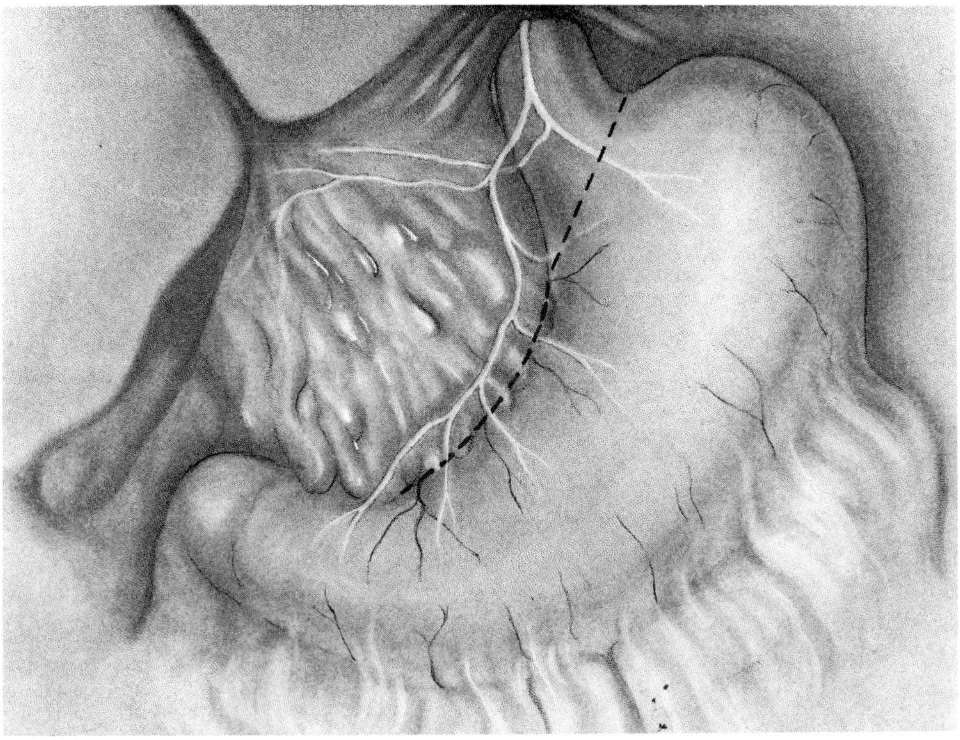

Fig. 13-1.

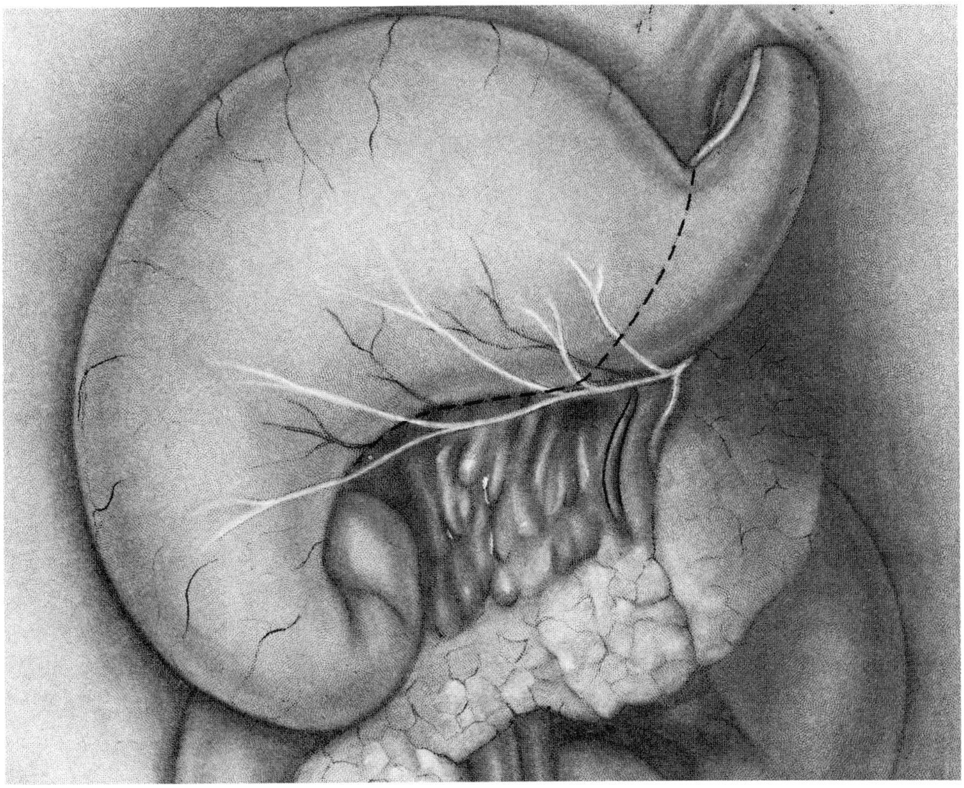

Fig. 13-2.

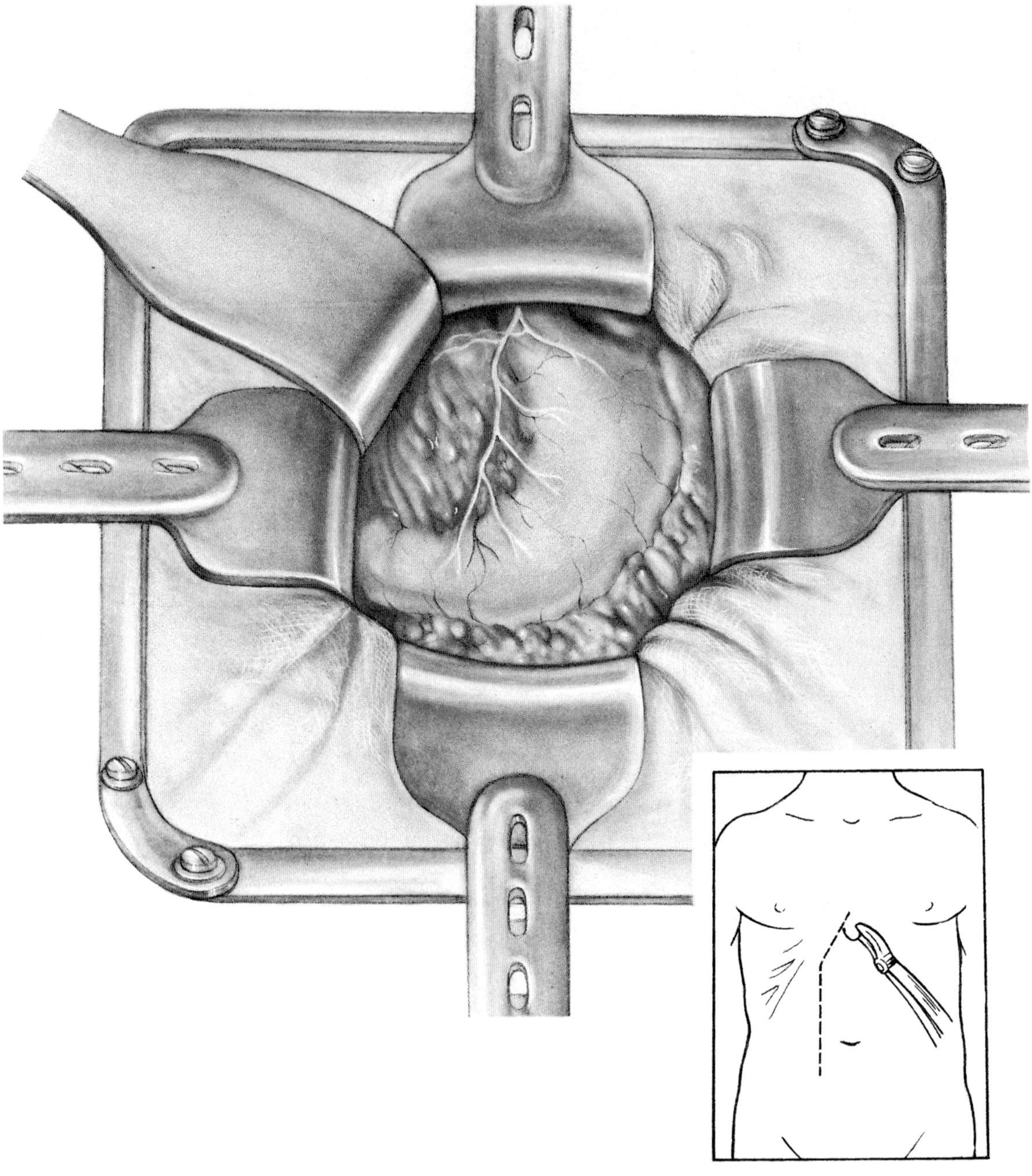

Fig. 13-3. Proximal gastric vagotomy technique, continued: The exposure. Essential to this procedure is some form of four-bladed retractor such as the one illustrated. The superior blade is pulled upward by a cord attached to its handle (not shown in this illustration). The *inset* shows the upper right paramedian incision with an extension to the midline that is used. The xiphisternum is excised if by so doing any greater exposure can be achieved.

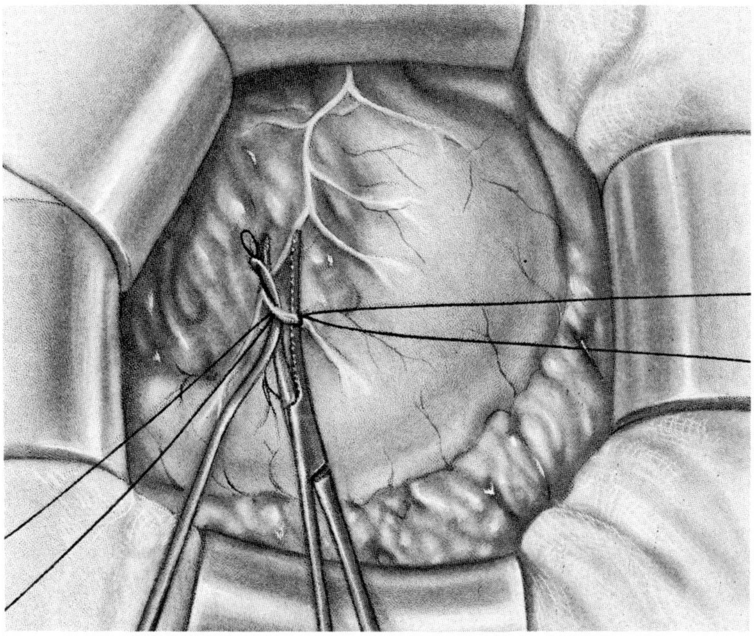

Fig. 13-4. Proximal gastric vagotomy technique, continued: The dissection is carried out by dividing the vessels between fine thread ligatures as they enter the lesser curvature of the stomach.

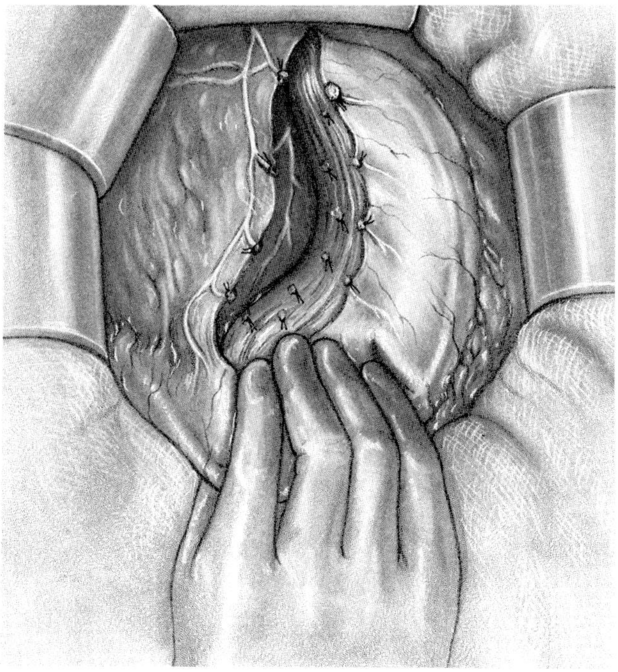

Fig. 13-5. Three layers of vessels enter the lesser curvature—an anterior, a posterior, and a rather irregular intermediate layer. The first part of the anterior dissection has been completed, and the anterior and intermediate vessels have been divided. Note that a nasogastric tube has been passed into the stomach and is being held by the first assistant, this being the most gentle and satisfactory way of drawing the stomach down into the field of vision. (From C. Wastell, Proximal gastric vagotomy. In L. M. Nyhus and R. J. Baker (eds.), *Mastery of Surgery*. Boston: Little, Brown, 1984.)

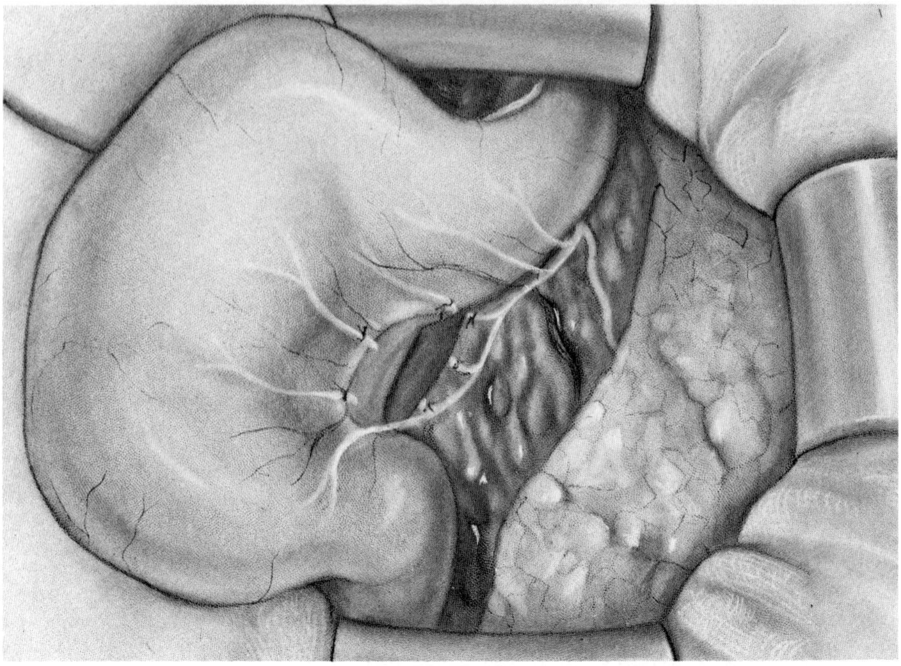

Fig. 13-6. Proximal gastric vagotomy technique, continued: The start of the posterior dissection. The lesser sac has been entered (one must take care not to injure the marginal artery running along the greater curvature of the stomach), and the dissection has been started from the same level as on the lesser curvature anteriorly. It is usually convenient to divide only two or three vessels from this aspect.

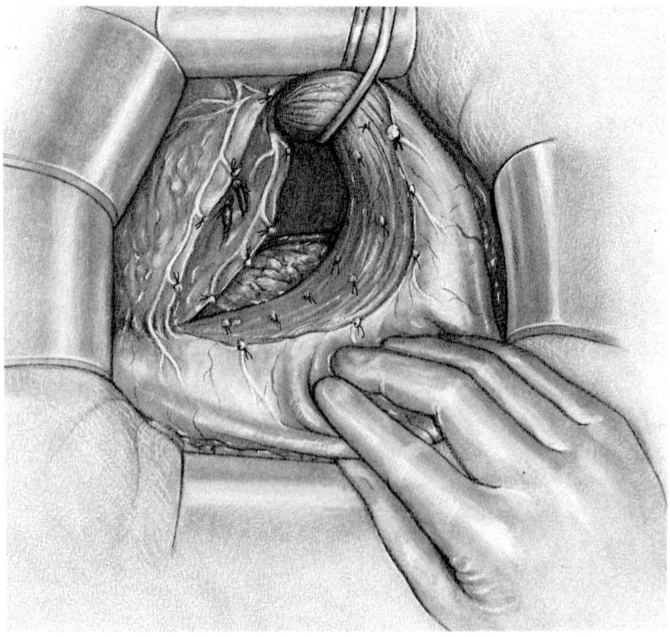

reported complication possibly related to ischemic necrosis of the lesser curvature of the stomach is the development of a gastric fistula [38]. Fortunately, the patient who had this complication was able to leave the hospital after the fistula had closed spontaneously.

Piasecki [78] described the existence of areas of mucosa along the lesser curvature of the stomach that are supplied by extramucosal arteries that do not anastomose with the submucosal plexus. It is possible that if too great an area of mucosa is supplied by these arteries, necrosis could result from their division. When necrosis with perforation does occur, the outcome is not necessarily fatal provided the condition is recognized and treated without delay [100]. Ischemia of the lesser curvature may also present with hemorrhage into the stomach [71].

Kennedy et al. [60] warn of the association between lesser curvature necrosis and a Nissen fundoplication. In 400 patients undergoing PGV, each of the three lesser curvature necroses were in patients who also had a Nissen fundoplication.

RECURRENCE

It is now more than a decade since the introduction of PGV, and the pattern of recurrence is becoming much clearer. Whereas in the early years reports suggested a recurrence rate of both duodenal and gastric ulcer of about 3 percent in patients operated on for duodenal ulcer, our recent review clearly indicates a rate of about 12 percent (Table 13-1).

This increase presumably has something to do with the passage of time from operation, although Christiansen et al. [15] found the risk of recurrence highest in the first three years after operation. The figures also reflect an awareness of the possibility of recurrence in the absence of symptoms: For example, Troidl et al. [88] found that the recurrent ulcer rate doubled if either endoscopy or barium meal were used on all patients rather than just those with symptoms.

Considering that the recurrent ulcer rate has been used to compare different procedures, it is extraordinary that the syndrome of recurrence has not been defined. The problem relates not to the patient with obvious severe recurrent ulceration, but rather to the person with transient symptoms who on endoscopy has only a shallow ulcer or perhaps duodenitis and who, on follow-up, is free of trouble perhaps for a long time. Should this situation be labeled for all time as "recurrence" and the patient confined within Visick grade IV? Clearly in some centers this is what happens, whereas in others it is not. Accepting that it is likely that most persons, at some time or another, suffer superficial duodenal ulceration but do not have the diathesis as such, a recurrence has several components. There should be an ulcer that as far as can be told both persists and penetrates to a level deep to the muscularis mucosa. The persistence of the ulcer is rather arbitrary, but if an average mucosal cell can be expected to survive for three to four days, an ulcer persisting for longer than one week is unlikely to be wholly superficial. Recurrence then has to be subdivided further according to whether or not there are symptoms. This discussion can of course be applied to the primary condition of chronic duodenal ulcer quite apart from the postoperative state.

Recurrence after operation can be treated, at least in most patients, with cimetidine [16], or if necessary by antrectomy [37].

Prevention of recurrence by accuracy of technique has been emphasized by Nyhus et al. [76]. Skandalakis et al. [83] provided a description of the distribution of the vagus

Fig. 13-7. With the stomach held downward by the first assistant grasping it around a nasogastric tube, the remainder of the dissection is performed from the front. When the esophagogastric junction is reached, a soft rubber tube is passed around the esophagus so that it can be held up and to the left. This makes the division of the last few strands of tissue passing to the righthand side of the esophagus easier. It is essential to lay bare at least 5 cm of the esophageal muscle and to visualize the posterior vagus nerve as it enters the abdomen between the crura during this part of the dissection. (From C. Wastell, Proximal gastric vagotomy. In L. M. Nyhus and R. J. Baker (eds.), *Mastery of Surgery*. Boston: Little, Brown, 1984.)

Table 13-1. Recurrent ulceration after proximal gastric vagotomy for duodenal ulcer

				Proved recurrent ulcer	
Author	Year	No. of patients	No. of years after operation	Duodenal (No.)	Gastric (No.)
Jordan [55]	1979	97	>2	5	
Koffman et al. [62]	1979	75	>1	6	
Makey et al. [68]	1979	115	1–5	6	3
Adami et al. [1]	1980	211	1–6	29	
Blackett and Johnston [11]	1981	233	5–12	29	6
Christiansen et al. [15]	1981	83	2–5	13	
Busman and Munting [14]	1982	229	1–8	22	
De Miguel [22]	1982	143	5–9	12	2
Mühe et al. [72]	1982	524	>5	73*	
Donahue et al. [23]	1984	40	4–12	8	
Graffner et al. [33]	1985	405	5	57	
Total		2155		260 (12%)	11 (0.6%)

*Includes asymptomatic recurrences.

nerves to the stomach on the basis of dissections on 100 cadavers. The antrum-corpus boundary was defined by Ahonen et al. [2] by means of a pH probe during operation, but when this method was compared with the more usual anatomical one, few advantages were found. Pendower [77] compared the Burge test with the Grassi test and concluded that the latter was more accurate, but Williams and Johnson [98] found that the price of intraoperative pH telemetry was a wound infection rate of 23 percent and an extra 20–40 minutes of operating time. Willie-Jørgensen and Jensen [97] showed that leukomethylene blue staining of vagal fibers at operation is of no value in helping to achieve a complete vagotomy. Donahue and Nyhus [24] have used the intraoperative Congo red test to the advantage of their patients.

The effect of individual surgeons' techniques has been considered in several reports [43]. In one of these the average recurrence rate after PGV was 8 percent when carried out by consultants and 16 percent when performed by senior registrars or lecturers, with a range from 2 percent for one surgeon to 28 percent for another [11]. However, Busman and Munting [14], while confirming between-surgeon variation, found the consultants to be less effective than the registrars, with 16 recurrences in 88 patients and 6 recurrences in 141 patients, respectively. Adami et al. [1] also found a range of recurrence—from 6.6 percent in 61 patients for one surgeon to 41.7 percent in 24 patients for another.

Various attempts have been made to define preoperatively the group of patients more likely to experience recurrence. Wastell et al. [92] found a greater tendency for men with a preoperative peak acid output (PAOp) greater than 45 mmol to suffer recurrence, and similar results were obtained by Joffe and Primrose [41]. However, a similar relationship could not be established either by Christiansen et al. [15] or by Blackett and Johnston [11].

DUMPING

One of the foremost theoretical reasons for advocating PGV was the hope that because the normal mechanism of gastric emptying was preserved, dumping would be prevented. The findings presented in Table 13-2 suggest that this hope has been fulfilled. Out of a collected 889 patients of both sexes, only 2 percent experienced dumping to a severe degree.

My associates' and my findings in this re-

Table 13-2. Dumping syndrome after proximal gastric vagotomy and proximal gastric vagotomy plus pyloroplasty

Author	Year	Patients No.	Patients Sex	No. of years after operation	Operation	Significant dumping (No.)
Holle et al. [42]	1972	338	M,F	1	PGV + P	0
Amdrup et al. [7]	1974	173	M,F	2–4	PGV	1
Wastell et al. [92]	1977	47	M	>1	PGV	0
		40	M	>1	PGV + P	2
Kronborg and Madsen [65]	1975	36	M	1	PGV	1
		14	F	1	PGV	
Jordan [55]	1979	23	M,F	>2	PGV	2
Koffman et al. [62]	1979	75	M,F	>1	PGV	2
Makey et al. [68]	1979	115	M,F	1–5	PGV	4
Adami et al. [1]	1980	211	M,F	1–6	PGV	3
De Miguel [22]	1982	143	M,F	5–9	PGV	0
Emås and Fernström [27]	1985	52	M,F	1–8	PGV	5
		56	M,F		PGV + P	14
Total		889	M,F		PGV	18 (2.0%)
		434	M,F		PGV + P	16 (3.7%)

spect [93] are of interest: After PGV with pyloroplasty, just over 25 percent had dumping and 5 percent experienced it to a severe degree. One of these patients was so crippled by symptoms as to require further surgical treatment. A 10-cm antiperistaltic jejunal loop was interposed between the stomach and duodenum, and six years postoperatively he remained free of symptoms. The difference between the two procedures with respect to dumping is significant and makes the addition of pyloroplasty to PGV unjustified, particularly since almost normal gastric emptying has been demonstrated after PGV without pyloroplasty [18, 56]. A possible reason for this difference may be the rapid emptying of which the innervated antrum is capable when there is a widely patent pyloroplasty. Our findings, however, are in sharp contrast to those of Holle et al. [42], who did not find dumping to be a serious problem after PGV with pyloroplasty.

DIARRHEA

Diarrhea is unusual and mild following PGV. Among the 846 patients listed in Table 13-3, only 1 had severe diarrhea; the total incidence of moderate-to-severe diarrhea was only 1.7 percent. If pyloroplasty is added to PGV, the percentage of patients with diarrhea (2.5 percent) [34, 93] is certainly not greater than after PGV alone, as might be expected from the work of McKlvey [70], who demonstrated "gastric incontinence" of fluid passing into the duodenum after pyloroplasty and suggested that this was a cause of diarrhea. These findings are in sharp contrast with the situation after truncal vagotomy and even after selective vagotomy with drainage. Almost complete absence of serious diarrhea is one of the great virtues of PGV.

BILE VOMITING

Vomiting of bile after PGV is rare (Table 13-4). Presumably duodenogastric reflux is not a problem when the innervated pylorus is preserved.

OTHER SYMPTOMS

Table 13-5 reviews other postoperative sequelae of PGV. The most common problem seems to be epigastric fullness experienced after

Table 13-3. Diarrhea after proximal gastric vagotomy

Author	Year	Patients No.	Patients Sex	No. of years after operation	Moderate-to-severe diarrhea (No.)
Amdrup et al. [7]	1974	108	M,F	2–4	0
Kronborg and Madsen [65]	1975	36	M	1	1
		14	F	1	
Wastell et al. [92]	1977	47	M	1	0
Jordan [55]	1979	97	M,F	>2	0
Koffman et al. [62]	1979	75	M,F	>1	2
Makey et al. [68]	1979	115	M,F	1–5	6
Adami et al. [1]	1980	211	M,F	1–6	5
De Miguel [22]	1982	143	M,F	5–9	0
Total PGV		846			14 (1.7%)

Table 13-4. Bilious vomiting after proximal gastric vagotomy

Author	Year	Patients No.	Patients Sex	No. of years after operation	Bilious vomiting (No.)
Amdrup et al. [7]	1974	108	M	2–4	4 (3.7%)
Kennedy et al. [59]	1975	36	M	1–4	1 (2%)
		14	F		
Wastell et al. [92]	1977	47	M	6	2 (4.3%)
Makey et al. [68]	1979	115	M,F	1–5	0
Total		320			7 (2.2%)

Table 13-5. Other symptoms after proximal gastric vagotomy

Symptom	No. of patients	All grades of severity (No.)
Food vomiting	320	19 (5.9%)
Fullness after meals	320	63 (19.7%)
Nausea	188	23 (12%)
Hypoglycemia-like attacks	108	7 (7%)
Flatulence	110	26 (24%)
Non-ulcer dyspepsia	115	21 (18.3%)
Heartburn	115	15 (13%)

Source: Data from Amdrup et al. [7]; Wastell et al. [93]; Kennedy et al. [59]; Kronborg and Madsen [65]; and Makey et al. [68].

meals. The highest recorded incidence was 29 percent in one series. This symptom is troublesome only if it results in such severe limitation of appetite as to interfere seriously with nutrition. The other symptoms are not generally of great importance since they do not interfere with the general well-being of the patient.

ACID SECRETION

Insulin Tests

The value of insulin tests after vagotomy is still a matter of debate. In 1946 and 1948 Hollander [39, 40] described qualitative tests in which an increase in acidity of the gastric juice by 20 mEq/L in one 15-minute sample following an intravenous dose of soluble insulin (over the acidity of the pooled, basal hour)

Table 13-6. Insulin response after proximal gastric vagotomy

Author	Year	No. of patients	Time after operation	Negative response (No.)	Late positive response (No.)	Early positive response (No.)
Imperati et al. [46]	1972	62	3 wk	50 (80%)	—	13 (20%)
Johnston et al. [52]	1973	100	1 wk	97 (97%)	3 (3%)	—
		53*	1 yr +	26 (49%)	17 (32%)	10 (19%)
Liavåg and Roland [66]	1973	238	2–3 wk	211 (89%)	23 (9%)	4 (2%)
		33*	1–2 yr	19 (58%)	—	14 (42%)
Kronborg and Madsen [65]	1975	36 M	10 days	12 (33%)	12 (33%)	12 (33%)
		14 F	10 days	9 (64%)	3 (21%)	2 (14%)

*These patients had a negative insulin response immediately after operation.

was considered positive, provided the blood sugar was reduced below 50 mg/100 ml. A positive result, it was suggested, indicated an incomplete vagotomy. This test has been extended to include a 2-hour collection of gastric juice after the insulin injection. If the criteria for a positive response were met in the first hour, this was termed *early positive* or *just positive,* and if the criteria were not met until the second hour, it was termed *late positive*. An early positive response was thought to represent a large, intact vagal component, and a late positive response, only a small vagal component. Since this time, various other criteria have been described in an attempt to relate the secretion stimulated by insulin to (1) the completeness or incompleteness of vagotomy and (2) the risk of recurrent ulceration. In a review of this subject, Baron [10] concluded that it is not possible to forecast with any degree of certainty the possibility of recurrence on the basis of the insulin response, and, moreover, that other or multiple criteria for the interpretation of the postinsulin gastric secretion are no better than those originally suggested by Hollander.

As Table 13-6 shows, negative responses to the Hollander test were found in from 33 to 97 percent of patients in the short term after operation. In patients who had a negative response up to three months after operation, however, a considerable number were found to have converted from a negative to a positive response. Thus at six months or more after operation, the proportion with a negative response had fallen to between 49 and 58 percent.

Stimulated Acid Responses

The reduction in the maximal or peak acid output to either histamine or pentagastrin can also be used to assess the effect of vagotomy. The degree of reduction, generally in the short term, is seen to be from 54 to 85 percent (Table 13-7), although most of the quoted data do not relate this reduction to the insulin response. This degree of reduction is similar to that seen after either truncal or selective vagotomy with drainage [19], in which loss of juice through either the pyloroplasty or the gastrojejunostomy during the test may occur and will have the effect of increasing the apparent reduction. Cowley et al. [19] found that the risk of recurrence increased sharply when the reduction was less than 60 percent, but as with insulin tests, the overlap was too great for accurate forecasting to be made. A similar correlation has been observed by Wittebol et al. [99].

Current Status of Proximal Gastric Vagotomy

Is it possible to claim that PGV is the operation of choice for the majority of patients with uncomplicated duodenal ulcer who require an operation? It is certainly the least disturbing

Table 13-7. Reduction in stimulated acid output after proximal gastric vagotomy

Author	Year	Patients		Insulin status	Time after operation	Mean acid output (mEq/hr)		Percent reduction
		No.	Sex			Preop.	Postop.	
Imperati et al. [46]	1972	63	M,F	Not stated	10 days	36.5[a]	11.4[a]	69
Holle et al. [42]	1972	30	M,F	Not stated	?	42.6[b]	6.6[b]	85
Johnston et al. [52]	1973	11	M,F	Various	1 yr +	42.0[c]	19.3[c]	56
		20	M,F	Various	1 yr +	39.2[c]	18.1[c]	54
Liavåg and Roland [66]	1973	246	M,F	Not stated	1–2 yr	—	—	56[d]
Wastell et al. [93]	1974	32	M	Negative response	2 wk	36.0[c]	15.0[c]	58
		7	M	Late positive response	2 wk	41.1[c]	20.2[c]	51
		8	M	Positive response	2 wk	41.0[c]	22.3[c]	44

[a]Maximum acid output to pentagastrin.
[b]Maximum acid output to human gastrin I (0.002 mg/gm).
[c]Peak acid output to pentagastrin.
[d]Peak acid output to augmented histamine.

Table 13-8. Visick grading after proximal gastric vagotomy

Author	Year	Patients		No. of years after operation	Visick grade			
		No.	Sex		I (%)	II (%)	III (%)	IV (%)
Amdrup et al. [7]	1974	108	M,F	2–4 yr + unit	71 (66)	24 (22)	8 (7)	5 (5)
Wastell et al. [88]	1974	32	M	1 yr	20 (62)	9 (28)	0	3 (10)
Kennedy et al. [56]	1975	50	M,F	1–4 yr + unit	30 (60)	18 (36)	1 (2)	1 (2)
Kronborg and Madsen [62]	1975	50	M,F	1 yr	34 (68)	5 (10)	1 (2)	10 (20)
Hopton et al. [42]	1976	25	Not stated	1 yr	15 (60)	5 (20)	3 (12)	2 (8)
Adami et al. [1]	1980	229	M,F	1–6 yr	84 (37)	75 (33)	24 (10)	46 (20)
Busman and Munting [14]	1982	229	M,F	1–8 yr	140 (61)	50 (22)	12 (5)	27 (12)
Emås and Fernström [27]	1985	52	M,F	1–8 yr	27 (54)	13 (26)	4 (8)	6 (12)
Total		775	M,F		421 (54)	199 (26)	53 (7)	100 (13)

procedure, from the point of view of both the effect on the physiology of the stomach and duodenum and the ease of early postoperative care. These factors are important when one is faced with the question of revision; although this stance may seem to acquiesce to the inevitability of severe postoperative sequelae in some patients, most surgeons would agree that there are few or no operations of this kind in which these sequelae do not occur. If revision is required, the field is left open in a way that it certainly is not after gastrectomy, for example. Proximal gastric vagotomy does seem to have dealt with the perennial problems of dumping and diarrhea—there is universal agreement on this point among the different series that have been published. In spite of anxiety about the safety of the procedure following reports of sloughing of the lesser curvature of the stomach, it would seem to be just as acceptable from this point of view as are other established procedures. Other symptoms such as bilious vomiting and epigastric fullness, although present do not seem likely to spoil the effectiveness of the procedure [4, 23, 53].

RECURRENCE OF ULCER

The debate about PGV will center around two vital issues. The first of these is recurrent or persistent ulceration.

Our forecast in the third edition of this book that the recurrent ulcer rate would rise has been shown to be true. Perhaps in some patients there is regeneration of vagal nerves. This has been shown to be a particularly vigorous process [73]. Attempts have been made to obstruct regeneration with either liver [93] or peritoneum [34]. Perhaps some patients have antral G-cell hyperplasia with an increased secretion of gastrin, although this has never been substantiated [17, 79], or perhaps some patients have a low duodenal mucosal resistance. Alternatively, there may be a combination of these and other factors.

Why recurrences occur in patients who apparently have had an adequate operation is obviously an important question and one that cannot be answered with certainty. Accepting for the moment that recurrent ulcers do occur, should this fact be allowed to dominate an approach to the problem of duodenal ulcer? Emphatically, it should not. It is important to aim for a population of postoperative patients who are free of serious side effects.

Recurrent ulceration after PGV can, as has been stated, be treated with an H_2-receptor blocker. If this is not effective, and there is a small group of patients who do not respond [16], a second operation may have to be performed. At the present time our approach is to carry out antrectomy with, if feasible, a Billroth I anastomosis.

TECHNICAL DIFFICULTY

The second vital issue regarding PGV is contained in the simple question: Is it worth it? Proximal gastric vagotomy is more time-consuming than other operations and is certainly more demanding of the surgeon. Truncal vagotomy and drainage achieve an 85 percent Visick I and II result in the medium term [31, 32, 90]; interestingly enough, this is 5 percent higher than the combined grades I and II after PGV (Table 13-8). The answer to this apparent inconsistency lies in the extraordinary intractability of postvagotomy diarrhea and dumping. These failures, when they occur, are often beyond help, whereas the failures after PGV due to recurrence can be treated and cured.

LONG-TERM RESULTS

The long-term results of these procedures are also important. It is hoped that PGV will not be attended by a severe nutritional defect such as occurs after gastrectomy [85] or vagotomy with either pyloroplasty or gastrojejunostomy [20, 89, 90, 95]. Time of follow-up is still too short for information about effects on nutrition, although it has been shown that the increase in fecal fat after operation is not as great as it is after either truncal or selective vagotomy with pyloroplasty [26].

Some attempts have been made to use PGV in patients with stenosis, acute perforation, or hemorrhage [49, 50, 75]. Numbers of patients so treated, however, are small, and it is still not possible to advocate its use for the complications of duodenal ulcer.

With these remarks in mind, it is concluded

that PGV may well offer the best compromise possible. Provided the recurrent ulceration rate does not rise, PGV is the procedure of choice for patients with uncomplicated duodenal ulcer.

Proximal Gastric Vagotomy for Gastric Ulcer

Naturally most of this chapter concerns the treatment of duodenal ulcer. The use of PGV for gastric ulcer should be mentioned, however, following the report by Reid et al. [81] of a series of patients an average of eight years after PGV with ulcer excision (PGVE). This procedure, by excising the ulcer for histopathologic study, deals with the objection to PGV alone in this condition—that the benign status of the ulcer could never be proved for certain.

Reid's trial concerned 56 patients randomly allocated to PGVE or Billroth (B-I) gastrectomy. At an average follow-up time of four years, there appeared to be no advantage for either procedure; however, another follow-up study four years later shows the balance has tipped decisively in favor of PGVE. Fifty-four patients were followed, and recurrent ulceration occurred in 6 after PGVE and 5 after BI gastrectomy. The difference really lies in the relative percentages of postoperative symptoms, excluding recurrence, which resulted in all the patients after PGVE being graded Visick I or II, compared with only 62 percent in these categories after B-I gastrectomy.

Clearly this study represents an interesting new approach to gastric ulcer; more patients treated in this way are required before a final assessment can be made.

References

1. Adami, H. O., Enander, L. K., Ingvar, C., and Rydberg, B. Clinical results of 229 patients with duodenal ulcer 1–6 years after highly selective vagotomy. *Br. J. Surg.* 67:29, 1980.
2. Ahonen, J., Hoepener-Hallikainen, D., Inberg, M., and Scheinin, T. M. The value of corpus-antrum border determinations in highly selective vagotomy. *Br. J. Surg.* 66:35, 1979.
3. Alexander-Williams, J. Current Practice. In J. Alexander-Williams and A. G. Cox (Eds.), *After Vagotomy*. London: Butterworth, 1969.
4. Amdrup, E., Andersen, D., and Jensen, H.-E. Parietal cell (highly selective or proximal gastric) vagotomy for peptic ulcer disease. *World J. Surg.* 1:18, 1977.
5. Amdrup, E., and Jensen, H.-E. Selective vagotomy of the parietal cell mass preserving innervation of the undrained antrum. *Gastroenterology* 59:522, 1970.
6. Amdrup, E., and Jensen, H.-E. One hundred patients five years after selective gastric vagotomy and drainage for duodenal ulcer. *Surgery* 74:321, 1973.
7. Amdrup, E., Jensen, H.-E., Johnston, D., et al. Clinical results of parietal cell vagotomy (highly selective vagotomy) two to four years after operation. *Ann. Surg.* 180:279, 1974.
8. Amdrup, E., and Johnston, D. Name of the new vagotomy. *Gastroenterology* 68:206, 1975.
9. Barnes, A. D., and Williams, J. A. The change of bowel habit following vagotomy and pyloroplasty. *Br. J. Surg.* 54:218, 1967.
10. Baron, J. H. Gastric Function Tests. In C. Wastell (Ed.), *Westminster Hospital Symposium on Chronic Duodenal Ulcer.* London: Butterworth, 1974.
11. Blackett, R. L., and Johnston, D. Recurrent ulceration after highly selective vagotomy for duodenal ulcer. *Br. J. Surg.* 68:705, 1981.
12. Burdette, W. J., Rasmussen, B. L., and Fitzpatrick, W. K. Management of duodenal ulcer by vagus resection and pyloroplasty. *Surg. Gynecol. Obstet.* 127:513, 1968.
13. Burge, H. W., Hutchinson, J. S. F., Longland, C. J., et al. Selective nerve section in the prevention of post-vagotomy diarrhoea. *Lancet* 1:577, 1964.
14. Busman, D. C., and Munting, J. D. K. Results of highly selective vagotomy in a non-university teaching hospital. *Br. J. Surg.* 69:620, 1982.
15. Christiansen, J., Jensen, H.-E., Ejby-Poulson, P., et al. Prospective controlled vagotomy trial for duodenal ulcer. *Ann. Surg.* 193:49, 1981.
16. Clark, C. G., Boulos, P. B., Haggie, S. J., and McDonald, A. M. H_2-antagonists in the treatment of recurrent ulceration after vagotomy. *Br. J. Surg.* 66:409, 1979.

17. Clark, C. G., Lewin, M. R., Stagg, B. H., and Wyllie, J. H. Effect of proximal gastric vagotomy on gastric acid secretion and plasma gastrin. *Gut* 14:293, 1973.
18. Clark, R. J., and Alexander-Williams, J. The effect of preserving antral innervation and of a pyloroplasty on gastric emptying after vagotomy in man. *Gut* 14:300, 1973.
19. Cowley, D. J., Spencer, J., and Baron, J. H. Acid secretion in relation to recurrence of duodenal ulcer after vagotomy and drainage. *Br. J. Surg.* 60:517, 1973.
20. Cox, A. G., Bond, M. R., Podmore, P. A., and Rose, D. P. E. Aspects of nutrition after vagotomy and gastrojejunostomy. *Br. Med. J.* 1:465, 1964.
21. Davies, J. A. L. Late results of vagotomy combined with gastrojejunostomy or pyloroplasty in the treatment of duodenal ulcer. *Br. Med. J.* 2:1086, 1956.
22. De Miguel, J. Late results of proximal gastric vagotomy without drainage for duodenal ulcer: 5–9 year follow-up. *Br. J. Surg.* 69:7, 1982.
23. Donahue, P. E., Bombeck, C. T., Condon, R. E., and Nyhus, L. M. Proximal gastric vagotomy versus selective vagotomy with antrectomy: Results of a prospective, randomized clinical trial after 4 to 12 years. *Surgery* 96:585, 1984.
24. Donahue, P. E., and Nyhus, L. M. The simplified endoscopic Congo red test for completeness of vagotomy. *Surg. Gynecol. Obstet.*, in press.
25. Dragstedt, L. R., Harper, P. V., Toree, E. B., and Woodward, E. R. Section of the vagus nerve to the stomach in the treatment of peptic ulcer. *Ann. Surg.* 126:687, 1947.
26. Edwards, J. P., Lyndon, J. P., Smith, R. B., and Johnston, D. Faecal fat excretion after truncal, selective and highly selective vagotomy for duodenal ulcer. *Gut* 15:521, 1974.
27. Emås, S., and Fernström, M. Prospective, randomized trial of selective vagotomy with pyloroplasty and selective proximal vagotomy with and without pyloroplasty in the treatment of duodenal, pyloric, and prepyloric ulcers. *Am. J. Surg.* 149:236, 1985.
28. Feggetter, G. Y., and Pringle, R. The long-term results of bilateral vagotomy and gastrojejunostomy for chronic duodenal ulcer. *Surg. Gynecol. Obstet.* 116:175, 1963.
29. Ferguson, D. J., Billings, H., Swensen, D., and Hoover, G. Segmental gastrectomy with innervated antrum for duodenal ulcer: Results at one to five years. *Surgery* 47:548, 1960.
30. Flynn, P. J., and Longmire, W. P. Subtotal gastrectomy with pyloric sphincter preservation. *Surg. Forum* 10:185, 1960.
31. Goligher, J. C., Irvin, T. T., Johnston, D., et al. Five to eight year results of truncal vagotomy and pyloroplasty for duodenal ulcer. *Br. Med. J.* 1:7, 1972.
32. Goodale, R. L., Tsung, M. S., Prevost, M., et al. Pylorus preserving gastrectomy (Maki): Effects upon antral function, gastric emptying and ulcerogenesis in the dog. *Arch. Surg.* 99:193, 1969.
33. Graffner, H. O., Liedberg, G. F., and Oscarson, J. E. A. Parietal cell vagotomy in the surgical treatment of chronic duodenal, pyloric and prepyloric ulcer disease. *Int. Surg.* 70:139, 1985.
34. Grassi, G. The technic of proximal selective vagotomy. *Chir. Gastroenterol.* 5:399, 1971.
35. Griffith, C. A., and Harkins, H. N. Partial gastric vagotomy: An experimental study. *Gastroenterology* 32:96, 1957.
36. Griffith, C. A., Stavney, L. S., Kato, T., and Harkins, H. N. Selective gastric vagotomy. *Am. J. Surg.* 105:13, 1963.
37. Hoffman, J., Meisner, S., and Jensen, H.-E. Antrectomy for recurrent ulcer after parietal cell vagotomy. *Br. J. Surg.* 70:120, 1983.
38. Hoile, R. W., and Turner, J. C. D. Gastric fistula after proximal gastric vagotomy. *Br. Med. J.* 2:282, 1975.
39. Hollander, F. The insulin test for the presence of intact nerve fibers after vagal operations for peptic ulcer. *Gastroenterology* 7:707, 1946.
40. Hollander, F. Laboratory procedures in the study of vagotomy. *Gastroenterology* 11:419, 1948.
41. Holle, F. *Spezielle Magenchirurgie*. Berlin: Springer, 1968. P. 508.
42. Holle, F., Bauer, H., Holle, G., et al. Clinical results of selective proximal vagotomy (SPV) in gastro-duodenal ulcer (GDU). *Langenbecks Arch. Chir.* 330:197, 1972.
43. Holst-Christensen, J., Hansen, O. H., Pedersen, T., and Kronborg, O. Recurrent ulcer after proximal gastric vagotomy for duodenal and pre-pyloric ulcer. *Br. J. Surg.* 64:42, 1977.
44. Holt, R. L., and Lythgoe, J. P. Treatment of chronic duodenal ulcer by vagotomy and anterior pylorectomy. *Br. J. Surg.* 52:27, 1965.
45. Hopton, D. S., Matheson, T. S., Hall, R., and Richards, B. Advantages and disadvantages of

highly selective vagotomy. *Br. Med. J.* 1:149, 1976.
46. Imperati, L., Natale, C., and Marinaccio, F. Acid fundic selective vagotomy of the stomach without drainage in the treatment of duodenal ulcer: Technique and results. *Br. J. Surg.* 59:602, 1972.
47. Joffe, S. N., and Primrose, J. N. A prospective study evaluating preoperative gastric secretion and choice of an operation for duodenal ulcer. *Surg. Gynecol. Obstet.* 152:421, 1981.
48. Johnston, D. Operative mortality and postoperative morbidity of highly selective vagotomy. *Br. J. Surg.* 62:160, 1975.
49. Johnston, D. Vagotomy for Complications. In J. H. Baron, J. Alexander-Williams, M. Allgöwer, C., Muller, and J. Spencer (Eds.), *Vagotomy in Modern Surgical Practice*. London: Butterworth, 1982. Pp. 216–47.
50. Johnston, D., Lyndon, P. J., Smith, R. B., and Humphrey, C. S. Highly selective vagotomy without a drainage procedure in the treatment of haemorrhage, perforation and pyloric stenosis due to peptic ulcer. *Br. J. Surg.* 60:790, 1973.
51. Johnston, D., and Wilkinson, A. R. Selective vagotomy with innervated antrum without drainage procedure for duodenal ulcer. *Br. J. Surg.* 56:626, 1969.
52. Johnston, D., Wilkinson, A. R., Humphrey, C. S., et al. Serial studies of gastric secretion in patients after highly selective (parietal cell) vagotomy without a drainage procedure for duodenal ulcer. I. Effect of highly selective vagotomy on basal and pentagastrin-stimulated acid output. II. The insulin test after highly selective vagotomy. *Gastroenterology* 64:1, 1973.
53. Jordan, P. H., Jr. A prospective study of parietal cell vagotomy and selective vagotomy-antrectomy for treatment of duodenal ulcer. *Ann. Surg.* 183:619, 1976.
54. Jordan, P. H., Jr. Current status of parietal cell vagotomy. *Ann. Surg.* 184:659, 1976.
55. Jordan, P. H. An interim report on parietal cell vagotomy versus selective vagotomy and antrectomy for treatment of duodenal ulcer. *Ann. Surg.* 189:643, 1979.
56. Kalbasi, H., Hudson, F. R., Herring, A., et al. Gastric emptying following vagotomy and antrectomy and proximal gastric vagotomy. *Gut* 16:509, 1975.
57. Kennedy, F., Mackay, C., Bedi, B. S., and Kay, A. W. Truncal vagotomy and drainage for chronic duodenal ulcer disease: A controlled trial. *Br. Med. J.* 2:72, 1973.
58. Kennedy, T. Selective Vagotomy. In C. Wastell (Ed.), *Westminster Hospital Symposium on Chronic Duodenal Ulcer.* London: Butterworth, 1974.
59. Kennedy, T., Johnston, G. W., Macrae, K. D., and Spencer, E. F. A. Proximal gastric vagotomy: Interim results of a randomised controlled trial. *Br. Med. J.* 2:301, 1975.
60. Kennedy, T., Magill, P., Johnston, G. W., and Parks, T. G. Proximal gastric vagotomy, fundoplication, and lesser curve necrosis. *Br. Med. J.* 1:1455, 1979.
61. Killen, D. A., and Symbas, P. N. Effect of the preservation of the pyloric sphincter during antrectomy on postoperative gastric emptying. *Am. J. Surg.* 104:836, 1962.
62. Koffman, C. G., Elder, J. B., Gillespie, I. E., et al. A prospective randomised trial of vagotomy in chronic duodenal ulceration. *Br. J. Surg.* 66:145, 1979.
63. Kraft, R. O., Fry, W. J., Wilhelm, K. G., and Ransom, H. K. Selective gastric vagotomy. *Arch. Surg.* 95:625, 1967.
64. Kronborg, O. Gastric acid secretion and risk of recurrence of duodenal ulcer within six to eight years after truncal vagotomy and drainage. *Gut* 15:714, 1974.
65. Kronborg, O., and Madsen, P. A controlled, randomised trial of highly selective vagotomy versus selective vagotomy and pyloroplasty in the treatment of duodenal ulcer. *Gut* 16:268, 1975.
66. Liavåg, I., and Roland, M. Selective proximal vagotomy in the treatment of gastroduodenal ulcers. *Scand. J. Gastroenterol.* 20(Suppl.):10, 1973.
67. Lygidakis, N. L. Surgical treatment of duodenal ulcers: When? How? Why? *Am. Surg.* 50:390, 1984.
68. Makey, D. A., Tovey, E. I., and Heald, R. J. Results of proximal gastric vagotomy over 1–5 years in a district general hospital. *Br. J. Surg.* 66:39, 1979.
69. Maki, T., Shiratori, T., Hatafuku, T., and Sugawara, K. Pylorus preserving gastrectomy as an improved operation for gastric ulcer. *Surgery* 61:838, 1967.
70. McKelvey, S. T. D. Gastric incontinence and post-vagotomy diarrhoea. *Br. J. Surg.* 57:741, 1970.
71. Moore, F. P., and Wyllie, J. M. Ischaemic necrosis of lesser curve after proximal gastric va-

gotomy. *Br. Med. J.* 3:328, 1975.
72. Mühe, E., Muller, C., Martinoli, S., et al. Five-Years' Results of a Prospective Multicentre Trial of Proximal Gastric Vagotomy. In J. H. Baron, J. Alexander-Williams, M. Allgöwer, C. Muller, and J. Spencer (Eds.), *Vagotomy in Modern Surgical Practice*. London: Butterworth, 1982. Pp. 176–86.
73. Murray, J. G. Regeneration of the Vagus. In J. Alexander-Williams and A. G. Cox (Eds.), *After Vagotomy*. London: Butterworth, 1969.
74. Newcombe, J. F. Fatality after highly selective vagotomy. *Br. Med. J.* 1:610, 1973.
75. Nouri, K. D. Pyloric stenosis treated by parietal cell vagotomy and gastrojejunostomy. *Proc. R. Soc. Med.* 64:1088, 1971.
76. Nyhus, L. M., Donahue, P. E., Krystosek, R. I., et al. Complete vagotomy: The evolution of an effective technique. *Arch. Surg.* 115:264, 1980.
77. Pendower, J. E. H. A comparison of the Burge and Grassi intraoperative tests for completeness of nerve section in parietal cell vagotomy. *Br. J. Surg.* 68:83, 1981.
78. Piasecki, C. Blood supply to the human gastroduodenal mucosa with special reference to the ulcer bearing areas. *J. Anat.* 118:295, 1974.
79. Pigott, H. W. S. Personal communication, 1975.
80. Pollock, A. V. Vagotomy in the treatment of peptic ulcer. *Lancet* 2:795, 1952.
81. Reid, D. A., Duthie, H. L., Bransom, C. J., and Johnson, A. G. Late follow-up of highly selective vagotomy with excision of the ulcer compared with Billroth I gastrectomy for treatment of benign gastric ulcer. *Br. J. Surg.* 69:605, 1982.
82. Schofield, P. F., Watson-Williams, E. J., and Sorrell, V. F. Vagotomy and pyloric drainage for chronic duodenal ulcer. *Arch. Surg.* 95:615, 1967.
83. Skandalakis, J. E., Gray, S. W., Soria, R. E., et al. Distribution of the vagus nerve to the stomach. *Am. Surg.* 56:130, 1980.
84. Smith, G. K., and Farris, J. M. Some observations upon selective gastric vagotomy. *Arch. Surg.* 86:716, 1963.
85. Stammers, F. A. R., and Williams, J. A. *Partial Gastrectomy: Complications and Metabolic Consequences*. London: Butterworth, 1963.
86. Stempien, S. J., Dagradi, A. E., Lee, E. R., and Simonton, J. H. Status of duodenal ulcer patients ten years of more after vagotomy-pyloroplasty (V-P). *Am. J. Gastroenterol.* 56:99, 1971.
87. Tanner, N. C. Drainage operations for vagotomy. *Proc. R. Soc. Med.* 60:21, 1967.
88. Troidl, H., Lorenz, W., Rohde, H., et al. Trends in der Chirurgie des chronischen ulcus duodeni; eins prospective Kontrallierte - aber nach immer nicht randomisierte -studie. *Chirurg* 50:285, 1979.
89. Walters, W., and Mobley, J. E. Five-to-ten year follow up of 162 cases of duodenal ulcer treated by vagotomy with and without associated gastric operations. *Ann. Surg.* 145:753, 1957.
90. Wastell, C. Long-term clinical and metabolic effects of vagotomy with either gastrojejunostomy or pyloroplasty. *Ann. R. Coll. Surg. Engl.* 45:193, 1969.
91. Wastell, C., Baron, J. H., and Alexander-Williams, J. Nomenclature of the new vagotomy. *Br. Med. J.* 1:482, 1973.
92. Wastell, C., Colin, J., Wilson, T., et al. Prospectively randomised trial of proximal gastric vagotomy either with or without pyloroplasty in treatment of uncomplicated duodenal ulcer. *Br. Med. J.* 2:851, 1977.
93. Wastell, C., Wilson, T., and Pigott, H. W. S. Proximal gastric vagotomy. *Proc. R. Soc. Med.* 67:41, 1974.
94. Weinberg, J. A. Vagotomy and pyloroplasty in the treatment of duodenal ulcer. *Am. J. Surg.* 105:347, 1963.
95. Wheldon, E. J., Venables, C. W., and Johnston, I. D. Late sequelae of vagotomy and gastroenterostomy. *Lancet* 1:437, 1970.
96. Whittaker, L. D., Judd, E. S., and Stauffer, M. H. Analysis of the use of vagotomy with a drainage procedure in the surgical management of duodenal ulcer. *Surg. Gynecol. Obstet.* 125:1018, 1967.
97. Wille-Jørgensen, P., and Jensen, H.-E. Leucomethylene blue staining during vagotomy. *Br. J. Surg.* 68:81, 1981.
98. Williams, R. S., and Johnson, A. G. Evaluation of an intraoperative test for the completeness of vagotomy. *Aust. N. Z. J. Surg.* 49:659, 1979.
99. Wittebol, P., Akkermans, L. M. A., and Hulstaert, P. F. Prognostic factors in surgery for duodenal ulcer. *Surg. Annu.* 17:235, 1985.
100. Wyllie, J. Complication of proximal gastric vagotomy. *Br. Med. J.* 2:561, 1974.

SPECIAL COMMENT
Nonresective Surgery for Gastroduodenal Ulcer
F. K. Holle

Pathophysiology

Development of the nonresective method proceeded from observations of fundectomies [2]. Proximal gastric resection is the most radical form of proximal denervation of the stomach. It causes a fluctuation in secretion behavior: Acid release occurs when the stomach is empty but not when it is full. Fullness triggers a severe gastric dilatation with a delay in emptying. Large quantities of food and gastric juice, which contain considerable acid concentrations, are retained. Larger meals are vomited after 2 to 8 hours. In this radical form, fundectomy is clinically impracticable. To determine the causes of this behavior, the proximal resection was omitted and the operation restricted to removal of the proximal nerves and blood vessels.

Only an adequate selective proximal vagotomy (a-SPV) produces the necessary acid reduction. The forms of vagotomy known before the introduction of selective proximal vagotomy (SPV)—truncal vagotomy (TV) and selective gastric complete vagotomy (SGV)—were unsatisfactory in this respect. A solution became apparent only with a radical removal of the vagus *and* vascular supply to the proximal stomach—the SPV. This operation was subjected to multiple efficiency tests by the recording of the most important standard factors: *secretion* (acid, gastrin) and *motility.*

Acid reduction is optimal after adequate a-SPV. Optimal acid reduction is achieved when the SPV extends from the cranial borderline nerves at the cardia through the angle of His and along the lesser curvature up to the distal ventral and dorsal borderline nerves of the antral innervation. This gives the greatest degree of acid reduction. This type of SPV—a-SPV—gives reliable success. Confirmation is made by the insulin and pentagastrin tests. The method should satisfy the O-theorem [7], i.e., after insulin stimulation, the basal acid output (BAO) postoperatively should not exceed 0.0 mEq/L, and the peak acid output (PAO) at 30 minutes should not exceed 0.0–0.6 mEq/L. Measured against this strict criterion or that of Emås [1], recurrences are 15 times more frequent after inadequate vagotomy than after a-SPV. Through a-SPV, a reduction in BAO of greater than 90 percent and of maximal acid output (MAO) of greater than 75 percent (± 2–3 percent in both instances) can be achieved even for hypersecretors (with the exception of those with Zollinger-Ellison syndrome). The acid reduction remains constant for longer than five years [1, 6]. Such a permanent acid exclusion cannot be achieved with any other therapy.

Gastrin determination is of special importance for excluding special instances. Special instances include hyperactive antrum, G-cell hyperplasia, and Zollinger-Ellison syndrome. After a-SPV, the basal gastrin level almost always increases. The operation causes hypergastrinemia in dogs and humans. Postprandially and after medical stimulation, a further increase in gastrin level of varying intensity and duration occurs. Since after a-SPV the parietal cells remain responsive to gastrin, it must be assumed that the postprandial acid production after a-SPV is caused by gastrin. The varying gastrin intensity depends on the number of existing gastrin cells and on their functional condition.

Gastric motility is used to check vagotomy. Antropyloric gastric motor function is to remain as intact as possible. The surgeon is faced with a dilemma here, since on the one hand he or she must denervate sufficiently distally to achieve optimal acid reduction, and on the other hand adequate motility of the antrum must be preserved. By means of muscle reduction plastic surgery—pyloroplasty appropriate to form and function (ff-Py), postprandial antral contractility can be lowered and the emptying adjusted to the standard [8, 9]. It is the responsibility of the surgeon to determine the correct extent of the plastic surgical correction.

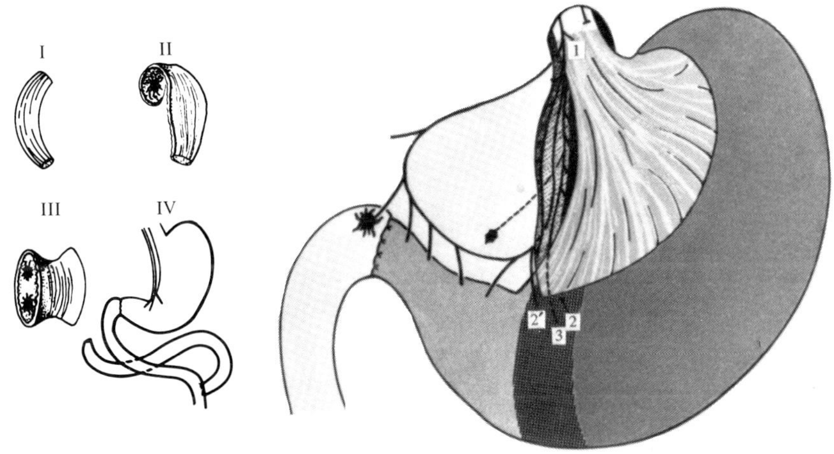

Fig. 13-8. Duodenal ulcer. Adequate selective proximal vagotomy (a-SPV): Cranial (1), proximal ventral (2), distal ventral (2′), and dorsal (3) borderline nerves. Pyloroplasty appropriate to form and function (ff-Py): I, submucosal ff-Py, seromuscular suture. II, open ff-Py (ulcer excision, direct closure). III, pylorectomy (total excision of the antropyloric "end segment" of the stomach with ulcers, gastroduodenostomy). IV, difficult duodenum (total excision of the end segment with part I–II of the duodenum, purse-string closure of the duodenum plus end-to-end gastrojejunostomy and end-to-side Roux-en-Y jejunojejunostomy).

Protective treatment is indispensable for the maintenance of adequate motility. The three most important areas (Figs. 13-8, 13-9) are located:

1. In the cardia sector (entrance of the cranial, ventral, and dorsal borderline nerves)
2. In the angle sector, or "crow's-foot" (entrance of the distal ventral and of the dorsal borderline nerves)
3. In the bulb sector (entrance of the hepatopyloric branches to the pylorus and duodenum)

The crow's-foot requires special attention. Here the entry points of the antral borderline nerves indicate the width of the "transition zone" in the middle of the stomach. The proximal border marks the proximal and the distal borderline nerves. The transition zone marks the transition of the mucosa of the corpus of the stomach into that of the antrum. The distribution of the vagal borderline nerves is variable. In every individual, its dimensions must be determined intraoperatively. These facts are of importance for selection of procedure and surgical technique.

Clinical checking of motility is most reliably made by the noninvasive method of esophagogastroduodenoscintigraphy [7]. Both the orthograde passage and emptying through the "bottlenecks"—cardia, antral sphincter, and pylorus (esophagus-stomach-duodenum)—as well as retrograde reflux (duodenum-stomach-esophagus) can be quantified in this way.

Clinical Application

Clinical application is based on perfect determination and selection, indication and choice of procedure, operation and technique, and checking and evaluation.

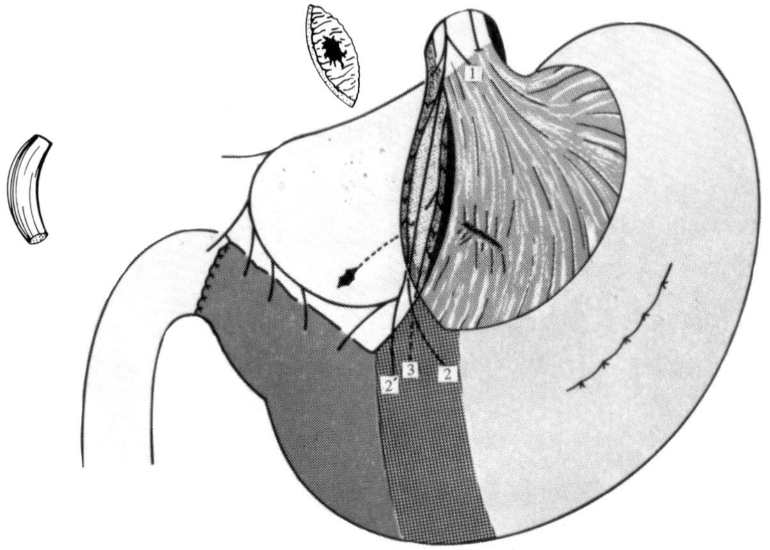

Fig. 13-9. Gastric ulcer. Selective proximal vagotomy: All borderline nerves preserved. Shown is a submucosal pyloroplasty appropriate to form and function. If this type of ff-Py cannot be performed, a resective procedure should be chosen.

A differential diagnostic regimen must consist of:

1. Outpatient examination (medical history, personal interview)
2. Roentgenographic examination (wall deformity, gastric passage, reflux)
3. Endoscopy (wall change, motility, successive biopsy)
4. Secretion studies (insulin/pentagastrin test, gastrin, basal levels); in suspicious instances, gastrin profiles (feeding, secretin level, calcium infusion)
5. Motility studies, scintigraphy
6. Psychological testing (in instances of suspected psychological abnormality)
7. Clinical conference
   Indication
   Clarification
   Scientific determination

The list contains most factors with a high degree of relevance for diagnosis of genuine ulcer disease. Only persons with genuine ulcer disease are operated on. We are able to select out candidates unacceptable for operation because of particularly rare disturbances of secretion or motility, or unusual anatomical form. Five standard situations can be differentiated (Table 13-9).

Operative Technique

The nonresective procedure (Figs. 13-8, 13-9) is performed as follows:

1. Removal of ulcer locally, denervating the proximal stomach up to the border points, 1, 2, 2′, 3
2. Protection of the lesser omentum as a whole and the antropyloric innervation and blood circulation
3. Normalizing of emptying and passage by ff-Py

Table 13-9. Indications for and suggested methods of operative treatment

I. Duodenal ulcer: Nonresective standard technique (95–98%)
- A. *Indications:* Vagal hypersecretion (pyloric stenosis), typical duodenal ulcer
  1. Secretion: BAO ↑ PAO ↑ ↑ PG/Ins ↑ ↑ Gastrin: basal →, feeding profile ↑
  2. Motility: passage ↑ ↑ (↓ in stenosis)
- B. *Technique:* a-SPV + ff-Py
  1. Submucosal pyloroplasty
  2. Open-ulcer excision
  3. Pylorectomy
  4. GJ (end-to-end), JJ (Roux-en-Y)

II. Gastric ulcer: Nonresective standard technique (40–50%)
- A. *Indication:* Typical gastric ulcer
  1. Secretion: BAO ↓ PAO → PG/Ins ↓ Gastrin: basal → or ↑, feeding profile → or ↑
  2. Motility: passage ↓
- B. *Technique:* SPV + ulcer excision (locally) + submucosal pyloroplasty (beware: preserve antral and pyloric innervation)

III. Duodenal ulcer: Primary resection (1–2%)
- A. *Indications:* Hyperactive antrum, duodenogastric reflux, gastritis, gastroesophageal reflux, esophagitis
  1. Secretion: BAO ↑ ↑ PAO ↑ PG/Ins ↑ ↑ Gastrin: basal ↑ ↑, feeding profile ↑ ↑ ↑ Secretin: paradoxical Calcium infusion: ↑ ↑ ↑
  2. Motility: passage ↑
- B. *Technique:* SV + 40% antrectomy + GJ + JJ (Braun)

IV. Gastric ulcer: Primary resection (~50%)
- A. *Indications:* Stasis, or suspicion of malignancy, duodenogastric reflux, gastritis, gastroesophageal reflux, or esophagitis
  1. Secretion: BAO ↓ PAO → or ↓ PG/Ins → or ↓ Gastrin: basal → or ↑, feeding profile ↑
  2. Motility: atonia (spontaneous denervation)
  3. Histology: suspicious for malignancy
- B. *Technique*
  1. Distal ulcer: SPV + pylorectomy + GD
  2. Medial ulcer: SV + 50–60% resection + GJ + JJ (Braun)
  3. Proximal ulcer (cardia involved): SPV + fundectomy + submucosal pyloroplasty

V. Multiple duodenal ulcers and gastric ulcers, Zollinger-Ellison syndrome (2–3%)
- A. *Indication:* Zollinger-Ellison syndrome
  1. Secretion: BAO ↑ ↑ ↑ PAO ↑ ↑ ↑ BAO/PAO, < 0.6 mEq Gastrin: basal ↑ ↑ ↑ Secretin: paradoxical Calcium infusion ↑ ↑ ↑
  2. Motility: passage ↑ ↑ ↑
  3. Computerized tomography: pancreatic tumors
  4. Histology: glandular hyperplasia
- B. *Technique:* Total gastrectomy, esophagojejunostomy (Roux, Longmire)

BAO = basal acid output; PAO = peak acid output; PG/Ins = pentagastrin/insulin; a-SPV = adequate selective proximal vagotomy; ff-Py = pyloroplasty appropriate to form and function; GJ = gastrojejunostomy; JJ = jejunojejunostomy; SPV = selective proximal vagotomy; SV = selective vagotomy; GD = gastroduodenostomy; ↑ = elevated; ↑ ↑ = moderately elevated; ↑ ↑ ↑ = greatly elevated; → = level or normal.

The technique adheres here to the rules of neurosurgical technique for ensuring an a-SPV for duodenal ulcer (Fig. 13-8) and an SPV for gastric ulcer (Fig. 13-9), and to the rules of plastic surgical technique for performance of an ff-Py.

As for the operation on the pylorus, all conventional pyloroplasties (Heineke-Mikulicz, Finney, Jaboulay, Weinberg) destroy form and interfere with function and are therefore unusable. The surgeon must learn how to remove the ulcer and the scars locally. Doing this will correct the functionally disturbed antral "end segment" through a muscle reduction plastic operation in such a manner that the antropyloric function resembles normal function as closely as possible.

My associates and I have described the techniques of a-SPV, and ff-Py has been described in detail in other publications [3, 5–7].

Through the correct combination of a-SPV and ff-Py, the opposite effects of the two measures are used to compensate for their disadvantages (increased danger of recurrence after inadequate SPV and increased retention hazard after adequate SPV alone) and to obtain the advantages of a maximal acid reduction and a timely passage of food after intake.

Results

The following represents the results from a study of my own patients, including 1456 who underwent SPV and ff-Py in the period from January 1, 1964 to March 31, 1980. Study of a consecutive series (1972–1977) included 503 (79.1 percent) of 636 patients operated on. The dumping syndrome occurred in 23 patients (4.5 percent). Dumping was of slight degree and was controlled with medicine and diet.

Seventeen of the 503 patients had recurrence (3.4 percent). The recurrence rate for duodenal ulcer alone was 2.7 percent and for gastric ulcer alone was 7.3 percent. The recurrence proportions fluctuated within the year's total. This fluctuation may cause confusion. In retrospective studies, at least five consecutive years should be collected. Here the same diagnostic regimen should be used pre- and postoperatively—the more roentgenographic and endoscopic examinations made, the more recurrences and persistent ulcers will be discovered. Questionnaires are useless.

Gastric ulcer recurs more frequently than duodenal ulcer. Consequently, the indications for nonresective procedures for gastric ulcer must be given special care. In doubtful situations, one should resect and anastomose "reflux free." In such an event, however, dumping complaints are probable for about 18 percent of patients. Ninety-five (± 2–3) percent of duodenal ulcers can be operated on without resection with lasting success. The remainder require resection. For gastric ulcer, the proportion of ulcers that can be treated surgically without resection lies between 40 and 50 percent.

Permanent success with nonresective surgical treatment of gastroduodenal ulcer, which is indicated in more than 95 percent of instances of duodenal ulcer and in approximately 50 percent of instances of gastric ulcer, can be expected only with a combination of an adequate selective proximal vagotomy with a pyloroplasty appropriate to form and function. As a result of this combination, disturbances of secretion and motility as well as the local foci are eliminated. Nonresective ulcer surgery is effective for cure if the method is employed in accordance with the described obligations [8].

Comment References

1. Bauer, H. *Nichtresezierende Ulcuschirurgie*. Berlin: Springer, 1980.
2. Holle, F. *Spezielle Magenchirurgie (235 Fälle)*. Berlin: Springer, 1968. Pp. 500–9.
3. Holle, F. Form- und funktionsgerechte Chirurgie des Gastro-Duodenal-Ulcus (580 Fälle). *Erg. Chir. Orth*. 54:1, 1970.
4. Holle, F. Nichtresezierende Chirurgie des Magen- und Zwölffinger-darmgeschwürs. In L. Demling (Ed.), *Klinische Gastroenterologie* (2nd ed.). Stuttgart: Thieme, 1984. Pp. 385–401.
5. Holle, F., and Andersson, S. *Vagotomy (910*

Fälle). Berlin: Springer, 1974.
6. Holle, F., Bauer, H., Andersson, S., et al. Die nichtresezierende Chirurgie des Gastro-Duodenal-Ulcus. I. Patho-physiologische Chirurgie. II. Indikation und Technik. III. Klinische Resultate (973 Fälle). *Munch. Med. Wochenschr.* 24:767, 1976.
7. Holle, F., and Holle, G. E. *Vagotomy and Pyloroplasty (1456 cases)*. Berlin: Springer, 1980.
8. Holle, F. K., and Holle, G. E. Selective proximal vagotomy and pyloroplasty. In H. W. Scott, Jr., and J. L. Sawyers (Eds.), *Surgery of the Stomach, Duodenum and Small Intestine*. Boston: Blackwell, in preparation.
9. Reiser, S. B., and Holle, G. E. Motor and electrical activity of the gastroduodenal junction before and after submucosal pyloroplasty in dogs. *World J. Surg*. 6:231, 1982.

SPECIAL COMMENT
The Problem of Recurrent Ulcer

Stephen N. Joffe

The incidence of recurrent ulceration after proximal gastric vagotomy (PGV) for peptic ulcer disease (PUD) was low in many of the initial reports. Reviewing six studies with at least a five-year follow-up time for all patients indicates a linear increase of recurrent peptic ulceration of 2 percent per year [5]. The cause of this recurrent ulceration is essentially unknown. Technical details shown to be important include adequate clearance of vagal fibers from the lower esophagus, dissection of the "crow's-foot" at the antropyloric junction, and division of the fundic nerve. Factors that may contribute include preoperative gastric hypersecretion, postoperative reduction in acid output, hypergastrinemia and autonomous-secreting gastrinomas, denervation hypersensitivity, ulcerogenic drugs, and mucosal cell proliferation; site of the primary ulcer may also be important.

After a PGV, a large number of patients convert from a "negative" to a "positive" insulin (Hollander) test. Immediately after operation, only 3–6 percent of patients tested are insulin-positive, but this figure increases to between 30 and 90 percent one to four years after the operation. Initially this conversion of the response to insulin was thought to be unimportant. There now appears to be a correlation between a positive Hollander test and the risk of recurrent peptic ulcer. Why a negative response to a Hollander test should convert to a positive response is unknown. Possible reasons include regeneration of vagal fibers, increased sensitivity of parietal cell mass to humoral stimuli, or a temporary neuropraxia. Faxen [1] showed that the acid response to insulin increased more rapidly with time after a PGV than after a selective vagotomy and postulated a reinnervation from the antrum to the body of the stomach. Hancock et al. [2], finding a significant reduction in the peak acid output using insulin discriminants when a PGV was combined with a rotational gastropexy, suggested that this prevented vagal nerve regeneration. All these suggestions, however, are purely hypothetical.

My associates and I developed a technique of producing duodenal ulcers in rats by the infusion of gastric secretagogues. These peptic ulcers can be prevented by various gastric antisecretory agents, truncal vagotomy, and PGV. In rats we found that a neurovascular parietal cell vagotomy prevented these experimental duodenal ulcers only temporarily—for 5 days—because of a gradual recovery of the parietal cell mass to stimulation [3]. Gastric ischemia could have partially accounted for this recovery. The technique of PGV was modified by dissecting the neurovascular bundle and dividing only the vagal nerve fibers to the body of the stomach while preserving the gastric blood vessels—a form of superselective PGV.

The aim was to examine some of the methods for assessing vagus nerve regeneration after a PGV in rats. This included measurement of gastric secretion and plasma levels of immunoreactive pancreatic polypeptide (PP) under basal conditions and following various stimulatory tests. The vagus nerve and its distribution in the stomach were examined by light microscopy using the methylene blue squash preparation technique and by electron microscopy at regular intervals after the PGV.

On *light microscopy,* nerves were identified in the muscle coat in all the rats not operated on and the rats having sham operations; the nerves were studied in both the muscularis mucosae and the mucosa. In the muscle coat, the nerves were clearly visible showing a plexiform arrangement of large-diameter beaded axons. The principal directions of the axons were parallel to the muscle fibers with branches running between the muscle fibers. The axons passed close to the interphase between the muscle coat and the connective tissue on the epithelial side of the muscle coat and then left the muscle coat to ramify in the connective tissue plane. In the connective tissue spaces on both sides of the muscularis mucosae, there were also beaded and unbeaded axons of equal or even slightly greater diameter, which usually ran in pairs beneath the muscularis mucosae. The variability of the beading was striking. Fine nerve fibers were barely discernible in the deepest part of the epithelium. One and two weeks after PGV, these nerve fibers were no longer identified in the muscle coat, muscularis mucosae, or mucosa. By 16 weeks, nerve fibers were identified that appeared to be identical to those seen in stomachs not operated on. In view of the greater specificity of electron microscopy, no further studies were done.

Electron microscopy showed that in all rats not operated on and those having sham operations, the nerve fibers in the mucosa were unmyelinated, with contact points found between axons and parietal cells. At one week after PGV, most of the axons were swollen and evacuolated, and contained an increased number of fibroblasts. Diameters of the axons were much more variable, with a large amount of collagen surrounding Schwann cells. These changes represented degeneration of the nerve fibers. Also present were isolated and randomly arranged but normal-appearing axons possibly indicating rapid regeneration. At two and three weeks after PGV, the axons were more densely packed with neurofilaments and less swollen. Plenty of collagen was still present around the axon groups. By the fourth and fifth weeks, a similar pattern was seen. There was a greater number of smaller and more normal-looking axons that were more densely packed with neurofilaments. Some swollen axons were still present but contained fewer fibroblasts in the Schwann cell processes. Enlarged Schwann cell processes were packed with axons in greater numbers than in the controls, and these axons appeared squashed rather than the normal circular shape.

In the sixth postoperative week, the Schwann cell processes contained numerous axons. Few swollen axons or collagen fibers could be found. However, two types of axons of differing diameter were now identified: a large axon, which was less densely packed with neurotubules, and a smaller axon containing two types of neurovesicles. One was a densely centered neurovesicle. The small axons were densely packed with neurotubules and filaments. By the seventh, eighth, and nineth weeks after PGV, the axons appeared similar to those found in control animals. The Schwann cell processes looked smaller and contained a smaller number of axons. Small nerve bundles containing both types of axons were found close to the gastric epithelial cells, and the remaining collagen was more mature. In the tenth and eleventh weeks postoperatively, the axons were still randomly arranged, and there was an increase in the number of contained vesicles. Specimens in the twelfth, thirteenth, and fourteenth weeks showed similar features. Naked axons were found, as were axons complete with a Schwann cell covering [4, 5].

Gastric Secretion

In rats that had sham operations the mean basal acid output (BAO) was 75 μmol/hr, and after secretagogue stimulation, the acid output had significantly increased to a mean of 164 μmol/hr ($p < .001$). On recovery from a PGV (day 0), the gastric juice was achlorhydric with a basal volume of 0.3 ml/hr. Stimulation with gastric secretagogues caused an increase in both volume (0.57 ml/hr) and acidity of gastric juice, and acid output was 26 μmol/hr. On the seventh day after a PGV, the basal and stimulated volume and acidity of gastric juice following secretagogue stimulation increased compared with the early postoperative results ($p < .001$). By the second and third weeks after PGV, the stimulated gastric acid output increased further and continued to increase with each week of testing. By the seventh week, the stimulated acid output was 93 percent higher than the preoperative level ($p < .001$), and by the ninth week was 12 times greater than that immediately after the PGV. On the first postoperative day, the BAO was 4.2 μmol/hr and after stimulation by insulin hypoglycemia was unchanged at 4.4 μmol/hr—similar to our previously obtained results following a bilateral subdiaphragmatic truncal vagotomy.

Pancreatic Polypeptide

Basal pancreatic polypeptide (PP) levels in the plasma were similar in rats not operated on and those having sham operations on the day of the insulin hypoglycemia test (mean 27 ± 2.2 pg/ml), the meal test (mean 26 ± 2.4 pg/ml), and after secretin challenge (mean 24 ± 3.2 pg/ml). In these same rats with sham or no operation, there was virtually no rise in plasma PP levels following insulin hypoglycemia and a meal test. Following the secretin challenge, there was a mean Δ% increase of the immunoreactive plasma PP levels of 58 percent at 2.5 minutes after the bolus injection of secretin; the levels rapidly returned to normal by 7.5 minutes. This increment was accounted for by a dramatic rise in plasma PP in only one rat, whereas in the remaining seven rats, there was virtually no change. With these negative results obtained following three stimulatory tests before a PGV, it was *not* considered worthwhile to repeat the experiments after PGV.

PGV with Antrectomy

At three days after PGV plus antrectomy, populations of normal and swollen axons were present in the mucosa and submucosa. Swollen axons contained relatively few neurotubules, attenuated cytoplasm, and phospholipid membranous debris. These axons were interpreted as degenerative. Many Schwann cells ensheathed a mixture of both normal and degenerating axons (Fig. 13-10). At three weeks the number of swollen axons appeared to be decreased. The division of axons into those that were large and less densely packed (as seen at six weeks in the previous PGV study) was already becoming apparent (Fig. 13-11). At each interval of three weeks, an increasing number of normal-appearing axon bundles was noted in the mucosa. These bundles were contained within Schwann cell sheaths. Naked axons, as found in the previous PGV study, were rarely seen in the first nine weeks of healing. Synaptic contact between nerve fibers and parietal cells was occasionally seen. Synaptic vesicles were clear and similar in morphology to cholinergic transmitter vesicles (Fig. 13-12).

Discussion

A PGV is currently the preferred treatment of chronic duodenal ulceration in many centers because of its efficiency in reducing gastric secretion without the sequelae of other operative procedures. There is, however, an unexplained and increasing incidence of recurrent peptic ulceration with each year of follow-up study. After a PGV, it has been shown that a large number of patients convert from a negative to a positive insulin hypoglycemia test. This conversion to a positive test was initially thought not to correlate with increased risk of recurrent peptic ulcer, but other evidence suggests there may be an association [6]. Possibilities for this insulin conversion include vagal nerve regeneration, increased sensitivity of the parietal cells, neuropraxis, or reinnervation. These studies in rats show the sequential neuropathological changes of nerve degeneration, regeneration, and functional reinnervation of the gastric mucosa with increased sensitivity of the parietal cell mass after parietal cell vagotomy.

Following PGV and antrectomy, there was

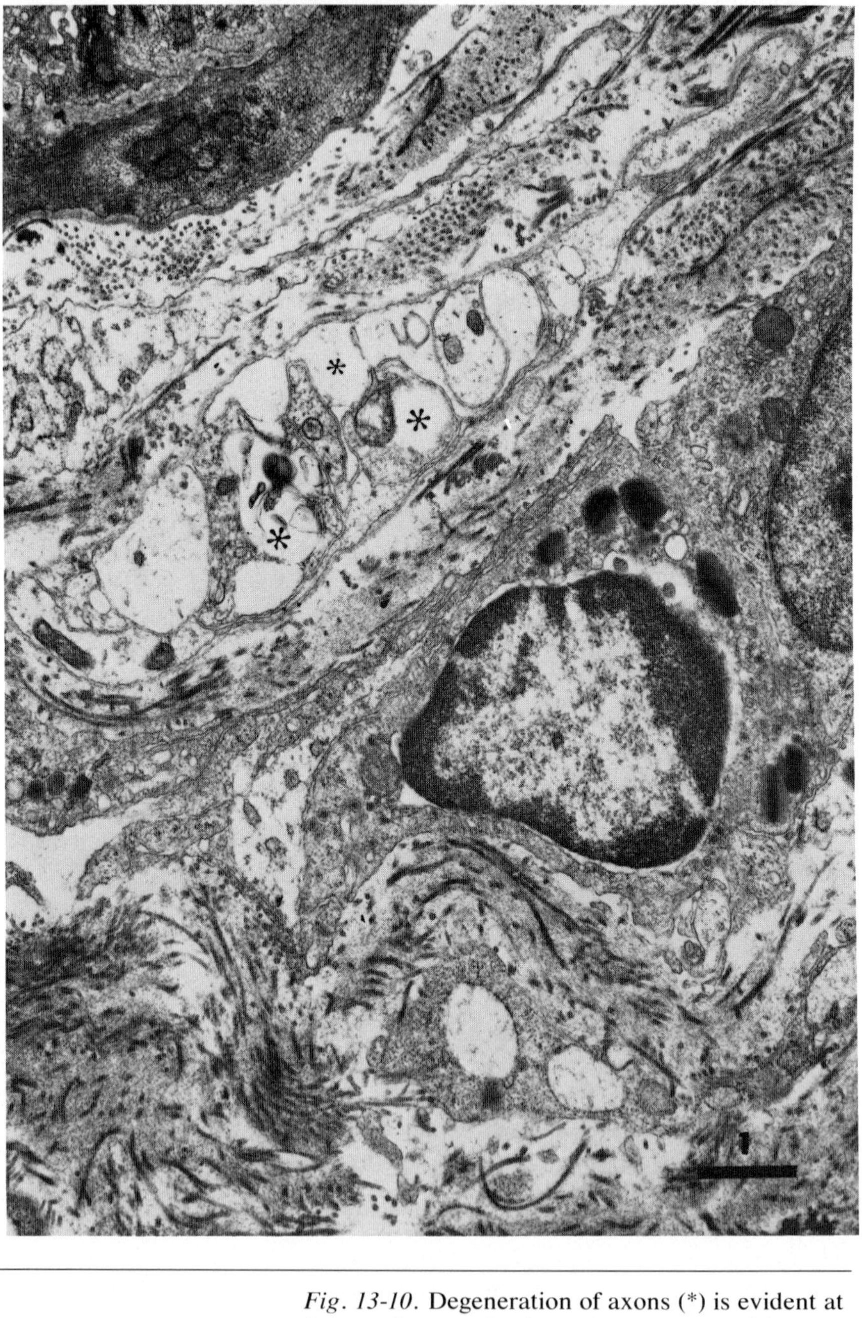

Fig. 13-10. Degeneration of axons (*) is evident at 3 days after proximal gastric vagotomy with antrectomy. Other axons within this Schwann cell appear swollen. Bar represents 1 micrometer.

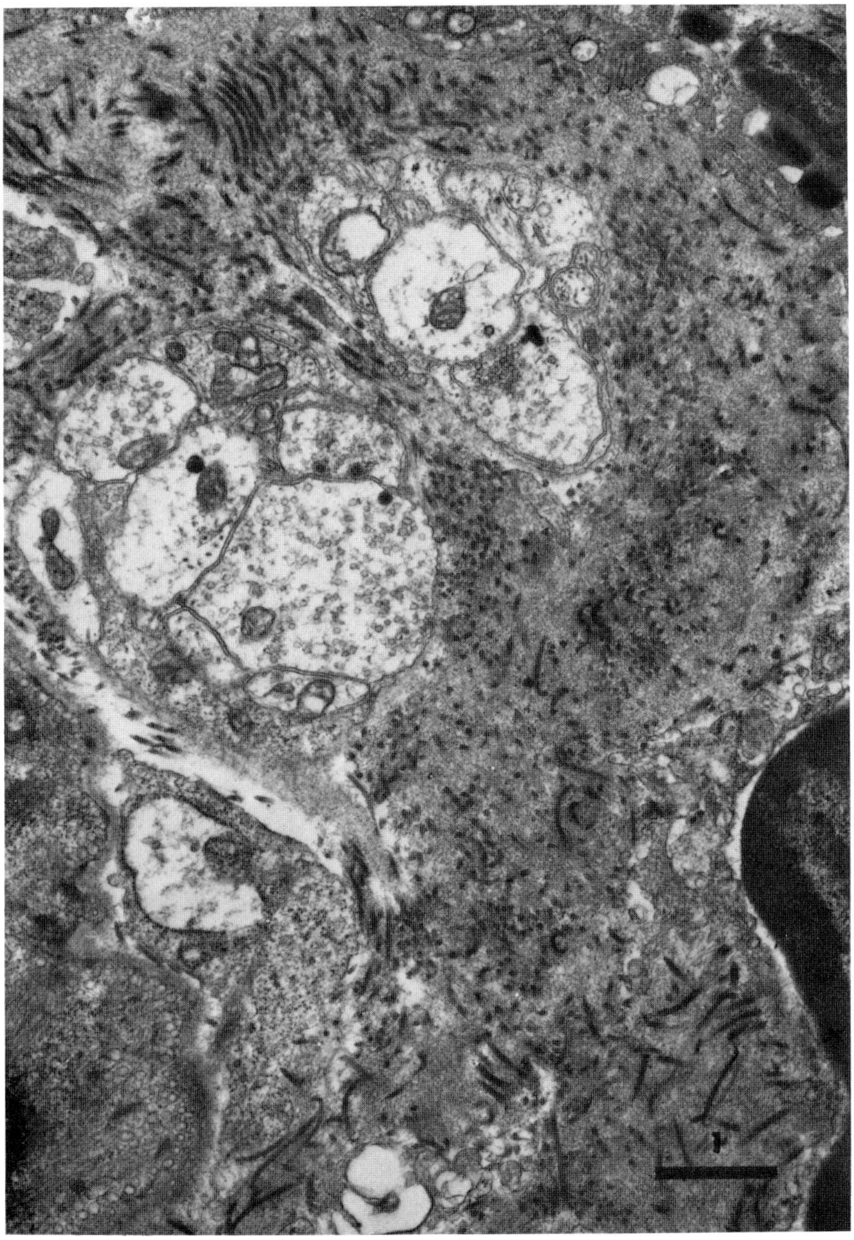

Fig. 13-11. The division of axons into small, densely packed axons with neurotubules and large, less densely packed axons is becoming apparent here at three weeks after PGV with antrectomy. Bar represents 1 micrometer.

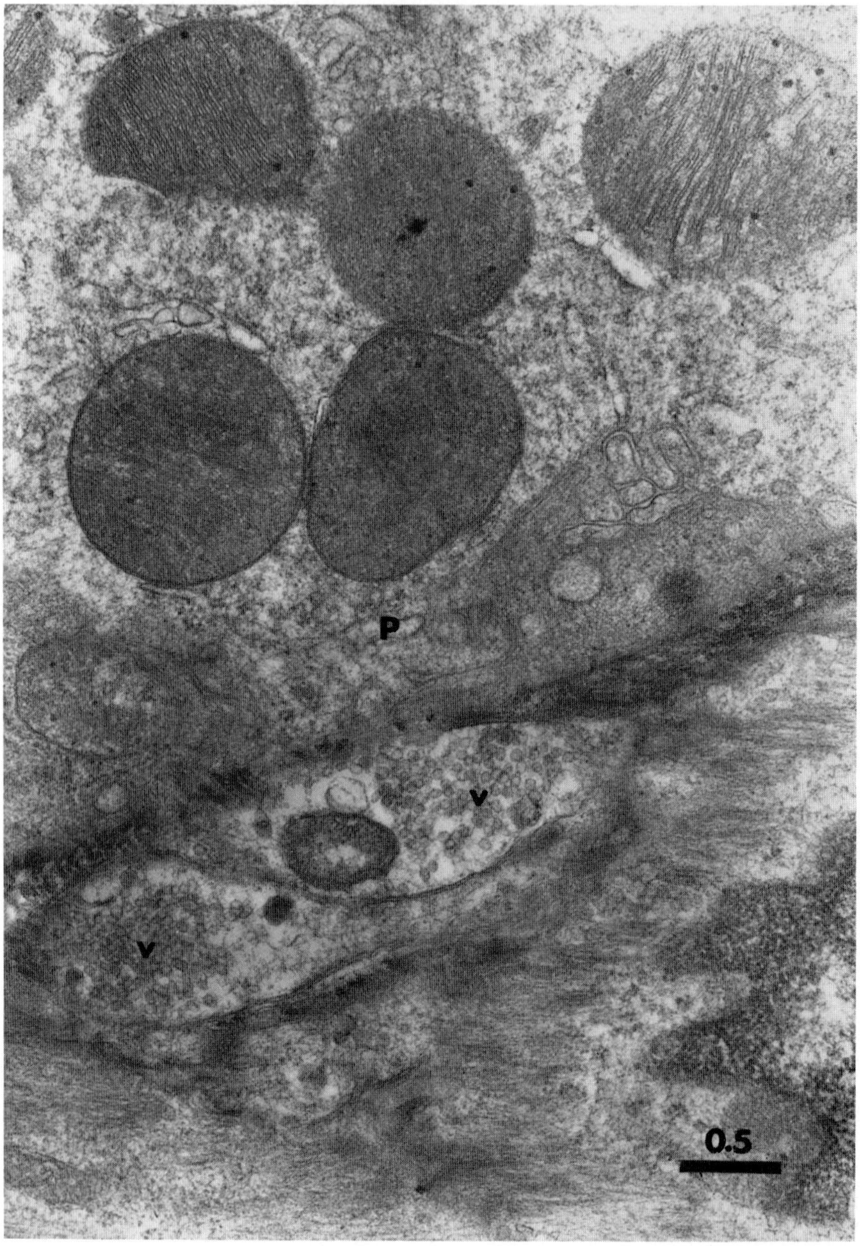

Fig. 13-12. Synaptic contact between nerve fibers and basal portion of parietal cell (P). Synaptic vesicles (v) are mostly small and clear-centered. Shown is PGV with antrectomy at 9 weeks. Bar represents 0.5 micrometer.

Table 13-10. Indications for proximal gastric vagotomy (applied by L. M. Nyhus)

Condition	Indicated	Alternative
Gastric ulcer	No	B-I antrectomy
Duodenal ulcer		
Uncomplicated	Yes	—
Pyloric stenosis	No	PGV + pylorotomy
Acute perforation	Yes	—
Massive hemorrhage	No	Ligation of bleeder; truncal vagotomy + pyloroplasty
High-risk patient	Yes	—
Antral G-cell hyperplasia	No	SV + A
Channel or prepyloric ulcer	No	SV + A
Zollinger-Ellison syndrome	No	Resection of gastrinoma and/or SV + A

B-I = Billroth I; PGV = proximal gastric vagotomy; SV = selective vagotomy; SV + A = selective vagotomy plus antrectomy.

an increase in the number of normal-appearing axons present in the mucosa, indicating extensive reinnervation. Further investigations are necessary to determine the exact nature and source of these nerve fibers, but it appears that they do not arise as an ingrowth from the antrum. If these changes are confirmed in the clinical situation, they may explain both insulin test conversion from negative to positive and the increased incidence of recurrent peptic ulceration. Furthermore, the finding may cast some doubt on the possible long-term effects of PGV in the treatment of chronic duodenal ulcers or at least suggest the need for alterations in the current operative technique.

Comment References

1. Faxen, A. Parietal cell vagotomy and selective vagotomy with pyloroplasty. *Scand. J. Gastroenterol.* 13:7, 1978.
2. Hancock, D. M., Sankar, M. Y., Old, J. M., et al. The combination of proximal gastric vagotomy with a rotational gastropexy for duodenal ulcer. *Br. J. Surg.* 65:706, 1978.
3. Joffe, S. N., and Bapat, R. D. The temporary effect of proximal gastric vagotomy on experimental duodenal ulcers and gastric secretion. *Br. J. Surg.* 66:234, 1979.
4. Joffe, S. N., Crocket, A., Chen, M., and Brackett, K. In Vitro and in Vivo Technique for Assessing Vagus Nerve Regeneration after Parietal Cell Vagotomy in the Rat. In J. G. Kral, T. L. Powley, and C. McC. Brooks (Eds.), *Vagal Nerve Function: Behavioral and Methodological Considerations.* Amsterdam: Elsevier North Holland, 1983.
5. Joffe, S. N., Crocket, A., and Doyle, D. Morphological and functional evidence of reinnervation of the gastric parietal cell mass following a parietal cell vagotomy. *Am. J. Surg.* 143:80, 1982.
6. MacLeod, R. S., and Cohen, Z. Highly selective vagotomy and truncal vagotomy and pyloroplasty for duodenal ulcer: A clinical review. *Can. J. Surg.* 22:113, 1979.

EDITOR'S COMMENT

Proximal gastric vagotomy continues to attract the attention of the surgical world. Our own results (*Surgery* 96:585, 1984) demonstrate an acceptable ulcer recurrence rate (12 percent). A number of prospective, controlled, comparative studies have now been published with the consensus that proximal gastric vagotomy can be performed with low risk for mortality and short- and long-term morbidity (Koo et al. *Ann. Surg.* 197:265, 1983; Elder et al. *Can. J. Surg.* 26:119, 1983;

Gleysteen et al. *Surgery* 94:15, 1983; Koffman et al. *Br. J. Surg.* 70:342, 1983).

The specter of a high recurrent ulcer rate figures prominently in discussions of this subject (Nyhus *Arch. Surg.* 118:1373, 1983). There is wide variation in the reported rate of ulcer recurrence. Within the references cited in the preceding paragraph, respected colleagues report a rate of ulcer recurrence ranging from 5 to 21 percent.

There is absolutely no question that this technique for vagotomy should be used. My view is to continue to search for the specific indications wherein this method of treatment clearly is superior to all other operative approaches. Herein lies the essence of the problem today. Table 13-10 summarizes my own approach to the selection dilemma as I face it daily. There is no need to expect proximal gastric vagotomy to be the operative panacea for all patients' complications subsequent to peptic ulcer disease. Proximal gastric vagotomy will find its place as a "pinch hitter" in the field of surgical gastroenterology and will not become that all-inclusive procedure we search for perennially.

L.M.N.

14

Vagotomy and Antrectomy

John L. Sawyers and John Lynwood Herrington, Jr.

Almost four decades have passed since bilateral subdiaphragmatic vagotomy combined with resection of the gastric antrum was introduced as a mode of definitive surgical therapy for control of complications of duodenal ulcer. The combined operation has unquestionably proved to be the most effective therapeutic procedure among the several operations employed today to control the ulcer diathesis. Even authorities who bitterly criticized the procedure during its infant years now agree concerning its extraordinary effectiveness. A large number of patients who have undergone this operation have now been followed for up to 35 years, and the incidence of recurrent ulceration has been about 1 percent. The recurrence rate has been less than that associated with two-thirds to three-fourths distal gastrectomy. Also, the undesirable side effects and long-range sequelae have been less pronounced than those associated with radical extirpation of the parietal cell mass. As a result of these observations and experiences, radical resection of the stomach for control of duodenal ulcer has lost much of its former prestige, popularity, and appeal in surgical centers throughout the world. Vagotomy has become the basis for the surgical treatment of duodenal ulcer. Controversy is not about vagotomy, but about which type of vagotomy—truncal, selective gastric, or proximal gastric—to use.

The concept of vagotomy and antral resection represents a sound physiological approach to the surgical treatment of duodenal ulcer. Subtotal gastric resection necessitates the extirpation of an extensive parietal cell mass in order to lower gastric acidity, while truncal vagotomy with antrectomy (TV-A) requires minimal sacrifice of gastric tissue. TV-A eliminates the two principal sources of gastric secretion, the cephalic or nervous phase mediated over the vagal pathways and the humoral or hormonal phase occurring as a result of release of gastrin from the antral mucosa.

It is somewhat ironic but interesting that the concept behind this combined operation is by no means new. In fact the procedure has evolved from physiological observations and experiments carried out many years ago [8, 9]. This is true of many of our modern-day clinical endeavors—that original experiments and pertinent facts were not put to clinical use for many decades following their original discovery.

Observations Regarding Vagotomy

In 1814 Sir Benjamin Brodie [10] first recorded his experiments on dogs demonstrating the importance of the vagus nerves in promoting gastric secretory activity. He showed that in dogs killed by the intravenous injection of arsenic, the stomachs contained copious quantities of mucus and watery fluids. In turn, if the vagus nerves were sectioned before the administration of a lethal dose of the drug, at autopsy the dog's stomach was found to be free of secretions. Claude Bernard [7] described a cessation of gastric contractions, an arrest in secretion, and abolition of sensitivity of the stomach following division of the vagi. Pavlov [116] noted in 1894 the absence of hydrochloric acid in the fasting gastric secretions of the dog following vagotomy, but he was able to induce a hydrochloric acid response with the subsequent introduction of bouillon. Almost two decades later he produced experimental evidence to show that the vagus nerves supply secretory fibers to the gastric glands and that they are the pathway for the stimuli that excite the cephalic or psychic phase of gastric secretion. He demonstrated that psychic stimuli cause a profuse flow of gastric juice lasting for several hours, or as long as an animal is sham-fed. On removal of the stimuli, gastric secretion was observed to continue for several hours.

Exner and Schwarzmann in 1914 [51] were perhaps the first to divide the vagus nerves in the human through the abdominal route. They reported 20 instances of gastric crisis, in 10 of which vagotomy proved beneficial. Exner clearly described gastric atony following vagotomy and advocated performing a gastrostomy over a tube passed through the pylorus into the duodenum to overcome this complication. Later he added gastroenterostomy to vagotomy. It was believed that the beneficial effects of vagotomy were due to a reduction in gastric hypersecretion as well as to a diminution in motility. The operation was done largely for functional disease of the gastrointestinal tract, but Latarjet [94] believed that vagotomy was indicated also in instances of gastric and duodenal ulcer. No doubt he was the first to combine pylorectomy with vagotomy in instances of pyloric obstruction. Schiassi [131] mentioned adding gastroenterostomy to vagotomy in instances of pyloric stenosis.

A. J. Carlson [15] demonstrated the presence of a more or less continuous secretion of gastric juice occurring during the fasting state in both humans and experimental animals. This was recognized as a normal phenomenon and was found to be influenced by emotional reactions. Likewise, Winkelstein [153] showed that the hypersecretion of gastric juice in the patient with duodenal ulcer was of nervous origin. He and Berg [154] advocated anterior vagal resection in combination with subtotal gastrectomy in patients who demonstrated hyperacidity. Klein [88] employed a similar operation.

From the early 1930s to 1943, little mention of vagotomy was made in the medical and surgical literature. The early writers apparently failed to publish follow-up data, and therefore the operation did not gain wide clinical acceptance. Also, several early reports had appeared of sectioning of the vagus nerves in the cervical region of experimental animals, with resultant death, and this no doubt was an argument against acceptance of the operation. In the United States during the 1920s and early 1930s, the rise in popularity of simple gastroenterostomy as treatment of duodenal ulcer tended to place vagotomy in the background.

In 1943 Dragstedt made a monumental contribution by arousing renewed interest in vagotomy, which has since made a lasting impact on the surgical world. He and Owens published an account of two patients with chronic duodenal ulcer treated successfully by transthoracic vagotomy [31]. This work confirmed without doubt the importance of the cephalic phase of gastric secretion in the patient with duodenal ulcer. In subsequent reports, Dragstedt [23] and co-workers [25, 26, 32, 34] stressed that the relief of ulcer distress following vagotomy was uniform and striking. Dragstedt also made the important observation that, although gastric secretion was reduced following the operation, it was by no means abolished [36]. The pH values of the gastric juice remained in the range of 1.9 to 3.7, which meant that considerable peptic activity still existed in spite of apparent complete nerve division. In the postoperative patients, the fasting free hydrochloric acid values ranged from 0 to 58 clinical units. Following vagotomy there was still some gastric secretory response to stimulants such as caffeine or histamine. Also, complete vagal interruption produced no significant effect on the total gastric secretory response when ingested food was used as a stimulant [150]. The microangiographic studies of Nylander and Olerud [107] relating to the effects of vagotomy in the rat are of interest. These studies indicate that in animals on which vagotomy has been performed, arteriolar filling was quite sparse in the mucosal and submucosal layers. This alteration may be related to the decreased acid secretion following vagotomy.

Schoen and Griswold [134] reported that complete vagotomy did not reduce peptic activity except to a minor degree. The basal secretory rate of six patients was reduced by an average of only 36 percent. They demonstrated that the vagotomized stomach was still capable of producing active gastric juice. These later findings subsequently assumed increasing significance, as follow-up data on patients who had undergone vagotomy revealed a rather high incidence of recurrent ulceration [13, 68, 77, 78, 103, 148, 152].

Soon after vagotomy was reintroduced in 1943, it became appreciated clinically that the procedure was followed by gastric hypotonicity and hypomotility and resulted in antral stasis, increased antral secretory activity, and subsequent gastric ulcer formation. In addition, the original duodenal ulcer all too often failed to heal or to remain healed. The addition of gastrojejunostomy as a complementary drainage procedure did much to obviate antral stasis, but still the recurrent ulcer rate ranged from 10 to 15 percent [1].

An appreciation of the importance of juxtapyloric gastroenterostomy with vagotomy to drain the antrum more adequately and diminish further the release of gastrin has resulted in a further lowering of the recurrent ulcer rate to between 5 and 15 percent. Of even greater importance has been the introduction of a patulous pyloroplasty as a drainage procedure in combination with vagotomy. The latter operation is more physiological than gastrojejunostomy in that it preserves gastroduodenal continuity. Using it as a drainage procedure in combination with vagotomy, the recurrent ulcer rate has been reduced to approximately 5 to 10 percent. Neither of the above operations, however, results in complete gastric achlorhydria, and significant acid-pepsin activity is still present.

It has become increasingly apparent through extensive experimental work that the vagus nerves exert an even more profound influence on gastric secretion than was originally believed [49, 105]. In addition to their role of mediating the interdigestive and nocturnal secretions of gastric juice, the vagus nerves are capable of producing the release of gastrin when the antrum is at an alkaline pH. Also the principal stimuli for pepsinogen secretion are mediated by the vagi. After vagal denervation there is a diminution in the release of antral gastrin and likewise a decreased secretory response of the parietal cell mass to histamine and parasympathomimetic drugs. The intact vagus potentiates the response of parietal cells to all stimuli. It has been shown that vagotomy of the main stomach has no significant effect on the augmented gastric phase of secretion produced by antral exclusion [16]. Vagotomy reduces the acid response to gastrin to a greater degree than it does to histamine [62].

There has also been recent emphasis on the extragastric effects of vagotomy. Experimental stimulation of the vagus nerve has been demonstrated to produce increased peristaltic activity of the entire small intestine and right half of the colon. After vagal section, motor activity of the denervated intestine has been shown to exhibit discoordinated and inadequate peristalsis. These effects, however, are inconstant and may vary from hypomotility with dilatation of the intestine to hyperactivity with decreased intestinal transit time. In most instances these changes are temporary, and they usually revert to normal after several weeks to months [17, 20]. Experiments [3, 4] have demonstrated that total vagotomy in dogs produces decreased fat absorption and a reduction in mucosal enzymes that may last for several months. Because of a decrease in HCl, an increase in bacterial flora of the small intestine has been observed along with an inflammatory response and atrophy of the small intestinal villi. The blood flow to the small intestine has been shown to decrease, also because of denervation. Each of these effects is again transitory and disappears in several weeks to months. Rudick, Guntheroth, and Nyhus [122] have shown that truncal vagotomy decreases gastric blood flow.

Stimulation of the vagi has also been observed to affect the biliary system by stimulating motor activity and increasing bile flow [123]. Heer et al. [69] showed experimentally that insulin-induced hypoglycemia produced a vagally mediated choleresis by stimulating the hepatic secretion of bile. This response was independent of the production of endogenous secretin and could be almost entirely inhibited by atropine. After complete truncal vagotomy, dilatation of the gallbladder has been a common observation along with a diminution in bile flow. Nielson [104] believes that there is a definite increase in the incidence of cholelithiasis among patients who have had previous truncal vagotomy.

Vagal stimulation also increases the enzymatic content of pancreatic juice; however, the effects of division of the vagi on pancreatic function are not well established. There are conflicting reports as to whether or not vagotomy reduces the volume and enzymal content of pancreatic secretions [99]. The pancreatic secretory response to gastric dilatation is abolished by vagotomy. Dreiling et al. [37] observed that after complete vagotomy the response of the pancreas to secretin was unaltered, but that the usual enzyme response to vagal stimulation produced by insulin hypoglycemia was abolished. They therefore believed that the diarrhea sometimes observed after vagotomy could not be explained on the basis of any alteration in pancreatic function.

Experimental and Clinical Review of the Gastric Antrum: Rationale of Vagotomy with Antrectomy

Pavlov [116] first noted the stimulating effect of food and water in the stomach on the secretion of hydrochloric acid. In 1906 Edkins [38, 39] isolated a substance from the pyloric mucosa of cats and dogs that caused a marked increase in the secretion of gastric juice when injected intravenously. He called this substance gastrin and elaborated his hypothesis of the humoral or gastric phase of secretion. His original work precipitated much controversy and conflicting experimental evidence for the three decades that followed [97, 98].

In the early 1940s Komarov [89–91] isolated gastrin from the pyloric mucosa of experimental animals and found it to be a proteinlike substance free of histamine. Uvnäs [144–146] confirmed Komarov's work, and employing different extraction methods, he increased the potency of the isolated gastrin. Uvnäs also extracted gastrin from the human pyloric mucosa, and Ferguson [55] demonstrated that the secretagogue recovered from patients with active duodenal ulcer was more than 4 times as potent as that extracted from patients with inactive duodenal ulcer. The original findings of Edkins and more eloquent elaborations of his work have been carried out by Dragstedt and his associates [24, 27, 28, 30, 35], Harkins and co-workers [67] and others [63, 108–110, 118, 121, 157, 160].

It has been shown that the release of gastrin from the antrum, with subsequent stimulation of gastric secretion, takes place in the presence of an alkaline or slightly acid medium. This stimulation continues until the acidity of the gastric juice approximates a pH of 1.5–3.0. Then further liberation of gastrin ceases, and the humoral phase of secretion becomes quiescent [96].

When 24-hour quantitative collections of

gastric secretions were made from animals with a Pavlov or Heidenhain pouch, complete removal of the gastric antrum with reconstruction of continuity by anastomosing the body of the stomach to the side of the duodenum produced a profound reduction in the gastric juice secreted by the isolated pouch. After complete vagotomy in dogs with a Pavlov pouch, subsequent removal of the antrum almost completely abolished the secretion of gastric juice from the isolated stomach pouch [156]. Thus it is believed that the vagus nerves and the gastric antrum contain the key to the secretory activity of the gastric glands. The secretory importance of the antrum was further exemplified by transplantation experiments [27, 28] in which the antrum was transplanted into the side of the duodenum or into the transverse colon as a diverticulum, with resultant augmentation of gastric secretion from a Pavlov pouch. After antral extirpation, these secretions were reduced. Schmitz et al. [133] concluded that gastric drainage procedures that permitted increased antral stimulation and alkali-acid rebound caused an increase in Heidenhain pouch hydrochloric acid secretions. The high incidence of recurrent ulceration following antral exclusion operations further attests to the importance of the gastric antrum as a potent source of acid stimulation [2, 48, 93, 132, 158].

Perhaps one of the most convincing experiments depicting the role of the antrum in the possible genesis of ulcer disease is the ingenious three-phase total parietal cell pouch devised by Sauvage et al. [125, 126]. Sauvage demonstrated that this procedure is a potent ulcerogenic preparation. Vagotomy alone did not decrease the incidence of ulceration in the pouch dogs in this experimental procedure, but antral extirpation did. Antrectomy combined with vagotomy offered a marked degree of protection against the development of stomal ulceration.

Storer et al. [142] showed that vagotomy and antral resection afforded protection against stomal ulceration in the Mann-Williamson preparation. Vagotomy alone afforded protection against ulceration in 55 percent of the animals; antral resection alone gave protection to two-thirds of the animals; but a combination of the two procedures offered complete protection to 83 percent of the animals.

A. W. Kay [86, 87] of Glasgow found that antrectomy reduced gastric secretion by 70 percent and that vagotomy alone likewise reduced the total acid output by some 60–70 percent. A combination of the two procedures resulted in a 95 percent reduction in acid output. Although the parietal cell population is virtually unaltered after antrectomy and vagotomy, the acid-secretory cells no doubt become considerably less responsive to histamine stimulation. After complete vagotomy and antral resection in patients with duodenal ulcer, achlorhydria occurs during the fasting state and after stimulation with a test meal. Most of the patients have no free hydrochloric acid response to histamine, and when a response is elicited it usually ranges from 5 to 15 clinical units [42, 53, 112]. The quantitative hourly secretory volumes of gastric juice obtained after the combined procedure usually range from 0 to 50 ml, and the hourly output of free hydrochloric acid is usually less than 1 mEq. Under these circumstances the patient theoretically should be protected against the development of recurrent ulceration.

Gregory and Tracy [61], by using extraction methods, were able to isolate gastrin I and gastrin II, each peptide having identical amino acid compositions but differing in electrophoretic and chromatographic properties. Each gastrin was many times more potent than histamine in stimulating acid secretion from a Heidenhain pouch. Both gastrins under experimental conditions not only stimulated acid secretion but also stimulated pepsin secretion, pancreatic flow, pancreatic enzyme secretion, and gastrointestinal motility [60]. These actions of gastrin are performed by the C-terminal tetrapeptide amide portion of the molecule.

Various mechanisms have been shown to be responsible for the release of gastrin from the pyloric antrum. The presence of food in the antrum, mechanical and chemical stimulation, vagal impulses, and pH content of the antrum are all important factors in exciting antral secretory activity. Dragstedt et al. [33] demonstrated that the antrum may undergo constant 24-hour stimulation with neutral liver extract without showing signs of decreased secretion from a Heidenhain pouch. Jordan [83] showed that gastrin is also present in the alimentary tract distal to the pylorus, and this extra-antral gastrin may be under vagal control. Gastrin within the antrum may come from the antral G cell, which is now immunohistologically and ultrastructurally well defined [21]. Extra-antral G cells have been found in the upper part of the duodenum and are said to be more frequent in patients with duodenal ulcer [117].

Woodward and co-investigators [156] demonstrated that antrectomy was followed by a 74 percent decrease in the volume of gastric output, a 51 percent drop in acid concentration, and an 86 percent reduction in total mEq of HCl from Heidenhain and Pavlov pouches. They also thought that partial antrectomy led to a proportionate diminution in acid output. Although there have been conflicting reports on the parietal cell response to histamine following antrectomy, Waddell [147] noted a profound reduction. Gillespie et al. [56], studying the effect of simple antrectomy in duodenal ulcer patients, noted a marked decrease in acid output. Palumbo [114] reported a 45 percent decrease in acid secretion after antrectomy.

The stimulatory phases of gastric acid secretion include direct stimulation of the parietal cells through the vagus nerve, through release of gastrin in response to vagal stimulation, through release of gastrin by local stimulation of the antrum, and through release of hormones by the intestinal mucosa. The operation of vagotomy and antrectomy removes all of these stimuli except the intestinal phase, which is thought to be of the least clinical importance. The effectiveness of the operation has been demonstrated by the very low recurrent ulcer rate.

Clinical Experience with Vagotomy and Antrectomy

In October, 1946, Smithwick of Boston operated on a patient in whom a marginal ulcer developed after a simple gastroenterostomy. He dismantled the anastomosis, resected the distal 50 percent of the stomach, performed a bilateral truncal vagotomy, and constructed a retrocolic Hofmeister anastomosis. Three months later, L. W. Edwards, unaware of Smithwick's contribution, operated on a physician with an obstructed duodenal ulcer at the Vanderbilt University Hospital. He performed a vagotomy with an estimated 40 percent distal resection and a classic Billroth II reconstruction [44]. Smithwick [139, 140] called his resection a *hemigastrectomy,* and Edwards used the term *antrectomy*. Both observers believed that the operative procedure represented a physiological approach to the surgical treatment of duodenal ulcer. Each subsequently reported excellent short-term follow-up results [40–43, 45, 46, 53, 54, 140]. Edwards [40] reviewed the excellent results obtained in 150 patients with duodenal ulcer treated by vagotomy with antrectomy, with a maximum follow-up time of nine years. Not a single incident of marginal or recurrent ulceration occurred in this group. As a result of this experience TV-A became the procedure of choice for complications of duodenal ulcer treated at Edwards-Eve Clinic and on the teaching services of the Vanderbilt University affiliated hospitals. It has been Edward's conviction that TV-A was founded on sound physiological principles, and that it has subsequently offered as much protection against recurrent ulceration as has radical subtotal resection, with fewer undesirable side effects [47, 127]. The usefulness of the operation has by no means been restricted to the patient who undergoes an elective operation for duodenal ulcer; it has also proved applicable to the patient with massive bleeding and has been used in selected patients with acute perforation. Reports by other authors have revealed satisfactory results with the combined procedure [5, 11, 12, 18, 52, 55, 59, 64, 65, 79–82, 100, 114, 115, 135, 137, 141, 143, 151, 159].

During the years 1947–1972 members of our surgical group at the Vanderbilt University affiliated hospitals and the Edwards-Eve Clinic performed vagotomy with antrectomy for duodenal ulcer disease on 3584 patients [76].

The youngest patient in the series was an 8-year-old boy who underwent operation for repeated hemorrhages, and the oldest patient was 94 years of age and likewise underwent operation to control massive bleeding. The ratio of men to women was 7 : 1. The average age was 47 years, and the length of ulcer history before surgical intervention averaged 12 years.

The indications for operation among the entire group of patients were those of chronic duodenal ulcer and its complications. Many patients had various combinations of these indications, but there was generally one principal indication necessitating operation. In 1828 patients (51 percent), the primary indication requiring operation was recurrent ulcer symptoms with persistent pain refractory to medical management. In 1146 patients (32 percent), a single massive hemorrhage or repeated minor hemorrhages constituted the reason for operation. Gastric outflow tract obstruction necessitated operation in 502 patients (14 percent), and a small group of 108 patients (3 percent) underwent operation for acute ulcer perforation. There was but 1 hospital death among the patients with ulcer perforation (Fig. 14-1).

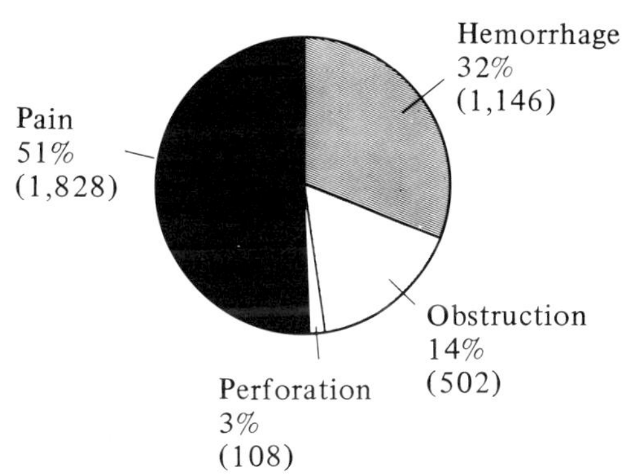

Fig. 14-1. Indications for operation in 3584 patients. (From J. L. Sawyers, J. L. Herrington, Jr., and H. W. Scott, Jr. Vagotomy and Antrectomy for Duodenal Ulcer. In J. S. Najarian and J. P. Delaney (Eds.), *Surgery of the Gastrointestinal Tract*. Miami: Symposia Specialists, 1974.)

The diagnosis of duodenal ulcer generally has been established not only by the patient's symptoms but also by the presence of an ulcer crater on upper gastrointestinal roentgenological studies. Since the fiberoptic flexible gastroscope has been so readily available, our patients have had both gastroscopic and roentgenological demonstrations of their duodenal ulcers. All patients with upper gastrointestinal hemorrhage undergo esophagogastroduodenoscopy as soon as their condition permits. This is usually done in the intensive care unit concurrent with whatever supportive or resuscitative measures are needed. Endoscopy is usually more accurate than upper gastrointestinal fluoroscopy and roentgenography in diagnosing bleeding duodenal ulcers, although the latter is also done for diagnostic purposes after the acute bleeding episode subsides. Acute perforation is usually diagnosed by history, physical findings, and roentgenographic demonstration of free air in the peritoneal cavity. In a review of 360 patients with perforated duodenal ulcer, pneumoperitoneum was demonstrated in 71 percent by chest or abdominal roentgenograms [129]. In all our patients undergoing vagotomy with antrectomy, either a duodenal ulcer crater or a duodenal deformity from scarring secondary to ulcer disease has been present.

Preoperative gastric acid secretory studies are not considered essential in all patients, but most of our patients have had acid secretion studies before and after operation because we wish to collect these data for evaluation studies. We use a 1-hour basal gastric acid secretion analysis followed by a maximum acid secretion test using betazole hydrochloride (Histalog). Coutsoftides and Himal [19] suggested that Oxo stimulation of the antrum preoperatively may allow selection of patients who have a significant antral component, and that these patients, therefore, must have an antrectomy as part of their operative procedure.

The follow-up study among the entire series has been 98 percent (71 patients lost to follow-up) and has consisted of frequent office and hospital outpatient visits, hospital readmissions when deemed necessary, and interviews by members of the surgical group. Some patients, of course, have subsequently died of unrelated causes since operation, particularly patients operated on in the early period of the study. Each was followed to the time of death, and the results have continued to be tabulated in the clinical study.

RESULTS

Clinical results have been tabulated as excellent, good, fair, or poor, or Visick I to IV. An excellent result (Visick I) indicates that the patient is in excellent nutritional condition and has no symptoms whatsoever referable to the gastrointestinal tract. A good result (Visick II) is attributed to those patients who have excellent gastrointestinal function with no ulcer symptoms and who are in a good state of nutrition, but who occasionally have epigastric fullness, mild dumping symptoms, or bouts of diarrhea. A fair result (Visick III) is listed if the patient has obtained benefit from the operation and is without residual ulcer symptoms. However, in this group abdominal fullness, postprandial diarrhea, or moderate dumping symptoms have been prominent sequelae. In the poor result category (Visick IV) are listed those patients with recurrent ulcer, nutritional difficulties, and postgastrectomy symptoms severe enough to interfere with regular employment.

According to these criteria, the clinical results have been excellent in 66 percent, good in 28 percent, fair in 5 percent, and poor in 1 percent. Thus 94 percent (3250) of the patients in the series are considered to have an entirely satisfactory result after vagotomy and antrectomy (Fig. 14-2).

Weight losses following operation have not posed a particular problem. Eighty percent of patients have maintained their weights in the preoperative or ideal range. Ten percent of the patients have noted weight gains since operation, and another 10 percent have lost weight postoperatively. It is unusual, indeed, for the postoperative weight loss to be in excess of 5 to 7 kg. Anemia has been a rare finding during the postoperative follow-up period.

More than 90 percent of patients undergoing postoperative betazole hydrochloride stimulation tests have no free hydrochloric acid. The hourly basal total acid output is usually 0.1–0.5 mEq, and the stimulated total acid output is less than 2 mEq.

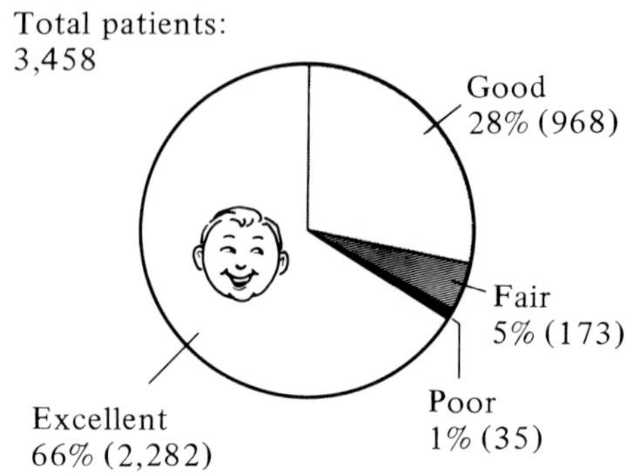

Fig. 14-2. Results of operation for the 3458 patients in the follow-up study. (From J. L. Sawyers, J. L. Herrington, Jr., and H. W. Scott, Jr. Vagotomy and Antrectomy for Duodenal Ulcer. In J. S. Najarian and J. P. Delaney (Eds.), *Surgery of the Gastrointestinal Tract.* Miami: Symposia Specialists, 1974.)

COMPLICATIONS

Delayed gastric emptying during the postoperative period was present in 138 patients (4 percent), and reoperation was necessary in 48 patients. No particular difference was noted between the Billroth I and Billroth II types of reconstruction with regard to emptying problems, but during the past 15 years the Billroth I anastomosis [71] has been employed far more frequently on our services. Leakage from the duodenal stump occurred in 18 patients and resulted in death in 12. This complication has not occurred during the past 10 years, since we do not attempt to remove a deeply imbedded posterior wall ulcer. A minor anastomotic leakage has been suspected in several patients undergoing a Billroth I reconstruction, but no deaths have resulted.

Hemorrhage during the early postoperative period, usually while the patient was still in the recovery room, occurred in a few instances. Iced saline irrigations administered through the nasogastric tube have served to control this complication on occasion, but frequently these patients require reoperation to arrest bleeding, which usually occurs from a small vessel in a suture line. In recent years we have stressed the importance of having a member of the operating room staff irrigate the gastric pouch with saline solution through the indwelling nasogastric tube before the abdomen is closed to be certain that all blood clots have been removed from the stomach. Any evidence of active hemorrhage may be discovered and tended to at this time. Operative injury to the spleen, esophagus, and common bile duct has occurred in rare instances but has been corrected without further difficulty. We have not encountered either dysphagia or cardiospasm as a complication of vagotomy.

Symptoms suggestive of the dumping syndrome have occurred in 25 percent of the patients. The symptoms have occurred with almost equal frequency in the Billroth I and Billroth II groups. In most instances the symptoms have been mild to moderate in degree, and in many instances they have improved with time or have been alleviated with a proper dietary regimen. In 1 percent of patients diarrhea has been severe and disabling, and several of these patients have undergone remedial operations.

Among the series of 3584 patients, 55 postoperative deaths occurred either in the hospital or within 30 days following dismissal (mortality, 1.6 percent). Most deaths (31) took place in patients operated on as an emergency procedure for the control of massive bleeding. Many of these patients were elderly and had cardiovascular or renal disease. Disabling associated disease, particularly chronic respiratory problems, accounted for the deaths of 7 patients during the early postoperative course, and 12 patients died as a result of a duodenal stump blowout. Several of these patients likewise had coexisting disease, which made it even more difficult to control their problems following the duodenal stump blowout. Three patients died of acute hemorrhagic pancreatitis, and 2 died as the result of uncontrollable rebleeding (Fig. 14-3).

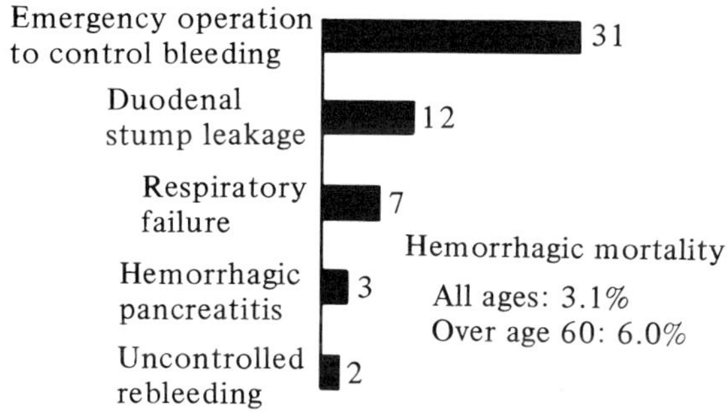

Fig. 14-3. Factors responsible for 55 deaths in 3584 patients (1.6 percent mortality). (From J. L. Sawyers, J. L. Herrington, Jr., and H. W. Scott, Jr. Vagotomy and Antrectomy for Duodenal Ulcer. In J. S. Najarian and J. P. Delaney (Eds.), *Surgery of the Gastrointestinal Tract.* Miami: Symposia Specialists, 1974.)

RECURRENT ULCERATION

The recurrent ulcer rate during the follow-up study has been astoundingly low. There have been 20 proved recurrent ulcers among the entire series (incidence of 0.6 percent). More than 1500 patients have been followed for longer than 10 years. The patients who subsequently died of disease unrelated to ulcer were followed until the time of death. Each of the 20 recurrent ulcers was manifested by recurrent ulcerlike pain, bleeding, or perforation that occurred within 24 months of operation.

Among the 20 recurrent ulcers observed to date, 4 resulted from a Zollinger-Ellison tumor unrecognized at the time of the original operation but proved either at subsequent operation or at autopsy. Thirteen patients had incomplete vagotomy at the original operation that was confirmed later by the Hollander test and at subsequent operation for correction of the recurrence. A functioning adrenal gland tumor was responsible for recurrence in 1 patient. Two additional patients with recurrence probably had incomplete vagotomy, but this was not proved (Fig. 14-4).

Of the 20 ulcer recurrences, 13 followed vagotomy with antrectomy and a Billroth I reconstruction, and 7 took place after a Billroth II-type anastomosis. It should be stressed that

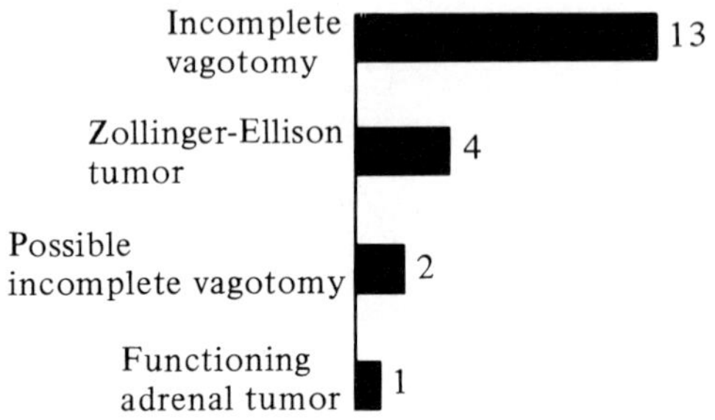

Fig. 14-4. Reasons for recurrent ulcer (0.6 percent) in 3458 patients having vagotomy with antrectomy for duodenal ulcer. (From J. L. Sawyers, J. L. Herrington, Jr., and H. W. Scott, Jr. Vagotomy and Antrectomy for Duodenal Ulcer. In J. S. Najarian and J. P. Delaney (Eds.), *Surgery of the Gastrointestinal Tract*. Miami: Symposia Specialists, 1974.)

the Billroth I anastomosis has been used more frequently than the Billroth II, particularly during the past 15 years.

ACCUMULATED DATA

Reports from other medical centers using vagotomy and antrectomy in the treatment of duodenal ulcer are shown in Table 14-1. Including our patients, the accumulated data comprise more than 5000 patients with follow-up studies extending to 26 years. The ulcer recurrence rate has generally been about 1 percent, which is much lower than the ulcer recurrence rate following other widely used operations for duodenal ulcer. The clinical results have been highly satisfactory. The only criticism of vagotomy with antrectomy expressed by the authors is that the procedure should not be employed for the treatment of massive hemorrhage in the high-risk patient, in the elderly patient with associated disease, or in the exceptional patient in whom duodenal pathology renders resection hazardous.

Operative Technique

VAGOTOMY

The technique of vagotomy and antrectomy is based on a meticulously performed bilateral subdiaphragmatic truncal vagotomy with a resection of the distal 40 percent of the stomach. The abdomen is usually entered through an upper midline incision that ends just to the left of the xiphoid process. A self-retaining retractor is used to elevate the xiphoid and the subcostal margin. The left hepatic lobe is elevated superiorly with a retractor without dividing the suspensory ligament of the liver. Moist laparotomy packs are used to protect the spleen against injury. The stomach is retracted downward, and the peritoneum overlying the abdominal esophagus is incised transversely. A previously placed indwelling nasogastric tube aids in identification of the esophagus. Traction is placed on the stomach pulling the organ to the left and caudally. This maneuver usually reveals the course of the anterior vagus nerve, hepatic branches, and anterior gastric nerve of Latarjet. The anterior vagal nerve trunk may be palpated. The layer of fibroareolar tissue investing the esophagus is divided transversely to expose the anterior wall of the esophagus. The anterior vagal trunk is then identified and elevated from the esophagus by a right-angle clamp or a long nerve hook. A 4- to 6-cm segment of the anterior vagal trunk is resected. The ends of the divided nerve trunks are secured with hemoclips or silk ligatures. Any other vagal branches that pass downward over the anterior esophageal wall are divided.

An empty sponge forceps is used to separate the right or medial wall of the esophagus from adjacent tissue. This action exposes the space bounded posteriorly by the aorta, laterally by the diaphragmatic crura, and anteriorly by the esophagus. With traction on the stomach, the posterior vagus nerve trunk is palpated by the surgeon's index finger and elevated by a right-angle clamp. A segment of the posterior vagal trunk is excised and the ends are secured (Fig. 14-5).

The esophagus is then encircled by the surgeon gently passing a finger from the patient's left to right side and placing a narrow Penrose drain around the esophagus. This maneuver is easy at this stage and should not be done as the initial procedure in performing a truncal vagotomy. No esophageal perforations have

Table 14-1. Vagotomy with antrectomy for duodenal ulcer: results from other medical centers

Author	No. of patients	Satisfactory results (%)	Complications (%) Ulcer recurrence	Mortality	Follow-up (yr)
Thoroughman [143][a]	504	91	0.4	1.6	2–14
Palumbo [113][a]	510	90	0.6	2.7	1–16
Smithwick [139][a]	719	93	1.5	1.9	1–26
ReMine [119]	223	90	1.3	0	7–17
Jordan [84][b]	90	89	1.1	0	1–8
Wolf [155][a]	547	90	0.6	1.1	1–10
Hubert [81][b]	466	95	0.7	1.1	13–25
Koo [92][b]	51	96	0	2	1–6
Donahue [22]	46	80	0	0	4–12

[a]Elective and emergency operations.
[b]Elective operations.

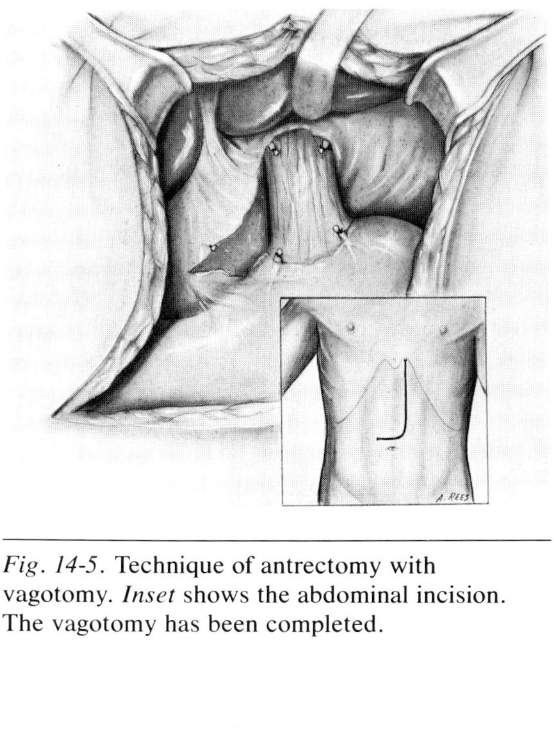

Fig. 14-5. Technique of antrectomy with vagotomy. *Inset* shows the abdominal incision. The vagotomy has been completed.

occurred in more than 2500 truncal vagotomies done using this technique.

The esophagus is retracted to the patient's right, and a careful search is made for vagal fibers passing to the posterior portion of the fundus (the criminal nerves). After these nerves are divided, the distal esophagus is carefully inspected circumferentially for intramuscular fibrils that course to the fundus. These vagal branches may be identified and divided by careful palpation with the distal esophagus under tension. A superficial circumferential division of the distal esophagus is an alternative method to divide these fibrils.

To perform truncal vagotomy demands more of the surgeon than simply identifying the anterior and posterior vagal trunks and excising a segment of each. The techniques of selective gastric and proximal gastric vagotomy have taught surgeons to be more meticulous in performing truncal vagotomy. Nyhus et al. [106] have emphasized the need for a rigorous technique with special attention to dividing all accessory nerve fibers.

ANTRECTOMY

Attention is next directed to removing the antrum of the stomach. Babcock forceps are placed on the greater curvature portion of the body of the stomach, and the organ is lifted up and forward. The arcade of vessels along the middle portion of the greater curvature is divided and ligated with silk. The lesser peritoneal cavity, thus widely opened, is explored, and all fibrous attachments between the posterior gastric wall and the pancreatic pseudocapsule are divided. At this point an excellent view of the pancreas is obtained, and the organ is again carefully inspected for possible adenoma or other pathology. The greater curvature is mobilized from the pylorus to a point midway to the fundus.

The dissection is carried several centimeters above the incisura angularis on the lesser curvature, and the vessels along the lesser curvature are likewise secured. The descending branch of the left gastric artery is divided and transfixed with silk.

With traction applied to the greater curvature by the use of several Babcock clamps, the mobilized stomach is fanned out and a point at the midway portion of the curvature is selected for division. This point is usually just to the right of the first of the vasa brevia. A similar site is selected on the lesser curvature just proximal to the midway point between the pyloric vein and the esophagogastric junction. This latter point is usually 3 to 4 cm above the termination of the gastric nerves of Latarjet (the crow's-foot).

Two Kocher or Allen clamps are placed at right angles to the long axis of the stomach along the greater curvature at the previously selected site. This is approximately the midway point between the pylorus and the fundus. The proximal clamp defines the size of the gastroenteric stoma that is to be constructed. This portion of the stomach, which approximates one-third of the width of the organ, is then divided. From this point of division straight clamps are placed obliquely along the lesser curvature up to the point previously selected for division. This is the technique originally described by Schoemaker of The Hague. This portion of the stomach is then transected and is closed with two inverted layers of fine catgut and a third layer of interrupted fine silk (Fig. 14-6).

The resulting gastric remnant assumes a tubular shape. The distal transected stomach is then reflected to the right. At this point the entire pancreas can again be fully visualized and examined. By applying traction to the distal transected stomach, the stomach can serve as a handle, and the dissection of the pylorus and duodenal bulb is thereby greatly facilitated. This method has proved much easier and more efficacious in our hands than other methods described in which the duodenum is mobilized before the division of the stomach. The division is carried distally on the duodenum far enough to remove all antral tissue.

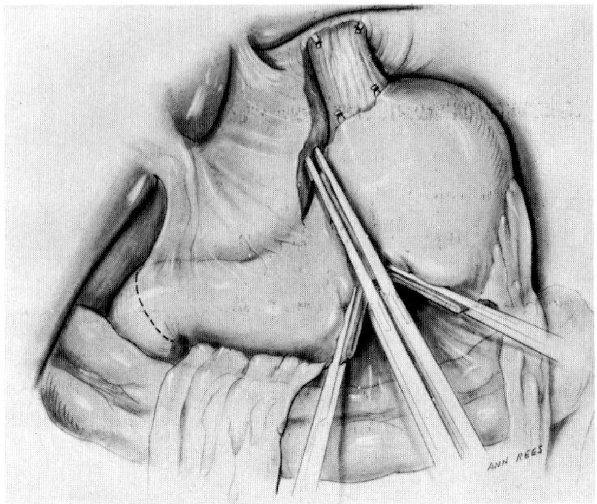

Fig. 14-6. Transection of the stomach being completed.

BILLROTH I RECONSTRUCTION

It was formerly our practice to use a Billroth I end-to-end gastroduodenostomy after vagotomy and antrectomy only when the ulcer could be easily excised and to use the Billroth II gastrojejunostomy when pathological changes in the duodenum indicated that excision of the ulcer might be technically difficult or hazardous. However, we have found that a Billroth I reconstruction is feasible in most of our patients who have had duodenal ulcer. Gastroduodenal continuity offers certain physiological advantages over gastrojejunostomy, since many nutritional studies have indicated diminished loss of fecal fat and nitrogen with gastroduodenostomy. Iron absorption is also enhanced by maintaining the duodenum in alimentary continuity. The incidence of reflux gastritis is diminished.

It is essential that a normally wide duodenal lumen without constriction at or beyond the ulcer be present or be surgically produced when end-to-end gastroduodenostomy is done. The Horsley longitudinal incision of the anterior duodenal wall may be employed to produce a satisfactory lumen if narrowing of the duodenum exists. With severe scarring and constriction of the first or second part of the duodenum associated with a deeply penetrating posterior bulbar or postbulbar ulcer, the Finney–von Haberer modification of the Billroth I procedure may be used advantageously to exclude the ulcer in the duodenal stump and to preserve gastroduodenal continuity.

It is not necessary to remove the ulcer if there is no evidence of cicatricial stenosis at or distal to the site of the ulcer in the duodenum. In one study [130] we found a lower morbidity in patients who did not have their duodenal ulcer excised. It is preferable to leave a difficult penetrating ulcer in situ rather than to be too aggressive in attempting to remove it. Unwarranted aggressive attempts to remove the duodenal ulcer may result in increased mortality and morbidity due to anastomotic leaks, infection, or pancreatitis. When a large, penetrating ulcer of the posterior wall is encountered and scarring extends about the entire circumference of the duodenum, particularly in an obese patient, we may elect to close the duodenal stump by using a long anterior-wall cuff of duodenum. This long cuff is buttressed to the bed of the ulcer using two inverting layers of catgut sutures, after which the pseudocapsule of the pancreas is approximated to the duodenal serosa with interrupted silk. A retrocolic Hofmeister reconstruction is then carried out using a short afferent loop (see Fig. 14-10).

We have seldom had occasion to resort to catheter drainage of the duodenal stump, but we realize that it is a safe and effective method in certain circumstances in which the duodenal tissue and the inflammatory tissue do not lend themselves to secure closure.

In performing end-to-end gastroduodenostomy, the duodenum is not as a rule kocherized except in unusual circumstances. Routine kocherization is neither necessary nor preferred. After mobilization of the distal stomach beyond the pylorus, the gastric pouch with the Kocher clamp still applied to the greater curvature is brought downward and to the right. The structures to be anastomosed can always be approximated without the slightest amount of tension. With the distal stomach still attached to the freed duodenum, a row of interrupted seromuscular silk sutures is placed between the posterior gastric and posterior duodenal walls below the ulcer site (Fig. 14-7). The sutures are rendered taut, and the first assistant approximates the gastric pouch to the posterior duodenal wall by gentle traction on these structures. The sutures are then tied by the operator, after which the specimen is removed.

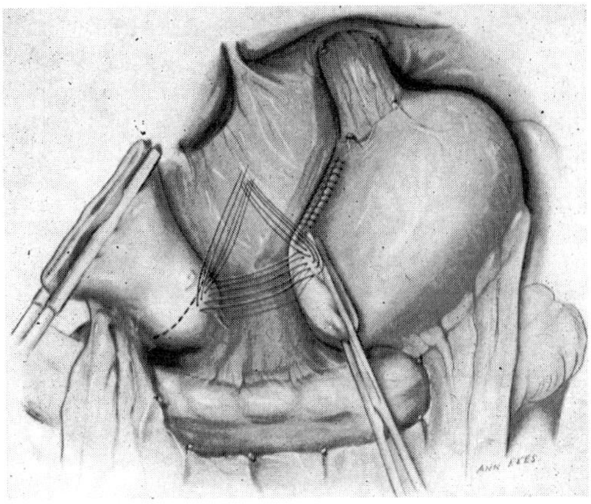

Fig. 14-7. The row of interrupted silk sutures between the opposing gastric and duodenal walls is being placed.

An inner layer of continuous 000 chromic catgut suture is now placed through the entire thickness of the posterior gastric and duodenal walls, which also serves to approximate the opposing mucosal surfaces. The previously placed seromuscular silk sutures are held elevated by an assistant as the continuous posterior catgut suture is being taken, since this maneuver allows for better visualization of the opposing gastric and duodenal mucosae. As the continuous catgut suture ad-

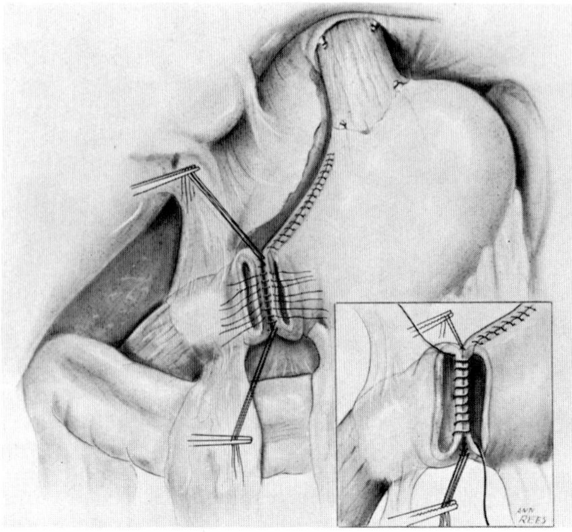

Fig. 14-8. The posterior layer of silk sutures has been placed and the gastric pouch and duodenum approximated. *Inset* shows the continuous catgut suture placed posteriorly, which will be continued anteriorly as an inverting suture.

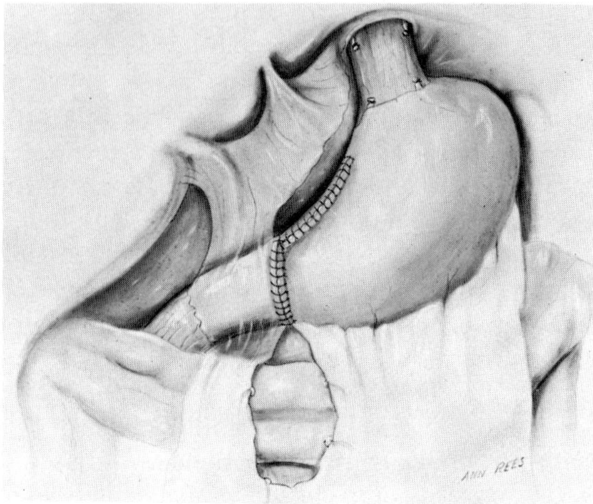

Fig. 14-9. Completed operation—bilateral vagotomy, antrectomy, and a Billroth I reconstruction.

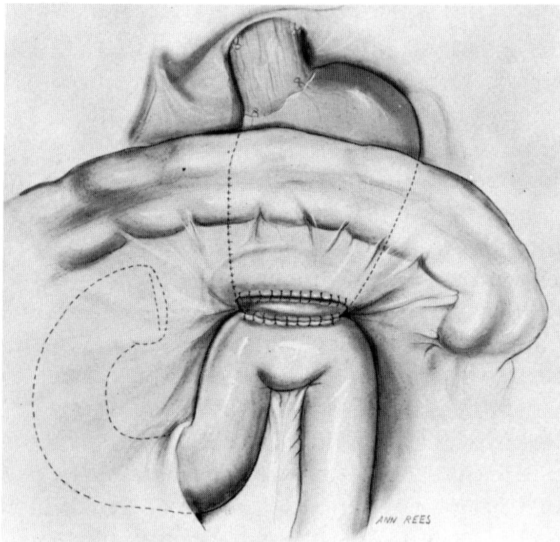

Fig. 14-10. Completed operation—bilateral vagotomy, antrectomy, and a retrocolic Hofmeister reconstruction.

vances, the interrupted sik sutures are cut close to the knots. The catgut suture is then continued anteriorly, inverting the opposing gastric and duodenal walls (Fig. 14-8). An outer layer of interrupted 4-0 silk completes the anastomosis. Care is taken that the critical angle is securely closed. If there is any appreciable discrepancy between the opposing structures to be anastomosed, the antimesenteric border of the duodenum may be divided for 1 to 2 cm before completing the anterior row of sutures (Horsley maneuver). The resulting gastroduodenal stoma will usually admit 1½ fingertips. It is important not to make it larger (Figs. 14-9, 14-10).

The nasogastric tube is then irrigated by a member of the operating room staff before the abdomen is closed to be sure that all blood clots have been removed from the gastric pouch. We prefer to remove the nasogastric tube after the first 24 hours, provided the operation has progressed smoothly. At present we remove the nasogastric tube early in approximately 75 percent of the patients [74]. When the operative procedure is carried out on an emergency basis, particularly for an acute ulcer perforation in which extensive peritoneal soiling is present, the tube is left in place for approximately 72 hours or until the patient expels flatus. Also, in some instances of massive bleeding in which the gastrointestinal tract is filled with blood, adynamic ileus may be anticipated postoperatively. These patients fare better with nasogastric suction for a few days.

During the postoperative period (the first 72 hours), the patient is given nothing but parenteral fluids. Small amounts of tap water are allowed on the fourth postoperative day, and a liquid diet is usually begun on the fifth day. A postgastrectomy diet is begun on the sixth or seventh day. Antibiotics are not given unless definitely indicated, and, of course, the patient gets out of bed and walks on the first postoperative day.

Discussion

A critical appraisal of the clinical data from several medical centers using vagotomy and antrectomy in the treatment of duodenal ulcer enforces the conclusion that this operation provides effective therapy for chronic duodenal ulcer and its complications [73]. Vagotomy with antrectomy appears to be the most accurate method thus far devised for control of the ulcer diathesis. The procedure is based on the sound physiological concepts of eliminating both cephalic and gastric sources of stimuli to excessive gastric acid secretion [29], while preserving an adequate gastric reservoir. Vagotomy with antrectomy is now the standard against which other operations for duodenal ulcer are compared.

MORTALITY

An analysis by Herrington et al. [75] of the etiological factors influencing operative mortality after vagotomy and antrectomy emphasized that the greatest risk of the procedure was encountered in its application to the management of massive bleeding from duodenal ulcer, especially in elderly, debilitated patients. The dissection of the diseased duodenum constitutes the most hazardous part of the operation for duodenal ulcer. Antrectomy should be replaced by a procedure of lesser magnitude when problems are encountered in performing the duodenal dissection. In an attempt to reduce the mortality, we have tended to use vagotomy and a drainage procedure, usually pyloroplasty, rather than antral resection in elderly, debilitated patients, especially those with massive bleeding and those with technical problems that increase the hazard of antral resection. Since we adopted this approach in 1964, the operative mortality in our entire series of patients has steadily dropped from a high of 3.1 percent in 1958 to 1.6 percent. Our overall mortality when operating for the control of bleeding has been 3.1 percent, including all ages. For patients older than 60 years of age, the mortality has been 6 percent.

Jordan and Condon [85] in a prospective randomized study comparing patients undergoing truncal vagotomy and antrectomy with patients undergoing truncal vagotomy and pyloroplasty on an elective basis found that the mortality after vagotomy with antrectomy was zero. A follow-up study by Jordan [84] supports the conclusions that vagotomy with antrectomy can be performed with a mortality as low as that usually reported for vagotomy and a drainage procedure and that vagotomy with antrectomy is superior to vagotomy and pyloroplasty because "it is associated with fewer recurrent ulcers without a significant difference in the severity of other postoperative gastrointestinal complaints." In his series recurrent ulcer developed and required reoperation in nine patients after truncal vagotomy and pyloroplasty (8.3 percent), while only one recurrent ulcer (1.1 percent) developed after vagotomy with antrectomy.

The proponents of both truncal vagotomy with pyloroplasty and truncal vagotomy with antrectomy are in essential agreement that the incidences of significant weight loss, diarrhea, and dumping are approximately equal following the two operations, and in most instances the sequelae are not severe.

Goligher et al. [58] in their classic Leeds/York study found that truncal vagotomy and pyloroplasty resulted in the poorest results according to the Visick grading. A follow-up study of these patients continues to show a significant advantage of vagotomy-antrectomy over vagotomy-pyloroplasty [57]. As in Jordan's study, however, patients were relegated to the vagotomy with drainage group if it was believed that gastric resection could not be performed with reasonable safety. One can conclude from this and other studies that patients can be treated by vagotomy and antrectomy with negligible mortality if vagotomy and drainage is used for patients in whom dissection of the duodenum may be unduly hazardous. Also, in the elderly, debilitated patient with associated systemic disease and in the elderly, massively bleeding patient, vagotomy with pyloroplasty is preferred; the higher ulcer recurrence rate following vagotomy and pyloroplasty is accepted in these few patients.

CLINICAL RESULTS

It is indeed gratifying to note that 94 percent of the group undergoing vagotomy with antrectomy experienced a satisfactory clinical result. It should be emphasized that many of the patients who had an unsatisfactory result benefited from the operative procedure, and except for the 20 patients in whom recurrent ulcerations developed, each was relieved of ulcer distress. The disadvantage of antrectomy is loss of the pylorus, which may result in dumping syndrome, diarrhea, or reflux gastritis. Proximal gastric vagotomy has almost eliminated postgastrectomy disorders but has a higher ulcer recurrence rate [128].

BILLROTH I VERSUS BILLROTH II OPERATION

Harkins et al. [66] were the first to employ vagotomy and distal gastrectomy with gastroduodenostomy for duodenal ulcer. They and others [50, 95] described improved metabolic factors following the procedure, including better secretory activation, better fat and iron absorption, and improved weight gain.

In our early experience the Billroth II reconstruction was employed exclusively. At present Billroth I reconstruction is being used in almost all patients. As experience with end-to-end gastroduodenostomy has increased, we have found it safe to adapt the principle to many of the large posterior wall ulcers. We have applied the procedure to postbulbar ulcers that had not bled preoperatively. It is our belief that for most deep, penetrating ulcers the classic Billroth I method can be employed. If there is any discrepancy in the size of the duodenal opening to be anastomosed to the gastric pouch, the Horsley maneuver of incising the antimesenteric duodenal border may be performed. As with any other type of operation, one becomes more proficient in its use as experience accumulates. It is extremely important, however, that one is able to recognize the extensive inflammatory duodenal ulcer process that will be better managed by other procedures.

Because of the increased incidence of reflux gastritis after a Billroth II operation, we now prefer a Roux-en-Y gastrojejunostomy rather than a Billroth II procedure in the few patients in whom a gastroduodenostomy cannot be performed.

EXTENT OF ANTRECTOMY

Much discussion has arisen about the anatomical extent of the distal resection necessary to ensure complete antral extirpation [70]. The limits of the antrum are variable, and antral mucosa is known to extend higher on the lesser curvature than on the greater curvature. In recent years several sophisticated methods of defining the antral limits at the time of operation have been described by Capper et al. [14], Osborne and Frederick [111], Moe et al. [101, 102], and Bergström and Broomé [6]. These methods employ staining and pH studies for the most part. Ruding and Hirdes [124], using histological techniques, found the antral glands to occupy as much as 80 percent of the lesser curvature and about 50 percent of the greater curvature. On occasion the antrum was demonstrated to extend 0.5 cm distal to the pyloric muscle. Earlier staining studies defining the antral limits were reported by Landboe-Christensen [93].

Our objective in removing the antrum has been to divide the stomach obliquely at the lesser curvature several centimeters above the angle and about midway along the greater curvature. If the Billroth II type of reconstruction is employed after vagotomy with antrectomy, it is imperative to remove the distal extent of the antrum because excluded antral tissue is a potent ulcerogenic preparation. The clinical observations of von Eiselsberg [48] regarding antral stimulation were brought to our attention through a patient in whom multiple recurrent ulcerations continued to develop despite a complete vagotomy and multiple resections of the gastric pouch performed elsewhere. At reexploration a very small antral cuff was found attached to the duodenum. After the cuff was removed, the marginal ulcer promptly healed [136]. If a cuff of proximal antral tissue is left after a Billroth I anastomosis, it is of far less importance, and to leave behind a small antral segment either proximally or distally after vagotomy with antrectomy and a classic Billroth I reconstruction probably creates no particular hazard. In the latter circumstance the small residual secretions of acid from the gastric fundus and the inhibitory action of the duodenum render innocuous any residual tissue left in continuity.

During the early postoperative period it is of extreme importance to instruct the patients about a proper dietary program. Most operative procedures in use for duodenal ulcer either interrupt or destroy the integrity of the pyloric sphincter, and all persons who undergo operation for duodenal ulcer are potential candidates for the dumping syndrome. The patients are placed on a high-protein, high-fat, low-carbohydrate intake consisting of small frequent feedings for the first four to six weeks following the operation. They are carefully instructed to take no liquids with meals but to drink them 30 minutes to an hour after eating. Symptoms associated with the dumping syndrome are carefully explained to each patient, along with measures to be taken should these symptoms occur. Usually after a period of several weeks after the operation the dietary measurement may be relaxed, with most patients having few, if any, dietary restrictions [120, 138, 149].

Vagotomy with antrectomy appears to have stood the test of time [72]. Many of its former critics are now among its staunchest supporters. The combined operation is currently the most effective operation at the surgeon's disposal to control the ulcer diathesis. The overall results are satisfactory, indeed, and nutritional problems have been minimal.

References

1. Allen, J. G. *The Physiology and Treatment of Peptic Ulcer.* Chicago: University of Chicago Press, 1959.
2. Bales, H. W., and Schilling, J. A. The role of the pyloric antrum in peptic ulcer. *Ann. Surg.* 143:531, 1956.
3. Ballinger, W. F., II, Aparite, I. J., Wirts, W. C., and Goldstein, F. Structure and function of the canine small intestine following total abdominal vagotomy. *Surg. Gynecol. Obstet.* 118:1305, 1964.
4. Ballinger, W. F., II., Padula, R. T., and Camishion, R. C. Mesenteric blood flow following total and selective vagotomy. *Surgery* 57:409, 1965.
5. Barber, K. W., Judd, E. S., and Stauffer, M. H. Hemigastrectomy and vagotomy in the treatment of complications of duodenal ulcer. *Arch. Surg.* 86:710, 1963.
6. Bergström, H., and Broomé, A. Preoperative determination of the boundary between gastric antrum and fundus. *Acta Chir. Scand.* 128:526, 1964.
7. Bernard, C. *Leçons sur la Physiologie et la Pathologie due Système Nerveux.* Paris: Balière, 1858.
8. Bircher, E. Die Resektion von Aesten der N. vagus zur Behandlung gastrischer Affektionen. *Schweiz. Med. Wochenschr.* 1:519, 1920.
9. Borchers, E. L. Anteil des Nervus vagus an der motorischen Innervation des Magens in Hinblick auf die operative Therapie von Magenkrankheiten Studien zur Physiologie und Pathologie der Magenchirurgie. *Beitr. Klin. Chir.* 122:547, 1921.
10. Brodie, B. C. Experiments and observations on the influence of the nerves of the eighth pair on the secretions of the stomach. *Philos. Trans. R. Soc. Lond.* 104:102, 1814.
11. Buchanan, L. C., Grady, E. D., Riccardi, L., and Martin, J. D., Jr. Hemigastrectomy and vagotomy. *South. Med. J.* 47:659, 1954.
12. Burdette, W. J., and Fitzpatrick, W. K. Objective evaluation of vagectomy-antrectomy for duodenal ulcer. *Ann. Surg.* 149:875, 1959.
13. Cameron, D. A. Vagotomy for peptic ulcer. *Am. J. Med. Sci.* 214:202, 1947.
14. Capper, W. M., Butler, T. J., Buckler, K. G., and Hallet, C. P. Variation in size of the gastric antrum: Measurement of alkaline area associated with ulceration and pyloric stenosis. *Ann. Surg.* 163:281, 1966.

15. Carlson, A. J. The secretion of gastric juice in health and disease. *Physiol. Rev.* 3:1, 1923.
16. Chapman, N. D., Nyhus, L. M., Devito, R. V., et al. Experimental evaluation of the concept of antral exclusion for the surgical treatment of duodenal ulcer. *Surgery* 51:378, 1962.
17. Clark, C. G., Murray, J. G., Slessor, I. M., and Wyllie, J. H. Complete vagotomy and its consequences: Follow-up of 146 patients. *Br. Med. J.* 2:900, 1964.
18. Coffey, R. J., and Lazard, E. J. Vagotomy and hemigastrectomy and gastroduodenostomy (Finney–von Haberer) in the treatment of duodenal ulcer. *Ann. Surg.* 141:862, 1955.
19. Coutsoftides, T., and Himal, H. S. The effect of vagotomy antrectomy or vagotomy pyloroplasty on the response of the antrum to meat extract in duodenal ulcer patients. *Ann. Surg.* 184:212, 1976.
20. Cox, A. G., Bond, M. R., Podmove, D. A., and Rose, D. P. Aspects of nutrition after vagotomy and gastroenterostomy. *Br. Med. J.* 1:465, 1964.
21. Creutzfeldt, W., Creutzfeldt, C., and Arnold, R. Gastrin-Producing Cells. In W. Y. Chey and F. P. Brooks (Eds.), *Endocrinology of the Gut.* Thorofare, N.J.:Slack, 1974.
22. Donahue, P. E., Bombeck, C. T., Condon, R. E., and Nyhus, L. M. Proximal gastric vagotomy versus selective vagotomy with antrectomy: Results of a prospective randomized clinical trial after 4 to 12 years. *Surgery* 96:585, 1984.
23. Dragstedt, L. R. Vagotomy for gastroduodenal ulcer. *Ann. Surg.* 122:973, 1945.
24. Dragstedt, L. R. The physiology of the gastric antrum. *Arch. Surg.* 75:552, 1957.
25. Dragstedt, L. R., Fournier, H. J., Woodward, E. R., et al. Transabdominal gastric vagotomy. *Surg. Gynecol. Obstet.* 85:461, 1947.
26. Dragstedt, L. R., Harper, P. V., Jr., Tovee, E. B., and Woodward, E. R. Section of the vagus nerves to the stomach in the treatment of peptic ulcer. *Ann. Surg.* 126:687, 1947.
27. Dragstedt, L. R., Oberhelman, H. A., Jr., and Smith, C. A. Experimental hyperfunction of the gastric antrum with ulcer formation. *Ann. Surg.* 134:332, 1951.
28. Dragstedt, L. R., Oberhelman, H. A., Jr., and Woodward, E. R. Physiology of gastric secretion and its relation to the ulcer problem. *J.A.M.A.* 147:1615, 1951.
29. Dragstedt, L. R., Oberhelman, H. A., Jr., Woodward, E. R., and Smith, C. A. Interrelationship between the cephalic and gastric phases of gastric secretion. *Am. J. Physiol.* 171:7, 1952.
30. Dragstedt, L. R., Oberhelman, H. A., Jr., Zubiran, J. M., and Woodward, E. R. Antrum motility as a stimulus for gastric secretion. *Gastroenterology* 24:71, 1953.
31. Dragstedt, L. R., and Owens, F. M., Jr. Subdiaphragmatic section of the vagus nerves for treatment of duodenal ulcer. *Proc. Soc. Exp. Biol. Med.* 53:152, 1943.
32. Dragstedt, L. R., Palmer, W. L., Schaefer, P. W., and Hodges, P. C. Supradiaphragmatic section of the vagus nerves in the treatment of duodenal and gastric ulcers. *Gastroenterology* 3:450, 1944.
33. Dragstedt, L. R., Quintana, R. B., de la Rosa, C., and Linares, C. A. The question of fatigue in the gastric mechanism. *Arch. Surg.* 89:1043, 1964.
34. Dragstedt, L. R., and Schaefer, P. W. Removal of the vagus innervation of the stomach in the gastroduodenal ulcer. *Surgery* 17:742, 1945.
35. Dragstedt, L. R., Woodward, E. R., Oberhelman, H. A., Jr., et al. Effect of transplantation of antrum of stomach on gastric secretion in experimental animals. *Am. J. Physiol.* 165:386, 1951.
36. Dragstedt, L. R., Woodward, E. R., Storer, E. H., et al. Quantitative studies on the mechanism of gastric secretion in health and disease. *Ann. Surg.* 132:626, 1950.
37. Dreiling, D. A., Druckerman, L. J., and Hollander, F. Effect of complete vagi section and vagal stimulation on pancreatic secretions in man. *Gastroenterology* 20:578, 1952.
38. Edkins, J. S. The chemical mechanism of gastric secretion. *J. Physiol.* (Lond.) 24:183, 1906.
39. Edkins, J. S., and Tweedy, M. J. The natural channels of absorption evoking the chemical mechanism of gastric secretion. *J. Physiol.* (Lond.), 38:263, 1909.
40. Edwards, L. W. Duodenal ulcer. *Am. Surg.* 20:8, 1954.
41. Edwards, L. W., and Herrington, J. L., Jr. Vagotomy and antral resection in the treatment of duodenal ulcer. *J. Tenn. Med. Assoc.* 46:8, 1953.
42. Edwards, L. W., and Herrington, J. L., Jr. Vagotomy and gastroenterostomy-vagotomy and conservative gastrectomy: A comparative study. *Ann. Surg.* 137:6, 1953.
43. Edwards, L. W., and Herrington, J. L., Jr.

The technic of vagus nerve resection. *Am. Surg.* 20:8, 1954.
44. Edwards, L. W., and Herrington, J. L., Jr. Efficacy of 40 per cent gastrectomy combined with vagotomy for duodenal ulcer. *Surgery* 41:346, 1957.
45. Edwards, L. W., Herrington, J. L., Jr., Cate, W. R., Jr., and Lipscomb, A. B. Gastrojejunal ulcer: Problems in surgical management. *Ann. Surg.* 143:2, 1956.
46. Edwards, L. W., Herrington, J. L., Jr., Cate, W. R., Jr., et al. Duodenal ulcer: Treatment by vagotomy and removal of the gastric antrum. *Ann. Surg.* 145:5, 1957.
47. Edwards, L. W., Scott, H. W., Jr., Edwards, W. H., et al. The surgical treatment of duodenal ulcer by vagotomy and antral resection. *Am. J. Surg.* 105:352, 1963.
48. Eiselsberg, A. von. Die chirurgische Behandlung des Magenulkus. *Acta Chir. Scand.* 59:71, 1925.
49. Emås, S., and Fyrö, B. Vagal release of gastrin in cats following reserpine. *Acta Physiol. Scand.* 63:358, 1965.
50. Everson, T. C. An experimental comparison of protein and fat assimilation after Billroth I and Billroth II reconstructions and segmental type of subtotal gastrectomy. *Surgery* 36:525, 1954.
51. Exner, A., and Schwarzmann, E. Gastrische Krisen und Vagotomie. *Mitt. Grenzgeb. Med. Chir.* 28:15, 1914.
52. Fallis, L. S., and von Barron, J. Haberer-Finney gastrectomy with vagotomy. *Arch. Surg.* 59:758, 1949.
53. Farmer, D. A., Howe, C. W., Porrell, W. J., and Smithwick, R. H. The effect of various surgical procedures upon the acidity of the gastric contents of ulcer patients. *Ann. Surg.* 134:319, 1951.
54. Farmer, D. A., and Smithwick, R. H. Hemigastrectomy combined with section of the vagus nerves. *N. Engl. J. Med.* 247:1097, 1952.
55. Ferguson, L. K., Bravo, J. L., and Nusbaum, M. Comparison of surgical treatment of duodenal ulcer: Results of 50% gastrectomy and vagotomy compared to results of 75% gastric resection for duodenal ulcer. *Arch. Surg.* 82:627, 1961.
56. Gillespie, I. E., Clark, D. H., Kay, A. W., and Tankle, H. I. Effect of antrectomy-vagotomy with gastrojejunostomy and antrectomy with vagotomy on the spontaneous and maximal gastric acid output in man. *Gastroenterology* 38:361, 1960.
57. Goligher, J. C., Feather, D. B., Hall, R., et al. Several standard elective operations for duodenal ulcer. *Ann. Surg.* 189:18, 1979.
58. Goligher, J. C., Pulvertaft, C. N., de Dombal, F. T., et al. Five- to eight-year results of Leeds/York controlled trial of elective surgery for duodenal ulcer. *Br. Med. J.* 2:781, 1968.
59. Grady, E. D. The case for hemigastrectomy and vagotomy in surgical treatment of duodenal ulcer. *Am. Surg.* 22:1052, 1956.
60. Gregory, R. Gastrin and the Zollinger-Ellison syndrome. *Ir. J. Med. Sci.* 6:443, 1964.
61. Gregory, R. A., and Tracy, H. J. The preparation and properties of gastrin. *J. Physiol.* (Lond.) 156:523, 1961.
62. Grossman, M. I., and Anderson, S. Effect of vagal denervation of pouches on gastric secretion in dogs with intact or resected antrums. *Gastroenterology* 48:449, 1965.
63. Grossman, M. I., Robertson, C. R., and Ivy, A. C. Proof of a humoral mechanism for gastric secretion: The humoral transmission of the digestive stimulus. *Am. J. Physiol.* 153:1, 1948.
64. Harkins, H. N., Chapman, N. D., Condon, R. E., and Jesseph, J. E. Combined operation: Vagotomy-antrectomy for gastroduodenal ulcer. *Arch. Surg.* 85:936, 1962.
65. Harkins, H. N., Jesseph, J. E., Stevenson, J. K., and Nyhus, L. M. The combined operation for peptic ulcer. *Arch. Surg.* 80:743, 1960.
66. Harkins, H. N., Schmitz, E. J., Harper, H. P., et al. A combined physiologic operation for peptic ulcer (partial distal gastrectomy, vagotomy, and gastroduodenostomy): A preliminary report. *West. J. Surg.* 61:316, 1953.
67. Harkins, H. N., Zech, R. K., Nyhus, L. M., et al. The relative effects of different gastric drainage procedures on the hormonal phase of gastric secretion. *Surg. Forum* 5:281, 1954.
68. Harper, P. V., Tovee, E. B., and Woodward, E. R. Section of the vagus nerves to the stomach in the treatment of peptic ulcer. *Ann. Surg.* 126:687, 1947.
69. Heer, F. W., Baldwin, J. N., Ruby, L., et al. Effect of vagal nerves on hepatic secretions of bile in humans. *Am. J. Surg.* 111:66, 1966.
70. Herrington, J. L., Jr. The pyloric antrum: The relative extent of distal gastrectomy necessary to insure its complete extirpation. *Surgery* 44:775, 1958.

71. Herrington, J. L., Jr., Classen, K. L., and Edwards, L. W. Experiences with a Billroth I reconstruction following vagotomy and antrectomy for duodenal ulcer. *Ann. Surg.* 153:575, 1961.
72. Herrington, J. L., Jr., and Edwards, L. W. Are we too rigid in our criteria in advising surgery for the complications of duodenal ulcer? *Surgery* 43:3, 1958.
73. Herrington, J. L., Jr., Edwards, W. H., and Edwards, L. W. Re-evaluation of the surgical treatment of duodenal ulcer. *Surgery* 49:540, 1961.
74. Herrington, J. L., Jr., Edwards, W. H., and Sawyers, J. L. Elimination of routine use of gastric decompression following operation for gastroduodenal ulcer. *Ann. Surg.* 159:807, 1964.
75. Herrington, J. L., Jr., Edwards, W. H., Sawyers, J. L., et al. Etiologic factors influencing the operative mortality following vagotomy and antrectomy for duodenal ulcer. *Am. J. Surg.* 107:289, 1964.
76. Herrington, J. L., Jr., Sawyers, J. L., and Scott, H. W., Jr. A 25-year experience with vagotomy-antrectomy. *Arch. Surg.* 106:469, 1973.
77. Hoerr, S. O. Duodenal ulcer treated by subdiaphragmatic vagus resection and posterior gastroenterostomy. *A.M.A. Arch. Surg.* 67:436, 1953.
78. Hoerr, S. O. Evaluation of vagotomy with gastroenterostomy performed for chronic duodenal ulcer. Report based on five-year follow-up of 145 patients. *Surgery* 38:149, 1955.
79. Hoerr, S. O. Preliminary observations on hemigastrectomy with subdiaphragmatic vagotomy for the average case of chronic duodenal ulcer. *Cleve. Clin. Q.* 22:172, 1955.
80. Howe, C. W., and Porrell, W. J. Effects of 50% gastrectomy alone and combined with vagotomy. *A.M.A. Arch. Surg.* 65:714, 1952.
81. Hubert, J. P., Jr., Kiernan, P. D., Beahrs, O. H., and ReMine, W. H. Truncal vagotomy and resection in the treatment of duodenal ulcer. *Mayo Clin. Proc.* 55:19, 1980.
82. Jordan, G. L., Jr., Quast, D., and Johnston, R. Hemigastrectomy and vagotomy for the treatment of duodenal ulcer. *Am. J. Gastroenterol.* 35:546, 1961.
83. Jordan, P. H., Jr. Relation of humoral mechanisms to ulcerogenesis. *Surg. Clin. North Am.* 46:297, 1966.
84. Jordan, P. H., Jr. A follow-up report of a prospective evaluation of vagotomy-pyloroplasty and vagotomy-antrectomy for treatment of duodenal ulcer. *Ann. Surg.* 180:259, 1974.
85. Jordan, P. H., Jr., and Condon, R. E. A prospective evaluation of vagotomy-pyloroplasty and vagotomy-antrectomy for treatment of duodenal ulcer. *Ann. Surg.* 172:547, 1970.
86. Kay, A. W. Gastrointestinal surgery and human physiology. *J. R. Coll. Surg. Edinb.* 7:275, 1962.
87. Kay, A. W. Personal communication, 1966.
88. Klein, E. Left vagus section and partial gastrectomy for duodenal ulcer with hyperacidity. *Ann. Surg.* 90:65, 1929.
89. Komarov, S. A. Gastrin. *Proc. Soc. Exp. Biol. Med.* 38:514, 1938.
90. Komarov, S. A. Studies on gastrin. I. Methods of isolation of a secretagogue from the pyloric mucous membrane. *Rev. Can. Biol.* 1:191, 1942.
91. Komarov, S. A. Studies on gastrin. I. *Phys. Prop. Sec.* 421:377, 1942.
92. Koo, J., Lam, S. K., Lee, N. W., et al. Proximal gastric vagotomy, truncal vagotomy with drainage and truncal vagotomy with antrectomy for chronic duodenal ulcer: A prospective, randomized controlled trial. *Ann. Surg.* 197:265, 1983.
93. Landboe-Christensen, E. The extent of the pylorus zone in the human stomach. *Acta Pathol. Microbiol. Scand.* 54(Suppl.):671, 1944.
94. Latarjet, A. Résection des nerfs de l'estomac. *Bull. Acad. Natl. Med.* (Paris) 87:681, 1922.
95. Lenninger, G. G., White, T. T., and Magee, D. F. Studies of pancreatic juice in the proximal loop after Billroth II gastrectomy. *Surg. Gynecol. Obstet.* 120:507, 1965.
96. Longhi, E. H., Greenlee, H. B., Bravo, J. L., et al. The question of an inhibitory hormone from the gastric antrum. *Am. J. Physiol.* 191:164, 1957.
97. Lowicki, E. M. Gastrin and its surgical implication. *Surgery* 57:602, 1965.
98. Lowicki, E. M. The discoverer of gastrin: John Sydney Edkins. *Surgery* 58:1044, 1965.
99. Magee, D. F. *Gastrointestinal Physiology.* Springfield, Ill.: Thomas, 1962.
100. Martin, G. H. The treatment of duodenal ulcer by vagotomy-antrectomy and Billroth I anastomosis. *Minn. Med. J.* 4:523, 1963.
101. Moe, R. E., Klopper, P. J., and Nyhus, L. M. Demonstration of the functional anatomy of

the common gastric antrum. *Am. J. Surg.* 111:80, 1966.
102. Moe, R. E., Nyhus, L. M., and Harkins, H. N. The use of dye for differentiating the gastric antrum from the gastric corpus. *Bull. Soc. Int. Chir.* 22:424, 1964.
103. Moore, F. D. Vagus resection for ulcer: An extensive evaluation. *Ann. Surg.* 126:664, 1957.
104. Nielson, J. R. Development of cholelithiasis following vagotomy. *Surgery* 56:909, 1964.
105. Nyhus, L. M., Chapman, N. D., and Harkins, H. N. The control of gastrin release: An experimental study illustrating a new concept. *Gastroenterology* 39:582, 1960.
106. Nyhus, L. M., Donahue, P. E., Krystosek, R. J., et al. Complete vagotomy: The evolution of an effective technique. *Arch. Surg.* 115:264, 1980.
107. Nylander, G., and Olerud, S. The vascular pattern of the gastric mucosa of the rat following vagotomy. *Surg. Gynecol. Obstet.* 112:475, 1961.
108. Oberhelman, H. A., Jr. The function of the gastric antrum. *Surg. Clin. North Am.* 46:269, 1966.
109. Oberhelman, H. A., Jr., Rigler, S. P., and Dragstedt, L. R. The significance of innervation in the function of the gastric antrum. *Surg. Forum* 7:353, 1956.
110. Oberhelman, H. A., Jr., Rigler, S. P., and Dragstedt, L. R. The significance of innervation in the function of the gastric antrum. *Am. J. Physiol.* 190:391, 1957.
111. Osborne, M. P., and Frederick, P. L. Precise resection of the gastric antrum: A simple method. *Surg. Gynecol. Obstet.* 121:592, 1965.
112. Palumbo, L. T., and Sharpe, W. S. Neurohumoral gastric secretory control in chronic duodenal ulcer. *Surgery* 56:1045, 1964.
113. Palumbo, L. T., Sharpe, W. S., Lulu, D. J., et al. Distal antrectomy with vagectomy for duodenal ulcer. *Arch. Surg.* 100:182, 1970.
114. Palumbo, L. T., Sharpe, W. S., Lulu, D. J., et al. Distal antrectomy with vagectomy. *Arch. Surg.* 89:637, 1964.
115. Palumbo, L. T., Sharpe, W. S., Lulu, D. J., et al. Antrectomy with vagectomy for chronic duodenal ulcer. *Surgery* 46:1005, 1959.
116. Pavlov, I. P. *The Work of the Digestive Glands* (2d ed., trans. W. H. Thompson). London: Griffin, 1910.
117. Polak, J. M., Stagg, B., and Pearse, A. G. E. Two types of Zollinger-Ellison syndrome: Immunofluorescent, cytochemical and ultrastructural studies of the antral and pancreatic gastrin cells in different clinical states. *Gut* 13:501, 1972.
118. Ragins, H., Rigler, S. P., Evans, S. O., et al. Studies on the physiology of the gastric antrum. *A.M.A. Arch. Surg.* 75:230, 1957.
119. ReMine, W. H. Personal communication, 1972.
120. Robinson, F. W., and Pittman, A. C. Dietary management of postgastrectomy dumping syndrome. *Surg. Gynecol. Obstet.* 104:529, 1957.
121. Rudick, J., Gajewski, A. K., Pitts, C. L., et al. Inhibition of gastric secretion by fractional lymph elaboration of gastrone-like substance during digestive phases in dogs. *Am. Surg.* 32:513, 1966.
122. Rudick, J., Guntheroth, W. G., and Nyhus, L. M. Recent Observations on Gastric Blood Flow and Acid Secretion. In R. C. Harrison (Ed.), *Gastric Secretion: Mechanism and Control.* Oxford, Engl.: Pergamon, 1966.
123. Rudick, J., and Hutchinson, J. S. F. Effects of vagal nerve section on the biliary system. *Lancet* 1:579, 1964.
124. Ruding, R., and Hirdes, W. H. Extent of gastric antrum and its significance. *Surgery* 53:743, 1963.
125. Sauvage, L. R., Schmitz, E. J., Storer, E. H., et al. The relation between the physiologic stimulatory mechanisms of gastric secretion and the incidence of peptic ulceration. *Surg. Gynecol. Obstet.* 96:127, 1953.
126. Sauvage, L. R., Schmitz, E. J., Storer, E. H., et al. A new operative preparation for production of peptic ulcer in the dog. *Proc. Soc. Exp. Biol. Med.* 79:436, 1952.
127. Sawyers, J. L., Edwards, L. W., Herrington, J. L., Jr., and Scott, H. W., Jr. Vagotomy and Antrectomy for Duodenal Ulcer. 20e Congrès de la Société Internationale de Chirurgie, September, 1961. Brussels: Imprimérie Médicale et Scientifique, 1963. P. 1022.
128. Sawyers, J. L., Herrington, J. L., Jr., and Burney, D. P. Proximal gastric vagotomy compared with vagotomy and antrectomy and selective gastric vagotomy and pyloroplasty. *Ann. Surg.* 186:510, 1977.
129. Sawyers, J. L., Herrington, J. L., Jr., Mulherin, J. L., et al. Acute perforated duodenal ulcer: An evaluation of surgical management. *Arch. Surg.* 110:527, 1975.
130. Sawyers, J. L., Scott, H. W., Jr., Wimberly,

J. E., and Green, J. W. Is it necessary to excise the duodenal ulcer with a Billroth I anastomosis? *Am. Surg.* 37:150, 1971.
131. Schiassi, B. M. The role of the pyloroduodenal nerve supply in the surgery of duodenal ulcer. *Ann. Surg.* 81:939, 1925.
132. Schilling, J. A., and Pearse, H. E. Re-evaluation of the role of the pyloric antrum in marginal peptic ulcers. *Surg. Gynecol. Obstet.* 87:225, 1948.
133. Schmitz, E. J., Kanar, E. A., Storer, E. H., et al. The effect of vagotomy of the main stomach on Heidenhain pouch secretions. *Surg. Forum* 3:17, 1952.
134. Schoen, A. M., and Griswold, R. A. The effect of vagotomy in human gastric function. *Ann. Surg.* 126:655, 1947.
135. Schuberth, O., and Westerholm, P. Vagotomy and antral resection in the surgery of duodenal ulcer. *Acta Chir. Scand.* 129:530, 1965.
136. Scott, H. W., Jr., Herrington, J. L., Jr., Edwards, L. W., and Shull, H. J. The hazards of antral exclusion with vagotomy in the surgical treatment of duodenal ulcer. *Ann. Surg.* 151:181, 1960.
137. Scott, H. W., Jr., Sawyers, J. L., Gobbel, W. G., Jr., et al. Vagotomy and antrectomy in surgical treatment of duodenal ulcer disease. *Surg. Clin. North Am.* 46:349, 1966.
138. Scott, H. W., Jr., Weidner, M. G., Shull, H. J., and Bond, A. G. The dumping syndrome: Further investigations in the etiology of patients and experimental animals. *Gastroenterology* 37:194, 1959.
139. Smithwick, R. H., Farmer, D. A., and Harrower, H. W. Hemigastrectomy and truncal vagotomy in the treatment of duodenal ulcer. *Am. J. Surg.* 127:631, 1974.
140. Smithwick, R. H., Harrower, H. W., and Farmer, D. A. Hemigastrectomy and vagotomy in the treatment of duodenal ulcer. *Am. J. Surg.* 101:325, 1961.
141. Stock, F. E., Hui, K. K. L., and Tinckler, L. F. Vagotomy and pylorectomy in the treatment of duodenal ulceration. *Surg. Gynecol. Obstet.* 102:358, 1956.
142. Storer, E. H., Woodward, E. R., and Dragstedt, L. R. The effect of vagotomy and antrum resection on the Mann-Williamson ulcer. *Surgery* 27:526, 1950.
143. Thoroughman, J. C., Walker, L. G., Jr., and Raft, D. A review of 504 patients with peptic ulcer treated by hemigastrectomy and vagotomy. *Surg. Gynecol. Obstet.* 119:257, 1964.
144. Uvnäs, B. The part played by the pyloric region in the cephalic phase of gastric secretion. *Acta Physiol. Scand.* 13(Suppl. 4):42, 1942.
145. Uvnäs, B. The gastric secretory excitant from the pyloric mucosa. *Acta Physiol. Scand.* 6:97, 1943.
146. Uvnäs, B. The presence of a gastric secretory excitant in the human gastric and duodenal mucosa. *Acta Physiol. Scand.* 10:97, 1945.
147. Waddell, W. R. The physiologic significance of retained antral tissue after partial gastrectomy. *Ann. Surg.* 143:520, 1956.
148. Walters, W., and Mobley, J. E. Five- to ten-year follow-up of 162 cases of duodenal ulcer treated by vagotomy with or without associated gastric operation. *A.M.A. Arch. Surg.* 68:163, 1956.
149. Weidner, M. C., Jr., Scott, H. W., Jr., Bond, A. G., and Shull, H. J. The dumping syndrome. I, Studies in patients after gastric surgery. *Gastroenterology* 37:188, 1959.
150. Weinstein, V. A., Colp, R., Hollander, F., and Jemerin, E. E. Vagotomy in the therapy of peptic ulcer. *Surg. Gynecol. Obstet.* 79:297, 1944.
151. Welch, C. E. Personal communication, 1963.
152. Wells, C. A report on the late complications of gastrectomy. *Ann. R. Coll. Surg. Engl.* 16:145, 1955.
153. Winkelstein, A. Some observations on the relationship of the vagus nerve to peptic ulcer. *J. Mt. Sinai Hosp. N. Y.* 9:859, 1942.
154. Winkelstein, A., and Berg, A. A. Vagotomy plus partial gastrectomy for duodenal ulcer. *Am. J. Dig. Dis.* 5:497, 1938.
155. Wolf, J. S., Bell, C. C., and Zimberg, Y. H. Analysis of ten years in experience with surgery for peptic ulcer disease. *Am. Surg.* 38:187, 1972.
156. Woodward, E. R., Bigelow, R. R., and Dragstedt, L. R. Effect of resection of antrum of stomach on gastric secretion in Pavlov pouch dogs. *Am. J. Physiol.* 162:99, 1950.
157. Woodward, E. R., Lyon, E. S., Landor, J., and Dragstedt, L. R. The physiology of the gastric antrum. *Gastroenterology* 27:766, 1954.
158. Woodward, E. R., and Tillmanns, V. C. Mechanism for ulcer recurrence following the antrum exclusion gastrectomy. *Surg. Forum* 6:301, 1955.
159. Zollinger, R. M., and Williams, R. D. Considerations in the surgical treatment of duodenal ulcer. *J.A.M.A.* 160:367, 1956.

160. Zubiran, J. M., Kark, A. E., Montalbetti, A. J., et al. Quantitative studies on the effect of gastrojejunostomy on gastric secretion. *Surg. Forum* 3:5, 1952.

EDITOR'S COMMENT

I am in complete agreement with the authors that "vagotomy with antrectomy is now the standard against which other operations for duodenal ulcer are compared." Of course I would modify the statement to reflect the use of selective vagotomy rather than truncal or total vagotomy. At least 40 percent of the operations performed in the United States today for complications of the duodenal ulcer diathesis are truncal vagotomies with antrectomy, a reflection of its general acceptance.

There has been a major swing away from the surgical treatment of duodenal ulcer toward the medical use of H_2 receptor blockers of acid secretion. It is now clear that this medical approach does not cure the ulcer diathesis. It offers palliation of the symptoms and short-term healing of the ulcer, but when the patient stops taking the medication, the ulcer recurs with its concomitant distress. Vagotomy plus antrectomy removes the ulcer diathesis permanently in 99 percent of patients who undergo the procedure. No intravenous or oral medication has been found to give this guarantee of cure. Surgeons must let patients and fellow physicians know of their ability to cure and not only to palliate duodenal ulcer disease.

I note that Drs. Sawyers and Herrington mention the nerves of Latarjet. That mention reminds me that I had searched for the origin of the eponym *nerves of Latarjet* without success. Professor C. Couinaud and his colleague Dr. Yves Janin of Paris made an analysis of my dilemma and presented the following solution:

> Based on the following facts, it is our opinion that the eponym "nerves of Latarjet" has been persistently suggested, in a subtle way, by Professor A. Latarjet's assistant, Professor P. Wertheimer, and then by Professor A. Latarjet himself.
>
> In his thesis of medicine, published in 1922 under the sponsorship of Professor A. Latarjet, Professor P. Wertheimer [4] is the first author to use Latarjet's name in the description of the anterior and posterior vagal branches to the gastric antrum. He wrote: "We called it the main anterior nerve of the lesser curvature (Latarjet) . . . which constitutes the main posterior nerve of the lesser curvature (Latarjet). . . ."
>
> This description was cited in its entirety by Professor A. Hovelacque [1] in his textbook on the anatomy of the cranial, peripheral, and autonomic nerves, which was published in 1927, and which has been and still is a standard reference on the anatomy of the peripheral nervous system. This is the first textbook in which Latarjet's name was directly associated with the designation of the vagal branches to the gastric antrum.
>
> Having been invited to edit the eighth [2] and ninth [3] editions of Professor L. Testut's textbook of anatomy, which is the most famous French reference book on human anatomy, Professor A. Latarjet implicitly associated his name with the designation of the vagal fibers that innervate the gastric antrum. He wrote: "The last is the most voluminous, it is the main anterior nerve of the lesser curvature (Latarjet). . . . It constitutes the main posterior nerve of the lesser curvature (Latarjet), homologous of the synonymous anterior nerve."
>
> The last edition of "The Testut" was published in 1949 [3], two years after the death of its last editor, Professor A. Latarjet. It was after this date that the eponym "nerves of Latarjet" started to be commonly used to describe the vagal fibers that innervate the gastric antrum.

L.M.N.

Comment References

1. Hovelacque, A. *Anatomie des nerfs craniens et rachidiens et du systeme grand sympathique*. Paris: G. Doin & Co., 1927. Pp. 243–4.
2. Testut, L., and Latarjet, A. *Traite d'anatomie humaine* (8th ed.), Vol. 3. Paris: G. Doin & Co., 1930. P. 186.
3. Testut, L., and Latarjet, A. *Traite d'anatomie humaine* (9th ed.), Vol. 3. Paris: G. Doin & Co., 1949. Pp. 182, 184.
4. Wertheimer, P. L'innervation et l'enervation gastriques: Etude anatomique, experimentale et clinique. *These Med.* 149:27, 1922.

V

Special Problems

15

Massive Upper Gastrointestinal Hemorrhage

Philip E. Donahue
Lloyd M. Nyhus

A pale, apprehensive 50-year-old man has just been admitted to the hospital ward. The patient has moist skin and a rapid pulse, and he has just soiled the clean bed linen with vomitus of bright red or coffee ground-colored liquid. A true medical emergency exists.

The literature is replete with suggestions as to the course of action, yet the mortality for medical and surgical management of this condition remains high. The overall mortality for massive hemorrhage from peptic ulcer treated by medical therapy alone is 10 percent, and although not entirely comparable, the mortality for early emergency surgical intervention (within the first 48 hours) is reported to be the same [36]. Not all authors would agree that the mortality figures are so similar; for example, Brown and his associates [20] reported that in a group of massive bleeders the mortality following medical treatment alone was 86 percent, while surgical treatment incurred a mortality of 18 percent. Likewise, Miller [147] found that medically treated patients who required blood transfusions had a mortality of 52.9 percent in contrast to a similar group of patients treated surgically, who had a mortality of 27.9 percent. Hemorrhage as a complication of peptic ulcer occurs in approximately 25 percent of instances [36] and is the most frequent cause of death from peptic ulcer, responsible for 46 percent of ulcer-related deaths [223].

Definition of Massive Hemorrhage

It is important to understand completely what is meant by massive hemorrhage. We consider massive hemorrhage to be present when the estimated rapid blood loss is in excess of 1000 ml (in an adult). For individuals of small body mass, the figure of 1000 ml is not absolute; anyone with a loss of 30 percent of his or her circulating blood volume has sustained massive hemorrhage. The average blood volume for adults is 70 ml per kilogram of ideal weight (80 ml per kilogram for young children).

Several factors indicate blood loss of the 30 percent magnitude: shock alone; severe orthostatic hypotension (a fall of 15 mmHg or more in the systolic blood pressure on assuming the upright position) [74, 192, 227]; and, of course, a large volume of blood passed by mouth or rectum measured directly. Specific laboratory data indicating hemorrhage would be a fall of the hematocrit or hemoglobin value (each 500 ml of blood lost will result in a fall of approximately 3 hematocrit points, or 1 gm of hemoglobin).

Diagnosis

SIMULTANEOUS DIAGNOSTIC AND THERAPEUTIC MEASURES

A complete history should be deferred until the immediate emergency is over, but all data pertinent to the illness causing bleeding must be obtained as early as possible. Of particular interest in the past medical history are symptoms of ulcer diathesis, alcohol abuse, cardiovascular disease, or bleeding tendency. A medication history is essential as well; increasing numbers of people are undergoing long-term anticoagulant therapy or therapy with drugs irritating to the mucosa, and treatment of the hemorrhage may be hampered unless the use of such drugs is taken into account.

Physical examination is performed as soon as feasible, with the patient in the supine position. A rapid systematic approach will establish the physiological status of the patient. The pulse rate and character, the blood pressure, the presence or absence of neck vein distention, and the state of peripheral capillary perfusion are noted in the first moments. These quickly provide information about the effective blood volume, which will guide the pace of further maneuvers. If marked abnormalities are present, the physician should hasten to begin resuscitation while completing the physical examination.

All clothing is removed with appropriate attention to the sensitivities of the patient. The patient's general physical condition, especially the peripheral vascular system, and any signs of vascular insufficiency, can be easily noted. The chest and heart are examined next; the presence of cardiac murmurs or extra heart sounds may be an indication of serious heart disease. The abdomen when examined may reveal clues to the underlying disorder: Ascites, spider nevi, hepatosplenomegaly, or masses are all important. Although a bruit in the epigastrium may be heard in healthy persons, it may signal a large abdominal aneurysm. Next, the genitalia and the rectum are examined. Bright red blood in the rectum often indicates rapid transit from the upper gastrointestinal tract, and it can appear within 15 minutes from a gastric source; in this setting auscultation of the abdomen would reveal continuous, vigorous peristaltic activity. Melena (tarry stools) indicates less rapid bleeding; the dark color is caused by degradation products of hemoglobin (at first hematin alone, then various porphyrin compounds) as it passes through the intestines.

As the physical examination is completed, enough blood for emergency studies and for crossmatching (30 ml) is drawn through a large-bore catheter. Fluids are transfused as the situation dictates; the best guide to fluid therapy is clinical experience in the care of such patients. The pressing need is restoration of blood volume, and the best solutions for this purpose are isotonic saline solutions; 2 units of albumin may be added initially for its colloid osmotic effect in debilitated patients.

A Foley catheter is inserted in any massively bleeding patient so that urine volumes can be measured precisely; in most hemorrhaging patients central venous pressure monitoring is also beneficial. We list the insertion of a nasogastric tube as the last of the diagnostic steps because the violent emesis that often ensues will further stress the patient, and it will be better tolerated if fluid resuscitation has already begun (actually two large intravenous routes should have been established, with care to ensure that they are not dislodged by any means).

When the nasogastric tube is being inserted, the decision about which tube to use depends on the situation: If bleeding is massive, an Ewald tube or similar large-bore tube will facilitate the evacuation of clots from the stomach. About 80 percent of individuals with massive bleeding will stop bleeding if the stomach can be adequately emptied of clots and ice-water lavage can be instituted. If coffee ground-colored emesis is the sign of bleeding, a smaller nasogastric tube will suffice for irrigating the stomach.

The Diagnostic Process

Thus resuscitation has begun; the pace of diagnostic and therapeutic maneuvers will vary as the rapidity of bleeding and response to initial therapy are seen. At this point, no matter what response is occurring, a tabular hemorrhage sheet as advocated by Elliot et al. [54] should be started (Fig. 15-1). A supply of these forms should be accessible in the emergency suite or in the intensive care unit.

WHICH PATIENTS STOP BLEEDING—HOW MANY CONTINUE?

In most patients the bleeding will cease after the measures outlined previously have been employed. However, of 1400 patients studied prospectively, 16.1 percent required emergency surgical treatment [159]; another series revealed that of 585 patients studied, 22 percent required operation [233]. Therefore, it is still true that many individuals with massive upper gastrointestinal bleeding will require operative therapy. Although it is not always possible to predict which patients will eventually require an operation, it is possible to determine with some accuracy the source of hemorrhage. The evolution of this diagnostic process is best appreciated by considering specific potential bleeding sites. The common causes of bleeding are mucosal or submucosal lesions relating to benign and malignant diseases (Fig. 15-2). The following section illustrates the mechanics of diagnosis. A consideration of the historical approach to upper gastrointestinal tract hemorrhage also is in order; this perspective shows the logic of current approaches to diagnosis and therapy.

The Patient's History

Maloney [135] reemphasized the old dictum that "70 percent of useful diagnostic information comes from the history, 20 percent from the physical exam, and only 10 percent from laboratory tests." Unfortunately for the diagnostician and the patient, a history of duodenal ulcer or even a history of previous bleeding from an ulcer does not exclude other possible causes of bleeding (Fig. 15-2).

Presence of Esophageal Varices

Even when the stigmata of portal hypertension, such as enlarged spleen or liver, abdominal wall venous collateral circulation, "liver" palms, or spider telangiectases are apparent on physical examination, there is no guarantee that known varices are actively bleeding. The barium meal examination does not provide evidence of the presence of varices in as many as 50 percent of patients later found to have definite varices. Hirschowitz et al. [92] pointed out the superiority of the flexible esophagoscope for this examination, and the flexible scopes have now become so refined that examination of the stomach and proximal duodenum can be accomplished routinely.

BIOCHEMICAL TESTS OF LIVER FUNCTION. The Bromsulphalein-retention liver function test has been suggested as a reliable method for determining liver disease severe enough to cause esophageal varices. Zamcheck et al. [235] in a group of 61 patients observed that normal Bromsulphalein (BSP) retention (5 percent or less) excluded the possibility of liver disease, and a high retention (15 percent or greater) indicated the possibility of serious liver disease. Enquist et al. [55] found much less correlation between the BSP test and liver disease. These authors used the test in 382 patients with upper gastrointestinal bleeding to detect unsuspected liver disease. Of 66 patients with abnormal tests, more than half had normal livers. When Belkin and Conn [10] studied both BSP retention and blood ammonia concentration in patients with upper gastrointestinal tract hemorrhage, they stated that "the concurrence of elevated blood ammonia and BSP levels (higher than 150 micrograms per 100 ml and 15 percent, respectively) was practically diagnostic of cirrhosis." These tests were of little value if only one determination was elevated and the other was normal.

At present, the Bromsulphalein test has no practical role in the acutely bleeding patient. The test itself is associated with a number of

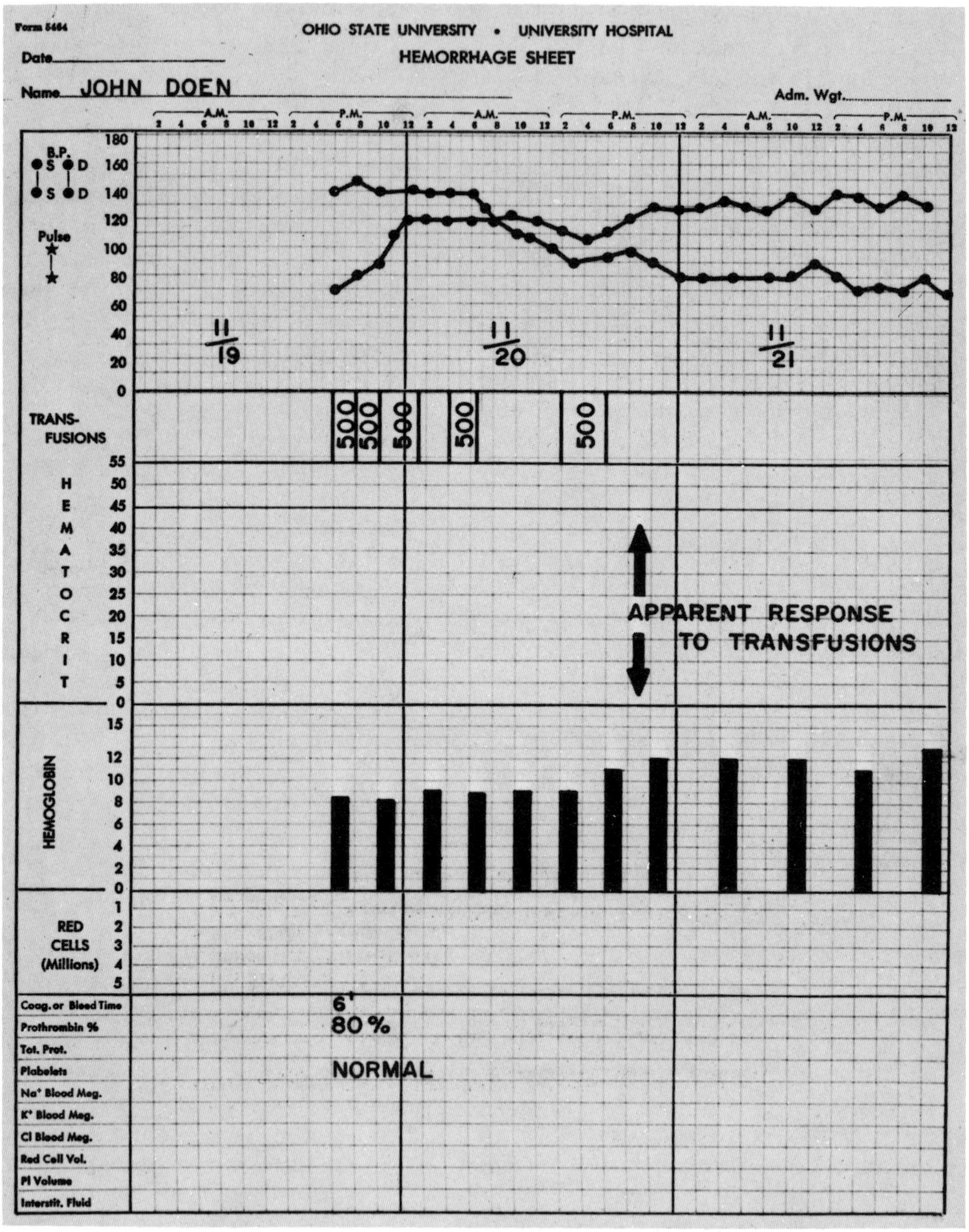

Fig. 15-1. A "Hemorrhage Sheet" helps in giving accurate replacement transfusions by combining, in one place, pulse rate, systolic blood pressure, pints of blood given and time when given, and hemoglobin response. The arrow points to first evidence of response to transfusion therapy. (From Elliott et al. [54]. Copyright 1958, American Medical Association.)

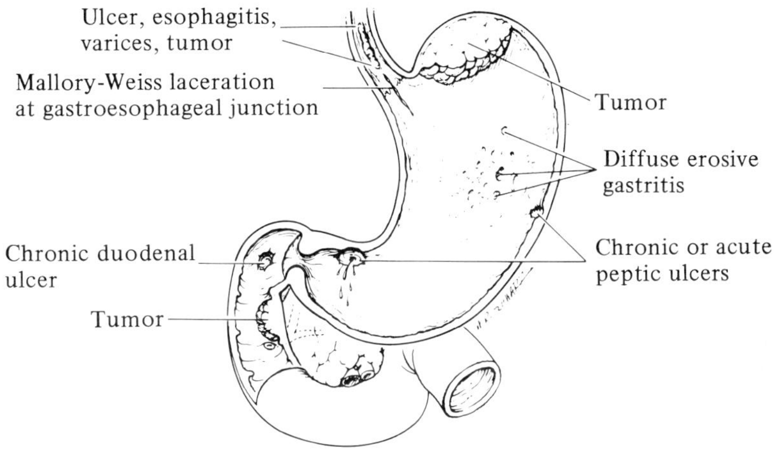

Fig. 15-2. Bleeding commonly originates in lesions visible through the flexible fiberoptic gastroscope. Even if no specific lesion is seen, valuable negative evidence is obtained, such as the absence of esophageal varices, diffuse gastritis, and duodenal ulcer. Endoscopy should be performed as a first priority.

disadvantages: Extravasation of dye may cause serious local inflammation; occasional allergic reactions may ensue; the test is so sensitive that there are many false positive findings; and, finally (in this context), it is only an indirect indication that varices may be present.

ESOPHAGOSCOPY. In contrast to all of these methods, the efficacy of modern endoscopes in establishing the presence or absence of esophageal varices is high; most important, the critical information as to whether or not they are the source of bleeding is obtained. Because of this fact, the diagnostic approach has shifted toward early endoscopy. Previously the demonstration that an early barium examination of the esophagus, stomach, and duodenum would not harm the patient [157] was considered an important advance. Emergency barium studies have led to the diagnosis in as many as 50 percent of the patients in whom the source of bleeding was in the stomach or the duodenum; however, 50 percent accuracy does not meet modern diagnostic standards. When gastroscopy before laparotomy was reported by Tanner and Desmond [213], the preoperative accuracy increased to 90 percent. Jones and King [108] showed the efficacy of gastroscopy in making a certain diagnosis of superficial gastric ulcers or mucosal lesions. Chandler et al. [24] were able to demonstrate mucosal abnormalities in 55 percent of patients suspected of bleeding from acute lesions. These are some of the earlier approaches that were applied in the diagnosis of upper gastrointestinal bleeding. Refinement and further evolution of these techniques are the cornerstone of the diagostic study of the patient with upper gastrointestinal hemorrhage.

Some Outmoded Approaches

Emergency splenic punctures for pressure studies [75, 183] had disparate results in attempting correlation between splenic pulp pressures and the site of bleeding; these are rarely used today. The Einhorn string test [52] as modified by Traphagen and Karlan [218] used a fluorescein marker injected intravenously, which would mark a swallowed umbilical tape at the bleeding site. Haynes and Pittman [83] and Reisberg and Haubrich [171] confirmed the efficacy of this test. Healey et al. [84] used radiophosphorous-labeled red cells plus Geiger-Müller counters placed in a Cantor tube. Another technique that employs the multi-lumen tube had been introduced, first with quadruple lumen [162] and then with triple lumen [151] tubes, but use of such tubes never became widespread; technical factors plus misinterpretations of the results combined to make these techniques of limited applicability for most practitioners.

Endoscopy—The First Priority
The history is helpful in only half the patients, and it may be misleading in others. Esophagoscopy and gastroscopy employed in selected patients [108] have shown that bleeding from superficial gastric erosions could be distinguished from gastric ulcer bleeding by use of the rigid endoscope. The next development, routine use of flexible fiberoptic endoscopes, might have been predicted to have an exciting impact on the diagnostic approach to upper gastrointestinal tract hemorrhage. It has lived up to these predictions, with many series of patients now reported in which there has been 90 percent (or better) accuracy in locating the source of gastrointestinal bleeding. A subgroup of patients has been identified in whom the risk of rebleeding is so high that endoscopic control [45, 88] of the potential bleeding point is recommended. The risk of rebleeding in these patients who have a visible vessel in the base of the ulcer is between 50 and 70 percent and warrants an aggressive plan of management [121, 161, 207]. When no bleeding point is seen, valuable negative information (e.g., regarding the presence of esophageal varices or diffuse gastric lesions) is obtained [149, 232].

It is recommended, therefore, that endoscopy of the upper gastrointestinal tract be performed as soon as feasible during the episode of bleeding; this examination takes precedence over the barium meal examination [219]. Upper gastrointestinal bleeding is one of the few indications for performing endoscopic examination before obtaining barium studies.

Finally, it must be recognized that routine endoscopic examinations may not influence the overall morbidity in a population of patients with massive upper gastrointestinal hemorrhage. Indeed, in several large studies in major medical centers this conclusion has been reached [28, 164]. Each study, however, has its own peculiarities, such as "escape clauses" and exclusions, and at present no conclusion can be universally supported. On the other hand, we are now aware of endoscopic findings that greatly influence management (the visible vessel) and are only beginning to see widespread application of the therapeutic techniques described later. Perhaps the major shortcoming of the previous studies was the failure to consider that endoscopic control of hemorrhage would become a practical reality.

Specific Problem Areas Aided by Endoscopic Data
Advances in the management of specific causes of hemorrhage have been heartening to the clinical surgeon. The surgeon is no longer obliged to do a blind subtotal gastrectomy for someone with undiagnosed bleeding, and he or she does not have to perform an urgent portacaval shunt on a patient with known esophageal varices who has bled from a duodenal ulcer. Both of these problems occurred typically before the development of endoscopy but now are routinely avoided if the bleeding point can be localized preoperatively.

In addition to identification of the bleeding lesion, the routine use of endoscopy has allowed us to assess the frequency of acute gastric mucosal lesions accompanying stressful situations of differing causes. In all these situations the advantages of endoscopic examination are obvious; in the few years since its introduction endoscopy has become indispensable.

Therapeutic Endoscopy
All of the presently successful endoscopic means of controlling hemorrhage function according to the same principle: that blood ceases to flow in a vessel once the local temperature exceeds a critical point [193]. The possible means of achieving this goal include monopolar and bipolar coagulation probes and several laser devices. At this time it is clear that each of these techniques can be effective and that surgical procedures that would have been necessary in the past are being postponed until the patient is in better condition,

or avoided altogether. The era of therapeutic endoscopy has matured so during the past five years that we generally recognize the efficacy and usefulness of this approach in the control of patients with upper gastrointestinal tract hemorrhage.

ELECTROCOAGULATION. The experimental reports of Blackwood and Silvis [15] demonstrated the feasibility of performing transendoscopic electrocoagulation without significant morbidity. Sugawa et al. [210] expanded this work experimentally by applying electrocoagulation to experimental bleeding sites, and they reported as well the successful clinical use of this technique in six patients (three with gastritis and one each with gastric ulcer, bleeding polyp, and Mallory-Weiss syndrome). Gaisford [67] reported a series of 20 patients with acute upper gastrointestinal hemorrhage treated with transendoscopic electrocoagulation, and Papp [160] successfully stopped hemorrhage in 55 of 58 patients, most of whom had duodenal or gastric ulcers (44 of 58) or Mallory-Weiss tears (11 of 58). The success of electrocoagulation in controlling bleeding has led to the current attitude that bleeding or visible vessels should be coagulated whenever encountered. It is true that coagulation does not cure ulcerations per se, but if a bleeding vessel can be stopped, an ulcer bed can eventually heal. Similarly, patients with acute gastric mucosal lesions that continue to bleed can be successfully coagulated; in these patients the primary problem, whether sepsis, stress, or hypotension, can be adequately treated in the interim. Since surgical procedures performed to control acute bleeding from the gastrointestinal tract have a high morbidity, especially in the elderly, these new techniques may become as much a part of therapy as fiberoptic endoscopy has become part of the diagnostic study [45, 88].

LASER COAGULATION. Cauterizing with laser light delivered by flexible fiberoptic systems has been shown to be effective experimentally in preliminary reports [50, 71, 222, 234] and has been applied in a few selected instances in human beings. It is hard to predict the eventual role of lasers in the control of gastrointestinal bleeding; while lasers offer an interesting technique, the results appear similar to those achieved with endoscopic cauterization. Perhaps further study of the capabilities of lasers and clinical trials will demonstrate their real merit in the next decade.

ENDOSCOPIC SCLEROTHERAPY FOR ESOPHAGEAL VARICES. As discussed in a later section, sclerosing solutions can be injected into the lumina of bleeding varicose veins of the esophagus. Injection techniques in these challenging patients have been extremely useful.

Selective Visceral Angiography

DIAGNOSIS OF BLEEDING. Angiographic demonstration of bleeding in the gastrointestinal tract has been widely applied since it was introduced by Nusbaum and Baum [153]. The technique is a sensitive one, and rates of bleeding between 0.5 ml and 2 ml per minute can be demonstrated. There are two categories of patients in whom angiography may be useful: First, there are those with obscure bleeding points; second, there are those who are not "fortunate" enough to bleed when an endoscopist is available. Anastomotic ulcers, or lesions in areas relatively "blind" for the endoscopist (such as the lesser curvature of the antrum, high on the lesser curvature of the stomach, or the medial portion of the proximal duodenum) may be difficult to demonstrate convincingly by other techniques and are routinely shown by angiography if they are bleeding sufficiently at the time of the study. (If the lesion has stopped bleeding at the time, it may be well to leave the catheter in place and to have it perfused for 24 hours to facilitate reexamination or infusion of vasopressin should further bleeding occur.) If endoscopists are not available to pinpoint the bleeding area before the operation, specific identification of the bleeding artery by angiography (e.g., the left gastric artery) can guide the surgeon to the pathology, especially if previous operations have obliterated tissue planes. Additionally, bleeding in certain areas may suggest the next therapeutic maneuver. For example, multiple small bleeding points in the distribution of the left gastric artery may suggest infusion of vasoconstricting agents as therapy, while a leaking aortoduodenal fistula is clearly an indication for surgical treatment.

Therapeutic Angiography
The Seldinger technique of percutaneous angiography was first developed as a diagnostic tool, but as experience with selective angiography grew, therapeutic applications were developed and tested. These applications comprise a valuable addition to the techniques available for caring for gastrointestinal bleeding problems.

VASOPRESSIN INFUSION. Variceal bleeding associated with portal hypertension has been successfully treated by systemically (intravenously) administered vasopressin [188, 191]. The ability of vasopressin to lower portal pressure has been established for many years, but adverse effects have been noted. These side effects—arrhythmias or decreased renal blood flow, or both—are largely avoided when the drug is given by selective visceral infusion [154]. (It should be noted that a paper [102] given to the American Surgical Association in March of 1977 reported that because of reduced complexity of administration, decreased morbidity, and equal efficacy in control of bleeding by the systemic route, vasopressin is best given by continuous peripheral intravenous administration for control of bleeding esophageal varices.)

While systemic vasopressin was initially used for the control of variceal bleeding, it was quickly recognized that bleeding from a variety of sources could be controlled by selective visceral infusion. Baum et al. [9], in treating 160 patients, were able to control bleeding from esophageal varices, esophagitis, esophageal tumors, gastric and duodenal ulcers, anastomotic ulcer, gastritis, and tumors of the stomach. No patient had to have the infusion stopped because of cardiac arrhythmia or clinical evidence of decreasing cardiac output. Although half the patients had four or more days of infusions, there was no thrombosis at the site of puncture. Rau et al. [168] successfully diagnosed 26 (63 percent) of 41 patients with acute gastrointestinal bleeding. Selective infusion of vasopressin was successful in treating 12 of the 18 patients in whom it was attempted. Frey et al. [66] had previously been able to control bleeding in 56 (58 percent) of 95 patients with bleeding from a variety of sources.

Although all investigators can relate a number of spectacular episodes in which vasopressin infusion has proved worthwhile, there has been some concern about its role in the management of patients with massive gastrointestinal hemorrhage. The prospective controlled trial of Conn et al. [31] nicely illustrated some of these concerns. For example, the survival rate of vasopressin-treated patients did not differ from the survival rate of those who received conventional treatment. Furthermore, 12 of 29 successfully treated patients bled again within one week of treatment, and 7 of these 12 died. The conclusion was drawn that intra-arterial infusion of vasopressin did not completely eliminate lethal hemorrhage, although it could provide temporary control that would convert an emergency situation to a semi-elective one. In Conn's study [31] the transfusion requirements of the vasopressin group were significantly less, which demonstrates another tangible benefit from infusion. Considering all the findings, however, it seems that infusion of vasoconstricting agents is not as completely effective a technique as was once hoped.

SELECTIVE EMBOLIZATION. Control of the bleeding point with infused vasopressin has been only temporarily effective in certain lesions and relatively ineffective in others, such as massively bleeding duodenal ulcers. An alternative technique for controlling hemorrhage is selective embolization of the bleeding vessel, which was first introduced in 1972 [178]. Clotted autogenous blood, small bits of Gelfoam [111], and other materials have been embolized in this manner with dramatic success at times, especially in areas such as the duodenum, where the success rate of vasopressin infusion is relatively low. Because the duodenum has a rich collateral blood supply, a selective embolization might be directed entirely into the liver, pancreas, or elsewhere, depending on local blood flow at the precise moment of injection. One ingenious method for dealing with this problem is to use an occluding balloon near the tip of the catheter to prevent the embolized material from traveling retrograde through the catheterized artery. Eisenberg and Steer [53] reported an incident of multiple hepatic infarcts complicating embolization of the gastroduodenal artery in their report of six patients with massive pyloroduodenal hemorrhage. Of interest is their note of caution regarding embolization of less richly vascularized areas. In one well-documented instance, gastric infarction complicated therapeutic embolization in a setting of compromised circulation to the gastric remnant [18]. Caution in application of this technique is certainly warranted, but the potential benefits of this approach in selected instances are obvious.

RADIONUCLIDE ANGIOGRAPHY. Technetium-labeled red blood cells have found an application in some unique situations. The usefulness of this method is related to the fact that the sensitivity of detecting bleeding is quite high, with rates of 0.2 ml/min routinely recorded in the laboratory, and, since labeled cells remain in the circulation for more than 24 hours, an intermittent source of bleeding can be discovered by serial scans of the abdomen [21, 145, 163]. McKusick et al. [145] reported an experience with 80 patients with varying degrees of gastrointestinal hemorrhage. Only 8 of the 51 positive studies became positive within 15 minutes, while 16 became positive within 12 to 24 hours. In McKusick's roentgenographic unit, furthermore, the radionuclide scan is so sensitive that it is used before any attempt at emergency selective angiography, based on the premise that a negative radionuclide scan indicates a nonactive bleeding site, which contraindicates emergent angiography.

Treatment

EMERGENCY MEASURES

1. The physical examination and initial assessment previously described must be completed (see page 422).
2. A large-bore needle (No. 16 or greater) is inserted into an available vein, and 30 ml of blood is withdrawn for emergency studies (see No. 6 below). Available plasma expanders are infused as dictated by the situation; saline solution, lactated Ringer's solution, fresh plasma, or serum albumin are ordinarily used while awaiting whole blood. If unable to find a vein, the physician must proceed to a cutdown or central venipuncture without delay; the primary physician must establish a large intravenous line without delay by the most effective technique with which he or she is familiar.
3. The rate of fluid infusion is important, and it will depend on the specific patient's condition; overt shock demands rapid infusion of 500–1000 ml of fluid (or more), with further treatment depending on the response to the first liter of fluid. Central venous pressure determinations are helpful in gauging the response, especially in the elderly, in those with history of myocardial infarction, or in those with concomitant chest pain [101].
4. If the patient is hypotensive, the legs are elevated on a folded blanket, or the foot of the bed is elevated. Hypotensive patients require expansion of the plasma volume by saline solution, albumin, or whole blood. The use of vasoconstrictors in this setting only aggravates an already serious problem.
5. Insertion of a Foley catheter is mandatory. There are so many possible problems that are avoided by the accurate measurement of urine output that the moderate risk of infection is acceptable. The urine output is the most reliable indicator of the state of hydration, and it serves as the guide to fluid therapy.
6. The 30 ml of blood is sent to the laboratories for typing and crossmatching; serum chemistries (at least sodium, potassium, chloride, carbon dioxide, creatinine, and glucose; bilirubin as indicated); prothrombin and partial thromboplastin time determinations; and platelet count. If any of the clotting studies are abnormal, the remaining blood specimen should be saved in the coagulation laboratory for future determinations of fibrinogen, fibrin split products,

or other special clotting factors as indicated. One tube of blood will remain, and this is saved as an additional tube for the blood bank if required and as a convenient, visible way of checking clot retraction.

7. The surgical team should be notified of the situation so that arrangements can be made for any necessary action. Coordination of the complex team required to care for massively bleeding patients is indeed a challenge for the most experienced clinicians; in most settings the general surgeon is the logical supervisor of these activities.
8. A portable chest roentgenogram and electrocardiogram should be obtained as soon as possible. The patient must *not* be sent off to the roentgenography department without continuous supervision of the intravenous infusions and the patient's condition. So many patients have their intravenous bottles go dry, begin bleeding again, or have other difficulties that it is probably unwise to send them anywhere except to an intensive care unit.
9. Blood pressure and pulse should be checked at least every 30 minutes. Shock must be avoided; the vital signs and urine output are the guides to success or failure of therapy.
10. Lavage of the stomach is begun with iced saline solution.

    If bleeding diminishes within 30 to 45 minutes, as it will in most patients, then a conservative approach is indicated; if bleeding is brisk, perhaps an emergency surgical procedure will be required.
11. Flexible fiberoptic endoscopic examination is the next logical step in the care of this patient. The procedure should be performed by someone who is expert in the total management of the bleeding patient and who can determine whether or not the bleeding lesion will require surgical therapy. Ideally, the equipment for sclerosis of esophageal varices or coagulation of an active bleeding point (or visible vessel) will be available.

    In many patients the efficacy of selective visceral angiography in controlling massive upper gastrointestinal hemorrhage has been impressive; Athanasoulis et al. [6] controlled such bleeding in 31 of 37 of their patients by using this method. Effective as it is, however, the personnel required for performance of these studies are not generally available in all hospitals on a 24-hour basis.

    Whichever technique is used, there is general agreement that barium has no place in the diagnosis of massive upper gastrointestinal bleeding. Barium in the stomach will hamper endoscopy and obscure angiography as well.
12. Administer blood as necessary to keep the hematocrit reading at 30 percent or higher and the blood pressure normal. At times it may be necessary to give type-specific or universal donor (type O, Rh negative) blood to a patient in extremis with catastrophic hemorrhage; these situations are unusual, but they occur from time to time. Only the physician who has defined for himself or herself the type of situation demanding this approach will have the courage to employ it.

CONSERVATIVE MANAGEMENT

Fortunately a high percentage (75 percent [215]) of patients with moderate or massive hemorrhage will stop bleeding on conservative management. Thus all patients presenting with these signs and symptoms should first be treated conservatively. While recognizing this as a general rule, we must also be thoroughly cognizant of the problems that may develop under medical management. Although many patients will stop bleeding, it must be remembered that the first hemorrhage is usually the most severe and is attended by the highest mortality of all bleeding episodes. Blackford and Williams [14] reported that in their autopsy series 78 percent of the deaths occurred during the first hemorrhage. Rosenak et al. [179] found the mortality of patients experiencing the initial hemorrhage to be 3 times that of patients having subsequent hemorrhages, and no deaths occurred in the group with third and fourth episodes of bleeding.

In 1959 Mandelbaum and Brackup [136]

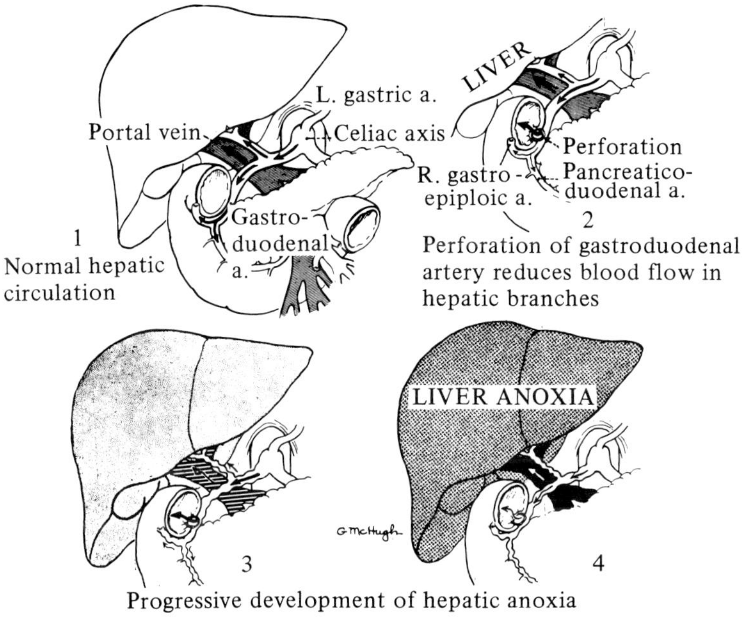

Fig. 15-3. The blood supply to the liver is illustrated. The rates of blood flow are indicated by the sizes of the arrows. The degree of oxygen desaturation in the portal vein and in the liver is indicated by the degree of blackness. When an ulcer erodes into the gastroduodenal artery, hemorrhage into the gastrointestinal tract occurs. The blood flow through the hepatic artery is selectively reduced. As the hemorrhage proceeds toward shock levels, there is a decrease in portal vein oxygen tension and a further reduction in the hepatic artery blood flow. The liver hypoxia is then apparent. Possible spasm of the hepatic artery contributes to the reduction in arterial blood flow. Liver anoxia eventually results from a further reduction in the oxygen saturation of portal vein blood and the almost complete cessation of hepatic arterial flow. (From LeVeen et al. [123]. By permission of *Surgery, Gynecology & Obstetrics.)*

clearly presented the danger of myocardial ischemia during gastrointestinal hemorrhage. They emphasized the frequency of cardiac complications in gastrointestinal hemorrhage and stressed the great importance of detecting these cardiac abnormalities early. Amendola [4] suggested that the epigastric pain associated with severe hemorrhage may well be angina related to the anemia. Experience at the Harper Hospital, Detroit, indicated that 64 percent of the deaths among 254 patients treated medically for upper gastrointestinal bleeding were caused by myocardial infarction or cerebrovascular accident [185].

LeVeen et al. [123] clearly defined another danger inherent in massive hemorrhage from a duodenal ulcer. They demonstrated experimentally that massive hemorrhage arising from the gastroduodenal artery or a large contiguous vessel selectively reduced the hepatic artery blood pressure and blood flow far in excess of that seen in more distal vessels. This reduction of blood flow was greatest when systemic blood pressures reached levels below 100 mmHg. They found that there was a reduction in the oxygen tension of the portal venous blood, which made oxygen from this source unavailable to the liver and resulted in hepatic anoxia (Fig. 15-3). It is their belief that hepatic anoxia is an important factor in the death of patients with massive hemorrhage, and they emphasize that every attempt should be made to maintain a good systemic pressure by transfusion or surgical procedure, or both.

Amaurosis has fortunately become a rare

complication following gastrointestinal hemorrhage. Jones [106] reported on two patients with this tragic complication. He pointed out that recurrent hemorrhage in an already anemic patient sets the stage; the generalized vasoconstriction may affect the optic artery, thus severely restricting the blood supply to the optic nerve. This complication has been stressed particularly in the British literature [80, 175, 215].

What possibility is there of future hemorrhage following the first episode? This consideration becomes most important in borderline situations when one is determining the therapeutic regimen to be employed. Subsequent massive hemorrhage may occur much more frequently than is generally believed. Wilkinson and Tracy [231] reported that 77 percent of all patients whose hemorrhages were managed on a medical regimen subsequently had a massive hemorrhage. Wenckert et al. [229] found that the frequency of recurrent bleeding was 46 percent in gastric ulcer and 53 percent in duodenal ulcer. Donaldson et al. [46] found that 34 (43 percent) of 80 patients living more than five years after the initial hemorrhage had recurrence of bleeding. Probably of more importance, only one-third (47 of 136) of the patients with gastrointestinal bleeding from duodenal ulcer escaped all the following events within five years from the time they were first examined: subtotal gastrectomy, recurrent hemorrhage, death.

Hemorrhage occurs after operative intervention. Boles et al. [16] reported a 15 percent incidence of further hemorrhage in patients surgically treated and followed for four years. Donaldson et al. [46] found that 20 percent of patients with a history of gastrectomy for bleeding had another bleeding episode within five years. Certain observers believe that patients who bleed from peptic ulceration have a definite propensity to bleed again, regardless of the type of therapy [118, 190]. It is stated that about one-third of patients treated by subtotal gastrectomy for exsanguination from peptic ulcer will bleed again in the next 5 to 10 years. This recurrent bleeding may have its source in any portion of the gastrointestinal tract.

All of these general statements attempt to evaluate the effect of discrete variables on the outcome of gastrointestinal hemorrhage. Since these situations are modified by so many variables, the effect of isolated factors is sometimes difficult to discern. We should be aware that computer-assisted comparisons can be helpful in sorting out some of our long-accepted clinical axioms [90, 98].

STEPS IN CONSERVATIVE MANAGEMENT

Feeding and Oral Medications

1. Give *nothing by mouth* if the patient is bleeding from esophageal varices; if he or she is very actively bleeding, is in shock, or is vomiting frequently; or if an early operation (i.e., within 3 hours) is seriously contemplated.
2. Otherwise, give antacids hourly in adequate doses. If bleeding is probably caused by peptic ulcer or erosive gastritis, antacids are indicated. The frequency of antacid administration may be decreased in some patients to 2-hour intervals at night. Milk and milk with cream are not efficient antacids. Unfortunately, the addition of 15(R)-15-methyl prostaglandin E to antacid therapy has no merit in the prophylaxis against gastrointestinal bleeding in seriously ill patients [197]. Therefore, its use in therapy for active bleeding is questioned.
3. Start oral feedings cautiously after 24 hours. If an operation is still being considered, it is best to order a liquid or clear liquid diet. As soon as possible give the patient a regular well-balanced diet, the only limitations being the exclusion of caffeine, alcohol, and of course, fibrous ingredients.
4. Avoid constipation and fecal impaction. Mineral oil or milk of magnesia may be given early. Avoid constipating antacids. After active bleeding has ceased, a gentle tap water enema may be given.

Accessory Medications

1. Morphine and meperidine should be avoided; they are relatively contraindicated because they produce spasm of the upper gastrointestinal tract.

2. Mild sedation is often desirable. Remember that restlessness may be an indication of continuing hemorrhage or anoxemia; therefore, do not oversedate when repair of hypovolemia is what is really needed.
3. Anticholinergic drugs are undesirable immediately after an acute hemorrhage. They are contraindicated in patients with severe cardiac disability, paralytic ileus, pyloric obstruction, prostatic hypertrophy, or glaucoma. Fecal impaction and gastric retention are common sequelae.

Miscellaneous Care

1. Strict bed rest is essential until after all signs of bleeding have ceased.
2. Fluid balance should be watched carefully; urine output should be measured and recorded.
3. A nasogastric tube is helpful in localizing the site of bleeding and can monitor for continuing active bleeding of gastric and esophageal lesions. Full diagnostic use involves proper placement of the tube and positioning of the patient to ensure that blood will be obtained if it is present in the stomach. The nasogastric tube is left in place both when surgical treatment is considered likely and when distention, obstruction, perforation, or signs of abdominal inflammation are present.

   The nasogastric tube is also a convenient route for irrigating the stomach with antacids to minimize the chances of further bleeding from gastritis or other focal mucosal lesions [37]. A typical regimen includes hourly instillation of 30–50 ml of antacid, clamping of the nasogastric tube for 30 minutes, and suctioning and rechecking the pH at the end of the hour. The cycle is then repeated using as much antacid as necessary to keep the pH at 6 or greater. A nasogastric tube is usually not left in place when the patient has esophagitis or gastritis; the presence of a nasogastric tube is always a threat to initiation or exaggeration of esophagitis. Medications and feedings may be given through the nasogastric tube, after which the tube should be clamped.
4. Lowering of the temperature locally may help bleeding to cease because of vasoconstriction, slowing of blood flow, and increasing blood viscosity. If upper gastrointestinal hemorrhage continues unabated for any appreciable time, the institution of local hypothermic measures is strongly recommended. Usually this treatment should be initiated with iced saline gastric lavage given through a round-tipped Ewald tube. At least 2 liters of iced saline solution should be infused and recovered per hour. After the stomach has been thoroughly cleaned of old clots by this procedure, more prolonged cooling is most conveniently accomplished by use of an inlying gastric hypothermic balloon, which may be left in from 20 to 40 hours. In the presence of bleeding varices, tamponade of the cardia can be effected simultaneously by this device if it is placed with proper tension [44, 176, 187]. Hypothermia has continued to be quite successful at times in the treatment of upper gastrointestinal bleeding [224]. Himal et al. [89] reported success in 22 of 26 patients that had acute gastric erosions of differing causes. Though successful, hypothermia is generally confused with gastric freezing and therefore summarily dismissed. Perhaps it should be more frequently employed.
5. By tamponading the bleeding point, the Sengstaken-Blakemore tube [189] has been effective in temporarily controlling acute variceal hemorrhage. Although the tube has been associated with major complications, modifications that minimize the risk of pulmonary aspiration have been developed; the use of these tubes in acutely hemorrhaging varices is the treatment of choice [165] provided the accuracy of diagnosis has been checked by endoscopic means. Use of the Linton tube [128] is another application of the technique of tamponade of bleeding points by intraluminal balloon. While tamponade techniques have been widely and successfully applied in the management of variceal bleeding and Mallory-Weiss tears, they have not been widely used for the control of bleeding from duodenal ulcer.

Guevara et al. [77] and Zimmon [236] have reported successful control of bleeding duodenal ulcer by the tamponade technique, and they suggest that it may be helpful in selected patients. Even though at present there is only a minor role for balloon compression of a bleeding point in the duodenum, one can easily envision a circumstance in which it might be helpful. The device consists of a triple-lumen tube equipped with two balloons. The distal balloon is inflated after being passed into the duodenum, and then it is pulled back. The second (proximal) balloon is inflated as the first is pulled taut against the pylorus, thereby preventing peristalsis from pulling the first balloon distally.

Continuing Hemorrhage

As previously mentioned, most of the patients stop bleeding; treatments are then directed at the primary source of bleeding if a precise diagnosis has been made. The record of modern upper gastrointestinal endoscopy in this area is impressive and gratifying, with 90–95 percent of bleeding sites correctly diagnosed after initial emergency endoscopy. The ability to apply specific, proper therapy for these problems is an advantage to all concerned.

If hemorrhage continues, endoscopic or angiographic capabilities (which vary widely with the institution) may provide invaluable assistance in the diagnostic and treatment plan. If these are not available, a more pragmatic approach must be taken, with the attendant difficulties in precise diagnosis.

OBSERVATIONS FOR POSSIBLE CONTINUING HEMORRHAGE.[1] The following measures are taken when continuing hemorrhage is possible:

1. Pulse and blood pressure are checked every 30 minutes, hourly, or every 2 hours for the first 24 hours in accordance with the condition of the patient, and thereafter at intervals as designated. Whereas these data are of the utmost importance, the attending physician's general clinical impression of the patient's condition may be of even greater value when further hemorrhage is suspected. Frequent abdominal auscultation is helpful. Persistence of turbulent peristalsis, apart from that which accompanies the taking of food or liquid, suggests continuing hemorrhage; absence suggests cessation of hemorrhage [72]. As the blood volume approaches normal, the blood pressure rises; the pulse slows; the peripheral venous pressure returns so that veins become more apparent; the blood pressure is maintained on sitting; and, finally, the patient can stand without symptoms or a marked fall in blood pressure. Once the blood volume has reached normal, changes in blood pressure and pulse are often the most sensitive indexes of further bleeding.
2. All stools and vomitus passed should be seen by a member of the house staff or by the attending physician. The amount and character of each should be recorded in the nursing notes.
3. The hematocrit reading should be repeated once or twice daily until stools are grossly normal in appearance and thereafter occasionally until the stools are negative by guaiac testing. Hematocrit changes are not an early indication of change in blood volume, since 6-10 hours may be required for significant dilution. However, serial hematocrit reading (e.g., every 6–12 hours) to denote trend are of definite value when properly interpreted. Remember that intravenously administered saline solution or plasma dilutes the hematocrit, while gastrointestinal fluid loss (saline) or inflammatory fluid loss (plasma) increases the hematocrit values.
4. Stools should be checked daily for occult blood by guaiac testing until they are consistently negative. Again, all findings must be regularly documented on the chart.
5. Until the patient is completely out of danger and his or her condition is well stabilized, a daily progress note summarizing the above points should be entered in the hospital record.
6. Overtransfusion is indicated by full neck veins, high venous pressure, and finally, congestive heart failure. It is *very* difficult

[1]Modified from Volwiler and Harkins [220].

to overtransfuse a person with a normal cardiovascular system. With severe heart disease a relatively small increase in blood volume can take a patient from apparent shock into congestive heart failure. This is especially likely to occur when blood loss has been chronic and the amount of acute bleeding has been overestimated. Great skill is required to maintain such a patient between shock and congestive failure, and the use of packed red cells may be indicated. Modern intensive care monitoring of pulmonary capillary wedge pressures, cardiac output, and peripheral resistance offers the most definitive means of determining when fluid therapy is optimal. Since we find that many of our patients with massive hemorrhage are elderly or have major systemic illnesses, it is apparent that many of these individuals must have optimal cardiovascular support.

WHEN IS SURGICAL INTERVENTION INDICATED?

The current recommendations for an emergency or elective operation reflect a combination of the classic criteria used by two generations of general surgeons and the increased ability to diagnose and treat specific lesions with newer modalities. Whereas the classic criteria dealt with the association of mortality with specific clinical signs, the modern approach entails a greater ability to individualize management problems. In the following outline of the classic versus the current approaches, the classic signs are still seen as valuable predictive criteria, and in the final analysis, they often provide the rationale for surgical therapy.

Classic Signs

The classic signs that favor urgent surgical therapy are as follows:

1. *Patient age.* The increasing mortality for major bleeding in patients over 60 years of age was noted by Jones [106], who found that patients less than 60 years old had less than a 6 percent mortality, while those over 60 had a mortality of 10–21 percent. Himal et al. [90], in a multiparametric analysis, found that age greater than 60 was a factor in increased mortality. Jensen et al. [100] found that up to age 70 the mortality for bleeding gastric ulcer was low, but was approximately 30 percent for those more than 70 years of age.
2. *Gastric ulcer.* The increased mortality for bleeding gastric ulcers was documented by Gordon-Taylor [73]; in addition, he showed that age greater than 50 or any narrowing of the gastric outlet bode unfavorably for cessation of bleeding and that recurrence of bleeding in a patient under good medical control was an indication for surgical treatment. A certain number of patients with gastric ulcer will stop bleeding shortly after admission. These individuals are at risk for a second hemorrhage at a later date if the ulcer fails to heal or recurs. Smith and Farris [200] found that 45 percent of such patients will have a second hemorrhage, will require operation, or will die of complications within five years, regardless of the age of the patient when the hemorrhage occurs.
3. *Duration of ulcer history.* It is clear that a chronic ulcer with excessive fibrous tissue surrounding the arteries that course below it has a propensity for repeated and protracted hemorrhage. The vessels in question are sclerotic, contract poorly, and commonly fail to stop bleeding.
4. *Visible vessel in ulcer base seen through the endoscope.* Either coagulation or surgical therapy should be planned.

General Approach

Finsterer [60] outlined a specific plan for particular patients. His approach has two major tenets.

1. If a patient is admitted with a massive gastroduodenal hemorrhage and is known to be suffering from a chronic peptic ulcer, immediate surgical intervention is undertaken.
2. If a patient is admitted with a massive gastroduodenal hemorrhage and has no history of chronic peptic ulceration, he or she is treated conservatively, but a repetition of

bleeding or persistent bleeding is an indication for surgical exploration.

Tanner and Desmond [213] lowered mortality from a high of 20 percent to 7 percent when they adopted Finsterer's approach in a series of 183 patients. Stewart et al. [205], in a well-controlled study, operated on every patient with accurately measured massive hemorrhage and reported a mortality of 11 percent. Since then Stewart [204] has used this approach routinely in more than 300 patients, with exceptional success. Read et al. [170] in a randomized study of massive bleeding from peptic ulceration, had no deaths among patients operated on early—within 5 hours (average) of hospital admission. Mortality in control group ulcer patients, operated on after a delay of 32 hours (average), was 23 percent (30 percent, surgical mortality).

Adequate Transfusion

This is the sine qua non of initial treatment. Emphasis must be placed on *adequate* transfusion, for there is a tendency for blood replacement to be given on the basis of the presence or absence of shock instead of attempting to raise the blood volume levels to nearly normal or to raise the hematocrit reading to 35–40 percent. To have a margin of safety in the event of increased hemorrhage or recurrence of hemorrhage, it is imperative that the patient be adequately transfused.

In a superb study by Weber et al. [226] it was conclusively shown that early replacement of lost blood is imperative. Under the conditions of their study, it was found that by giving sufficient blood to restore the circulating red cell mass rapidly (caution being taken in patients suspected of having limited cardiac reserve), significant improvement in the end result could be attained.

Costello [35] clearly demonstrated the value of adequate blood transfusions. He reported a 25 percent mortality in 300 patients who had been given extremely small quantities of blood. Subsequently, 70 patients were adequately transfused; the mortality was only 4 percent, and 49 (70 percent) of these 70 patients had reached or passed the fifth decade of life. Devitt et al. [42] studied 50 consecutive fatal instances of bleeding peptic ulcer at the Ottawa Civic Hospital. In 44 of the 50 patients inadequate transfusion, both in volume and rate, was found to be a prime causative factor.

The condition of most patients treated with adequate transfusion will temporarily stabilize. If after the rapid transfusion of 1500–2000 ml of whole blood the patient remains in a state of shock or borderline shock, the difficult decision must be made as to whether surgical intervention should be accomplished posthaste. Fortunately, this is an infrequent problem. When a decision is made to operate under these conditions, the patient should be taken to the operating room and two vein cutdowns using No. 15 polyethylene catheters should be performed, and whole blood should be given under pressure. At the same time that the vein cutdowns are performed, the abdomen should be aseptically prepared and draped. When these procedures are followed, it is rare indeed for the blood pressure not to return to nearly normal, and the operation may then begin under conditions that give the best chance for survival. Although patients have been saved by operation before stabilization of the blood pressure, this approach has caused the death of more patients than it has saved. Under the most dire circumstances, consideration might be given to the use of circumferential pneumatic compression (G suit) of the abdomen [69]. Gardner and Storer [69] suggest that the G-suit technique shunts blood from below the diaphragm to vital structures above it, and they state that the encircling force overcomes the tangential tension in the blood vessel wall, which is the prime factor in the continuation of the bleeding.

The most common and also the most difficult decision to be made involves the patient whose condition has stabilized initially but who continues to bleed. In general, if any patient, regardless of age, needs more than 1500 ml of whole blood in any given 24-hour period after the initial stabilizing replacement, he or she should be operated on. Failure to stop bleeding after 48 hours, regardless of replacement need, or an instance of rebleeding under treatment places the patient in an operative category. Many reports indicate that operative intervention after 48 hours doubles or even triples the operative mortality [59, 87, 206].

Hematemesis after initial stabilization in the hospital is also an indication for operation [212]. Jones [107] compared the mortality among 1061 patients without recurrent bleeding after admission with the mortality among 353 patients who bled after admission, and the results were striking—1.7 percent versus 21.6 percent, respectively. Jones further found that among patients older than 60 years of age, the mortality for recurrent bleeding in the hospital from either chronic gastric or duodenal ulcer was about 43 percent.

In summary, the course of action in the presence of an established diagnosis of ulcer should be as outlined in the following list.

1. Conservative medical treatment at the outset
   a. Adequate and rapid replacement of deficient blood volume
   b. Early endoscopy in patients without a known source of hemorrhage
2. Absolute indications for operative approach
   a. After initial stabilization, need for over 1500 ml of whole blood transfusion in any 24-hour period
   b. Bleeding continuing for more than 48 hours from onset (in patients over 60, bleeding continuing for more than 24 hours from onset)
   c. Bleeding recurring after initial cessation while the patient is under hospital medical treatment
   d. Coincident perforation and hemorrhage
3. Relative indications for operative approach
   a. Patient over 60 years of age [148]
   b. History of hematemesis during the current episode
   c. History of chronic ulcer disease or previous hemorrhages
   d. History of severe pain preceding the hemorrhage or pain persisting during the hemorrhage
   e. Gastric ulcer
   f. Shortage of available whole blood
   g. The visible vessel in an ulcer as seen endoscopically

CURRENT RECOMMENDATIONS

These recommendations are based on the ability of the gastrointestinal bleeding team to assess accurately the cause of bleeding in 90–95 percent of instances, which allows for more individualized therapy. The course of action when endoscopic or angiographic capabilities are not present may require modification in particular instances; transfer of a patient to another medical facility is often precluded by the patient's condition, but it should be considered for the patient whose condition stabilizes under conservative management.

The decision to operate will be made in the following situations:

1. When there are lesions that invariably continue bleeding (aortoduodenal fistula) or lesions that have a high chance of recurrent hemorrhage (e.g., gastric ulcer)
2. When there are neoplastic growths
3. When the sources of hemorrhage are undiagnosed (by all available techniques) and the classic criteria are met (see p. 435)
4. When all available nonoperative therapy to control hemorrhage has failed even in situations carrying 50 percent or greater risk of death.

The last group includes patients with acute gastric mucosal lesions and bleeding esophageal varices; the extremely high surgical mortality for acute procedures in this group of patients has made the advent of selective infusion of vasopressin and endoscopic techniques of particular interest. Conn et al. [31] showed that vasopressin infusion was effective in stopping hemorrhage but not in prolonging life in a series of patients who had 60 episodes of bleeding followed prospectively. This is a partial explanation for the high mortality for patients with these lesions: The hemorrhage is merely the "last straw."

OPERATIVE APPROACH

We have emphasized the need for adequate blood replacement both in conservative treatment and in preparation for surgical intervention.

An upper abdominal, vertical midline incision is favored. This is particularly true when the diagnosis is in question. When the lesion is easily found, rapid control of the bleeding point is imperative. As soon as this is achieved, the elected definitive technique can generally be undertaken without need for excessive haste.

A technique described by Illingworth [97] has much merit for the bleeding duodenal ulcer. This technique takes advantage of the fact that most of these ulcers penetrate posteriorly into the head of the pancreas. The lesser sac is entered by incision through the gastrocolic omentum. Preferably with the surgeon on the left side of the table, the stomach is lifted anteriorly placing slight tension on the junction of the duodenum and pancreas. The thumb of the right hand is forcibly pressed against the indurated wall of the duodenum, adjacent to the penetrating ulcer. The edematous area is very friable, and the ulcer is readily broken into. The bleeding source is thus rapidly visualized, and one or two sutures of No. 1 silk will suffice to transfix the bleeding vessel (Fig. 15-4). This technique may also be used in posterior penetrating gastric ulcers in the region of the antrum or lesser curvature. If the patient has a stable blood pressure, if evidence of continued bleeding is absent, and if an obvious duodenal or gastric ulcer is present, the surgeon may proceed with an unhurried elective procedure.

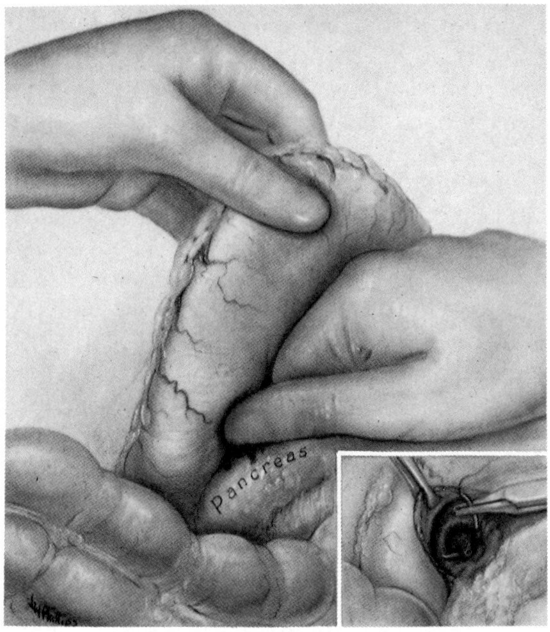

Fig. 15-4. Illingworth maneuver [95] for rapid control of hemorrhage from duodenal ulcer. The lesser sac is rapidly entered through the gastrocolic omentum. Anterior traction on the stomach permits visualization of gastropancreatic edema near a posterior penetrating duodenal ulcer. Pressure of the thumb on the operator's right hand will easily break into the ulcer bed. Transfixion of the bleeding vessel with nonabsorbable suture is then easily accomplished.

Course of Action when the Source of Bleeding is Unknown

Frequently it is necessary to explore hemorrhaging patients when the diagnosis is still in question. Exploration alone will reveal the cause of hemorrhage in a high percentage of instances. Small gastric ulcers on the lesser curvature that cannot be palpated may be suspected when enlarged lymph nodes are felt in the gastrohepatic omentum [99]. Subserosal hemorrhage at the gastroesophageal junction suggests Mallory-Weiss syndrome [65]. The small intestine should be inspected carefully for the presence and level of intraluminal blood. Although blood can reflux high into the small intestine from colonic hemorrhage, in general the higher the level of blood in the small intestine, the greater the chance that the source of bleeding is the esophagus, stomach, or duodenum. Evidences of portal hypertension include cirrhosis, splenomegaly, and dilated veins, particularly in the region of the porta hepatis and gastrohepatic omentum. Excessive bleeding while the abdominal incision is being made should also alert the surgeon to the possibility of portal hypertension.

Loe [129] has recommended the use of a sigmoidoscope for visualization of the stomach,

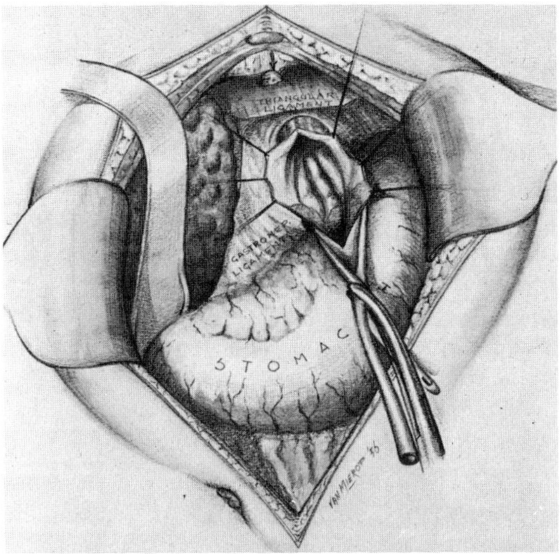

Fig. 15-5. Abdominal approach for ligation of varices. Midline incision of the abdomen is used, and the xiphoid process is resected. The triangular suspensory ligament of the left lobe of the liver has been depressed downward and to the right, exposing the esophageal hiatus. The esophagus has been mobilized, and a tourniquet has been placed around the esophagogastric junction. The esophagus and stomach have been opened for 9 cm, exposing the varices within the lumen. After the varices have been oversewn, the esophagus and stomach are closed longitudinally. (From Welch [228]. Reprinted, by permission, from *The New England Journal of Medicine* 255:677, 1956.)

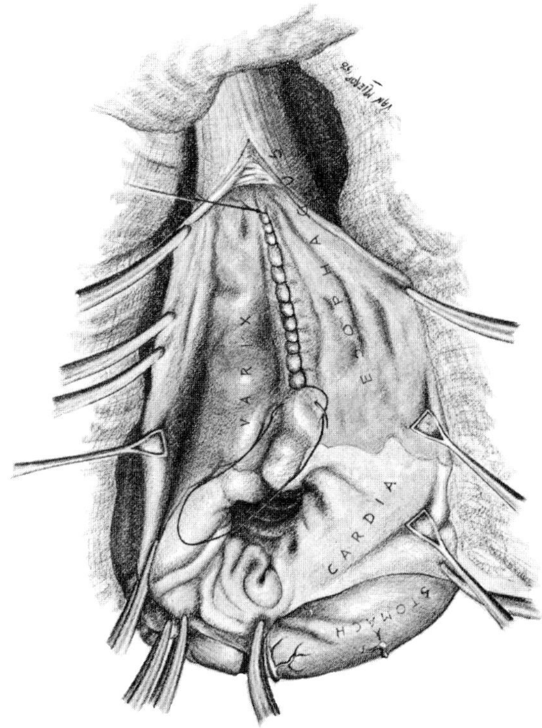

Fig. 15-6. Details of abdominal approach for suture ligation of esophageal varices. Three groups of varices can be identified. The stomach must be adequately opened to ensure oversewing of the varices into the cardia and particularly over the cardioesophageal junction. (From Welch [228]. Reprinted, by permission, from *The New England Journal of Medicine* 255:677, 1956.)

lower esophagus, and duodenum. The technical difficulties of this procedure have prevented it from being universally used. The use of a long gastrotomy incision has been advocated [135, 202, 203]. This enables a positive diagnosis in a high percentage of instances. We believe that gastrotomy should be undertaken before consideration of a blind gastric resection, for resection will be "blind" in very few patients if a wide gastrotomy is performed; furthermore, with present diagnostic aids the need for gastrotomy will diminish. Visualization of the lower esophagus is relatively easy by the abdominal approach [228], after which suture ligature of the esophageal bleeding source may be performed (Figs. 15-5, 15-6).

One of the major considerations is the specific operation to be used. Certainly in the high-risk patient, the most attractive technique is gastrotomy or duodenotomy followed by suture ligation of the bleeding point [1]. Unfortunately, this has not proved to be a satisfactory method. Heuer [87], Baker [7], and Allen and Oberhelman [2] indicated that ligation of the bleeding point is not a reliable procedure and is associated with a fairly high incidence of recurrent bleeding. In experienced hands, however, this technique when performed with pyloroplasty and vagotomy has proved particularly efficacious [57, 64, 144, 150, 200]. When suturing the bleeding point through the pyloroplasty, the presence of multiple anastomoses of the bleeding ulcer (in the bed of the ulcer) should be anticipated; a U-shaped stitch technique [13] is effective in preventing further bleeding from such an anastomotic vessel.

Considerable interest has developed in the use of vagotomy, pyloroplasty, and suture ligation in the treatment of massive hemorrhage from duodenal ulcer. It has become apparent that an inordinately high mortality accompanies the use of subtotal gastric resection in patients who are critically ill from hemorrhaging [63, 214]. Although early recurrent bleeding has been a problem following vagotomy, pyloroplasty, and suture ligation, the overall mortality is much improved over that of subtotal gastric resection. Because of this well-demonstrated and indeed dramatic improvement in mortality statistics, vagotomy, pyloroplasty, and suture ligation must be considered the procedure of choice. Dorton [47] advocates a similar approach for the bleeding chronic gastric ulcer; we emphasize, however, that effective treatment of bleeding gastric ulcers requires resection.

When gastric resection accompanies vagotomy or is used alone, the question of duodenal exclusion arises. Although Baker et al. [8] and Warren and Lanman [225] have expressed the opinion that exclusion of a duodenal ulcer is a satisfactory procedure, provided the duodenum itself is transected and provided the bleeding from the ulcer has been controlled, we have been loath to follow this practice. The use of the Strauss maneuver [208] will allow removal of most duodenal ulcers under the severest conditions.

Special Considerations

ESOPHAGEAL VARICES

The mortality for the first massive hemorrhage from esophageal varices in patients with *intra*hepatic portal bed block is about 17 percent; however, the mortality from variceal bleeding in patients with *infra*hepatic portal bed block, i.e., portal vein thrombosis, is about 3 percent [146]. Whereas the initial treatment for the latter group consists generally of whole blood transfusions, patients with intrahepatic portal bed block present such a complex management problem that even the most astute clinician is often perplexed as to the proper course of action.

In general, the patient with infrahepatic portal bed block is in the younger age group. A liver profile will reveal normal parenchymal function; confirmation of the varices and site of portal circulation block may be made by endoscopy and portography, respectively.

Portography accomplished by the splenic or arterial routes gives invaluable information about the portal circulation. While arterial portography has largely replaced splenic puncture, splenic puncture portography is the standard used for comparison of other techniques [182]. The mortality for venovenous shunts in cirrhotic patients approximates 20 percent for most series. Thus prophylactic portal-systemic vein shunts are not indicated before the first hemorrhage, even though one fully recognizes that the first hemorrhage carries a mortality of at least 17 percent. Sandblom [186] would perform a prophylactic portacaval shunt in patients with proven varices and evidence of good liver function. The mortality in his experience under these conditions has been about 4 percent. Similarly, the 8 percent operative mortality reported by Drapanas et al. in 1975 [49] suggests that the H-shaped shunt might be considered for prophylactic decompression of the portal system. The report of 48 patients treated by Galambos et al. [68] that compared two therapeutic shunts (distal splenorenal versus H grafts) indicates that both of these can be performed with a low hospital fatality (2 of 48 patients). The distal splenorenal shunt had a much lower incidence of postoperative encephalopathy in this series.

Nonoperative Treatments

These include tamponade of the bleeding point, injection of sclerosing agents, and infusion of vasopressin.

TAMPONADE OF THE BLEEDING POINT. There is little argument that the first therapeutic approach after beginning blood volume replacement is tamponade with an esophageal balloon. Novis et al. [152] reported initial control in 87 percent of their patients, although rebleeding occurred in more than one-half of the patients after removal of the Sengstaken-Blakemore tube; thus balloon compression was the final, definitive means of stopping hemorrhage in 46 percent of the patients. Unfortunately, the lethal character of these tubes has received scant attention [26, 32]. Sudden rupture of one of the balloons while in position within the esophagus leads to a calamitous situation; the counterweight used for traction will pull the remaining intact balloon suddenly into the oropharynx, with asphyxiation of the patient [11]. The Sengstaken-Blakemore tube must not be used unless the patient is constantly attended. Kulick and Rousselot [115] perfected an apparatus for accurate pressure control of balloon tamponade with an automatic signaling device that is set off when there is a sudden decrease in either gastric traction force or esophageal balloon pressure. According to the authors, this apparatus has greatly reduced the hours of nursing supervision usually required by these patients.*

INJECTION OF SCLEROSING AGENTS. If the bleeding cannot be controlled by tamponade, there are other modes of treatment available. The first of these, transendoscopic injection of sclerosing agents, is a technique that deserves further consideration and application in the management of variceal hemorrhage. Although not without morbidity, the procedure has been successful in 80 percent of instances in a 15-year series of 130 patients who had 297 instances of bleeding [104]. More than 80 percent of the patients were successfully treated by Raschke and Paquet in another series [167]. The material injected was a mixture of fatty acids and benzyl alcohol, and was injected through the rigid esophagoscope. Sclerosis has been adapted to the flexible endoscope, with encouraging results [124, 196, 211]. The results of injections with the flexible technique are comparable with or better than those reported with the use of rigid endoscopes, with the important advantage that general anesthesia is not employed. The debate now revolves around the type of sclerosant, the use of temporary tamponade after injection, and the use of radiographic techniques to verify the position of the needle before injection [211].

INFUSION OF VASOPRESSIN. The selective infusion of vasopressin into the superior mesenteric artery (this site of injection results in greater lowering of the portal pressure) is gaining popularity as a means of treating variceal hemorrhage. While systemic vasopressin (20 units given intravenously over 20 minutes) is often effective in the first attempts to control hemorrhage [29], selective infusion is even more effective in controlling hemorrhage and should be employed. However, if vasopressin for infusion purposes is unavailable for any reason, it may be necessary to proceed directly to the next step in management—a surgical procedure.

Operative Treatment

DIRECT SUTURE LIGATION. Direct suture ligation has had many advocates [19, 95, 127], but there is some debate about the best operative approach. Since an abdominal exploration allows evaluation of associated abdominal pathology, it had been our first choice (Figs. 15-5, 15-6) until the advent of the devascularization procedures described in the following section. Bleeding esophageal or gastric varices can be adequately treated in this manner [228] as can an unsuspected bleeding duodenal ulcer. This last problem is largely avoided with the use of preoperative endoscopy; the surgeon must be aware, however, that endoscopy is not 100 percent effective in the evaluation of upper gastrointestinal bleeding and that there may be a previously unrecognized lesion that might be the source of the bleeding. By retaining a high index of suspicion and performing endoscopy on all bleeding patients (preferably by the surgeon who will operate on the patient), the number of diagnostic errors will be minimized.

DEVASCULARIZATION OF THE LOWER ESOPHAGUS AND PROXIMAL STOMACH. The efficacy of devascularization of the gastroesophageal junction, the target area for bleeding varices, has now been demonstrated in several medical

*The apparatus is illustrated in a book on portal hypertension by H. R. Liebowitz [126].

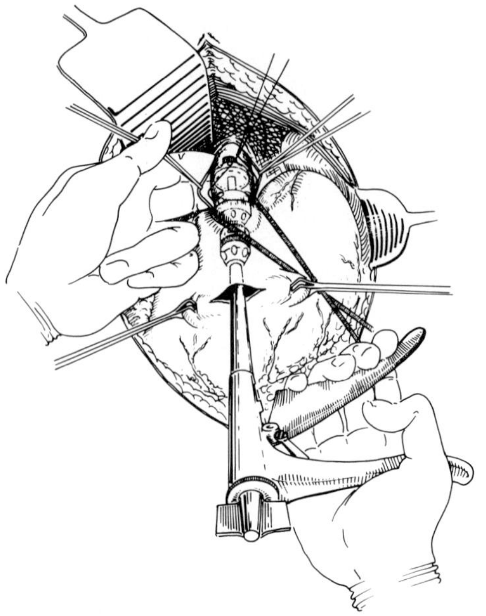

Fig. 15-7. After ligation of all venous collaterals of the proximal lesser curvature of the stomach and the distal 5 cm of the esophagus, the vagus nerves are carefully identified. A stapling device is inserted through a gastrotomy until the cartridge straddles the esophagogastric junction.

centers [91, 103]. The procedure must be considered an alternative to emergency shunts, and has the desirable feature of preserving portal flow to the liver. The experience at the Royal Victoria Hospital in Belfast reported by Johnston is illustrative of this fact: In 61 patients with varices who were unfit for shunt procedures, bleeding was controlled with a 14 percent hospital mortality, and late variceal bleeding occurred in only 4. A total of 69 percent of these individuals lived for three years after the procedure. When the procedure was done as an emergency, 31 percent of 19 patients died. The operation performed includes ligation of the left gastric vein (Figs. 15-7 and 15-8), ligation of all periesophageal venous collaterals for 5 cm, and transection of the esophagus at the gastroesophageal junction with a circular stapling device. The vagus nerves are carefully preserved, and splenectomy is performed only if thromboycytopenia is present [103].

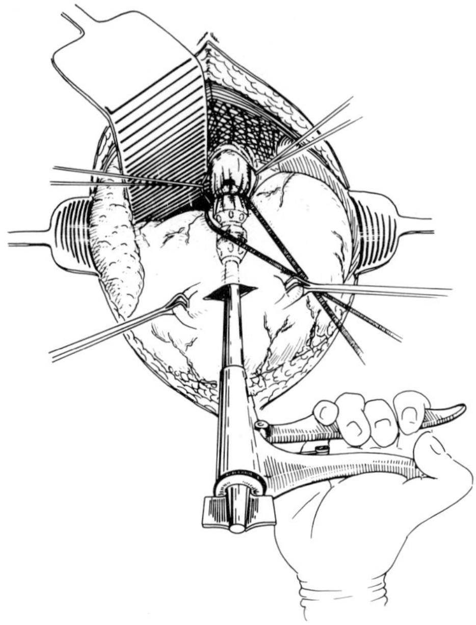

A

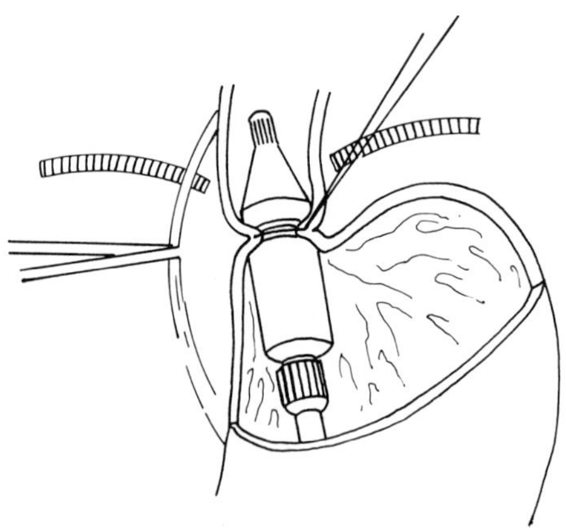

B

Fig. 15-8. With the cartridge in place (A), an 00 silk tie is tightened to compress the distal esophagus (B), incorporating the intramural veins within the tissue to be transected. After stapling, the instrument is removed and the doughnut-shaped mass is inspected; the gastrotomy is then closed. (From Dudley, H. (ed.). *Rob and Smith's Operative Surgery: Alimentary Tract and Abdominal Wall* (4th ed.). London, Butterworths 1983.)

EMERGENCY PORTACAVAL SHUNTING. Emergency portacaval shunting is not routinely employed because the associated mortality is so high. Orloff et al. [158] suggested that rapid assessment of the clincal status of the patient be followed by emergency portacaval shunt, without a trial of therapy with balloon tamponade. By performing a shunt procedure within 8 hours (mean of 8.5 hours) in 138 consecutive unselected patients, Orloff was able to achieve a 50 percent survival rate.

Another operation that achieves the desired decrease in portal pressure with a relatively simpler operative approach is the mesocaval shunt [25]. The modified technique, which interposes a 20- to 22-mm prosthetic device between the vena cava and the mesenteric vein (Fig. 15-9), achieves a 95 percent patency rate when done electively, with a small risk of further bleeding [48]. Although mesocaval shunt procedures have been most frequently used in elective situations, the surgeon should consider their use for the emergency situation as well.

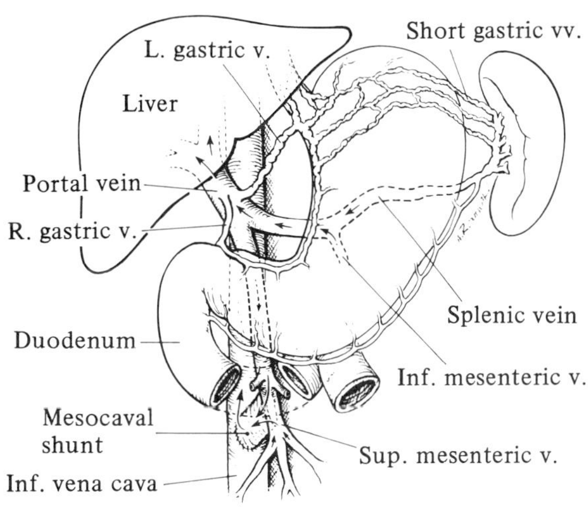

Fig. 15-9. This portal-systemic shunt has the advantages of ease and rapidity of performance and has been quite successful both in preventing recurrent variceal hemorrhaging and in maintaining perfusion of the liver (thereby minimizing hepatic encephalopathy).

Despite the fact that variceal bleeding is most often associated with portal hypertension, esophageal varices may arise from different mechanisms not associated with portal hypertension, for example, thrombosis of the splenic vein. If such a patient is operated on for bleeding varices, and atypical findings (not suggestive of portal hypertension) are seen, the surgeon should consider possible alternative explanations. In the example mentioned (splenic vein thrombosis), the operative findings of splenomegaly, distended varices along the greater curvature and gastroesophageal junction, and a grossly normal liver would suggest that splenectomy be considered as the appropriate (and curative) procedure [184]. Bleeding varices that are related to splenic vein thrombosis would be treated definitively by splenectomy.

Bleeding Varices in Children

Since bleeding in most children with varices will stop with conservative therapy, surgical treatment is reserved for the patient with repeated and frequent episodes. If the child's splenic vein is 1.0 cm in diameter, the splenorenal shunt [5] would be of potential value. This shunt does not completely decompress the liver, so the incidence of encephalopathy is low. Although associated hypersplenism would be effectively treated by splenectomy during the procedure, it must be emphasized that splenectomy is not the operation of choice in this situation.

Other innovative procedures that may be applicable for children include the mesocaval shunt [25], which entails transection of the infrarenal vena cava with end-to-side anastomosis of the distal vena cava to the superior mesenteric vein. Drapanas [48] began a prospective analysis of a modified (interposition) mesocaval graft in 1968 (Fig. 15-9). The advantages of this type of graft are that all of the vessels involved remain in situ, the Dacron graft that is interposed is capable of long-term patency, recurrent hemorrhage is infrequent, and the operative mortality and the incidence of encephalopathy are low [49]. By 1975 80 patients had been so treated, with an 8 percent operative mortality, and 11 percent incidence of encephalopathy, and excellent five-year survival statistics (100 percent in low-risk patients, 65 percent in high-risk patients). Although much of the data have been obtained from adults with intrahepatic block and portal hypertension, the mesocaval graft approach has much to recommend it, from a theoretical point of view, when considering the treatment of children with variceal hemorrhage.

Since it is impossible to predict which patients with portal hypertension will hemorrhage, it is impossible to preselect those patients at risk for preventive treatment. While prophylactic portacaval shunting usually prevents further hemorrhage, the controlled studies show no difference in long-term survival rates between shunted and nonshunted individuals [27, 30, 172].

STRESS GASTRITIS

The gastric mucosa has long been recognized as a target organ of stress resulting from a number of causes. These stressors include central nervous system (CNS) trauma, burns, trauma, sepsis, shock, and various chemical agents. Specific studies implicating acid production, back-diffusion of acid, alterations in blood flow, and the mucosal barrier are of great interest. These studies show that the incidence of stress gastritis is greater than recognized previously. Lucas et al. [130] studied 42 trauma patients (who subsequently bled) by serial photographs of the gastric mucosa taken with a flexible fiberoptic gastrocamera and documented sequential changes in the mucosa of these patients within 24 hours of the injury as well as the progression of these changes until hemorrhage occurred. They stressed the early onset of these changes and the concept that associated sepsis, pulmonary insufficiency, and other pathology must be treated aggressively to minimize the progression of these changes. Silen et al. [194] emphasized the need to clarify the predisposing factors in any so-called stress ulcer so that those with clearly differing mechanisms (such as ulcers occurring after CNS trauma) could be excluded. Ulcers occurring after CNS trauma are associated with high serum gastrin and high acid production.

Incidence

Whatever the cause, the increasing use of endoscopy in the diagnosis of acute upper gastrointestinal hemorrhage has demonstrated the frequent occurrence of stress gastritis. Wolff and Shinya [232] found that 18.7 percent of 471 patients with upper gastrointestinal hemorrhage had gastritis; Himal et al. [89] reported that 12 percent of 630 bleeding patients had acute gastric erosions. That all patients in whom acute mucosal lesions develop do not bleed is attested to by the prospective studies of Czaja et al. [38], who found acute lesions in more than 80 percent of individuals with large burns, and acute bleeding episodes in a small minority.

Management of Mucosal Lesions

In patients with established mucosal lesions or in those at risk, treatment of the basic medical problem, whether it is shock, infection, or toxic agents, is the first priority. Specific controlled prospective trials of ancillary measures, such as control of pH of gastric secretions and gastric hypothermia, are not in evidence, but guarded conclusions regarding their use appear justified. By eliminating an acid environment in the stomach, Curtis et al. [37] controlled progressive hemorrhage in 21 of 22 patients; Simonian and Curtis [195] later reported control of massive hemorrhage in 44 of 49 patients. Furthermore, many clinicians are of the opinion that the incidence of stress ulcers has markedly diminished since the use of antacids in seriously injured patients has become routine [194]. Hypothermia has been largely discarded in this country, but in Canada Himal et al. [89] reported an 84 percent success rate with hypothermia in the control of acute bleeding from gastric erosions; unfortunately, the absence of controls makes interpretation of these data difficult, since 75 percent or more of these patients may stop bleeding spontaneously.

Operative and Nonoperative Treatment of Massive Hemorrhage

The surgical approach to bleeding gastritis has been associated with a devastating mortality.

Most authors report a 40 percent or greater mortality [89, 131, 232]. The best results are found when vagotomy with drainage is performed in conjunction with oversewing of bleeding points; the probable mechanism accounting for the efficacy of vagotomy is decreased mucosal blood flow [155]. Although gastric resection has been advocated, the associated mortality makes this approach unappealing as an initial procedure.

The selective infusion of vasopressin is useful in control of acute hemorrhage, although it may not reduce the mortality of associated illness. It is a useful alternative to surgical treatment, however, in patients with gastritis. Another new technique, the transendoscopic electrocoagulation of bleeding points, may prove useful if initial favorable reports continue [67].

PERFORATION AND HEMORRHAGE

The simultaneous occurrence of the severe complications of perforation and hemorrhage may not be as rare as was previously thought. Gordon-Taylor [72] has placed the incidence of ulcer perforation in patients with massive hemorrhage at about 2–3 percent. Olson and Norgore [156] reported the high incidence of 13 percent in their series, and Martinis et al. [138], using more liberal criteria for bleeding than those used in other series, found the incidence to be 16.9 percent.

Gordon-Taylor classified patients with these associated complications into three groups: (1) those with concomitant hemorrhage and perforation; (2) those with hemorrhage following a recently treated perforation; and (3) those with initial hemorrhage followed by early perforation.

The prognosis is usually best when the hemorrhage and perforation occur simultaneously. In general, the perforation is readily diagnosed, and the patient remains in fair condition. The time sequence (delay) becomes the paramount consideration in dealing with patients in groups 2 and 3 and affords an explanation for the dismal results of these complications. The patient has been extremely ill for a longer period of time and has a decreased reserve to fight the new insult. In addition, diagnosis of the perforation is usually delayed because of masking of the clear-cut signs and symptoms of perforation by the state of shock or exsanguination.

The treatment for concomitant hemorrhage and perforation is emergency partial gastrectomy [72, 81, 199]. Hemorrhage with subsequent perforation is treated similarly, but, as indicated, the results will not be as good. As in all situations, treatment must be determined on an individual basis. This probably is most essential in patients who hemorrhage after surgical repair or resection of a perforated ulcer. A conservative medical regimen should be initially attempted for such patients, with surgical intervention considered in accordance with the general policy outlined previously.

MALLORY-WEISS SYNDROME

The Mallory-Weiss syndrome, first described by Mallory and Weiss in 1929 [134], has received considerable attention [39, 65, 110, 112]. The syndrome is characterized by gastrointestinal hemorrhage caused by two or more linear tears in the mucosa of the esophagogastric junction following repeated emesis. Unfortunately this diagnosis is frequently made at autopsy. Although increasing awareness of this entity as well as greater use of endoscopy should allow for better diagnosis, the failure of a significant number of patients to indicate previous vomiting is most misleading. The single most impressive observation made to help the operating surgeon was noted by Freeark and colleagues [65]. Subserosal hemorrhage was noted at the esophagogastric junction at an early phase of the abdominal exploration.

Recent success of conservative medical treatment of such tears at the gastroesophageal junction and the success of electrocoagulation of such lesions make it obvious that only a small percentage of patients with Mallory-Weiss bleeding will eventually require operative repair [67, 132, 209]. The treatment of choice for patients who continue bleeding under conservative management is direct suture repair of the lacerated mucosa through a generous anterior gastrotomy. Truncal vagotomy may facilitate operative exposure of the gastroesophageal junction in certain instances by allowing greater mobilization of the distal esophagus.

ESOPHAGEAL, GASTRIC, DUODENAL, AND JEJUNAL DIVERTICULA

Hemorrhage from esophageal diverticula is unusual, but it does occur [105]. True gastric diverticula of congenital origin are relatively rare. Feldman [58] found an incidence of only 0.2 percent at autopsy. He reported the incidence on roentgenogram in 136,000 collected instances to be about 0.4 percent. There are few reported instances in which diverticula have been incriminated as the source of massive hemorrhage [119]. Cosman et al. [34] pointed out that the diagnosis of massive hemorrhage from gastric diverticular disease is made by inference and exclusion and that exploratory laparotomy is necessary to rule out the presence of other lesions. The treatment of choice is excision of the offending diverticula [217]. Duodenal diverticula are more common, and although exceedingly rare, massive hemorrhage can occur from duodenal diverticula [17, 86]. The exact incidence of this complication is unknown; however, Forrest [61] found a significant positive correlation between gastrointestinal bleeding and the incidence of duodenal diverticula. If the diagnosis can be confirmed, the treatment is excision of the diverticulum.

Massive hemorrhage from jejunal diverticula is also rare, but it is a well-documented entity [41, 140]. In patients with repeated massive hemorrhage of uncertain origin, the surgeon must consider jejunal diverticulosis in the differential diagnosis.

RETROGRADE JEJUNOGASTRIC INTUSSUSCEPTION

Retrograde jejunogastric intussusception is a rare entity [62, 133, 137, 166]. It has occurred after simple gastroenterostomy in a majority of instances; however, several instances of this complication after partial gastrectomy have been reported. Foster [62] summarized the salient features of diagnosis as follows: "Any patient who has had gastric surgery and who subsequently develops (1) severe epigastric pain, (2) persistent vomiting (either bile-stained or bloody), (3) a palpable epigastric mass, (4) tenderness over the epigastrum, or (5) any combination of the preceding signs or symptoms should be suspected of having jejunogastric intussusception until proven otherwise." Foster further states, "The diagnosis should also be seriously considered in cases of massive upper gastrointestinal bleeding following gastric surgery whether with or without pain, whether with or without a palpable mass, but almost certainly if accompanied by both pain and a mass." The treatment for this complication is operative intervention; nonoperative therapy carries a mortality of 100 percent.

HEREDITARY ELASTODYSTROPHY (GRÖNBLAD-STRANDBERG SYNDROME)

Hereditary elastodystrophy is a systemic disease characterized by widespread degeneration of elastic tissue, particularly in the skin, eyes, and viscera. Massive upper gastrointestinal hemorrhage has occurred as a complication of elastodystrophy [12, 23, 109, 142, 173]. Unfortunately, valid documentation that impairment of the elastic tissues per se plays the ultimate role in producing gastric hemorrhage is minimal. Kaplan and Hartman [109] demonstrated that gastric hemorrhage was secondary to degeneration of the elastic tissue in gastric arterial vessels, with formation of microaneurysms, and to internal obliterative sclerosis, with formation of calcified plaques. The presence of angioid streaks of the retina should suggest the diagnosis. The combination of massive upper gastrointestinal hemorrhage and pregnancy should also suggest the possibility that hereditary elastodystrophy is present [142]. The therapeutic course to be followed is not well delineated. Antiulcer regimens as well as partial gastrectomy have been used with moderate success.

HEREDITARY HEMORRHAGIC TELANGIECTASIA (OSLER-WEBER-RENDU DISEASE)

Hereditary hemorrhagic telangiectasia is characterized by repeated hemorrhages from groups of abnormally dilated capillaries and veins. Most mucous membrane surfaces of the body have been reported as presenting these dilated vessels. Bleeding from the upper gastrointestinal tract may be chronic or acute and massive [116]. The diagnosis is confirmed by gastroscopy [141]. Kushlan [116] described the gastroscopic appearance of these lesions as rather large (1–10 mm in diameter) superficial mucosal purpuric hemorrhages, which on close examination were seen to have fingerlike projections. In addition he noted a few small, bright red, raised "cherry angiomata" diffusely scattered about the stomach. These areas were basically identical with the red spots seen on the skin and mucous membranes of these patients. Nonoperative treatment for the hemorrhage has generally been the rule; however, one can readily envisage a situation in which resection may be necessary [51].

PREVIOUS VASCULAR OPERATIONS

If an aortofemoral, aortorenal, or other vascular reconstruction has been performed, there is a subsequent risk of massive hemorrhage where the graft passes beneath the duodenum. Some of these patients present with a "herald-bleed" and signs of sepsis and are admitted to the hospital for evaluation. If endoscopic examination is normal and there is definite evidence of an upper gastrointestinal source, urgent operative exploration of the graft may be the only way of ascertaining whether a graft-enteric fistula is present. Occasionally the endoscopist may see the ribbed vascular prosthesis or an intramural duodenal hematoma that might be present. These lesions are related to either physical trauma or graft sepsis, and adequate treatment can only be achieved surgically. If untreated and managed "expectantly," a fatal rebleeding episode is not unusual [180]. The situation in which a normal examination prompts surgical exploration is unique.

MISCELLANEOUS CONDITIONS

Massive upper gastrointestinal hemorrhage has been reported in association with the following conditions:

1. Thrombotic thrombocytopenic purpura [85].
2. Recklinghausen's disease [56]
3. Primary polyarteritis nodosa [122]
4. Leiomyoma of the duodenum [22]; (see also Chap. 21)
5. Abdominal aortic aneurysm [33, 43, 114, 120, 198, 221]
6. Ingestion of aspirin [3, 117, 181]
7. Duodenal varices [96, 230]
8. Heterotopic pancreatic tissue of the stomach and esophagus [94, 169]
9. Trauma, operations, and neurosurgical procedures [40, 70, 139, 174]
10. Schönlein-Henoch purpura [125]
11. Intragastric rupture of splenic artery aneurysm [177, 201]
12. Crohn's disease of the stomach and duodenum [113]
13. Gastric carcinoid tumor [93]
14. Hematobilia [76, 79, 82, 143]
15. Renal transplantation [78]

References

1. Albright, H. L., and Kerr, R. C. Suture control of bleeding duodenal ulcer. *A.M.A. Arch. Surg.* 71:803, 1955.
2. Allen, J., and Oberhelman, H. A. The problem of the bleeding peptic ulcer. *Surgery* 37:1019, 1955.
3. Alvarez, A. S., and Summerskill, W. H. J. Gastrointestinal hemorrhage and salicylates. *Lancet* 2:920, 1958.
4. Amendola, F. H. Surgical intervention in massive gastroduodenal bleeding. *Surgery* 31:340, 1952.
5. Arcari, F. A., and Lynn, H. B. Bleeding esophageal varices in children. *Surgery* 112:101, 1961.
6. Athanasoulis, C. A., Baum, S., Waltman, A. C., et al. Control of acute gastric mucosal hemorrhage: Intra-arterial infusion of posterior pituitary extract. *N. Engl. J. Med.* 290:597, 1974.

7. Baker, C. Bleeding peptic ulcer. *Guy's Hosp. Rep*. 96:1, 1947.
8. Baker, J. W., Boyd, R. S., and Foster, R. A. Gastric resection with exclusion of complicated duodenal ulcer: An analysis of 122 cases. *Ann. Surg*. 142:519, 1955.
9. Baum, S., Athanasoulis, C. A., Waltman, A. C., and Ring, E. J. Gastrointestinal hemorrhage: Angiographic diagnosis and control. *Adv. Surg*. 7:95, 1973.
10. Belkin, G. A., and Conn, H. O. Blood ammonia concentration and bromsulfalein retention in upper gastrointestinal hemorrhage. *N. Engl. J. Med*. 260:530, 1959.
11. Bennett, H. D., Baker, L., and Baker, L. A. Complications in use of esophageal compression balloons (Sengstaken tube). *A.M.A. Arch. Intern. Med*. 90:196, 1952.
12. Berlyne, G. M. Pseudoxanthoma elasticum. *Lancet* 1:77, 1960.
13. Berne, C. J., and Rosoff, L. Peptic ulcer perforation of the gastroduodenal artery complex. *Ann. Surg*. 169:141, 1969.
14. Blackford, J. M., and Williams, R. H. Fatal hemorrhage from peptic ulcer. *J.A.M.A*. 115:1774, 1940.
15. Blackwood, W. D., and Silvis, S. E. Gastroscopic electrosurgery. *Gastroenterology* 61:305, 1971.
16. Boles, R. S., Jr., Cassidy, W. J., and Jordan, S. M. Medical versus surgical management for the complication of hemorrhage in duodenal ulcer. *Gastroenterology* 32:52, 1957.
17. Bradham, G. B., and Martin, J. B. Massive bleeding from a polyp in a duodenal diverticulum. *Ann. Surg*. 156:81, 1962.
18. Bradley, E. B., III, and Goldman, M. L. Gastric infarction after therapeutic embolization. *Surgery* 79:421, 1976.
19. Britton, R. C., and Crile, G., Jr. Late results of transesophageal suture of bleeding esophageal varices. *Surg. Gynecol. Obstet*. 117:10, 1963.
20. Brown, J. R., Meyers, S. G., Posch, J. L.,and Deneen, O. Massive hemorrhage from the upper gastrointestinal tract: A study of three hundred and twenty-four cases observed at the Detroit Receiving Hospital over a nine-year period. *Arch. Surg*. 61:767, 1950.
21. Bunker, S. R., Brown, J. M., McAuley, R. J., et al. Detection of gastrointestinal bleeding sites: Use of in vitro technetium Tc 99m–labeled RBCs. *J.A.M.A*. 247:789, 1982.
22. Butler, M. F. Severe melaena due to a leiomyoma of the duodenum. *Br. J. Surg*. 46:367, 1959.
23. Carlborg, U. Studies of circulatory disturbances, pulse wave velocity and pressure pulses in larger arteries in cases of pseudoxanthoma elasticum and angioid streaks: A contribution to the knowledge of the function of elastic tissue and smooth muscles in larger arteries. *Acta Med. Scand*. 151:1, 1944.
24. Chandler, G. N., Cameron, A. D., Nunn, A. H., and Street, D. F. Early investigation of haematemesis. *Gut* 1:6, 1960.
25. Clatworthy, H. W., and Boles, T., Jr. Extrahepatic portal bed block in children: Pathogenesis and treatment. *Ann. Surg*. 150:371, 1959.
26. Conn, H. O. Hazards attending the use of esophageal tamponade. *N. Engl. J. Med*. 259:701, 1958.
27. Conn, H. O. Therapeutic portacaval anastomosis: To shunt or not to shunt. *Gastroenterology* 67:1065, 1974.
28. Conn, H. O. To scope or not to scope. *N. Engl. J. Med*. 304:967, 1981.
29. Conn, H. O., and Dalessio, D. J. Multiple infusions of posterior pituitary extract in the treatment of bleeding esophageal varices. *Ann. Intern. Med*. 57:804, 1962.
30. Conn, H. O., Lindenmuth, W. W., and May, C. J. Prophylactic portacaval anastomosis: A tale of two studies. *Medicine* 51:27, 1974.
31. Conn, H. O., Ramsby, G. R., Storer, E. H., et al. Intraarterial vasopressin in the treatment of upper gastrointestinal hemorrhage: A prospective controlled clinical trial. *Gastroenterology* 68:211, 1975.
32. Conn, H. O., and Simpson, J. A. Excessive mortality associated with balloon tamponade of bleeding varices. *J.A.M.A*. 202:135, 1967.
33. Cordell, A. R., Wright, R. H., and Johnston, F. R. Gastrointestinal hemorrhage after abdominal aortic operations. *Surgery* 48:997, 1960.
34. Cosman, B., Kellum, J., and Kingsbury, H. Gastric diverticula and massive gastrointestinal hemorrhage. *Am. J. Surg*. 94:144, 1957.
35. Costello, C. Massive hematemesis: Analysis of 300 consecutive cases. *Ann. Surg*. 129:289, 1949.
36. Crohn, B. B. Need for aggressive therapy in massive upper gastrointestinal hemorrhage. *J.A.M.A*. 151:625, 1953.
37. Curtis, L. E., Simonian, S., Buerk, C. A., et al. Evaluation of the effectiveness of controlled pH in the management of massive up-

per gastrointestinal bleeding. *Am. J. Surg.* 125:474, 1973.
38. Czaja, A. J., McAlhany, J. C., and Pruitt, B. A., Jr. Acute gastroduodenal disease after thermal injury: An endoscopic evaluation of incidence and natural history. *N. Engl. J. Med.* 291:925, 1974.
39. Dagradi, A. E., Broderick, J. T., Juler, G., et al. The Mallory-Weiss syndrome and lesion. *Am. J. Dig. Dis.* 11:710, 1966.
40. Davis, R. A., Wetzel, N., and Davis, L. Acute upper alimentary tract ulceration and hemorrhage following neurosurgical operations. *Surg. Gynecol. Obstet.* 100:51, 1955.
41. Denkewalter, F. R., Molnar, W., and Horava, A. P. Massive gastrointestinal hemorrhage in jejunal diverticulosis. *Ann. Surg.* 148:862, 1958.
42. Devitt, J. E., Brown, F. N., and Beattie, W. G. Fatal bleeding ulcer. *Ann. Surg.* 164:840, 1966.
43. Diethrich, E. B., Campbell, D. A., and Brandt, R. L. Gastrointestinal hemorrhage: Presenting symptom of aortoduodenal fistulization. *Am. J. Surg.* 112:903, 1966.
44. Dollinger, M. R., and Morgan, L. R. Local cooling in the management of acute upper gastrointestinal bleeding. *Am. J. Surg.* 111:651, 1966.
45. Donahue, P. E., Mobarhan, S., Layden, T. J., and Nyhus, L. M. Endoscopic control of upper gastrointestinal hemorrhage with a bipolar coagulation device. *Surg. Gynecol. Obstet.* 159:113, 1984.
46. Donaldson, R. M., Jr., Handy, J., and Papper, S. Five-year follow-up study of patients with bleeding duodenal ulcer with and without surgery. *N. Engl. J. Med.* 259:201, 1958.
47. Dorton, H. E. Vagotomy, pyloroplasty, and suture for bleeding gastric ulcer. *Surg. Gynecol. Obstet.* 122:1015, 1966.
48. Drapanas, T. Interposition mesocaval shunt for treatment of portal hypertension. *Ann. Surg.* 176:435, 1972.
49. Drapanas, T., LoCicero, J., III, and Dowling, J. B. Hemodynamics of the interposition mesocaval shunt. *Ann. Surg.* 181:523, 1975.
50. Dwyer, R. M., Haverback, B. J., Bass, M., and Cherlow, J. Laser-induced hemostasis in the canine stomach. *J.A.M.A.* 231:486, 1975.
51. Ecker, J. A., Doane, W. A., Dickson, D. R., et al. Gastrointestinal bleeding in hereditary hemorrhagic telangiectasia. *Am. J. Gastroenterol.* 33:411, 1960.
52. Einhorn, M. A new method of recognizing ulcers of the upper digestive tract and of localizing them. *Med. Rec.* 75:549, 1909.
53. Eisenberg, H., and Steer, M. L. The nonoperative treatment of massive pyloroduodenal hemorrhage by retracted autologous clot embolization. *Surgery* 79:414, 1976.
54. Elliott, D. W., Harlte, R., Marshall, F., and Zollinger, R. M. Response to transfusion as guide in management of upper gastrointestinal hemorrhage. *A.M.A. Arch. Surg.* 77:386, 1958.
55. Enquist, I. F., Dennis, C., Fierst, S. M., and Karlson, K. E. Validity of the bromsulphalein test in patients with acute severe upper gastrointestinal hemorrhage. *Am. J. Surg.* 107:306, 1964.
56. Farrar, T., and Chappel, F. W. Severe gastrointestinal hemorrhage resulting from Recklinghausen's disease. *A.M.A. Arch. Surg.* 79:106, 1959.
57. Farris, J. M., and Smith, G. K. Vagotomy and pyloroplasty: A solution to the management of bleeding duodenal ulcer. *Ann. Surg.* 152:416, 1960.
58. Feldman, M. *Clinical Roentgenology of the Digestive Tract* (4th ed.). Baltimore: Williams & Wilkins, 1957. P. 176.
59. Finsterer, H. Surgical treatment of acute profuse gastric hemorrhages. *Surg. Gynecol. Obstet.* 69:291, 1939.
60. Finsterer, H. Der Wert der Fruhoperation bei akuten Magenblutungen aus einen chronischen Ulkus. *Wien. Med. Wochenschr.* 97:3, 1947.
61. Forrest, A. D. Incidence of bleeding in duodenal diverticula. *Gastroenterology* 33:800, 1957.
62. Foster, D. G. Retrograde jejunogastric intussusception: A rare cause of hematemesis. *A.M.A. Arch. Surg.* 73:1009, 1956.
63. Foster, J. H., Hall, A. D., and Dunphy, J. E. Surgical management of bleeding ulcers. *Surg. Clin. North Am.* 46:387, 1966.
64. Foster, J. H., Hickok, D. F., and Dunphy, J. E. Changing concepts in the surgical treatment of massive gastroduodenal hemorrhage. *Ann. Surg.* 161:968, 1965.
65. Freeark, R. J., Norcross, W. J., Baker, R. J., and Strohl, E. L. The Mallory-Weiss syndrome. *Arch. Surg.* 88:882, 1964.
66. Frey, C. F., Renter, S. R., and Bookstein, J. Localization of gastrointestinal hemor-

rhage by selective angiography. *Surgery* 67:548, 1970.
67. Gaisford, W. D. A new prototype 2-channel upper gastrointestinal operating fiberscope. *Gastrointest. Endosc.* 22:148, 1976.
68. Galambos, J. T., Warren, W. D., Rudman, D., et al. Selective and total shunts in the treatment of bleeding varices. A randomized controlled trial. *N. Engl. J. Med.* 295:1089, 1976.
69. Gardner, W. J., and Storer, J. The use of the G suit in control of intra-abdominal bleeding. *Surg. Gynecol. Obstet.* 123:792, 1966.
70. Goldfarb, I., and Saltzstein, H. C. Massive hemorrhage from peptic ulcer following operation or trauma. *Gastroenterology* 31:525, 1956.
71. Goodale, R. L., Okada, A., Gonzales, R., et al. Rapid endoscopic control of bleeding gastric erosions by laser radiation. *Arch. Surg.* 101:211, 1970.
72. Gordon-Taylor, G. The problem of the bleeding peptic ulcer. *Br. J. Surg.* 25:403, 1937.
73. Gordon-Taylor, G. The present position of surgery in the treatment of bleeding peptic ulcer. *Br. J. Surg.* 33:336, 1946.
74. Green, D. M., and Metheny, D. The estimation of acute blood loss by the tilt test. *Surg. Gynecol. Obstet.* 84:105, 1947.
75. Greene, L., Weisberg, H., Rosenthal, W. S., et al. Evaluation of esophageal varices in liver disease by splenic-pulp manometry, splenoportography, and esophagogastroscopy: Diagnostic discrepancies. *Am. J. Dig. Dis.* 10:284, 1965.
76. Grove, W. J. Biliary tract hemorrhage as a cause of hematemesis. *Arch. Surg.* 83:67, 1961.
77. Guevara, A. V., Lizaraso, F. C., DelAquila Hoyos, L., et al. Hemostatic catheter by compression in antral and duodenal bleeding ulcers. *Enfermed. App. Dig.* 28:509, 1969.
78. Haffner, J. F. W., Jakobsen, A., and Flatmark, A. L. Upper gastrointestinal bleeding in renal transplant recipients: The role of prophylactic surgery. *World J. Surg.* 7:738, 1983.
79. Harlaftis, N. N., and Akin, J. T. Hemobilia from ruptured hepatic artery aneurysm. *Am. J. Surg.* 133:229, 1977.
80. Harris, L. Loss of vision following haemorrhage. *Br. Med. J.* 1:871, 1941.
81. Harvey, H. D. Emergency gastric resection for bleeding and perforation. *Arch. Surg.* 86:557, 1963.
82. Hawes, D. R. Traumatic hematobilia. Angiographic diagnosis. *Am. J. Dis. Child.* 125:130, 1973.
83. Haynes, W. F., Jr., and Pittman, F. E. Application of the fluorescein string test in 32 cases of upper gastrointestinal hemorrhage. *Gastroenterology* 38:690, 1960.
84. Healey, W. V., Riggins, R. C., White, R. L., et al. An experimental method for localizing the source of intestinal bleeding. *Surg. Gynecol. Obstet.* 112:285, 1961.
85. Hellstrom, H. R., Nash, E. C., and Fisher, E. Thrombotic thrombocytopenic purpura as a cause of massive gastrointestinal hemorrhage. *Gastroenterology* 36:132, 1959.
86. Herrington, J. Massive hemorrhage resulting from benign ulceration in a primary duodenal diverticulum. *Surgery* 43:340, 1958.
87. Heuer, G. J. Surgical aspects of hemorrhage from peptic ulcer. *N. Engl. J. Med.* 235:777, 1946.
88. Himal, H. S. Endoscopic control of upper gastrointestinal bleeding. *Can. J. Surg.* 28:305, 1985.
89. Himal, H. S., Watson, W. W., Jones, C. W., and MacLean, L. D. The management of bleeding acute gastric erosions: The role of gastric hypothermia. *Br. J. Surg.* 62:221, 1975.
90. Himal, H. S., Watson, W. W., Jones, C. W., et al. The management of upper gastrointestinal hemorrhage: A multiparametric computer analysis. *Ann. Surg.* 179:489, 1974.
91. Hirashima, T., Hara, T., Takeuchi, H., et al. Transabdominal esophageal mucosal transection for the control of esophageal varices. *Surg. Gynecol. Obstet.* 151:36, 1980.
92. Hirschowitz, B. I., Luketic, G. C., Balint, J. A., and Fulton, W. F. Early fiberscope endoscopy for upper gastrointestinal bleeding. *Am. J. Dig. Dis.* 8:816, 1963.
93. Honig, L. J., and Weingarten, G. A gastric carcinoid tumor with massive bleeding. *Am. J. Gastroenterol.* 61:40, 1974.
94. Hudock, J. J., Wanner, H., and Reilly, C. J. Acute massive gastrointestinal hemorrhage associated with pancreatic heterotopic tissue of the stomach. *Ann. Surg.* 143:121, 1956.
95. Hunt, A. H. Haematemesis in portal hypertension. *Br. J. Surg.* 51:749, 1964.
96. Hwang, P., Joergenson, E. J., Anspach, P., and Brown, A. F. Fatal hemorrhage from duodenal varix. *J. Int. Coll. Surg.* 31:414, 1959.
97. Illingworth, C. F. W. *Peptic Ulcer.* Edinburgh: Livingstone, 1953.
98. Irvin, G. L., and Zeppa, R. Predicted survival

in peptic ulcer patients based on computer analysis of preoperative variables. *Ann. Surg.* 183:594, 1976.

99. Jamieson, A. Personal communication, 1956.
100. Jensen, H. E., Amdrup, E., Christiansen, P., et al. Bleeding gastric ulcer: Surgical and nonsurgical treatment of 225 patients. *Scand. J. Gastroenterol.* 7:535, 1972.
101. Johnson, H. D. Venous pressure: Its physiology and pathology in haemorrhage, shock and transfusion. *Br. J. Surg.* 51:276, 1964.
102. Johnson, W. C., Widrich, W. C., and Nabseth, D. C. Control of bleeding varices by vasopressin: A prospective randomized study. Paper presented to the American Surgical Association, Boca Raton, Florida, March 24, 1977.
103. Johnston, G. W. Six years experience of oesophageal transection for oesophageal varices using circular stapling gun. *Gut* 23:770, 1982.
104. Johnston, G. W., and Rodgers, H. W. A review of 15 years' experience in the use of sclerotherapy in the control of acute haemorrhage. *Br. J. Surg.* 60:797, 1973.
105. Jonasson, O. M., and Gunn, L. C. Midesophageal diverticulum with hemorrhage. *Arch. Surg.* 90:713, 1965.
106. Jones, F. A. Haematemesis and melaena: With special reference to bleeding peptic ulcer. *Br. Med. J.* 2:477, 1947.
107. Jones, F. A. Hematemesis and melena: with special reference to causation and to the factors influencing the mortality from bleeding peptic ulcers. *Gastroenterology* 30:166, 1956.
108. Jones, F. A., and King, W. E. A study of acute gastric ulcers causing haemorrhage. *Aust. Ann. Med.* 2:179, 1953.
109. Kaplan, L., and Hartman, S. W. Elastica disease: Case of Grönblad-Strandberg syndrome with gastrointestinal hemorrhage. *A.M.A. Arch. Intern. Med.* 94:489, 1954.
110. Katz, D., Freud, M., and McKinnon, W. M. P. The Mallory-Weiss syndrome: Evaluation by early endoscopy of its clinical picture and its incidence in upper gastrointestinal hemorrhage. *Am. J. Dig. Dis.* 10:314, 1965.
111. Katzen, B. T., and McSweeney, J. Therapeutic transluminal arterial embolization for bleeding in the upper part of the gastrointestinal tract. *Surg. Gynecol. Obstet.* 141:523, 1975.
112. Kendall, R. W. Mallory-Weiss syndrome. *Northwest. Med.* 62:261, 1963.
113. Kim, U.-S., Zimmerman, M. J., and Weiss, M. Massive upper gastrointestinal hemorrhage associated with Crohn's disease of the stomach and duodenum: A case report. *Am. J. Gastroenterol.* 59:244, 1973.
114. Kubota, N., and Moragues, V. Ruptured abdominal aortic aneurysm with massive gastrointestinal hemorrhage. *Am. Heart J.* 58:547, 1959.
115. Kulick, G., and Rousselot, L. M. Combined pressure control and signal apparatus for safer emergency management of bleeding esophagogastric varices. Exhibit presented at Clinical Session, American College of Surgeons, Atlantic City, N.J., 1959.
116. Kushlan, S. D. Gastro-intestinal bleeding in hereditary hemorrhagic telangiectasia: Historical review and case report with gastroscopic findings and rutin therapy. *Gastroenterology* 7:199, 1946.
117. Lamphier, T. A., and Young, W. A. Bleeding from the upper part of the gastrointestinal tract secondary to ingestion of acetylsalicyclic acid (aspirin). *J. Int. Coll. Surg.* 29:395, 1958.
118. Langman, M. J. S. Relationship between preoperative bleeding and perforation and bleeding after operations for duodenal ulcer. *Gut* 6:134, 1965.
119. Lapin, R., Kamath, M., Engler, J., and Friedman, H. Massive gastrointestinal hemorrhage from duodenal diverticula. *Am. J. Gastroenterol.* 61:185, 1974.
120. Law, S. W., Garrett, H. E., and De Bakey, M. E. Gastrointestinal hemorrhage due to rupture of abdominal aortic aneurysm: Report of a successfully treated case. *Gastroenterology* 43:680, 1962.
121. Leading Article. Bleeding ulcers: Scope for improvement? *Lancet* 1:715, 1984.
122. Lee, H. C., and Kay, S. Primary polyarteritis nodosa of the stomach and small intestine. *Ann. Surg.* 147:714, 1958.
123. LeVeen, H.H., Mulder, A. G., and Prokop, F. The physiological mechanism for death in massively bleeding peptic ulcer. *Surg. Gynecol. Obstet.* 94:433, 1952.
124. Lewis, J., Chung, R. S., Allison, J., and Callahan, R. J. Sclerotherapy of esophageal varices. *Arch. Surg.* 115:476, 1980.
125. Lindenauer, S. M., and Tank, E. S. Surgical aspects of Henoch-Schönlein's purpura. *Surgery* 59:982, 1966.
126. Liebowitz, H. R. *Bleeding Esophageal Varices, Portal Hypertension.* Springfield, Ill.: Thomas, 1959. P. 803.
127. Linton, R. R. The emergency and defini-

tive treatment of bleeding esophageal varices. *Gastroenterology* 24:1, 1953.

128. Linton, R. R. The treatment of esophageal varices. *Surg. Clin. North Am.* 46:485, 1966.
129. Loe, R. H. Massive hemorrhage in the upper part of the gastrointestinal tract. *Arch. Surg.* 61:183, 1950.
130. Lucas, C. E., Sugawa, C., Riddle, J., et al. Natural history and surgical dilemma of "stress" gastric bleeding. *Arch. Surg.* 102:266, 1971.
131. Lulu, D. J., and Dragstedt, L. R., II. Massive bleeding due to acute hemorrhagic gastritis. *Arch. Surg.* 101:550, 1970.
132. Mackie, D. B., and Gent, A. E. Management of upper gastrointestinal hemorrhage. *Ann. R. Coll. Surg. Engl.* 59:56, 1977.
133. Madding, G. F., McLaughlin, B. F., and DeRiemer, R. Jejunogastric intussusception. *Am. J. Surg.* 92:636, 1956.
134. Mallory, G. K., and Weiss, S. Hemorrhages from lacerations of cardiac orifice of stomach due to vomiting. *Am. J. Med. Sci.* 178:506, 1929.
135. Maloney, J. V., Jr. Diagnosis and management of the rare causes of gastrointestinal hemorrhage. *J.A.M.A.* 168:1604, 1958.
136. Mandelbaum, R. A., and Brackup, A. H. Myocardial infarction during gastrointestinal hemorrhage. *N.Y. State J. Med.* 59:2896, 1959.
137. Marshall, S. F., and Kornegay, R. D. Jejunogastric intussusception: Report of a case. *Lahey Clin. Bull.* 11:194, 1960.
138. Martinis, A. J., Olson, H. H., and Harkins, H. N. The treatment of perforated peptic ulcer: A report of four hundred and thirty-seven surgical cases. *West. J. Surg.* 65:72, 1957.
139. Marvel, J. A. Interrelationship between brain damaging processes and peptic ulceration, perforation and hemorrhage. *Henry Ford Hosp. Med. Bull.* 7:73, 1959.
140. Mayo, C. W., Baskin, R. H., Jr., and Hagedorn, A. B. Hemorrhagic jejunal diverticulitis. *Ann. Surg.* 136:691, 1952.
141. McCafferty, T. D., Jr., and Lilly, J. O. Hereditary telangiectasia manifested as gastrointestinal bleeding without external visible telangiectasia. *Am. J. Gastroenterol.* 63:327, 1975.
142. McCaughey, R. S., Alexander, L. C., and Morrish, A. The Grönblad-Strandberg syndrome. *Gastroenterology* 31:156, 1956.
143. McGehee, R. N. Traumatic hemobilia. *Ann. Surg.* 179:311, 1974.
144. McGregor, D. B., Savage, L. E., and McVay, C. B. Massive gastrointestinal hemorrhage: A twenty-five year experience with vagotomy and drainage. *Surgery* 80:530, 1976.
145. McKusick, K. A., Froelick, J., Callahan, R. J., et al. 99m Tc red blood cells for detection of gastrointestinal bleeding. *Am. J. Radiol.* 137:1113, 1981.
146. Merendino, K. A., and Volwiler, W. Medical and surgical aspects of portal hypertension: A report of twelve cases. *Northwest. Med.* 52:724, 1953.
147. Miller, H. R. Mortality factors of gastrectomy or medical treatment in upper gastrointestinal bleeding. *Am. J. Surg.* 111:202, 1966.
148. Morris, D. L., Hawker, P. C., Brearley, S., et al. Optimum timing of surgery for bleeding peptic ulcers (abstract). *Br. J. Surg.* 71:382, 1984.
149. Morris, D. W., Levine, G. M., Soloway, R. D., et al. Prospective randomized study of diagnosis and outcome in acute upper gastrointestinal bleeding: Endoscopy versus conventional radiography. *Am. J. Dig. Dis.* 20:1103, 1975.
150. Mustard, R. A. Massive gastro-duodenal haemorrhage: A plan for management. *Can. Med. Assoc. J.* 85:1, 1961.
151. Nachlas, M. M. The use of a triple-lumen single-balloon tube in the diagnosis and treatment of massive upper gastrointestinal hemorrhage. *Surgery* 38:667, 1955.
152. Novis, B. H., Duys, P., Barbezat, G. O., et al. Fiberoptic endoscopy and the use of the Sengstaken tube in acute gastrointestinal haemorrhage in patients with portal hypertension and varices. *Gut* 17:258, 1976.
153. Nusbaum, M., and Baum, S. Radiographic demonstration of unknown sites of gastrointestinal bleeding. *Surg. Forum* 14:374, 1963.
154. Nusbaum, M., Baum, S., Sakiyalak, P., and Blakemore, W. S. Pharmacologic control of portal hypertension. *Surgery* 62:299, 1967.
155. Nyhus, L. M., and Rudick, S. The Treatment of Massive Gastroduodenal Hemorrhage: Vagotomy and Pyloroplasty. In F. Holle (Ed.), *Spezielle Magenchirurgie*. New York: Springer, 1968. Pp. 406–13.
156. Olson, H. H., and Norgore, M. Perforated gastroduodenal ulcers: A study of 166 cases. *Ann. Surg.* 124:479, 1946.
157. Oneal, W. J., and Hirsh, M. A. Emergency barium study of severe hematemesis. *Surgery* 52:592, 1962.

158. Orloff, M. J., Crane Carters, A., III, Chandler, J. G., et al. Portacaval shunt as emergency procedure in unselected patients with alcoholic cirrhosis. *Surg. Gynecol. Obstet.* 141:59, 1975.
159. Palmer, E. D. Vigorous diagnostic approach to upper gastrointestinal tract hemorrhage: A 23-year prospective study of 1400 patients. *J.A.M.A.* 207:1477, 1969.
160. Papp, J. P. Endoscopic electrocoagulation of actively bleeding arterial upper gastrointestinal lesions. *Am. J. Gastroenterol.* 71:516, 1979.
161. Papp, J. P. Endoscopic electrocoagulation in the management of upper gastrointestinal tract bleeding. *Surg. Clin. North Am.* 62:797, 1982.
162. Patton, T. B., and Johnston, C. G. A method for control of bleeding from esophageal varices. *Arch. Surg.* 59:502, 1949.
163. Pavel, D. G., Zimmer, A. M., and Patterson, V. N. In vivo labeling of red blood cells with Tc 99m: A new approach to blood pool visualization. *J. Nucl. Med.* 18:305, 1977.
164. Peterson, W. L., Barnett, C. C., Smith, H. J., et al. Routine early endoscopy in upper gastrointestinal tract bleeding: A randomized, controlled trial. *N. Engl. J. Med.* 304:925, 1981.
165. Pitcher, J. L. Safety and effectiveness of the modified Sengstaken-Blakemore tube: A prospective study. *Gastroenterology* 61:291, 1971.
166. Prohaska, J. V., Govostis, M. C., Harms, H. P., and Evans, S. O. Jejunogastric intussusception following subtotal gastrectomy. *Am. J. Surg.* 94:776, 1957.
167. Raschke, E., and Paquet, K. T. Management of hemorrhage from esophageal varices using the esophagoscopic sclerosing method. *Ann. Surg.* 177:99, 1973.
168. Rau, R. M., Thompson, R. J., Jr., Simmons, C. R., et al. Selective visceral angiography in the diagnosis and treatment of gastrointestinal hemorrhage. *Am. J. Surg.* 128:160, 1974.
169. Razi, M. D. Ectopic pancreatic tissue of esophagus with massive upper gastrointestinal bleeding. *Arch. Surg.* 92:101, 1966.
170. Read, R. D., Huebl, H. C., and Thal, A. P. Randomized study of massive bleeding from peptic ulceration. *Ann. Surg.* 162:561, 1965.
171. Reisberg, I. R., and Haubrich, W. S. Localizing obscure upper gastrointestinal bleeding by the fluorescein string test. *Henry Ford Hosp. Med. Bull.* 13:265, 1965.
172. Resnick, R. H., Chalmers, T. C., and Ishihara, A. M. A controlled study of the prophylactic portacaval shunt: A final report. *Ann. Intern. Med.* 70:675, 1969.
173. Revell, S. T. R., Jr., and Carey, T. N. Pseudoxanthoma elasticum as a disseminated disease. *South. Med. J.* 41:782, 1948.
174. Risholm, L. Acute upper alimentary tract ulceration and haemorrhage following surgery or traumatic lesions. *Acta Chir. Scand.* 110:275, 1955.
175. Robertson, C. K. Sudden blindness following gastrointestinal haemorrhage. *Edinb. Med. J.* 48:414, 1941.
176. Rodgers, J. B., Older, T. M., and Stabler, E. V. Gastric hypothermia: A critical evaluation of its use in massive upper gastrointestinal bleeding. *Ann. Surg.* 163:367, 1966.
177. Rogers, J. B. Intragastric rupture of a splenic artery aneurysm. *Med. Ann. D.C.* 42:14, 1973.
178. Rösch, J., Dotter, C. T., and Brown, M. J. Selective arterial embolization: A new method for control of acute gastrointestinal bleeding. *Radiology* 102:303, 1972.
179. Rosenak, B. D., Moser, R. H., Fisch, C., et al. Hemorrhage from peptic ulcer: An analysis of 223 cases. *Gastroenterology* 20:272, 1952.
180. Rosenthal, D., Deterling, R. A., Jr., O'Donnell, T. F., Jr., and Callow, A. D. Positive blood culture as an aid in the diagnosis of secondary aortoenteric fistula. *Arch. Surg.* 114:1041, 1979.
181. Roth, J. L. A., Valdes-Dapena, A., Pieses, P., and Buchman, E. Topical action of salicylates in gastrointestinal erosion and hemorrhage. *Gastroenterology* 44:146, 1963.
182. Rousselot, L. M., and Burchell, A. R. Splenic and Arterial Portography and Hemodynamics in Portal Hypertension. In L. Schiff (Ed.), *Diseases of the Liver.* Philadelphia: Lippincott, 1975.
183. Rousselot, L. M., Gilbertson, F. E., and Panke, W. F. Severe hemorrhage from esophagogastric varices: Its emergency management with particular reference to portacaval anastomosis. *N. Engl. J. Med.* 262:269, 1960.
184. Salam, A. A., Warren, W. D., and Tyras, D. H. Splenic vein thromboses: A diagnosable and curable form of portal hypertension. *Surgery* 74:961, 1973.
185. Saltzstein, H. C., Mahlin, M. S., and Scheinberg, S. R. Bleeding peptic ulcer. *A.M.A. Arch. Surg.* 67:29, 1953.
186. Sandblom, P. Personal communication, March 17, 1960.

187. Schaller, R. T., Jr., Hessel, E. A., II, King, L. T., Jr., and Stevenson, J. K. Gastric hypothermia for massive upper gastrointestinal hemorrhage: Experience with 24 patients and a review of literature. *Arch. Surg.* 92:707, 1966.
188. Schwartz, S. I., Bales, H. W., Emerson, G. L., and Mahoney, E. B. The use of intravenous pituitrin in treatment of bleeding esophageal varices. *Surgery* 45:72, 1959.
189. Sengstaken, R. W., and Blakemore, A. H. Balloon tamponade for the control of hemorrhage from esophageal varices. *Ann. Surg.* 131:781, 1950.
190. Serebro, H. A., and Mendeloff, A. I. Late results of medical and surgical treatment of bleeding peptic ulcer. *Lancet* 2:7462, 1966.
191. Shaldon, S., and Sherlock, S. The use of vasopressin (Pitressin) in the control of bleeding from oesophageal varices. *Lancet* 2:222, 1960.
192. Shenkin, H. A., Cheney, R. H., Govons, S. R., et al. On the diagnosis of hemorrhage in man: A study of volunteers bled large amounts. *Am. J. Med. Sci.* 208:421, 1944.
193. Sigel, B., and Dunn, M. R. The mechanisms of blood vessel closure by high frequency electrocoagulation. *Surg. Gynecol. Obstet.* 121:823, 1965.
194. Silen, W., and Skillman, J. J. Stress ulcer, acute erosive gastritis and the gastric mucosal barrier. *Adv. Intern. Med.* 19:195, 1974.
195. Simonian, S. J., and Curtis, L. E. Treatment of hemorrhagic gastritis by antacid. *Ann. Surg.* 184:429, 1976.
196. Sivak, M. V., Jr., Stout, D. J., and Skipper, G. Endoscopic injection sclerosis (EIS) of esophageal varices. *Gastrointest. Endosc.* 27:52, 1981.
197. Skillman, J. J., Lisbon, A., Long, P. C., and Silen, W. 15(R)-15-Methyl prostaglandin E_2 does not prevent gastrointestinal bleeding in seriously ill patients. *Am. J. Surg.* 147:451, 1984.
198. Skromak, S. J., O'Neill, J. F., Ciccone, E. F., and Snyder, R. J. Aneurysm of the abdominal aorta. *Gastroenterology* 33:575, 1957.
199. Slater, N. S. Associated perforation and haemorrhage in peptic ulcers. Treatment by immediate gastrectomy. *Br. Med. J.* 2:1257, 1951.
200. Smith, G. K., and Farris, J. M. Rationale of vagotomy and pyloroplasty in management of bleeding duodenal ulcer. *J.A.M.A.* 166:878, 1958.
201. Soeno, T., Kakizaki, G., Fujiwara, Y., et al. Massive hemorrhage into the upper digestive tract due to rupture of splenic artery aneurysm into the pancreas. *Am. J. Gastroenterol.* 61:55, 1974.
202. Spencer, F. C., and Maloney, J. V., Jr. The examination of the gastric mucosa through a large gastrotomy in the diagnosis of intestinal hemorrhage of obscure origin. *Surgery* 40:904, 1956.
203. Starzl, T. E., and Sanders, R. J. A maneuver for detection of the site of gastric hemorrhage. *Surg. Gynecol. Obstet.* 116:121, 1963.
204. Stewart, J. D. Personal communication, May 12, 1960.
205. Stewart, J. D., Sanderson, G. M., and Wiles, C. E., Jr. Blood replacement and gastric resection for massively bleeding peptic ulcer. *Ann. Surg.* 136:742, 1952.
206. Stewart, J. D., Schaer, S. M., Potter, W. H., and Massover, A. J. Management of massively bleeding peptic ulcer. *Ann. Surg.* 128:791, 1948.
207. Storey, D. W., Bown, S. G., Swain, C. P., et al. Endoscopic prediction of recurrent bleeding in peptic ulcers. *N. Engl. J. Med.* 305:915, 1981.
208. Strauss, A. A., Strauss, S. F., Schwartz, A. H., et al. Results of subtotal gastrectomy for gastric and duodenal ulcers since 1917. *J.A.M.A.* 149:1095, 1952.
209. Sugawa, C., Benishek, D., and Walt, A. J. Mallory-Weiss syndrome: A study of 224 patients. *Am. J. Surg.* 145:30, 1983.
210. Sugawa, C., Schier, M., Lucas, C., and Walt, A. Electrocoagulation of bleeding in the upper part of the gastrointestinal tract: A preliminary experimental clinical report. *Arch. Surg.* 10:975, 1975.
211. Takase, Y., Ozaki, A., Nagoshi, K., et al. Injection sclerotherapy of esophageal varices for patients undergoing emergency and elective surgery. *Surgery* 92:474, 1982.
212. Tanner, N. C. Personal communication, March 14, 1956.
213. Tanner, N. C., and Desmond, A. M. The surgical treatment of haematemesis and melaena. *Postgrad. Med. J.* 26:253, 1950.
214. Thorne, F. L., and Nyhus, L. M. Treatment of massive upper gastrointestinal hemorrhage: A ten-year review. *Am. Surg.* 31:413, 1965.
215. Tidey, H. L. Loss of vision following haemorrhage. *Br. Med. J.* 1:774, 1941.
216. Todd, M. H. Massive bleeding from peptic ul-

cer. *Va. Med.* 83:55, 1956.
217. Tracey, M. L., and Colcock, B. P. Gastric diverticulum: Diagnosis and indications for surgical excision. *Gastroenterology* 18:165, 1951.
218. Traphagen, D. W., and Karlan, M. Fluorescein string test for localization of upper gastrointestinal hemorrhage. *Surgery* 44:644, 1958.
219. Villar, H. V., Fender, H. R., Watson, L. C., and Thompson, J. C. Emergency diagnosis of upper gastrointestinal bleeding by fiberoptic endoscopy. *Ann. Surg.* 185:367, 1977.
220. Volwiler, W., and Harkins, H. N. *Suggested Management for the Patient with Massive Upper Gastrointestinal Hemorrhage at the King County Hospital* (brochure). Seattle, Wash.: King County Hospital, 1967.
221. Voyles, W. R., and Moretz, W. H. Rupture of aortic aneurysms into gastrointestinal tract. *Surgery* 43:666, 1958.
222. Waitman, A. M., Spira, I., Chryssanthou, C. P., and Stenger, R. J. Fiberoptic-coupled argon laser in the control of experimentally produced gastric bleeding. *Gastrointest. Endosc.* 22:78, 1975.
223. Wangensteen, O. H. The surgical treatment of peptic ulcer. *J. Iowa Med. Soc.* 44:365, 1954.
224. Wangensteen, O. H., Salmon, P. A., Griffen, W. O., et al. Studies of local gastric cooling as related to peptic ulcer. *Ann. Surg.* 150:346, 1959.
225. Warren, R., and Lanman, T. H. Surgery in bleeding peptic ulcer: Urgent operation and principle of exclusion. *Surg. Gynecol. Obstet.* 87:291, 1948.
226. Weber, R. A., Schroeter, M. M., and Riddell, O. The management of bleeding peptic ulcer. *Surg. Gynecol. Obstet.* 106:199, 1948.
227. Wechsler, R. L., Roth, J. L. A., and Bockus, H.L. The use of serial blood volumes and head-up tilts as important indicators of therapy in patients with bleeding from the gastrointestinal tract. *Gastroenterology* 30:221, 1956.
228. Welch, C. S. Ligation of esophageal varices by the transabdominal route. *N. Engl. J. Med.* 255:677, 1956.
229. Wenckert, A., Borg, I., and Lindblom, P. Review of medically treated bleeding gastric or duodenal ulcers. *Acta Chir. Scand.* 120:66, 1960.
230. Wheeler, H. B., and Warren, R. Duodenal varices due to portal hypertension from arteriovenous aneurysm. *Ann. Surg.* 146:229, 1957.
231. Wilkinson, S. A., and Tracy, M. L. The history of hemorrhage in peptic ulcer. *Gastroenterology* 7:450, 1946.
232. Wolff, W. I., and Shinya, H. Modern endoscopy of the alimentary tract. *Curr. Probl. Surg.* Chicago: Year Book, January, 1974, monograph.
233. Yajko, R. D., Norton, L. W., and Eiseman, B. Current management of upper gastrointestinal bleeding. *Ann. Surg.* 181:474, 1975.
234. Yellin, A. E., Dwyer, R. M., Craig, J. R., et al. Endoscopic argon-ion laser phototherapy of bleeding gastric lesions. *Arch. Surg.* 111:750, 1976.
235. Zamcheck, N., Chalmers, T. C., White, F. W., and Davidson, C. S. The bromsulphalein test in the early diagnosis of liver disease in gross upper gastro-intestinal hemorrhage. *Gastroenterology* 14:343, 1950.
236. Zimmon, D. S. A device for balloon tamponade of the duodenal bulb at endoscopy. *Gastrointest. Endosc.* 20:31, 1973.

EDITOR'S COMMENT

One of the disappointing aspects of this subject is the persistently high mortality in spite of all the modern improvements in patient care. One small series by Hunt and colleagues [2] does report a reduction in mortality to only slightly more than 3 percent in 93 patients treated by a "planned" approach. This included a prospective system with an active policy of early endoscopy, an operation, and a regular audit.

Part of the problem is related to the need to carry out what is a major abdominal procedure in a patient who is unfit by virtue of hemorrhage, is often old, and usually has other diseases. As the authors of this chapter mention, to stop the hemorrhage using an endoscopic method is attractive, and an argon laser used in conjunction with a gastroscope is capable of closing a vessel up to 1 mm in diameter; only a few bleeding gastric ulcers have vessels of diameter greater than this. The use of the argon laser in 60 patients bleeding from either a gastric ulcer or a duodenal ulcer has been described, in which 25 out of 36 spurting vessels seen at endoscopy were controlled [4]. Nevertheless, the evidence from controlled series is more controversial. Swain et al. [6] reported that in 52 patients with a visible vessel 8 of 24 rebled without a death, whereas 17 of 28 in the control group rebled, 7 of whom died. In 1981 Vallon and colleagues [7] carried out a randomized trial using an argon laser and found no difference between the treatment and control groups in terms of rebleeding, the need for surgical treatment, and death.

The neodymium YAG laser penetrates more deeply than does the argon laser. In a controlled and randomized study Ihre and colleagues [3] found that its use made no difference to the outcome. This was in distinction, however, to the study by Rutgeerts and colleagues [5], who found that although the YAG laser was more successful than conservative treatment at stopping the bleeding from nonspurting vessels, it had no effect on mortality as compared with the controls.

It seems, therefore, that massive upper gastrointestinal hemorrhage, occurring as it does in a progressively older age group, is associated with an inherent mortality, the bleeding often merely an event within a patient's more general decline.

I do not wish to end this comment on such a negative note. Progress has been made. Greenburg and his colleagues have defined patterns of disease and age-related operative and mortality rates [1]. For example, the recognition of severe stress after trauma, shock and sepsis and vigorous treatment of the stress with prophylactic H_2 receptor blockers has caused the near disappearance of stress mucosal hemorrhage in these patients. A more assertive policy for surgical intervention has decreased operative mortality in all age groups. Attention to the details of patient management presented in this chapter will undoubtedly serve to improve overall results in treating this acute and clinically difficult problem. C. W.

Comment References

1. Greenburg, A. G., Saik, R. P., Bell, R. H., and Collins, G. M. Changing patterns of gastrointestinal bleeding. *Arch. Surg.* 120:341, 1985.
2. Hunt, R. S., Korman, M. G., Hansky, J., et al. Bleeding duodenal ulcer: Reduction in mortality with a planned approach. *Br. J. Surg.* 66:633, 1979.
3. Ihre, T., Johansson, C., Saligson, V., and T'Orgren, S. Endoscopic YAG laser treatment in massive upper gastrointestinal bleeding: Report of a controlled randomised study. *Scand. J. Gastroenterol.* 16:633, 1981.
4. Laurence, B. H., Vallon, A. G., Cotton, P. B., et al. Endoscopic laser photocoagulation for bleeding peptic ulcers. *Lancet* 1:124, 1980.
5. Rutgeerts, P., van Trappen, G. M., Broeckaert, L., et al. Controlled trial of YAG laser treatment of upper digestive haemorrhage. *Gastroenterology* 83:410, 1982.
6. Swain, C. P., Bown, S. G., Storey, D. S., Kirkham, J. G., Northfield, T. D., and Salmon, P. R. Controlled trial of argon laser photocoagulation in bleeding peptic ulcers. *Lancet* 2:1313, 1981.
7. Vallon, A. G., Cotton, P. B., Laurence, B. H., et al. Randomised trial of argon laser photocoagulation in bleeding peptic ulcers. *Gut* 22:228, 1981.

16

Acute Perforation of Peptic Ulcer

Leonard Rosoff, Sr.
Clarence J. Berne

Surgery has been made safe for the patient, and we must now make the patient safe for surgery.
Lord Moynihan, Harveian Oration, 1926

The magnitude of the abdominal holocaust that follows free perforation of a peptic ulcer is determined by the amount and causticity of the spilled material. Optimal management of this very acute situation requires full knowledge of peptic ulcer disease, the natural history of the perforation, the abdominal and systemic effects of the spillage, and the various operative procedures from which a choicc must be made under emergency conditions.

Since the first successful operative closure of a perforated peptic ulcer in 1891 [65], there has been a steady increase in the number of methods available for controlling the perforation and the spillage effects. These methods include nonoperative as well as a variety of operative procedures. Disparate opinions still exist relative to preferred methods of management, and the treatment of this disease is far from uniformly successful [11, 30, 52, 55, 60, 61, 70, 72, 82, 88, 89, 99, 103].

Incidence

A marked decrease in mortality and hospital admissions for duodenal ulcer disease was noted in the United States, England, Wales, and Scotland during the 1960s and 1970s. In the United States hospital admissions for duodenal ulcer to short-term, nonfederal hospitals between 1970 and 1978 decreased by 43 percent [32]. A decline in hospitalization for duodenal ulcer perforation also occurred, but it was much smaller than that for uncomplicated ulcers, and the decrease was not considered statistically significant. In Australia between 1979 and 1981 there was a 35 percent drop in the number of patients admitted to hospitals with peptic ulcers [1]. From 1958 to 1977 a similar reduction in hospital admissions for peptic ulcer occurred in England and Wales. Additionally, perforated ulcers became less common in young men and more common in middle-aged and elderly women [17]. The cause of these changes remains obscure. The use of H_2-receptor antagonists was not a factor as they were generally unavailable until 1977. It is unknown whether there has been a true decrease in the incidence of duodenal ulcer or whether the condition has become more benign in nature. Nevertheless, peptic ulcer disease continues to be a prevalent medical problem with a relatively high mortality. Most deaths are caused by perforation.

History

The first publication reporting on a group of patients with acute free perforation of peptic ulcer was by Benjamin Travers in 1817 [97]. The report included a clear, brief description of the signs and symptoms of this condition. In 1843 Edwards Crisp [22] reported 50 cases and accurately summarized the clinical aspects of perforation. According to Cope [21], he also suggested the possibility of operative closure.

The earliest attempt at surgical control of perforation was by Mikulicz in 1884, and it was unsuccessful [73]. The first successful closure of a perforated gastric ulcer was achieved by Heusner in 1891 [65], and Dean successfully closed a perforated duodenal ulcer in 1894 [24]. Postoperatively Dean's patient was "fed solely per rectum by nutrient enemata and suppositories for seventeen days." In the United States the first successful closure was achieved in the same year by Atherton [37].

At the turn of the century other technical procedures were added to that of simple closure. In 1897 Braun added posterior gastroenterostomy, which was widely used in this situation for the next 40 years [13]. In 1902 Keetley initiated immediate gastrectomy [62]; this use was greatly developed in the next 30 years in central Europe.

In the middle of the present century Dragstedt [27] added vagotomy as a method for curing ulcer, thus greatly extending the potential for cure of peptic ulcer disease in elective operations. In the same time period, planned nonoperative treatment of acute perforations evolved as a definitive method of management, largely through the contributions of Taylor [95].

The Perforated Ulcer

A 3 : 2 ratio of deaths due to perforation compared to hemorrhage from gastroduodenal ulcers was found in a study several years ago of more than 31,000 necropsies at the Los Angeles County-University of Southern California Medical Center. At this hospital, the ratio of perforated duodenal ulcer to gastric ulcer was approximately 14 : 1. The mortality from perforation of gastric ulcer is higher than that from duodenal ulcer [12, 18, 26], with an average rate greater than 20 percent for gastric ulcer perforation and 10–12 percent for perforation of duodenal ulcer. Results of studies by the Commission on Professional and Hospital Activities indicate that the median percentage of death from complications of peptic ulcer disease from 1970 to 1978 was approximately 3.5 percent for hemorrhage, 9 percent for perforated duodenal ulcers, and 13 percent for perforated gastric ulcers [32]. The wide variation in reported mortality frequently correlates with the difference in the average age and socioeconomic status of the patients treated.

Associated hemorrhage is reported to occur in approximately 10–15 percent of patients, and if severe, it greatly increases the mortality [74, 105]. Usually in such circumstances the perforation occurs in one ulcer, and the bleeding is from a second ulcer. Frequently a chronic posterior duodenal ulcer coexists with an anterior duodenal ulcer [9]. If the anterior ulcer perforates, associated hemorrhage is usually due to the posterior "kissing" ulcer. In such instances the anterior ulcer is often acute, perhaps in association with acute ulceration of a chronic posterior ulcer. Occasionally a saddle ulcer produces both perforation and hemorrhage. Such an ulcer lies transversely across the superior border of the duodenum or lesser curvature of the stomach.

Concurrent hemorrhage and perforation may produce a hemoperitoneum, which may be large.

Taylor [96] stated that if perforation dyspepsia is of less than three months' duration, acute ulcer should be considered to be the probable cause of acute gastroduodenal perforation. The accuracy of the diagnosis of acute ulcer is much greater if three desiderata coexist; a very brief period of antecedent dyspepsia, a small perforation, and the absence of callosity of the ulcer at the time of operation. Such an acute ulcer has relatively little tendency to become chronic, and a curative operation for the ulcer is believed by many to be undesirable for this condition. It must be recognized that a positive ulcer history may be obtained at the time of discharge, following recovery from acute perforation, even though such a history was not obtainable at the time of admission. Conversely, despite a truly negative or brief antecedent history of dyspepsia, a perforated calloused ulcer may be present.

Many studies show that following recovery from routine simple closure of all perforated peptic ulcers, approximately 70 percent of patients have continued activity of their ulcer disease [44, 56], and half of these require operative treatment. With few exceptions such data include unidentified proportions of acute ulcers [29]. If the follow-up time of patients with perforation of proven chronic ulcer is adequate in length, considerably more than 70 percent of patients will subsequently have ulcer symptoms [43, 56, 77]. As a prognostic event in chronic peptic ulcer disease, perforation indicates that subsequent progression of the process is highly probable.

Natural History of the Perforation

Acute free perforation of a peptic ulcer can occur only when it penetrates a free serosal surface following acute or chronic transmural ulceration. The size of the perforation is usually proportional to the duration of the ulcer. Local antecedent tissue response near the chronic ulcer is strikingly absent, which suggests that the perforative phase is quite rapid, just as it is in the acute ulcer. The greater omentum is only occasionally a factor in spontaneous sealing of the perforation. Much fibrin is produced in response to peptic ulcer perforation, and when spontaneous sealing occurs, it is usually by fibrinous fusion of the duodenum to the liver. The first portion of the duodenum lies against the quadrate lobe of the liver in the recess between the gallbladder and the falciform ligament. Because the undersurface of the quadrate lobe of the liver is contiguous with the anterosuperior surface of the distal antrum and proximal duodenum, it becomes a major factor in the local events following perforations in this area. Frequent spontaneous sealing is provided by the foregoing factors. With perforated gastric corpus ulcers along the lesser curvature, the contiguity factor in self-sealing is determined by the extent of overlap of the left lobe of the liver. An additional favorable factor is a perforation of small size; however, large perforations also may seal spontaneously. The term *duodenal ulcer* is here used to include, in addition to duodenal ulcers, those perforated ulcers just proximal to the duodenum in the pylorus and distal antrum. The exact anatomical location of perforation in this area relative to the pylorus is difficult to ascertain because of the pathological changes usually present.

Occasionally sealing is not total, leaving a small pocket adjacent to the perforation. Radiologically this may appear as an extraluminal gas pocket, or, when filled with contrast media, this pocket may simulate a diverticulum. Such a gas pocket may also be caused by a minute perforation that has sealed [36].

Free perforation of gastric ulcer into the lesser sac is uncommon. With a patent foramen of Winslow, the clinical features may be similar to those of anterior perforations. When the spillage is confined to the lesser sac, the symptoms and findings are deceivingly milder than those found with perforation into the peritoneal cavity [35]. Appropriate roentgenographic studies of gas-fluid levels and the use of intragastric contrast media are needed to establish the diagnosis.

Spillage collections are usually absorbed. When absorption is incomplete and bacteria are present, abscess formation occurs. Clinically important abscesses of this type are usually subphrenic or pelvic, but they may occur near the perforation. Such abscesses are now infrequent, probably because of early intensive antibiotic therapy following perforation.

Spillage Effects

In the surgical literature, perforations of gastric and of duodenal ulcers are nearly always considered as a single subject. This may be because of the usual impossibility of making a bedside distinction among free perforations of gastric carcinoma, gastric peptic ulcer, and duodenal ulcer, because clinically identical and even maximal abdominal effects may occur whether the perforative spill is from a nonacid-secreting stomach, from a low-acid-secreting, stomach, or from the limited area distal to a hypersecreting stomach. In many patients with acute perforation of chronic duodenal ulcer, study of the gastric aspirate immediately after admission fails to reveal free hydrochloric acid, and hypersecretion of acid is again present after recovery. Therefore, although acid is often an initial component of the spillage, the spillage must contain a peritoneal irritant other than acid. Food seldom constitutes an important component of the spillage. Perforative spillage may contain oral microflora that have survived passage through any acid barrier present. Aerobic cultures of gastric aspirate are commonly sterile, even though the pH is not low. In instances of in-hospital perforation, any swallowed antibiotic-resistant nosocomial flora may constitute a factor in the known higher lethality of this situation, in which coexistent disease is usually the major factor.

In addition to gastric fluid spillage, effluent from the papilla of Vater also escapes into the peritoneal cavity through perforated gastric or duodenal ulcers (Fig. 16-1). This effluent, consisting of bile and pancreatic juice, initially has a short period of exposure to duodenal enterokinase for enzyme activation, and therefore

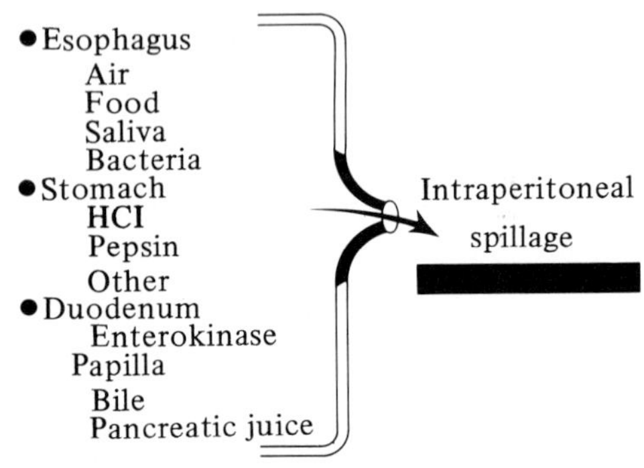

Fig. 16-1. The substances in the spillage through a perforated peptic ulcer. These may be qualitatively and quantitatively similar in gastric and duodenal perforations.

relatively small amounts of trypsin and chymotrypsin are present. As paralytic ileus develops, enteric stasis increases, and regurgitation of duodenojejunal contents occurs. This secondary regurgitative phase delivers increasing amounts of bile, active pancreatic enzymes, and any existing proximal enteric flora into the peritoneal cavity through the gastric or duodenal perforation. In advanced disease with large amounts of peritoneal fluid, the fluid is usually green, indicative of the presence of bile peritonitis. The amylase content of the peritoneal fluid is an index of the amount of papilla effluent present in the spill (Fig. 16-2). Peculiarly, fat necrosis is rarely seen.

The role of pancreatic enzymes in the peritonitis is not established. When brown peritoneal fluid is present, its amylase content is often very high, indicating the presence of much papilla effluent even in the absence of the characteristic green color. This brown fluid constitutes a covert bile peritonitis in which the cholic acid is the principal peritoneal irritant. Perforated peptic ulcer is probably the most frequent cause of bile peritonitis. The great lethality of bile peritonitis was well established in the classic study by Harkins et al. [51] and was later verified by Moretz and Erickson [75]. Studies regarding the foregoing matters are few [54, 106]. Relevant experimental studies are those regarding the intense

Peritoneal fluid

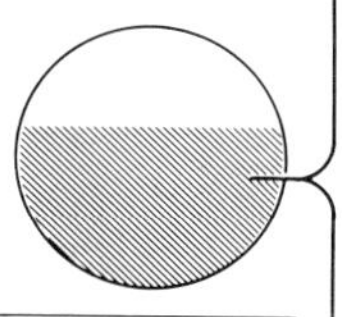

Combined acid	14	mEq/L
Free acid	0	
Bilirubin	2.0	mg%
Cholate	?	
Amylase	9600	units
Trypsin	5.8	γ/ml
Albumin / Globulin	2.8	gm%
Sodium	136	mEq/L
Potassium	5.2	mEq/L
Chloride	108	mEq/L
Bicarbonate	26	mEq/L

Gastric juice	
Free acid	0
pH	4.5
Amylase	50

Fig. 16-2. The chemical and enzymatic findings, with concurrent determination of gastric acidity in a leaking perforated duodenal ulcer. Amylase concentration is an index of the proportional amount of bile in the peritoneal fluid.

pulmonary injury consequent to the aspiration of vomitus [49, 67]; however, in most of these studies only hydrochloric acid has been used as the pulmonary irritant.

After 6–12 hours of leakage, the proliferation of spilled oral microflora and any intestinal flora added by regurgitation superimposes a bacterial peritonitis, the severity of which is extremely variable. At the time of operation, peritoneal fluid should always be taken for aerobic and anaerobic bacteriological studies and direct antibiotic sensitivity tests. Cultures of such fluid taken early after the perforation usually will be sterile, but if they are obtained later they are often positive [4, 23]. Routine culture methods do not give an index of the bacterial population, which will be revealed by Gram stain of the peritoneal fluid. Streptococci are the most commonly found organisms, and gram-negative bacilli also are often present.

The extent and intensity of the acute chemical-enzymatic-bacterial peritonitis, which can be considered a peritoneal burn, are directly proportional to the character, amount, and duration of the spill. The irritating qualities of the spillage are manifested by the large amounts of fibrin characteristically present in the upper abdomen, especially in the region of the perforation. The intra-abdominal effects of the spillage also include an acute reactive effusion of moderately dilute plasma [20] into the peritoneal cavity and juxtaperitoneal areolar tissues. Further, the consequent inhibitive ileus is associated with the pooling of intraluminal and mural enteric fluids. Also sequestered is the fluid spilled through the perforation. All of these fluids are preempted from the circulating blood by the peritonitic lesion [101]. These spill effects continue dynamically for many hours after the spontaneous or operative closure of the perforation, and they may be manifested clinically as postoperative shock and may be revealed by reelevation of a previously corrected hematocrit value.

Intense hyperemia is a component of the peritonitis. Studies indicate that arteriovenous shunting may accompany this peritonitis, as evidenced by a high cardiac output and rapid circulation time [87]. The intense upper abdominal pain and consequent thoracoabdominal splinting result in severe impairment of respiratory excursion, which interferes markedly with bronchial and parenchymal pulmonary function. These pulmonary sequelae are greatly aggravated by a large pneumoperitoneum, sizable peritoneal effusion, and intestinal distention.

Clinical Features

In the usual situation, the patient has had symptoms of peptic ulcer for some time, and commonly, for a few days preceding perforation there has been an increase in symptoms associated with a decreased food intake. It is uncommon for perforation to occur sooner than 2–4 hours after the ingestion of a meal.

Usually the perforation is heralded by sudden, intense upper abdominal pain, which soon becomes excruciating. The pain is constant, unrelenting, and spreads throughout the abdomen, and, if subphrenitis evolves, pain is felt at the top of the shoulder. Back pain is rare. Severe nausea is uncommon, and similarly, vomiting is seldom a prominent feature.

On examination the profoundly distraught, agonized patient is found lying immobile with grunting, shallow respirations. The abdominal muscles are maximally contracted, presenting a boardlike rigidity. Tenderness is marked, especially in the epigastrum, and bowel sounds are strikingly absent. Shortly after the onset a temporary partial abatement of symptoms may occur, occasionally the classically described lull. With the development of a large pneumoperitoneum, the abdomen becomes barrel-shaped and parietal peritoneal irritation decreases.

Variations from the usual are also seen frequently. One such variation is based on early cessation of leakage. In a perforation with a small spill and early self-sealing, the patient experiences upper abdominal pain of short duration and the abdominal findings are not severe and disappear rapidly. In such instances an aborted perforation should be suspected. A diagnosis of forme fruste perforation [92] is verifiable by the demonstration of pneumoperitoneum. Another variation is seen when, with somewhat greater leakage, the duodenal spillage is deflected by the falciform ligament and descends along the right paracolic gutter to the cecal fossa. The initial upper abdominal phenomenon may be replaced by right lower quadrant pain, tenderness, and rigidity, thereby closely simulating acute appendicitis (Fig. 16-3). Under these circumstances roentgenographic studies should be made to demonstrate the presence or absence of pneumoperitoneum. If present, pneumoperitoneum strongly suggests the true diagnosis of perforated duodenal ulcer, although on very rare occasions it may occur with perforated appendicitis. The foregoing pseudoappendicitis syndrome may occur either with self-sealing or with continued slow leakage.

Early in the postperforation period, the patient is normovolemic. With progressive peritoneal transudation of vascular fluid, the plasma volume decreases, with consequent hemoconcentration. Intravascular shifting of the body's interstitial fluid partially compensates for this plasma loss. After 6–8 hours of continued sizable spillage, the sequestering process creates important hypovolemia not revealed by the brachial arterial pressure, which is maintained at normal levels by compensatory vasomotor constrictive response. With

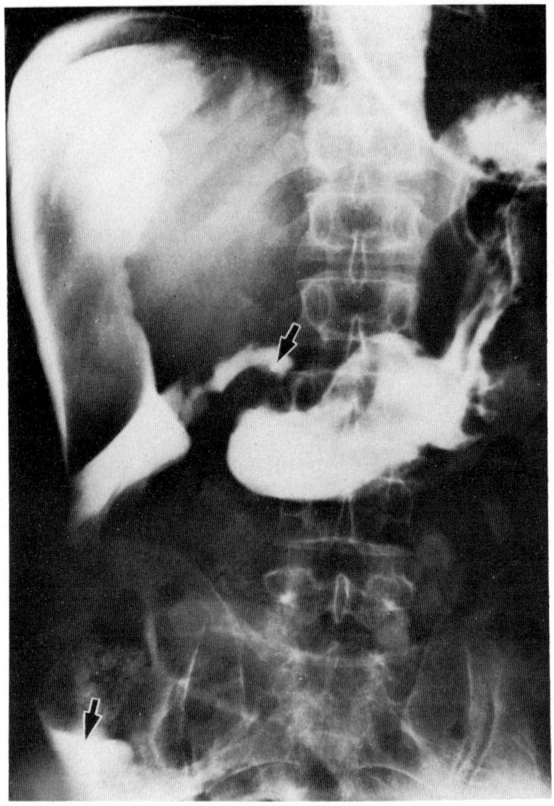

Fig. 16-3. Gastroduodenogram demonstrating spill of Hypaque from a perforated duodenal ulcer. Spillage is entirely to the right with accumulation around the right hepatic lobe and in the cecal fossa. The *upper arrow* indicates the duodenal ulcer, and the *lower arrow* indicates a collection in the cecal fossa.

this normotensive hypovolemia, the pulse volume is decreased and the ankle and foot veins are contracted. As the hypovolemia increases, there is proportionate progressive upward cooling of the lower extremities [7]; also, the hourly urine output begins to decrease abruptly. When the blood volume has been reduced by about 25 percent, the arterial pressure falls and decompensated shock ensues.

There are no laboratory test results that are pathognomonic of perforated peptic ulcers. A moderate neutrophilic leukocytosis is usually present. The decreased plasma volume caused by major spillage of gastroduodenal fluids results in hemoconcentration and elevation of the hematocrit value. If the preperforation hematocrit reading is known, the inherent postperforation elevation constitutes a direct index of the reduced plasma volume and therefore the proportionate reduction in blood volume. However, the hematocrit and hemoglobin levels may be highly deceptive. When the postperforative admission hematocrit value is normal, previous or concurrent bleeding should be suspected. In such instances a normal hematocrit reading represents a moderate preexisting anemia, and a reading moderately below normal indicates the existence of a severe anemia at the time of perforation.

Because of the violence of the abdominal disturbance, acute pancreatitis is often suspected; serum amylase determinations are therefore obtained. In patients with perforated gastric or duodenal ulcers a moderate hyperamylasemia may be found [2]. Values higher than 200 Somogyi units are encountered in 15 percent of instances. Only rarely do the values exceed 600 units, and when in the latter range, the mortality is exceedingly high [83]. Peritoneal fluid obtained by diagnostic peritoneal tap may yield amylase values as high as 80,000 Somogyi units. In such situations the serum amylase level may be only moderately elevated or even normal, and the urinary diastase values may be in the normal range.

Initial Management

In the initial diagnostic studies an intense effort should be made to obtain information regarding preexisting ulcer disease, the use of antacids, prior ulcerlike dyspepsia, or the occurrence of melena. Recent melena has been found to occur in 10 percent of patients.

The immediate specific therapeutic objective is to arrest spillage by providing intraluminal suction as near as possible to the site of perforation. This requires the passage of a nasogastric tube into the stomach for evacuation and continuous aspiration. Intragastric suction will maintain decompression of the stomach, but uniform decompression of the duodenum is not achieved. Polymicrobial antibiotic therapy should be instituted promptly, and pain should be treated immediately. A major benefit of pain reduction is the proportionate reduction of the intense grunting respirations, which amount to a semisustained Valsalva maneuver and impair venous return into the chest as well as pulmonary ventilation.

A relatively young person who is otherwise healthy and has a very recent perforation seldom presents problems in adjuvant therapy. The major lethal factors are hypovolemia [16], serious concurrent disease, and senescence. With uncontrolled leakage, hypovolemia increases rapidly from the sixth to twelfth hours and beyond. The "12-hour rule" is a tragic fallacy. Patients with uncorrected hypovolemia should never be rushed to the operating room to have an operation before 12 hours, since operation in the presence of hypovolemia increases lethal risk. Prevention or correction of hypovolemia should be initiated promptly on admission and continued during subsequent diagnostic studies. Dextrose-free lactated Ringer's and albumin solutions, given concurrently, specifically substitute for the vascular and interstitial fluid preempted by the abdominal lesion. Anemia should be corrected only when mandated by its severity. Except in early favorable situations, an indwelling urethral catheter is essential for the monitoring of hourly urine output as an index of renal blood flow [86]. A sustained hourly output of 30 ml or more of sugar-free urine indicates correction of hypovolemia to a degree that will largely preclude hypovolemic hypotension after the induction of anesthesia.

Cardiopathy demands an electrocardiogram and Swan-Ganz catheterization monitoring [94]. This monitoring is desirable in all patients who are seriously hypovolemic to ascertain their tolerance of rapidly given intravenous fluids. If the equipment and staff needed for Swan-Ganz catheterization monitoring are not available, central venous pressure determinations by simple catheter may provide useful information regarding the permissiveness of the heart to accept the intravenous fluids necessary for resuscitation [86]. Elderly hypovolemic patients constitute a special high-risk category because of the great likelihood that coronary and cerebrovascular thrombosis will occur because of decreased blood flow and, if hemoconcentration is present, because there may be increased blood viscosity. Initial rapid repletion with dextrose-free saline solution is specifically indicated for these patients to correct the hypovolemia and hemoconcentration.

Peritoneal tap, at times useful for diagnosis, may also provide benefit by decompressing a large pneumoperitoneum. A patient with a distended abdomen who does not respond to repletion therapy may improve markedly with sump drainage of the right upper quadrant. This may be accomplished by using local anesthesia and withdrawing large amounts of gas and fluid from the abdominal cavity, thereby greatly improving pulmonary function.

Roentgenographic Studies

Diagnostic roentgenographic studies are secured when the circulatory status of the patient permits. Chest roentgenograms and plain roentgenograms of the abdomen are obtained. A left lateral decubitus view of the abdomen is essential, and for this to be accomplished the patient should be kept in this well-tolerated position for at least 5 minutes. Keeping the patient in this position for this amount of time, which is often not possible when taking upright chest roentgenograms, greatly increases the frequency of detection of pneumoperitoneum. We then obtain a roentgenographic study of the upper gastrointestinal tract, specifically an esophagogastroduodenogram, using Hypaque for the contrast medium [57]. The use of other aqueous radiopaque material for such studies has been reported also [40, 104]. The sequential enterogram available in this study may disclose intestinal abnormalities accompanying or simulating perforated peptic ulcer. A peptic ulcer if present will be demonstrated by the foregoing method in a high percentage of patients. An unsealed perforation is revealed by the leakage of Hypaque (Fig. 16-3). In the absence of pneumoperitoneum, such leakage establishes the diagnosis of peptic ulcer with perforation, eliminating concern regarding other diagnostic possibilities such as acute pancreatitis and strangulation obstruction. In the presence of pneumoperitoneum, a demonstrable peptic ulcer, and no spill of Hypaque, a presumptive diagnosis of sealed perforated ulcer is made. However, in all instances of pneumoperitoneum without spill of Hypaque, even if a duodenal ulcer is demonstrated, infrequent causes of pneumoperitoneum, such as a perforated appendix, ruptured sigmoid diverticulum, or other colonic lesion, must be excluded. This is usually not difficult on clinical grounds. Occasionally severe pylorospasm or pyloric stenosis may be present, preventing visualization of the duodenum with the contrast medium. This precludes conclusions regarding the presence or absence of duodenal leakage.

Operative Treatment

The first successful operation for perforated peptic ulcer was performed in the last decade of the nineteenth century and consisted of simple closure, lavage, and drainage [37]. At the end of that decade, gastrojejunostomy was added to the foregoing. During the next 30 years, immediate gastric resection for perforation was extensively developed by central European surgeons [108]. This evolved in their geographic area largely because of the high frequency of associated gastritis and multiple ulcers as well as the early appreciation of the unsatisfactory results of gastrojejunostomy [46, 81, 100]. During the same period of time, nearly all North American and British surgeons adhered to the principle that the operative procedure should be limited to the closure of the perforation [25, 45].

Since the 1940s the concept of an immediate ulcer curative operation has been applied with increasing frequency. Excellent results of partial gastrectomy [10, 34, 93], some with vagotomy [47, 59, 88], have been reported. Highly selective vagotomy without drainage with simple closure or omental patch of the perforation has also been used on a small, selected group of patients [31, 58]. The long-term results reported by Jordan et al. [59] merit consideration of this procedure as an excellent method of definitive treatment of perforated duodenal ulcer.

For leaking perforated duodenal ulcer, our preference remains pyloroplasty with excision of the ulcer (Fig. 16-4A) and vagotomy [9, 50, 61, 63, 80]. This operation is of lesser magnitude than any other curative procedure for ulcer, and it avoids most of the sequelae observed in gastrectomies with subtotal resections. However, many surgeons still prefer simple closure only for all patients [12, 28, 71], and even proponents of curative operations for ulcers prefer simple closure for high-risk patients [11].

When an operation is planned for perforation of peptic ulcer, certain biological considerations relative to the ulcer are determinative [7]. Because of the minimal tendency toward chronicity, simple closure appears to be preferable for perforation of an acute ulcer. When chronic ulcer disease is present, especially if there has been previous perforation or hemorrhage, and when the patient's condition permits it, a curative operation is desirable. More than simple closure also will be demanded by pyloric obstruction or by concurrent bleeding. These criteria for curative operations for ulcer are now well established.

Perforated juxtapyloric gastric ulcers and pyloric ulcers are best treated as instances of duodenal ulcer disease, since all three are pathophysiologically similar. A perforation of the stomach may be caused by a peptic ulcer that is acute or chronic or by a carcinomatous ulcer. If only simple suture of a gastric ulcer perforation is feasible because of the patient's condition, a biopsy of the ulcer should be done, preferably by excision. The biopsy must at least consist of a full-thickness wedge. If the latter fails to show carcinoma, appropriate follow-up examination by barium studies is essential because of the possibility of a false negative biopsy. Conservative gastric resection is the optimal surgical procedure for most gastric corpus perforations caused by chronic peptic ulcer [41]. Such resectional treatment is mandatory if the ulcer is large or if there is seri-

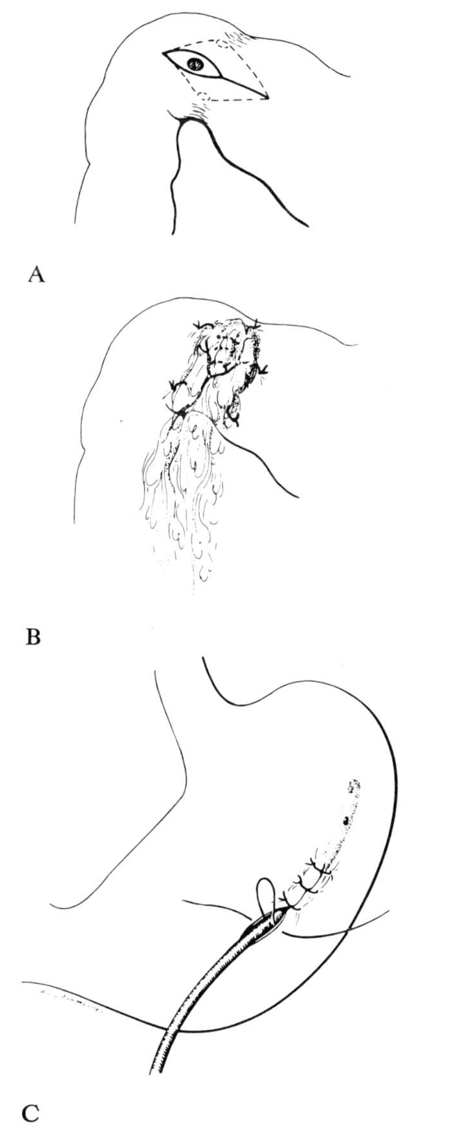

Fig. 16-4. Operative control of the perforation. (A) Heineke-Mikulicz pyloroplasty with incision modified to include excision of the perforated ulcer. (B) Simple closure reinforced by a pedicled omental patch, sutured at the margin to avoid ischemia. (C) A Witzel-Marwedel tunnel maintains the position of the gastrostomy catheter in the dependent portion of the stomach in the supine patient.

ous concurrent bleeding. Vagotomy should be added if there is evidence of concomitant duodenal ulcer disease. Its routine use has been recommended [66]. Mediastinitis as a complication of vagotomy has not been reported. The curative potential of vagotomy, pyloroplasty, and ulcer excision for perforated primary gastric corpus ulcer has not been established.

Reperforation in the immediately postoperative period is a hazard whenever simple suture is done, particularly if the peritonitis is severe. The seroserosal closure of perforations should be reinforced with a locally available fat tab or omentum, which is placed over the line of closure as a pedicle patch and its edges stiched to the serosa of the duodenum (Fig. 16-4B). Unlike free fat grafts or omentum over which sutures are tied, this living patch, with its blood flow intact, delivers additional fibrin to aid in the sealing. When the perforation is large, excision of the ulcer with pyloroplasty and vagotomy provides a much safer means of closure than simple suture. In such situations, when the duodenum is immobile, its mobilization by the Kocher method will relieve undesirable tension.

Peritoneal lavage was used extensively in the past, but now it is seldom advised. Its use deserves reevaluation. Papilla effluent, because of its cholic acid and pancreatic enzyme content, should not be left in the peritoneal cavity. A saline washout of such fluid will complement suction aspiration of the peritoneal cavity. Lavage also assists the peritoneal toilet when food is present. Drainage of the peritoneal cavity was practiced for many years but is now seldom recommended.

Postoperative intragastric suction is valuable because it retards further distension of the intestine, prevents aspiration pneumonitis from vomiting, and assists in the maintenance of the closure of a perforation. When a nasogastric tube is objectionable because of intolerance to it preoperatively, asthenia with poor cough ability, coexisting cardiac or pulmonary disease, or the anticipated need for prolonged gastric suction, a temporary gastrostomy is preferable. It is critical that the gastrostomy catheter be directed toward the fundus of the stomach. A Witzel-Marwedel tunnel will maintain the tube in the proper position (Fig. 16-4C). Failure to drain the bottom of the gastric pool that collects in the fundus of the stomach with the patient in the dorsal decubitus position may be followed by vomiting and fatal aspiration pneumonitis.

Nonoperative Treatment

Crisp, in his report on perforation of the stomach in 1843 [22], noted that "occasionally the aperture is filled up by adhesion of the stomach to some of the surrounding viscera, and in these instances the contents of the stomach do not escape into the peritoneum." Battams [5] in 1883 described two fatal cases of perforated gastric ulcer in which the perforations were found at autopsy to be sealed by fibrin. Hall [48] in 1892 reported six collected cases of spontaneous recovery following gastric ulcer perforation and added one of his own. In spite of such early recognition of the potential for spontaneous recovery, no planned therapeutic policy evolved based on this potential for self-sealing until Wangensteen's report in 1935 [102]. He treated nine patients nonoperatively using nasogastric suction. Ten years later Bedford-Turner [6] reported six consecutive cases successfully treated by a planned nonoperative program, the central feature of which consisted of frequent aspiration of the stomach using an indwelling nasogastric tube. In the same year Taylor [95] presented the first of a series of important reports in which conservative treatment was successfully applied to the management of perforated peptic ulcer. Taylor's analysis of his patients added greatly to our understanding of the difference between the natural history of acute versus chronic ulcer following perforation. Others [43, 78] have concurred that acute ulcer with perforation does not subsequently tend to become chronic, but some disagree [53]. Taylor [96] advised that conservative treatment be limited to perforation of acute ulcers, which he defines as those in patients with "no history of indigestion longer than, say, three months." Additionally, he advised that certain patients who are "too ill for surgery" should be similarly treated. This latter indication, first stated by Wangensteen, has been quite universally accepted [98]. An extensive study of nonoperative management is that of Fontaine et al. [39], who reported that approximately 80 percent of all patients recovered without operation, paralleling the finding of Taylor and others [33, 42, 90]. In these reports optional elective nonoperative management is based on efficient nasogastric suction.

There is an almost complete lack of knowledge concerning whether self-sealing is induced by nasogastric suction or occurs independently but concurrent with it. Proponents require precise roentgenographic positioning of the tube in the stomach and similar roentgenographic proof of effective gastric evacuation. They have not suggested duodenal intubation for perforated duodenal ulcer. Failure of abdominal findings to lessen within 3 to 5 hours [39], demonstration of increasing pneumoperitoneum, obvious severe aerophagia, or deterioration after a period of improvement are considered indications for discontinuation of nonoperative treatment.

Wide acceptance of nonoperative treatment has not developed because of the all-too-frequent tragic instances of death caused by continued leakage from the perforation. Visible proof of the persistence of the hole at the site of the perforated peptic ulcer can be established precisely by the roentgenographic method using aqueous Hypaque. This is shown by leakage of Hypaque, which establishes a precise diagnosis and the need for emergency operation. In the presence of pneumoperitoneum and absence of leakage, failure to visualize the duodenum with Hypaque and inability to exclude other causes of pneumoperitoneum are indications for emergency operation.

In 1958 the use of Hypaque for emergency upper gastrointestinal roentgenographic studies was proposed and instituted by one of us (C. J. B.) [8] at the Los Angeles County–University of South California Medical Center to determine the presence or absence of continuing leakage from perforated peptic ulcers. Spontaneous sealing is only rarely detected by operating surgeons [19] because the seal is usually disrupted in exposing the perforation. In more than 350 perforated duodenal ulcers examined by the Hypaque method, over 40 percent were found to be sealed at the time of the patient's admission to our hospital. Relatively few of these were instances of the well-known overt forme fruste perforation [92], in which spillage is minimal. The abdominal findings in most of these self-sealed instances were similar to those in which sealing had not occurred. The foregoing establishes that self-sealing after perforation with sizable, diffuse spill is a clinical entity and is commonly encountered. This constitutes a covert forme fruste or covertly aborted perforation. In the presence of pneumoperitoneum, self-sealing is established by the absence of Hypaque leakage, the demonstration of a peptic ulcer, and a firm clinical diagnosis.

We have managed all cases of self-sealing without operation. Unsealing has been exceedingly infrequent, and excellent results have been obtained. These patients have been treated as in the Taylor method using nasogastric suction, parenteral fluids, and antibiotics. In the rare instances in which the abdominal findings do not begin to improve after 4–6 hours, an operation is done. Otherwise, this regimen is continued for a minimum of three days. If abdominal findings have not normalized at that time, the treatment is continued until they have. Some patients with demonstrated active leakage who were considered to be prohibitive operative risks have been treated with this method, and they have demonstrably experienced spontaneous sealing and have recovered (Table 16-1).

There is no evidence that the results of non-operative—or operative—treatment of perforated peptic ulcer have been significantly affected by the use of H_2-receptor antagonists.

Perforation of Rarer Types of Peptic Ulcer

DISTAL ESOPHAGUS

Perforations in the distal esophagus are uncommon. Histologically the causative ulcer may be one of three types of epithelium: ec-

Table 16-1. Summary of Treatment of Acute Perforation of Chronic Peptic Ulcer

Type of Disease	Treatment
Sealed perforation	
No concurrent disease, mild spillage effects	Operation optional (ulcer curative)
Severe concurrent disease, severe spillage effects	No emergency operation; maintain seal
Leaking perforation	
No concurrent disease, mild spillage effects	Prompt operation (ulcer curative)
Severe concurrent disease, severe spillage effects	Restoration, tolerable operation
Very severe concurrent disease	Induce sealing
Very severe spillage effects	RUQ sump drainage

Note: RUQ = right upper quadrant.

topic gastric mucosa (Barrett's ulcer), epithelium that is regenerative and gastric in type [76], or stratified squamous epithelium. Such ulcers may be located above or below the diaphragmatic esophageal hiatus, and therefore the perforation may be into the chest or abdomen. Cardiac incompetence, usually secondary to hiatal hernia, is a predisposing factor to the ulceration. Occasionally, as in perforated peptic ulcer of the jejunum, the mechanism may be the intense gastric hypersecretion of the Zollinger-Ellison syndrome. Lower esophageal ulcer perforations simulate effort rupture (Boerhaave's syndrome), which occurs in the same area. The operative approach for these lesions is thoracotomy or celiotomy. With the latter, a bilateral vagotomy allows the esophagus to be drawn down for operative closure of the perforation. Any needed chest drainage can be provided by an intercostal tube.

STOMAL ULCER DISEASE

With the present infrequent use of gastroenterostomy for treatment of duodenal ulcer, perforations of stomal ulcer, previously unusual, will become even more rare [69]. Vagotomy added to gastroenterostomy or gastric resection has not eliminated this complication [15, 107]; stomal ulcer disease is often manifested within one year following such operations, and barium studies fail to reveal the ulcer in 50 percent of instances. When perforation occurs and the gastrojejunostomy is antecolic, the irritation of the anterior abdominal parietes will be much greater than when the anastomosis is retrocolic. In most instances simple closure of a perforated gastrojejunal ulcer is the preferred method of treatment, with the addition of vagotomy or revision of a previous vagotomy. A search for ulcerogenic islet-cell tumor should be made, but it seldom should involve pancreatic mobilization. If gastrectomy was done at the initial operation and the patient's condition permits, any antral remnant must be eliminated.

MECKEL'S DIVERTICULUM

Meckel's diverticulum of the ileum occurs in 1–3 percent of the population, and although most frequently located within 30 cm of the ileocecal valve, it may be as distant as 90 cm. Ectopic gastric mucosa is frequently present in the fundus of the diverticulum and may produce peptic ulceration of the ectopic gastric mucosa or of the nearby ileal mucosa. Free perforation of such an ulcer occasionally occurs and, when the diverticulum is in its usual location, simulates acute appendicitis with perforation. Whenever an operation is done for acute appendicitis and the appendix is found to be normal, perforation of a Meckel's diverticulum is among the conditions to be sought [79]. The presence or absence of ectopic tissue can be detected only by microscopical examination. Therefore, when considering prophylactic diverticulectomy during an operation for some other lesion, the surgeon should be guided by the fact that complications caused by ectopic gastric mucosa decrease steadily with increasing age.

PERFORATION OF STEROID ULCER

The frequency and virulence of steroid-induced ulcers are influenced by the disease for which the steroid therapy is given [84]. Rheumatoid arthritis is the most common major disease and chronic ulcerative colitis the least common in which peptic ulcers develop during treatment with steroids. Aspirin, which is often included in therapy for rheumatoid arthritis, is an additional ulcerogenic factor. Patients with malignant disease compose the second large group in which ulcer disease develops as a complication of steroid therapy.

The virulence and frequency of steroid ulcer disease are proportional to the dosage of steroids. With high daily dosages, such as 200 mg of prednisone, multiple ulcers, most often gastric ulcers, are likely. When the process is severe, the ulcerative lesions are similar to those found in many instances of acute stress ulcer [14, 38]. The duodenum is frequently involved, and ulcerations may also occur in the esophagus or jejunum.

Patients with steroid ulcer tend to have few symptoms from the ulcer, and when perforation occurs, the peritoneal response to spillage is less than that occurring with perforation of nonsteroid ulcers. The perforation is evidenced by only mild or moderate pain and tenderness, often with preservation of bowel sounds. In some instances perforation is initially almost asymptomatic. In such instances roentgenographic studies using Hypaque may be of special value in establishing the diagnosis.

Little is known regarding self-sealing of steroid ulcer perforations. Steroid-induced ulcer perforations are best treated by simple closure and placement of a pedicled fat patch. Hemorrhage is often associated with such perforations, and in such instances gastric resection may be necessary. Treatment of perforation of a steroid-aggravated peptic ulcer should include ulcer curative surgery when feasible.

PERFORATIONS IN YOUNG PATIENTS

Peptic ulcer perforations in newborn infants are believed to be caused by acute stress ulcer, birth constituting the stress mechanism. Because of the brevity of the stress, successful simple closure usually terminates the ulcer disease. Acute stress ulcer complicating serious disease is the usual type of ulceration occurring in infants. In newborns and infants perforated ulcer is associated with a very high mortality, improvement of which is largely dependent on earlier diagnosis [3, 68, 91].

After the first year of life, acute peptic ulcer becomes more frequent, and after school age is reached, chronic ulcer disease appears. The acute stress ulcer and the acute ulcer are usually reported to produce hemorrhage much more frequently than they produce perforation [64]. When perforation occurs, most often it is in a child undergoing treatment for ulcer hemorrhage. In some series perforation has been noted to occur more frequently [85]. Simple closure is preferred for treatment of children with perforations of the acute type. Perforation of chronic duodenal ulcer, which is encountered in older children, is best treated by pyloroplasty and vagotomy.

References

1. Adler, J., Ingram, D., and Hause, T. Perforated peptic ulcer: A seasonal disease? *Aust. N.Z. J. Surg.* 54:59, 1984.
2. Amerson, J. R., Howard, J. M., and Vowles, K. D. J. The amylase concentration in serum and peritoneal fluid following acute perforation of gastroduodenal ulcers. *Ann. Surg.* 147:245, 1958.
3. Arrants, J. E., Brogdon, B. G., and Jurkiewicz, M. J. Neonatal gastric perforation. *Am. Surg.* 31:96, 1965.
4. Bach-Nielsen, P., and Amdrup, E. Preoperative bacteriologic examination of the stomach and duodenum. *Acta Chir. Scand.* 129:521, 1965.
5. Battams, J. S. Two cases of perforating ulcer of the stomach: Death: Necropsy. *Br. Med. J.* 1:862, 1883.
6. Bedford-Turner, E. W. Conservative treatment of duodenal ulcer. *Br. Med. J.* 1:457, 1945.
7. Berne, C. J. Diagnosis of compensated hypovolemic shock. *Am. J. Surg.* 103:412, 1962.
8. Berne, C. J., and Mikkelsen, W. P. Management of perforated peptic ulcer. *Surgery* 44:591, 1958.
9. Berne, C. J., and Rosoff, L. Cine Clinic. Vagotomy and pyloroplasty for bleeding and for perforated duodenal ulcer. Film presented at American College of Surgeons Clinical Congress, 1963.

10. Bisgard, J. D. Subtotal gastric resection for acute perforated peptic ulcers. *J.A.M.A.* 160:363, 1956.
11. Boey, J., Wong, J., and Ong. G. B. A prospective study of operative risk factors in perforated duodenal ulcers. *Ann. Surg.* 195:265, 1982.
12. Booth, R. A. D., and Williams, J. A. Mortality of perforated duodenal ulcer treated by simple suture. *Br. J. Surg.* 58:42, 1971.
13. Braun, H. Ueber den Verschluss eines perforierten Magen-geschwurs durch Netz. *Zentralbl. Chir.* 24:739, 1897.
14. Bryant, L. R., and Griffen, W. O. Vagotomy and pyloroplasty: An inadequate operation for stress ulcers? *Arch. Surg.* 93:161, 1966.
15. Cleator, I. G. M., Holubitsky, I. B., and Harrison, R. C. Perforated anastomotic ulcer. *Ann. Surg.* 177:436, 1973.
16. Clowes, G. H., Jr., Vucinic, M., and Weidner, M. G. Circulatory and metabolic alterations associated with survival or death in peritonitis: Clinical analysis of 25 cases. *Ann. Surg.* 163:866, 1966.
17. Coggon, A., Lambert, P., and Langman, M. J. S. 20 years of hospital admissions for peptic ulcer in England and Wales. *Lancet* 1:1302, 1981.
18. Cohen, M. M. Treatment and mortality of perforated peptic ulcer: A survey of 852 cases. *Can. Med. Assoc. J.* 105:263, 1971.
19. Cohn, R., and Mathewson, C. The place of the nonoperative treatment in the therapy of perforated peptic ulcer. *Calif. Med.* 69:351, 1948.
20. Cope, O., and Wight, A. Metabolic derangements imperiling the perforated ulcer patient. VI. The plan of therapy. *Arch. Surg.* 72:571, 1956.
21. Cope, Z. *A History of the Acute Abdomen.* London: Oxford University Press, 1965. P. 47.
22. Crisp, E. Cases of perforation of the stomach, with deductions therefrom relative to the character and treatment of that lesion. *Lancet* 2:639, 1843.
23. Davison, M., Aries, L. J., and Pilot, I. A bacteriological study of the peritoneal fluid in perforated peptic ulcers. *Surg. Gynecol. Obstet.* 68:1017, 1939.
24. Dean, H. P. A case of perforation of a chronic ulcer of the duodenum successfully treated by excision. *Br. Med. J.* 1:1014, 1894.
25. DeBakey, M. Acute perforated gastroduodenal ulceration. *Surgery* 8:852, 1028, 1940.
26. Donaldson, G. A., and Jarrett, F. Perforated gastroduodenal ulcer disease at the MGH from 1952 to 1970. *Am. J. Surg.* 120:306, 1970.
27. Dragstedt, L. R., Harper, P. V., Jr., Tovee, E. B., and Woodward, E. R. Section of the vagus nerves to the stomach in the treatment of peptic ulcer. *Ann. Surg.* 126:687, 1947.
28. Drury, J. K., McKay, A. J., Hutchinson, J. S. F., and Jaffe, S. N. Natural history of perforated duodenal ulcers treated by suture closure. *Lancet* 2:749, 1978.
29. Duhamel, P. A., Black, M. A., and Haubrick, W. S. Are benign gastric ulcers really benign? *Arch. Surg.* 87:391, 1963.
30. Editorial. Treatment of perforated peptic ulcer. *Lancet* 1:36, 1951.
31. Eisenberg, M. M. Physiologic approach to the surgical management of duodenal ulcer. *Curr. Probl. Surg.* January, 1977.
32. Elashoff, J. D., and Grossman, M. I. Trends in hospital admissions and death rates for peptic ulcer in the United States from 1970 to 1978. *Gastroenterology* 78:280, 1980.
33. Elliott, J. L., and Lane, J. D. Perforated peptic ulcer treated by the nonoperative method. *Am. J. Dig. Dis.* 4:950, 1959.
34. Emmett, J. M., and Williams, H. L. Gastric resection: A definitive treatment for perforated peptic ulcer. *Am. Surg.* 23:993, 1957.
35. Feldman, M. Peptic ulcer perforation into the lesser peritoneal sac. I. A statistical study of 57 collected cases. *Am. J. Dig. Dis.* 17:333, 1950.
36. Feldman, M. A review of some unusual forms of perforation complicating benign peptic ulcer. *Rev. Gastroenterol.* 18:89, 1951.
37. Finney, J. T. Perforating ulcer of the stomach. *Ann. Surg.* 32:1, 1900.
38. Fletcher, D. G., and Harkins, H. N. Acute peptic ulcer as a complication of major surgery, stress or trauma. *Surgery* 36:212, 1954.
39. Fontaine, R., Hiebel, G., Lang, G., and Barth, G. The continuing aspiration in the manner of Taylor for perforated gastroduodenal ulcer in generalized peritonitis. *Lyon Chir.* 59:682, 1963.
40. Fraser, G. M., and Fraser, I. D. Gastrografin in perforated duodenal ulcer and acute pancreatitis. *Clin. Radiol.* 25:397, 1974.
41. Gall, W. J., and Talbot, C. H. Perforated gastric ulcer. *Br. J. Surg.* 51:500, 1964.
42. Giani, E. Considerations on continuing suction technique in perforated gastroduodenal ulcer. *Reforma Med.* 75:457, 1961.
43. Gilmour, J. Prognosis and treatment in acute

perforated peptic ulcer. *Lancet* 1:870, 1953.
44. Glenn, F., and Harrison, C. S. Acute free perforation of peptic ulcer: Complication of ulcer diathesis: 139 consecutive cases. *Arch. Surg.* 65:795, 1952.
45. Graham, R. R. The treatment of perforated duodenal ulcers. *Surg. Gynecol. Obstet.* 64:235, 1937.
46. Graves, A. M. Perforated peptic ulcer in German clinics: An analysis of 4,402 cases. *Ann. Surg.* 98:197, 1933.
47. Gray, J. G., and Roberts, A. K. Definitive emergency treatment of perforated duodenal ulcer. *Surg. Gynecol. Obstet.* 143:1, 1976.
48. Hall, W. W. Case of perforating gastric ulcer: Peritonitis: Recovery. *Br. Med. J.* 1:64, 1892.
49. Hamelberg, W., and Bosomworth, M. D. Aspiration pneumonitis: Experimental studies and clinical observations. *Anesth. Analg.* (Cleve.) 43:669, 1964.
50. Harbrecht, P. J., and Hamilton, J. E. Vagotomy and emptying procedure in the treatment of acute perforated duodenal ulcer. *Arch. Surg.* 85:174, 1962.
51. Harkins, H. N., Harmon, P. H., and Hudson, J. E. Lethal factors in bile peritonitis. I. "Surgical shock." *Arch. Surg.* 33:576, 1936.
52. Heslop, T. S., Bullough, A. S., and Brun, C. The treatment of perforated peptic ulcer: A comparison of two parallel unselected series. *Br. J. Surg.* 40:52, 1952.
53. Hofkin, G. A. Course of patients with perforated duodenal ulcers. *Am. J. Surg.* III:193, 1966.
54. Howard, J. M., and Singh, L. M. Peritoneal fluid pH after perforation of peptic ulcers: The myth of "acid-peritonitis." *Arch. Surg.* 87:483, 1963.
55. Hoyer, A. Perforating gastric and duodenal ulcers: A compilation of 2,224 cases from 16 Scandinavian hospitals. *Acta Chir. Scand.* 113:282, 1957.
56. Illingworth, C. F. W., Scott, L. D. W., and Jamieson, R. A. Progress after perforated peptic ulcer. *Br. Med. J.* 1:787, 1946.
57. Jacobson, G., Berne, C. J., Meyers, H. I., and Rosoff, L. The examination of patients with suspected perforated ulcer using a water-soluble contrast medium. *Am. J. Roentgenol.* 86:37, 1961.
58. Johnston, D., Lyndon, P. J., Smith, R. B., and Humphrey, C. S. Highly selective vagotomy without a drainage procedure in the treatment of haemorrhage, perforation, and pyloric stenosis due to peptic ulcer. *Br. J. Surg.* 60:790, 1973.
59. Jordan, G. L., Jr., Angel, R. T., and DeBakey, M. E. Acute gastroduodenal perforation: Comparative study of treatment with simple closure, subtotal gastrectomy and hemigastrectomy and vagotomy. *Arch. Surg.* 92:449, 1966.
60. Jordan, P. H. Proximal gastric vagotomy without drainage for treatment of perforated duodenal ulcer. *Gastroenterology* 83:179, 1982.
61. Kay, P. H., Moore, K. T. H., and Clark, R. G. The treatment of perforated duodenal ulcer. *Br. J. Surg.* 65:801, 1978.
62. Keetley, C. B. The surgery of nonmalignant gastric ulcer and perforation. *Lancet* 1:885, 955, 1902.
63. Kirkpatrick, J. R., and Bouwman, D. L. A logical solution to the perforated ulcer controversy. *Surg. Gynecol. Obstet.* 150:683, 1980.
64. Krasna, I. H., Schneider, K. M., and Becker, J. M. Surgical management of stress ulcerations in childhood: Report of five cases. *J. Pediatr. Surg.* 6:301, 1971.
65. Kriege, H. Ein Fall von einem frei in die Bauchhöhle perforirten magengeschwür Laparotomie. Naht der Perforationsstelle. Heilung. *Berl. Klin. Wochenschr.* 29:1244, 1892.
66. Landor, J. H., Manouchehr, F., and Clark, J. M. Emergency operation for complicated gastric ulcer: Considerations in the choice of a definitive procedure. *Am. J. Surg.* 111:483, 1966.
67. Lawson, D. W., Defalco, A. J., Phelps, J. A., et al. Corticosteroids as treatment for aspiration of gastric contents: An experimental study. *Surgery* 59:845, 1966.
68. Leix, F., and Greaney, E. M. Surgical experience with peptic ulcer in infancy and childhood. *Am. J. Surg.* 106:173, 1963.
69. Lynch, F. P., Coppinger, W. R., Sawyer, R. B., and Sawyer, K. C. Free perforation of marginal ulcers. *Arch. Surg.* 100:97, 1970.
70. Martinis, A. J., Olson, H. H., and Harkins, H. N. The treatment of perforated peptic ulcer. *West. J. Surg.* 65:72, 1957.
71. McEwan, A. J., and Milligan, G. F. The place of a definitive operation in the treatment of perforated duodenal ulcer. *Scott. Med. J.* 15:19, 1970.
72. Mikal, S., and Morrison, W. R. Acute perforated peptic ulcer: Criteria for operation and analysis of 500 cases. *N. Engl. J. Med.* 247:119, 1952.
73. Mikulicz, J. Ueber Laparotomie bei Magen-

und Darmperforation. *Samml. Klin. Vortr.* (Leipzig) 262 (Chir. No. 83):2307, 1885.
74. Moore, S. W., and Fuller, F. W. Multiple simultaneous complications of peptic ulcer. *Am. J. Surg.* 97:184, 1959.
75. Moretz, W. H., and Erickson, W. G. Neutralization of HCl in the peritoneal cavity. *Arch. Surg.* 75:834, 1957.
76. Mossberg, S. M. The columnar-lined esophagus (Barrett syndrome): An acquired condition? *Gastroenterology* 50:671, 1966.
77. Nemanich, G. J., and Nicoloff, D. M. Perforated duodenal ulcer: Long-term followup. *Surgery* 67:727, 1970.
78. Noordijk, J. A. Perforated peptic ulcer: The results of treatment in the Netherlands (1934–1950), an analysis of 2,551 cases. *Arch. Chir. Neerl.* 5:252, 1953.
79. Passaro, E., Jr., Richmond, D., and Gordon, H. E. Surgery for Meckel's diverticulum in the adult. *Arch. Surg.* 93:315, 1966.
80. Pierandozzi, J. S., Hinshaw, D. B., and Stafford, C. E. Vagotomy and pyloroplasty for acute perforated duodenal ulcer: A report of 75 cases. *Am. J. Surg.* 100:245, 1960.
81. Portis, S. A., and Jaffe, R. H. A study of peptic ulcer based on necropsy records. *J.A.M.A.* 110:6, 1938.
82. Rees, J. R., Swan, K. G., and Thorbjarnarson, B. Perforated duodenal ulcer. *Am. J. Surg.* 120:775, 1970.
83. Rogers, F. A. Elevated serum amylase: A review and an analysis of findings in 1,000 cases of perforated peptic ulcer. *Ann. Surg.* 153:228, 1961.
84. Roseman, D. L., and Economous, S. G. Treatment of complications of gastroduodenal "steroid ulcers." *Arch. Surg.* 90:488, 1965.
85. Rosenlund, M. L., and Koop, C. E. Diagnosis and treatment: Duodenal ulcer in childhood. *Pediatrics* 45:283, 1970.
86. Rosoff, L., and Berne, C. J. Oliguira in surgical patients. *Calif. Med.* 95:1, 1961.
87. Rosoff, L., Weil, M., Bradley, E. C., and Berne, C. J. Hemodynamic and metabolic changes associated with bacterial peritonitis. *Am. J. Surg.* 114:180, 1967.
88. Sawyers, J. L., Herrington, J. L., Jr., Mulherin, J. L., et al. Acute perforated duodenal ulcer. *Arch. Surg.* 110:527, 1975.
89. Schmitz, E. J., Harkins, H. N., Olson, H. H., et al. Perforated peptic ulcer: A study of 136 cases in a county hospital. *Ann. Surg.* 138:689, 1953.
90. Seeley, S. F., and Campbell, D. Nonoperative treatment of perforated peptic ulcer: A further report. *Surg. Gynecol. Obstet.* 102:435, 1956.
91. Shaw, A., Symonds, F., Bush, J., and Wardlaw, L. Surgical management of Curling's ulcer in children. *J.A.M.A.* 197:922, 1966.
92. Singer, H. A., and Vaughan, R. T. Treatment of the forme fruste type of perforated peptic ulcer. *Surg. Gynecol. Obstet.* 54:945, 1932.
93. Skarstein, A., and Høisaeter, P. A. Perforated peptic ulcer: A comparison of long term results following partial gastric resection or simple closure. *Br. J. Surg.* 63:700, 1976.
94. Swan, H. J. C., Ganz, W., Forrester, J., et al. Catheterization of the heart in man with use of a flow-directed balloon tipped catheter. *N. Engl. J. Med.* 283:447, 1970.
95. Taylor, H. Peptic ulcer perforation treated without operation. *Lancet* 2:441, 1946.
96. Taylor, H. The non-surgical treatment of perforated ulcer. *Gastroenterology* 33:353, 1957.
97. Travers, B. Additional observations on a report of rupture of the stomach by Crampton, J. *Med. Chir. Trans.* 8:228, 1817.
98. Vaughan, R. H., and Warren, B. Perforated peptic ulcer: A study of the indications for nonsurgical treatment in selected cases. *N. Engl. J. Med.* 244:898, 1951.
99. Visick, A. H. Conservative treatment of patients with acute perforated peptic ulcer. *Br. Med. J.* 2:941, 1946.
100. von Haberer, H. Zur Therapie akuter Geschwürsperforationen des Magens und Duodenums in die freie Bauchhöhle. *Wien. Klin. Wochenschr.* 32:413, 1919.
101. Walker, G. R., and Hardy, J. D. Fluid shifts in peritonitis. *Am. Surg.* 28:451, 1962.
102. Wangensteen, O. H. Non-operative treatment of localized perforations of the duodenum. *Minn. Med.* 18:477, 1935.
103. Watson, J. H. Acute perforating duodenal and gastric ulcers. *Br. Med. J.* 2:169, 1930.
104. Wellwood, J. M., Wilson, A. N., and Hoplinson, B. R. Gastrografin as an aid to the diagnosis of perforated peptic ulcer. *Br. J. Surg.* 58:245, 1971.
105. Winters, W. L., and Egan, S. The incidence of hemorrhage occurring with perforation in peptic ulcer. *J.A.M.A.* 113:2199, 1939.
106. Worman, L. W. The role of fluid sequestration in the pathogenesis of mediastinitis. *Am. J. Surg.* 111:813, 1966.
107. Wychulis, A. R., Priestley, J. T., and Foulk, W. T. A study of 360 patients with gastroje-

junal ulceration. *Surg. Gynecol. Obstet.* 122:89, 1961.
108. Yudine, S. S. Etude sur lels ulcères gastriques et duodenaux perfores. *J. Int. Chir.* 4:219, 1939.

EDITOR'S COMMENT

A modest controversy continues relative to simple closure of a perforated ulcer versus performance of a definitive procedure aimed at curing the ulcer diathesis. This is not an either-or situation, because each patient presents with a unique set of intrinsic factors that should sway the surgeon in the proper direction. For example, Sirinek and colleagues (*Arch. Surg.* 116:591, 1981) demonstrated that advanced age and a delay in treatment of more than 30 hours are factors suggesting that simple closure of the ulcer is propitious. When I was an intern, simple closure of the perforation was the only method of treatment. At about the midpoint in my surgical training, however, the Harkins group of Seattle wrote the following: "Primary subtotal gastric resection would appear to be the treatment of choice in individuals coming to operation early who have had previous failures of treatment, previous perforation, or are known to be uncooperative, and who are in condition to withstand a major operative procedure" (Schmitz et al. *Ann. Surg.* 138:689, 1953). From that point forward, I have been a devotee of the definitive operation, using good sense in applying the proper indications for a given patient. I have not been sorry in these 33 years for espousing this selective approach to the patient with a perforated duodenal ulcer.

L.M.N.

EDITOR'S COMMENT

There can of course be little doubt that when a patient has a perforated duodenal ulcer, lapartomy is indicated, perhaps mainly to achieve peritoneal lavage. There does remain, however, a small proportion of patients who are elderly, perhaps with intercurrent disease, whom it would be safer to treat without a laparotomy. Berne, Rosoff et al. [1] demonstrated the efficacy of a water-soluble gastroduodenogram to detect the presence of continuing leakage after perforation. This approach may be used to prevent an operation in poor-risk patients.

Another area for debate is the question of definitive surgical intervention. It remains my prejudice that simple suture and peritoneal lavage result in the lowest possible mortality. Any of the other procedures, for example, truncal vagotomy and pyloroplasty [2], will inevitably be followed in approximately 15 percent of these patients by undesirable and severe postoperative sequelae such as diarrhea, dumping, or bilious vomiting—and only about 50 percent of patients who have had an acute perforation can be expected to require further surgical treatment.

It would seem that the decline in incidence of perforation previously noted and commented on by the authors of this chapter continues, and McKay and McArdle [3] have found a continuing reduction in the numbers of perforated peptic ulcers in the west of Scotland. A similar result was found by Watkins et al. [4] in the Oxford region of England. They comment that most perforations occurring in their region were of acute ulcers, and they speculated that therefore improved therapy for chronic peptic ulceration is unlikely to result in a greater reduction in incidence. In addition, the trend in the direction of equality between the sexes, also noted in this chapter, was confirmed in that the male-to-female ratio, initially 4.9 : 1 in 1965–1970, fell to 1.9 : 1 between 1977 and 1982. This drop was caused not only by a reduced incidence of perforation in men but by an increase in incidence in women, which simply confirms that everything has its price.

C.W.

References

1. Jacobson, G., Berne, C. J., Harvey, I., and Rosoff, L. The examination of patients with suspected ulcer using a water-soluble contrast medium. *Am. J. Roentgenol.* 86:37, 1961.
2. Kirkpatrick, J. R., and Bouwman, B. L. A logical solution to the perforated ulcer controversy. *Surg. Gynecol. Obstet.* 150:683, 1980.
3. McKay, A. J., and McArdle, C. S. Cimetidine and perforated peptic ulcer. *Br. J. Surg.* 69:319, 1982.
4. Watkins, R. M., Dennison, A. R., and Collin, J. What has happened to perforated peptic ulcer? *Br. J. Surg.* 71:774, 1984.

17

Pyloric Stenosis

Harold Ellis

From the standpoint of pathology, the term *pyloric stenosis*, referring to the adult patient, is usually inaccurate; this is because the site of the obstruction is rarely the pylorus itself but more often immediately proximal to the sphincter, where the diagnosis of carcinoma is most probable, or more distally in the duodenal bulb, where the cause is almost invariably a duodenal ulcer. It would be more accurate to use the term *gastric outlet obstruction*, but the term *pyloric stenosis* is now so well established that it is unlikely to be uprooted for some time to come.

Criteria vary for accepting a diagnosis of pyloric stenosis. This lack of uniformity accounts to some extent for the differences one may find in reports of the incidence and clinical features from different centers. The criteria that we accept in our own studies are as follows:

1. Clinically, one or more of the following features—projectile vomiting (especially if food is identified as having been eaten the previous day), a gastric splash heard 3–4 hours after the last meal, visible gastric peristalsis, or a palpably distended, hypertrophied stomach
2. A gastric residue of 500 ml or more
3. Roentgenographic evidence of gastric outlet obstruction
4. Demonstration at operation or autopsy of gross narrowing of the gastric outlet

Causes of Obstruction

The most common cause of obstruction is peptic ulceration, usually duodenal, but occasionally pyloric, prepyloric, or even extending into the body of the stomach. Second to this comes carcinoma of the gastric antrum. Other causes are numerous but rare; they include adult hypertrophy of the pylorus [31, 52], gastroduodenal tuberculosis [48], benign tumors of the pylorus, Hodgkin's disease and leukemic infiltration of the stomach [11], heterotopic pancreatic tissue at the pylorus [58], invasion of the duodenum from an adjacent carcinoma of the pancreas, a prepyloric mucosal diaphragm [10, 23], or fibrous adhesions between the duodenum and an inflamed gallbladder or to the liver bed following cholecystectomy [22]. The causes of pyloric stenosis in a consecutive series of 100 patients admitted to Westminster Hospital were as follows [36]: duodenal ulcer, 56; carcinoma of the antrum, 36; gastric ulcer, 4; adult hypertrophy of the pylorus, 2; Hodgkin's disease, 1; heterotopic pancreatic nodule, 1.

Balint and Spence [2], in 118 consecutive cases of pyloric obstruction at the Central Middlesex Hospital, London, reported the following causes: duodenal ulcer, 95 (including prepyloric and pyloric ulcers); gastric ulcers remote from the pylorus, 7; antral carcinoma, 13; adhesions to chronically inflamed gallbladder, 2; congenital diaphragm, 1.

When stenosis is caused by a duodenal ulcer, the obstruction is rarely produced by fibrous scar tissue alone. In most instances the obstruction occurs in the presence of an active ulcer, and the associated inflammation, edema, and pylorospasm add considerably to the narrowing produced by the scar tissue. Indeed, healing of the ulcer by intensive medical treatment considerably ameliorates the clinical features of obstruction and may even give long-term relief [6].

Benign peptic ulcers of the antrum or of the pyloric channel itself may obstruct the gastric outlet by a combination of pathological effects similar to those of duodenal ulceration. As one might expect, ulcers in the pyloric channel are often associated with gastric retention, and this occurred in 46 of 100 consecutive patients with this lesion reported by Ruffin et al. [53]. Less easy to explain is the gastric retention that is sometimes seen in association with gastric ulcers remote from the prepyloric or pyloric region. This is often attributed loosely to pylorospasm, but Hinds and Harper [27] have pointed out that the lesser curvature of the stomach may undergo considerable shortening in association with gastric ulceration. Frequently they found residue to be present 24 hours after a barium meal examination within a pouch formed by the inferior portion of the stomach when the patient was standing in the erect position. Stomach emptying did not take place in these patients unless they were laid on the right side in a semiprone position. Hinds and Harper recorded 10 such patients, all men; 9 of these had vomited, and all 10 showed roentgenographic evidence of gastric retention.

THE COMPENSATED AND DECOMPENSATED PHASES OF PYLORIC STENOSIS

In the early stages of obstruction, emptying of the stomach may be normal or nearly normal and is associated with the presence of giant peristaltic waves on the barium meal examination. This has been appropriately termed the *compensated phase of pyloric stenosis* [55]. This excessive gastric peristalsis results in hypertrophy of the stomach wall, which not infrequently extends upward to include even the lower esophagus. In long-standing obstruction the stomach enters a phase of decompensation in which it becomes grossly dilated and relatively atonic. This may be compared with cardiac muscle decompensation, which occurs in stenotic valvular disease of the heart and which precipitates cardiac failure. The exact cause of this decompensation of the musculature is obscure, but it may be dependent on intracellular shifts of potassium or magnesium. The clinical signs of effortless and profuse vomiting in the late stages of gastric outlet obstruction may well be caused more by this failure in gastric peristalsis than by the degree of stenosis itself.

Metabolic Effects

Profound metabolic disturbances may take place as a result of the loss of gastric juice in the vomitus or even its sequestration within the dilated stomach.

Originally the illness that may accompany the stenosis was attributed to some toxic substance secreted by the obstructed stomach. In 1918 McCann [40] demonstrated both tetany and alkalosis after pyloric obstruction in dogs. MacCallum et al. [39] showed that gastric tetany could be correlated with loss of gastric juice. A year later Hastings, Murray, and Murray [25] reported on the changes in blood chemistry after experimental pyloric stenosis in the dog. They noted alkalosis, a marked decrease in plasma chloride, and, to a lesser extent, a decrease in plasma sodium.

In 1925 Gamble and Ross [21] clearly defined the loss of sodium and chloride and the increase in bicarbonate in plasma in experimental pyloric stenosis in the dog, and they demonstrated the beneficial effect of saline replacement. It was comparatively recently that the importance of potassium loss also became recognized [5, 37], and indeed it is only in the last few years that the intense metabolic changes associated with pyloric stenosis have been fully analyzed. Simple quantitative analysis of the amount of fluid and electrolytes lost in the gastric secretion does not alone explain all the effects, since they are complicated by consequent alterations in renal function [9, 28, 47].

Gastric juice in pyloric stenosis contains an average of 100 mEq/L chloride, 45 mEq/L sodium, and 10 mEq/L potassium, although it should be noted that these figures vary widely. The initial disturbance is caused by the vomiting of fluid containing chloride in excess of sodium and potassium, and the excess is lost as HCl. The hydrogen ion is derived from H_2CO_3, the residual HCO_3 passing into the extracellular fluid. The first disturbance is therefore a fall in plasma chloride and a rise in plasma bicarbonate. In the early stages this alkalotic tendency is compensated for by renal excretion of excess sodium bicarbonate, which maintains the pH within normal limits. It is of interest that there is little evidence of respiratory compensation by excretion of this excess of CO_2 in the expired air [1, 28].

In this early stage the urine is concentrated and diminished in volume (because of dehydration), its chloride content is diminished and then obliterated in response to an increasing chloride deficit, and it is alkaline.

As the situation progresses, a large sodium deficit develops partly because of losses in the vomitus and partly because of the still greater amount excreted in the urine. This is a consequence of the increased bicarbonate excretion in the urine, which must be accompanied by cation (mainly in the form of sodium and, to a lesser extent, potassium). This loss of sodium leads to a diminution in the extracellular fluid volume, which may be great enough to produce peripheral circulatory failure. As the plasma volume contracts, so glomerular filtration diminishes, urea clearance falls, and the blood urea level rises.

The body attempts to conserve its depleting sodium reserves by substituting hydrogen and potassium ions for the sodium as cation to be excreted with the bicarbonate. This accounts for the paradox in the advanced case in which the patient with alkalosis excretes an acid urine. This loss of H^+ and K^+ not only aggravates the extracellular alkalosis by further loss of hydrogen ions in the urine but also accentuates the potassium deficit that is already developing as a result of the loss of potassium in the vomitus. The potassium loss, like the sodium loss, is actually greater in the urine than in the vomitus. As potassium is lost from the cells it is replaced in part by sodium and in part by hydrogen. This shift produces an intracellular acidosis and aggravates still further the extracellular alkalosis [54].

In the advanced case, tetany results from a shift of the weakly alkaline ionized calcium phosphate to its un-ionized form in an attempt to reduce the alkalosis. There is thus a consequent fall in the concentration of calcium ions in the plasma, although the total calcium concentration is not reduced.

To sum up the metabolic disturbances, the patient is dehydrated and has a raised hematocrit reading. The serum chloride, sodium, and potassium levels are lowered, and plasma bicarbonate and urea concentrations are increased. The serum ionized calcium level falls. Urine is small in amount, it is initially alkaline but then becomes acid, and its chloride content is greatly reduced or absent.

Because of the dehydration, the concentration of electrolytes tends to increase, and in some instances rehydration causes a fall in both serum potassium and serum chloride levels. Because of this, Clark and Norman [9] suggest that the degree of metabolic alkalosis reflected by the level of standard bicarbonate provides a better index of the total metabolic disturbance than does the electrolyte pattern alone.

Correction of the metabolic disturbance described depends primarily on replacement with isotonic saline solution. Administration of the solution restores the volume of extracellular fluid and of plasma and hence restores a normal renal blood flow. It provides chloride in excess of its plasma concentration, thus replacing the chloride deficit, and the sodium enables the kidney to excrete an alkaline urine. Potassium supplements are indicated in the severe situation.

Incidence

Published results for the incidence of gastric outlet obstruction caused by peptic ulceration are highly variable. Discrepancies are caused by differences in definitions of stenosis and by disparity of populations being analyzed statistically.

Thus Portis and Jaffe [49] found an 11.8 percent incidence of stenosis in a postmortem study of 339 peptic ulcers found in 9171 consecutive autopsies at the Cook County Hospital, Chicago. This was similar to a figure of 11.7 percent given by Emery and Monroe [19] in a clinical study of 1435 inpatients and outpatients with peptic ulcer at the Peter Bent Brigham Hospital, Boston.

Hurst and Stewart [29] reviewed 5000 consecutive autopsies at Leeds, England; there were 403 peptic ulcers, 63 of which had stenosis (15.6 percent).

In operative series, Moynihan [46] had 56 examples of stenosis in his 288 duodenal ulcer patients undergoing surgical treatment (19.5 percent). Half a century later Moody, Cornell, and Beal [44] reviewed 70 cases of pyloric obstruction in 242 surgically treated patients with duodenal ulcer (28.9 percent). Berkman [4] found a 22.6 percent incidence of gastric retention in 97 gastric ulcers and 16 percent in 582 duodenal ulcers operated on in the Mayo Clinic.

Balint and Spence [2], estimating the incidence of pyloric stenosis in the ulcer population of their area of north London, concluded that it would be in the region of 2 percent.

There have been some excellent reviews of large hospital populations with peptic ulcer that deal with the incidence of stenosis. Haubrich [26] found that 7 percent of 4971 patients with duodenal ulcer at the Henry Ford Hospital had some degree of pyloric obstruction, compared with a 16.1 percent incidence of hemorrhage and a 3.1 percent incidence of perforation. The most exhaustive report published to date is that of Kozoll and Meyer [32], who presented a detailed survey of 8451 patients admitted to the Cook County Hospital between 1936 and 1955 who had gastroduodenal peptic ulceration. In this series there were 885 examples of obstructing gastroduodenal ulcer (10.5 percent). Of these, 226 were caused by gastric ulcer and 659 by duodenal ulceration. Gastric ulcer constituted 28.8 percent of all ulcers treated, and obstruction occurred in 8.9 percent. Duodenal ulcer comprised 17.2 percent of the entire series, and obstruction occurred in 11.1 percent of these patients. In this series it is particularly interesting that of 226 gastric ulcers, 71 were pyloric and 37 were situated in the antrum. The others were on the lesser curvature, on the anterior or posterior wall, and even (rarely) at the cardia or on the greater curvature. Thus in over two-thirds of instances the gastric ulcer was situated away from the gastric outlet.

Clinical Features

HISTORY: PAIN

The patient with gastric outlet obstruction caused by a benign peptic ulcer usually has a long preceding story of ulcerlike pain; we found this to be of 10 years' or longer duration in half our patients at Westminster. A short history should make one consider a malignant obstruction (in nearly two-thirds of our patients with cancer, it was under one year), and complete absence of pain (present in nearly one-third of our cancer patients) makes the likelihood of cancer extremely high. Balint and Spence [2] also found that about half of their peptic ulcer patients with stenosis had a history of pain of 10 years or more. Of 14 of their patients with a history of less than one year, 9 had carcinoma of the stomach; 7 of their 13 patients with malignant obstructions had no pain. Moody, Cornell, and Beal [44] noted an average length of history of 12 years in their 70 patients with stenosis caused by duodenal ulcer, but in 4 of these it was less than one year. Occasionally a patient will present with painless vomiting and will be found to have a benign obstructing ulcer. Usually the patient is a placid individual of low intelligence, with a high pain threshold.

As stenosis progresses and as the stomach becomes both dilated and decompensated, the actual character of the pain may alter. It may become more generalized upper abdominal discomfort that builds up during the day as the stomach fills and is then relieved by a massive vomit, which may well be self-induced.

Vomiting is an important feature, occurring in about 90 percent of patients with pyloric obstruction [33]. Typically the vomiting is projectile and large in amount and contains particles of food that have been eaten many hours or even two or three days previously.

When vomiting is copious and frequent, the patient may also complain of anorexia, coated tongue, an unpleasant taste in the mouth, thirst, and weakness (the last indicative of electrolyte disturbance). Rarely there may be tetanus, mental disturbance, convulsions, and even coma. In a series of 100 consecutive patients with pyloric stenosis [36], only 5 were admitted in a clinically obvious state of electrolyte imbalance—ill, dehydrated, weak, and, in one instance, irrational and tetanic.

Occasionally a patient will have gross pyloric stenosis and gastric dilatation that are readily detected both clinically and roentgenographically without having had a single episode of vomiting.

OTHER SYMPTOMS

Weight loss is a prominent feature in both benign and malignant pyloric obstruction and is an obvious sequela of the anorexia and vomiting. Recent constipation, presumably as a result of dehydration and absence of roughage in the diet, is a common complaint. Less frequent is diarrhea, a feature that was stressed by Balint and Spence [2], who noted this in 23 of their 118 patients (19 percent). In 6 it was severe enough to be one of the presenting symptoms. About 7 percent of Kozoll and Meyer's [33] 885 patients had diarrhea, and we noted it in 6 of 100 consecutive patients. Its cause is a matter for conjecture.

A history of previous gastrointestinal bleeding is obtained in about one-fourth of the patients with benign obstruction and may occur, although less frequently, in malignant disease. A history of repair of perforation is not unusual in the benign group but is extremely rare in the malignant group of obstructions.

Occasionally fermentation of retained gastric contents may be responsible for foul-smelling eructations. Analysis of the gas in the stomach reveals that it contains carbon dioxide, hydrogen, and methane, a highly inflammable mixture. There have been several instances of this gas exploding when the patient has lighted a cigarette or pipe. Victims have singed their beards, eyebrows, lips, and fingers in this dangerous occurrence [15]. Tydd and Dyer [60] reported two patients, both with obstructing carcinomas of the stomach, who presented with halitosis and malodorous belching.

EXAMINATION

Examination of the patient as a whole and of the abdomen in particular is of great importance in the diagnosis of gastric outlet obstruction and of not inconsiderable value in establishing its cause.

It is obvious that the "typical ulcer facies" of the old clinical textbooks applies to many patients with pyloric stenosis caused by peptic ulceration; many are thin (approximately two out of three in our series), and it is unusual to see a patient with this condition who is overweight. Dehydration and signs of electrolyte disturbance, as mentioned earlier, may be present but are fortunately not often encountered in modern practice.

Abdominal examination may reveal one of three stages of progressive enlargement of the stomach described by the late Sir James Walton of the London Hospital in his clinical teaching: "The stomach you can hear, the stomach you can see, and the stomach you can feel." First, a gastric splash may be detected by shaking the patient's trunk vigorously; this is important if heard 3 to 4 hours after the last meal or drink. As the stomach dilates and hypertrophies, a visible swelling appears in the upper abdomen, and visible peristalsis passing from the left to the right is observed. This peristalsis can be accentuated by giving the patient a drink of soda water [38]. Finally, the grossly dilated stomach, weighed down by its retained gastric contents, may be not only audible and visible but also palpable.

In 56 consecutive patients with stenosing duodenal ulcer we found a splash to be present in 36 (64 percent). Visible peristalsis was obvious in 9, of whom 4 had gastric distention great enough to produce a palpable mass.

Carcinoma of the stomach in most instances produces obstruction more rapidly than do peptic ulcers, often not allowing time for gastric hypertrophy and dilatation to take place to the same degree as in benign stenosis. Thus only 5 of our 36 patients with malignant obstruction had a splash (14 percent), and only 1 of these had visible peristalsis. In no patient was the distended stomach palpable.

The presence of a mass in the pyloric region is suggestive of a carcinoma and is found in about half the patients with cancer. Rarely, a peptic ulcer produces an inflammatory mass with the head of the pancreas, the adjacent omentum, or the hepatic flexure of the colon that is large enough to produce a tender, palpable swelling. Not surprisingly, this is usually mistaken for a malignant tumor.

The clinical differences between benign peptic ulcers and gastric carcinomas that result in gastric outlet obstruction are summarized in Table 17-1.

Table 17-1. Comparison of benign and malignant gastric outlet obstruction

History and physical findings	Peptic ulcer	Carcinoma
Length of history	Long	Short
Pain	Usually typical of ulcer	May be completely absent
Signs of gastric enlargement (splash, peristalsis)	Common	Unusual
Mass at pylorus	Unusual	Common

Roentgenographic Appearances

The roentgenographic signs of pyloric stenosis fall into two groups—those indicating an obstruction at the gastric outlet and those demonstrating its site and possible nature.

The plain roentgenogram itself may show evidence of gastric stasis by the presence of a large gastric shadow with retained food particles that appear as patchy translucencies. An erect roentgenogram will show a large high gastric fluid level.

SIGNS OF OBSTRUCTION AT THE GASTRIC OUTLET

There are a number of signs on barium meal examination that indicate obstruction at the gastric outlet. The *presence of excessive fasting gastric juice* is immediately evident as the first mouthful of barium is observed entering the stomach. Instead of running down the lesser curvature and parting the opposed gastric walls, the particles of barium are observed to sink through a layer of fluid and come to rest at the bottom of the greater curvature to produce a saucerlike appearance. The roentgenogram taken in the erect position shows three layers—air, gastric juice, and barium—separated from each other by two fluid levels (Fig. 17-1).

In the compensated phase of pyloric obstruction, *giant peristaltic waves* are seen, which indent the greater and lesser curvatures simultaneously (Fig. 17-2). When compensation fails, however, these waves fade away after a variable period of between 1 and 3 hours; thus although there is good initial emptying of the stomach through the stenosed

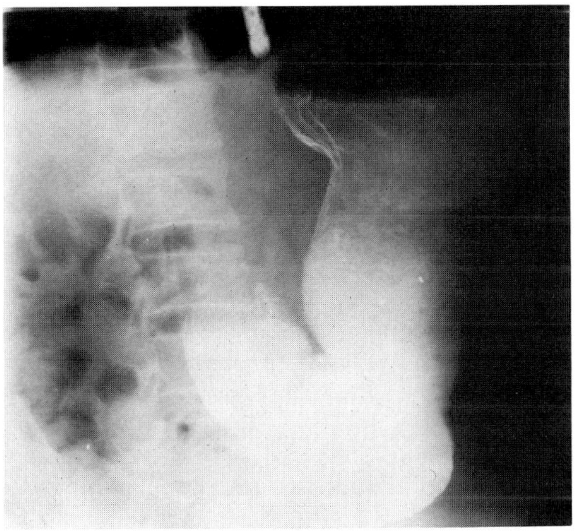

Fig. 17-1. Gastric outlet obstruction caused by a stenosing duodenal ulcer. As barium enters the stomach in the presence of excessive gastric juice, three layers of media are demonstrated—barium, gastric juice, and air—together with the two intervening fluid levels.

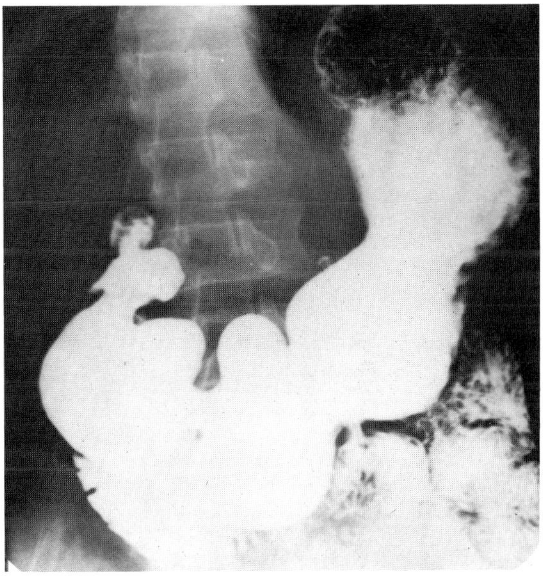

Fig. 17-2. Giant peristaltic waves in the compensated phase of gastric outlet obstruction that was caused, in this patient, by a penetrating posterior duodenal ulcer. At this stage no barium was present in the stomach at the 6-hour roentgenogram. Four months later the patient was readmitted in the decompensated phase, and a further barium meal examination demonstrated a large atonic stomach.

area, a considerable amount of barium remains in the stomach at 4–6 hours.

Eventually in the decompensated phase the stomach appears as a large, atonic bag. This is more commonly seen in obstruction caused by duodenal ulcer than with malignant lesions, and it fits with the clinical observation we have already mentioned that the very large stomach is usually associated with benign obstruction (Fig. 17-3).

The normal stomach empties in about 2 hours, although occasionally a small residue may be seen after 4–6 hours, which is diluted by gastric secretion. In pyloric stenosis, however, there is *more than a 50 percent retention* of the barium sulfate in the 4- to 6-hour roentgenogram. It is important to distinguish obstructive lesions in the lower duodenum or uppermost jejunum, where considerable delay in emptying may be found. Pylorospasm can be distinguished by administering intravenous propantheline bromide, after which normal gastric emptying will take place.

When the obstruction is situated beyond the pylorus, *abnormal dilatability of the pyloric canal* may be seen either on screening or by studying serial roentgenograms. The canal may dilate up to 2.5 cm in width and then contract down again to its usual size (Fig. 17-4). Kreel and I have found this to be a reliable sign of duodenal bulb obstruction [36]. This appearance may also occur in obstructive lesions placed more distally in the duodenum, e.g., carcinoma.

SIGNS INDICATING SITE AND TYPE OF OBSTRUCTION

That the pyloric stenosis is produced by a duodenal ulcer is indicated first by the presence of an active ulcer crater and second by the demonstration of scarring of the duodenal cap. The ulcer is often of the penetrating type and

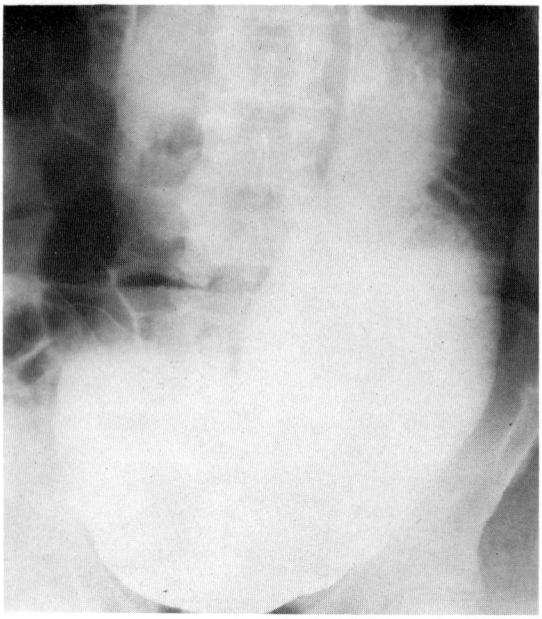

Fig. 17-3. The decompensated phase of pyloric obstruction; the stomach is large and atonic. The obstruction is caused by a long-standing active stenosing duodenal ulcer. Satisfactory recovery followed vagotomy and posterior gastrojejunostomy.

most frequently occurs on the posterosuperior aspect of the duodenum. This type of crater gives the appearance of an irregular diverticulum that remains constant in size. Scarring of the duodenal cap may be central, producing an irregular, star-shaped appearance, or eccentric, with the formation of a prestenotic diverticulum; the latter appearance is more common.

If the obstruction is situated at the gastric antrum, the most likely diagnosis is of a carcinoma of the stomach. The roentgenographic signs are rigidity of the antral wall with irregular contour and lack of peristalsis. The antrum may give a tapered appearance, and there may be a filling defect caused by carcinomatous ulcer. Occasionally the granulation tissue that surrounds a penetrating posterior wall gastric ulcer produces a similar appearance, and more rarely antral obstruction may be caused by corrosives or chronic inflammatory lesions. Occasionally the malignant process arises outside the stomach; for example, pancreatic carcinoma or Hodgkin's disease involving the adjacent lymph nodes.

Lesions occurring at the pyloric canal itself may produce obstruction, but in fact this is the least common site of obstruction of the gastric outlet. There may be an active pyloric ulcer with a visible ulcer niche, but more commonly the obstruction results from scarring around such an ulcer, in which case the canal becomes narrowed and elongated.

Adult hypertrophic pyloric stenosis is recognized by the bulbous intrusion into the base of the cap. A rare finding is the presence of heterotopic pancreatic tissue encircling the pyloric canal. The clue to its presence lies in the demonstration of a thin streak of barium that communicates with the pyloric lumen and represents the duct of the ectopic pancreas.

Of course the important practical point is the differentiation between obstruction caused by a stenosing duodenal ulcer and obstruction caused by a carcinoma of the stomach (Fig. 17-5 A and B). Malignant disease involving the antrum rarely encroaches on the duodenal cap; moreover, antral carcinoma is distinctly rare in association with active duodenal ulceration. Deformity proximal to the duodenal bulb is therefore strongly suggestive of malignant disease, whereas deformity of the duodenal cap itself greatly suggests benign obstruction.

Endoscopy

It might be imagined that the introduction of fiberoptic gastroscopy has revolutionized diagnosis in pyloric stenosis. Unfortunately, this has not proved to be so. It is true that in early pyloric obstruction it is possible to clear the mucosa sufficiently by lavage to obtain adequate views of the region, identify the pathology of the obstruction, and obtain biopsy material for histological examination. In severe instances, however, the gross contamination of stale food (and often residual barium) and the impossibility of removing all the fluid residue in the stomach make adequate visualiza-

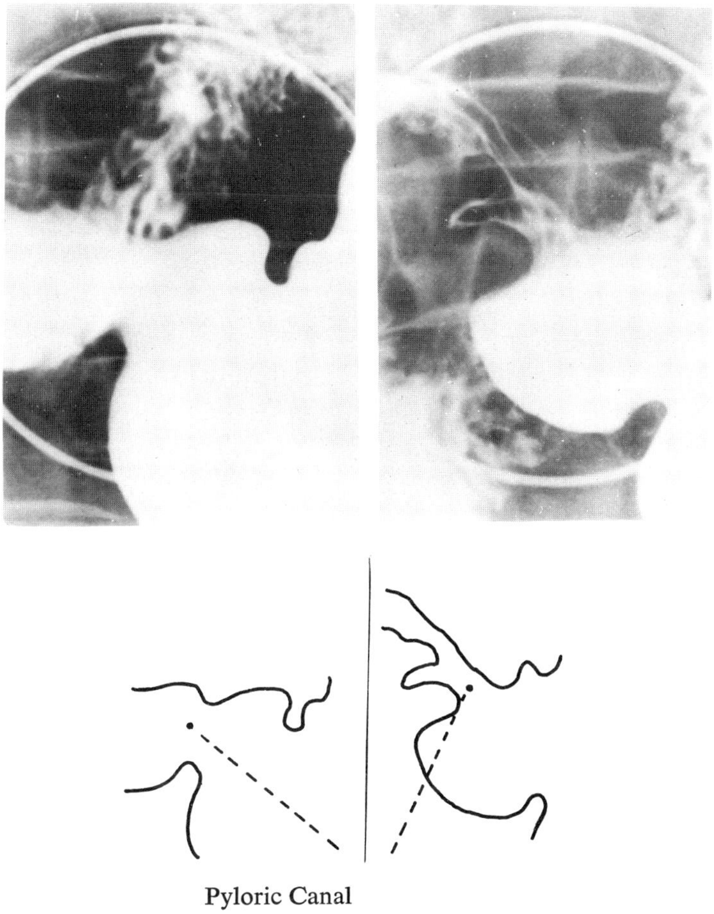

Fig. 17-4. Two adjacent spot roentgenograms from a series, showing abnormal dilatability of the pylorus proximal to a stricture of the midportion of the duodenal bulb produced by a stenosing duodenal ulcer. The accompanying tracings of the roentgenograms demonstrate the wide range in the width of the pyloric canal that can be observed during screening.

tion of the crucial pyloric region impossible. Roentgenographic examination, therefore, remains the mainstay of our special investigations.

Treatment

PREOPERATIVE TREATMENT

The treatment of established pyloric stenosis caused by duodenal ulceration is inevitably surgical, but it must be preceded by a period of meticulous medical preparation [59], the aims of which are decompression of the dilated stomach, control of the activity of the ulcer, correction of fluid and electrolyte imbalance, and improvement in the general condition of the patient.

Twice-daily gastric aspirations are carried out, using a wide-bore tube; the gastric residue is measured and the stomach washed out with normal saline solution. Plain water must not be used, since further electrolyte loss will occur as a dialysate into the lavage fluid. Once the residue has fallen to below 250 ml, lavage can be reduced to once a day. During this time there is no need to restrict fluids; indeed, hourly milk drinks are encouraged. Administration of cimetidine 400 mg twice daily is started. The belladonna alkaloids should not

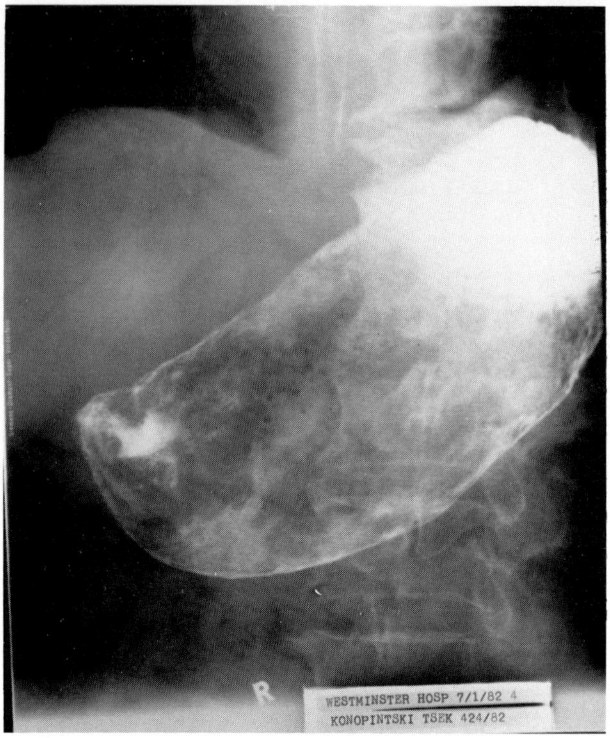
R
WESTMINSTER HOSP 7/1/82 4
KONOPINTSKI TSEK 424/82

A

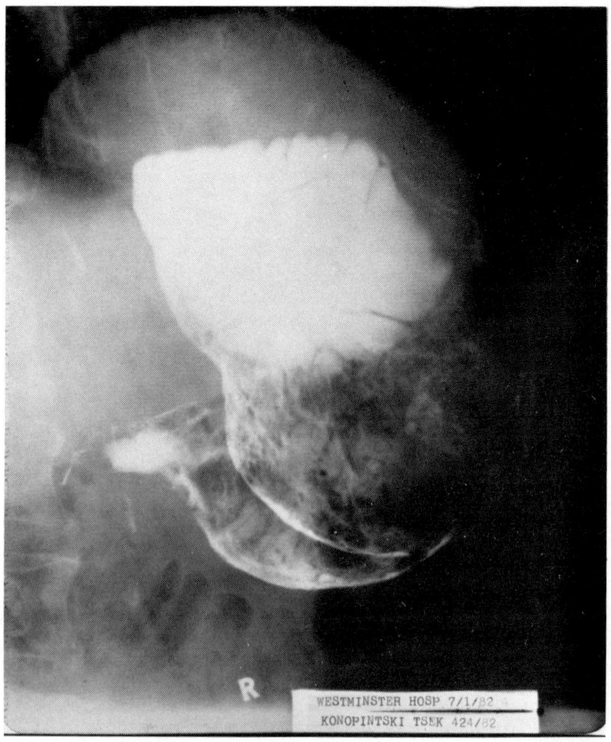
R
WESTMINSTER HOSP 7/1/82
KONOPINTSKI TSEK 424/82

B

be prescribed; they inhibit peristalsis and aggravate the degree of gastric retention [35].

Within a very few days the ulcer begins to heal, the adjacent tissue becomes less edematous, and the associated gastritis subsides; the degree of obstruction lessens, and considerable amounts of fluids can be taken readily by mouth. Solid food is forbidden, since particles will certainly clog the narrowed gastric outlet. Ascorbic acid is given by injection, since often these patients are incipiently scorbutic because of a long period of dietary restriction.

If the blood biochemistry is undisturbed, no intravenous replacement is usually needed, but if electrolyte depletion has occurred or if the patient is obviously dehydrated, intravenous replacement therapy is necessary as already described.

Anemia below 80 percent hemoglobin should be corrected by blood transfusion. The low hemoglobin may become manifest only when the dehydration has been corrected; an initial artificially high level may reflect diminished plasma volume. Any dental caries should receive attention, and preoperative breathing exercises together with active general physiotherapy are initiated.

Usually 7 or even 10 days are required to prepare a patient with severe stenosis for the operation, but this is time well spent and will convert what is perhaps a seriously ill, anemic, dehydrated, and electrolyte-depleted patient into one fit for a major operation.

OPERATION OF CHOICE

The conventional operation for the stenosing duodenal ulcer is a high partial gastrectomy with some type of gastrojejunal reconstruction. Vagotomy and antrectomy with gastroduodenal anastomosis are difficult procedures because of the gross duodenal scarring, whereas the stenosis actually makes closure of the duodenal stump delightfully easy. The duodenum is mobilized just distally to the stenosed area and divided through its narrowest part; closure by means of a series of pursestring sutures can then be performed with complete safety.

Although vagotomy combined with gastric drainage is now a well-established procedure in the surgical attack on duodenal ulceration, it was suggested by a number of authorities that it should not be employed when pyloric stenosis exists [7, 24, 34, 42, 45]. It has been argued that the decompensated musculature of the stomach that has been dilated as a result of the pyloric obstruction may be more susceptible to the atonic effect of the vagotomy and that prolonged gastric stasis is likely to follow this operation. Bergin and Jordan [3] found that 8 of their 32 patients with stenosis treated by vagotomy combined with drainage had gastric retention for more than 10 days following operation, but there was not a single example of this complication in 42 similar cases treated by gastric resection only. Kraft, Fry, and DeWeese [34] compared patients with duodenal ulceration who had been treated by gastrectomy, by vagotomy combined with hemigastrectomy, and by vagotomy and drainage. The patients were divided into those who did not have an obstruction and those with established pyloric stenosis. In the patients without an obstruction the incidence of postoperative gastric retention that existed for 14 days or more was, respectively, 3 percent, 9 percent, and 5 percent in the three procedures. In the patients with pyloric stenosis, the incidence was zero, 9 percent, and 27 percent, respectively, in the three procedures. Because of the high incidence of gastric retention following vagotomy, these authors strongly advised against vagotomy in the surgical management of such patients.

In contrast, Smith [56] noted uniformly satisfactory results in his 27 patients treated by vagotomy and pyloroplasty for stenosis and

Fig. 17-5. Typical barium meal appearances of an obstructing carcinoma of the antrum. (A) The obstructed stomach, which is less dilated than in a typical benign occlusion. The site of the obstruction lies proximal to the duodenum. (B) The patient has now been tipped slightly head-down. This enables the radiologist to demonstrate quite clearly the irregular neoplastic narrowing of the antrum.

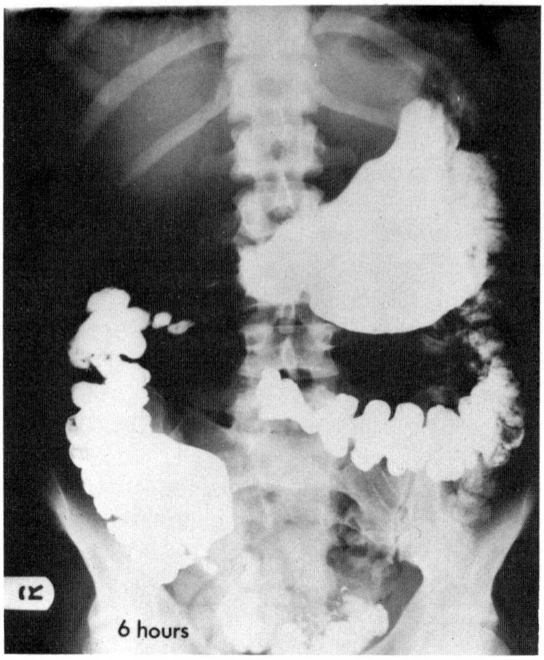

Fig. 17-6. Gastric outlet obstruction caused by stenosing duodenal ulcer with gross gastric retention; there is considerable residue on this 6-hour film.

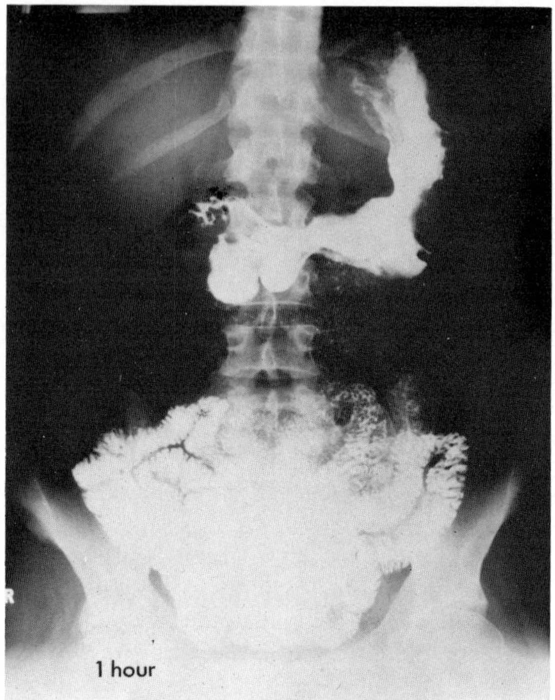

Fig. 17-7. Barium meal examination of the same patient one year after vagotomy and pyloroplasty of the Weinberg type. The stomach has regained its normal size, tone, and emptying ability, as shown on this roentgenogram taken 1 hour after the ingestion of barium.

encountered no problems of postoperative gastric retention. Feggetter and Pringle [20] found no differences in their long-term follow-up results between patients operated on because of failed medical treatment and those with stenosis, both groups having been treated by vagotomy and gastrojejunostomy.

My colleagues and I have reported a clinical and roentgenographic study of 21 patients with gross pyloric stenosis treated by vagotomy and either pyloroplasty or gastrojejunostomy and followed for nine months to five years [18]. This study showed uniformly good immediate and late long-term results. Postoperative gastric retention did not occur in any of the patients, and none required postoperative gastric aspiration. All had good functional results, and subsequent barium meal studies showed return of the dilated stomachs to normal size and tone with satisfactory emptying (Figs. 17-6, 17-7).

By 1972 we were able to report on 56 patients treated by this technique [17], and at present our total has reached 180 patients. To date (apart from 1 patient in whom a stomal ulcer has developed and who has required conversion to a partial gastrectomy) the results have been uniformly satisfactory, and our findings even suggest that stenosis represents an indication rather than a contraindication to vagotomy and drainage.

The last decade has seen the acceptance of this philosophy in many parts of the world. From the United States, Rachlin [50] reported clinically uncomplicated postoperative progress in eight patients who had vagotomy and Heineke-Mikulicz pyloroplasty for moderate-to-complete pyloric obstruction caused by duodenal ulcer. De Matteis and Hermann [13] gave an account of their 60 patients with stenosing duodenal ulcer treated by vagotomy and a variety of drainage procedures. Postoperative gastric atony was not a problem, although nasogastric intubation was used for one to eight days postoperatively. The best long-term results were achieved with vagotomy and Finney pyloroplasty. Davis and Williams [12] from Birmingham, England, reported a satisfactory postoperative course and long-term follow-up studies in 15 patients reviewed one to six years after vagotomy and pyloroplasty. In Cairo, El-Katib and Mashhoor [16] treated 13 patients with stenosis by means of proximal gastric vagotomy and gastrojejunostomy. Nasogastric suction was used for up to 72 hours postoperatively, and the short-term follow-up results were satisfactory. In Spain, Miguel [43] treated a group of 16 patients with severe pyloric stenosis by vagotomy and pyloroplasty [12] or vagotomy and gastroenterostomy [4]. Postoperative decompression was not required in any of these patients. From Dakar, in North Africa, Chabal and his colleagues [8] reported an interesting series of 76 patients with stenosis treated by vagotomy and drainage. Three had associated gastric resection, 67 had gastroenterostomy, and 3 had plastic enlargement of the pyloric canal using the serosal patch technique in which the loop of the proximal jejunum is brought up and its serosal surface used to cover the defect in the opened pylorus.

Johnston [30] in 1974 reported the treatment of 15 consecutive patients with pyloric stenosis secondary to duodenal ulcer by proximal gastric vagotomy combined with digital dilation of the stricture through a small gastrotomy incision. The follow-up barium meal examinations performed one year or more after operation showed that gastric emptying was satisfactory and the patients were progressing well clinically. In 1976 the same group in Leeds [41] increased the series to 23 patients followed from four months to five years. They were able to compare this group with 23 similar patients treated by vagotomy and drainage by other surgeons during the same period. Two patients in each group required further drainage procedures, although the functional results were better in the group that underwent highly selective vagotomy. White and his colleagues [61] treated 12 patients with stenosis secondary to duodenal ulceration by proximal gastric vagotomy and either a duodenoplasty or, if this was not possible, retrograde dilation through a duodenotomy. Two of these patients had transient stasis but all had satisfactory gastric emptying at three months.

Although there seems little doubt that this technique results in satisfactory gastric emptying, it is now well recognized that the recurrence rate following proximal gastric vagotomy is high. For example, from University College Hospital in London, Storey and his colleagues [57] report a follow-up study of 93 patients treated by proximal gastric vagotomy from five to nine years previously. The confirmed recurrence rate was no less than 16 percent. In addition there were patients with transient recurrent ulceration and a group with persistent dyspeptic symptoms but in whom no ulcer was demonstrated. Similarly, Donahue and his co-workers [14] in a prospective, randomized study of proximal gastric vagotomy versus selective vagotomy and antrectomy with a 4- to 12-year follow-up period found the rate of recurrent ulcer to be 20 percent in the patients who underwent proximal gastric vagotomy, yet the postoperative morbidity for selective vagotomy and antrectomy was of such consequence that the former procedure seemed to be an acceptable operation. The surgeon needs to weigh the undoubtedly high proportion of excellent functional results following this most conservative of vagotomies against the undoubtedly higher incidence of recurrent ulceration.

Gastroenterostomy alone, once a standard treatment for pyloric stenosis [51], still has a place in the treatment of the ill and elderly patient. However, by meticulous preoperative treatment, many of these patients can be rendered fit to withstand the comparatively slight addition of vagotomy to the drainage procedure.

The treatment of other causes of pyloric obstruction, such as benign and malignant gastric antral ulceration and adult pyloric hypertrophy, are discussed in other chapters.

References

1. Aber, G. M., Sampson, P. A., Whitehead, T. P., and Brooke, B. N. The role of chloride in the correction of alkalosis associated with potassium depletion. *Lancet* 2:1028, 1962.
2. Balint, J. A., and Spence, S. Pyloric stenosis. *Br. Med. J.* 1:890, 1959.
3. Bergin, W. F., and Jordan, P. H. Gastric atonia and delayed gastric emptying after vagotomy for obstructing ulcer. *Am. J. Surg.* 98:612, 1959.
4. Berkman, D. M. Gastric retention: Its treatment and surgical mortality. *Coll. Papers Mayo Clin.* 15:92, 1923.
5. Black, D. A. K., and Jepson, R. P. Electrolyte depletion in pyloric stenosis. *Q. J. Med.* 23:367, 1954.
6. Brown, C. H. Duodenal ulcer complicated by obstruction: Results of medical treatment. *Am. J. Dig. Dis.* 4:940, 1959.
7. Capper, W. M. Alimentary Disease. In R. B. Scott and R. M. Walker (Eds.), *Medical Annual.* Bristol, Eng.: Wright, 1965. P. 54.
8. Chabal, J., Ballon, C., and Croizat, B. Le traitement des sténoses pyloriques. *Lyon Chir.* 63:680, 1967.
9. Clark, R. G., and Norman, J. N. Metabolic alkalosis in pyloric stenosis. *Lancet* 1:1244, 1964.
10. Conway, N. Pyloric antral mucosal diaphragm. *Br. Med. J.* 1:970, 1965.
11. Cornes, J. S., and Jones, T. G. Leukaemic lesions of the gastrointestinal tract. *J. Clin. Pathol.* 15:305, 1962.
12. Davis, N. P., and Williams, J. A. Duodenal ulcer stenosis with gastric dilatation: Treatment by vagotomy and pyloroplasty. *Am. J. Surg.* 121:260, 1971.
13. De Matteis, R. A., and Hermann, R. E. Vagotomy and drainage for obstructing duodenal ulcers. *Am. J. Surg.* 127:237, 1974.
14. Donahue, P. E., Bombeck, C. T., Condon, R. E., and Nyhus, L. M. Proximal gastric vagotomy versus selective vagotomy with antrectomy: Results of a prospective randomized clinical trial after 4 to 12 years. *Surgery* 96:585, 1984.
15. East, T. An explosive eructation. *Lancet* 2:252, 1934.
16. El-Katib, Y., and Mashhoor, N. Highly selective vagotomy and drainage for duodenal ulcer stenosis. *Br. J. Surg.* 61:241, 1974.
17. Ellis, H. Pyloric Stenosis due to Duodenal Ulceration. In C. Wastell (Ed.), *Chronic Duodenal Ulcer.* London: Butterworth, 1974. P. 251.
18. Ellis, H., Starer, F., Venables, C. W., and Ware, C. C. Clinical and radiological study of vagotomy and gastric drainage in the treatment of pyloric stenosis due to duodenal ulceration. *Gut* 7:671, 1966.
19. Emery, E. S., and Monroe, R. T. Peptic ulcer: Nature and treatment based on a study of 1435 cases. *Arch. Intern. Med.* 55:271, 1935.
20. Feggetter, G. Y., and Pringle, R. The relationship between the severity of duodenal ulceration and the results of bilateral vagotomy and gastrojejunostomy. *Br. J. Surg.* 52:691, 1965.
21. Gamble, J. L., and Ross, S. G. The factors in the dehydration following pyloric obstruction. *J. Clin. Invest.* 1:403, 1925.
22. Ger, R. Postoperative extrinsic pyloric stenosis. *Br. Med. J.* 2:294, 1964.
23. Gerber, B. C. Prepyloric diaphragm: An unusual abnormality. *Arch. Surg.* 90:472, 1965.
24. Harper, F. B. Gastric dysfunction after vagectomy. *Am. J. Surg.* 112:94, 1966.
25. Hastings, A. B., Murray, C. D., and Murray, H. A. Certain chemical changes in the blood after pyloric obstruction in dogs. *J. Biol. Chem.* 46:223, 1921.
26. Haubrich, W. S. Obstruction At or Near the Pylorus. In H. L. Bockus (Ed.), *Gastroenterology* (2d ed.), Vol. 2. Philadelphia: Saunders, 1963.
27. Hinds, S. J., and Harper, R. A. K. Shortening of the lesser curvature in gastric ulcer. *Br. J. Radiol.* 25:451, 1952.
28. Howe, C. T., and LeQuesne, L. P. Pyloric stenosis: The metabolic effects. *Br. J. Surg.* 51:923, 1964.
29. Hurst, A. F., and Stewart, M. J. *Gastric and Duodenal Ulcer.* London: Oxford University Press, 1929.
30. Johnston, D. A New Look at Vagotomy. In L. M. Nyhus (Ed.), *Surgery Annual,* 1974. New York: Appleton-Century-Crofts, 1974. P. 125.
31. Keynes, W. M. Simple and complicated hypertrophic pyloric stenosis in the adult. *Gut* 6:240, 1965.
32. Kozoll, D. D., and Meyer, K. A. Obstructing gastroduodenal ulcers. *Arch. Surg.* 88:793, 1964.
33. Kozoll, D. D., and Meyer, K. A. Obstructing gastroduodenal ulcer: Symptoms and signs. *Arch. Surg.* 89:491, 1964.
34. Kraft, R. O., Fry, W. J., and DeWeese, M. S. Postvagotomy gastric atony. *Arch. Surg.* 88:865, 1964.

35. Kramer, P. The adverse effects of belladonna alkaloids in benign pyloric obstruction: An experimental study. *N. Engl. J. Med.* 251:600, 1954.
36. Kreel, L., and Ellis, H. Pyloric stenosis in adults: A clinical and radiological study of 100 consecutive patients. *Gut* 6:253, 1965.
37. Lans, H. S., Stein, I. F., and Meyer, K. A. Electrolyte abnormalities in pyloric obstruction resulting from peptic ulcer and gastric carcinoma. *Ann. Surg.* 135:441, 1952.
38. Lees, F. Clinical diagnosis of pyloric obstruction: The soda water test. *Br. Med. J.* 1:1016, 1956.
39. MacCallum, W. G., Lintz, J., Vermyle, H. N., et al. The effect of pyloric obstruction in relation to gastric tetany. *Bull. Johns Hopkins Hosp.* 31:1, 1920.
40. McCann, W. S. A study of the carbon dioxide combining power of the blood plasma in experimental tetany. *J. Biol. Chem.* 35:553, 1918.
41. McMahon, M. J., Greenall, M. J., Johnston, D., and Goligher, J. C. Highly selective vagotomy plus dilatation of the stenosis compared with truncal vagotomy and drainage in the treatment of pyloric stenosis secondary to duodenal ulceration. *Gut* 17:471, 1976.
42. Mialaret, J. Indications et Contre-indications de la Vagotomie dans le Traitement chirurgical de l'Ulcère duodénal. In A. G. Weiss and L. F. Hollender (Eds.), *La Vagotomie dans l'Ulcère Gastro-Duodéno-Jéjunal.* Paris: Expansion Scientifique Française, 1964. P. 89.
43. Miguel, J. Vagotomia y drenaje gástrico en las formas estenosantes de la ulcera duodenal. *Cir. Ginecol. Urol.* 21:104, 1967.
44. Moody, F. G., Cornell, G. N., and Beal, J. M. Pyloric obstruction complicating peptic ulcer. *Arch. Surg.* 84:462, 1962.
45. Moore, F. D., Chapman, W. P., Schulz, M. D., and Jones, C. M. Resection of the vagus nerves in peptic ulcer: Physiological effects and clinical results with a report of two years' experience. *J.A.M.A.* 133:341, 1947.
46. Moynihan, B. G. A. *Duodenal Ulcer* (2d ed.). Philadelphia: Saunders, 1912.
47. Parsons, F. M., and Watkinson, G. The treatment of pyloric stenosis in peptic ulceration. *Postgrad. Med. J.* 30:145, 1954.
48. Picardi, N. Pyloric stenosis of rare aetiology: Gastro-duodenal tuberculosis. *Chir. Gastroenterol.* 7:287, 1973.
49. Portis, S. A., and Jaffe, R. H. Study of peptic ulcer based on necropsy records. *J.A.M.A.* 110:6, 1938.
50. Rachlin, L. Vagotomy and Heineke-Mikulicz pyloroplasty in the treatment of pyloric stenosis. *Am. Surg.* 36:251, 1970.
51. Reid, H., and Marcus, R. Posterior gastroenterostomy for organic pyloric stenosis. *Br. J. Surg.* 35:304, 1948.
52. Riesenfeld, G. Primary stenosing hypertrophy of the pylorus in the adult. *J. Isr. Med. Assoc.* 86:239, 1974.
53. Ruffin, J. M., Johnston, D. H., Carter, D. D., and Baylin, G. J. Clinical picture of pyloric channel ulcer: Analysis of 100 consecutive cases. *J.A.M.A.* 159:668, 1955.
54. Saunders, S. J., Irvine, R. O. H., Crawford, M. A., and Milne, M. D. Intracellular pH of potassium-deficient voluntary muscle. *Lancet* 1:468, 1960.
55. Shanks, S. C., and Kerley, P. J. *A Text-Book of X-Ray Diagnosis* (3d ed.), Vol. 3. London: H. K. Lewis, 1958. P. 128.
56. Smith, G. K. Post-vagotomy atony. *Arch. Surg.* 88:872, 1964.
57. Storey, D. W., Boulos, P. B., Ward, M. W. N., and Clark, G. C. Proximal gastric vagotomy after five years. *Gut* 22:702, 1981.
58. Tonkin, R. D., Field, T. G., and Wykes, P. R. Pancreatic heterotopia as a cause of dyspepsia. *Gut* 3:135, 1962.
59. Turner, F. P. Hyperalimentation in management of pyloric obstruction with comments on certain theoretical relationships between protein deficiency and peptic ulcer. *Gastroenterology* 29:1061, 1955.
60. Tydd, T. F., and Dyer, N. H. Pyloric stenosis presenting with halitosis. *Br. Med. J.* 3:321, 1974.
61. White, C. M., Harding, L. K., Keighley, M. R. B., et al. Gastric emptying after treatment of stenosis secondary to duodenal ulceration by proximal gastric vagotomy and duodenoplasty or pyloric dilatation. *Gut* 19:783, 1978.

EDITOR'S COMMENT

Pyloric obstruction as a complication of duodenal ulcer disease will always be a clinical entity. Although new and improved drugs have decreased the necessity for operation in this patient population, there is a recurrent ulcer problem unless patients are placed on a lifelong medication regimen. Each sequence of exacerbation or recurrence and healing moves the patient closer and closer to symptomatic pyloric obstruction.

Lunde, Liavag, and Roland (*World J. Surg.* 9:165, 1985) obtained excellent results in a 13-year experience treating patients with duodenal ulcer and pyloric stenosis by proximal gastric vagotomy plus pyloroplasty (PGV + P). They reported a recurrent ulcer rate of only 1.3 percent. When I first read Lunde's article, it seemed obvious that the good results reported were caused by "burned out" ulcer disease. For many years we taught that patients with pyloric stenosis had a low gastric acid output and that almost any operation to relieve the obstruction would cure the disease. Thus simple gastrojejunostomy frequently was used for "cure." Fortunately, the authors performed both basal and maximal acid output determinations on their patients preoperatively and postoperatively. It was clear that their patients were hypersecretors. Rather than having "burned out" ulcer disease, the patients had the same gastric acid profile as a control group of patients with duodenal ulcer without pyloric stenosis. Whereas the former group of patients was treated with proximal gastric vagotomy and Heineke-Mikulicz pyloroplasty, the patients serving as controls were treated with proximal gastric vagotomy alone (PGV). The difference in recurrent ulcer rates following these rather similar procedures is striking—1.3 percent for PGV + P and 11.4 percent for PGV.

How can we explain this difference between the two operations in terms of recurrent ulceration? There is no certain explanation. Yet I find it interesting that the recurrent ulcer rate of 1.3 percent for PGV + P mirrors the 1.5 percent recurrence following selective proximal vagotomy plus pyloroplasty (SPV + P) in 1318 patients reported by Holle (*World J. Surg.* 1:26, 1977). For the purpose of this discussion, the selective proximal vagotomy of Holle is considered identical to proximal gastric vagotomy. The results are exceptional when pyloroplasty is added to PGV in the presence of gastric outlet obstruction, as reported by Lunde and co-workers, and when pyloroplasty is added (SPV + P), as reported by Holle, in patients without pyloric obstruction. Is there an underlying canon hidden in these observations?

Holle related his clinical studies to a lifetime of observations in the experimental laboratory. He has summarized the compensatory effect of pyloroplasty appropriate to form and function as diminution of postprandial acid concentration, diminution of postprandial gastrin release, and normalization of disturbances to motility (Holle, F., In F. Holle and G. Holle (Eds.), *Vagotomy and Pyloroplasty: Advances 1975–1980*. Berlin: Springer, 1980).

The work of Holle and the observations of Lunde et al. suggest a need to reopen the issue stated in the question, "Should PGV be performed with or without pyloroplasty?"
L.M.N.

18

The Zollinger-Ellison Syndrome

Robert M. Zollinger
Helene P. Ayres

Three decades have passed since a direct relationship between non-beta islet-cell tumors of the pancreas and gastric hypersecretion was first suggested in 1955 [93]. The classic ulcerogenic tumor syndrome is characterized by massive gastric hypersecretion, peptic ulceration, and a non-beta islet-cell tumor of the pancreas or duodenum. Diarrhea may be the initial and only complaint, but more commonly ulceration of the duodenum or upper jejunum recurs despite repeated traditional surgical procedures. A second important characteristic is the presence of adenomas of other endocrine glands, particularly the parathyroid glands, which may occur in a familial pattern. The association of the non-beta islet cell tumor of the pancreas and fulminating gastric hypersecretion has been known as the Zollinger-Ellison syndrome, the islet-cell ulcerogenic syndrome, and, more recently, the gastrinoma syndrome.

Since 1960 it has been known that ulcerogenic tumors and their metastases can produce 35–45 times more gastrin than a similar weight of porcine gastric antrum [30]. Direct measurement of gastrin in serum and tissues, made possible by the brilliant development of the gastrin radioimmunoassay [54], has made the diagnosis of the ulcerogenic tumor syndrome easier and more certain. This technique has also permitted assessment of the immediate results of surgical treatment and has aided in the monitoring of postoperative patients for indications of recurrence of the disease.

Etiology

PANCREAS-INDUCED ULCER

The possibility of a relationship between the pancreas and peptic ulceration was the object of studies by gastrointestinal physiologists and surgeons for many years. Exalto [25] and later Mann and Williamson [51] demonstrated chronic progressive ulcerations in animals following isolation of the duodenum and drainage of its secretions into the lower intestine. Others [24] confirmed this finding in dogs prepared with external pancreatic fistulas. In 1942 Dragstedt [19] reported that the incidence of experimental ulceration following ligation of the internal pancreatic ducts was 29 percent, whereas it was only 1.2 percent following pancreatectomy.

Six years later, Poth et al. [63] reported a study in which they injected dogs with a histamine-in-beeswax preparation after total pancreatectomy, after ligation of the pancreatic ducts, and after producing diabetes with alloxan. Fulminating ulcerations developed when the pancreatic secretions were diverted from the duodenum. While pancreatectomy itself did not seem to produce ulcers, the result of subsequent histamine stimulation suggested a strong predisposition to ulcer formation after extirpation of the gland. Poth concluded that "both the internal and external secretions of the pancreas may be implicated in ulcer formation."

Many isolated clinical reports pointed out an association between peptic ulceration and supposedly nonfunctioning islet-cell tumors, but this association was regarded as mere coincidence. The hereditary polyglandular syndrome of Wermer [85] and others [56, 79] was likewise associated with peptic ulcerations in several patients. Wermer stated in 1954 [85] that this syndrome is caused by a dominant autosomal gene with a high degree of penetrance and that the peptic ulcers of the stomach and duodenum are merely another expression of the abnormal gene.

A direct causal relationship between nonbeta islet-cell tumors of the pancreas and peptic ulcer disease was not advanced until 1955 [93]. The original report was based on two patients with severe primary peptic ulcerations in the jejunum that were characterized by enormous gastric hypersecretion and continued ulcer recurrences until total gastrectomy became mandatory. In both patients a nonspecific islet-cell tumor was found, even though neither one presented clinical or laboratory evidence of hyperinsulinism. Therefore an *ulcerogenic* humoral factor of pancreatic islet origin was postulated.

The existence of the syndrome gained considerable support from hundreds of reports that appeared in the literature. Additional evidence of a relationship between ulcer and pancreatic tumor was obtained in rare instances in which total tumor removal was possible [18, 22, 50, 58]. Such patients had prompt relief of ulcer symptoms and a dramatic reduction in gastric hypersecretion.

Failure to identify either the responsible hormone or the islet cell or origin led to alternative conclusions about the syndrome in the five years between 1955 and 1960. Associated abnormalities of other endocrine organs in 28 percent of the reported patients were thought to play a role in the ulcer diathesis. Rudolf et al. [66] reported on a patient with adrenal hyperplasia and adenomas, islet-cell adenomas, gonadal hypoplasia, amphophilic hyperplasia of the anterior pituitary gland, and parietal cell hyperplasia. They suggested that failure of secretion of one of the target endocrine organs brought about neoplastic changes in the pituitary gland. Peptic ulcer resulted either directly from parietal cell hyperplasia or indirectly as a by-product of secretions from one of the involved endocrine glands. Other investigators singled out a primary disorder of the hypothalamus as an explanation for both the gastric hypersecretion and the high incidence of associated endocrine adenomas.

In 1960 Osborne and colleagues [59] extracted a possible gastric secretagogue from an ulcerogenic islet-cell tumor. They reported that the substance was not identified with histamine, glucagon, or insulin; that it quickly effected acid secretion from an isolated Heidenhain pouch of a dog that had undergone vagotomy when given intravenously; and that it was not present in control preparations of human pancreas or liver.

In the same year, Gregory et al. [38] described a "gastrin-like secretagogue" found in an ulcerogenic tumor removed from a patient by Professor Stammers and colleagues in Birmingham, England. Using the picric acid technique that had been successful in obtaining gastrin from porcine antrum, they extracted a substance with 35–45 times greater secretagogue properties. Grossman et al. [43] and later Friesen et al. [30] and Code et al. [13] found a similar gastrinlike substance in metastases of an ulcerogenic islet-cell tumor. This proof that the metastases were as potent as the "mother tumor" lent strong support to the original suggestion that total gastrectomy should be performed in these patients. Verification for the first time of a potent extra-antral source of gastrin stimulated great interest in this polypeptide and its physiological properties.

It had been known for many years that extracts of gastric antrum, but not extracts of fundus, would stimulate gastric acid secretion; but this capability was ascribed to histamine rather than to gastrin or the "gastric secretion" described by Edkins in 1906 [21]. In 1938 Komarov [48] verified gastrin as a proteinlike substance distinct from histamine, and Grossman et al. [42] subsequently demonstrated a *circulating* stimulant of acid secretion in dogs with totally denervated gastric pouches. In 1964 Gregory and Tracy [35] completed the purification of porcine gastrins I and II, permitting the determination of the complete sequence of the 17 amino acid residues and the synthesis of the entire molecule [32, 34, 35]. Two years later the purification, structural determination, and synthesis of gastrin obtained from human antral mucosa was achieved [3, 4, 39]. Evidence was obtained that the amino acid content and structure of ulcerogenic tumors and of human antral gastrin were identical and that the peptides produced by enzymatic degradation of gastrin from tumors were identical with those of human antral gastrin [33, 37].

The availability of semipurified and purified human and porcine gastrin led to the development of radioimmunoassay systems for gastrin, and the gastrin radioimmunoassay was first introduced into clinical practice in 1968 by McGuigan and Trudeau [55]. The now widely available radioimmunoassay is commonly used in many patients with gastric complaints and in most patients with gastric or duodenal ulceration or an unexplained fulminating diarrhea.

MOLECULAR FORMS OF GASTRIN

A family of gastrin species existing in both a nonsulfated (I) and a sulfated (II) form is now recognized. The known members of this family, in ascending order of complexity, are C-4, minigastrin, little gastrin, big gastrin, component I (Rehfeld), and big-big gastrin. Yalow and Berson [89] named the largest component *big-big gastrin*. It is present in relatively small amounts in patients with gastrin-producing tumors, but it may be especially abundant in the serum after partial gastrectomy [90]. The biological activity and chemical structure of this material are yet unknown.

The principal form of circulating gastrin in the fasting state is big gastrin [6]. Gregory and Tracy [36] purified big gastrin from ulcerogenic tumors and determined that it is composed of 34 amino acids [82]. Little gastrin is the heptadecapeptide originally isolated from antrum as gastrin. It is released into the circulation by antral stimulation. Its 17 amino acid residues are well characterized structurally, and the substance is commercially available as synthetic human gastrin I. Another form identified in the serum is minigastrin [64]. This material appears to be identical with the C-terminal 14 amino-acid sequence of little gastrin. Little is known about the activity of minigastrin, but it has been identified in extracts of antrum mucosa and from ulcerogenic tumors [82]. C-4, the terminal tetrapeptide, has been identified in cerebrospinal fluid and may modulate neural control of the stomach.

The Gastrinoma Syndrome

The passage of three decades has made knowledge of the ulcerogenic tumor syndrome (Zollinger-Ellison syndrome, gastrinoma) virtually universal. It presents classically as a fulminating ulcer diathesis, with or without diarrhea, in the presence of massive and intractable gastric hypersecretion. The patient secretes enormous amounts of gastric juice from an unobstructed stomach or very soon after a radical gastric resection, which may have included vagotomy. Additional signs that should immediately suggest the presence of an ulcerogenic tumor include (1) a primary ulceration in the jejunum beyond the ligament of Treitz; (2) ulcer symptoms associated with hypercalcemia or other evidence of multiple endocrine involvement, especially hyperparathyroidism;

(3) an ulcer diathesis occurring for the first time in a very young or elderly patient; (4) severe ulcer symptoms, with hemorrhage or perforation, that occur in the immediately postpartum period or soon after a standard operation for ulcer; and (5) diarrhea of obscure origin associated with marked gastric hypersecretion [70].

The symptoms of the ulcerogenic tumor syndrome vary and exhibit a wide range of severity. It is possible to categorize patients into at least four clinical groups: those with borderline gastrin levels, those with associated hyperparathyroidism, those with an iatrogenic ulcer diathesis, and those with the classical ulcerogenic tumor syndrome. The disease can be virulent or it may be borderline, with the symptoms approximating those seen in the typical peptic ulcer patient. There have been long delays in the diagnosis, especially when symptoms were not life-threatening; surprisingly, patients are still encountered with sagas of intractable peptic ulceration, having undergone multiple gastric resections for recurrences before the diagnosis was confirmed by a gastrin radioimmunoassay.

CLINICAL MANIFESTATIONS

The ulcerogenic tumor syndrome has been encountered in patients ranging from 7 to 90 years of age. The development of ulcer symptoms in the very young or in the elderly for the first time should strongly suggest the presence of an ulcerogenic tumor. In contrast to the patient with an ordinary peptic ulcer in whom the age of occurrence is well below 40 years, the peak of the ulcerogenic syndrome appears to occur at about the fifth decade. There is no clear sex predominance; about 60 percent of the reported patients are men.

Symptomatically the ulcerogenic tumor syndrome is dominated by a fulminating ulcer diathesis in only about 59 percent of patients. Common complications associated with the ulcer include intractability to treatment (43 percent), hemorrhage (32 percent), perforations (23 percent), and obstruction (7 percent). The low incidence of obstruction may be related to the fulminating nature of the ulcer diathesis, which does not allow time for healing with scar formation followed by recurrence as seen in ordinary peptic ulcer disease. About 8 percent of patients have had multiple perforations, with 6 percent of these occurring in the jejunum beyond the ligament of Treitz. The finding of an active or perforated jejunal ulcer in this location in a patient who has not undergone a previous gastric operation should be considered pathognomonic of an ulcerogenic tumor.

Approximately 30 percent of patients have an ulcer as well as diarrhea. The remaining 5–10 percent have diarrhea and marked gastric hypersecretion. The absence of peptic ulceration may be explained on the basis of increased mucosal resistance to the acid or excessive pancreatic hypersecretion, or both. Patients with excessive pancreatic hypersecretion must be distinguished from patients who have fulminating watery diarrhea and achlorhydria associated with islet-cell tumor production of the vasoactive polypeptide [96]. Steatorrhea has also been reported in many instances of gastrinoma, but its true prevalence has never been statistically determined.

The diarrhea in the ulcerogenic tumor syndrome is associated with gastric hypersecretion and can be relieved by nasogastric suction or H_2-receptor antagonist therapy, or abolished by total gastrectomy. It is believed to be caused by multiple factors, including excessive gastric acid in the duodenum, damage to the small intestinal mucosa by the acid gastric juice, decreased small intestinal absorption, and increased intestinal motility caused by the hypergastrinemia. The steatorrhea associated with the ulcerogenic syndrome is thought to result from inactivation of lipase and mucosal damage produced by the low pH in the lumen of the small intestine.

ASSOCIATED ENDOCRINE ADENOMAS

Associated endocrine tumors occur in the ulcerogenic syndrome in about 25 percent of patients [92]. Hyperparathyroidism is the most common associated endocrine abnormality (22–28 percent) with adenoma or hyperplasia of the pituitary, thyroid, and adrenal glands each occurring in approximately 10 percent of patients. The multiple endocrine neoplasia

(MEN) syndrome type I also known as Wermer's syndrome [85], consists in neoplasia or hyperplasia of pancreatic islet cells, the parathyroid glands, and the pituitary gland. The MEN II, or Sipple, syndrome consists in involvement by pheochromocytoma, thyroid carcinoma, parathyroid adenoma, or hyperplasia, and occasionally, mucosal neurofibromatosis. There is enough overlap, however, to warrant considering adrenal involvement in MEN I and pancreatic islet-cell tumors in MEN II. Cameron and Spiro [10] reported a patient having a gastrinoma associated with the MEN II syndrome.

Friesen et al. [27] studied members of two families with proven multiple endocrine adenomatosis (MEA) syndrome and found antral G-cell hyperplasia in all of the members of one family who had antral biopsies, which suggests that these changes may precede the development of active endocrine disease. Hyperplasia of antral G cells has also been noted in patients with gastric hypersecretion, duodenal and gastric ulcer with pyloric obstruction, hyperparathyroidism caused by adenoma or hyperplasia, or acromegaly, as well as in some patients with the ulcerogenic tumor who do not have associated endocrine adenomas [14, 60–62, 73]. A diagnosis of antral G-cell hyperplasia is suggested when the fasting gastrin levels are elevated. These levels may be doubled after eating, but there is no change in gastrin levels in response to the secretin push test. This test is helpful in differentiating antral G-cell hyperplasia from a gastrinoma, since the latter causes gastrin levels to rise in response to the secretin push.

The unusually high incidence of hyperparathyroidism associated with the ulcerogenic tumor syndrome is of great interest. Kaplan and colleagues [47] emphasized the role of systemic metabolic alkalosis in the causation of the hyperparathyroidism seen in some patients with the ulcerogenic syndrome. This was also observed by Trudeau and McGuigan [77]. It has been speculated that a greater or more prolonged decrease in calcium level associated with the extreme metabolic alkalosis seen in some patients with the ulcerogenic tumor syndrome may result in more intense stimulation of the parathyroid glands. Hypercalcemic hyperparathyroidism may occur later and is called *tertiary hyperparathyroidism*.

Investigators at the University of Chicago [46] and at the Mayo Clinic [72] have demonstrated that some ulcerogenic tumor patients have elevated concentrations of circulating parathyroid hormone (PTH) despite low or normal serum calcium levels. Surgical excision of the ulcerogenic tumors and correction of the gastric hypersecretory state was followed by a decrease in PTH level and a rise in serum calcium level, both to normal. On the other hand, it has been reported that correction of the hyperparathyroidism by resection of one or more parathyroid adenomas markedly improved the symptoms of peptic ulcer disease and decreased the gastric acid secretion when an ulcerogenic tumor was also present [78]. This beneficial effect is related to correction of the hypercalcemia.

Diagnosis

GASTRIC ANALYSIS

The finding that suggests the presence of an ulcerogenic tumor is copious and intractable gastric hypersecretion. Patients produce 100–200 ml of gastric juice per hour with a free acid content of 100–300 mEq/L. In addition, the 1-hour basal secretion may be greater than 15 mEq [1]. Ruppert et al. [67] found that the ratio of basal to maximal acid concentration after histamine stimulation is selective for an ulcerogenic tumor when it is greater than 0.6. Many investigators, however, have called attention to the vagaries of interpreting acid secretory findings [83, 88], and in general the main role of the gastric analysis has become one of identifying patients who should be further evaluated by radioimmunoassay of gastrin. The finding of free hydrochloric acid rules out many other causes of hypergastrinemia, such as pernicious anemia, gastric polyposis, and atrophic gastritis.

GASTRIN RADIOIMMUNOASSAY

One of the most brilliant recent advances in medicine is the development of the immunoassay technique for measuring circulating polypeptides and other biologically active materials. The concept was first developed by Berson and Yalow in 1958 [5] as a result of their studies with radioiodine-labeled insulin in insulin-treated diabetics. They reasoned that the process that bound injected, labeled insulin to the circulating insulin antibodies in these patients could be developed into a highly specific and sensitive immunoassay system. McGuigan and Trudeau [55] first successfully adapted this concept to gastrin, and the gastrin radioimmunoassay has become an integral part of the routine automated biochemical screening done in almost all modern hospitals. Just as the routine use of serum calcium determinations disclosed many patients with asymptomatic hypercalcemia and increased the number of parathyroid adenomas diagnosed, routine gastrin determinations should disclose many ulcerogenic tumors before their symptoms become life-threatening.

Gastrin radioimmunoassay should be performed in all patients who have peptic ulcer disease and acid hypersecretion, as well as those who have recurrent ulcer symptoms following gastric resection or vagotomy. In addition, it should be part of the screening of patients who have severe diarrhea of unknown cause. Table 18-1 lists the circumstances that cause either slight-to-moderate or moderate-to-marked increases in serum gastrin level.

A fasting serum gastrin level greater than 500 pg/ml in a patient with free hydrochloric acid in the gastric juice generally indicates the presence of a gastrinoma, and many such patients will have fasting levels well in excess of 1000 pg/ml. Jaffe et al. [45] described four patients who had serum gastrin concentrations in the ulcerogenic tumor range but in whom no tumors were found initially. Subsequently, small duodenal tumors were demonstrated, emphasizing the value of gastrin radioimmunoassay in discovering occult ulcerogenic tumors.

As in other endocrine syndromes, elaboration of the offending hormone is neither steady nor uniform. Day-to-day variations in gastrin level have occurred in some patients, with values ranging from diagnostic to merely suggestive. Likewise, it is not uncommon in a large series of duodenal ulcer patients to find a few with serum gastrin levels of 150–250 pg/ml, overlapping the lowest values for some patients with an ulcerogenic tumor. Faced with this clinical challenge, the surgeon must turn to provocative stimulation tests using secretin, calcium gluceptate, or magnesium sulfate.

The provocative secretin push test is decisive in confirming or disproving the diagnosis of gastrinoma, especially in the presence of borderline elevations of gastrin level (Fig. 18-1). The test is performed in a fasting patient who does not show a positive reaction to intradermally injected secretin (gastric inhibitory hormone GIH). A heparin venous well is inserted, and 2 clinical units of secretin per kilogram of body weight are injected within 30 seconds. Serum samples are taken promptly at 1, 3, 5, 7, 10, 15, and 30 minutes. A positive test for gastrinoma is an elevation of the secretin level to at least 200 pg above the fasting level. The secretin push does not elevate the

Table 18-1. Circulating Gastrin Levels[a]

Slight-to-moderate increases[b]
Gastric ulcer
Vagotomy (truncal, selective, proximal gastric)
Billroth I
Obstructed duodenal ulcer
Carcinoma of gastric antrum
Moderate-to-marked increases[b]
Ulcerogenic tumor
Pernicious anemia
Retained gastric antrum
Carcinoma of gastric corpus
Gastritis (hyperplasia of antral G cells)
Short bowel syndrome
Chronic renal failure
Borderline area: 250–500 pg/ml
Challenge with infusion of secretin (2 clinical units per kilogram of body weight injected intradermally within 30 seconds)

[a]Normal, 20–180 pg/ml (mean, 40); after protein meal, 50–150% increase.
[b]Fasting and postprandial.

Secretin Diagnostic Test
Fasting gastrin
Secretin (GIH)
 2 clinical units per kg
 Injection within 30 seconds
 Measure gastrin q2min ×5
 Positive test: 200 pg/ml above basal level

Fig. 18-1. The secretin diagnostic test is performed by injecting secretin (GIH), 2 clinical units per kg body weight within 30 seconds, and measuring gastrin at 1, 3, 5, 7, 10, 15, and 30 minutes. A positive test is 200 pg/ml above basal fasting gastrin level.

gastrin levels from other causes, e.g., antral G-cell hyperplasia, retained gastric antrum, small bowel syndrome, renal failure, the ingestion of food.

A positive secretin test establishes the diagnosis of gastrinoma earlier than it could otherwise be documented. It provides supportive evidence for surgical exploration and enables the surgeon to take appropriate steps to control the enormous gastric hypersecretion, even when a tumor is not found at the time of operation. Blind resection of the left half of the pancreas is no longer advocated.

The secretin push test is also valuable in follow-up evaluations of patients with fasting gastrin levels under 1000 pg. The maximum levels of gastrin within 3–7 minutes can be compared to previous results. Secretin has largely replaced calcium gluconate and magnesium sulfate as a diagnostic test for gastrinoma.

ROENTGENOLOGICAL FINDINGS

Barium contrast studies of the upper gastrointestinal tract often lend important support to a suspected diagnosis of ulcerogenic tumor, and some clinicians have suggested that the diagnosis is primarily the roentgenologist's responsibility [91]. Characteristically there are huge gastric folds caused by mucosal hyperplasia and large amounts of gastric juice in the stomach unless the patient has been undergoing H_2-receptor antagonist therapy. An ulcer in the duodenal bulb or immediately postbulbar area is seen in many patients. Other findings are evidence of duodenitis, megaduodenum, and irregularity of the duodenal wall from edema, which may be mistaken for Crohn's disease. The mucosa of the first portion of the duodenum may have a cobblestone appearance from hyperplasia of the Brunner glands. A primary jejunal ulcer beyond the ligament of Treitz is considered pathognomonic of an ulcerogenic tumor, but it occurs in only about 20–25 percent of patients. Postresectional ulcerations are deep, penetrating, and multiple, and generally are found on the mesenteric border of the efferent loop rather than in the usual marginal location [12]. The ulcerogenic tumors themselves are usually so small that such indirect signs as organ displacement or invasion of the stomach and duodenal C-loop are rarely detected. However, patients have been observed who demonstrated a niche in the duodenum thought to be an ulcer but found at operation to be a duodenal wall tumor.

It should be pointed out that this well-known catalog of characteristic signs has been revised because ulcerogenic tumors are diagnosed earlier and the classical findings may be altered in patients receiving long-term cimetidine therapy.

The value of arteriography and radioisotopic scanning in the preoperative diagnosis of the ulcerogenic tumor syndrome has, in general, been minimal. There have been reports in which angiography has been successful. Arteriograms can be useful as a means of detecting metastatic tumors in the liver and in monitoring the progress of therapy when metastatic nodules have been found at operation. Because the gastrinoma tends to be multiple and relatively small, the diagnostic value of echograms and computerized tomographic (CT) scans is often disappointing. However, percutaneous transhepatic portal and splenic venous sampling, drawing from various anatomical divisions of the pancreas, i.e., head, neck, body, and tail, has provided tumor localization in some patients, especially if the tumor is a solitary one [9, 20, 70] (Fig. 18-2).

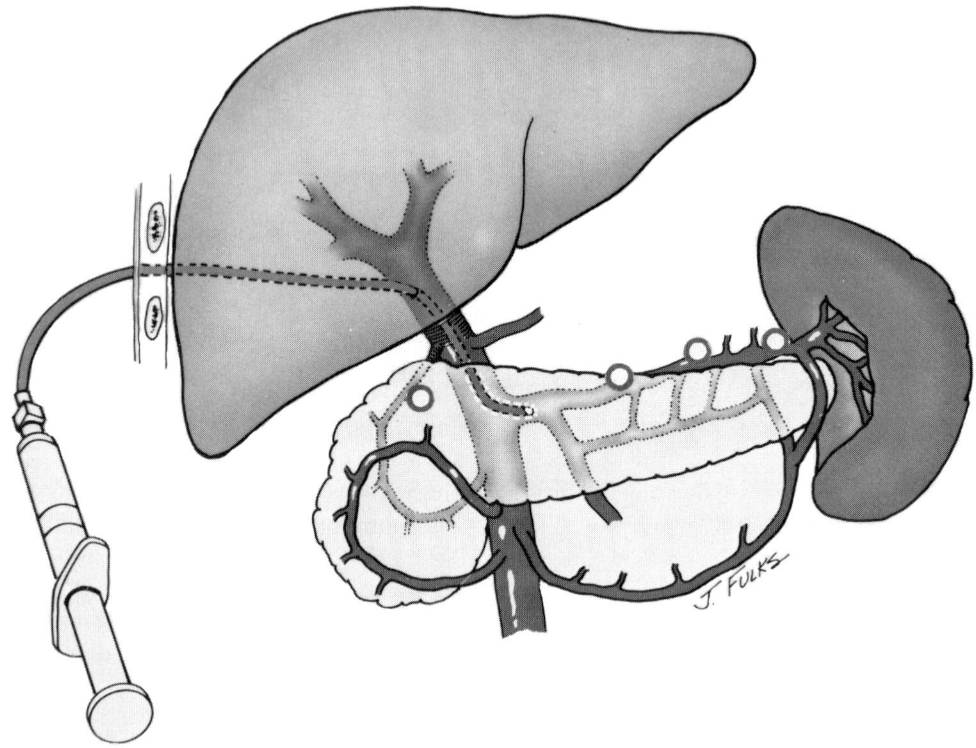

Fig. 18-2. Percutaneous venous sampling may be used to localize a pancreatic endocrine tumor. The frequency of multiple gastrinomas with functioning metastases reduces the localization potential in comparison with other endocrine tumors such as insulinoma.

Treatment

GENERAL PRINCIPLES

During the first 25 years after the ulcerogenic islet-cell tumor syndrome was postulated, the accepted treatment was total gastrectomy. This provided the only means of controlling the severe gastric hypersecretion. Currently, however, there are other therapeutic options since the effective H_2-receptor antagonist, cimetidine, has become widely used. The acid factor can be controlled by cimetidine while diagnostic studies are made and surgical intervention considered.

Cimetidine is well tolerated and has infrequent and minor side effects. It is usually taken orally in a dosage of 300 mg with meals and at bedtime, but it can be taken intravenously or in rectal suppositories. The maximal concentration occurs in 1–1½ hours, and it is effective for approximately 4 hours. Most of the drug is excreted in the urine within 24 hours, but some is excreted in the bile. It crosses the placental barrier and may be found in mothers' milk.

Given the usual doses, cimetidine inhibits not only fasting secretion but secretion induced by sham feeding, pentagastrin, fundic distention, insulin, caffeine, and eating [31]. The drug is also effective in depressing the cephalic vagal phases of gastric secretion. The volume of gastric juice is reduced, as are hydrogen ion concentration and pepsin. While it has no effect on basal gastrin levels, it may increase the postprandial concentration of gastrin. It does not appear to have an effect on lower esophageal sphincter pressure, gastric emptying, or pancreatic secretion. Some patients have antiandrogenic effects, such as gynecomastia, decreased potency, and reduced sperm count. Of much greater concern is the occurrence of mental confusion, especially in the elderly or those requiring large doses. The dosage should be decreased and the interval of administration doubled when the BUN or creatinine concentration is elevated. Cimetidine also has been shown to modify the rate of liver blood flow; therefore, drugs metabolized in the liver are generally contraindicated. These can include vasodilators (theophylline), antidepressants (diazepam), anticoagulants (warfarin), and beta-blocking drugs such as propranolol.

An occasional patient does not respond to cimetidine, and some do not accept the necessity of taking the drug regularly around the clock without a single day of interruption. Others may require anticholinergic or antacid therapy, especially at bedtime, in addition to the 300 mg of cimetidine with meals and at bedtime to ensure freedom from discomfort before morning.

Because the H_2-receptor antagonists are so effective in providing relief, there may be a tendency to delay further investigation. But as the patient becomes comfortable, further studies are indicated to confirm the suspicion of a gastrinoma (Fig. 18-3). Fasting serum gastrin and calcium levels should be repeated as upper gastrointestinal barium studies are performed. If the calcium level is elevated, parathormone levels should be determined and a search made for other endocrine tumors, as of the adrenal glands and the pituitary gland. When the gastrin levels are elevated to less than 1000 pg, the secretin push test should be performed. An elevated gastrin level in response to this test should be considered confirmation of a gastrinoma, since the gastrin levels are not elevated in other disorders associated with a modest elevation in the fasting gastrin level in the presence of free hydrochloric acid.

Both patient and physician may be so gratified by the effective pain control given by cimetidine that due consideration may not be allowed to the fact that the gastrinoma is a malignant lesion. Some hold the opinion that as long as the patient seems to be doing well, there is no need to consider surgical intervention, since the gastrinoma tends to grow so slowly. The fact that metastasis occurs and that cimetidine does not hinder the continued tumor growth of this unusual neoplasm tends to be overlooked.

Initial Management
- Cimetidine, 300 mg ×4
  - Symptom-free
  - Confirm diagnosis
    - Barium studies
    - Secretin push
    - Calcium, parathormone
    - Other endocrine tumors?

Fig. 18-3. Adequate cimetidine therapy provides relief from pain and complications during preoperative evaluation and preparation.

There are three general areas of consideration in the management of the gastrinoma. The first is the initial management, which has been discussed; the second is the medical choice, which includes conservative surgical treatment; and the third is the surgical choice, which includes aggressive tumor excision and total gastrectomy.

There is general agreement that H_2-receptor antagonist therapy is worthwhile in improving the surgical risk. The danger of serious complications from massive gastric hypersecretion is avoided, and the inflammatory reaction about the ulcerations is retarded. Diarrhea is controlled, and ulcerations tend to heal. If hyperparathyroidism has been proved, all parathyroid glands should be explored, and any enlarged glands removed because of the tendency toward later recurrence of hyperparathyroidism. A muscular implant of parathyroid tissue may be performed on rare occasions.

Regardless of how well the patient does taking medication, every patient should undergo surgical exploration when the maximal improvement of surgical risk has been attained (Fig. 18-4). The argument has been presented that only by surgical exploration can the diagnosis be microscopically proved, the extent of the tumor determined, and, in approximately 20 percent of patients, the syndrome

Medical Choices
Cimetidine: Improve surgical risk
Parathyroidectomy?
Conservative, exploration
  Vagotomy, pyloroplasty
    No tumor
    Solitary tumor excised
  Poor risk, elderly
Cimetidine, lifetime

Fig. 18-4. A conservative medical-surgical option as an alternative to routine total gastrectomy in certain selected patients combines vagotomy with tumor excision followed by lifelong H_2-receptor antagonist therapy.

Surgical Choices
For minimal disease:
Choices: Vagotomy
  Pyloroplasty
Indications: Negative exploration
  Poor risk
  Elderly
For maximal disease:
Choices: Aggresive tumor excision
  Total gastrectomy
Indications: Extensive tumor
  Metastases
  Drug failure
  Young patient

Fig. 18-5. In addition to the option of a conservative surgical approach, aggressive tumor resection is indicated followed by a Roux-en-Y anastomosis in patients with multiple tumors, proved metastasis, or probable residual tumor, also when response to medication has failed, and in the very young patient.

corrected by the removal of a solitary tumor. Confirmation of the diagnosis by microscopical examination is a requirement for subsequent chemotherapy. The attainment of cure by finding and removing a solitary tumor has relatively increased, but should not be considered the major indication for surgical exploration. Some insist that since that acid factor can be controlled by the H_2 receptor antagonist, there is no longer a need to consider total gastrectomy. The medical choice of therapy, if it includes surgical exploration, involves less than a total gastrectomy.

When less than a total gastrectomy is performed, vagotomy should be added. Vagotomy was reported by Ellison in 1956 to lower the 72-hour overnight volume of secretion by 50 percent, with a corresponding gastrin decrease in the total milliequivalents of free hydrochloric acid in a patient with gastrinoma operated on by Zollinger in 1947 [23]. Richardson et al. [65] emphasized the potential benefit of vagotomy in managing several patients with gastrinoma. The H_2 receptor antagonist can be far more effective after a vagotomy. This conservative surgical approach can be considered in patients who refuse total gastrectomy or in those in whom no tumor is found during a thorough examination of a mobilized pancreas. A blind resection of the left half of the pancreas in a valiant search for a small, hidden gastrinoma is no longer considered justifiable. The conservative approach may also be favorably considered when the surgeon believes he or she has removed the only tumor present, i.e., from the submucosa of the first portion of the duodenum or from the left half of the pancreas. Very high-risk patients or elderly patients who have always been well below their ideal weight may be candidates for less than a total gastrectomy. Most patients in this group, however, will be committed to a lifetime of H_2-receptor antagonist therapy or eventual total gastrectomy.

The third method of treatment is a surgical choice (Fig. 18-5). In contrast to former years, the surgeon can now take time to improve the surgical risk without fear of catastrophic complications. There is a better understanding of the bizarre and unpredictable growth habits of the gastrinoma. The surgeon searches for and hopes to find only a solitary tumor that can be removed, with cure of the patient and microscopical confirmation of the diagnosis. Surgeons are no longer hesitant to perform a minimal surgical procedure such as truncal vagotomy and pyloroplasty when no gross tumor is found or in a high-risk, elderly, or emaciated patient. However, they have learned it is justifiable to perform aggressive tumor resection, including metastases, as demonstrated by an improved five-year survival rate [94]. Tumor removal takes precedence over an initial and routine total gastrecomy [2, 17, 50]. However, when multiple tumors are verified in the pancreas, positive metastases proved in the adjacent lymph nodes, or a metastasis found in the liver, a total gastrectomy along with aggressive tumor resection ensures an improved five-year survival rate. A number of total gastrectomies will also be required either because cimetidine does not control the clinical symptoms or because the patient cannot or will not adhere to the rigid discipline required by cimetidine therapy [16, 74, 76, 96].

Total gastrectomy should be considered when proven gastrinoma is found in a very young or teenage patient because of the possibility of years of clinical management with medication every 4 to 6 hours. Young patients develop normally despite total gastrectomy. Patients with gastrinoma do far better after total gastrectomy than those undergoing this procedure for cancer of the stomach. Perhaps the trophic effects on the small intestinal mucosa from the hypergastrinemia have a beneficial effect. Certainly, total gastrectomy can be done with a satisfactory mortality and morbidity. The patients eventually enjoy three meals a day; three-fourths of them approach their calculated ideal weight.

The five-year survival rate following total gastrectomy approximates 50 percent but is increased to 68 percent if the tumor is removed by hemipancreatectomy. The patient described in the original report [93] underwent total gastrectomy with removal of metastatic tumor in two lymph nodes adjacent to the pancreas in November 1954 and was still living after 27 years. She observed no dietary restrictions, and her weight remained above the ideal. She had two children, born five and seven years after she underwent total gastrectomy. During the intervening years, she underwent cholecystectomy and left-sided pancreatectomy, and later, a panhysterectomy. A small adenoma was found in the resected pancreas at the time of cholecystectomy, but there was no evidence of metastasis 10 years after the total gastrectomy. Careful follow-up study has shown her gastrin levels to be rising slowly after 25 years. Her survival for 27 years shows that a patient with an ulcerogenic tumor with lymph node metastasis can live for many years after total gastrectomy. She received no chemotherapy but does receive a monthly injection of vitamin B_{12}.

PREOPERATIVE PREPARATION

Patients should be informed of the pros and cons of both medical and surgical treatment. The fact that they do not have symptoms may imply to the patients as well as the physician that the growth of the tumor has subsided. They should be informed that this is usually a slow-growing tumor but one with a definite malignant potential. The longer surgical treatment is delayed, the greater is the chance for metastasis and the less the chance of complete removal of the tumor. On the other hand, there is little evidence that total gastrectomy has any effect on tumor growth, although Friesen [28] has collected case studies supporting this concept. The chance that a solitary tumor will be found is probably less than 5 in 20 and thus supports the argument favoring an operation. The patient should know of the surgical possibilities, including vagotomy, total gastrectomy, hemipancreatectomy, splenectomy, and removal of adjacent lymph nodes or solitary hepatic metastases.

Patients in recent years are coming to operation earlier than before because of earlier diagnosis, and they are in better condition because of the efficacy of the H_2-receptor antagonists. There are fewer patients with previous gastric surgical failure.

Control of hypersecretion by H_2-receptor antagonists ensures a patient better prepared than formerly. An inflammatory reaction in the upper gastrointestinal tract is less evident, and healing of the ulcerations may have taken place. Of special importance is the correction of the excessive loss of fluids by gastric aspiration or diarrhea. Formerly it was necessary to replace large volume losses from gastric secretion as well as diarrhea. The blood volume should be restored and the patient evaluated as a reasonable risk for a major upper abdominal operation. Blood should be availabe for transfusion.

SURGICAL TECHNIQUE

If the patient has undergone no previous operation on the upper abdomen, the preliminary exploration is performed through a midline incision extending well over the xiphoid process and well below the umbilicus on the left side. The incision may need to be altered in the presence of one or more scars from previous operations. The xiphoid process should be removed to a level that is as high as possible. Great care must be taken in opening the peritoneal cavity, especially in patients who have had a previous operation, because of the frequent presence of penetration of a stomal ulceration against the anterior parietes. Evidence of duodenal ulcerations may or may not be found; however, the finding of a primary ulcer beyond the ligament of Treitz is considered pathognomonic of an ulcerogenic tumor.

The type of definitive surgical procedure needed can be determined only after meticulous exploration of the entire pancreas, duodenum, and gastric antrum. Regional lymph nodes (peripancreatic, periduodenal, and mesenteric) and the liver are also carefully examined for evidence of metastases. These patients often present the surgeon with a variety of perplexing problems in judgment that may challenge his or her surgical acumen. Based on experience, it appears that the problems revolve around findings such as a negative exploration, a solitary tumor in the duodenal wall, a tumor in children, liver metastases in the elderly, excision of the metastasis, excision of the solitary pancreatic tumor, and total gastrectomy when residual tumor remains.

SURGICAL JUDGMENT PROBLEMS

Negative Exploration

The first and second portions of the duodenum are first freed up by a Kocher maneuver, which permits inspection of the anterior and posterior walls and direct palpation of the head of the pancreas and the area around the portal vein. Stabile and co-workers [75] emphasize the importance of mobilizing the head of the pancreas in a search for tumor in the area they refer to as the "gastrinoma triangle." They found a 37 percent long-term cure rate after excision of occult tumor from this triangle. The wall of the duodenum, particularly along the mesenteric border, is carefully palpated for tumorous nodules arising from an aberrant pancreas. Subsequent to a negative exploration, the pylorus may be split and the lumen of the first and second portions of the duodenum explored digitally for intramural adenomas. The omentum is next reflected upward, and the upper jejunum is surveyed for some distance because of the high incidence of primary jejunal ulcerations occurring beyond the ligament of Treitz.

The greater omentum is next separated from the hepatic to the splenic flexure of the colon to obtain complete exposure of the pancreas. The greater omentum is reflected upward while downward traction is maintained on the transverse colon, the omentum is separated by sharp dissection, and the lesser sac is entered. The stomach is retracted upward, and the entire body and tail of the pancreas are inspected. Since these tumors are usually quite small, they may not be apparent from gross palpation. The surgeon must mobilize the body and tail of the pancreas for direct palpation. It is doubtful that the body and tail of the pancreas can be completely and satisfactorily explored without complete mobilization of the spleen and the body and tail of the pancreas toward the midline and up into the wound. Any enlarged lymph nodes or small nodules over the pancreas should be excised and submitted for frozen section examination.

One of the greatest challenges facing the surgeon is what should be done when, despite a firm preoperative diagnosis, no tumor is found at surgical exploration. If the patient has undergone a previous operation for ulcer, the surgeon must determine that no iatrogenic causes of recurrent ulcer are present. These include an overlooked vagus nerve (particularly the posterior one), antral distention from failure to place the gastrojejunostomy sufficiently near the pylorus (3–4 cm), a modest gastric resection without vagotomy, a long-loop gastrojejunostomy following the Billroth II procedure, and, more rarely, a retained gastric antrum. While the fasting gastrin levels are elevated in the presence of gastrinoma in response to secretin stimulation, such is not the case in the presence of a retained antrum [49] or antral G-cell hyperplasia. This is why it is so important to have the information provided by a secretin push.

Before the widespread availability of the gastrin radioimmunoassay, it was common, when no tumor could found, to mobilize the spleen and left side of the pancreas into the wound before ligation of the major splenic vessels and to divide the pancreas a short distance to the left of the portal vein. Such "blind" resections occasionally uncovered a small adenoma grossly or diffuse microadenomatosis observed by pathological examination. The incidence of complications was increased by this procedure, however, which was carried out because microscopical proof of tumor was believed to be essential before considering a total gastrectomy. Blind resection of the pancreas has been discontinued since the hypersecretion can be controlled by an H_2-receptor antagonist. In the face of a negative exploration, the surgeon has several choices. Although he or she may proceed with a total gastrectomy, the trend is toward avoiding total gastrectomy in the absence of gross tumor and performing instead a pyloroplasty and vagotomy. The duodenum can be carefully palpated and inspected for evidence of a small submucosal tumor.

Duodenal Wall Tumors

Wilson and colleagues [44] have found that duodenal wall tumors occur in about 13 percent of patients with the ulcerogenic syndrome. In more than half the patients, multiple tumor sites were found. The occult nature of the adenoma was illustrated by the fact that these tumors were found and removed at the first operation in only 22 percent of the patients. Oberhelman [57, 58] and others [80, 81, 84] have long championed local or radical tumor excision as a desirable alternative to total gastrectomy, and they have recorded favorable results in their series. Wilson, too, found that of 43 patients who underwent local excision, subsequent ulcerations developed in 19 patients, requiring total gastrectomy or pancreatectomy. This constitutes a 44 percent failure rate of local tumor excision and reflects the high incidence of multiple undetected tumor sites. Of Wilson's 103 patients, 38 percent had malignant lesions in the form of tumor metastases or vascular or lymphatic invasion. Only 2 patients died of metastatic disease.

Gastrin-producing tumors in the submucosa of the first portion of the duodenum are commonly reported as carcinoid tumors. When no gross tumor is found in the pancreas and a vagotomy has been performed, it is desirable to explore the mucosa digitally on either side of the pylorus. These tumors are sometimes so small that the pathologist has difficulty finding the lesion even when the first portion of the duodenum is resected. It is a clinical impression that the duodenal tumors are not as malignant as gastrinomas elsewhere and may be more common in patients with the MEN I syndrome.

Solitary Pancreatic Tumors

In exceptional situations the surgeon can remove all the gastrin-producing tissue without resorting to total gastrectomy. This is especially tempting when a small tumor is verified in the submucosa of the duodenum or what seems to be a solitary tumor is found in the left half of the pancreas. Since the long-term results expected from what appears to be a solitary tumor are so often disappointing, the surgeon should consider an additional conservative procedure, such as truncal vagotomy and pyloroplasty. Some have advocated a Whipple procedure [68], especially when venous sampling has implicated the head of the pancreas as the location of a probable solitary tumor.

Ulcerogenic Tumors in Children

Tumors occur in every age group, and ulerogenic islet-cell tumors are no exception. Among the recorded cases, approximately 20 patients were diagnosed as having an ulcerogenic tumor before their sixteenth birthday, and each has been followed closely by Wilson and associates [86, 87]. All the children had gastrointestinal hemorrhage or perforation at some time during the course of the disease. In 5 the symptoms were present for one to two years before the first surgical procedure. Interestingly, there was not one instance of an associated endocrine adenoma, even though 2 of the patients had a family history positive for ulcer disease and pancreatic tumors. The response to operation in this group of young patients was particularly striking. Those who underwent total gastrectomy lived and continued to develop normally. None was on a special diet, although most snacked or ate extra meals. Analysis of their dietary habits indicated that the youngest patients adapted to total gastrectomy. In contrast, all of the children who had less than total gastrectomy died. The surgeon, therefore, should not hesitate to remove the entire stomach regardless of the youthful age of the patient. Although it may seem tempting to treat these patients with a lesser surgical procedure and cimetidine rather than with total gastrectomy, it is doubtful the children will take medication on the required basis for the rest of their lives. Total gastrectomy does not interfere with growth and development in the young.

Gastrinoma in the Elderly

At the other end of the age spectrum are elderly patients in whom a fulminating ulcer diathesis develops for the first time. This diathesis should strongly suggest the presence of an ulcerogenic tumor. The H_2-receptor antagonist can provide immediate and usually lasting relief of discomfort to this elderly group. In contrast to former years, when total gastrectomy was routinely advised because of the high incidence of fatal complications, a more conservative approach is warranted. Even if the patient fails to respond adequately to cimetidine, a conservative surgical procedure consisting of vagotomy, pyloroplasty, and excision of readily available tumor and metastases should be considered. Cimetidine therapy should be more effective after vagotomy, and the risk of an operation should be minimized.

RESECTION IN THE CLASSICAL ULCEROGENIC SYNDROME

Total gastrectomy remains the most effective means for long-term control of gastric hypersecretion in the presence of extensive tumor involvement of the pancreas with metastases to the liver and regional lymph nodes. The patient's age, general condition, life expectancy, family commitments, type of work, and acceptance or rejection of long-term frequent medication are some of the factors to be considered in the pros and cons of total gastrectomy. Certainly, total gastrectomy should be considered when cimetidine fails to provide relief. This radical approach has been suggested as the best mode of therapy in the long term for the very young. Specific problems such as alcoholism or failure to comprehend the importance of frequent long-term medication are other reasons for considering total gastrectomy. The risk of total gastrectomy should be no greater than that of any other major abdominal procedure, since catastrophic complications and previous surgical failures have been dramatically decreased as a result of earlier diagnosis with the gastrin immunoassay and control of hypersecretion by cimetidine.

Once the decision to perform total gastrectomy is made, the right gastric and gastroepiploic vessels are doubly ligated and the duodenum divided. The lumen of the duodenum is palpated digitally for evidence of a small submucosal tumor nodule. The ring of excised duodenum should be fixed to ensure the pathologist the opportunity to study the entire circumference in search of a submucosal islet-cell tumor. The duodenal stump is then closed with a layer of interrupted 4-0 silk and an inversion layer of interrupted 00 silk mattress sutures. The left gastric artery is doubly ligated, and the uppermost portion of the gastrohepatic ligament is likewise divided and transfixed on both sides with 00 silk. The spleen usually has been separated from the stomach as part of the mobilization of the spleen and the tail of the pancreas for complete exploration.

The lower end of the esophagus must be exposed with great care to avoid fraying the nonperitonealized, muscular esophageal wall. It is also important that the left lobe of the liver be freed up and mobilized toward the midline to ensure adequate exposure of the esophagogastric junction. The gastrohepatic ligament, which contains a branch of the inferior phrenic artery, is clamped and ligated. After both vagi have been resected, the esophagus will descend at least 5–6 cm into the abdominal cavity, but it will retract into the mediastinum unless it has been anchored at several points to the crus of the diaphragm. The esophageal wall can be given further substance at the point of division by placing a series of interrupted encircling mattress sutures of 4-0 silk horizontally. Such fixation prevents fraying of the muscle and affords a firm cuff for the anastomosis. Placement of medial and lateral angle sutures will also help to maintain proper orientation and will prevent rotation of the esophagus as the anastomosis is carried out.

TOTAL GASTRECTOMY RECONSTRUCTION

Every surgeon has his or her own preference for reestablishing gastrointestinal continuity after total gastrectomy. Some prefer to interpose a segment of jejunum between the ends of the esophagus and the duodenum, while others create a pouch type of gastrojejunostomy such as in the Poth, Longmire-Beal, or Hunt-Lawrence procedure [92]. When it is performed end-to-side to the jejunum, with the end of the jejunum directed to the left, the Roux-en-Y reconstruction has been satisfactory from the standpoint of minimizing subsequent alkaline esophagitis if the arm of jejunum is at least 15–20 cm beyond the jejunojejunostomy. The jejunum is anchored to the diaphragm posterior to the esophagus before starting the two-layer anastomosis between the esophagus and jejunum (Fig. 18-6).

After the two-layer posterior anastomosis has been completed, a large Einhorn stomach tube can be inserted alongside the Levin tube into the jejunum. The large tube serves as a stent to facilitate proper placement of the anterior row of sutures, and at the same time it should ensure as large an anastomotic lumen as possible.

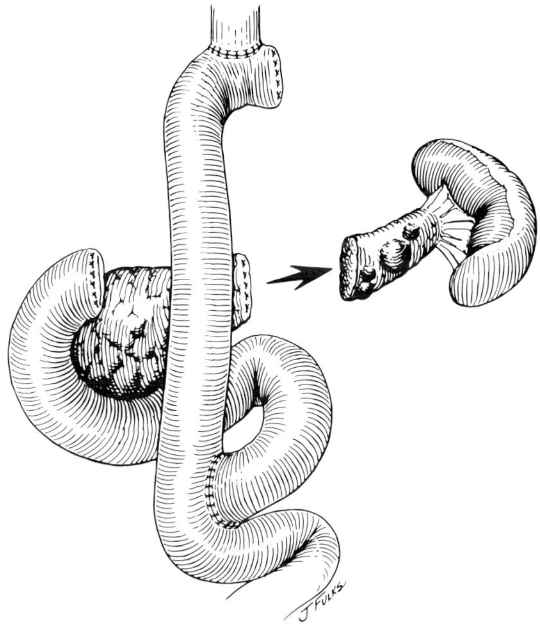

Fig. 18-6. The Roux-en-Y type of reconstruction follows aggressive tumor resection, which may include hemipancreatectomy as well as excision of metastatic lymph nodes and liver metastases. Tumors within the head of the pancreas may be locally excised. A Whipple procedure is rarely performed because of the multicentric locations of gastrinoma.

Pathology

Ulcerogenic tumors of the pancreas are usually small, and both the primary and metastatic tumors may be difficult to locate during an operation. They are malignant in fully 60 percent of instances, however, and are multiple in many. They can be located equally in the head, body, or tail of the pancreas and can occur as microadenomatosis [92]. As noted, duodenal wall tumors occur in 13 percent of patients [44] and are often described as carcinoid tumors.

Excessive production of gastrin from islet-cell tumors may be associated with hyperplasia, adenoma, or carcinoma; in some patients, it may be associated with a combination of these lesions [69]. Microscopically the tumor cells are arranged in tubules or rosettes, which may assume a trabecular, or ribbonlike arrangement. The appearance is often similar to that of carcinoid tumors [84]. The various histological patterns have not been correlated with the functional capacity of the tumor. Bloodworth and Elliott [7] many years ago emphasized that benign and malignant tumors demonstrate a similar morphological pattern. Thus the pathologist must rely on findings of venous or arterial invasion or actual evidence of metastatic spread before an unequivocal diagnosis of a malignant tumor can be established. Using routine histological stains, islet-cell tumors arising from any of the cell types are almost identical [69]; however, modern methods of histochemistry have been helpful in differentiating them.

The cells of most endocrine tumors of the foregut have been shown to develop in common from precursor neuroectodermal cells that have migrated from the neural crest [11, 62]. Pearse and Polak [61] have shown that most of the cells in the foregut endocrine system share common cytochemical properties, including their ability to take up and decarboxylate certain amino acids that are the precursors of fluorogenic amines (*a*mine *p*recursor *u*ptake and *d*ecarboxylation, or APUD cells). These endocrine cells are located in the human foregut from the anterior pituitary gland to the middle of the duodenum and the pancreas, and also in the loci of the neuroendocrine systems of the adrenal medulla, paraganglionic tissues, and other mesodermal areas [61]. They may elaborate a variety of polypeptides, including insulin, gastrin, adrenocorticotropic and melanocyte-stimulating hormones, glucagon, vasoactive intestinal polypeptide, somatostatin, serotonin, a secretinlike substance, and others [71, 92], and they produce a variety of unusual clinical syndromes.

Greider and McGuigan [41, 53] have demonstrated by immunohistological methods that the normal human pancreas contains gastrin in cytoplasmic granules of a population of islet cells interspersed along the periphery of the islets. The cells that reacted with fluorescent antigastrin resembled the classic delta cell of Bloom [8] and were argyrophilic with the Davenport staining method [40]. Argyrophil cells, which are morphologically similar to the delta cells of the pancreas, have been demonstrated in the antral-pyloric region of the stomach [73]. These gastrin cells are primarily distributed in the gastric antrum and by immunofluorescence have been shown to store gastrin [52, 53]. McGuigan and Greider [53], in studies of 10 ulcerogenic tumors, found that the staining characteristics were similar to those of the antral G cell. However, considerable confusion still remains about the precise islet cell of origin in the ulcerogenic tumor, as well as its relation to the delta cell of the pancreas and the G cell of the gastric antrum. The gastrin-producing tumor cells have been referred to as *argyrophil-metachromatic islet cells,* a term that encompasses the delta cell, alpha-1 argentaffin cells, F cells, and G cells [43].

Follow-Up Care

The postoperative clinical course of these patients may be altered by the extent of tumor and metastasis found at operation, as well as by the procedure performed (total gastrectomy or vagotomy and pyloroplasty). Patients who have had total gastrectomy require monthly injections of Vitamin B_{12} for the rest of their lives. It is advisable to rehospitalize these patients at intervals of three to six months for several years to survey their dietary habits as well as to confirm the adequacy of the esophageal anastomosis. Digestive complaints may be the result of partial stenosis of the esophagojejunal anastomosis that requires dilation. Sometimes cholelithiasis and cholecystitis develop during the follow-up period. Symptoms may recur when less than a total gastrectomy has been performed and the patient does not respond to H_2-receptor antagonist therapy. Total gastrectomy may be required.

The follow-up study of the patient with gastrinoma may extend over many years. Fasting serum gastrin levels and the response to a secretin push should be evaluated every year. The gastrin levels tend to fall after many surgical procedures, raising false hope of a complete cure, but over the ensuing months and years there is usually a steady rise in gastrin levels. A secretin push should be performed if the fasting gastrin level is less than 1000 pg/ml. Gastrin levels may reach surprisingly high levels in patients who have no symptoms. When there is laboratory evidence of increased tumor activity, a liver-spleen scan as well as a computerized tomographic scan or echogram may demonstrate evidence of metastasis. Unlike carcinoma of the pancreas, islet-cell tumors may involve the pancreas extensively without producing either local or distant discomfort. Hyperparathyroidism tends to recur despite the previous removal of a parathyroid adenoma, and blood calcium levels should be checked every time gastrin levels are taken.

Chemotherapy using streptozocin or chlorozocin either alone or in combination with other drugs should be considered in the presence of extensive residual tumor in the pancreas or liver, or both. Treatment is started three weeks after operation. A dose of chlorozocin (200 mg/sq m) is given every six weeks if the patient is younger than 65 years of age. Evidence suggests that occasionally the islet-cell tumor will respond to chemotherapy, and perhaps chemotherapy should be given more routinely when obvious residual tumor is present.

In general neither the clinical history, extent of tumor found at operation, nor level or trend of serum gastrin levels provides a reliable prognostic sign for the individual patient.

EFFECT OF TREATMENT ON TUMOR

Friesen [27, 29] and others have reported regression of metastatic tumor and decrease in serum gastrin level after total gastrectomy. The frequency of this phenomenon and the mechanisms that produce it are not known. Friesen [27] has postulated a mechanism based on malfunction of the gastropituitary axis that does not take place in the absence of the stomach. In a report by Fox et al. [26], only 4 of 157 patients had clearly documented regression of metastatic tumor following total gastrectomy. In addition, there was *presumptive* regression of primary tumors in 7 patients, 5 of whom underwent total gastrectomy. However, Davis and Vansant [15] in 1979 reported a 20-year survival time in a patient with regression of metastasis to the liver.

LONG-TERM SURVIVAL

Since 1955 a series of 44 patients has been studied for longer than five years after operation, and it has been found that a direct and aggressive surgical approach to the tumor improves long-term survival rates. The five-year survival rate was 76 percent in patients having complete resection of all gross tumor from the pancreas, duodenum, lymph nodes, or liver, in contrast to 21 percent in those in whom complete tumor resection was not possible. When all identified tumor was excised, the duration of survival increased by an average of six years.

To establish the long-term contribution of the H_2-receptor antagonists, with or without vagotomy, will require more than five years of follow-up observation. Sufficient time has not yet elapsed to evaluate survival of patients having less than a total gastrectomy and requiring continued H_2-receptor antagonist therapy for relief. A surprising number of patients seem to do well with less than a total gastrectomy, while others eventually require total gastrectomy.

The myriad complexities of hormone-secreting tumors of the pancreas demand explanations of mechanisms and development of guidelines for managing individual patients. The ability of the gastrin radioimmunoassay combined with widespread recognition of the symptoms has led to earlier diagnosis of the ulcerogenic tumor syndrome, with improved rates of morbidity and mortality. The effectiveness of the H_2-receptor antagonists in control of fulminating gastric hypersecretion has brought about dramatic improvement in the care of these patients: These agents have provided time for safely establishing the diagnosis, improved the surgical risk, and, in a few selected patients, permitted less than a total gastrectomy provided that vagotomy is performed. The gastrinoma is a solid intraabdominal tumor, however, with a potential for metastasis in approximately three-fourths of patients. Only by surgical excision can the microscopical diagnosis and extent of the disease be determined and some patients be cured while others have their lives extended. A combination of H_2-receptor-antagonist therapy and vagotomy may be used in the management of selected patients, but total gastrectomy with Roux-en-Y reconstruction combined with aggressive tumor resection should remain the treatment of choice in most patients with gastrinoma.

References

1. Aoyagi, T., and Summerskill, W. H. J. Gastric secretion with ulcerogenic islet cell tumor. *Arch. Intern. Med.* 117:667, 1966.
2. Barreras, R. F., Mack, E., Goodfriend, T., and Damm, M. Resection of gastrinoma in the Zollinger-Ellison syndrome. *Gastroenterology* 82:953, 1982.
3. Beacham, J., Bentley, P.H., and Gregory, R. A. Synthesis of human gastrin I. *Nature* 209:585, 1966.
4. Bentley, P. H., Kenner, G. W., and Shepard, R. C. Structures of human gastrins I and II. *Nature* 209:583, 1966.
5. Berson, S. A., and Yalow, R. S. Isotopic tracers in the study of diabetes. *Adv. Biol. Med. Phys.* 6:350, 1958.
6. Berson, S. A., and Yalow, R. S. Nature of immunoreactive gastrin extracted from tissues of gastrointestinal tract. *Gastroenterology* 60:215, 1971.
7. Bloodworth, J. M. B., Jr., and Elliott, D. W. The histochemistry of pancreatic islet cell lesions. *J.A.M.A.* 183:1011, 1963.
8. Bloom, N. New type of granular cell in islets of Langerhans in man. *Anat. Rec.* 49:363, 1931.
9. Burcharth, F., Stage, J. G., Stadil, F., et al. Localization of gastrinomas by transhepatic portal catheterization and gastrin assay. *Gastroenterology* 77:444, 1979.
10. Cameron, D., and Spiro, H. M. Zollinger-Ellison syndrome with multiple endocrine adenomatosis type II (letter). *N. Engl. J. Med.* 299:152, 1978.
11. Carvalheira, A. F., Welsch, N., and Pearse, A. G. E. Cytochemical and ultrastructural observations on the argentaffin and argyrophil cells of the gastro-intestinal tract in mammals and their place in the APUD series of polypeptide-secreting cells. *Histochemie* 14:33, 1968.
12. Christoforidis, A. J., and Nelson, S. W. Radiological manifestations of ulcerogenic tumors of the pancreas. *J.A.M.A.* 198:511, 1966.
13. Code, C. F., Hallenbeck, G. F., and Summerskill, W. H. J. Extraction of a gastric secretagogue from primary and metastatic islet cell tumor in two cases of the Zollinger-Ellison syndrome. *J. Surg. Res.* 2:136, 1962.
14. Creutzfeldt, W., Arnold, R., Creutzfeldt, C., et al. Gastrin and G cells in the antral mucosa of patients with pernicious anaemia, acromegaly and hyperparathyroidism and in a Zollinger-Ellison tumour of the pancreas. *Eur. J. Clin. Invest.* 1:461, 1971.
15. Davis, C. E., and Vansant, H. J. Spontaneous regression of advanced intra-abdominal metastases with 20 year survival. *Ann. Surg.* 189:620, 1979.
16. Deveney, C. W., and Deveney, K. E. Medical treatment of peptic ulcers. *Surg. Annu.* 17:219, 1985.
17. Deveney, C. W., Deveney, K. E., Stark, D., et al. Resection of gastrinomas. *Ann. Surg.* 198:546, 1983.
18. Donaldson, R. M., Jr., vom Eigen, P. R., and Dwight, R. W. Gastric hypersecretion, peptic ulceration, and islet-cell tumor of the pancreas (the Zollinger-Ellison syndrome). *N. Engl. J. Med.* 257:965, 1957.
19. Dragstedt, L. R. Pathogenesis of gastroduodenal ulcer. *Arch. Surg.* 44:438, 1942.
20. Dunn, E., and Stein, S. Percutaneous transhepatic pancreatic vein catheterization in localization of insulinoma. *Arch. Surg.* 116:232, 1981.
21. Edkins, J. S. The chemical mechanism of gastric secretion. *J. Physiol.* (Lond.) 34:133, 1906.
22. Eiseman, B., and Maynard, R. M. Non-insulin producing islet cell adenomas associated with progressive ulceration (Zollinger-Ellison syndrome). *Gastroenterology* 31:296, 1956.
23. Ellison, E. H. The ulcerogenic tumor of the pancreas. *Surgery* 40:147, 1956.
24. Elman, R., and Hartman, A. F. Spontaneous peptic ulcers of duodenum after continued loss of pancreatic juice. *Arch. Surg.* 23:1030, 1931.
25. Exalto, J. Ulcus jejuni nach Gastroenterosto-

mie. *Mitt. Granzgeb. Med. Chir.* 23:13, 1911.

26. Fox, P. S., Hogmann, J. W., DeCosse, J. J., and Wilson, S. D. The influence of total gastrectomy on survival in malignant Zollinger-Ellison tumors. *Arch. Surg.* 180:558, 1974.
27. Friesen, S. R. A gastric factor in the pathogenesis of the Zollinger-Ellison syndrome. *Ann. Surg.* 168:483, 1968.
28. Friesen, S. R. Zollinger-Ellison syndrome. *Curr. Probl. Surg.* April, 1972.
29. Friesen, S. R., Bolinger, R. E., Pearse, A. G. E., and McGuigan, J. E. Serum gastrin levels in malignant Zollinger-Ellison syndrome after total gastrectomy and hypophysectomy. *Ann. Surg.* 172:504, 1970.
30. Friesen, S. R., Tracy, H. J., and Gregory, R. A. Mechanism of the gastric hypersecretion in the Zollinger-Ellison syndrome: Successful extraction of gastrin-like activity from metastases and primary pancreaticoduodenal islet cell carcinoma. *Ann. Surg.* 155:167, 1962.
31. Goodman, L. S., Gilman, A. (Eds.). *The Pharmacological Basis of Therapeutics* (6th ed.). New York: Macmillan, 1980.
32. Gregory, R. A. The isolation and chemistry of gastrin (memorial lecture). *Gastroenterology* 51:953, 1966.
33. Gregory, R. A., Grossman, M. I., Tracy, H. J., and Bentley, P. H. Nature of the gastric secretagogue in Zollinger-Ellison tumours. *Lancet* 2:543, 1967.
34. Gregory, H., Hardy, P. M., Jones, D. S., et al. The antral hormone gastrin: Structure of gastrin. *Nature* 204:931, 1964.
35. Gregory, R. A., and Tracy, H. J. The constitution and properties of two gastrins extracted from hog antral mucosa. I. The isolation of two gastrins from hog antral mucosa. *Gut* 5:103, 1964.
36. Gregory, R. A., and Tracy, H. J. The isolation of two "big gastrins" from Zollinger-Ellison tumours. *Lancet* 2:797, 1972.
37. Gregory, R. A., Tracy, H. J., Agarwal, K. L., and Grossman, M. I. Amino-acid constitution of two gastrins isolated from Zollinger-Ellison tumour tissue. *Gut* 10:603, 1969.
38. Gregory, R. A., Tracy, H. J., French, J. M., and Sircus, W. Extraction of a gastrin-like substance from a pancreatic tumour in a case of Zollinger-Ellison syndrome. *Lancet* 1:1045, 1960.
39. Gregory, R. A., Tracy, H. J., and Grossman, M. I. Isolation of two gastrins from human antral mucosa. *Nature* 209:583, 1966.
40. Greider, M. H., Benscome, S. A., and Lechago, J. The human pancreatic islet cells and their tumors. *Lab Invest.* 22:344, 1970.
41. Gredier, M. H., and McGuigan, J. E. Cellular localization of gastrin in the human pancreas. *Diabetes* 20:389, 1971.
42. Grossman, M. I., Robertson, C. R., and Ivy, A. C. The proof of a hormonal mechanism for gastric secretion: The humoral transmission of the distention stimulus. *Am. J. Physiol.* 153:1, 1948.
43. Grossman, M. I., Tracy, H. J., and Gregory, R. A. Zollinger-Ellison syndrome in a Bantu woman with isolation of a gastrin-like substance from the primary and secondary tumors. II. Extraction of gastrin-like activity from tumors. *Gastroenterology* 41:87, 1961.
44. Hofmann, J. W., Fox, P. S., and Wilson, S. D. Duodenal wall tumors and the Zollinger-Ellison syndrome: Surgical management. *Arch. Surg.* 107:334, 1973.
45. Jaffe, B. M., Peskin, G., and Kaplan, E. L. Diagnosis of occult Zollinger-Ellison tumors by gastrin radioimmunoassay. *Cancer* 29:694, 1972.
46. Jaffe, B. M., Peskin, G. W., and Kaplan, E. L. Serum levels of parathyroid hormone in the Zollinger-Ellison syndrome. *Surgery* 74:621, 1973.
47. Kaplan, E. L., Peskin, G. W., Deveney, C. et al. Ulcer disease, metabolic alkalosis and hyperparathyroidism: A mechanism of interrelationship? *Ann. Surg.* 180:549, 1974.
48. Komarov, S. A. Gastrin. *Proc. Soc. Exp. Biol. Med.* 38:514, 1938.
49. Korman, M. G., Scott, D. F., Hansky, J., and Wilson, H. Hypergastrinemia due to excluded gastric antrum: A proposed method for differentiation from Zollinger-Ellison syndrome. *Aust. N.Z. J. Med.* 2:266, 1972.
50. Landor, J. H. Control of the Zollinger-Ellison syndrome by excision of primary and metastatic tumor. *Am. J. Surg.* 147:486, 1984.
51. Mann, F. C., and Williamson, C. S. The experimental production of peptic ulcer. *Ann. Surg.* 77:409, 1932.
52. McGuigan, J. E. Gastric mucosal intracellular localization of gastrin by immunofluorescence. *Gastroenterology* 55:315, 1968.
53. McGuigan, J. E., and Greider, M. H. Correlative immunochemical and light microscopic studies of the gastrin cell of the antral mucosa. *Gastroenterology* 60:223, 1971.
54. McGuigan, J. E., and Trudeau, W. L. Immu-

nochemical measurement of elevated levels of gastrin in the serum of patients with pancreatic tumors of the Zollinger-Ellison variety. *N. Engl. J. Med.* 278:1308, 1968.
55. McGuigan, J. E., and Trudeau, W. L. Studies with antibodies to gastrin: Radioimmunoassay in human serum and physiological studies. *Gastroenterology* 58:319, 1970.
56. Moldawer, M. P., Nardi, G. L., an Raker, J. W. Concomitance of multiple adenomas of the parathyroids and pancreatic islets with tumor of the pituitary: A syndrome with familial incidence. *Am. J. Med. Sci.* 228:190, 1954.
57. Oberhelman, J. A., Jr. Excisional therapy for ulcerogenic tumors of the duodenum. *Arch. Surg.* 104:447, 1972.
58. Oberhelman, H. A., Jr., Nelsen, T. S., and Dragstedt, L. R. Peptic ulcer associated with tumors of the pancreas. *Arch. Surg.* 77:402, 1958.
59. Osborne, M. P., Brown, M. E., and LeCompte, P. M. Ulcerogenic non-beta cell pancreatic islet carcinoma: Studies on the extraction and assay of a possible gastric secretagogue. *Am. J. Surg.* 100:48, 1960.
60. Pearse, A. G. E., and Bussolati, G. Immunofluorescence studies of the distribution of gastrin cells in different clinical states. *Gut* 11:646, 1970.
61. Pearse, A. G. E., and Polak, J. M. Neural crest origin of the endocrine polypeptide (APUD) cells of the gastrointestinal tract and pancreas. *Gut* 12:783, 1971.
62. Polak, J. M., Bussolati, G., and Pearse, A. G. E. Cytochemical immunofluorescence and ultrastructural investigations of the antral G cells in hyperparathyroidism. *Virchows Archir.* (Cell Pathol.) 9:187, 1971.
63. Poth, E. J., Manhoff, L. H., and DeLoach, A. W. The relation of pancreatic secretion to peptic ulcer formation: Effect of pancreatectomy, ligation of pancreatic ducts and diabetes on the production of histamine-induced ulcers in the dog. *Surgery* 24:62, 1948.
64. Rehfeld, J. F., and Stadil, F. Gel filtration studies on immunoreactive gastrin in serum from Zollinger-Ellison patients. *Gut* 14:369, 1973.
65. Richardson, C. T., Feldman, M., McClelland, R. N., Dickerman, R. M., Kumpuris, D., and Fordtran, J. S. Effect of vagotomy in Zollinger-Ellison syndrome. *Gastroenterology* 77:682, 1979.
66. Rudolf, L. E., Dammin, G. F., and Moore, F. D. Intractable peptic ulcer and endocrine adenomas with pituitary amphophilic hyperplasia. *Surgery* 48:170, 1960.
67. Ruppert, R. D., Greenberger, N. J., Beman, F. M., and McCullough, F. M. Gastric secretion in ulcerogenic tumors of the pancreas. *Ann. Intern. Med.* 67:808, 1968.
68. Sailer, S., and Zinninger, M. M. Massive islet cell tumor of the pancreas without hypoglycemia. *Surg. Gynecol. Obstet.* 82:301, 1946.
69. Schein, P. S. Islet cell tumors: Current concepts and management (National Institutes of Health Conference). *Ann. Intern. Med.* 79:239, 1973.
70. Sigel, B., Kraft, A. R., Nyhus, L. M., et al. Identification of a parathyroid adenoma by operative ultrasonography. *Arch. Surg.* 116:234, 1981.
71. Sircus, W. Peptide-secreting tumors with special reference to the pancreas. *Gut* 10:506, 1969.
72. Sizemore, G. W., Go, V. L. W., Kaplan, E. L., et al. Relationships of calcitonin and gastrin in the Zollinger-Ellison syndrome and medullary carcinoma of the thyroid. *N. Engl. J. Med.* 228:641, 1973.
73. Solcia, E., Capella, C., and Vassalo, G. Endocrine cells of the stomach and pancreas in states of gastric hypersecretion. *Gastroenterology* 2:147, 1970.
74. Stabile, B. E., Ippoliti, A. F., Walsh, J. H., and Passaro, E., Jr. Failure of histamine H_2-receptor antagonist therapy in Zollinger-Ellison syndrome. *Am. J. Surg.* 145:17, 1983.
75. Stabile, B. E., Morrow, D. J., and Passaro, E., Jr. The gastrinoma triangle: Operative implications. *Am. J. Surg.* 147:25, 1984.
76. Thompson, J. C., Lewis, B. G., Wiener, I., and Townsend, C. M., Jr. The role of surgery in the Zollinger-Ellison syndrome. *Ann. Surg.* 197:594, 1983.
77. Trudeau, W. L., and McGuigan, J. E. Effects of calcium on serum gastrin levels in the Zollinger-Ellison syndrome. *N. Engl. J. Med.* 281:862, 1969.
78. Turbey, W. J., and Passaro, E., Jr. Hyperparathyroidism in the Zollinger-Ellison syndrome. *Arch. Surg.* 105:62, 1972.
79. Underdahl, L. O., Woolner, L. B., and Black, B. M. Multiple endocrine adenomas: Report of 8 cases in which the parathyroids, pituitary and pancreatic islets were involved. *J. Clin. Endocrinol.* 13:20, 1953.
80. Waddell, W. R., Coppinger, W. R., and Lough-

ery, R. W. Pancreaticoduodenectomy for Zollinger-Ellison syndrome. *Ann. Surg.* 168:641, 1968.
81. Waddell, W. R., Leonskins, A. V., and Zuidema, G. D. Gastric secretory and other laboratory data on two patients with Zollinger-Ellison syndrome. *N. Engl. J. Med.* 260:56, 1959.
82. Walsh, J. H. Radioimmunoassay of Gastrin. In B. Rothfeld (Ed.), *In Vitro Nuclear Medicine*. Philadelphia: Lippincott, 1974.
83. Way, L., Goldman, L., and Dunphy, J. E. Zollinger-Ellison syndrome: An analysis of twenty-five cases. *Am. J. Surg.* 116:293, 1968.
84. Weichert, R. F., III, Roth, L. M., Krementz, E. T., et al. Carcinoid-islet cell tumors of the duodenum. *Am. J. Surg.* 121:195, 1971.
85. Wermer, P. Genetic aspects of adenomatosis of endocrine glands. *Am. J. Med.* 16:363, 1954.
86. Wilson, S. D., and Ellison, E. H. Total gastric resection in children with the Zollinger-Ellison syndrome. *Arch. Surg.* 91:165, 1965.
87. Wilson, S. D., Schulte, W. J., and Meade, R. C. Longevity studies following total gastrectomy: In children with the Zollinger-Ellison syndrome. *Arch. Surg.* 103:108, 1971.
88. Winship, D. H., and Ellison, E. H. Variability of gastric secretion in patients with and without the Zollinger-Ellison syndrome. *Lancet* 1:1128, 1972.
89. Yalow, R. S., and Berson, S. A. And now, "big-big" gastrin. *Biochem. Biophys. Res. Commun.* 48:391, 1973.
90. Yalow, R. S., and Wu, N. Additional studies on the nature of big big gastrin. *Gastroenterology* 65:19, 1973.
91. Zollinger, R. M. Non-beta islet cell tumors of the pancreas and the alimentary tract. *Am. J. Surg.* 129:102, 1975.
92. Zollinger, R. M., and Coleman, D. W. *The Influences of Pancreatic Tumors on the Stomach*. Springfield, Ill.: Thomas, 1974.
93. Zollinger, R. M., and Ellison, E. H. Primary peptic ulcerations of the jejunum associated with islet cell tumors of the pancreas. *Ann. Surg.* 142:709, 1955.
94. Zollinger, R. M., Ellison, E. C., Fabri, P. J., et al. Primary peptic ulcerations of the jejunum associated with islet cell tumors: Twenty-five year appraisal. *Ann. Surg.* 192:422, 1980.
95. Zollinger, R. M., Ellison, E. C., O'Dorisio, T. M.,and Sparks, J. Thirty years' experience with gastrinoma. *World J. Surg.* 8:427, 1984.
96. Zollinger, R. M., Tompkins, R. K., Amerson, J. R., et al. Identification of the diarrheogenic hormone associated with non-beta islet cell tumors of the pancreas. *Ann. Surg.* 168:502, 1968.

SPECIAL COMMENT

The Use of Operative Ultrasound to Localize Endocrine Tumors of the Pancreas

Bernard Sigel

The ideal surgical management of the Zollinger-Ellison syndrome is complete removal of the causative gastrinoma. This is usually not possible, however, because of metastases, a multifocal primary tumor, or inability to locate the tumor definitively at operation. For this reason, complete removal of the end-organ of acid secretion by means of a total gastrectomy is frequently the procedure used to contain this problem. We have had preliminary experience with a new technique for endocrine tumor localization at operation using imaging ultrasound. Operative ultrasonography has the potential for helping the surgeon find endocrine tumors within the pancreas. This could increase the number of resections of the primary lesion and reduce the need for total gastrectomy.

Operative ultrasonography is an imaging technique that uses real-time B-mode ultrasonic scanning during a surgical procedure. A sterile ultrasonic probe is placed in the operative field and maneuvered to reveal tissue structures. B-mode ultrasound is two-dimensional imaging. Real-time processing permits instant display of sections showing image changes caused by motion within the tissue.

Two factors have facilitated the use of ultrasound in the detection of pancreatic endocrine tumors at operation. These are recent developments in ultrasonic technology and the characteristic ultrasonic appearance of endocrine tumors.

Technological advances have now provided us with real-time ultrasonic equipment that is compact and simple to operate and that produces high-resolution images. The newer

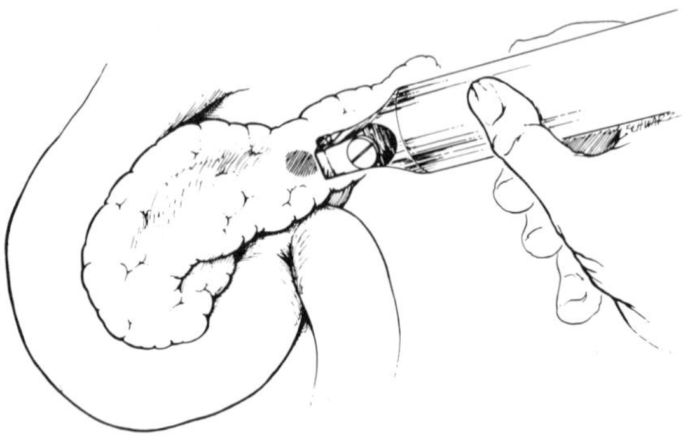

Fig. 18-7. Ultrasonic scanner head over the exposed pancreas. The scanner head is held 5–10 mm from the surface of the gland and moved along longitudinal scan paths. (By permission of *Surgery, Gynecology & Obstetrics.*)

equipment has produced far better images, which more closely resemble anatomical and pathological structures than instruments available only a few years ago. Small ultrasonic probes may be used directly in the operative field by the surgeon to scan the exposed pancreas. Pancreatic ducts, arteries, and veins may be readily discerned by surface scanning with real-time ultrasound. Lesions beneath the pancreatic capsule or within the substance of the gland also may be recognized by this examination.

Endocrine tumors usually produce a characteristic appearance on ultrasonic scanning. Endocrine tumors of the pancreas and at other sites, whether seen on regular body scanning or by operative ultrasound, most often are hypoechogenic. Hypoechogenicity is a reduction in the number and intensity of internal echos produced by a tissue. The decrease in echos of endocrine tumors makes them quite distinguishable from surrounding structures. The reason for the hypoechogenicity of endocrine tumors is not known. A possible explanation may be related to a greater and more homogeneous cellularity with less stromal elements and ducts. Figure 18-7 shows the scanning technique during operation, and Figure 18-8 demonstrates a directly scanned islet-cell tumor of the pancreas.

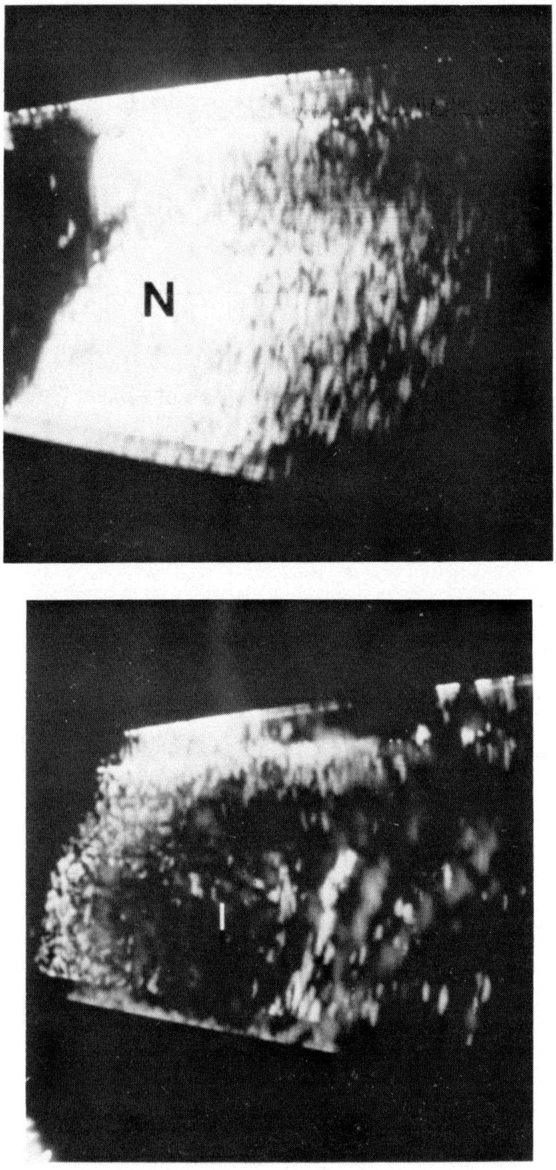

Fig. 18-8. Two sonograms obtained from the same pancreas. The view on the top shows normal pancreatic tissue (N). The view on the bottom illustrates an insulinoma (I) with a thin covering rim of normal pancreas. The insulinoma is less echogenic than the normal pancreas. (By permission of *Surgery, Gynecology & Obstetrics.*)

Ultrasonography during pancreatic surgery for Zollinger-Ellison tumors may assist the surgeon by confirming the presence of tumor in suspicious nodules found on routine exploration or by finding lesions otherwise not detected by inspection or palpation. Operative ultrasound may assist the surgeon by strengthening the likelihood of a diagnosis by revealing a nodule to consist of hypoechogenic tissue. Such a finding is particularly helpful in situations in which multiple nodules of the pancreas are found. When no external abnormalities of the pancreas are evident, operative ultrasound may locate lesions or rule out their presence within the substance of the pancreatic gland.

My colleagues' and my experience with pancreatic islet-cell tumors is limited [1, 2]. We have, however, been able to establish the presence of tumors in nodules as small as 4 mm. This has increased the certainty of diagnosis and facilitated the search process for endocrine tumors of the pancreas.

Comment References

1. Sigel, B., Coelho, J. C. U., Nyhus, L. M., et al. Detection of pancreatic tumors by ultrasound during surgery. *Arch. Surg.* 117:1058, 1982.
2. Sigel, B., Duarte, B., Coelho, J. C. U., et al. Localization of insulinomas of the pancreas at operation by real-time ultrasound scanning. *Surg. Gynecol. Obstet.* 156:145, 1983.

EDITOR'S COMMENT

It is of course extremely difficult to comment on a chapter written by an eponymous author and his colleague. However, with care not to trespass, there are perhaps one or two things to add to this marvelously clear and well-written chapter.

It is interesting that the young people with Zollinger-Ellison syndrome did so extraordinarily badly if treated with anything less than a total gastrectomy. This has been ascribed in part at least to the difficulty of localizing the tumor and to the great tendency for the gastrin-producing cells to be in multiple sites. There is, however, another curious feature: Even if all the tumor or tumors are apparently removed and the postoperative gastrin falls to normal levels, there is a tendency for these gastrin levels to rise some years later in some patients. The reason for this is not understood but could perhaps be related to the fact that the definition of a benign gastrinoma on histopathological grounds is difficult.

H_2-receptor blockade with either cimetidine or ranitidine has become the accepted method of medical management in this syndrome, but there are, unfortunately, some patients whose hypersecretion cannot be controlled in this way. For this reason the new Na-K-ATP-ase inhibitor omeprazole is of particular interest concerning its capacity to inhibit 24-hour intragastric acidity and, in particular, overnight gastric secretion [1, 4]. Indeed omeprazole has been found to be effective therapy in the Zollinger-Ellison syndrome [2, 3]. It is unfortunate, therefore, that some toxicological studies in rats have resulted in a suspension of clinical trials at the present time, although the drug does continue to be used for patients with the Zollinger-Ellison syndrome.

Richardson et al. [5] studied a medical-surgical approach in 22 patients with the Zollinger-Ellison syndrome. The patients were treated initially with cimetidine or ranitidine. A laparotomy was performed to remove easily resectable tumors and to carry out a proximal gastric vagotomy. Tumors were found in nine patients, and all visible tumors were removed from six of the nine patients. Fasting serum gastrin concentrations and serum gastrin responses to intravenous secretin were normal six weeks after the operation in each of the patients from whom all visible tumors were resected and were normal in four patients from six weeks to five years after the operation. Acid secretion was reduced after vagotomy in each patient even when tumors were not found or were completely resected. Thus, vagotomy decreased the acid secretory response to endogenous hypergastrinemia. In addition, vagotomy augmented the inhibitory effect of H_2-receptor blockers on acid secretion. The follow-up periods ranged from six weeks to six years (median, two years). Follow-up studies showed that (1) dosages of cimetidine or ranitidine were reduced, compared with preoperative amounts, in all but one patient; (2) two patients were taking no antisecretory drugs; (3) only three patients had occasional symptoms of ulcer disease; (4) complications such as bleeding, perforation, or obstruction did not occur in any patient. Endoscopy was performed in all patients to estimate the point prevalence of active ulcers, and an ulcer was found in one patient.

Richardson's is a fascinating and important study. The combined therapeutic approach to patients with the Zollinger-Ellison syndrome merits further study.

C.W.

Comment References

1. Attzel, D. J., and Shearman, D. J. C. Omeprazole inhibition of overnight gastric secretion in patients with duodenal ulcer disease. *Gastroenterology* 86:1112, 1984.
2. Lamers, C. B. H., Lind, T., Moberg, S., et al. Omeprazole in Zollinger-Ellison syndrome. *N. Engl. J. Med.* 310:758, 1984.
3. McArthur, K. E., Collen, M. J., Cherner, J. A., et al. Omeprazole as a single daily dose is effective therapy in Zollinger-Ellison syndrome. *Gastroenterology* 63:1178, 1984.
4. Naesdal, J., Bodemar, G., and Walan, A. Omeprazole: 24-hour intra-gastric acidity and plasma concentrations in peptic ulcer patients. *Gastroenterology* 86:1192, 1984.
5. Richardson, C. T., Peters, M. N., Feldman, M., et al. Treatment of Zolliger-Ellison syndrome with exploratory laparotomy, proximal gastric vagotomy, and H_2-receptor antagonists: A prospective study. *Gastroenterology* 89:357, 1985.

19

Recurrent Ulcer

Charles M. Sheaff
Lloyd M. Nyhus

Until 30 years ago (1955) the term *recurrent ulcer* carried the connotation of gastrojejunal or jejunal ulcer following some form of gastrojejunal anastomosis. However, recurrent ulcer may refer as well to recurrent duodenal ulcer disease subsequent to a Billroth I reconstruction after gastrectomy, vagotomy and pyloroplasty, vagotomy and antrectomy, mucosal antrectomy with vagotomy, suprapyloric antrectomy with vagotomy, selective proximal vagotomy with drainage (Holle procedure), or proximal gastric vagotomy without drainage. A wealth of knowledge is available about gastrojejunal ulceration, whereas many facts concerning recurrent ulcer following the procedures retaining duodenal continuity remain to be elucidated. *Recurrent, anastomotic, stomal,* and *marginal* are synonymous terms in this presentation, each connoting return of the ulcer problem.

The recurrence of an ulcer after surgical treatment is primarily a problem after treatment of a duodenal ulcer. Fortunately, if a gastric ulcer is properly removed, usually by subtotal gastrectomy, recurrent ulceration is rare. Of all recurrent ulcers, about 95 percent occur after surgical intervention for duodenal ulcer; only 2–4 percent occur after operations for gastric ulcer [67]. The individual risk of a recurrent ulcer developing after an operation for gastric ulcer, as long as it is away from the pylorus, is only 2 percent [12].

Etiology

Recurrent ulcers result generally from inadequate surgical therapy, that is, insufficient resection of the parietal cell mass during subtotal gastrectomy or incomplete vagotomy. This fact should not preclude the investigation of other, less common, causes of recurrent ulceration before reoperative therapy. Simple gastroenterostomy seems to have an intrinsic adverse effect on gastric secretion apart from the original factors of the ulcer diathesis [45]. In recent years much attention has been focused on the Zollinger-Ellison syndrome as an etiological mechanism for recurrent ulceration (see Chap. 18). We must also be sure not to

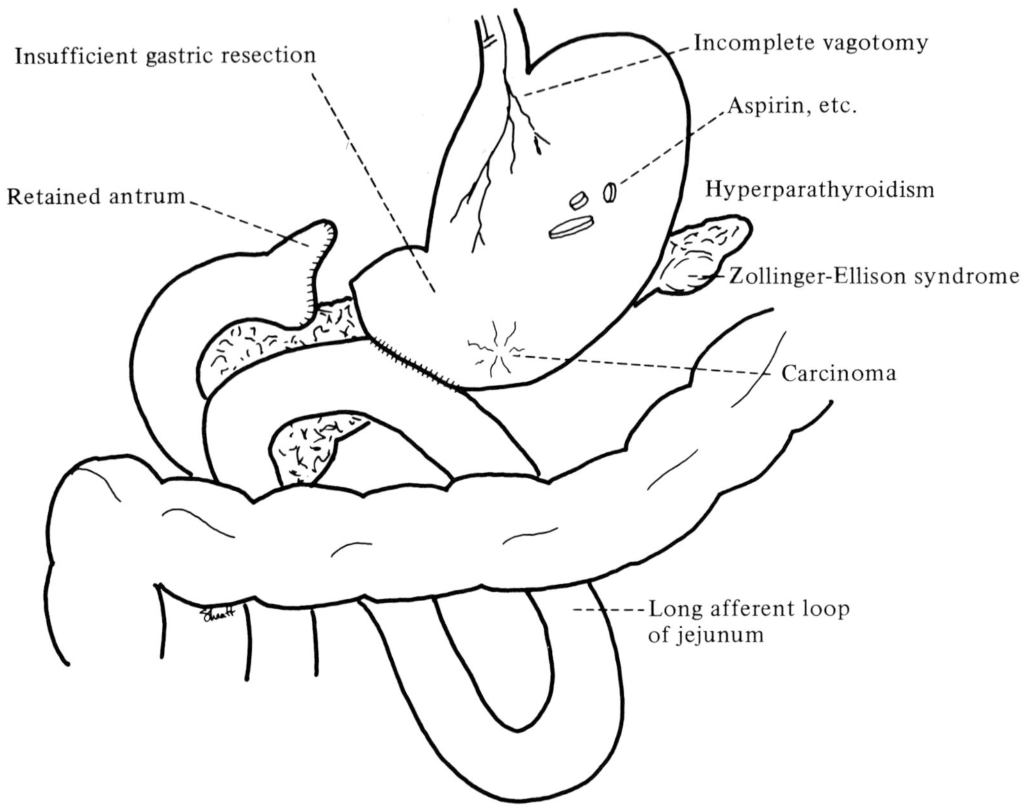

Fig. 19-1. Summary of common causative factors resulting in stomal ulceration.

forget hypercalcemia, smoking, ulcerogenic drug abuse, and development of carcinoma as etiological factors (Fig. 19-1).

The importance of inadequate gastric resection has been demonstrated in several animal and clinical studies. Lannin et al. [57] and Baronofsky et al. [10] demonstrated in dogs that a minimum of 75 percent gastric resection was necessary to prevent histamine-provoked ulceration. It has been clearly shown that the recurrence rate in duodenal ulcer patients is directly correlated with the amount of stomach resected [40]. These observations reinforce the need for quantitative evaluation of the amount of stomach resected [76]. The surgeon's estimate of amount of resection is usually not sufficient. Most surgeons have never quantified residual stomach and thus have no basis for an "educated guess" of the percentage of stomach resected. Although these comments are more germane to the era of extended distal gastrectomy, the antrectomist of today may wish to document accurately the percentage of the resection.

The length of the afferent loop has also been shown to be of great importance. For many years the expression "intrinsic sensitivity of the jejunum to acid" was commonly heard. The classical experiments of Kiriluk and Merendino [50, 51] proved that this concept is without basis. These authors demonstrated that the buffering capacity of bile and pancreatic juice decreases in direct proportion to the distance from their entrance into the duodenum. This factor of buffering capacity, rather than intrinsic jejunal sensitivity to acid, was shown to be the important aspect of jejunal ulceration. These experiments succinctly demonstrated why gastrojejunostomy should be performed with an afferent limb as short as possible, and they also confirmed the previous work of Merendino et al. [70], which demonstrated in dogs that a short afferent duodenal loop (Billroth II resection) protected against anastomotic ulceration when the preparation was challenged with ulcerogenic doses of histamine in beeswax.

The prime mechanism for development of an anastomotic ulcer after operative procedures using vagotomy is failure to sever all the vagus fibers. Vagal fibers begin to arborize at the distal end of the esophagus, so a concerted search must be made in every instance for more than two major vagal trunks. An intraoperative test for completeness of vagotomy is needed. The Grassi method of measuring gastric mucosal pH appears reliable and effective but requires opening the stomach [35]. Kusakari et al. [55] presented an endoscopic technique that seems to hold considerable promise. Saik and colleagues [88] modified the method slightly and have been very satisfied with its use.

Some ulcer operations are intrinsically ulcerogenic. Simple gastroenterostomy was already briefly alluded to as an example of such a procedure. This is documented by reported recurrence rates ranging from 34 to 60 percent [60]. Another ulcerogenic operation is the antral exclusion operation of Von Eiselsberg [102] and Devine [25], because of stimulation of the gastrin mechanism. Many modifications of the exclusion procedure have failed [73, 75]. Removal of the antral mucosa as suggested by Wilmanns [111], Bancroft [9], and Plenk [83] is the only modification of the antral exclusion operation that has not been intrinsically ulcerogenic.

The constant stimulation of a pouch of retained antrum in continuity with the duodenum produces a "gastrin factory." The endogenous levels of gastrin can make differentiation from a gastrinoma difficult. Radioisotopic scanning has been useful in several reported instances for delineating the retained antrum [21, 97, 108]. It is believed that the pertechnetate ion used in these scans is secreted by the gastric mucous cells, thus allowing the antrum to be visualized in spite of a paucity of parietal cell mass. Combining this scanning technique with a secretin-stimulated gastrin measurement has proved to be an elegant method of documenting retained antrum and excluding gastrinoma [108, 116]. In 1976 White and Harrison [109] reported the use of hypotonic duodenography to outline the afferent loop and retained antrum, if present.

A racial propensity to marginal ulcer has been reported [103, 113]. It was suggested that only Jewish persons suffered from an increased incidence of anastomotic ulceration following gastroenterostomy. This has been completely disproved by Tanner [98] and Lewisohn [60], who showed that racial considerations are of no importance. The propensity of recurrent ulcer to develop in patients with blood group O has been well documented by Peebles Brown et al. [78], Doll et al. [26], Cleator et al. [22], Blegvad [16], and Small [93]. The full significance of this observation is not known, particularly since Blegvad [17] found no relationship between ABO blood groups and gastric acidity. Smoking almost certainly has an effect on recurrence of ulceration: Smokers have been found to have a higher ulcer incidence, slower healing, lowered ratio of response to cimetidine, more ulcer-related complications, and a higher ulcer-related death rate. The relationship of smoking to ulcer disease has been studied and reviewed by Piper et al. [82].

Occasionally recurrent ulceration actually represents the occurrence of carcinoma. This complication is most frequent after Billroth II reconstruction or gastroenterostomy and is probably related to alkaline reflux bathing the gastric mucosa. In humans many investigators have observed an increased incidence of gastric stump cancer following Billroth II operation [19, 27, 65]. The incidence appears to be approximately 3 percent, with a median time of occurrence of 15–20 years, although a study from the United States gives a much lower relative risk [90].

Additional etiological factors include heavy use of salicylates, hypercalcemia, gastrinomas, poor antral drainage, suture-induced granulomas, and other ulcerogenic drug use. Such factors have been reviewed [14, 34, 96].

Incidence

Recurrent ulcers are more common than is generally believed. The surgeon who does only an occasional operation for duodenal ulcer because of lack of volume has no conception of his or her recurrent ulcer potential. Probably of more importance is the inability to follow these patients adequately for a long time postoperatively, not because of lack of interest but because of lack of time. These same considerations hold as well for other long-term complications after gastric operations, such as dumping and weight loss. An acceptable recurrent ulcer rate for any type of operative approach for duodenal ulcer would be about 3 percent. A procedure that cannot protect against recurrent ulceration to this degree must have some extenuating factor to allow its perpetuation. A summary of reported recurrent ulcer rates is shown in Table 19-1.

Although the recurrent ulcer rate after vagotomy and a drainage procedure is above the acceptable level of 3 percent, the low operative mortality associated with these operations may outweigh this criticism. Surgeons who use this procedure report a mortality near 0.5 percent. This figure must be contrasted with an average mortality of about 2 percent for resectional therapy. This means that for every 10,000 operations for duodenal ulcer, approximately 50 patients will die after vagotomy and a drainage procedure and 200 patients will die after gastric resection. In view of these striking mortality figures, it may be well to accept the complication of recurrent ulcers in 500 of the 10,000 patients treated by vagotomy and a drainage procedure. If the mortality of reoperation were 5 percent, the total patient mortality of 75 per 10,000 patients treated would still be a significant improvement. It should be pointed out that these mortality figures represent the results of experienced surgeons.

Proximal gastric vagotomy appears to have one of the higher recurrent ulcer rates. Reports vary from 1 to 25 percent [10, 44, 74, 86]. Selking [92] compared proximal gastric vagotomy to vagotomy and pyloroplasty and found twice the recurrent ulcer rate with proximal gastric vagotomy (16 percent compared to 8 percent) and twice the symptomatic failure rate with proximal gastric vagotomy (25 percent Visick grade IV compared to 13 percent). This is in sharp contradistinction to almost all other reports, in which postvagotomy syndromes and symptomatic failures after proximal gastric vagotomy are negligible [101]. Many surgeons still prefer a proximal gastric vagotomy in selected patients because of the incredibly low incidence of dumping and diarrhea as well as decreased mortality in spite of the increased recurrent ulcer rate [28].

Diagnosis

MAJOR SYMPTOMS

Epigastric pain is the most common complaint of patients with recurrent ulcer. The pain may be similar to that present before an operation, but it is not uncommon for the pain to present in bizarre ways. By using discriminant analysis and weighted tables to analyze questionnaires from patients with symptoms, Keighley et al. [48] were able to predict the presence of recurrent ulceration with 85 percent accuracy. Weight was given to the presence of moderate-to-severe pain that could be relieved by food. The diagnosis was weighted against food-provoked sickness, and moderate-to-severe or bilious vomiting more often suggested the diagnosis of alkaline reflux gastritis. Other disease entities can of course cause postoperative symptoms, including cholelithiasis, efferent or afferent loop syndromes, and reflux esophagitis. All patients with symptoms should be evaluated by barium meal, cholecystography, and endoscopy.

Hemorrhage occurs as a complication of recurrent ulcer in 50–70 percent of patients. Massive hemorrhage may occur, but the bleeding is usually of a more chronic nature, with anemia prominent in the presenting symptom complex [94]. Sudden development of diarrhea and associated weight loss subse-

Table 19-1. Incidence of recurrent ulcer

Author	Year	Operation	Recurrent ulcer (%)	Comments
Lewisohn [59]	1925	Simple gastroenterostomy	34	Constant observation
Harkins and Nyhus [39]	1956	Three-quarter gastrectomy, Billroth I	3.5	Others report higher recurrence rate following operation for duodenal ulcer
Marshall and Reinstine [69]	1955	Three-quarter gastrectomy, Billroth II	2.3	A standard observation
Harkins [38]	1960	Vagotomy + antrectomy	0.5	A standard observation
Burge [20]	1959	Vagotomy + gastrojejunostomy	3.8	Slightly lower than other reports
Burge [20]	1959	Vagotomy + pyloroplasty	3.1	Slightly lower than other reports
Wangensteen [106]	1957	Segmental resection	0	Relatively early in follow-up
Wangensteen [106]	1957	Tubular resection	2	Small number of cases; Wangensteen rejects as operative procedure
Allen and Welch [5]	1942	Exclusion operation (von Eiselsberg)	80	A universal finding
Griffith et al. [37]	1972	Selective vagotomy + pyloroplasty	0.97	One of 103 patients followed 4–9 years
Bauer et al. [11]	1976	Selective proximal vagotomy with drainage (Holle)	1.5	1339 selective proximal vagotomies in a 12-year period
Anderson et al. [7]	1982	Selective vagotomy + pyloroplasty	9	5-year rate for duodenal ulcer disease
			14	5-year rate for pyloric ulcer disease
		Parietal cell vagotomy (PGV)	15	5-year rate for duodenal ulcer disease
			33	5-year rate for pyloric ulcer disease
Fischer [32]	1984	Three-quarter gastrectomy (Billroth II)	2.6	1025 patients followed 22–30 years
Grassi et al. [35]	1980	Proximal selective vagotomy	1	1202 selective proximal vagotomies
Donahue et al. [28]	1984	Proximal gastric vagotomy	20	4–12 year follow-up study
Donahue et al. [28]	1984	Selective vagotomy + antrectomy	0	Randomized with PGV, above

quent to gastroenterostomy should alert the examiner to the possibility of gastrojejunocolic fistula.

TIME INTERVAL BETWEEN OPERATION AND ONSET OF SYMPTOMS

It is generally believed that symptoms of marginal ulcer appear earlier after gastric resection for duodenal ulcer than after gastroenterostomy; however, Beal [13] found in a series of 204 patients with marginal ulceration that the peak incidence for secondary ulceration after both partial gastrectomy and gastroenterostomy was within one year of the primary procedure. Ivy et al. [42] stated that 70 percent of marginal ulcers developed within two years. Walters et al. [104] found that the mean interval between a previous partial gastric resection and the operation for treatment of gastrojejunal ulcer was 3.7 years, while in patients with gastrojejunal ulcer following gastroenterostomy, the mean interval was 11.2 years. Postlethwait [85] found an average interval to reoperation for recurrent ulcer of 15.4 years for gastroenterostomy, 3.2 years for gastric resection, and 2.5 years for vagotomy and gastroenterostomy. There is no good explanation for the short time between the first operation and the development of a marginal ulcer after vagotomy plus gastroenterostomy. One would expect failures of this operation to be caused by incomplete vagotomy. This being the case, the procedure performed would then be a gastroenterostomy and should have the same failure pattern—continued recurrences for many years. This is not an isolated observation. Wychulis et al. [115] found the average interval between initial operation and symptoms of recurrent ulceration to be 7.4 years after gastroenterostomy, 1.9 years after gastric resection, 1.7 years after gastroenterostomy and vagotomy, and 1.1 years after gastric resection and vagotomy.

Although a well-defined interval has not been worked out for recurrence of ulcers after either selective vagotomy plus drainage or proximal gastric vagotomy, it would be expected that the time is short, as with other vagotomies. In a report in which the recurrence rate was as high as 42 percent after proximal gastric vagotomy, all the failures but one occurred within the first three years of observation [84]. On the other hand, a report from Aarhus, Denmark, suggests that the cumulative recurrence rate after proximal gastric vagotomy is 15 percent at 5 years and continues to rise [7]. In the Donahue et al. study [28], the interval from operation ranged from 1 to 16 years. It is clear that there is no consensus in the literature regarding the final recurrence rate or the time interval to recurrence after proximal gastric vagotomy.

GASTRIC ACID DETERMINATIONS

Gastric acid determinations are not diagnostic of ulcer recurrence or even of the risk of ulcer recurrence, when done postoperatively [52, 54]. Virtually the same mean basal and stimulated acid levels are present in patients with and without recurrent ulcers. On the other hand, results of preoperative acid testing can predict the risk of recurrent ulceration. Hood et al. [41] found a 1.4 percent risk of recurrence when preoperative basal acid secretion was under 2 mEq/hr and an 18.5 percent risk of recurrence when basal acid secretion was greater than 10 mEq/hr. Wittebol and colleagues [112] have made similar observations. This does not suggest that postoperative acid testing should not be done when recurrent ulcer is suspected. There is great value in postoperative acid testing in the evaluation of each individual situation, in terms of directing further diagnostic studies or choosing therapy.

Another laboratory determination that parallels gastric acid secretions is the serum pepsinogen I level [89]. This determination is probably related to uropepsin levels, which were reported by Nyhus [72] to correlate with symptoms caused by recurrent ulceration after gastrojejunostomy. Hyperpepsinogenemia I has been found in some families to act as a genetic marker for the development of ulcer disease [87]. Elevated serum pepsinogen I levels not only mark duodenal ulcer patients, but also, if very elevated, predict a poor response to cimetidine therapy [81].

PALMER TEST

In 1927 Palmer [77] described a method of differentiating between ulcer pain and gastritis.

A solution of 200 ml of 0.5 percent hydrochloric acid is introduced through a tube into the empty stomach. In a patient with anastomotic ulcer, immediate severe ulcer pain may be produced—a pain quickly relieved by aspiration of the acid. Ivy et al. [42] pointed out that occasionally this pain response is seen in patients with gastritis; therefore, the test as outlined should be followed by the introduction of 0.36 percent sodium bicarbonate solution, which will not cause pain in the ulcer patient but usually will cause distress in patients with gastritis. Warshaw [107] rediscovered this test, which showed great potential in predicting relief with surgical treatment. A similar maneuver was proposed by Alexander-Williams [2], who suggested collecting the nasogastric drainage of patients. If this drainage was bile stained it was then reinfused through the nasogastric tube. If this action provoked symptoms, the diagnosis was reflux gastritis.

GASTROSCOPY

The fiberoptic endoscopes have revolutionized the diagnostic approach to recurrent ulcer. Although anatomical changes secondary to an operation make visualization of postanastomotic ulcers difficult, the procedure is mandatory in all patients who have symptoms. When gastroscopy is positive for an anastomotic ulcer, the results are, of course, definitive. Often other pathology is encountered that explains the symptoms on a basis other than ulcer recurrence [29]. When gastroscopy is negative, other investigations are warranted to search further for ulcer recurrence.

ROENTGENOLOGICAL STUDIES

Although the upper gastrointestinal series is a mainstay for the diagnosis of gastric and duodenal ulcer, the same cannot be said of roentgenological studies for the diagnosis of recurrent ulcer [1]. Walters et al. [104] reported that a positive roentgenological diagnosis of gastrojejunal ulcer was made in only 50 percent of patients with gastrojejunal ulcer after gastric resection and in 37 percent of patients after gastroenterostomy. Thompson [99] in his series found that a positive diagnosis of gastrojejunal ulcer on roentgenological evidence was made in 27 percent of instances. On the basis of this low rate of diagnosis the surgeon may be "often compelled to make a diagnosis in spite of a negative roentgenogram, providing the patient has previously undergone gastric surgery, and has bled or has persistent ulcer-like pain or a combination of both symptoms" [99]. Fortunately, we are now more aware that the symptoms of gastrojejunal ulcer and reflux alkaline gastritis are similar. Because of this and because gastroscopy with biopsy is now available, we are no longer compelled to make the diagnosis of recurrent ulcer blindly.

Experienced roentgenologists can make the diagnosis of anastomotic ulcer without actually demonstrating an ulcer niche. Stomal tenderness and excessive stomal irritability as indicated by stomal spasm on palpation are two of the most common signs they use.

Normal postgastrectomy stomal folds or niches may be confused with stomal ulcers. This occurred several times in our early experience with the Billroth I gastric resection. With the addition of vagotomy to resection, roentgenological examination is not feasible in the early postoperative period because of moderate gastric stasis, and we now obtain a roentgenological examination of the stomach routinely at about six to eight weeks after the operation. Since adopting this policy we have not been troubled with operative artifacts of the stoma in patients with questionable recurrent ulcer. It is possible that roentgenological examination is more helpful in sorting out recurrence after vagotomy and pyloroplasty than it is after other operative procedures [3].

Treatment

The patient with a recurrent ulcer, the internist who originally referred the patient for operative treatment, and the surgeon who did the gastric operation are all displeased with the development of recurrent ulceration. The patient and internist are loath to accept recommendations for further operations, whereas the surgeon, if he or she is fortunate enough to see the patient again, is prone to recommend another surgical attack on the ulcer diathesis. Therefore, emotions of the interested persons may play a major role in making decisions for further care and may prevent a course of action based on knowledge gleaned from past experience or facts available at the time. The experience with various modalities of treatment for recurrent ulcer is described in the following discussion.

MEDICAL APPROACH

One might expect that various operations for ulcer disease would remove a portion of the acid-stimulatory mechanism and that the addition of antacid therapy would suffice to control the resurgent disease. Unfortunately, this has not been the finding. In a review of this problem, Everson and Allen [30] found that only 11 of 39 patients treated by special diets, frequent feedings, and antacids responded in a satisfactory manner. There was a 15 percent mortality among the patients treated medically, with 2 patients dying of perforation, 2 of exsanguinating hemorrhage, and 2 of gastrojejunocolic fistulas. This mortality, as pointed out by Everson, is well above that which might be expected from operations performed by competent surgeons on reasonably low-risk patients. Similarly, Beal [13] noted an 11.3 percent mortality in 44 patients treated without operation, and only 4 of the survivors remained free of ulcer symptoms.

The H_2 antagonists have been examined and found to have a better success rate than the methods of the aforementioned studies but still have the problem of high relapse rates unless cimetidine is continued in high doses. Berstad et al. [15] reported 90 percent success in healing recurrent ulcers with six weeks of cimetidine, but 33 percent of the patients with successful results had relapses while taking 400 mg per day maintenance dosages. A second course achieved healing in all the patients who relapsed, and they were then maintained successfully on 800 mg per day of cimetidine to be continued indefinitely. Kennedy and Spencer [49] compared the efficacy of cimetidine to placebo for recurrent ulcers and found no differences, with the ulcers of only 7 of 12 patients treated with cimetidine healing with those of 5 of 12 placebo-treated patients in six weeks. Festen et al. [31] found that recurrent ulcers healed with cimetidine (86 percent), but even on 800 mg per day maintenance, there was a 16 percent relapse rate in one year. Koo and associates [53] found that although a 92 percent healing rate could be achieved with cimetidine, relapse occurred in 71 percent of patients within six months of stopping the cimetidine. On the basis of these results it appears that nonsurgical therapy for recurrent ulcers is inferior.

There have been several new approaches to medical therapy for primary ulcer disease that may be as effective as cimetidine. Coating the ulcer bed appears to be the mechanism of action of sucralfate. Prostaglandins of the E and I groups stimulate mucous production. Tricyclic antidepressants inhibit gastrin release, and new antimuscarinic agents show some promise. In addition newer, more potent H_2 antagonists are being evaluated. None of these therapies has yet been tested on patients with recurrent ulcers, so while our hopes remain high for the development of an effective medical regimen in the future, we must currently advocate surgical treatment as the best approach.

SURGICAL APPROACH

It is widely held that recurrent ulceration is the product of an ill-advised or poorly executed primary operation [24]. The usual technical factor incriminated is completeness of vagotomy, and for this reason revagotomy is proposed as the usual solution. If such a simple analysis were correct, then early postoperative acid secretion should correlate with risk of development of recurrent ulcer. In fact the correlation has been weak or nonexistent. Of much greater value is the *preoperative* acid study which correlates well with the risk of recurrence [41, 54, 112]. This would tend to indicate that there is a class of patients who are more difficult to treat because of a more severe ulcer diathesis. It would also indicate that a cautious analysis of the individual problem is warranted rather than just revagotomy when a postoperative acid analysis and insulin

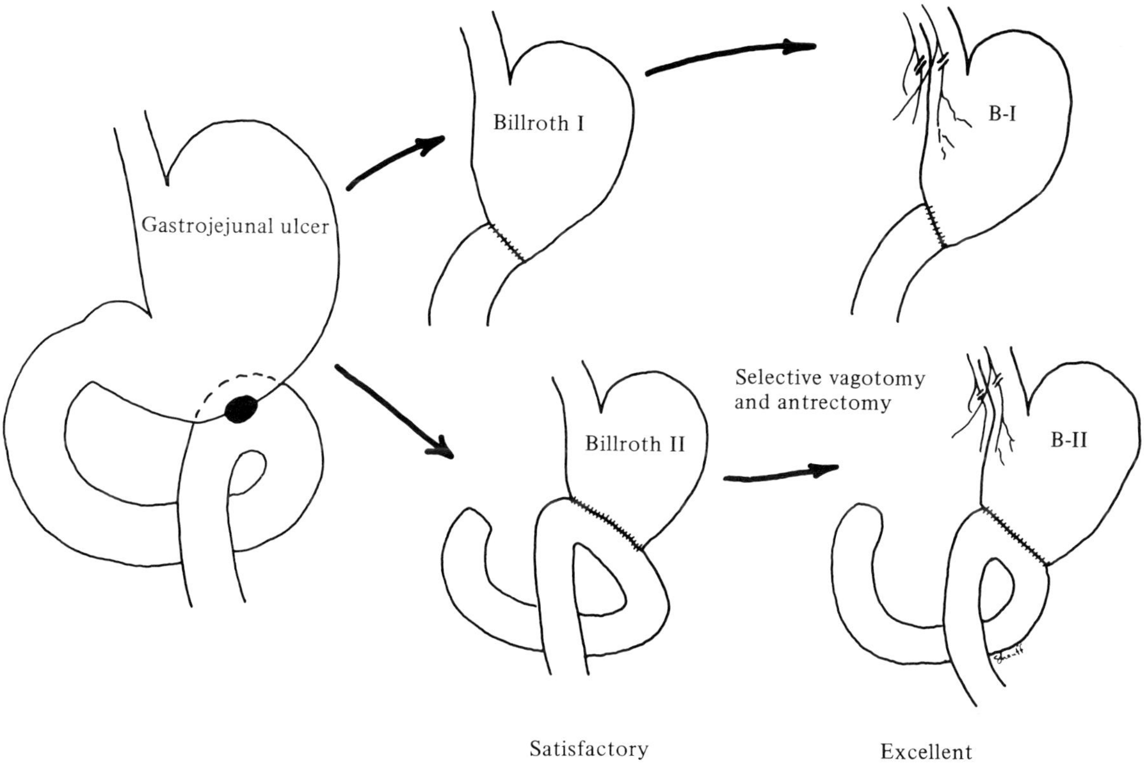

Fig. 19-2. Stomal ulceration after gastroenterostomy may be treated by antrectomy. Adding a selective vagotomy may be advantageous.

test point toward insufficient vagotomy. Each case must be individualized based on the previous operation, the diagnostic analysis, and the patient's condition. The importance of choosing the most effective reoperation is highlighted by mortalities that rise with each succeeding operation. In large series, mortalities of second operations range from 4 to 9 percent if a gastric resection is part of the operation [14, 22, 71, 96]. Vagotomy alone is much safer than vagotomy plus gastric resection, and it is undoubtedly logical in the face of evidence indicating an incomplete vagotomy. But when vagotomy has already failed once, another attempt results in an incomplete vagotomy 30 percent of the time, with recurrent ulcers developing 20 percent of the time [77]. The difficulty in choosing the safest operation in terms of mortality and recurrence is evident in the large variety of operations used for this problem [8]. Apparently in instances in which an incomplete vagotomy can be demonstrated and additional resection is not indicated, a transthoracic approach can offer lower morbidity and a higher success rate for completeness of vagotomy than a transabdominal approach [58].

Anastomotic Ulcer After Gastroenterostomy

Gastric resection appears to be the treatment of choice when an anastomotic ulcer develops after gastroenterostomy (Fig. 19-2). The recurrence rate can probably be reduced somewhat further by the addition of a vagotomy. The most elegant theoretical approach is to close the stoma and perform a proximal gastric vagotomy without drainage. The experience with this approach is meager and not en-

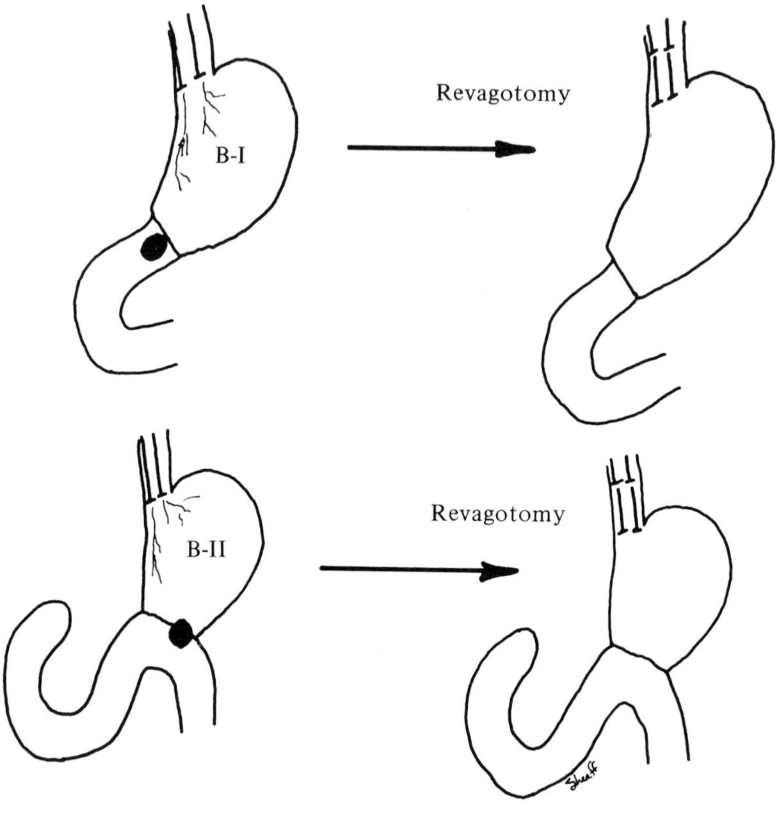

Fig. 19-3. Stomal ulceration after a standard subtotal gastrectomy is best treated by vagotomy. The transthoracic route is preferable.

couraging. Green et al. [36] report an early recurrence of two patients in a total of five so treated. This probably reflects the same problem that leads to a recurrence rate of 24 percent when vagotomy alone is used [96].

Anastomotic Ulcer After Gastric Resection

Vagotomy alone is superior in this situation (Fig. 19-3), giving a recurrence rate of about 12 percent [22, 61]. Although re-resection and vagotomy can reduce the rate to 8 percent, the improvement is bought with a disproportionate rise in mortality. All this presupposes a preoperative series of studies to exclude the problem of retained antrum. This is especially important in patients who have had a Billroth II gastrectomy; they may have an incidence of 40 percent of some retained antrum [18]. For this reason Thompson [99] recommended unfolding the inverted stump to make sure this ulcerogenic mechanism was not in action. Scott et al. [91] reported on a patient who had three operations for anastomotic ulcer before retained antrum was discovered in the duodenal stump and excised.

Recurrent Ulcer After Vagotomy and Drainage

When a previous vagotomy has failed, even if there is excellent evidence indicating an incomplete vagotomy, another attempt will be met with failure 30 percent of the time. For this reason resectional therapy should be used in the approach to this problem, with revagotomy added when insulin testing or a Kusakari test demonstrates an incomplete vagotomy.

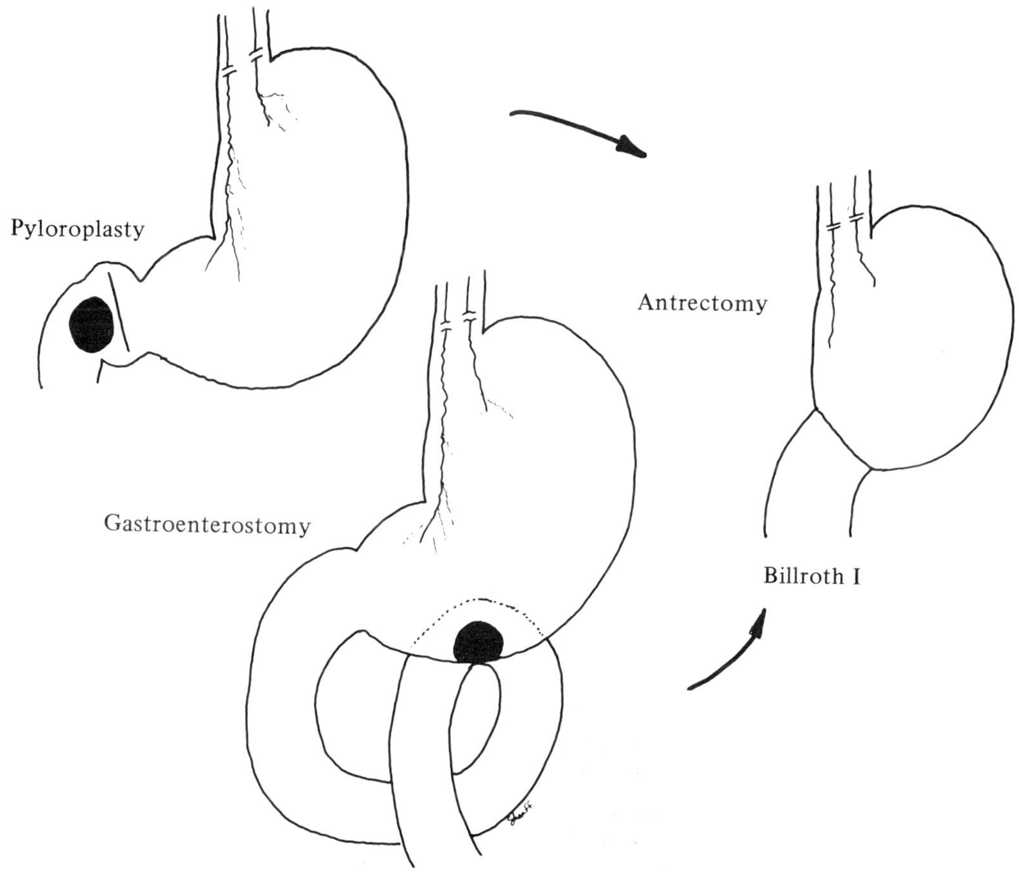

Fig. 19-4. Stomal ulceration after vagotomy and drainage is best treated by antrectomy plus reexploration for intact vagal fibers.

Since accurate preoperative testing demonstrates an incomplete vagotomy 78 percent of the time [47], a revagotomy will be added quite often. The amount of stomach it is necessary to resect is not known. Antrectomy (35 percent resection) is probably satisfactory [71] as shown in Figure 19-4.

Recurrent Ulcer After Proximal Gastric Vagotomy

With the rise in popularity of proximal gastric vagotomy and the relatively high recurrence rates reported from some centers, this problem promises to become more common. The most common practice is to perform this operation without a drainage procedure, and for this reason transthoracic vagotomy should be avoided. Indeed any attempt at revagotomy will be accompanied by a high incidence of gastric retention in the absence of a drainage procedure. The logical choice in this situation is an antrectomy with addition of a vagotomy if preoperative testing indicates a need (Fig. 19-5).

Complications

HEMORRHAGE

The problem of hemorrhage is seen much more often with an anastomotic ulcer than with gastric or duodenal ulcers. As previously mentioned, the incidence approximates 60 percent of all patients with this disease entity.

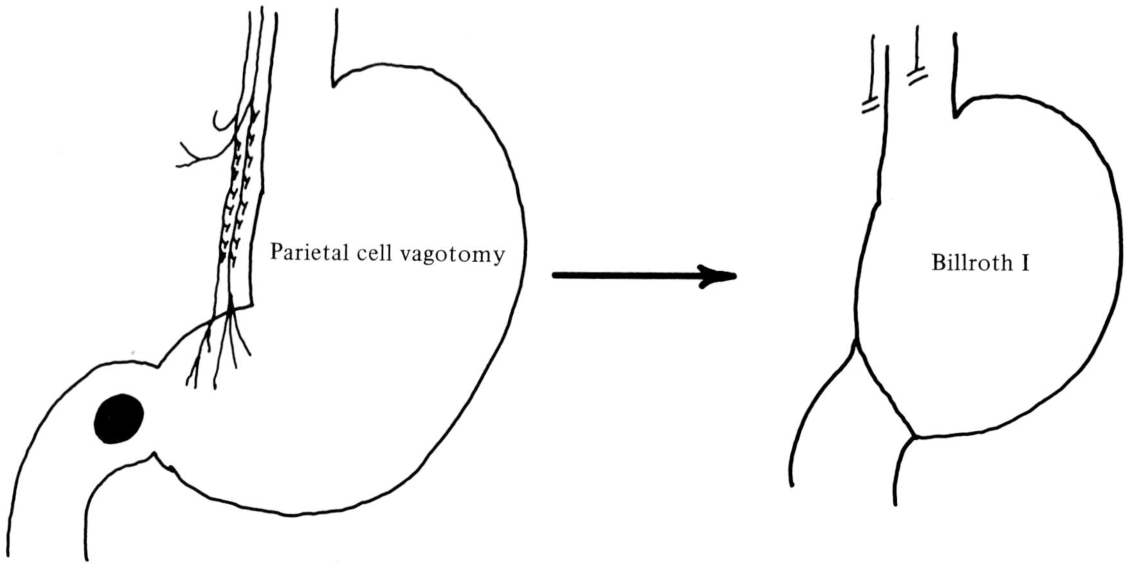

Fig. 19-5. Ulceration after parietal cell vagotomy must be treated with at least an antrectomy and most of the time a revagotomy. Vagotomy alone would leave stasis problems.

Although the bleeding is usually of a chronic nature, true massive hemorrhage can occur, necessitating emergency operative measures. The indications for emergency operative intervention are essentially the same as those outlined in Chapter 15. Resectional therapy is indicated under these circumstances.

PERFORATION

The complication of perforation may be seen in as many as 10 percent of all patients presenting with marginal ulceration [95]; however, most series report a lower incidence than this. The presenting symptoms and physical findings in this catastrophe differ little from those seen after perforation of duodenal or gastric ulcers. In general, the precepts of treatment follow the outline presented previously in this chapter; that is, the definitive procedure for the ulcer diathesis should be performed (see also Chap. 16). Simple closure of the perforation or gastric tube aspiration should be reserved for the occasional high-risk patient who will not tolerate the definitive operation, since 89 percent of the survivors of aspiration or closure will suffer from another recurrent ulcer [100].

ANTERIOR ABDOMINAL WALL ABSCESS

A complication seen occasionally after an antecolic gastrojejunostomy is an anterior abdominal wall mass or abscess, whereas after a retrocolic anastomosis, gastrojejunocolic fistula is prone to occur. The presence of an abdominal wall mass plus a history of a prior operation for ulcer disease should alert the observer to the diagnosis of gastrojejunal ulcer with anterior perforation. The treatment after diagnosis consists of abscess drainage and subsequent operative approach to the basic problem, which is gastrojejunal ulcer [33].

ZOLLINGER-ELLISON SYNDROME

For a complete discussion of this complication, see Chapter 18.

GASTROJEJUNOCOLIC FISTULA

Gastrojejunocolic fistula is encountered infrequently today. A modicum of proximity of the organs involved is necessary for development

Table 19-2. Incidence of gastrojejunocolic fistula with gastrojejunal ulcer

Author	Year	Percent
Judd and Hoerner [46]	1935	8.7
Wright [114]	1935	8.7
Lahey [56]	1936	11.0
Allen [4]	1937	14.0
Walters and Clagett [105]	1939	13.6
Lowdon [63]	1948	22.4
Marshall and Knud-Hansen [68]	1957	15.1
Amlicke and Ponka [6]	1964	8.6
Wychulis et al. [115]	1966	5.0
Cody et al [23]	1975	18.0

of the fistula, a spatial situation that is ideally present after retrocolic gastroenterostomy. Simple gastroenterostomy has been almost abandoned as a primary operation for patients with duodenal ulcer; thus the incidence of gastrojejunocolic fistula should fall significantly. It must be noted, however, that fistula into the colon has been reported after essentially every operation devised for the treatment of peptic ulcer disease.

Incidence

The incidence of gastrojejunocolic fistula (Table 19-2) associated with marginal ulcer has ranged from 5 percent [115] to a high of 22.4 percent [64]. The disease is primarily seen in men: Of more than 400 fistulas reported to 1953, only 5 occurred in women [68].

Diagnosis

A triad of symptoms has been defined—diarrhea, weight loss, and fecal breath or vomiting. Diarrhea with subsequent weight loss is usually the predominant presenting complaint. Pain may be present, but frequently it subsides with progression of diarrhea. The diarrhea is severe and debilitating.

Originally the diarrhea was considered a result of dumping of gastric content into the colon. Pfeiffer and Kent [80] were the first to postulate that the diarrhea was caused by the presence of feces in the jejunum. This concept was proved correct by the remarkable improvement in these patients' conditions after proximal colostomy or ileosigmoidostomy, and the theory has been substantiated experimentally [43].

The symptoms of fistula formation may develop at any time subsequent to the initial operative procedure. Marshall and Knud-Hansen [68] found the average time lapse to be about six years. Physical findings usually include emaciation and evidence of fluid and electrolyte imbalance. Abdominal tenderness, distention, and borborygmi may be present; about 50 percent of the patients, however, present no abdominal findings.

The most reliable diagnostic measure is the barium enema. The upper gastrointestinal series has been recognized as a poor method for demonstrating the presence of a fistula. Whenever this symptom complex develops, a faulty anastomosis—gastroileal or gastrocolic—must also be considered and ruled out. An upper gastrointestinal series has been recommended as a better method to delineate a faulty anastomosis if one exists. The time interval from initial operation to the pronounced symptoms of abnormal intestinal connection is usually much shorter following faulty anastomosis than it is for fistula formation.

Treatment

The evolution of the proper treatment for gastrojejunocolic fistula is interesting (Fig. 19-6). The mortality for this complication before 1930 was appalling. Two concepts had to evolve before the proper therapeutic regimen could be initiated. The first giant step forward was the recognition of the fecal irritation of the jejunum with the concomitant debilitating diarrhea. Wilkie of Edinburgh [110] first recommended exclusion of the involved loop of colon as a first-stage operation; however, the true problem was not clarified until the work of Pfeiffer and Kent [80]. They recommended ascending colostomy as a first stage to divert the fecal stream away from the jejunum (we prefer proximal transverse colostomy to ascending colostomy). Pfeiffer [79], using this approach, reported only 1 death in a series of 15 patients—a remarkable advance.

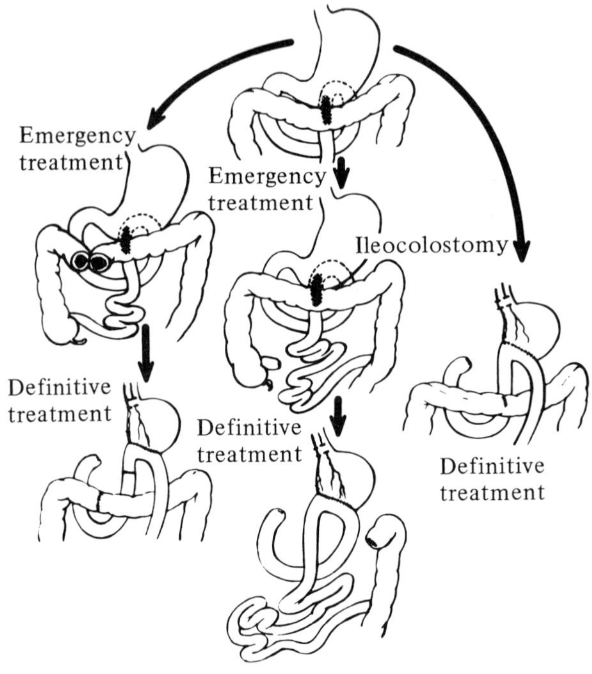

Fig. 19-6. Treatment of gastrojejunocolic fistula. Emergency treatment consists of either a proximal transverse colostomy (our preference) or an ileosigmoidostomy. These temporizing procedures must be followed by a definitive attack on the ulcer diathesis, e.g., vagotomy plus antrectomy. In the low-risk patient the definitive operation may be performed as a primary procedure.

At about the same time, Lahey [56] used another type of defunctionalizing procedure: ileosigmoidostomy. As a second stage he performed an en bloc resection of the fistula, the distal two-thirds of the stomach, and the right and transverse portions of the colon. This extensive secondary procedure presents a definite disadvantage to ileosigmoidostomy as a primary treatment. However, the work of Lahey and others brought into focus the other factor important in treatment, namely, the recognition of a dire need to treat the ulcer diathesis vigorously. Localio et al. [62] reviewed reports of 115 patients in the literature and found a recurrent ulcer rate of 50 percent in patients in whom only the fistula was eliminated, compared with a 4 percent recurrent ulcer rate when efforts were made to correct the ulcer diathesis. As recently as 1957, MacLeod and Galloway [66] proposed that ileosigmoidostomy be the definitive procedure if the patient continued to have no symptoms. This is a dangerous recommendation. The basic ulcer disease must be treated by definitive methods.

The final step in the evolution of the current approach was the development of the one-stage operation. The refinements in preoperative and postoperative care, particularly intravenous hyperalimentation with correction of fluid and electrolyte imbalances (potassium and calcium depletion), have made the one-stage procedure feasible. In gastrojejunocolic fistula following gastroenterostomy, the specific operation to control the ulcer diathesis should be distal gastrectomy with or without vagotomy. The procedure to be undertaken when a fistula develops after one of the current standard operative procedures for treatment of peptic ulcer should in general follow the precepts outlined previously in this section.

A word is necessary concerning care of the colonic fistula. Lowdon [64] clearly defined the approach:

When the anastomosis and the fistula have been defined by dissection it is advisable to deal with the colon first. Separation of the fistula from the colon usually results in an opening which can be repaired transversely, but the surgeon should be satisfied that there is no stenosis resulting from previous scarring or from the excision and repair; occasionally resection of a portion of the colon is advisable. In either case the presence of a proximal colostomy is an added safeguard.

References

1. Ahmad, W., and Harbrecht, P. J. Recurrent duodenal ulcer disease. *Arch. Surg.* 108:428, 1974.
2. Alexander-Williams, J. Alkaline reflux gastritis: A myth or a disease? *Am. J. Surg.* 143:17, 1982.
3. Alexander-Williams, J., and Toye, D. K. M. Recurrent ulcer after vagotomy and pyloroplasty: The x-ray appearances and their value in diagnosis. *Gut* 11:405, 1970.
4. Allen, A. W. Aseptic technique applicable to gastrojejunocolic fistula. *Surgery* 1:338, 1937.
5. Allen, A. W., and Welch, C. E. Gastric resection for duodenal ulcer. *Ann. Surg.* 115:530, 1942.
6. Amlicke, J. A., and Ponka, J. L. Gastrocolic and gastrojejunocolic fistulas: A report of 16 cases. *Am. J. Surg.* 107:744, 1964.
7. Andersen, D., Amdrup, E., Hostrup, H., and Sorensen, F. H. The Aarhus County vagotomy trial: Trends in the problem of recurrent ulcer after parietal cell vagotomy and selective gastric vagotomy with drainage. *World J. Surg.* 6:86, 1982.
8. Andros, G., Donaldson, G. A., Hedberg, S. E., et al., Anastomotic ulcer. *Ann. Surg.* 165:955, 1967.
9. Bancroft, F. W. Modification of Devine operation of pyloric exclusion for duodenal ulcer. *Am. J. Surg.* 16:223, 1932.
10. Baronofsky, I., Lannin, B. G., Lanchez-Palomera, E., and Wangensteen, O. H. Billroth I gastric resection: Extent necessary to protect against histamine-provoked ulcer. *Proc. Soc. Exp. Biol. Med.* 59:229, 1945.
11. Bauer, H., Bruckner, W., Welsche, K. H., and Holle, F. Die night-resezierende Chirurgie des Gastro-Duodenal Ulkus. III. Klinische Resultate. *Munch. Med. Wochenschr.* 118:785, 1976.
12. Beahrs, O. H. Surgical management of peptic ulceration recurring postoperatively. *Surg. Clin. North Am.* 51:879, 1971.
13. Beal, J. M. The surgical treatment of marginal ulcer. *Am. Surg.* 25:1, 1959.
14. Becker, H. D., and Caspary, W. F. Recurrent Peptic Ulceration. In H. D. Becker and W. F. Caspary (Eds.), *Postgastrectomy and Post-Vagotomy Syndromes*. Berlin: Springer, 1980.
15. Berstad, A., Aadland, E., and Bjerke, K. Cimetidine treatment of recurrent ulcer after proximal gastric vagotomy. *Scand. J. Gastroenterol.* 16:891, 1981.
16. Blegvad, B. ABO blood groups and stomal ulcer. *Dan. Med. Bull.* 7:72, 1960.
17. Blegvad, B. ABO blood groups and gastric acidity. *Dan. Med. Bull.* 7:73, 1960.
18. Boles, R. S., Jr., Marshall, S. F., and Bersoux, R. V. Follow-up study of 127 patients with stomal ulcer. *Gastroenterology* 38:763, 1960.
19. Brollon, A., Velisig, M., DiBonito, L., and Bianchi, C. High relative risk of gastric stump cancer in young gastric resection patients. *Minerva Med.* 79:1921, 1981.
20. Burge, H. Discussion on the surgical management of chronic duodenal ulcer. *Proc. R. Soc. Med.* 52:839, 1959.
21. Chaudhuri, T. K., Chaudhuri, T. K., Shirazi, S. S., and Condon, R. E. Radioisotopic scan: A possible aid in differentiating retained gastric antrum from Zollinger-Ellison syndrome in patients with recurrent peptic ucer. *Gastroenterology* 65:697, 1973.
22. Cleator, I. G. M., Holubitsky, I. B., and Harrison, R. C. Anastomotic ulceration. *Ann. Surg.* 179:339, 1974.
23. Cody, J. H., DiVincenti, F. C., Cowick, D. R., and Mahanes, J. R. Gastrocolic and gastrojejunocolic fistulae: Report of twelve cases and review of the literature. *Ann. Surg.* 181:376, 1975.
24. Cohen, M. M. Practical management of recurrent peptic ulcer. *Can. J. Surg.* 21:21, 1978.
25. Devine, H. B. Basic principles and supreme difficulties in gastric surgery. *Surg. Gynecol. Obstet.* 40:1, 1925.
26. Doll, R., Swynnerton, B. F., and Newell,

A. C. Observations on blood group distribution in peptic ulcer and gastric cancer. *Gut* 1:31, 1960.
27. Domellof, L., Eriksson, S., and Janunger, K. G. Carcinoma and possible precancerous changes of the gastric stump after Billroth II resection. *Gastroenterology* 73:462, 1977.
28. Donahue, P. E., Bombeck, C. T., Condon, R. E., and Nyhus, L. M. Proximal gastric vagotomy versus selective vagotomy with antrectomy: Results of a prospective randomized clinical trial after 4 to 12 years. *Surgery* 96:585, 1984.
29. Donahue, P. E., and Nyhus, L. M. Surgeon-endoscopists and the assessment of postoperative patients. *South. Med. J.* 75:1570, 1982.
30. Everson, T. C., and Allen, M. J. Gastrojejunal ulceration. *A.M.A. Arch. Surg.* 69:140, 1954.
31. Festen, H. P. M., Lamers, C. B. H., Driessen, W. M. M., and Van Tongern, J. H. M. Cimetidine in anastomotic ulceration after partial gastrectomy. *Gastroenterology* 76:83, 1979.
32. Fischer, A. B. Twenty-five years after Billroth II gastrectomy for duodenal ulcer. *World J. Surg.* 8:293, 1984.
33. Foster, J. H., and Carlson, R. I. Gastrojejunal ulcer presenting as a mass in the abdominal wall. *Surgery* 44:1034, 1958.
34. Fromm, D. Recurrent Peptic Ulcer. In *Complications of Gastric Surgery.* New York: Wiley, 1977.
35. Grassi, G., Orecchia, C., Grassi, G. B., Jr., and Defidio, L. The importance of determining the distal limit of vagal resection in proximal selective vagotomy. *Int. Surg.* 65:291, 1980.
36. Green, W. E. R., Kennedy, T., Hassard, T., and Spencer, E. F. A. Management of recurrent peptic ulceration. *Br. J. Surg.* 65:422, 1978.
37. Griffith, C. A., Leyse, R. M., Davis, D. R., and Magoon, C. C. Mortality and recurrent ulcer after selective vagotomy plus pyloroplasty. *Am. Surg.* 38:504, 1972.
38. Harkins, H. N. Discussion of Hutchinson, W. B., and Kiriluk, L. B. Billroth I gastric resection for chronic duodenal ulcer. *Am. J. Surg.* 100:253, 1960.
39. Harkins, H. N., and Nyhus, L. M. A comparison of the Billroth I and Billroth II procedures: Clinical and experimental studies. *Bull. Soc. Int. Chir.* 15:111, 1956.
40. Holst-Christensen, J., Hansen, O. H., Pedersen, T., and Kronborg, O. Recurrent ulcer after proximal gastric vagotomy for duodenal and pre-pyloric ulcer. *Br. J. Surg.* 64:42, 1977.
41. Hood, J. M., Spencer, E. F. A., Macrae, K. D., and Kennedy, T. Value of perioperative acid tests in predicting recurrent ulceration after vagotomy. *Br. J. Surg.* 62:8, 1975.
42. Ivy, A. C., Grossman, M. I., and Bachrach, W. A. *Peptic Ulcer.* Philadelphia: Blakiston, 1950.
43. Jew, P. W., Jr., Lavowitz, B. S., and Fisher, B. Alteration of the effects of jejunocolic fistula: An experimental study. *Ann. Surg.* 155:175, 1962.
44. Johnston, D. Surgical Options and Duodenal Ulcer. In K. H. Holtermuller and J. R. Malagelada (Eds.), *Advances in Ulcer Disease.* Amsterdam: Excerpta Medica, 1980.
45. Jones, T. W., DeVito, R. V., Nyhus, L. M., and Harkins, H. N. A prime physiologic mechanism for the failure of gastrojejunostomy in the treatment of peptic ulcer disease. *Surgery* 43:781, 1958.
46. Judd, E. S., and Hoerner, M. T. Jejunal ulcer. *Ann. Surg.* 102:1003, 1935.
47. Juler, G. L., Dagradi, A. E., Stempien, S. J., and Combs, R. C. Evaluation of recurrent duodenal ulcer after vagotomy-pyloroplasty. *Am. J. Surg.* 132:243, 1976.
48. Keighley, M. R. B., Hoare, A. M., Horrocks, J. C., et al. A symptomatic discriminant to identify recurrent ulcer in patients with dyspepsia after gastric surgery. *Lancet* 2:278, 1976.
49. Kennedy, T., and Spencer, A. Cimetidine for recurrent ulcer after vagotomy or gastrectomy: A randomized controlled trial. *Br. Med. J.* 1:1242, 1978.
50. Kiriluk, L. B., and Merendino, K. A. An experimental study of the buffering capacity of the contents of the upper small bowel. *Surgery* 35:532, 1954.
51. Kiriluk, L. B., and Merendino, K. A. The comparative sensitivity of the mucosa of the various segments of the alimentary tract in the dog to acid-peptic action. *Surgery* 35:547, 1954.
52. Kjaergaard, J., Jensen, H., and Allermand, H. Inadequately reduced acid secretion after vagotomy for duodenal ulcer. *Ann. Surg.* 192:711, 1980.
53. Koo, J., Lam, S. K., and Ong, G. B. Cimetidine versus surgery for recurrent ulcer after

gastric surgery. *Ann. Surg.* 195:406, 1982.
54. Kronborg, O. The value of the insulin test in predicting recurrence after vagotomy and drainage for duodenal ulcer. *Scand. J. Gastroenterol.* 6:471, 1971.
55. Kusakari, K., Nyhus, L. M., Gillison, E. W., and Bombeck, C. T. An endoscopic test for completeness of vagotomy. *Arch. Surg.* 105:386, 1972.
56. Lahey, F. H. Experiences with postoperative jejunal ulcer and gastrojejunocolic fistula. *Am. J. Dig. Dis.* 2:673, 1936.
57. Lannin, B. G., Hay, L. J., Judd, E. S., and Wangensteen, O. H. Evaluation of a satisfactory operation for ulcer. *Proc. Soc. Exp. Biol. Med.* 56:231, 1944.
58. Lehr, L., and Pichlmayr, R. Low risk thoracic vagotomy for anastomotic ulceration. *World J. Surg.* 6:93, 1982.
59. Lewisohn, R. The frequency of gastrojejunal ulcer. *Surg. Gynecol. Obstet.* 40:70, 1925.
60. Lewisohn, R. Frequency of gastrojejunal ulcer following simple gastroenterostomy for duodenal ulcers. *J.A.M.A.* 154:1301, 1954.
61. Lindenauer, S. M., and Dent, T. L. Management of the recurrent ulcer. *Arch. Surg.* 110:531, 1975.
62. Localio, S. A., Stone, P., and Hinton, J. W. Gastrojejunocolic fistula. *Surg. Gynecol. Obstet.* 96:455, 1953.
63. Lowdon, A. G. R. Gastrojejunal ulceration. *Edinb. Med. J.* 55:533, 1948.
64. Lowdon, A. G. R. Gastrojejunocolic fistula. *Br. J. Surg.* 41:113, 1953.
65. Lygidakis, N. J. Gastric stump carcinoma after surgery for gastroduodenal ulcer. *Ann. R. Coll. Surg. Engl.* 63:203, 1981.
66. MacLeod, R. G., and Galloway, J. P. A trial of ileosigmoidostomy in the treatment of gastrojejunocolic fistula. *Surg. Gynecol. Obstet.* 105:545, 1957.
67. Maddock, W. G. Current concepts of the treatment of gastrojejunal ulcer. *Proc. Inst. Med. Chic.* 21:111, 1956.
68. Marshall, S. F., and Knud-Hansen, J. Gastrojejunocolic and gastrocolic fistulas. *Ann. Surg.* 145:770, 1957.
69. Marshall, S. F., and Reinstine, H. W., Jr. The role of the pyloric antrum in the production of gastrojejunal ulcer following gastrectomy. *Surg. Clin. North Am.* 35:711, 1955.
70. Merendino, K. A., Lannin, B. G., Kolouch, F., Jr., et al. Length of afferent duodenojejunal loop in gastric resection, a factor in stomal ulcer. *Proc. Soc. Exp. Biol. Med.* 58:226, 1945.
71. Neustein, C. L., Bushkin, F. L., Weinshelbaum, E. I., and Woodward, E. R. Reoperation for postsurgical peptic ulcer recurrence. *Ann. Surg.* 185:169, 1977.
72. Nyhus, L. M. Uropepsin excretion: Its relation to duodenal ulcer disease in diagnosis and therapy. *Surgery* 41:406, 1957.
73. Nyhus, L. M. The role of the antrum in the surgical treatment of peptic ulcer. *Gastroenterology* 38:21, 1960.
74. Nyhus, L. M. Proximal gastric vagotomy: Gold or dross? *Arch. Surg.* 118:1373, 1983.
75. Nyhus, L. M., Chapman, N. D., DeVito, R. V., and Harkins, H. N. Experimental studies of gastric secretion following antrum exclusion and vagotomy. *Bull. Soc. Int. Chir.* 20:23, 1961.
76. Olch, P. D., and Harkins, H. N. Quantitative assessment of extent of gastric resection: Comparison of pattern-planimeter and pattern-weight methods. *Surgery* 48:437, 1960.
77. Palmer, W. L. The "acid test" in gastric and duodenal ulcer. *J.A.M.A.* 88:1778, 1927.
78. Peebles Brown, D. A., Melrose, A. G., and Wallace, J. The blood groups in peptic ulceration. *Br. Med. J.* 2:135, 1956.
79. Pfeiffer, D. B. The surgical treatment of gastrojejunocolic fistula. *Surg. Gynecol. Obstet.* 72:282, 1941.
80. Pfeiffer, D. B., and Kent, E. M. The value of preliminary colostomy in the correction of gastrojejunocolic fistula. *Ann. Surg.* 110:659, 1939.
81. Pikkarainen, P., Vuoristo, M., and Tarpila, S. Ulcer healing and serum pepsinogen I in cimetidine and glycopyrrolate treated duodenal ulcer patients. *Ann. Clin. Res.* 13:81, 1981.
82. Piper, D. W., McIntosh, J. H., Grieg, M., and Shy, C. M. Environmental factors and chronic gastric ulcer. *Scand. J. Gastroenterol.* 17:721, 1982.
83. Plenk, A. Zur Technik der Resection zur Ausschaltung. *Zentralbl. Chir.* 63:3019, 1936.
84. Poppen, B., and Delin, A. Parietal cell vagotomy for duodenal and pyloric ulcers. *Am. J. Surg.* 141:323, 1981.
85. Postlethwait, R. W. Marginal Ulcer. In R. W. Postlethwait (Ed.), *Results of Surgery for Peptic Ulcer.* Philadelphia: Saunders, 1963.
86. Romeo, G., Giovinetto, A., Sanfilippo, G., et al. Follow-up study in 402 patients after pari-

etal cell vagotomy for duodenal ulcer. *Int. Surg.* 66:303, 1981.
87. Rotter, J. I., Wong, F. L., Samloff, I. M., et al. Evidence for a major dominance component in the variation of serum pepsinogen I levels. *Am. J. Hum. Genet.* 34:395, 1982.
88. Saik, R. P., Greenburg, A. G., and Peskin, G. W. The Congo red test to determine completeness of vagotomy. *Am. J. Surg.* 144:518, 1982.
89. Samloff, I. M., Secrist, D. M., and Passaro, E., Jr. Serum group I pepsinogen levels and their relation to gastric acid secretion in patients with and without recurrent ulcer. *Gastroenterology* 70:309, 1976.
90. Schafer, L. W., Larson, D. E., Melton, L. J., III, et al. The risk of gastric carcinoma after treatment for benign ulcer disease. *N. Engl. J. Med.* 309:1210, 1983.
91. Scott, H. W., Jr., Herrington, J. L., Jr., Edwards, W. H., and Shull, H. J. The hazards of antral exclusion with vagotomy in the surgical treatment of duodenal ulcer. *Ann. Surg.* 151:181, 1960.
92. Selking, O., Krause, U., Nilsson, F., and Thoren, L. Parietal cell vagotomy and truncal vagotomy as treatment of duodenal ulcer. *Acta Chir. Scand.* 147:561, 1981.
93. Small, W. P. The recurrence of ulceration after surgery for duodenal ulcer. *J. R. Coll. Surg. Edinb.* 9:255, 1964.
94. Small, W. P., Smith, A. N., Ruckley, C. V., et al. The continuing problem of jejunal ulcer. *Am. J. Surg.* 121:541, 1971.
95. Smith, L., and Strang, V. M. Marginal ulcer: An analysis of twenty cases and a case presentation in which adenocarcinoma occurred at a gastroenterostomy site. *Surgery* 39:441, 1956.
96. Stabile, B. E., and Passaro, E., Jr. Recurrent peptic ulcer. *Gastroenterology* 70:124, 1976.
97. Sugawara, S., Nakamura, M., Sawai, Y., Yamazaki, T., and Ouchi, A. A case report of retained antrum syndrome diagnosed by ^{99m}Tc-pertechnetate scintigraphy. *Rinsho Hoshasen* 25:943, 1980.
98. Tanner, N. C. Discussion of the surgical management of chronic duodenal ulcer. *Proc. R. Soc. Med.* 52:840, 1959.
99. Thompson, J. E. Stomal ulceration after gastric surgery. *Ann. Surg.* 143:697, 1956.
100. Thoroughman, J. C., Walker, L. G., Jr., Taylor B. G., and Dunn, T. Free perforation of anastomotic ulcers. *Ann. Surg.* 169:790, 1969.
101. Trout, H. H. Ulcer recurrence, morbidity, and mortality after operations for duodenal ulcer. *Am. J. Surg.* 144:570, 1982.
102. Von Eiselsberg, A. Zur Behandlung des Ulcus ventriculi et duodeni. *Arch. Klin. Chir.* 114:539, 1920.
103. Walters, W., and Chance, D. P. Vagotomy as a prophylactic and curative procedure in peptic ulcer. *J.A.M.A.* 153:993, 1953.
104. Walters, W., Chance, D. P., and Berkson, J. A comparison of vagotomy and gastric resection for gastrojejunal ulceration: A follow-up study of 301 cases. *Surg. Gynecol. Obstet.* 100:1, 1955.
105. Walters, W., and Clagett, O. T. Gastrojejunocolic ulcer and fistula. *Am. J. Surg.* 46:94, 1939.
106. Wangensteen, O. H. Segmental gastric resection: An acceptable operation for peptic ulcer; tubular resection unacceptable. *Surgery* 41:686, 1957.
107. Warshaw, A. L. Intragastric alkali infusion: A simple, accurate provocative test for diagnosis of symptomatic alkaline reflux gastritis. *Ann. Surg.* 194:297, 1981.
108. Webster, M. W., Barnes, E. L., and Stremple, J. F. Serum gastrin levels in the differential diagnosis of recurrent peptic ulceration due to retained gastric antrum. *Am. J. Surg.* 135:248, 1978.
109. White, T. T., and Harrison, R. C. Late complications of gastric surgery: Diagnosis and treatment. *Surg. Annu.* 8:197, 1976.
110. Wilkie, D. P. D. Jejunal ulcer: Some observations on its complications and their treatment. *Ann. Surg.* 99:401, 1934.
111. Wilmanns, R. Resectio praepylorica bei Ulcus duodeni. *Zentralbl. Chir.* 53:1874, 1926.
112. Wittebol, P., Akkermans, L. M. A., and Hulstaert, P. F. Prognostic factors in surgery for duodenal ulcer. *Surg. Annu.* 17:235, 1985.
113. Woolsey, G. The question of gastroenterostomy in duodenal ulcer. *Surg. Gynecol. Obstet.* 42:90, 1926.
114. Wright, G. Collective inquiry by fellows of Association of Surgeons into gastrojejunal ulceration. *Br. J. Surg.* 22:433, 1935.
115. Wychulis, A. R., Priestly, J. T., and Foulk, W. T. A study of 360 patients with gastrojejunal ulceration. *Surg. Gynecol. Obstet.* 122:89, 1966.
116. Zollinger, R. M., Ellison, E. C., O'Dorsio,

T. M., and Sparks, J. Thirty years' experience with gastrinoma. *World J. Surg.* 8:427, 1984.

EDITOR'S COMMENT

Many physicians believe that the question of recurrent ulceration after operations for duodenal ulcer has been somewhat overemphasized. The problem of deciding between supereffective ulcer-curing operations such as vagotomy and antrectomy and other, less effective procedures, such as proximal gastric vagotomy has often been solved in favor of the "safety" of the ulcer-curing operation, come what may. Two occurrences have influenced this decision: The first is the development of H_2-receptor blockers and the second is the apparent increase in the recurrence rate following proximal gastric vagotomy. To emphasize this point, I cite a paper by Hoffman and his colleagues from Copenhagen, who reported a recurrence rate after proximal gastric vagotomy of just over 30 percent in 79 patients.

With the use of H_2-receptor blockers, a recurrent duodenal ulcer diathesis can be controlled and therefore does not represent the surgical disaster previously encountered. The rise in the reported recurrence rate after proximal gastric vagotomy is not accepted as inevitable by all, for example, Johnston [2]. In my series of patients treated either by proximal gastric vagotomy or by selective vagotomy and antrectomy, depending on the preoperative peak and output, the recurrence rate appears to be low. It would seem important to me to limit as far as possible the number of patients who have such complications as dumping, bilious vomiting, and diarrhea, which so often defy all methods of treatment and control; limiting complications remains, therefore, a powerful argument in favor of proximal gastric vagotomy.

Apart from the question of etiology, we should perhaps address ourselves to two further problems. The first is one of definition. It is too simple to look down an endoscope, see a breach in the mucosa, and thereafter forever label a patient as having a recurrent duodenal ulcer. For one thing, there is a well-known tendency for endoscopists to overdiagnose gastroduodenal mucosal ulceration, and for another, the patient who carries the label of duodenal ulceration in the absence of any other symptoms, signs, or pathological evidence is familiar to all of us. Unfortunately, histological study cannot help, although some estimate of the depth of an ulcer is fundamental to the question of definition. Deeper ulcers tend to be more persistent. The second problem is the now widely recognized fact that many patients do not suffer symptoms in spite of the presence of an ulcer in the duodenum. Mühe and associates are correct when they quote two recurrence rates, the first in patients with symptoms, and the second (lower) in patients who have no symptoms and whose recurrent ulcer is diagnosed by routine endoscopy. Perhaps a duodenal ulcer or recurrent duodenal ulcer of importance should be defined as an ulcer in the mucosa at least as deep as the muscularis that is present on two separate occasions separated by at least two weeks. The point of the time separation is that if the ulcer is superficial, of lesser importance, and mucosal only, it is likely to heal before the second endoscopy.

The debate will continue as reports from more and more centers in the United States, Europe, Scandinavia, and other parts of the world come in. There will be no final answer because of change in the disease itself, the continued development of new techniques [4], and the time it takes for a controlled clinical trial to be set up and allowed to mature. One thing is certain, however: A patient presenting in 1986 with a duodenal ulcer has a very much better chance of a satisfactory outcome as a result of treatment than ever before.

C.W.

Comment References

1. Hoffman, J., Jensen, H. E., Schulz, E. S., Poulsen, P. E., and Christiansen, J. Prospective con-

trolled vagotomy trial for duodenal ulcer: Results after five years. *Br. J. Surg.* 71:582, 1984.
2. Johnston, D. Personal communication, 1984.
3. Mühe, E., Muller, C., Martinoli, S., Schacht, U., Fielder, L., Engelke, B., Zumtobel, V., and Marrie, A. Five Year Results of a Prospective Multi-Centre Trial on Proximal Gastric Vagotomy. In J. H. Baron, et al. (Eds.), *Vagotomy in Modern Surgical Practice*. London: Butterworth, Pp. 176–86.
4. Oostvogel, H. J., and van Vroonhoven, J. M. V. Anterior seromyotomy and posterior truncal vagotomy: Technique and early results of a randomized trial. *Netherlands J. Surg.* 37:69, 1985.

20

Remedial Operations

John Lynwood Herrington, Jr.
John L. Sawyers

Operations used currently to control the complications of gastroduodenal ulcer disease provide satisfactory long-term results in approximately 75–80 percent of patients. In the remaining 20–25 percent, undesirable side effects take place resulting largely from ablation of gastric tissue and from removal, bypass, or alteration of the pyloric sphincter mechanism, which plays a vital role in regulating gastric emptying. In addition, both truncal and selective gastric vagotomy, important components of many operations currently done for duodenal ulcer, may at times produce physiological aberrations resulting in unpleasant long-term symptoms. Fortunately, these sequelae are usually mild to moderate in degree, and many disappear with time. The relatively new operation of proximal gastric vagotomy alters gastric emptying but little and is associated with an almost negligible rate of long-term ill effects.

During the past two decades widespread use of fiberoptic endoscopy and increased knowledge and application of gastric physiology have provided both surgeon and gastroenterologist with a better understanding of the various postgastrectomy problems. The postgastrectomy syndrome may be broken down into disorders of a *pathophysiological* nature, most of which may be managed satisfactorily with nonmedical measures, and *mechanical* disorders, which may at times require reoperation for correction (Table 20-1).

In diagnosis of the various postgastrectomy disorders a carefully taken history is of utmost importance in delineating the particular problem that the patient is experiencing. It is not unusual for a patient to present with more than one postgastrectomy disorder. For example, a patient may suffer from alkaline reflux gastritis in combination with dumping, or may experience severe dumping and postvagotomy diarrhea. The particular syndrome or set of disorders must be accurately defined when contemplating a remedial operation.

Pathophysiological Disorders

ALKALINE REFLUX GASTRITIS

Bilious vomiting was recognized shortly after the introduction of gastroenterostomy in 1881,

Table 20-1. Postgastrectomy syndrome

PATHOPHYSIOLOGICAL DISORDERS
Alkaline gastritis
Reflux esophagitis
Reflux gastritis and delayed gastric emptying
Early dumping
Late dumping
Postvagotomy diarrhea
Dumping and postvagotomy diarrhea
Dumping and reflux gastritis
Postvagotomy diarrhea and reflux gastritis
Dumping, reflux, diarrhea
Malabsorption
Bezoar formation
Motility and emptying problems—gastric remnant carcinoma
Small gastric pouch syndrome
MECHANICAL DISORDERS
Acute afferent loop obstruction
Chronic afferent loop obstruction
Acute efferent loop obstruction
Chronic efferent loop obstruction
Internal herniation
Late gastroduodenal obstruction

and a few years later was observed as a complication of gastric resection with a Billroth II reconstruction. In the decades that followed, surgeons devised various methods of gastrointestinal reconstruction with gastric resection in an attempt to correct the problem because bilious vomiting was associated with appreciable morbidity and mortality. It was the erroneous belief during this period that bile vomiting after gastroenterostomy alone was caused by the passage of gastric chyme into the afferent jejunal limb and back into the stomach through a patent pylorus (circulus vitiosus). Bile regurgitation after a Billroth II reconstruction was believed to result from gastric chyme entering the afferent loop: When the loop became filled to the closed duodenal stump, an increase in loop pressure took place and bile regurgitation occurred. This disturbing complication continued in spite of repeated attempts by surgeons to modify the technical aspects of gastroenterostomy and gastric resection [100]. The complication was also observed after gastric resection with gastroduodenostomy, but the Billroth I technique lost favor throughout Europe rather early after its inception because of the frequent complication of anastomotic leakage at "the angle of sorrow." The procedure was rarely used in the United States until the late 1940s, when it was repopularized by Henry Harkins et al. [30]. Later Harkins added vagotomy and used a more conservative distal resection with gastroduodenostomy.

In 1958 Lees and Grandjean [64] were among the first to suggest that abdominal pain and bile vomiting after gastric resection might result from an inflammatory insult to the gastric mucosa produced by regurgitant afferent loop contents. A few years later Toye and Williams [106] studied endoscopically a patient who presented with constant epigastric pain and bile vomiting following gastric resection with a Billroth II reconstruction for ulcer disease. The gastric mucosa appeared bile stained, and an area of erythema, friability, and inflammation was noted. At subsequent cholecystectomy a balloon catheter was placed in the patient's afferent jejunal limb, and long-term studies showed that withdrawal and reinstallation of afferent loop content into the stomach remnant produced pain and gastric inflammatory changes. Withdrawal of the afferent loop content through the catheter resulted in subsidence of pain and resolution of gastric inflammatory changes.

It is well known that many patients who do not have symptoms after gastric operations have bile and duodenal content in the gastric remnant with or without the presence of gastric mucosal inflammatory changes. Indeed in a small percentage of healthy patients who have never undergone a gastric operation, bile may be observed in the stomach. There is no correlation between the degree and extent of gastric mucosal inflammatory changes and the patient's symptoms. Only a small percentage of patients have symptoms as a result of alkaline reflux, and there is no clear explanation at present of why this small percentage of patients is susceptible to mucosal injury.

Alkaline reflux gastritis is likely to occur more often after a Billroth II reconstruction than after a Billroth I repair, but it may be observed after a Billroth I and even after pyloroplasty and simple gastroenterostomy. In patients with symptoms, burning epigastric pain is a constant finding and is quite different from the discomfort of the original ulcer disease. Bile vomiting is a constant feature, and weight loss may occur in up to 50 percent of patients. The intake of food usually accentuates the discomfort, and caloric intake may be restricted. Anemia is not uncommon, and overt gastrointestinal bleeding may occur in a small percentage of patients.

The diagnosis is made by a carefully taken history and a complete gastrointestinal survey. Endoscopy is of vital importance in combination with multiple biopsy specimens taken along the extent of the gastric mucosa. Endoscopy alone is insufficient because the gross presence of gastric mucosal edema, erythema, and friability does not necessarily correlate with the findings of microscopic gastric mucosal inflammatory changes. Gastric analysis usually shows either hypoacidity or achlorhydria. Diffuse inflammatory changes along the extent of the gastric remnant are usually necessary to substantiate the diagnosis of reflux gastritis, not changes limited to the peristomal area alone. Histological studies throughout the gastric mucosa may vary, showing the presence of acute and chronic inflammatory infiltrates, hemorrhage, loss of height of the mucosal column, diminution of parietal cell mass, and increase in mucin cells and frank mucosal ulcerations.

The medical treatment of reflux gastritis consists of diet and therapy with antispasmodics, antacids, and cholestyramine. Cholestyramine, however, has not been proved effective. Metoclopramide also has not resulted in substantial improvement of symptoms, and anticholinergic drugs are contraindicated. Total parenteral nutrition has been of benefit in preparing the malnourished patient for a remedial operation. If symptoms are sustained and not relieved by medical therapy, a remedial operation should be given serious consideration.

For the very small percentage of patients who require surgical intervention, the only operation that has proved effective is a Roux-en-Y procedure, which diverts the total duodenal content away from the gastric remnant. It is important to divert the alkaline content at least 45–60 cm below the gastroenterostomy site. Most patients who demonstrate severe reflux have originally undergone gastric resection with either a Billroth II or a Billroth I reconstruction along with vagotomy. At the time of reoperation it is important to be sure that the original vagotomy was complete and that at least 40–50 percent of the distal stomach was removed. If the first operation was vagotomy and pyloroplasty, the gastric antrum must be excised: Both the neural and hormonal phases of gastric secretion must be eliminated because the Roux-en-Y in itself is ulcerogenic (Fig. 20-1).

While significant gastric mucosal inflammatory changes may be present in patients without symptoms, and minimal inflammatory changes may exist in patients with appreciable subjective symptoms, it is difficult at times to accept the diagnosis of reflux and even more frustrating to decide which patient is in need of surgical correction. Unfortunately, the outcome of surgical treatment cannot be predicted from current preoperative evaluations, most of which are in large part subjective. In spite of this confusion, however, many surgeons have noted that Roux-en-Y diversion has resulted in improvement in from 60 to 80 percent of patients (Table 20-2). Seventy-five of our 88 patients were available for long-range follow-up studies. Forty-one had excellent clinical results and 19 had good results [39, 91]. These figures are in accord with those reported in the literature [8, 15, 23, 33, 54, 58, 67, 81, 86, 103, 105].

In an attempt to define the patient selection procedure and to improve the postoperative success rate, several authors have stressed the importance of preoperative objective data as guidelines (Table 20-3). According to Hoare et al. [41] measurement of bile acids in the fasting gastric aspirate is useful in predicting the outcome of surgical treatment. Provocative testing with autologous duodenal content and

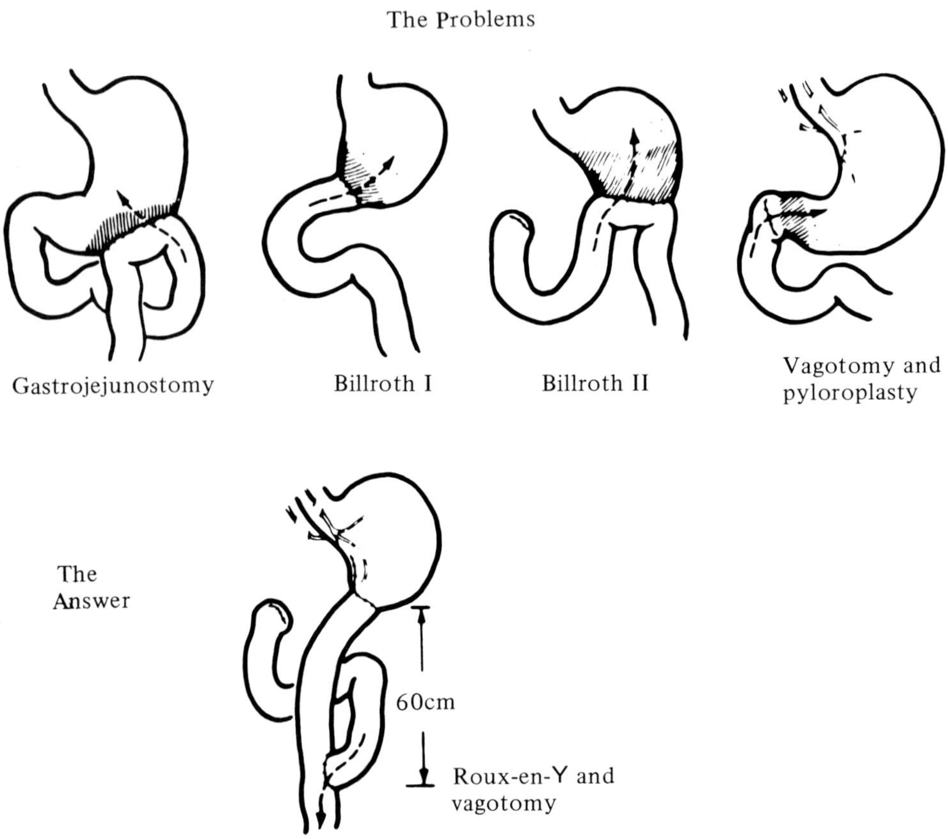

Fig. 20-1. Severe reflux gastritis following gastrojejunostomy alone or following vagotomy and pyloroplasty is treated by removal of the gastric antrum and conversion to a Roux-en-Y anastomosis. Reflux gastritis following gastric resection with either a Billroth I or a Billroth II type of reconstruction is treated by simple Roux-en-Y diversion. (Vagotomy is mandatory to prevent recurrent ulceration when Roux-en-Y diversion is used.)

intragastric alkali infusion have been used in patient selection [2, 108]. Quantitative assessment of reflux and further breakdown of bile acid products are being studied as possible culprits [26, 42, 73, 87, 94]. These new methods may define the precise constituents of the duodenal content responsible for gastric mucosal injury, along with the biological and chemical mechanisms by which these constituents produce that injury.

REFLUX GASTRITIS AND ESOPHAGITIS

A small percentage of patients, less than 5 percent of those with severe reflux gastritis, may also on endoscopy and biopsy demonstrate varying degrees of esophagitis. Such patients may present with an associated sliding esophageal hiatal hernia or demonstrate a low distal esophageal sphincter pressure measurement. A Roux-en-Y diversion will eliminate both the gastric and esophageal mucosal changes, but the patient may continue to have symptoms from regurgitation of gastric chyme into the incompetent distal esophagus. Such patients are treated with the addition of an antireflux operation, usually Nissen fundoplication.

REFLUX GASTRITIS AND DELAYED GASTRIC EMPTYING

Davidson and Hersh [16, 17] reported only 47 percent satisfactory results among 59 patients

Table 20-2. Long-term results of Roux-en-Y diversion for alkaline reflux gastritis

Author	Country and Year	No. of patients	Results	
DeMol	(Belgium, 1977)	20	Excellent 80%	
Way	(U.S.A., 1980)	46	Good 65%	
Van Heerden	(U.S.A., 1981)	92	Good 75%	
Moseman	(Switzerland, 1981)	16	Satisfactory 94%	
Hellen	(Sweden, 1981)	11	Excellent 90%	
Kennedy	(Ireland, 1981)	27	Excellent 85%	
Fiore	(U.S.A., 1982)	23	Good 90%	
Tasse	(Canada, 1982)	23	Excellent 90%	
Lygidakis	(Greece, 1982)	28	Excellent 100%	
Vogel	(U.S.A., 1983)	97	Excellent 29% Good 30% Fair 18%	77%

Table 20-3. Objective preoperative assessment of alkaline reflux gastritis

1. Intragastric 0.1 N NaOH infusion
2. Autologous upper intestinal content infusion
3. Intragastric bile acid concentration
4. Net bile acid reflux per unit of time
5. Assessment of reflux volume (HIDA)
6. Gastric emptying—isotope labeling
7. Lysolecithin content of bile acids
8. Pancreatic phospholipase A-2 measurement
9. Intragastric pH and bacterial content
10. Intragastric deoxycholic acid content
11. Intragastric bilirubin and sodium concentrations

undergoing Roux-en-Y diversion for reflux gastritis. Thirty-seven percent of the 59 patients underwent preoperative gastric emptying studies, and 60 percent of this group demonstrated delayed emptying. Those with poor emptying as a rule had unsatisfactory results after Roux-en-Y diversion. Hocking et al. [43] in a sophisticated animal study showed that the Roux-en-Y diversion in itself produced delayed gastric emptying, but with vagotomy and a high subtotal gastrectomy (Roux-en-Y) gastric emptying was less impaired compared to vagotomy plus antrectomy (Roux-en-Y).

On preoperative evaluation of patients with reflux after vagotomy and antrectomy, Billroth II or Billroth I, we have likewise demonstrated delayed gastric emptying in a small percentage of patients using barium food meal and isotope-labeled studies. If such patients are treated for reflux by Roux-en-Y diversion alone, severe and symptomatic gastric emptying may persist postoperatively. Such patients are now being treated by a more extensive gastric resection (80–90 percent) in combination with Roux-en-Y diversion. The explanation for the gastric emptying is not clear. The vagotomy effect may be a factor along with preexisting gastric motility disturbances. Currently on our service all patients with severe alkaline reflux gastritis who are considered possible candidates for a remedial operation undergo gastric emptying studies (Fig. 20-2). Additional investigations in this field are currently being carried out by Vogel and associates [107].

EARLY DUMPING

The common denominator in instances of the dumping syndrome is ablation or bypass of the pyloric sphincter mechanism permitting the rapid passage of food and fluids into the duodenum or proximal jejunum and resulting in physiological disturbances of both a vasomotor and gastrointestinal nature. Complex neu-

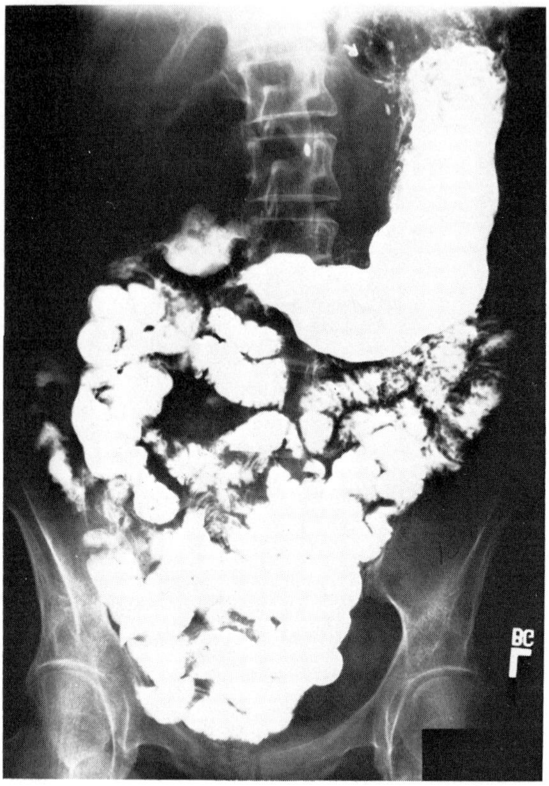

Fig. 20-2. Preoperative barium meal study in a patient who had previously undergone truncal vagotomy and pyloroplasty for duodenal ulcer disease. The patient now has marked reflux gastritis with inflammatory changes occupying the entire stomach. In addition, the barium meal shows a marked delay in gastric emptying. This patient should be treated with an extensive (80–90%) subtotal gastric resection along with Roux-en-Y diversion. Antrectomy with Roux-en-Y diversion would correct the alkaline reflux gastritis, but a 40–50% distal resection would not correct the gastric emptying problem.

rohormonal mechanisms also play a role in the pathophysiology of this disorder. Although dumping was recognized around the turn of the century, Charles L. Mix [78] in 1922, an internist at the Mercy Hospital in Chicago, was responsible for coining the term *dumping stomach*.

Dumping occurs to some extent after all gastric operations and is least encountered after proximal gastric vagotomy. The syndrome is probably more common after a Billroth II–type reconstruction. Symptoms consist of sweating, weakness, palpitations, nausea, vomiting, borborygmus, and diarrhea and occur in from 1 to 50 percent of postoperative patients. Fortunately, in most instances symptoms are mild to moderate and may disappear with time. Control of this unpleasant complication can usually be obtained with a low carbohydrate diet, frequent small feedings, and elimination of fluid intake with meals. Patients may assume a recumbent position for 30 minutes after meals, and this may at times provide relief by slowing the osmotic load presented to the proximal small intestine. For more persistent instances, drug therapy consisting of anticholinergic agents may at times provide a delay in intestinal transit, and adrenergic agents may reduce vasomotor symptoms. Serotonin antagonists have also been used, but in general drug therapy has not resulted in universal improvement. Symptoms may be severe and refractory to medical management in 1 percent of patients or less. Such patients may lose a considerable amount of weight, become malnourished, and have anemia. Under these circumstances a remedial operation should be given serious consideration. The objective of a corrective operation is to restore in part or whole the reservoir function of the gastric remnant and thus delay the rapid passage of food into the proximal small intestine.

Surgical Treatment

The early operative procedures designed to correct the dumping syndrome consisted of diminishing the size of the gastroenterostomy stoma, converting a Billroth II reconstruction to a Billroth I repair, and replacing a Pólya reconstruction by a Hofmeister anastomosis. Reconstruction of the pylorus after pyloroplasty has also been used. Each of these procedures has been directed toward an attempt to provide a delay in gastric emptying. Unfortunately, none of these methods has pro-

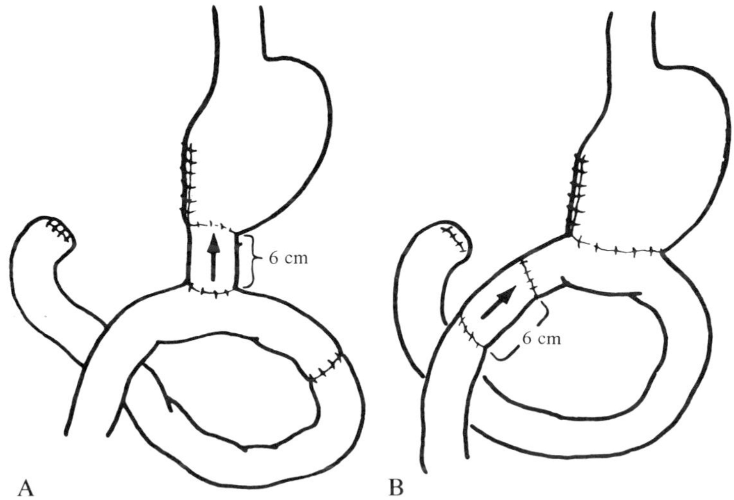

Fig. 20-9. A single reversed jejunal segment as described by Jordan (A) and the single reversal advocated by Christeas (B).

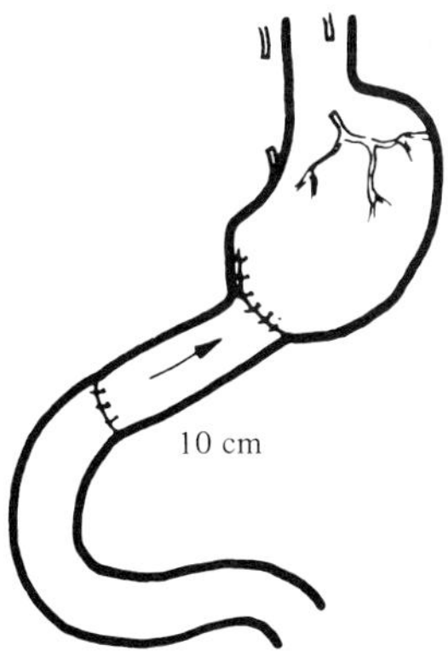

Fig. 20-10. Single reversed jejunal segment interposed between the gastric remnant and duodenum. This segment must be short, no longer than 10 cm. Longer segments will not produce a physiologic delay in emptying but will result in a true outlet obstruction.

pouch. Lygidakis states that such a reconstruction provides for normal pouch motility, produces delayed gastric emptying, and does not result in pouch dilatation or stasis. He further states that the emptying time of the pouch is approximately the same as in healthy controls. Excellent results were obtained in 25 of 28 patients available for follow-up study. Additional experience with and future reports on this procedure will be of interest (Fig. 20-8).

JEJUNAL REVERSAL. Christeas et al. [11] performed the first antiperistaltic jejunal transfer for dumping, the reversed segment being placed in the proximal efferent limb in a patient who had previously undergone a Billroth II–type reconstruction. Jordan [51] in both experimental and clinical studies revised a short jejunal segment between the gastric remnant and the gastrojejunostomy after a Billroth II reconstruction (Fig. 20-9). A short (8- to 10-cm) reversed jejunal segment placed between the gastric remnant and the duodenum was first used in the United States during the late 1950s and early 1960s by Poth [84], Schlicke [93], and Jordan [52] (Fig. 20-10). Each observer reported satisfactory results with the procedure. Alexander-Williams [1] and Fink [22] recorded excellent results with the single reversal. Benedini et al. [7] recently reported

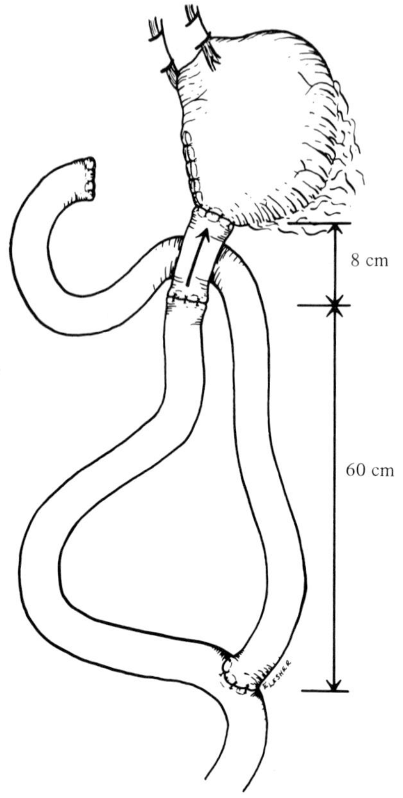

Fig. 20-11. The method described by Kennedy consisting of a short jejunal reversal constructed at the apex of a Roux-en-Y limb.

success with 11 of 18 patients. On the other hand Miranda et al. [77] experienced disappointment with 5 patients using the antiperistaltic segment.

During the past 20 years we have used a single reversed jejunal segment interpolated between the gastric remnant and the duodenum in 50 patients. Truncal vagotomy was a part of each procedure. During the follow-up period one patient was found to have an ulcer in the reversed segment, one had stenosis of the reversal, and a third patient had no improvement. As patients were followed longer an additional 6 were found to have alkaline reflux gastritis necessitating reoperation with a Roux-en-Y diversion. Thus our failure rate has been 18 percent. Eighty-two percent of patients have had either excellent or good results or have received benefit from the remedial operation.

In an effort to improve the overall results of dumping and to prevent alkaline reflux gastritis, Kennedy and Green [58] used a Roux-en-Y diversion with a short (8- to 10-cm) reversed jejunal segment placed between the gastric remnant and the Roux-en-Y limb (Figs. 20-11, 20-12). We have also performed this procedure on five patients during the past few years, with satisfactory results obtained in four (Figs. 20-13, 20-14). In one patient the reversal produced gastric stasis necessitating removal of the reversed segment. Miranda et al. [77] reported using the operation in five patients, but in three the reversal necessitated removal.

Miranda et al. [77] also reported 10 patients with severe dumping treated by Roux-en-Y diversion alone. *(It is imperative to perform complete vagotomy and antral resection when using the Roux principle or marginal ulceration may take place.)* Miranda made the fortuitous observation that most of his patients who underwent a Roux-en-Y gastroenterostomy for whatever reason had delayed gastric emptying, and dumping symptoms did not pose a postoperative problem (Fig. 20-15). He postulated that bypass of the duodenal and proximal jejunal pacemakers (in Roux-en-Y diversion) may have a negative influence on the peristaltic activity of the small intestine anastomosed to the gastric remnant. The group at the University of Florida at Gainesville [107] has now done the procedure in 17 patients with dumping, with a failure rate of only 7 percent, and the mean follow-up time is 68 months. During the past three years we have treated 4 patients in this manner with excellent short-term results. Currently, we are pursuing our interest in the Roux-en-Y diversion alone for treatment of the patient with dumping symptoms refractory to medical management.

LATE DUMPING (REACTIVE HYPERGLYCEMIA)

A small percentage of postgastrectomy patients experience either mild, moderate, or se-

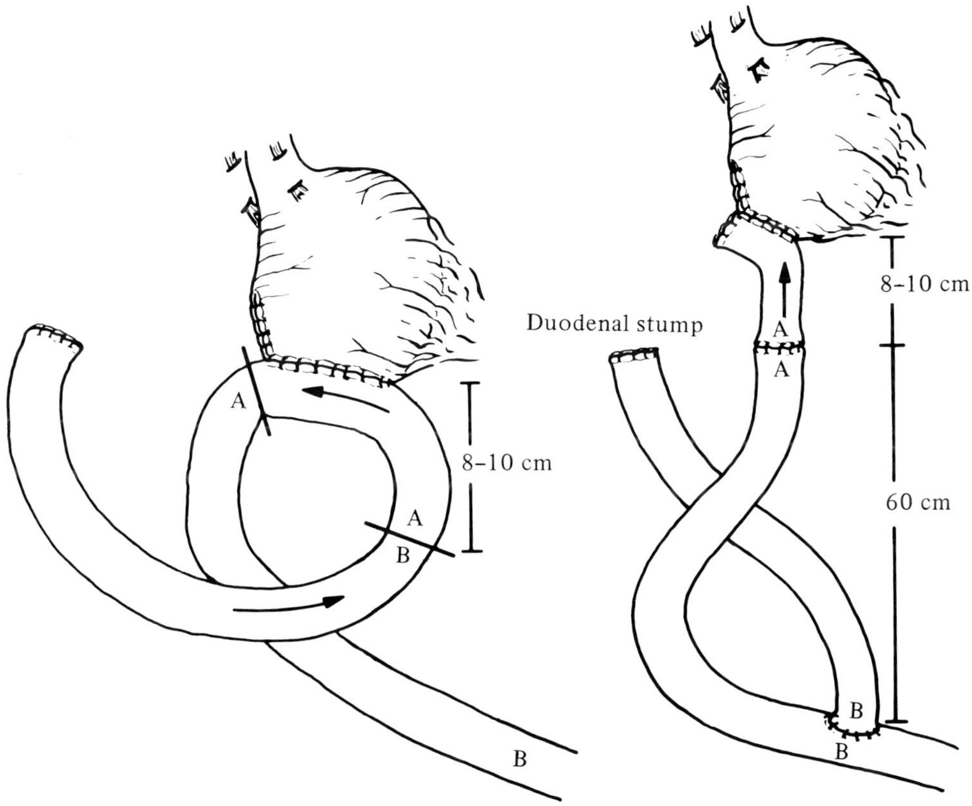

Fig. 20-12. A method of constructing a single short reversed segment at the apex of a Roux limb in a patient who had originally undergone vagotomy with resection and a Billroth II type reconstruction. The distal 8–10 cm of the afferent jejunal limb serves as the reversal. The distal afferent limb is divided and left attached to the gastric remnant. The long efferent limb is divided at the gastrojejunostomy and the distal end closed. The long efferent limb is then anastomosed end-to-end to the 8–10 cm jejunal reversal. The proximal end of the afferent jejunal limb is anastomosed side-to-end to the efferent limb in Y manner 60 cm distal to the short reversed segment.

vere vasomotor attacks 2–4 hours after the intake of food. When tested immediately after meals, these patients invariably show an initial hyperglycemia, but it is unusual also to observe early vasomotor phenomena in patients who demonstrate these clinical manifestations during the late postprandial period. Gastrointestinal symptoms usually do not accompany the late dumping syndrome. It is believed that the systemic symptoms are caused by an insulin response, resulting from an initial hyperglycemia. Individual hypersensitivity to insulin may also play a role. It is unusual for clinical symptoms to develop unless the insulin level falls below 60 mg/100 ml.

After gastric operations in which the pyloric sphincter mechanism is either altered or removed, there occurs a change in carbohydrate metabolism in terms of diminished tolerance

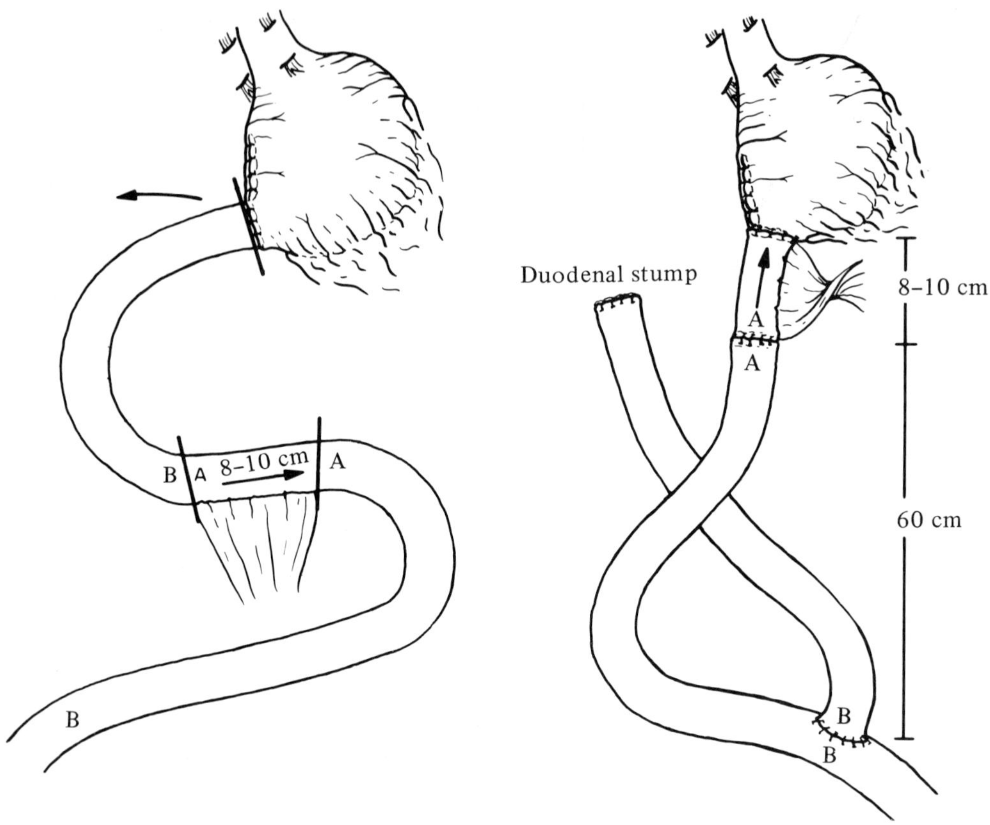

Fig. 20-13. Construction of a jejunal reversal at the apex of a Roux-en-Y limb in a patient who originally underwent vagotomy with antrectomy and a Billroth I reconstruction. The gastroduodenostomy is dismantled and the duodenal stump closed. The proximal jejunum is divided several inches beyond the ligament of Treitz and the distal efferent limb is brought up to the gastric pouch. A short jejunal reversal is then constructed at this point and anastomosed to the gastric remnant. The afferent jejunal limb containing the biliary and pancreatic contents are shunted into the efferent limb 60 cm distal to the short jejunal reversal.

for both oral and intravenous glucose. Schultz et al. [95] postulated that the activation of an intestinal enzyme system, possibly glucagon, might in part explain the initial hyperglycemia followed by excess insulin release in postoperative patients. Hypoglycemia acts as a homeostatis stimulus to the adrenal medulla, and the sudden outpouring of epinephrine into the circulation may explain the late postprandial symptoms.

Treatment of reactive hypoglycemia in most instances consists of conservative management directed toward decreasing the carbohydrate content of the diet with an increase in protein elements. The intervals between meals may be shortened, and attacks may be aborted by the intake of small quantities of glucose-containing foods. In the patient with rather marked symptoms, insulin administered be-

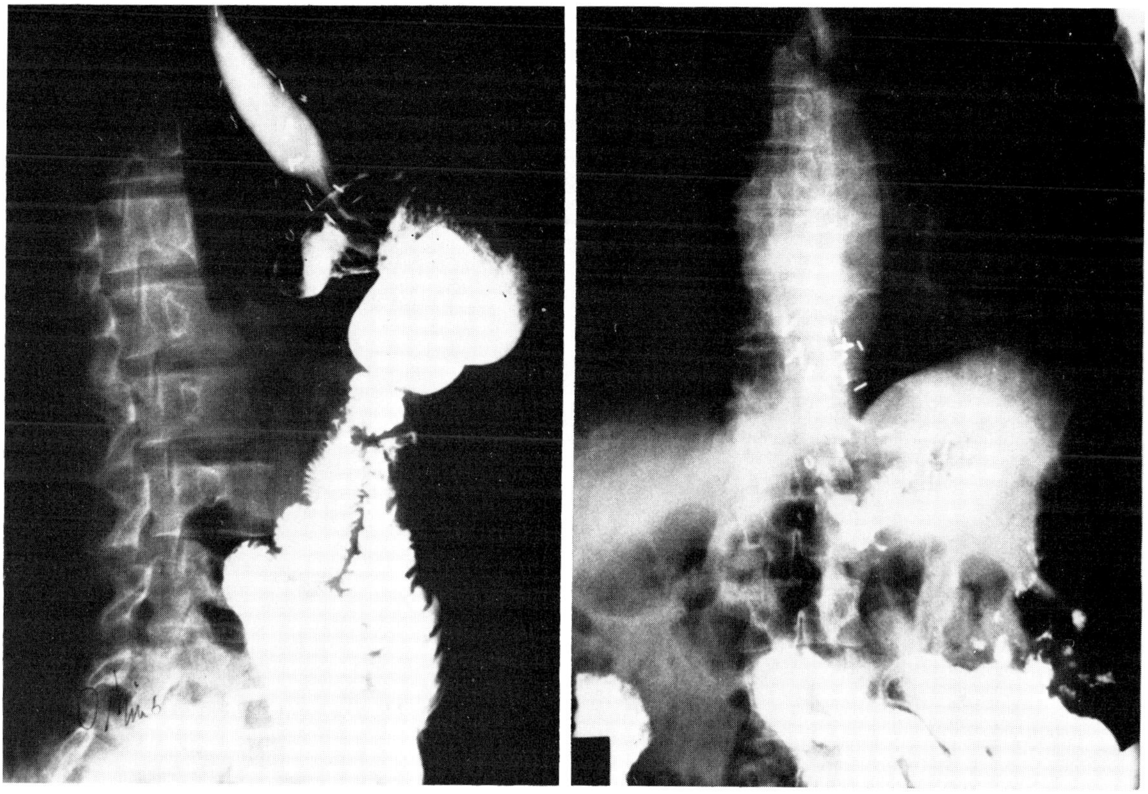

Fig. 20-14. Postoperative barium meal showing normal emptying in a patient who has undergone vagotomy with antrectomy with Roux-en-Y diversion with reversal of a short jejunal segment at the gastric remnant site. After 2½ hours the gastric remnant is empty and the mucosal pattern and transit throughout the small intestine is within normal limits.

fore meals presumably corrects or prevents hyperglycemia and facilitates glucose absorption by the small intestine. Antihyperglycemic agents such as tolbutamide have been followed by subjective improvement without change in glucose tolerance curves or plasma volume [96]. Foods containing guar or pectin—unabsorbable vegetable carbohydrates—reduce glycemia and prevent late hypoglycemia in healthy and diabetic persons [47].

Remedial operations to control symptoms of reactive hypoglycemia have rarely been resorted to. Should operation become necessary, one may choose a procedure for correction of early dumping symptoms as outlined. We have had no experience with a remedial operation for management of late dumping syndrome.

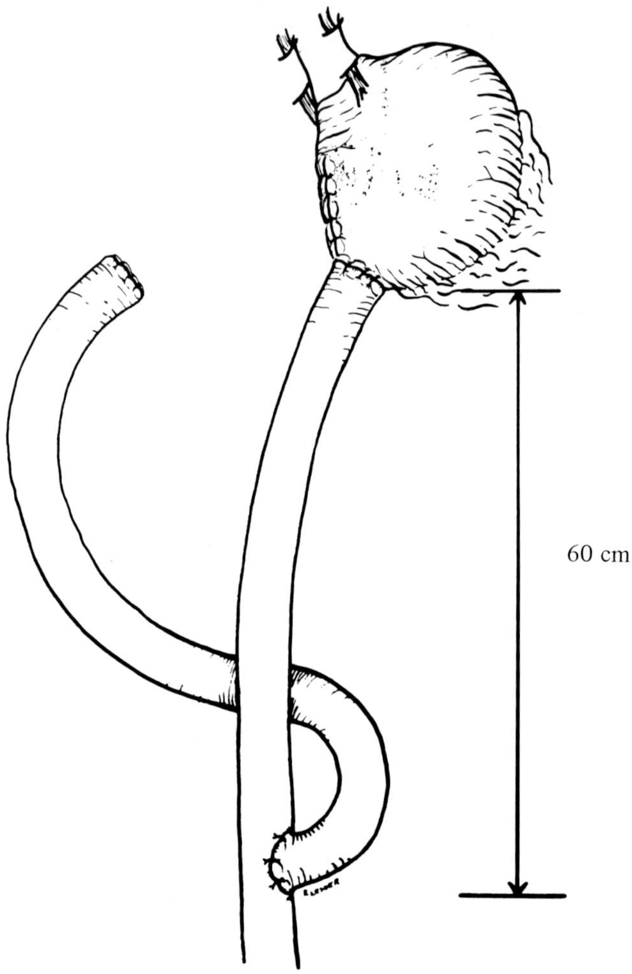

Fig. 20-15. Vagotomy-antrectomy with Roux-en-Y diversion alone is currently proving effective for treatment of the dumping syndrome as reported by the group at the University of Florida at Gainesville.

POSTVAGOTOMY DIARRHEA

Some alteration in bowel habit may take place in up to 70 percent of patients who undergo truncal vagotomy, but on the average only 10–25 percent of patients experience this change. The alteration may vary from constipation to normal movements in some patients, while in others several loose stools may occur over a 24-hour period. In only a small percentage of patients, usually less than 1 percent, is diarrhea a major problem. Diarrhea may occur with meals in association with the vasomotor symptoms of dumping and also may take place in intervals between meals. Our results show that after truncal vagotomy some change in bowel habit occurs in approximately 20 percent of patients, after selective gastric vagotomy in 3 percent, and after proximal gastric vagotomy in less than 1 percent [20, 38]. In unusual circumstances after truncal vagotomy, diarrhea may prove to be severe and incapacitating with up to 10–20 movements in 24 hours. Such patients may experience weight loss, extreme weakness, and anemia and may be considered candidates for a remedial operation. We have not encountered severe diarrhea after selective gastric vagotomy or after proximal gastric vagotomy.

After truncal vagotomy with drainage or antral resection, an alteration in gastric emptying takes place, and the duodenal regulation of gastric evacuation is lost [55, 75, 76]. Both truncal vagotomy and pyloric sphincter alteration or removal are doubtless conducive to gastric incontinence, but the exact role contributed by each procedure is poorly understood.

The cause of postvagotomy diarrhea remains poorly defined. Gastric stasis with hypoacidity, small intestinal dysmotility, impaired biliary and pancreatic function, changes in the intestinal villi and enzyme content of the mucosal epithelium, and reduction in splanchnic blood flow have each been incriminated. Malabsorption, bacterial colonization of the proximal small intestine, and increased fecal excretion of bile salts and acids are thought perhaps to be factors [3, 4, 5, 9].

Medical Treatment

The treatment of postvagotomy diarrhea begins with the reduction of carbohydrate and milk products in the diet. The use of foods low in fluid and elimination of fluid intake with meals has proved useful. Employment of neomycin or tetracycline in short courses may also at times be of benefit. Codeine, diphenoxylate with atropine (Lomotil), and cholestyramine therapy have each had some measure of success.

Surgical Treatment

The surgical treatment of postvagotomy diarrhea is based on the experimental work of Hammer et al. [29], who showed that death from electrolyte losses could be prevented in animals undergoing massive small intestinal resection by the simple reversal of a short segment of the remaining small intestine. The initial contribution to this disabling problem was the work of Madding et al. [71], who reversed a short jejunal segment in the proximal small intestine in a patient suffering disabling diarrhea from a spruelike syndrome. He later adapted the procedure for the treatment of severe postvagotomy diarrhea. Madding believed that the reversal should be constructed 90–100 cm below the ligament of Treitz. He reasoned that if the bolus of food could be temporarily arrested or slowed at this level in the intestine, there would result a better mixing with the biliary and pancreatic juices, and the optimum interluminal pH would be maintained. He also believed that the reversed segment might break the rapid wave of peristaltic movements frequently observed roentgenographically in patients with postvagotomy diarrhea. Madding reasoned that if the reversal were constructed at a higher level in the small intestine or low in the ileum, there would be less optimal mixing of the gastric chyme with intestinal enzymes. Both Hammer and Madding were careful to construct a short reversed jejunal segment to produce a physiological delay because animal experiments by both Kirstein [61] and Mall [74] over the five previous decades using long segments invariably ended in failure caused by obstruction and perforation.

During the past 18 years we have treated 16 patients with disabling postvagotomy diarrhea by the reversal of a 10- to 15-cm jejunal segment constructed 90–100 cm distal to the ligament of Treitz. Fourteen patients have done well, with diarrhea either completely eliminated or improved. Obstruction developed in one patient during the follow-up period as a result of the reversal, and at reoperation the segment was shortened with satisfactory results obtained. One patient had marked hypertrophy and elongation of the reversed segment, requiring its removal. The reversed segment on cinefluoroscopy with contrast media may demonstrate a to-and-fro movement, thus producing a physiological delay in the passage of contents through the reversed seg-

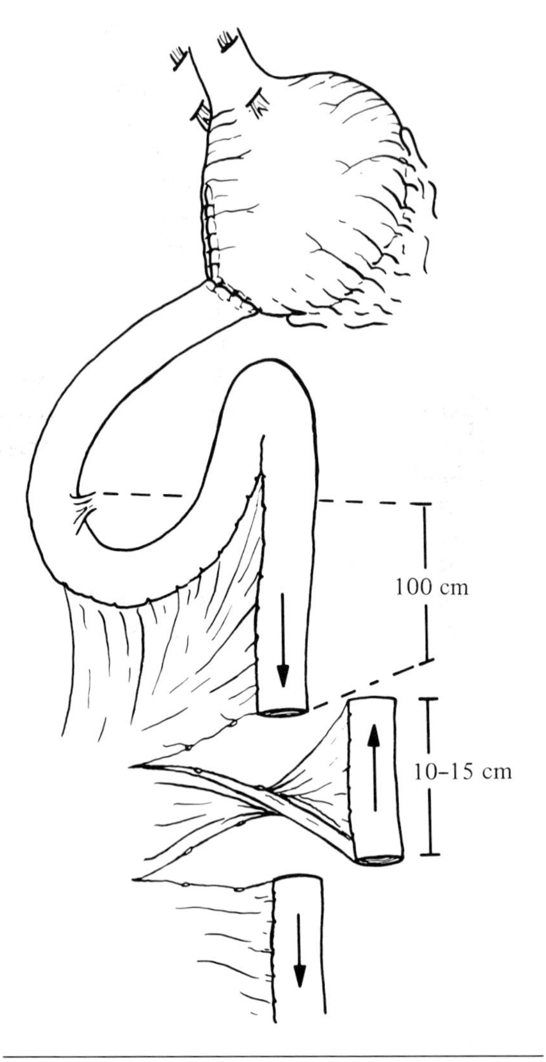

Fig. 20-16. Method of constructing a short jejunal reversal 100 cm distal to the ligament of Treitz for treatment of post-truncal-vagotomy diarrhea.

ment. The reversed segment continues to retain its original polarity over the years.

In constructing a jejunal reversal 100 cm distal to the ligament of Treitz the 10- to 15-cm segment is isolated, divided, and rotated counterclockwise through 180 degrees and reanastomosed in continuity using two layers of suture material. The small mesenteric defects at the end of the reversal are closed with interrupted silk sutures (Fig. 20-16). One possible disadvantage of this type of reversal is that it requires a slight twist of the mesenteric pedicle during construction, and one must be careful that the twist does not interfere with the mesenteric blood supply to the segment. As an alternative method of construction, we have used a modification of the procedure described by Poth [84], in which the autostapling apparatus is employed. At the 100-cm level below the ligament of Treitz a 20-cm segment of jejunum is isolated and divided with the GIA apparatus. The jejunum proximal to the isolated segment is anastomosed to the distal extremity of the isolated segment in a side-to-side manner again using the gastrointestinal stapler, creating a 5-cm stoma. The jejunum distal to the isolated segment is anastomosed to the proximal extremity of the isolated segment in a similar side-to-side manner. The isolated segment is now physiologically reversed instead of being anatomically reversed. With this method the mesenteric vessels are neither twisted nor rotated (Figs. 20-17, 20-18). We have had no clinical experience with the reversal methods described by Chrysospathis [12] and by Rygick and Nasarov [89] (Figs. 20-19, 20-20).

DUMPING AND POSTVAGOTOMY DIARRHEA

A carefully taken history may reveal a combination of dumping and postvagotomy diarrhea in a patient. Patients who have undergone a jejunal reversal constructed 90–100 cm distal to the ligament of Treitz for treatment of postvagotomy diarrhea have been studied on our metabolic unit to ascertain the effects of the reversal on the vasomotor and gastrointestinal symptoms of dumping. When such patients are challenged with oral hypertonic solutions, the clinical and physiological effects of dumping may be readily induced. Thus the reversal in the proximal jejunum in our experience affords no protection against the dumping syndrome. The results of our studies also show that a jejunal reversal placed between the gastric remnant and the duodenum or a Roux-en-Y reconstruction alone, although ef-

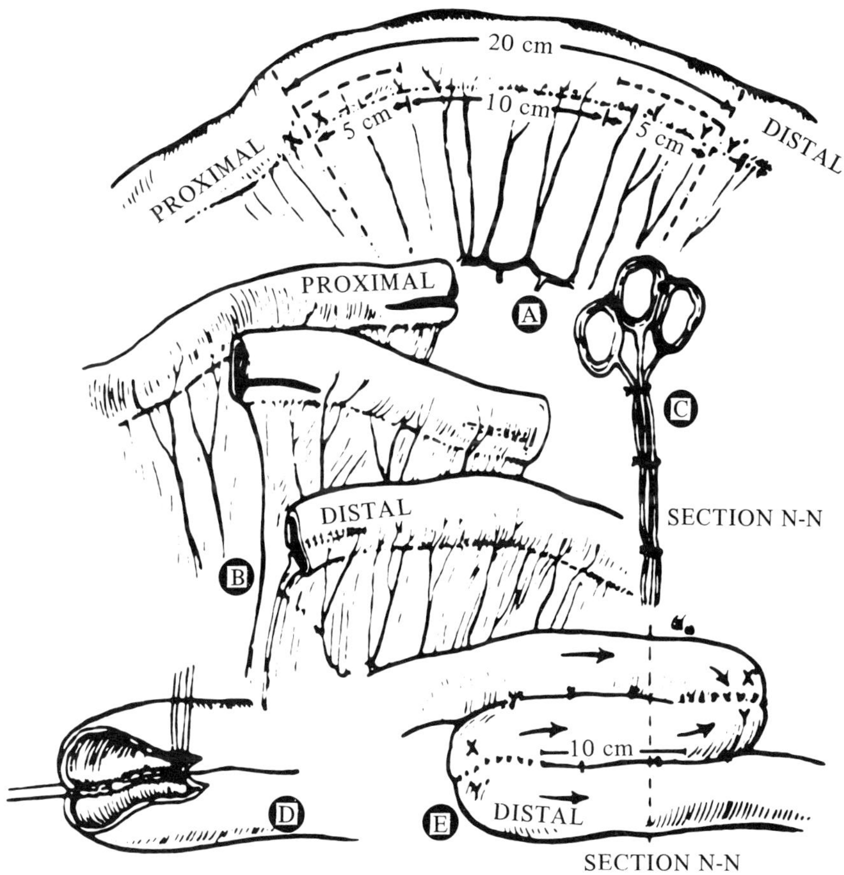

Fig. 20-17. Poth's method of constructing a jejunal reversal for treatment of postvagotomy diarrhea. With this method the mesenteric vessels are not distorted or twisted. (Courtesy of Dr. Edgar Poth.)

fective in alleviating or improving the symptoms of dumping, will not benefit the patient suffering from postvagotomy diarrhea [90]. For the patient with both severe dumping and postvagotomy diarrhea, therefore, it is our current practice to treat the symptoms of dumping with a Roux-en-Y reconstruction and also to reverse a short jejunal segment 100 cm distal to the ligament of Treitz (Figs. 20-21, 20-22, 20-23).

DUMPING AND REFLUX GASTRITIS

Alkaline reflux gastritis may also exist in a patient who is experiencing symptoms of the dumping syndrome. Formerly such patients were treated on our service by takedown of the original Billroth I or II anastomosis and conversion to a Roux-en-Y anastomosis. In addition, a short (8- to 10-cm) segment of jejunum at the Roux-en-Y gastrojejunostomy was reversed, or else a short segment several

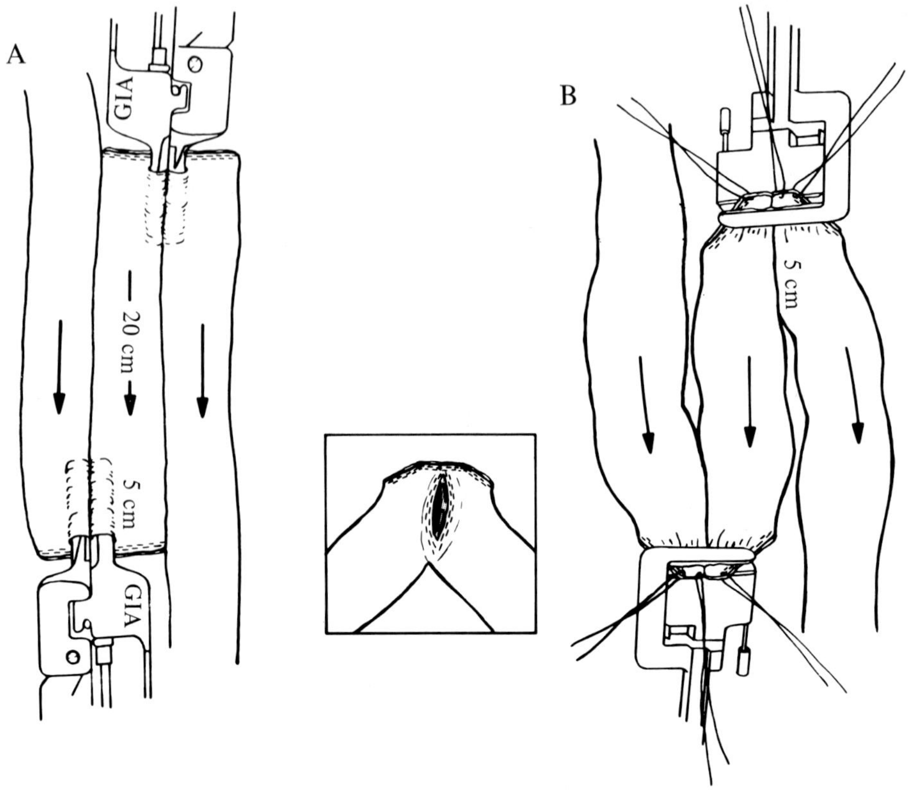

Fig. 20-18. A modification of the Poth method of constructing a jejunal reversal using autostapling instruments.

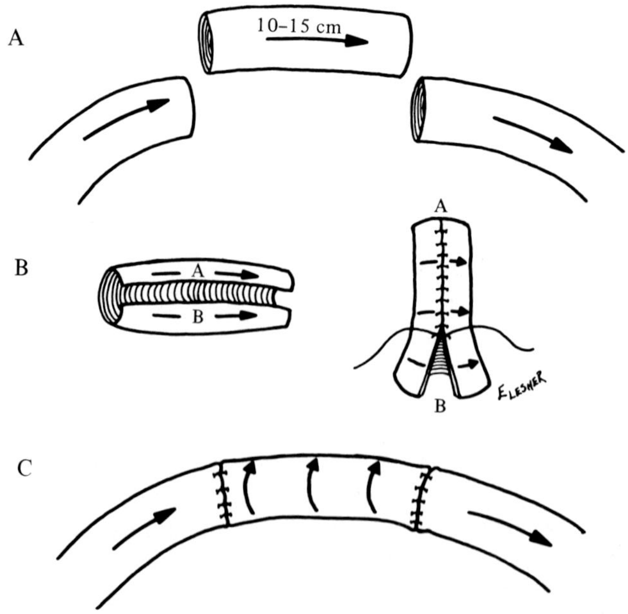

Fig. 20-19. Method of constructing a jejunal reversal originally described by Chrysospathis.

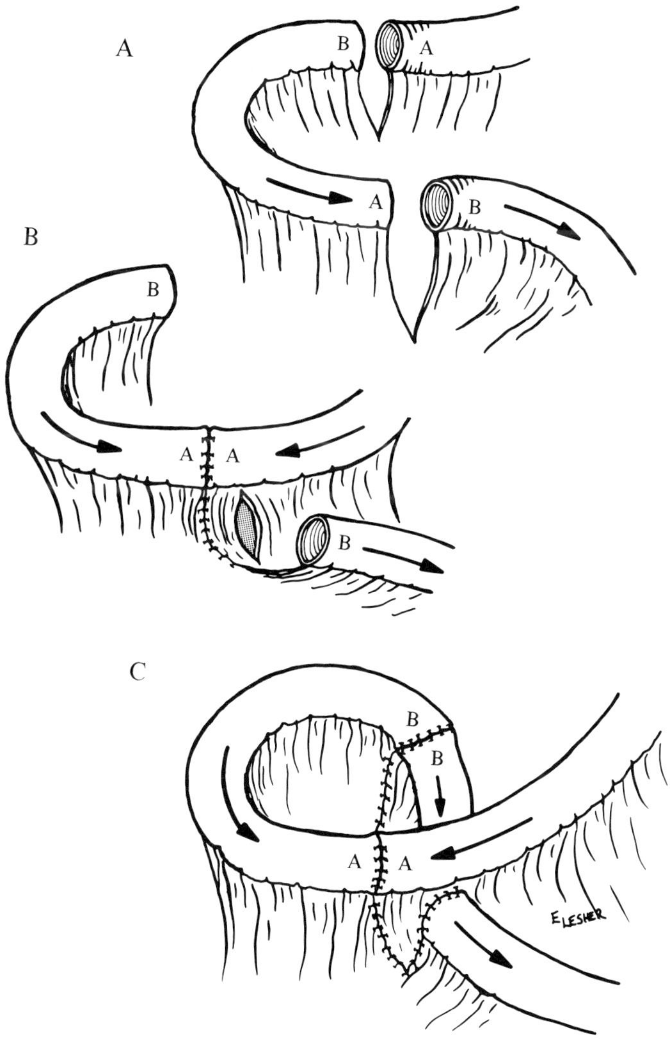

Fig. 20-20. Rygick's method of constructing a jejunal reversal. This technique also avoids a twist of the vascular pedicle. (Modified from Rygick and Nasarov [89]).

inches below the Roux-en-Y gastrojejunostomy was reversed and reanastomosed in continuity. These procedures have been described by both Coppinger et al. [15] and Kennedy and Green [58]. The jejunal reversal would serve to alleviate the symptoms of dumping, and the Roux-en-Y limb was effective in diverting the alkaline jejunal contents from the gastroenterostomy stoma, thus correcting reflux gastritis. Since it is currently appreciated that a Roux-en-Y alone not only is effective in alleviating alkaline reflux gastritis but also produces de-

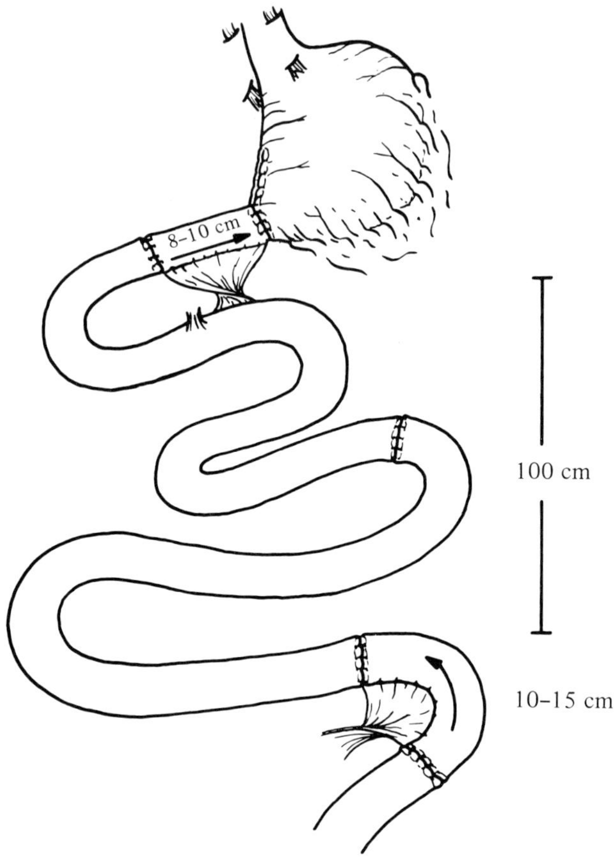

Fig. 20-21. Method formerly used to treat the patient with a combination of dumping and postvagotomy diarrhea. Although the reversal placed between the gastric remnant and the duodenum provided satisfactory results in 82% of patients, 18% had unsatisfactory results because of obstruction or alkaline reflux gastritis.

layed gastric emptying, we now use the Roux-en-Y principle alone to treat the patient who presents with both alkaline reflux gastritis and the dumping syndrome.

REFLUX GASTRITIS AND POSTVAGOTOMY DIARRHEA

For treatment of reflux gastritis in combination with severe postvagotomy diarrhea, the original Billroth I or Billroth II anastomosis is taken down and a Roux-en-Y reconstruction done to control reflux gastritis. The Y limb of the Roux is placed 60 cm distal to the gastrojejunostomy. Approximately 40 cm distal to the Y anastomosis, a 10- to 15-cm segment of jejunum is isolated, divided, reversed, and reanastomosed in continuity to control the associated diarrhea. This is the same procedure used to control dumping and postvagotomy diarrhea. During the past several years we have treated four such patients with satisfactory results.

REFLUX GASTRITIS, DUMPING, AND POSTVAGOTOMY DIARRHEA

Such a combination of events may occur in an occasional postgastrectomy patient and can be identified with a carefully taken history and appropriate studies. Such patients are treated

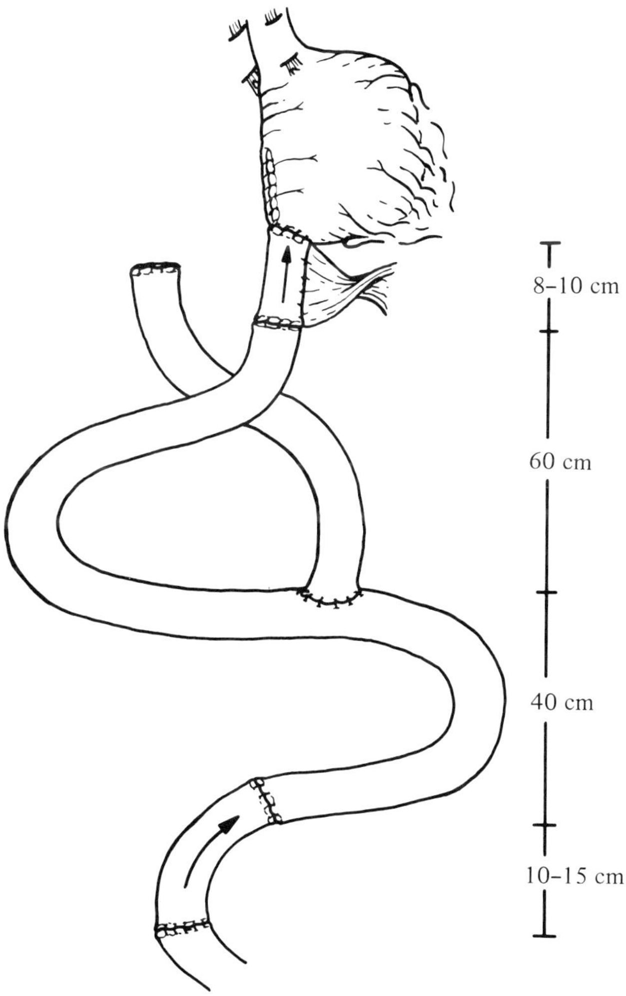

Fig. 20-22. The proximal and distal reversals used to treat a patient who presents with both disabling dumping and postvagotomy diarrhea. One of 5 patients treated in this manner on our service had poor results.

by takedown of the original Billroth I or Billroth II anastomosis with establishment of a Roux-en-Y diversion. The anatomical intestinal arrangement is conducive to improvement in the dumping syndrome and is highly effective in controlling reflux gastritis. In addition, a short reversed jejunal segment constructed 40 cm distal to the end-to-side jejunal (Y) anastomosis will benefit or alleviate the severe postvagotomy diarrhea.

MALABSORPTION

Excessive weight loss, fatigue, and anemia with or without diarrhea may occur in the postoperative patient in the absence of dumping symptoms [59, 65, 109]. A slender, asthenic female patient is more likely to have this array of symptoms, particularly if the indications for the primary operation were minimal or borderline. At times symptoms of

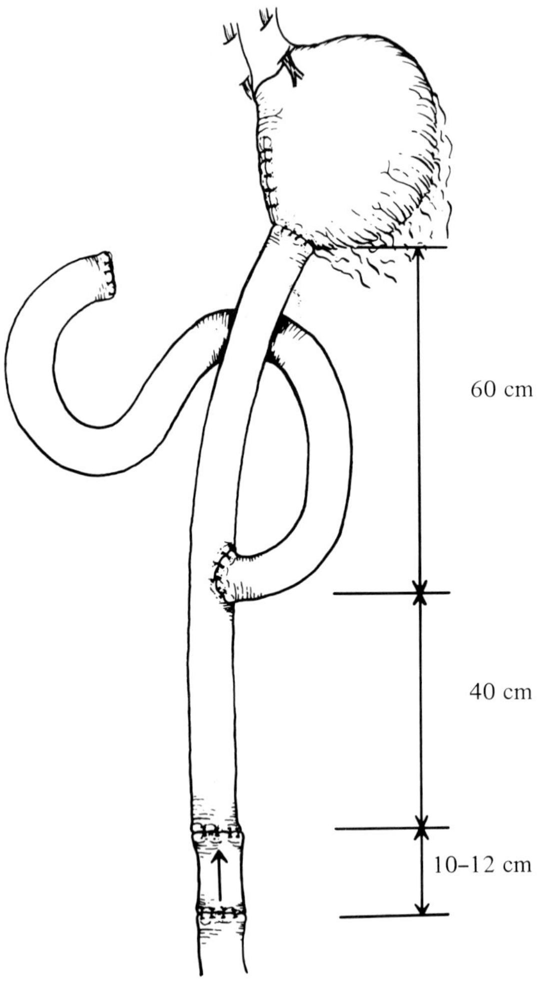

Fig. 20-23. The remedial procedure currently used to treat patients with severe dumping and postvagotomy diarrhea. The Roux-en-Y reconstruction has been effective thus far in controlling symptoms of dumping. The distal reversal placed 100 cm beyond the ligament of Treitz has been effective in controlling postvagotomy diarrhea.

dumping and other postgastrectomy sequelae may also occur [24].

Malabsorption is more likely to occur after a Billroth II reconstruction, particularly if a long afferent limb has been constructed, but such problems may also appear after a Billroth I anastomosis or pyloroplasty. With afferent loop stasis, fat absorption is impaired and an overgrowth of bacteria may be demonstrated in the afferent loop [6]. The pancreatic insufficiency that results is caused by ineffective enzyme mixing of food from delayed evacuation of contents from the afferent loop. A short course of tetracycline therapy along with pancreatic enzyme supplements results in improvement in many instances, thus confirming the clinical and laboratory impressions. If the patient is considered an acceptable surgical risk, such patients are candidates for a remedial operation, which consists of removal of the afferent loop with conversion to either a Billroth I anastomosis or a Roux-en-Y diversion. The results in highly selected patients have been rewarding. If dumping appears to be a coexisting problem, the Roux-en-Y conversion usually alleviates or markedly improves the situation. Patients with malabsorption defects as the result of primary pancreatic disease or lactase deficiency are not candidates for a remedial operation.

Gluten enteropathy, which produces absorption defects, may be unmasked by gastric resection. Janssen et al. [46] stated that, in the presence of steatorrhea, a fatty feeding preceding meals may serve as a secretagogue for pancreatic juice and bile. Therapy with folic acid, iron, and vitamin B_{12}, together with calcium and vitamin D, if such deficiencies are present, may be of value in the presence of malabsorption. Fortunately, patients currently presenting with malabsorption problems may have the benefit of extensive study and treatment on the metabolic wards of our medical centers. Currently, gastroenterologists are doing much for these debilitated patients. With the exception of the strict indications cited previously, remedial operations are rarely indicated for the treatment of malabsorption following operations on the stomach.

BEZOAR FORMATION

Bezoars may consist of mixtures of hair (trichobezoar), fruits or vegetables (phytobezoar), or both (trichophytobezoars). Gastric bezoars are more common after a Billroth I–type reconstruction or pyloroplasty than after other procedures and may result from preexisting gastric motility dysfunction, vagotomy effect, and stomal narrowing. Despite the size of bezoars, they rarely produce gastric obstruction. They may appear in the early postoperative period or may not present for many years following gastric procedures. Infrequently, the bezoar may produce symptoms of bleeding, perforation, and malnutrition. Treatment consists of oral agents such as gastroenterase or papase to digest the fiber mixture [99]. On occasion endoscopy may be used to crush and remove bezoars not responding to orally administered agents. Only on rare occasions is surgical intervention necessary to extract the bezoar. Long-term treatment consists in the use of low fiber diets and gastric wall musculature stimulants, which may prove effective in preventing recurrences.

MOTILITY AND EMPTYING PROBLEMS

Yamagishi and Debas [114] studied the emptying of solids and liquids in animals after gastric operations to differentiate the effect of vagotomy from that of gastric resection. Vagotomy alone was shown to delay the emptying of both liquids and solids in an intact stomach. After antrectomy, vagotomy was found to accelerate the emptying of liquids and delay the emptying of solids. Pyloroplasty produced a minor acceleration of the emptying of liquids, and when vagotomy was added, liquids emptied more rapidly without change in the emptying of solids. Antrectomy or pyloroplasty caused little change in the emptying of liquids. The rapid emptying of liquids after vagotomy is caused by the inability of the fundus to undergo receptive relaxation, resulting in an increase in transmural gastric pressure. Donovan [19] studied the emptying of liquids and solids after truncal vagotomy with antrectomy and proximal gastric vagotomy. There was little difference in the emptying of liquids with both operations, and both delayed the late phase of emptying of solids. Early emptying of liquids and solid meals was quicker after truncal vagotomy. Delayed gastric emptying after truncal vagotomy is perplexing and difficult to treat. Bethanechol chloride (Urecholine), an anticholinergic drug, may on occasion improve gastric emptying [68]. Metoclopramide, a smooth muscle stimulant of the gastrointestinal tract, has probably been more effective [18]. Coherin peptide isolated from bovine neurohypophysis has a regulating effect on electromotor activity [14]. This drug has been used with success in 17 patients [40]. Unfortunately, present surgical treatment has nothing to offer the patient with primary gastric motility disturbances. In the future "gastric pacing" may be developed to a degree that it will be of value. Gastric stasis after proximal gastric vagotomy is infrequently mentioned, but it does occur and is not easy to treat [110].

CARCINOMA OF THE GASTRIC REMNANT

Although carcinoma of the gastric remnant does not represent a true postvagotomy syndrome, it constitutes a long-range complication after gastric operations. It was once thought to be a rare occurrence and was all too frequently overlooked and misdiagnosed. Carcinoma of the gastric remnant is now being recognized with greatly increased frequency [79, 92]. Whether the incidence of tumors is rising or tumors are detected more frequently through more careful follow-up examinations including endoscopy is not clear at present. The lesion is apparently more common after a Billroth II–type reconstruction than after other operations but has been reported after a Billroth I procedure, after a gastroenterostomy, and even after gastric operations for lesions other than benign ulcer disease. Reflux gastritis resulting in deconjugation of bile salts has been suggested as a possible cause. Vagotomy also has been implicated, along with bacterial reduction of nitrates to nitrosamines [49]. Apparently individuals are at risk 10 or more years after gastric resection, and the current incidence of this disease ranges as high as 5 percent. Patients 10 or more years postgastrectomy should have an annual gastrointestinal series performed, along with a thorough gastroscopic examination including biopsies. The prognosis in this disease has been poor because of the delay in diagnosis on the part of both patient and physician. Also, some of these lesions have been misdiagnosed on roentgenograms and endoscopy as representing a marginal ulcer, and such patients have undergone prolonged medical therapy. The treatment of this condition is complete removal of the gastric remnant, including wide nodal dissection.

SMALL GASTRIC REMNANT SYNDROME

Seventy-five to eighty percent distal gastrectomy, advocated by some surgeons during the 1940s for the treatment of both benign gastric ulcer and duodenal ulcer, is fortunately seldom used today. Radical subtotal gastric resection for treatment of duodenal ulcer disease is currently looked on by many surgeons as being of historical interest only and has essentially been replaced by operations aimed at preserving gastric tissue, usually accompanied by some type of vagotomy. Many experienced surgeons currently prefer to treat high-lying benign gastric ulcers by less radical procedures such as the Kelling-Madlener operation or a Pouchet- or Belcher-type gastrectomy [57, 70, 72, 101–104].

It is generally recognized that after extensive resections of the stomach, the patient is likely to have dumping, fullness, epigastric distress, weight loss, early satiety, and nutritional defects. Indeed, many surgeons believe that the abdominal distress aggravated by the intake of food, resulting in a diminished caloric intake, is largely responsible for the metabolic deficiencies observed after extensive resection.

Medical Management

Treatment of patients with the small gastric remnant syndrome is largely conservative and consists in frequent small feedings and therapy with iron, pancreatic enzyme supplements, vitamins, and antispasmodic drugs. Total parenteral nutrition may at times prove beneficial. Such patients, however, can by no means be totally rehabilitated, although many may show weight gain and correction of anemias. Remedial operation plays a very small role in the management of these patients. On rare occasions, however, the severe symptoms may be uncontrollable in spite of intensive medical treatment, and a remedial operation should be strongly considered.

Surgical Treatment

The purpose of a remedial operation is to restore totally or in part the reservoir function of the gastric remnant and promote intestinal absorption, thus preventing the unpleasant complications associated with gastric incontinence.

Many complicated and sophisticated pouches have been described to replace the entire stomach or to be connected to a small gastric remnant. Many of these pouches were described in detail in the second edition of this book, Chapter 30, and will not be repeated here [37]. Over the years we have favored the Hunt-Lawrence pouch or the Tanner-Roux 19 over all others [45, 63, 103]. In the construction of a Hunt-Lawrence pouch following a high Billroth II–type of resection, the afferent jejunal limb is divided 10–12 cm from the intact gastrojejunostomy. The end of the 10- to 12-cm segment is closed and anastomosed side-to-side to the efferent jejunal limb, thus creating a double-limb pouch just distal to the gastrojejunostomy. The proximal divided afferent jejunal limb is then anastomosed to the efferent jejunal limb. (Roux-en-Y) 60 cm distal to the gastrojejunostomy.

If the original operation was a high Billroth I–type reconstruction, the gastroduodenostomy is dismantled and the duodenal stump closed. The jejunum is divided approximately 15 inches distal to the ligament of Treitz and the distal end closed. The long efferent jejunal limb is folded back on itself, and the two adjacent limbs are converted into a single receptacle approximately 10–12 cm in long. The pouch is brought up and anastomosed to the small gastric remnant. The afferent jejunal limb is anastomosed end-to-side to the efferent jejunal limb approximately 60 cm below the pouch.

A modification of the Hunt-Lawrence pouch popularized by Tanner has also been employed by us as a remedial operation following extensive gastric resection with a Billroth II–type reconstruction. The afferent jejunal limb is divided in its midportion, and the distal divided end is anastomosed end-to-side to the efferent jejunal limb 10–15 cm beyond the gastrojejunostomy. Thus a circular loop in-

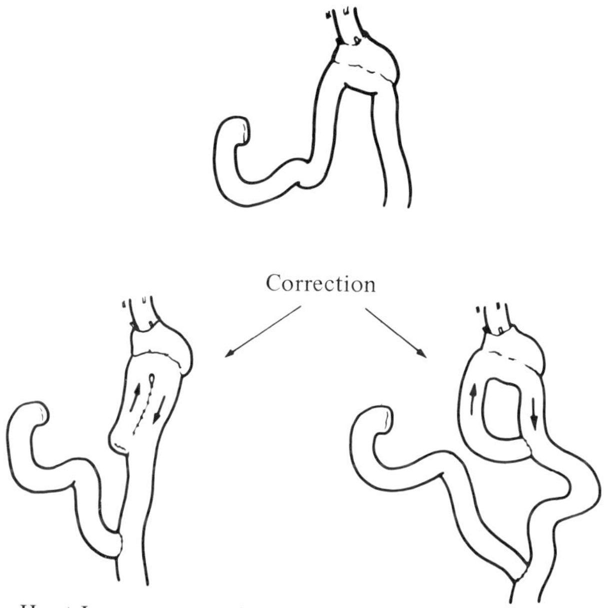

Fig. 20-24. The Hunt-Lawrence pouch and the Tanner–Roux 19 procedure have been used in a small number of patients suffering from the small gastric remnant syndrome.

stead of a pouch is created. The proximal divided end of the afferent jejunal limb is anastomosed (Roux-en-Y) into the side of the efferent jejunal limb 60 cm distal to the gastrojejunostomy (Fig. 20-24).

Mechanical Disorders

ACUTE AFFERENT LOOP OBSTRUCTION

Acute obstruction occurring along the course of a long afferent jejunal loop or at the gastrojejunostomy site in patients who have undergone a Billroth II–type reconstruction may at times be encountered. This complication may present in the early postoperative period or may become manifest weeks, months, or even years after the operation. Symptoms and signs are usually abrupt, consisting of severe upper abdominal discomfort, fever, tachycardia, nausea, vomiting, abdominal tenderness, and even shock. Such symptoms result from complete or near complete obstruction of the long afferent loop as the result of either an acute twist, volvulus, intussusception, or internal herniation. Such an array of symptoms in any patient who has undergone a gastric resection with a Billroth II reconstruction should arouse suspicion regarding the diagnosis. With distention of the obstructed afferent loop, venous pressure in the loop is soon exceeded; as further pressure accumulates, bile and pancreatic duct pressures are exceeded, and a rise in serum amylase level may occur. The surgeon should not be misled into the diagnosis of acute pancreatitis—an obstructive process exists that demands an immediate operation. Water-soluble contrast studies of the upper gastrointestinal tract and endoscopy may be of value in the diagnosis. Technetium 99m HIDA hepatobiliary scanning has been found effective in helping to differentiate the several causes of this symptom complex [98]. The presence of a dilated jejunal loop in the upper abdomen also should arouse suspicion. Operation consists in release of the obstruction and measures to prevent its recurrence [25, 28, 36, 44, 50, 60, 97].

At laparotomy if the obstructed afferent loop is found to be viable, the loop may be detached near the gastroenterostomy, the distal end closed and the afferent loop anastomosed to the efferent loop in a Roux-en-Y manner. If the patient's condition is precarious, a simple enteroenterostomy between the obstructed afferent loop and the normal efferent loop distal to the gastric remnant may prove simple and lifesaving. Operative procedures consisting of shortening of the afferent loop, conversion from a Billroth II to a Billroth I anastomosis, and suspending and anchoring the redundant afferent loop to the abdominal parietes are seldom used.

In a small number of patients with acute afferent loop obstruction in which there has been a delay in diagnosis, a portion of the afferent loop or the entire loop may be found at operation to be gangrenous. Treatment consists of removal of the nonviable area of intestine with either end-to-end anastomosis or conversion to a Roux-en-Y principle, depending on the findings. In rare situations the entire afferent loop may be found gangrenous, necessitating pancreaticoduodenectomy and Roux-en-Y reconstruction.

CHRONIC AFFERENT LOOP OBSTRUCTION

Before the introduction of fiberoptic endoscopy, many patients thought to be suffering from symptoms related to an afferent loop problem after a Billroth II reconstruction were actually experiencing symptoms due to alkaline reflux gastritis. The afferent loop syndrome and reflux gastritis are now recognized as separate and distinct syndromes (Table 20-4). During the 1930s, 1940s, and early 1950s surgeons were accustomed to making a long afferent jejunal loop when carrying out gastric resection with a Billroth II–type reconstruction. Not infrequently patients would have an intermittent obstruction along the course of the long redundant loop as the result of a twist, volvulus, intussusception, or kink at the gastrojejunostomy site. The obstruction was usually low grade and recurring, with a tendency to correct itself spontaneously as bile and duodenal secretions accumulated in the loop, resulting in sufficient intraluminal pressure to release the obstructive force with resultant projectile bilious vomiting [48, 111]. Several operations, consisting of suspension of the redundant loop, shortening of the loop, and jejunojejunostomy [13], were devised for correction. Currently more definitive operations are used, such as conversion to a Billroth I anastomosis or a Roux-en-Y reconstruction. Currently the chronic afferent loop problem is rarely encountered because surgeons for the past two decades have been using a short afferent jejunal loop with a Billroth II reconstruction. Also, current operations such as proximal gastric vagotomy, vagotomy and drainage, and Billroth I reconstruction are not associated with an afferent jejunal loop.

Table 20-4. Features that distinguish chronic afferent loop syndrome from alkaline reflux gastritis

Chronic afferent loop syndrome	Reflux gastritis
Mechanical obstruction	No obstruction
Pain related to meals	Constant pain
Pain relieved by vomiting	Pain unrelieved by vomiting
Vomitus containing bile	Vomitus containing bile and food
Projectile vomiting	Non-projectile vomiting
Bleeding and anemia (unusual)	Bleeding and anemia (not unusual)

ACUTE AND CHRONIC EFFERENT LOOP OBSTRUCTION

Efferent loop obstruction occurring weeks, months, or years after a Billroth II–type reconstruction is infrequently encountered. On unusual occasions symptoms may be ushered in abruptly with sudden and acute abdominal pain, necessitating an emergency operation. In most instances, however, the obstruction is mild, intermittent, and recurrent. The cause of the blockage is usually an adhesive band partially or totally occluding the efferent jejunal loop, a twist involving the loop, or an internal hernia [53]. The patient usually complains of vomiting bile-stained material, and roentgenographic study may demonstrate a partial delay in passage of contrast media in the proximal efferent loop, usually just below the gastroenteric stoma. Treatment at times may be relatively simple, consisting merely of lysis of the adhesive band and suture of the efferent loop to the adjacent abdominal parietes. At times procedures of greater magnitude may be indicated, such as conversion of a Billroth II reconstruction to a Billroth I repair or takedown of the gastrojejunostomy along with the proximal obstructed efferent limb with conversion to a Roux-en-Y reconstruction. Surgical findings will largely dictate the remedial procedure to be used.

INTERNAL HERNIA

Internal or retroanastomotic herniation may occur as an early postoperative complication following a Billroth II resection or simple gastrojejunostomy. Perhaps 50 percent of such problems, however, develop during the long-term follow-up period. Such hernias may involve either the afferent or the efferent jejunal loop, and on occasion both loops may be implicated. This complication was frequently encountered three to four decades ago, but with increasing use of the Billroth I reconstruction, vagotomy with pyloroplasty, short loop gastrojejunostomy, and proximal gastric vagotomy, as well as current emphasis on sound surgical technique, the problem is now rarely encountered [88].

After antecolic gastrojejunostomy, one large potential hernial space is created posterior to the stomach and the gastroenterostomy stoma. It is therefore imperative that after a Billroth II reconstruction or gastrojejunostomy alone the jejunal loop be anchored to the abdominal parietes, as advocated by Gray [28] and later by Morton et al. [80]. This maneuver is still frequently ignored by many surgeons.

Afferent loop herniation is more likely to occur after antecolic gastrojejunostomy if a long afferent loop is sutured to the lesser gastric curvature, with the anastomosis directed right-to-left. As a general rule, it is best to perform a gastrojejunostomy in a left-to-right direction, with the afferent loop sutured to the greater gastric curvature, because the ligament of Treitz lies to the left of the midline in 90 percent or more of patients. Thus the afferent loop is directed cephalad in almost a vertical plane, with the resulting anastomosis lying in a dependent and anatomical position. Efferent loop herniation after antecolic gastrojejunostomy is less frequently encountered, but it may occur if the efferent loop has been sutured to either the greater or the lesser gastric curvature (Fig. 20-25).

With a retrocolic gastrojejunostomy, two potential hernial spaces are created, one located cephalad to the transverse mesocolon and the other caudad, with the latter being of greater surgical importance. Both afferent and efferent loop hernias, however, are less frequently encountered after a retrocolic anastomosis, and an afferent loop hernia is more likely to occur if the afferent loop has been sutured to the lesser gastric curvature, since the loop of necessity must be made longer to reach the level of the lesser curvature from its origin at the ligament of Treitz to the left of the midline. With retrocolic anastomoses it is generally preferable to suture the afferent jejunal limb to the greater gastric curvature, with anastomoses directed left-to-right (Fig. 20-26).

Retroanastomotic hernias may present symptoms and signs of acute proximal intestinal obstruction demanding immediate operation. In many instances, however, symptoms are less severe and may be intermittent and recurring, not necessitating an emergency operation. The diagnosis of a retroanastomotic hernia is usually suspected on the basis of the history as well as endoscopic and barium examinations of the upper gastrointestinal tract. With afferent loop blockage, bile is usually absent from the vomitus and roentgenographic examination may reveal a soft tissue shadow in the upper abdomen along with a distended gastric remnant. With efferent loop obstruction, barium studies may at times show a normal afferent loop with some degree of obstruction along the course of the efferent loop.

During the operation, after reduction of the hernia the surgeon has several options to prevent recurrence. For the high-risk patient, reduction of the herniation, simple closure of the

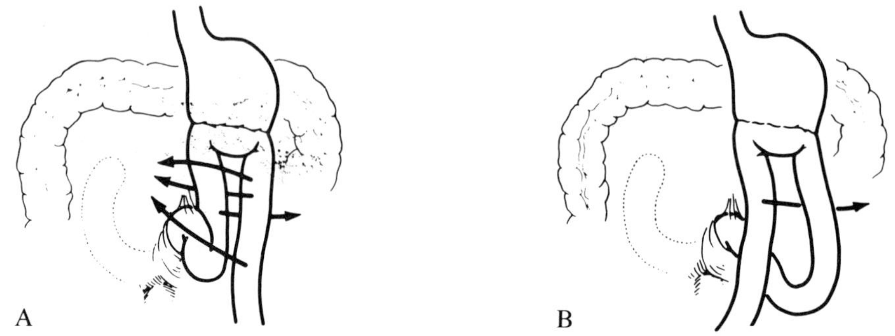

Fig. 20-25. With antecolic gastrojejunostomy (an anterior anastomosis), afferent limb herniation may occur unless sound surgical principles are executed. Efferent limb obstruction after antecolic gastrojejunostomy is infrequent. An antiperistaltic anastomosis is shown in A and an isoperistaltic anastomosis in B.

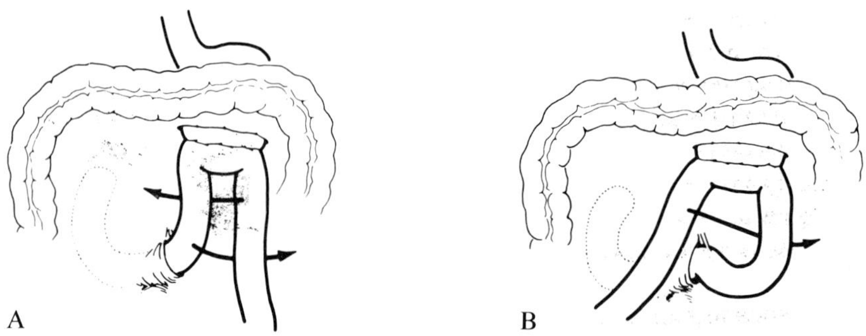

Fig. 20-26. Internal herniation may likewise occur after posterior gastrojejunostomy, but it is less frequently encountered than with an antecolic anastomosis. An antiperistaltic anastomosis is shown in A and an isoperistaltic anastomosis in B.

anastomotic traps with interrupted silk sutures, and suture of the afferent and efferent jejunal limbs to the posterior parietes are indicated. More definitive operations are used for the low-risk patient, consisting of reduction of the hernia, closure of all traps, and preferably, conversion to a Roux-en-Y diversion procedure.

LATE GASTRODUODENAL OBSTRUCTION

Gastroduodenal obstruction of a mechanical or functional nature following a Billroth I anastomosis is not an uncommon complication in the early postoperative period. Also, during the long-range follow-up period after a Billroth I reconstruction, one may occasionally encounter a patient in whom obstructive symptoms gradually develop [35]. The patient may have enjoyed a symptom-free interval lasting weeks to months before having signs of gastric outlet obstruction. In the absence of recurrent ulcer, such an obstruction may result from one of several causes. Extensive duodenal disease encountered at the time of the Billroth I reconstruction may be responsible for the insidious development of scarring and fibrosis around the anastomotic site. An anastomotic leak occurring at the time of operation may later result in periduodenal scarring sufficient to cause a gradual narrowing of the anastomotic site. Acute pancreatitis occurring in the early postoperative period and intraperitoneal hematoma may be causative factors. We have encountered gastroduodenal obstruction in which the gastroduodenal suture line was found to be adherent to the undersurface of the right lobe of the liver in patients in whom concomitant cholecystectomy was performed. It is indeed rare for alkaline reflux gastritis to result in stomal obstruction.

In the absence of a recurrent ulcer, gastroduodenal obstruction may be treated by one of several methods. A new Billroth I reconstruction may be performed, or the addition of simple gastrojejunostomy alone may be effective treatment. Takedown of the Billroth reconstruction with conversion to a Roux-en-Y anastomosis has also been used in recent years. The use of gastrostomy with instrumental dilation of the Billroth I anastomosis or employment of plastic procedures at the stomal site are fraught with failure and should be avoided. The treatment of choice in the final analysis depends on the judgment and experience of the surgeon.

References

1. Alexander-Williams, J. Gastric reconstructive surgery. *Ann. R. Coll. Surg. Engl.* 52:1, 1973.
2. Alexander-Williams, J. Alkaline reflux gastritis: A myth or a disease? *Am. J. Surg.* 143:17, 1982.
3. Ballinger, W. F. The extra gastric effects of vagotomy. *Surg. Clin. North Am.* 46:455, 1966.
4. Ballinger, W. F. Postvagotomy changes in the small intestine. *Am. J. Surg.* 114:382, 1967.
5. Ballinger, W. F., Tadular, T., and Camishion, R. C. Mesenteric blood following total and selective vagotomy. *Surgery* 57:409, 1965.
6. Barrett, C. R., Jr., and Holt, T. R. Postgastrectomy blind loop syndrome: Megaloblastic anemia secondary to malabsorption of folic acid. *Am. J. Med.* 41:629, 1966.
7. Benedini, E., Bertuccio, F., Mossini, A., and Viotto, A. Surgical treatment of the dumping syndrome after gastroduodenal resection. *Int. Surg.* 65:5, 1980.
8. Boren, C. H., and Way, L. W. Alkaline reflux gastritis: A reevaluation. *Am. J. Surg.* 140:40, 1980.
9. Browning, G. C., Cuchin, K. A., and MacKay, C. Small bowel flora and bowel habits studied at intervals following vagotomy/drainage. *Br. J. Surg.* 59:908, 1972.
10. Bushkin, F. L., Woodward, E. R., and O'Leary, J. P. Experience with the jejunal loop interposition in the treatment of postgastrectomy disorders. *Am. Surg.* 43:101, 1977.
11. Christeas, N., Kotlahis, G., Perimenis, A., and Megalooeconomore, A. Experimental study of the rate of evacuation of gastrectomized stomach, segmental antiperistaltic position of the efferent loop. *Acta Chir. Belg.* 6:4, 1960.
12. Chrysospathis, P. Technique chirurgicale. *Nouv. Presse. Med.* 8:15, 1972.
13. Conyers, J. H., Hall, R. A., Laning, D., et al. The use and abuse of the Roux-en-Y anastomosis in the relief of postgastrectomy symptoms. *Br. J. Surg.* 47:533, 1960.
14. Cooperman, A. M. Postgastrectomy syndromes. *Surg. Annu.* 13:139, 1981.
15. Coppinger, W. R., Job, H., Delauro, J. E., et al. Surgical treatment of reflux gastritis and esophagitis. *Arch. Surg.* 106:463, 1973.
16. Davidson, E. D., and Hersh, T. Bile reflux gastritis: Contribution of inadequate gastric emptying. *Am. J. Surg.* 130:514, 1975.
17. Davidson, E. D., and Hersh, T. The surgical treatment of bile reflux gastritis. *Ann. Surg.* 192:175, 1980.
18. Davidson, E. D., Hersh, T., Llaum, C., and Brooks, W. S. Use of metoclopramide in patients with delayed gastric emptying following gastric surgery. *Am. Surg.* 43:40, 1977.
19. Donovan, I. A. The different components of gastric emptying after gastric surgery. *Ann. R. Coll. Surg. Engl.* 58:368, 1976.
20. Emås, S., and Fernstrom, M. Prospective, randomized trial of selective vagotomy with pyloroplasty and selective proximal vagotomy

with and without pyloroplasty in the treatment of duodenal, pyloric, and prepyloric ulcers. *Am. J. Surg.* 149:236, 1985.
21. Fenger, H. J. L. Clinical and experimental studies of dumping disposition: A method for preoperative evaluation of individual dumping disposition. *Acta Chir. Scand.* [Suppl.] 371:1967.
22. Fink, W. J. Personal communication, 1983.
23. Fiore, A. C., Malangoni, M. A., Broadie, T. A., et al. Surgical management of alkaline reflux gastritis. *Arch. Surg.* 117:689, 1982.
24. Fischer, A. B., Knop, J., and Graem, N. Late mortality following Billroth II resection for duodenal ulcer. *Acta Chir. Scand.* 151:43, 1985.
25. Frey, C. F., and Coon, W. W. Afferent loop obstruction. *Am. J. Surg.* 115:730, 1968.
26. Gadacz, T. R., and Zuidema, G. D. Bile acid composition in patients with and without symptoms of postoperative reflux gastritis. *Am. J. Surg.* 135:48, 1978.
27. Grassi, G. The surgical therapy of postcibal and nutritional syndromes after gastrectomy. Presented to the 70th Congress of the Societa Italiana di Chirugia, Rome, October 14–16, 1968.
28. Gray, H. M. W. A cause of intestinal obstruction after gastroenterostomy. *Lancet* 2:526, 1904.
29. Hammer, J. M., Seay, T. H., Johnston, R. L., et al. The effect of antiperistaltic bowel segments on intestinal emptying time. *Arch. Surg.* 79:537, 1959.
30. Harkins, H. N., Schmitz, E. J., Nyhus, L. M., et al. The Billroth I gastric resection: Experimental studies and clinical observations on 109 cases. *Ann. Surg.* 140:405, 1954.
31. Hedenstedt, S. Gastrectomy with jejunal replacement. *Acta Chir. Scand.* 117:295, 1959.
32. Hedenstedt, S. Experiences with gastric resection with transposition of the jejunum and vagotomy. *Acta Chir. Scand.* 125:518, 1960.
33. Hellers, G., and Ewerth, S. Roux-en-Y loop reconstruction as remedial operation for reflux gastritis after gastric resection. *Acta Chir. Scand.* [Suppl.] 482:6, 1978.
34. Henley, F. A. Gastrectomy with replacement. *Ann. R. Coll. Surg. Engl.* 13:141, 1953.
35. Herrington, J. L., Jr. Consideration of factors responsible for stomal obstruction following a Billroth I anastomosis. *Ann. Surg.* 157:83, 1963.
36. Herrington, J. L., Jr. Experience with the surgical management of the afferent loop syndrome. *Ann. Surg.* 164:797, 1966.
37. Herrington, J. L., and Sawyers, J. L. Remedial Operations. In H. N. Harkins and L. M. Nyhus (Eds.), *Surgery of the Stomach and Duodenum* (2d ed.). Boston: Little, Brown, 1969. Chap. 30.
38. Herrington, J. L., Jr., and Sawyers, J. L. Results of elective duodenal ulcer surgery in women: Comparison of truncal vagotomy and antrectomy, gastric selective vagotomy and pyloroplasty, proximal gastric vagotomy. *Ann. Surg.* 187:576, 1978.
39. Herrington, J. L., Jr., and Sawyers, J. L. Surgical management of alkaline reflux gastritis and esophagitis. *Surg. Annu.* 13:341, 1981.
40. Hiatt, R. B., and Goodman, I. Peptide treatment of postgastrectomy obstruction. *Arch. Surg.* 111:997, 1976.
41. Hoare, A. M., Keighley, M. R. B., Starkey, B., and Alexander-Williams, J. Measurement of bile acids in fasting gastric aspirates: An objective test for bile reflux after gastric surgery. *Gut* 19:166, 1978.
42. Hoare, A. M., McLeish, A., Thompson, H., and Alexander-Williams, J. Selection of patients for bile diversion surgery: Use of bile acid measurement in fasting gastric aspirates. *Gut* 19:163, 1978.
43. Hocking, M. P., Vogel, S. B., Falasca, C. A., and Woodward, E. R. Delayed gastric emptying of liquids and solids following Roux-en-Y diversion. *Ann. Surg.* 194:494, 1981.
44. Hoyte, F. C. Afferent loop strangulation following partial gastrectomy. *Lancet* 1:93, 1957.
45. Hunt, C. J., and Colt, J. S. Modified technique for total gastrectomy with formation of a food pouch from the jejunum. *Am. Surg.* 18:85, 1952.
46. Janssen, B., Jr., Tyor, M. P., Owen, E. E., and Ruffin, J. M. Absorption of I^{131}-labeled lipids after intraduodenal administration: Effect of lipid prefeeding. *Gastroenterology* 38:211, 1960.
47. Jenkins, D. J. A., Gassull, M. A., and Leeds, A. R. Effect of dietary fiber on complications of gastric surgery: Prevention of postprandial hypoglycemia by pectin. *Gastroenterology* 73:215, 1977.
48. Johnson, M. Delayed afferent loop obstruction following partial gastrectomy. *Br. J. Surg.* 48:556, 1961.

49. Jones, S. M., Davies, P. W., and Savage, A. Gastric juice nitrate and gastric cancer. *Lancet* 1:1355, 1978.
50. Jordan, G. L., Jr. The afferent loop syndrome. *Surgery* 38:1027, 1955.
51. Jordan, G. L., Jr. The postgastrectomy syndromes. *J.A.M.A.* 163:1485, 1957.
52. Jordan, G. L., Jr. Surgical management of postgastrectomy problems. *Arch. Surg.* 102:251, 1971.
53. Jordan, G. L., Jr., and Walker, L. L. Severe problems with gastric emptying after gastric surgery. *Ann. Surg.* 177:660, 1973.
54. Keighley, M. R. B., Asquith, T., and Alexander-Williams, J. Duodenogastric reflux: A cause of gastric mucosal hyperemia and symptoms after operations for peptic ulceration. *Gut* 16:28, 1975.
55. Kelly, K. A. Gastric motility after gastric operations. *Surg. Annu.* 6:103, 1974.
56. Kelly, K. A., Becker, J. M., and Van Heerden, J. A. Reconstructive gastric surgery. *Br. J. Surg.* 68:687, 1981.
57. Kelling, G. Ueber die operative Behanblung des chronischen Ulcus Ventriculi. *Arch. Klin. Chir.* 109:775, 1918.
58. Kennedy, T., and Green, R. Roux diversion for bile reflux following gastric surgery. *Br. J. Surg.* 65:323, 1978.
59. Kinds, J. D., Hoffband, A. V., and Mollin, D. L. The hematologic complications following partial gastrectomy. *Am. J. Med.* 43:555, 1967.
60. King, H. A., Tucker, J. W., and Williamson, J. W. Afferent loop volvulus. *Am. Surg.* 23:161, 1957.
61. Kirstein, A. Experimentells zur pathologie des ileus. *Dtsch. Med. Wochenschr.* 15:1000, 1889.
62. Kradinov, A. I., and Volobuev, N. N. Nekotorye kliniko-retgenologicheskie paralleli pri dempingsindrome bo i posle eiunogastroplastiki (Reduodenizatsii) *Klin. Med.* (Mosk.) 44:75, 1966.
63. Lawrence, W. J., Jr., Kim, M., Isaacs, M., and Randall, H. T. Gastric reservoir construction for severe disability after subtotal gastrectomy. *Surg. Gynecol. Obstet.* 119:1219, 1964.
64. Lees, F., and Grandjean, L. C. The gastric and jejunal mucosae in healthy patients after partial gastrectomy. *Arch. Intern. Med.* 101:943, 1958.
65. Lloyd, D. A., and Valberg, L. S. Serum ferritin and body iron status after gastric operations. *Am. J. Dig. Dis.* 22:598, 1977.
66. Lygidakis, N. J. New surgical technique eliminates the dumping syndrome that often follows gastric surgery. *Ann. R. Coll. Surg. Engl.* 63:411, 1981.
67. Lygidakis, N. J. The value of revisional surgery for the treatment of postoperative alkaline reflux gastritis. *World J. Surg.* 6:226, 1982.
68. Machella, T. E., Lorber, S. H. Gastrointestinal motility following vagotomy and the use of Urecholine for the control of certain undesirable phenomena. *Gastroenterology* 11:426, 1948.
69. Mackie, C. R., Hall, A. W., Clark, J., et al. The effect of isoperistaltic jejunal interposition upon gastric emptying. *Surg. Gynecol. Obstet.* 153:813, 1981.
70. MacQueen, D. G. The Belcher gastrectomy for peptic ulcer. *Can. Med. J. Surg.* 57:741, 1970.
71. Madding, G. F., Kennedy, P. A., and McLaughlin, R. T. Clinical use of antiperistaltic bowel segments. *Ann. Surg.* 161:601, 1965.
72. Madlener, M. Uber, pyorektomie, bie pylorusfernem magengeschwur. *Zentralbl. Chir.* 15:1313, 1923.
73. Malagelada, J. R., Phillips, S. F., and Higgins, J. A. A prospective evaluation of alkaline reflux gastritis: Bile acid binding agents and Roux-en-Y diversion. *Gastroenterology* 76:1192, 1979.
74. Mall, F. Reversal of the intestine. *Bull. Johns Hopkins Hosp.* 1:993, 1896.
75. McKelvey, S. T. Gastric incontinence and postvagotomy diarrhea. *Br. J. Surg.* 57:741, 1970.
76. McKelvey, S. T., Cornell, A. M., and Kennedy, T. L. Gastric emptying and transit time as factors in postvagotomy dumping diarrhea. *Gut* 10:1047, 1969.
77. Miranda, R., Steffes, B., O'Leary, J. P., and Woodward, E. R. Surgical treatment of the postgastrectomy dumping syndrome. *Am. J. Surg.* 139:40, 1980.
78. Mix, C. L. Dumping stomach following gastrojejunostomy. *Surg. Clin. North Am.* 2:617, 1922.
79. Morgenstern, L., Yamakaws, T., and Seltzer, D. Carcinoma of the gastric stump. *Am. J. Surg.* 125:29, 1973.
80. Morton, C. H., Alrich, M., and Hill, L. D. In-

ternal hernia after gastrectomy. *Ann. Surg.* 141:759, 1955.
81. Mosimann, R., Loup, P., Fontolliet, C., and Mosimann, F. Postoperative reflux gastritis: Results of surgical treatment. *Scand. J. Gastroenterol.* [Suppl.] 67:237, 1981.
82. Nagel, C. B., and Farris, J. M. Clinical experiences with corrective surgery for the dumping syndrome. *Am. J. Surg.* 116:229, 1968.
83. Poth, E. J. The dumping syndrome and its surgical management. *Am. J. Surg.* 23:1097, 1957.
84. Poth, E. J. Surgical correction of severe dumping and postgastrectomy nutrition. A therapeutic and diagnostic test. *Ann. Surg.* 160:488, 1964.
85. Poth, E. J., and Smith, L. B. Gastric pouches: Their evaluation. *Am. J. Surg.* 112:721, 1966.
86. Reber, H. A., and Way, L. W. Surgical treatment of late postgastrectomy syndromes. *Am. J. Surg.* 129:71, 1975.
87. Ritchie, W. P. Alkaline reflux gastritis. An objective assessment of its diagnosis and treatment. *Ann. Surg.* 192:288, 1980.
88. Rutledge, R. H. Retroanastomotic hernias after gastrojejunal anastomosis. *Ann. Surg.* 177:547, 1973.
89. Rygick, A. N., and Nasarov, L. U. Antiperistaltic displacement of an ileo loop without twisting its mesentery. *Dis. Colon Rectum* 12:409, 1969.
90. Sawyers, J. L., and Herrington, J. L., Jr. Antiperistaltic jejunal segments for control of the dumping syndrome and postvagotomy diarrhea. *Surgery* 69:263, 1971.
91. Sawyers, J. L., Herrington, J. L., Jr., and Buckspan, G. S. Remedial operation for alkaline reflux gastritis and associated postgastrectomy syndromes. *Arch. Surg.* 115:519, 1980.
92. Schafer, L. W., Larson, D. E., Melton, L. J. M., III., et al. The risk of gastric carcinoma after surgical treatment for benign ulcer disease: A population-based study in Olmsted County, Minnesota. *N. Engl. J. Med.* 309:1210, 1983.
93. Schlicke, C. T. Complications of vagotomy. *Am. J. Surg.* 106:206, 1963.
94. Schoon, I. M., Anderson, H., Faxen, A., and Olbe, L. Gastric bile acids before and after Roux-en-Y transposition for bile reflux gastritis and in asymptomatic controls. *Scand. J. Gastroenterol.* 14:969, 1979.
95. Schultz, K. T., Eelon, F. A., Nilsen, I. B., and Lebovits, H. E. Mechanism of postgastrectomy hypoglycemia. *Arch. Intern. Med.* 128:240, 1971.
96. Sigstad, H. Effect of tolbutamide on dumping syndrome. *Scand. J. Gastroenterol.* 4:227, 1969.
97. Sisler, G. E., Haims, B. W., and Spencer, F. C. Postgastrectomy afferent loop volvulus and gangrene. *Am. J. Surg.* 114:932, 1967.
98. Sivelli, R., Farinon, A. M., Sianesi, M., et al. Technetium-99m HIDA hepatobiliary scanning in evaluation of afferent loop syndrome. *Am. J. Surg.* 148:262, 1984.
99. Staten, A., and Peters, H. E., Jr. Enzymatic dissolution of phytobezoars development. *Am. J. Surg.* 130:259, 1975.
100. Steinberg, M. E. A Brief History of Gastric Surgery and the Recognition of Duodenal Ulcer. In *Gastric Surgery: Errors, Safeguards and Management of Malfunction Syndromes.* New York: Appleton-Century-Crofts, 1963. Chap. 1.
101. Tanner, N. C. Restival symposium on peptic ulcer. *Br. Med. J.* 2:47, 1951.
102. Tanner, N. C. Nonmalignant affections of the upper stomach. *Ann. R. Coll. Surg. Engl.* 10:541, 1952.
103. Tanner, N. C. Result of operations for postgastrectomy symptoms. *Gastroenterology* 92:146, 1959.
104. Tanner, N. C. Disabilities which may follow the peptic ulcer operation. *Proc. R. Coll. Med.* 59:362, 1966.
105. Tasse, D., Ghosn, A., Gagnon, M., Martin, F., Morgan, S., Poitris, P., and Bernard, D. Alkaline reflux gastritis: Roux-en-Y diversion is effective. *Can. J. Surg.* 25:337, 1982.
106. Toye, D. S. M., and Williams, J. A. Postgastrectomy bile vomiting. *Lancet* 2:524, 1965.
107. Vogel, S. Personal communication, 1984.
108. Warshaw, A. L. Intragastric alkali infusion: A simple, accurate provocative test of symptomatic alkaline reflux gastritis. *Ann. Surg.* 94:297, 1981.
109. Wheldon, E. J., Venables, C. W., and Johnston, I. D. A. Late metabolic sequelae of vagotomy and gastroenterostomy. *Lancet* 1:437, 1970.
110. Wittebol, P., Akkermans, L. M. A., and Hulstaert, P. F. Prognostic factors in surgery for duodenal ulcer. *Surg. Annu.* 17:235, 1985.
111. Woodward, E. R. The pathophysiology of afferent loop syndromes. *Surg. Clin. North Am.* 46:411, 1966.
112. Woodward, E. R. Personal communication, 1984.

113. Woodward, E. R., and Hastings, N. Surgical treatment of the postgastrectomy dumping syndrome. *Surg. Gynecol. Obstet.* 115:420, 1960.
114. Yamagishi, T., and Debas, J. T. Control of gastric emptying: Interaction of the vagus and pyloric antrum. *Ann. Surg.* 187:91, 1978.

SPECIAL COMMENT

Terence Kennedy

Most experienced gastric surgeons would agree that the three cardinal problems after gastric operations are dumping, postvagotomy diarrhea, and bile reflux. Most of the problems discussed by Herrington and Sawyers followed gastrectomy, but today, at least in Europe, most ulcer operations are vagotomy and drainage without gastric resection. Treatment of the side effects of gastric operations is difficult—far more difficult than treatment of recurrent ulcer—so it is not surprising that many surgeons shun these unfortunate patients, whose disease they regard as incurable. This attitude is of course far too defeatist; my associates and I have now reoperated on more than 150 such patients, with just one postoperative death.

It is most important that none of these operations be undertaken until at least one year has elapsed since the original operation, and in all instances, completeness of vagotomy must be demonstrated.

Roux loop diversion is particularly valuable, and indeed easy to perform, after Billroth II gastrectomy; after vagotomy and drainage, antrectomy is required, making it a rather major procedure. During the past 15 years we have used a Roux-en-Y diversion procedure in 57 patients, and 51 have now been followed for 1–12 years (mean 5.1 years) (Table 20-5, Roux loop diversion). The success rate (Visick grades I and II) was 78 percent; failures were caused by jejunal ulcer in three early patients, in whom the need for vagotomy was not appreciated, and uncontrolled reflux in three patients whose loop was too short. We now know that the loop should be at least 45 cm in length, and some surgeons would say 60 cm.

Duodenogastric reflux is often associated with dumping and diarrhea. Hobsley [2] has produced evidence that all three symptoms have a common cause—precipitate gastric emptying with massive transfer of fluid from the circulation into the intestine. In postgastrectomy patients who have dumping or diarrhea in addition to bile reflux, it is possible to reverse a 10-cm jejunal segment at the gastric end of the Roux loop [4]. Our experience is limited to six patients. Four patients did very well, in one the result was moderate, but one patient died as a result of breakdown of the reversal anastomosis, a well-recognized hazard. Miranda and his colleagues [6] reported poor results with a Roux loop with reversal procedure.

In patients whose primary operation has been a truncal or selective vagotomy and gastrojejunostomy, it is a simple matter to close the gastrojejunostomy to prevent uncontrolled and precipitate gastric emptying. Provided at least one year has elapsed, the stomach will have regained enough tone to empty almost normally. The results of this simple operation have been most rewarding (Table 20-5, Closure of gastrojejunostomy).

The most common primary operation for duodenal ulcer is probably truncal vagotomy and pyloroplasty, and here reconstruction of the pylorus can be attempted [1, 5]. We have now reconstructed the pylorus in 13 patients, with good results in only about half (Table 20-5, Reconstruction of pylorus). The results are disappointing, but because the operation is safe and harmless it is perhaps worth a trial. Similar lack of success with closure of Jaboulay gastroduodenostomies has been reported [3].

We have tried conversion of a Billroth II to a Billroth I anastomosis and interposed iso- and antiperistaltic loops in a number of patients, but the results have been poor, and we believe that in general reconstructive surgery should be limited to the three aforedescribed procedures.

It is perhaps of some interest to look at the individual symptoms and the effect of the

Table 20-5. Long-term results of three repair procedures

Procedure	No. of patients or operations	Follow-up	Visick Grade I	II	III	IV	Causes of failure
Roux loop diversion	57	51 patients followed 1–12 yr (mean 5.1 yr)	20	20	6	5	Jejunal ulcer, 3 Reflux, 3
			78%		22%		
Closure of gastrojejunostomy	42	38 patients followed > 1 yr (mean 4.2 yr)	16	16	5	1	Recurrent ulcer, 1
			84%		16%		
Reconstruction of pylorus	14	13 patients followed > 1 yr (mean 3.8 yr)	Successes: 7 (54%)				Recurrent ulcer, 2 Roux for reflux, 3

Table 20-6. Effect of operations on symptoms

	Roux loop (n = 51)		Gastrojejunostomy closure (n = 38)		Pyloroplasty reconstruction (n = 13)	
	Relieved	Improved	Relieved	Improved	Relieved	Improved
Bile reflux	76%	14%	81%	11%	64%	0%
Dumping	58%	33%	52%	43%	45%	18%
Diarrhea	64%	9%	63%	25%	26%	22%

three advocated operations in the control of each symptom (Table 20-6). It is clear that bile reflux gastritis is the most easily treated and that gastrojejunostomy closure and Roux diversion are almost equally effective. These results suggest that there is undoubtedly a place for gastrojejunostomy closure and Roux diversion. Pyloroplastic reconstruction must at the present time remain sub judice. Our overall success rate for the three procedures has been 73 percent, a worthwhile result in these difficult problems.

Comment References

1. Christiansen, P. M., Hart-Hansen, O., and Pedersen, T. Reconstruction of the pylorus for post-vagotomy diarrhoea and dumping. *Br. J. Surg.* 61:519, 1974.
2. Hobsley, M. Dumping and diarrhoea. *Br. J. Surg.* 68:681, 1981.
3. Hoffman, J., Fischer, A., and Jansen, H.-E. Unsuccessful experience with closure of Jaboulay gastroduodenostomies in the treatment of post-vagotomy dumping and diarrhea. *Ann. Surg.* 198:142, 1983.
4. Kennedy, T., and Green, R. Roux diversion for bile reflux following gastric surgery. *Br. J. Surg.* 65:323, 1978.
5. Martin, C. J., and Kennedy, T. Reconstruction of the pylorus. *World. J. Surg.* 6:221, 1982.
6. Miranda, R., Steppes, B., O'Leary, J. P., and Woodward, E. R. Surgical treatment of the post-gastrectomy dumping syndrome. *Am. J. Surg.* 139:40, 1980.

21

Disorders of the Stomach and Duodenum

Robert E. Condon

Discussions of various less common surgical diseases of the stomach and duodenum are collected in this chapter to permit editorial emphasis elsewhere in the book on major surgical afflictions. Not all the entities discussed here are rare or esoteric. But even the rare lesions are of importance, since they often pose problems of diagnosis or management.

Tumors of the Stomach (Other Than Adenocarcinoma)

The discovery of any stomach tumor presents a problem in diagnosis. It is important that an accurate differentiation of these lesions be made so that a large sarcoma, for example, is not erroneously considered an untreatable and inoperable carcinoma.

CLASSIFICATION. For practical purposes, tumors of the stomach other than adenocarcinoma can be considered in two broad groups, *mucosal lesions* and *intramural lesions*. Within the mucosal group of tumors, the only relatively common entity is the benign gastric adenoma or polyp; it may present a wide variety of clinical appearances.

The intramural tumors are of diverse cell types, but they present basically similar gastroscopic, roentgenographic, and gross appearances. In most instances intramural tumors also tend to produce similar clinical symptoms and complications. Within the group of intramural tumors, those originating from connective tissues are the most important. They may be benign but equally often are malignant sarcomas. Cystic lesions of the gastric wall mimic a solid tumor.

INCIDENCE. The reported incidence of various gastric tumors varies with the source of the statistical material. Autopsy material can show an amazingly high incidence of benign tumors if minute masses are carefully sought. Meissner [238], for example, found leiomyomas in 46 percent of stomachs carefully examined at autopsy. More routine necropsy figures indicate that 75 percent of the more obvious tumors are carcinomas, 10 percent are adenomas, and 15 percent are benign intramural tumors [91, 384].

a suspicious polyp. A typical benign adenoma appears as a discretely demarcated, orange-red tumor with a smooth and intact mucosa, arising from a bed of atrophic grayish gastric mucosa. If the mucosa of the polyp is nodular, deeply ulcerated, or discolored by gray to white streaks, malignancy should be strongly suspected. Cytological study of gastric mucosal cells also can be valuable in differentiating benign from malignant gastric polyps.

Although small gastric adenomas having benign clinical, roentgenographic, gastroscopic, and cytological characteristics may be observed, especially in older or high-risk patients, periodic competent reappraisal of such lesions is absolutely necessary. It must be emphasized that the frequent association of gastric adenomas with anacidity, pernicious anemia, and adenocarcinoma requires constant vigilance if resection of the polyp is not performed.

Both patients and physicians are more comfortable with early resection of a polyp [37]. Simple endoscopic polypectomy should be done only for polyps less than 2 cm in diameter that have a definite stalk. Care must be taken to cauterize the stalk of the polyp away from the gastric wall. Polyps also can be removed through the gastroscope under emergency conditions to avert an abdominal operation in elderly patients [41].

Segmental gastric resection should be performed for sessile polyps and all lesions greater than 2 cm in diameter [189]. Histological verification of the benign nature of the resected polyp must be obtained by frozen section examination in all instances. If either in situ or invasive foci of carcinoma are discovered in a lesion that appeared to be clinically benign, adequate gastric resection must be carried out. The recommendation for gastric resection holds even if only carcinoma in situ is discovered, since the risk of inapparent concurrent or of subsequent adenocarcinoma is appreciable [295].

FAMILIAL GASTROINTESTINAL POLYPOSIS

PEUTZ-JEGHERS SYNDROME. Spotty mucocutaneous melanin pigmentation together with gastrointestinal polyposis that involves the entire length of the gastrointestinal tract are the hallmarks of Peutz-Jeghers syndrome, a disease transmitted as a non-sex-linked dominant trait [167, 351]. As is true of polyps elsewhere in the gastrointestinal tract in this disorder, the lesions are hamartomas. About one-fourth of affected patients have polyps in the stomach [23]. A related syndrome, a familial juvenile polyposis, also has been reported to exhibit gastric lesions [358]. Unlike the typical gastric adenoma associated with achlorhydria, there is no causal association of Peutz-Jeghers syndrome with development of carcinoma either of the stomach or of the colon [50, 212, 351].

FAMILIAL POLYPOSIS COLI. In this dominantly transmitted disorder, there is dense adenomatosis involving the entire length of the colon. The colonic polyps have a high incidence of carcinomatous degeneration. Gastric polyps occur infrequently in familial polyposis, although their incidence is greater than that of the normal population [167, 351].

Multiple gastric adenomas may be found in an occasional patient who has no familial tendency toward tumor formation. Two patients with apparent nonhereditary multiple gastric polyps associated with parathyroid adenomas have been reported [35]. Carcinoma of the stomach has been reported in association with gastric polyposis in 10–40 percent of instances [36]; gastric cancer also has been reported in association with colonic polyposis [209]. Since gastric polyps rarely are located in the fundus, distal subtotal gastrectomy effectively removes all the multiple adenomas. Occasionally total gastrectomy may be required in a patient with polyposis to remove all gastric polyps [299].

Benign Intramural Tumors

All the benign intramural gastric tumors have many features in common. They are solid, usually submucosal masses; they occur in middle-aged and older patients; and they show no predilection for either sex. Most of these tumors are mesenchymal or mesothelial in origin. Their incidence approximates that of gastric adenomas, that is, they comprise about 2 percent of surgically resected tumors and

21

Disorders of the Stomach and Duodenum

Robert E. Condon

Discussions of various less common surgical diseases of the stomach and duodenum are collected in this chapter to permit editorial emphasis elsewhere in the book on major surgical afflictions. Not all the entities discussed here are rare or esoteric. But even the rare lesions are of importance, since they often pose problems of diagnosis or management.

Tumors of the Stomach (Other Than Adenocarcinoma)

The discovery of any stomach tumor presents a problem in diagnosis. It is important that an accurate differentiation of these lesions be made so that a large sarcoma, for example, is not erroneously considered an untreatable and inoperable carcinoma.

CLASSIFICATION. For practical purposes, tumors of the stomach other than adenocarcinoma can be considered in two broad groups, *mucosal lesions* and *intramural lesions*. Within the mucosal group of tumors, the only relatively common entity is the benign gastric adenoma or polyp; it may present a wide variety of clinical appearances.

The intramural tumors are of diverse cell types, but they present basically similar gastroscopic, roentgenographic, and gross appearances. In most instances intramural tumors also tend to produce similar clinical symptoms and complications. Within the group of intramural tumors, those originating from connective tissues are the most important. They may be benign but equally often are malignant sarcomas. Cystic lesions of the gastric wall mimic a solid tumor.

INCIDENCE. The reported incidence of various gastric tumors varies with the source of the statistical material. Autopsy material can show an amazingly high incidence of benign tumors if minute masses are carefully sought. Meissner [238], for example, found leiomyomas in 46 percent of stomachs carefully examined at autopsy. More routine necropsy figures indicate that 75 percent of the more obvious tumors are carcinomas, 10 percent are adenomas, and 15 percent are benign intramural tumors [91, 384].

Sarcomas of the stomach, although not often tabulated in autopsy material, are clinically significant and represent about 2.5 percent of surgically resected gastric neoplasms. Sarcomas, then, may slightly exceed in incidence both benign adenomas and other intramural tumors in surgical material.

Excellent reviews of noncarcinomatous neoplasms of the stomach are those of Pack [268], Beard et al. [24], Naqvi et al. [255], and Burgess et al. [46, 47].

BENIGN GASTRIC ADENOMA

This is a benign proliferative tumor of the gastric mucosa that projects into the lumen of the stomach from a pedunculated or sessile base. Polyps can be classified as *hyperplastic* or *adenomatous*. Hyperplastic polyps are randomly distributed in the stomach, whereas adenomatous polyps are predominantly antral in location. Adenomatous polyps are more commonly associated with chronic atrophic gastritis and gastric carcinoma. Adenomatous polyps may be precursors of invasive gastric carcinoma, whereas morphological evidence for an association of hyperplastic polyps with gastric cancer is virtually nonexistent [344].

So-called pseudopolyps represent either hyperplastic regenerative overgrowth of mucosa occurring in chronic atrophic gastritis or surface nodularity of the mucosa caused by an underlying inflammatory reaction [154, 196]. An unusual case of hereditary hemorrhagic telangiectasia producing a gastric polypoid lesion has been reported [338].

Intramural tumors arising within the wall of the stomach also may present as pseudopolyps if their growth results in bulging of the tumor mass into the lumen of the stomach. Such lesions may even become pedunculated, but they usually remain covered by normal gastric mucosa.

True adenomas may be single or multiple and may occur in all parts of the stomach, although they show a predilection for the antrum [140, 227]. Adenomas are found in about 0.4 percent of routine autopsies, in 0.7 percent of roentgenographic examinations, and in 1.5 percent of gastroscopic examinations [227, 320].

The importance of selection in the reported frequency of gastric adenomas must be emphasized. If patients with achlorhydria are selected, 2–5 percent will have benign adenomatous polyps in the stomach [367], while if the patient has pernicious anemia, the incidence of polyps rises to 5–8 percent [99, 151, 289]. The lesions most commonly are only a few millimeters in diameter, but occasionally they are several centimeters in size.

The patient is most often between 60 and 80 years of age. Nearly 50 percent of the patients do not have symptoms; in the others, symptoms are nonspecific. A history of variable epigastric distress or pain can be elicited from slightly more than half of the patients who have a gastric adenoma; 30 percent have nausea or vomiting, and hematemesis or melena occurs in 20 percent. Anemia is a variable finding; it may be hypochromic because of bleeding, or it may be macrocytic pernicious anemia [102].

The most striking laboratory finding in gastric adenoma is achlorhydria, which is reported in 80–90 percent of patients. Antibodies against the microsomal fraction of gastric parietal cells are present in more than half the patients. Correlated with these findings is a high incidence of atrophic gastritis. Hay [140] found moderate-to-severe atrophic gastritis in 48 of 50 surgical specimens and in 52 of 64 patients examined by gastroscopy. Yarniss et al. [384] considered 38 of 42 patients with gastric adenomas to have atrophic gastritis on gastroscopic examination.

These statistics support the concept that atrophic gastritis provides a fertile bed for adenoma formation if it is not actually a precursor of adenomatosis. Because of the high incidence of achlorhydria and chronic atrophic gastritis in patients with gastric adenomas, demonstration of high acid values in a patient suggests that a diagnosis of adenomatous polyp is incorrect.

VILLOUS ADENOMA. These are rare lesions, usually forming an irregular, lobulated mucosal mass, which may have a lacy, "soap-bubble" appearance on barium contrast studies (Fig. 21-1). Villous adenomas have their peak incidence in the seventh decade of life.

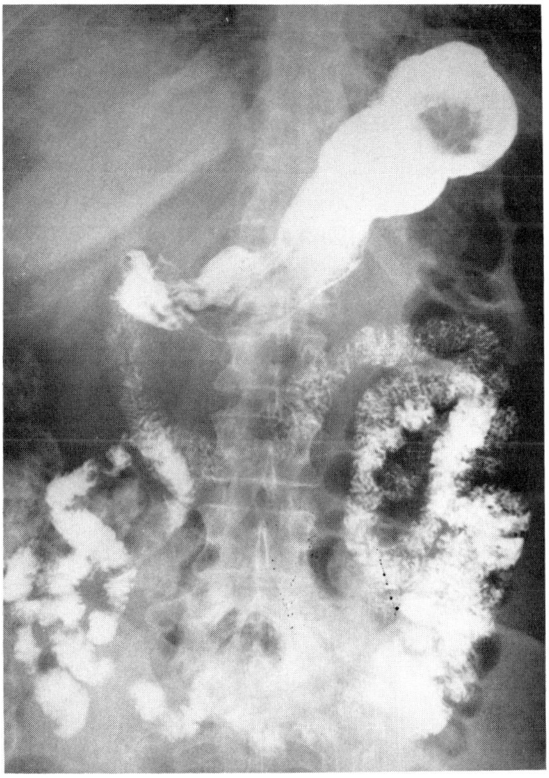

Fig. 21-1. A large villous adenoma appearing as a polyp in the gastric fundus. (Courtesy of Dr. J. Lynwood Herrington.)

There are no specific symptoms or findings, although some degree of anemia often is present. Carcinomatous change is frequent, particularly in lesions larger than 4 cm [48].

Brunner's gland adenomas of the stomach are both benign and rare. They are differentiated from more common gastric polyps only by histological examination of a biopsy or of the excised tumor.

An instance of *cystic mucosal hyperplasia* resulting in a polypoid lesion that prolapsed and obstructed a gastroenterostomy has been reported [213].

Adenoma and Carcinoma

The malignant potential of gastric polyps is still a subject of controversy. The presence of polyps in the stomach may be a harbinger of gastrointestinal malignancy. Goldman and Appelman [124] noted that 39 percent of patients with gastric polyps harbored a carcinoma somewhere in the gastrointestinal tract. There is little doubt that adenomas are associated with a high incidence of gastric carcinoma, as high as 51 percent in a study by Brunn and Pearl [44], but certainly many polyps never degenerate or become associated with malignancy. Carcinoma in situ was found in 10 percent of 153 patients with adenomatous polyps of the stomach reported by Monaco et al. [244]. A similar incidence has been noted in other studies [295].

The size of the polyp is important in determining whether or not malignant change has occurred. The study by Bonfield et al. [38] indicated that small polypoid gastric lesions less than 1 cm in diameter were very likely to be benign. In the studies of Hay [140, 141], only one of 81 polyps less than 2 cm in diameter had malignant change, while in polyps larger than this, 6 of 14 showed foci of malignancy. Similar findings were noted in the studies of Eklof et al. [99] and Tomasulo [344]. These observations are similar to those concerning the behavior of adenomatous polyps elsewhere in the gastrointestinal tract, particularly in the colon.

Management of Gastric Adenomas

When a polypoid lesion is demonstrated, attention is first directed toward determining whether the lesion is benign or malignant. Clinically the absence of gastric symptoms suggests an innocent lesion. Bleeding, which may be a feature in the history or may be discovered by guaiac examination of the stool, may occur with either benign or malignant lesions but is more prominent in carcinoma. Significant weight loss and weakness suggest the presence of a cancer. Roentgenographically, benign adenomatous polyps are small, smooth, and sharply etched; the wall surrounding the polyp is pliable; and the polyp is often pedunculated. The incidence of malignancy is increased if the polyp is sessile or irregular, or if the tumor or the nearby gastric wall is rigid [227] (Fig. 21-1).

A competent gastroscopist often is able to characterize the benign or malignant nature of a suspicious polyp. A typical benign adenoma appears as a discretely demarcated, orange-red tumor with a smooth and intact mucosa, arising from a bed of atrophic grayish gastric mucosa. If the mucosa of the polyp is nodular, deeply ulcerated, or discolored by gray to white streaks, malignancy should be strongly suspected. Cytological study of gastric mucosal cells also can be valuable in differentiating benign from malignant gastric polyps.

Although small gastric adenomas having benign clinical, roentgenographic, gastroscopic, and cytological characteristics may be observed, especially in older or high-risk patients, periodic competent reappraisal of such lesions is absolutely necessary. It must be emphasized that the frequent association of gastric adenomas with anacidity, pernicious anemia, and adenocarcinoma requires constant vigilance if resection of the polyp is not performed.

Both patients and physicians are more comfortable with early resection of a polyp [37]. Simple endoscopic polypectomy should be done only for polyps less than 2 cm in diameter that have a definite stalk. Care must be taken to cauterize the stalk of the polyp away from the gastric wall. Polyps also can be removed through the gastroscope under emergency conditions to avert an abdominal operation in elderly patients [41].

Segmental gastric resection should be performed for sessile polyps and all lesions greater than 2 cm in diameter [189]. Histological verification of the benign nature of the resected polyp must be obtained by frozen section examination in all instances. If either in situ or invasive foci of carcinoma are discovered in a lesion that appeared to be clinically benign, adequate gastric resection must be carried out. The recommendation for gastric resection holds even if only carcinoma in situ is discovered, since the risk of inapparent concurrent or of subsequent adenocarcinoma is appreciable [295].

FAMILIAL GASTROINTESTINAL POLYPOSIS

PEUTZ-JEGHERS SYNDROME. Spotty mucocutaneous melanin pigmentation together with gastrointestinal polyposis that involves the entire length of the gastrointestinal tract are the hallmarks of Peutz-Jeghers syndrome, a disease transmitted as a non-sex-linked dominant trait [167, 351]. As is true of polyps elsewhere in the gastrointestinal tract in this disorder, the lesions are hamartomas. About one-fourth of affected patients have polyps in the stomach [23]. A related syndrome, a familial juvenile polyposis, also has been reported to exhibit gastric lesions [358]. Unlike the typical gastric adenoma associated with achlorhydria, there is no causal association of Peutz-Jeghers syndrome with development of carcinoma either of the stomach or of the colon [50, 212, 351].

FAMILIAL POLYPOSIS COLI. In this dominantly transmitted disorder, there is dense adenomatosis involving the entire length of the colon. The colonic polyps have a high incidence of carcinomatous degeneration. Gastric polyps occur infrequently in familial polyposis, although their incidence is greater than that of the normal population [167, 351].

Multiple gastric adenomas may be found in an occasional patient who has no familial tendency toward tumor formation. Two patients with apparent nonhereditary multiple gastric polyps associated with parathyroid adenomas have been reported [35]. Carcinoma of the stomach has been reported in association with gastric polyposis in 10–40 percent of instances [36]; gastric cancer also has been reported in association with colonic polyposis [209]. Since gastric polyps rarely are located in the fundus, distal subtotal gastrectomy effectively removes all the multiple adenomas. Occasionally total gastrectomy may be required in a patient with polyposis to remove all gastric polyps [299].

Benign Intramural Tumors

All the benign intramural gastric tumors have many features in common. They are solid, usually submucosal masses; they occur in middle-aged and older patients; and they show no predilection for either sex. Most of these tumors are mesenchymal or mesothelial in origin. Their incidence approximates that of gastric adenomas, that is, they comprise about 2 percent of surgically resected tumors and about 0.5 percent of gastric tumors noted during routine autopsy examinations.

Palmer [270] summarized the characteristics of 1660 benign intramural tumors reported in the world literature. It should be emphasized that Palmer's review, as summarized in Table 21-1, pertains only to intramural tumors. If all benign tumors of the stomach are considered, polypoid adenoma is the most frequent; if interest is confined only to intramural tumors, then leiomyoma is the most frequent [314].

INCIDENCE. The recorded relative incidence of benign intramural tumors in the literature is misleading, since rare tumors tend to be reported whenever they are encountered, while less rare lesions are neglected. An example of this phenomenon is the report of gastric xanthoma, a small yellow submucosal nodule or macule that histologically demonstrates abundant lipid-laden histocytes [158]; this is a very rare lesion. By assessing clinical and autopsy material from several sources, a rough approximation of the true relative incidence of benign intramural gastric tumors has been calculated and is recorded in the last column of Table 21-1.

Table 21-1. Statistical analysis of 1660 benign intramural tumors of the stomach reported in the world literature

Tumor	No. of reported cases	Percent of total no. of reported cases	Probable percent of all benign intramural tumors
Leiomyomas (excluding tiny lesions)	610	37	56
Fibroma	289	17	30
Neurogenic tumors	263	16	5
Aberrant pancreas tumors	215	13	5
Fatty tumors	103	6	2
Vascular tumors	93	6	1
Cystic tumors	87	5	1
Total	1660	100	100

Source: Modified from Palmer [270].

CLINICAL FEATURES. Many benign intramural tumors are asymptomatic and are discovered only at autopsy. The majority of tumors discovered clinically, however, are symptomatic; therefore surgical removal of the lesion for the relief of symptoms (rather than for diagnosis or prophylaxis) is generally acceptable to all concerned—patient, physician, and surgeon. If the patient represents a high surgical risk or if the lesion is only minimally symptomatic, however, competent determination of the benign nature of the lesion by endoscopic biopsy will permit continuation of a program of nonoperative observation.

When an operation is indicated, local excision or a small gastric resection generally is adequate; mortality and morbidity of treatment of these benign gastric lesions thus can be kept acceptably low. The potential for malignancy always must be a factor in decisions regarding management, and the benign nature of the resected tumor should be histologically verified by frozen-section diagnosis in every instance. In tumors with known malignant potential, particularly angiomas and carcinoids, somewhat wider margins of resection probably are indicated than for other benign lesions. Of course, more radical gastric resection is appropriate for all tumors in which a histological diagnosis of malignancy is made at the time of initial operative treatment.

Leiomyoma

Even if minute leiomyomas are ignored, leiomyomas are the most common benign submucosal and intramural gastric tumors. Ninety percent are single and are found in the distal two-thirds of the stomach. Growth may occur toward the lumen (about 60 percent) or outward from the serosal surface [313]. Leiomyomas most often are spheroidal, but they may form hourglass or ringlike masses. Pedunculation is common. Ulceration of the overlying mucosa is usual in symptomatic instances (Fig. 21-2).

Symptoms are diverse, but the most common presenting complaint is gross gastric

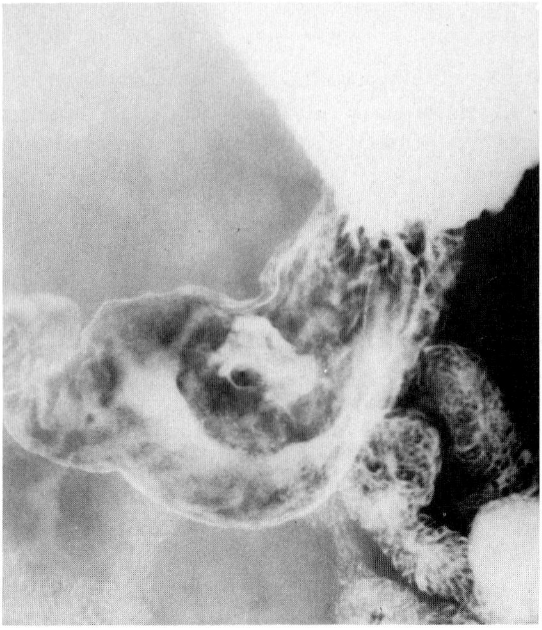

Fig. 21-2. A large gastric leiomyoma in a typical location. The large central ulcer had led to hematemesis.

hemorrhage [247]. About a third of patients complain of some abdominal distress, and 10 percent have episodic vomiting. Weight loss and weakness are rare. The tumor usually is demonstrable by roentgenographic studies and endoscopy. While exact diagnosis requires histological examination, the benign nature of leiomyomas generally can be established preoperatively.

It should be kept in mind that an occasional leiomyoma that is perfectly benign clinically may appear quite malignant on histological examination. Such a hypercellular lesion is called a *leiomyoblastoma,* and it can be differentiated from leiomyosarcoma by the absence of an increased incidence of mitosis [80, 246, 326].

Adenomyoma

These are rare benign lesions occurring in the distal antrum or at the pylorus. They are composed of hypertrophic smooth muscle enclosing cysts or glandular structures lined by tall columnar cells, Brunner glands, or sometimes, pancreatic tissue [199].

Fibromas and Fibromyomas

These tumors resemble leiomyomas in shape, size, clinical appearance, and complications. Unlike leiomyomas, they show no preference for the distal stomach. About half of these lesions histologically are "pure" fibromas, and the remainder are myofibromas, containing a mixture of smooth muscle and other connective tissue cells. Such differentiation is of no clinical importance. When the lesions are symptomatic, patients complain of abdominal pain and hemorrhage.

Neurogenic Tumors

Seventy percent of these tumors are neurilemomas (schwannomas) arising from nerve sheath, one-fourth are neurofibromas, and the remainder are a variety of tumors most often arising from the sympathetic nervous system (neuroblastoma, periganglioneuroma). Neurogenic tumors appear to be clinically more symptomatic, since more than 90 percent of reported instances have been found at operation rather than at autopsy; this preponderance of surgical diagnosis does not occur with any other benign intramural gastric tumor [270].

Schwannomas are generally single, spherical tumors occurring along the lesser curvature in the distal two-thirds of the stomach. Neurofibromas, on the other hand, often are multiple and occur in all parts of the stomach. Neurofibromas also may be associated with generalized neurofibromatosis (Recklinghausen disease). Superficial ulceration of neurogenic tumors is common, and hemorrhage is reported by a third of patients with symptoms. Other symptoms are usually vague, but pain is reported by one-fourth of the patients. Inflammatory fibroid polyps of the antrum recently have been interpreted as being neurogenic in origin [125].

Lipomas and Other Fatty Tumors

These are unusual gastric tumors [294]. More than 90 percent of these lesions are pure lipomas, the remainder being a variety of mixed types. Typically a lipoma is a single ulcerated sphere that is several centimeters in diameter. Usually lipomas are sessile, but pedunculated lesions also occur. Symptoms are related to superficial ulceration producing hemorrhage (47 percent) or to gastric outlet obstruction by a pedunculated tumor (20 percent).

Vascuar Tumors
These tumors are quite rare, but they are of particular clinical interest because of their tendency to bleed massively and because of their propensity to malignant change [98]. This group of tumors includes angiomas (60 percent) and endotheliomas (40 percent) of either blood vessel or lymphatic origin [58, 65, 225]. Ulceration of these tumors is frequent and leads to severe hemorrhage as the presenting complaint in 40 percent of the patients. If the hemangioma is very large, an extensive gastric resection occasionally may be required [336].

The *glomus tumor* of the stomach represents another special variety of vascular tumor. These benign neoplasms arise from capillary pericytes present in arteriovenous shunts in the gastric wall. Ulceration is common and will not heal with nonsurgical therapy [10, 225].

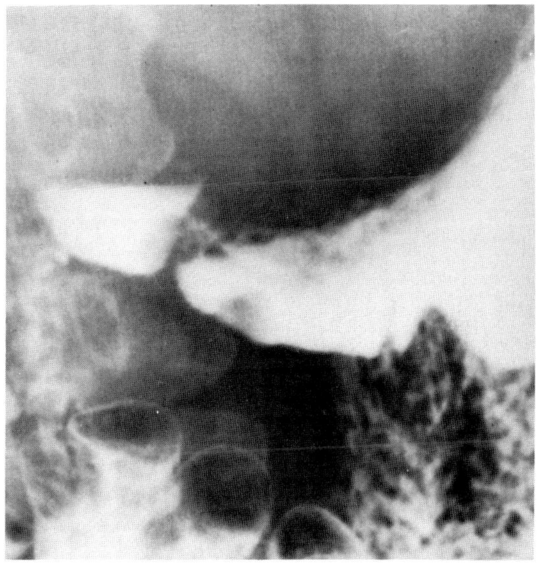

Fig. 21-3. Spot roentgenogram demonstrating a filling defect along the greater curvature in the antrum. At exploration there was a 1.5 cm subserosal hard mass, which was removed by wedge excision. Histological examination confirmed the presence of heterotopic pancreatic tissue. The patient made an uneventful recovery and has remained symptom-free. (Courtesy of Dr. Harry D. Fein.)

Heterotopic Pancreas
Pancreatic rests constitute by far the most common form of gastric heterotopia or hamartoma. An interesting instance of a nonpancreatic gastric hamartoma has been reported by Gruhn et al. [130]. Aberrant pancreas characteristically forms a solitary nodule that is usually less than 3 cm in diameter and is located in the antrum, most often along the greater curvature (Fig. 21-3). Unusual locations and multiple foci have been reported [79].

The prominent identifying characteristic is a small, central duct orifice that can be seen gastroscopically and that may even fill with barium [293, 325]. Detachment of a portion of the dorsal pancreatic primordium is the embryological basis for this lesion [21]. The tumor mass consists of densely packed pancreatic acini.

Aberrant pancreas usually causes no symptoms and is discovered incidentally during an operation for another disorder. When symptoms are present (25 percent of patients), they are related to partial pyloric obstruction or interference with gastric emptying [16, 113]. Less often, ectopic pancreas may be associated with ulceration, bleeding, and moderate dyspepsia. Even in patients in whom such symptoms are present, the symptoms are not necessarily caused by the heterotopic pancreas [89]. Local excision of the tumor is indicated if it is discovered incidentally intraoperatively or if it is identified preoperatively in a patient with symptoms.

Carcinoid Tumors
Tumors originating from argentaffin cells are unusual gastrointestinal neoplasms and are

very rare in the stomach. More than 70 instances of gastric carcinoid have been recorded in the literature [61]. These lesions behave differently clinically from their counterparts in the lower part of the small intestine and colon. Gastric carcinoids are often malignant in the sense that they show a propensity to metastasize, but long-term relief from symptoms is reported in patients in whom obvious tumor masses have been excised [1, 200, 305]. Gastric carcinoids usually are not associated with the carcinoid syndrome, although occasional instances are reported [292]. Stromal ossification may occur within these tumors [107, 305].

The relationship between carcinoid tumors and gastrointestinal ulceration remains unsettled. Typical duodenal ulcers occur in about one-fourth of patients with carcinoid tumors, and a giant duodenal ulcer associated with a gastric carcinoid has been reported by McCraken and Davenport [236]. Serotonin does not have intrinsic ulcerogenic properties, but high blood levels of serotonin have been alleged to act as a stimulus to histamine release. Complicating the situation is the histological resemblance of carcinoid tumors to pancreatic and duodenal adenomas, which are known to have ulcerogenic properties [114, 363, 365].

Gastric Teratoma

These are very rare lesions, 17 having been reported in the literature [77]. All of the lesions reported in association with the stomach have been in male patients and have been benign. Excision, which may involve an extensive gastric resection, is indicated.

SARCOMAS OF THE STOMACH. These malignant tumors comprise 2–5 percent of all gastric tumors and about 2 percent of all gastric cancers coming to operation [46, 144, 288, 348]. Sarcomas of the stomach rarely are reported in autopsy series of primary gastric tumors, probably because by the time the patient reaches autopsy many of these tumors are widely disseminated and are therefore classified as sarcomatosis. Sarcomas may develop from any of the mesenchymal elements in the gastric wall, but malignant lymphoma and leiomyosarcoma are by far the most common tumors of this group, comprising 95 percent of all gastric sarcomas (Table 21-2).

Table 21-2. Primary gastric sarcomas

Tumor type	Percent of all primary gastric sarcomas	
Lymphoma		75
Giant follicular	2	
Hodgkin	3	
Reticulum cell	25	
Lymphosarcoma	45	
Leiomyosarcoma		23
All others (fibrosarcoma, angiosarcoma, liposarcoma, neurogenic sarcoma, etc.)		2

A male preponderance is often reported for all gastric sarcomas, but the ratios are quite variable. Many statements suggest that sarcomas occur in a younger age group (by about one decade) than does carcinoma. Most important for clinical differentiation between carcinoma and sarcoma is the observation [229] that bulky malignant tumors occurring in young people tend to be sarcomas rather than carcinomas. Gastric sarcoma has a better prognosis than adenocarcinoma [25]. Sarcomas tend to remain localized for relatively long periods, thus allowing curative resection even of very bulky tumors.

Lymphoma

Most patients with gastric lymphoma are those in whom involvement of the stomach is secondary to disseminated disease. Such tumors rarely present diagnostic problems, and surgical therapy is required only occasionally to control complications such as acute massive gastrointestinal hemorrhage.

Less often the stomach is the site of a primary lymphoma arising from submucosal lymphoid tissue. There is a definite male preponderance in such instances [46]. Most frequently, primary gastric lymphomas are lymphosarcomas; less frequently they are reticulum cell sarcomas; and infrequently they are giant follicular lymphomas or primary Hodgkin disease lesions [215, 255, 366]. Dull epigastric pain and anorexia and weight loss are common symptoms. Bleeding has been reported in various amounts, but it is relatively frequent and in one series [288] occurred in half the patients with lymphomas. Coexisting ulcer disease occurs in a small percentage of patients, but achlorhydria is the more typical situation.

Primary lymphomas occur in all parts of the stomach. They are often large, bulky, and rubbery in consistency rather than hard; characteristically they show extensive surface ulceration. Athough at times they are polypoid or multilobulated, most often they present as a flat, intraluminal mass. Rarely they present as a diffusely infiltrative tumor of the gastric wall. An association between exposure to asbestos and gastrointestinal lymphoma has been suggested [296].

There may be considerable difficulty in differentiating grossly among malignant lymphoma, carcinoma, hypertrophic gastritis, and gastric pseudolymphoma. Pseudolymphoma has been associated with long survival periods because it is not a malignant lesion [14, 147, 232, 328, 359]. Nodular lymphoid hyperplasia of the stomach is another lesion that on occasion can be confused with lymphoma. Nodular lymphoid hyperplasia usually is limited to the small intestine, but occasionally the stomach is involved. Patients with the disorder have impaired humoral immunity caused by immunoglobulin deficiencies, with consequent susceptibility to infections, especially giardiasis [249].

Surgical exploration is indicated in all patients in whom a primary lymphoma appears to be confined to the stomach. Resection of the tumor, with wide margins, should be carried out whenever feasible. Despite their large bulk, most of these lesions have not metastasized at the time of exploration, and resection is possible in a high proportion of instances with good five-year survival rates. Total gastrectomy is indicated if it will permit complete removal of the tumor. The five-year survival rate of gastric lymphoma resected for cure is about 65 percent [66, 265].

Postoperative radiotherapy should be given to all patients, particularly those in whom the margins of resection have been close or inadequate or in whom the tumor has been incompletely removed. Postoperative radiation therapy also should be used in patients with tumors that are found at exploration not to be resectable.

Leiomyosarcoma

Leiomyosarcomas show some predilection for the distal stomach [228]. Since their growth is expansive rather than infiltrative, they tend to be well circumscribed and often present as pedunculated intragastric or exogastric tumors. The overlying mucosa is usually thinned out and ulcerated, often with a deep punched-out crater.

Symptoms are quite variable [210]. Pain, while common, usually is less severe than with other varieties of gastric sarcoma and may be confused with the pain of a peptic ulcer, since relief often is obtained with antacids [59]. Unlike ulcer pain, discomfort with leiomyosarcoma lacks periodicity. Significant weight loss and chronic bleeding are reported in about half of the patients with this lesion. Severe, acute hemorrhage is particularly characteristic of leiomyosarcoma, in contrast to other gastric sarcomas [368]. A majority of patients will demonstrate a palpable epigastric mass. Gastric analysis frequently shows hypochlorhydria or achlorhydria.

Clinically, leiomyosarcomas and other forms of gastric sarcoma mimic carcinoma and are generally so diagnosed preoperatively. Clues to a more precise diagnosis reside in the degree of general symptomatology. Sarcoma is more likely if the patient does not show severe anemia or cachexia, particularly when a rather large tumor mass is demonstrable. A large gastric tumor in a young person probably should be considered a sarcoma.

Adequate facilities for gastric cytological study [51] make exact diagnosis possible in a high percentage of instances, and endoscopic visualization of the tumor with direct biopsy often will establish the exact diagnosis. The occurrence together of a gastric leiomyosarcoma, a paraganglioma, and a chondroma has been reported as a new gastric tumor syndrome [54].

Leiomyosarcomas generally are isolated, well-localized tumors. Metastatic or invasive extension occurs comparatively late. Golden and Stout [121] have suggested that the behavior of these tumors is so relatively benign that they should be called *malignant leiomyomas*.

Leiomyosarcomas are more often resectable than lymphomas and generally require less radical surgical procedures. The extent of resection required must be determined at the time of exploration. Simple excision may be curative, but most leiomyosarcomas are best resected by a partial gastrectomy. Total gastrectomy is indicated if it permits complete removal of the lesion. Prolonged survival also has been recorded, even when it has been necessary to cut across tumor attached to the diaphragm or other adjacent structures to permit resection of the main tumor mass.

If the tumor is unequivocally nonresectable, a biopsy specimen should be obtained so that the diagnosis of sarcoma can be confirmed. If the lesion is not resectable or is incompletely removed, irradiation therapy should be given postoperatively. Leiomyosarcomas generally are regarded as radioresistant, but prolonged survival times have been recorded following treatment by irradiation [172].

Other Gastric Sarcomas

These are extremely rare tumors, and they exhibit histological characteristics compatible with the cell type of origin (fibrosarcoma, angiosarcoma, liposarcoma, neurogenic sarcoma). Lack of the usual palisaded appearance of regularly oriented muscle spindles and nuclei differentiate these sarcomas from leiomyosarcoma. Beyond this, these lesions frequently cannot be identified as to cell type of origin and are recorded simply as undifferentiated sarcoma. In comparison with leiomyosarcoma, these lesions tend to be associated more frequently with clinical symptoms. Their growth pattern within the gastric wall tends to be more infiltrative. The principles of treatment as outlined for leiomyosarcomas also apply to this group of tumors.

Primary Gastric Plasmacytoma

This is an extremely rare tumor. It is a focal variant of multiple myeloma, and in all reported instances it behaves as a malignant tumor with lymph node metastases and recurrence. The tumor is radiosensitive, and if identified and found to be confined to the stomach, it should be treated by gastric resection followed by irradiation. Steroids and chemotherapy are helpful in management of disseminated lesions [132].

Prognosis of Gastric Sarcoma

If results of all reports are analyzed, the five-year survival rate for patients with lymphoid tumors is about 15 percent and for those with leiomyosarcoma, about 25 percent. When the data are corrected, however, and patients who have had a gastric resection and have been followed for five years or more are considered, the five-year survival rate approaches 50 percent for primary lymphosarcoma, is about 40 percent for other lymphomas, and exceeds 60 percent for leiomyosarcoma [46, 161, 173, 210, 255, 348].

Most of the lymphoma survivors have been treated by gastrectomy of varying extent combined with postoperative irradiation therapy. The single factor that most influences the prognosis is the size of the tumor [46]. When resection is feasible, a reasonable cure rate can be expected. Even with extensive tumors, irradiation can save many patients.

In spite of the optimistic flavor of the foregoing figures, one must realize that not all series of gastric sarcomas show such a gratifying response to treatment. Palmer's report [271] on 21 patients seen in six years at the Walter Reed Hospital shows that in spite of a short time lapse from the onset of symptoms to institution of therapy (average four months), the longest survival time was 57 months and the average survival time only 15 months. While three of Palmer's patients had disseminated disease when first seen, the remainder had been considered candidates for cure. It is possible that the rampant course seen in this group of sarcoma patients is a reflection of their relative youth (15 of the 21 were younger than 40 years of age).

In any case, the usual experience with a gastric sarcoma is gratifyingly better than that with gastric adenocarcinoma. Therapy directed at cure is indicated for all of these lesions in spite of size and local extension when first seen. Postoperative irradiation should be used in every patient with primary gastric lymphoma and probably should be used in patients with leiomyosarcoma or other gastric sarcomas when any doubt exists as to complete extirpation of the primary lesion.

Carcinoma Metastatic to the Stomach

This syndrome is not as rare as might be thought. Metastases from the breast, for example, are not infrequent. Hartmann and Sherlock [137] reported that in an autopsy series of 204 patients who died of carcinoma of the breast, 38 had metastases involving the stomach (18 percent). Metastases were 6 times as frequent in patients who were receiving steroid therapy. If a patient with a carcinoma of the breast receiving adrenal steroid therapy has clinical signs of gastric bleeding, there is a 50 percent chance that the source will be a metastasis from the breast carcinoma rather than primary ulcer disease.

Other Rare Malignancies

SQUAMOUS CELL CARCINOMA OF THE STOMACH. This is a rare malignant tumor arising in gastric mucosa. Squamous metaplasia secondary to gastritis has been implicated as a possible precursor. In two instances reported by Eaton and Tennekoon [95], squamous cell carcinoma of the stomach followed a corrosive acid burn, a situation reminiscent of the development of Marjolin ulcer. Adenoacanthoma is another variant of gastric squamous cell carcinoma [70]. The clinical signs and symptoms and treatment of these lesions are the same as for adenocarcinoma of the stomach.

PRIMARY GASTRIC CHORIOEPITHELIOMA. This rare lesion has been reported 20 times [226, 349]. These tumors show both the gross and histological characteristics of genital chorioepitheliomas, and they usually exhibit systemic endocrine activity (gynecomastia, pituitary cytological changes, positive urine test for chorionic gonadotropin). Of the 20 reported patients, 12 were male. Whether the tumor arises in a teratoma or a germinal rest or represents a bizarre retrodifferentiation of adenocarcinoma is uncertain, although the last hypothesis is most attractive.

CARCINOSARCOMA. This is a very rare malignant neoplasm composed of both epithelial and nonepithelial elements [334]. The tumor should be treated in the same manner as an adenocarcinoma, that is, with resection with wide margins for all lesions confined to the stomach and immediately adjacent lymph nodes.

Gastric Diverticula, Duplications, and Cysts

DIVERTICULA OF THE STOMACH

Diverticula can be classified as false (acquired, traction, pseudo) or true (congenital, pulsion). Most false diverticula are secondary to benign ulceration, which leads to blind outpouching of the gastric wall following localized perforation or deep penetration of the ulcer. Central necrosis or ulceration of intramural tumors and defects at gastric anastomotic suture lines also may produce false diverticula [272].

True gastric diverticula are uncommon lesions, but more than 500 have been reported [103]. True diverticula often are thought to be caused by pulsion forces applied at areas of muscular weakness, but all layers of the gastric wall are found to be present on microscopical examination.

Gastric diverticula rarely are demonstrated before adulthood. They usually are single, are located high on the posterior gastric wall or the lesser curvature within 2 or 3 cm of the esophagogastric junction, and may be up to 5 cm in diameter. The diagnosis is made by roentgenographic examination (Fig. 21-4). The recent increase in the frequency of roentgenographic diagnosis is ascribable to more routine employment of maneuvers to demonstrate hiatal hernia, since these techniques also best show gastric diverticula [340].

Since 65 percent of patients in a collected series had their diverticula discovered in the

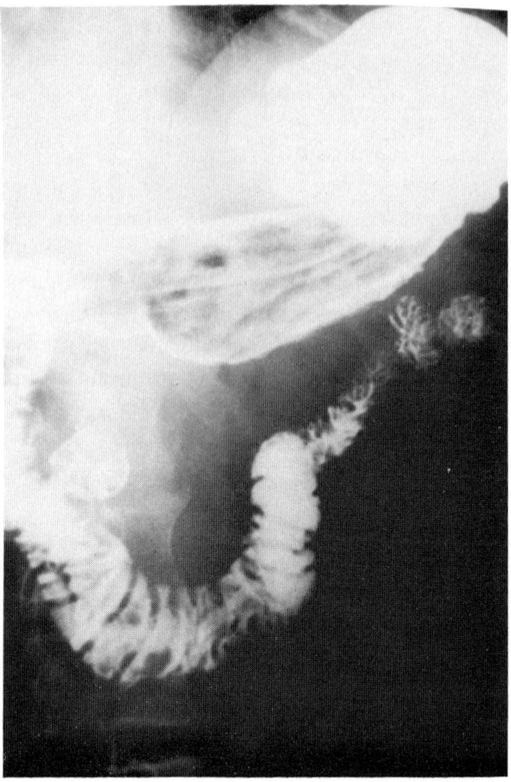

Fig. 21-4. Gastric and duodenal diverticula in typical locations. The gastric diverticulum arises from the upper lesser curvature; the duodenal diverticulum arises adjacent to the ampulla of Vater.

course of investigation for abdominal complaints, it would appear that these lesions can be associated with symptoms [103, 272, 318]. Half of the patients with symptoms complain of intermittent, nonradiating upper abdominal pain aggravated by meals, and another third have more vague dyspeptic complaints. Significant hemorrhage may occur [127].

Modification of eating habits will produce adequate relief in most patients with symptomatic gastric diverticula. The remainder may require surgical treatment if symptoms are persistent and relatively disabling. The surgical procedure of choice is amputation of the sac; invagination has resulted in ball-valve obstruction by the intragastric mass and should be avoided. Because the usual position of the diverticulum is high and posterior, a transthoracic approach has been advocated [276]. However, adequate exposure for resection of the diverticulum and closure of the gastric wound usually can be obtained through an abdominal approach.

DUPLICATION OF THE STOMACH

A true gastric duplication is a hollow structure lined with gastrointestinal epithelium and possessing a smooth muscular coat. The epithelium is usually gastric mucosa, although other types of intestinal mucosa occasionally may be found within the duplication. Duplications are intimately adherent to or are an integral part of the musculature of the normal stomach wall. About one-sixth of gastric duplications communicate with the lumen of the normal stomach, but the majority are blind structures.

It is quite difficult or impossible to separate a true gastric duplication from the wall of the normal stomach without injuring the stomach wall. This feature serves to differentiate a true gastric duplication from a dorsal enteric cyst, a lesion that is structurally similar but is not so intimately adherent to the stomach [129]. Gastric duplications also need to be differentiated from simple enterogenous cysts (see following section).

The stomach is the least common site in which duplications of the alimentary tract are found. Despite the fact that these are congenital lesions, they do not always produce symptoms early in life, and in up to 30 percent of the affected patients the diagnosis is not made until after 12 years of age.

Duplications have been found attached to every part of the stomach, but most are contiguous with the greater curvature [22]. The most frequent presenting symptoms and signs are a palpable abdominal mass, vomiting, weight loss or failure to thrive, and intermittent abdominal pain [11]. Anemia is present less often; melena and hematemesis are infrequent. Roentgenographically, an extramucosal mass bulging into the lumen of the barium-filled stomach is readily demonstrable.

The simplest treatment of gastric duplication is excision together with the part of the stomach to which the duplication is attached [371]. In very large or multiple duplications, the septum between the cyst and the main stomach may be excised, thereby converting the separate cyst and gastric cavities into one continuous structure [63, 138, 139, 259]. Brodie et al. [43] reported an instance of gastric duplication associated with duodenal ulcer in a young girl. The possibility of excessive gastrin production by the cystic duplication has been suggested [85] as a factor leading to duodenal ulceration in this situation.

CYSTS OF THE STOMACH WALL

More than half of the reported gross gastric cystic lesions are enterogenous cysts; about a third are echinococcal cysts, and the remainder are dermoids [270]. All of the cystic gastric lesions can be managed by adequate local excision. Enterogenous cysts and echinococcal cysts can be removed by submucosal enucleation if their large size demands an undesirable extent of resection.

An *enterogenous cyst* is a thin-walled, generally unilocular, fluid-filled sac lined with gastric mucosa most often found in the wall of the distal stomach. Although it may have a muscularis mucosa, an enterogenous cyst does not have a well-defined muscular wall and does not communicate with the lumen of the main stomach; these two features serve to differentiate an enterogenous cyst from a true gastric duplication.

These cysts are generally asymptomatic until they attain sufficient size to cause obstruction or a palpable epigastric tumor mass [281, 298]. Adenocarcinoma arising within a gastric enterogenous cyst is exceedingly rare, but it has been reported [234].

An *echinococcal cyst* is generally exogastric in location, probably because it is secondary to rupture or extension from a hydatid cyst of the liver, spleen, or kidney. Some cysts may drain into the stomach; they have been diagnosed by recovery of daughter cysts or larval fragments in gastric aspirate.

Dermoid cysts, like dermoids elsewhere, are composed of diverse tissues and may present as exogastric or intragastric masses.

Lesions Producing Obstruction

We are concerned here with those lesions, other than carcinoma and ulcer, that produce obstruction, typically at the pylorus or in the distal antrum. The major acquired lesion is gastric volvulus. Lesions that are of congenital origin but do not produce symptoms until adult life include pyloric and antral mucosal diaphragms, transpyloric mucosal prolapse, and adult hypertrophic pyloric stenosis. The major functional lesion is postvagotomy gastric atony.

GASTRIC VOLVULUS

Strictly speaking, the term *volvulus* implies complete obstruction, but modern definitions include a variety of clinical abnormalities brought about by torsion of the stomach with varying degrees of obstruction. The inclusion of nonstrangulating and nonobstructing varieties of abnormal gastric torsion as varieties of gastric volvulus and the more frequent and earlier application of operative therapy have increased our clinical understanding of this entity.

The stomach normally is held in place and torsion is resisted by several points of fixation. The most fixed anchor is the esophagus and its hiatus. The pylorus also is relatively fixed by the attachments of the postbulbar duodenum to the pancreas and portal triad. The lesser curvature is anchored to some degree by the left gastric artery and remnants of the dorsal mesentery. The greater curvature is held less firmly by the short gastric vessels and the peritoneal attachments of the spleen and transverse colon.

Some instances of volvulus or torsion may be idiopathic, but most of the time volvulus is secondary to an identifiable predisposing factor. Relaxation or loss of the ligamentous support of the stomach must be present in every instance of volvulus, since the normal stomach cannot be rotated through 180 degrees unless the gastrosplenic or gastrocolic ligaments are cut. In about 20 percent of patients with volvulus, there is a defect in the diaphragm (hiatal hernia, eventration) or a hernia of the abdominal wall into which the stomach rotates.

Types of Volvulus

Two planes of rotation in volvulus classically are described—mesenterioaxial and organoaxial. *Mesenterioaxial volvulus* is the most common type and usually is associated with chronic symptoms. In this situation the stomach rotates about the axis crossing the stomach transversely from the lesser to the greater curvature. Mesenterioaxial rotation can occur if there is loss of pyloric fixation, allowing the pylorus and antrum to double up toward the fundus. Less frequently, loss of splenic fixation allows the fundus and upper greater curvature to rotate distally into the right subhepatic area. In both situations the esophagogastric junction eventually comes to lie close to or even distal to the pylorus (Fig. 21-5).

Organoaxial volvulus occurs about the long cardiopyloric axis of the stomach. The entire body of the stomach may be involved in the twisting process, producing a picture resembling a wrung-out rag. More commonly, only a portion of the stomach body is involved or the twisting occurs either at the cardioesophageal or pyloric end only. Organoaxial rotation is the true volvulus, produces complete obstruction, and usually is associated with acute symptoms.

Mixed types of volvulus also occur. They usually begin as mesenterioaxial torsions producing approximation of the pyloric and cardioesophageal portions of the stomach. The unfixed stomach is predisposed thereby to further twisting in the organoaxial mode. With all types of volvulus, the rotating part may pass ventral or dorsal to the normal portion of the stomach, so that rotation can be considered to be either *anterior* or *posterior.*

Patients with Ehlers-Danlos syndrome are prone to gastric torsion and volvulus [211]. Other predisposing factors include defects in the anterior abdominal wall (hernia, omphalocele), which provide space into which the stomach may twist. Large gastric tumors may, because of their mass, lengthen gastric ligamentous attachments and create a tendency for the tumor to be "flipped," producing a volvulus. Other causes of volvulus include acute or chronic dilatation of the stomach and gastric ulcer, which, by creating adhesions to adjacent structures, may provide a fixed point for rotation of the remainder of the stomach.

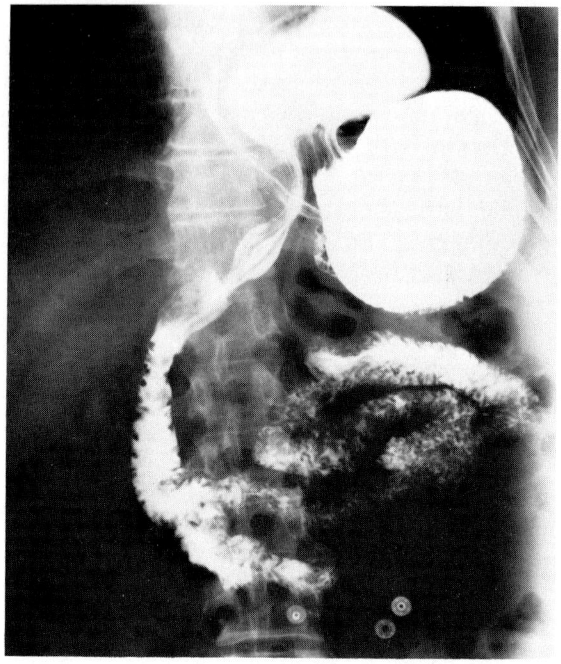

Fig. 21-5. Mesenterioaxial volvulus of the stomach has allowed the antrum and pylorus to herniate into the chest as a "paraesophageal" hernia. Volvulus is a common complication of all forms of hiatal hernia with intrathoracic stomach.

Clinical Symptoms

Two patterns of clinical symptoms occur. *Chronic volvulus* presents intermittent episodes of variable epigastric or substernal distress, which usually remit spontaneously [81]. In some patients who have torsion caused by a large diaphragmatic hernia, the complaints also include symptoms of impaired ventilation and dyspnea on exertion. Surgical therapy is directed at correcting the precipitating factors and anchoring the rotating part of the stomach. In high-risk patients, symptomatic control of chronic volvulus sometimes can be obtained with antacids, a bland diet, and elevation of the head of the bed.

Acute gastric volvulus is characterized by the sudden onset of severe epigastric pain followed by vomiting, which gives way to ineffectual retching associated with inability to pass a nasogastric tube. Abdominal distention and tenderness soon follow if the stomach is within the abdomen. But if most of the stomach has migrated into the chest (Fig. 21-5), there may be minimal abdominal findings [55]. The triad of repeated unsuccessful emetic attempts, circumscribed epigastric pain, and inability to pass a tube into the stomach (Borchardt-Lenormant triad) is pathognomonic [126]. If the volvulus is believed to be secondary to an associated lesion such as a hiatal hernia (and it usually is), removal or repair of the offending lesion can be performed at the primary operation if the risk involved is reasonable. Extensive correction should be reserved for a later date if any question exists concerning the patient's ability to tolerate the procedure.

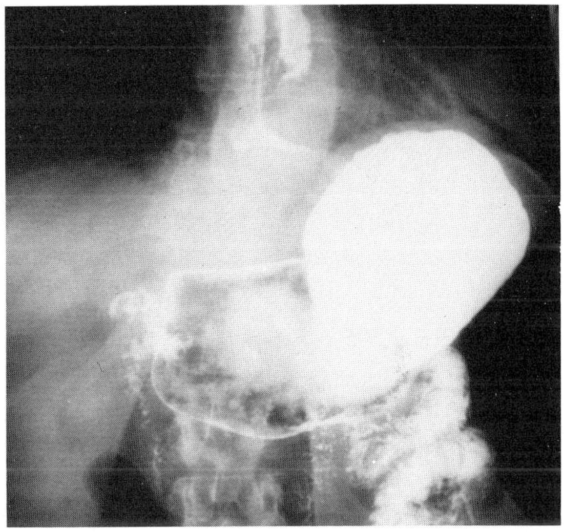

Fig. 21-6. Antral mucosal diaphragm. At operation there was a tiny eccentric orifice that just admitted the tip of a small hemostat. Despite this, the patient had grown normally and was somewhat overweight when the lesion was first demonstrated at the age of 54.

PYLORIC AND ANTRAL MUCOSAL DIAPHRAGM

More than 100 instances of these unusual lesions have now been reported [133, 274, 381]. The lesion is a thin diaphragm, consisting entirely of mucosa and submucosa, found either at the pylorus or in the antrum within 3 cm of the pylorus. Pyloric mucosal diaphragms are more common (70 percent of reported instances) and tend to be familial [18, 252, 332].

In adults a small orifice, usually situated eccentrically, is always present in the diaphragm. The edge of this orifice is soft and free of fibrosis, but it is of sufficient strength to resist dilation [298]. The lesion probably represents failure of recanalization of the embryonic gastrointestinal tube and is similar to congenital diaphragms and stenoses found elsewhere in the intestine. Indeed, anomalies elsewhere in the intestine should be sought whenever a pyloric or antral diaphragm is identified [135].

In adults, symptoms usually do not begin until middle age. This late onset has been explained as being caused by a progressive decrease in gastric tonus with advancing age [330]. The usual symptoms are nausea and vomiting following meals; pain and weight loss invariably are present. Some patients have reported relief with antacids. Gastric ulcers have been present in many reported instances and may be caused by antral retention producing excessive secretion of gastrin [315]. Hiatal hernia and reflux esophagitis also may be associated.

The roentgenographic appearance (Fig. 21-6) of this lesion is striking and diagnostic [119, 274]. The thin mucosal diaphragm produces a constant, knifelike filling defect transecting the distal antrum or the pylorus. Gastric retention is marked.

Gastrectomy has been the treatment usually carried out in these situations. Resection, however, seems illogical for this simple congenital deformity; treatment should be limited in most instances to simple excision of the membrane, perhaps combined with pyloroplasty [30, 274, 346].

TRANSPYLORIC PROLAPSE

This is a roentgenographic observation. In instances in which gastric mucosa prolapses through the pylorus, there is a mushroomlike defect in the base of the duodenal bulb with rugal folds extending through the pylorus. Benign or malignant pedunculated gastric tumors also may prolapse through the antrum to produce obstruction [165]. Prolapse of gastric mucosa is much more common than tumor prolapse.

Mucosal prolapse is demonstrated most commonly in men in their fifth and sixth decades of life, often in association with other gastric or duodenal disease. By far the most commonly associated lesion is duodenal ulcer. Hypertrophic or superficial chronic gastritis is also recorded as a frequent concomitant finding.

The existence of other gastrointestinal or hepatobiliary disease processes as a basis for any symptoms must be considered, and adequate diagnostic studies should be performed. Since prolapse may simulate a benign polypoid gastric tumor [72, 208], this possibility must be evaluated by endoscopic examination. If other lesions accompanying mucosal prolapse are identified, appropriate treatment of those lesions should be carried out.

If mucosal prolapse is an isolated finding, the roentgenographic observation should be ignored. Gastric mucosa normally is mobile in relation to the muscular gastric wall. Therefore, it is difficult to ascribe any symptoms to the peristaltic sweep of normally mobile mucosa transiently through the pylorus. Nonspecific management of ill-defined epigastric symptoms may be instituted in the form of a bland diet, mild sedatives, antacids, and antispasmodics. Surgical therapy is unnecessary in the management of mucosal prolapse.

ADULT PYLORIC HYPERTROPHIC STENOSIS

This lesion is characterized by the thickening of the circular pyloric muscle to 2 to 3 times normal size with a variable fusiform extension of the muscular hypertrophy proximally into the wall of the antrum. In adults, in contrast to children, the muscular hypertrophy may be focal and incomplete [188].

Although the onset of major symptoms occurs in middle age, in about one-fourth of the patients a history extending back to childhood is obtained. Patients complain of varying degrees of epigastric distress and bloating culminating in pernicious vomiting [219]. Roentgenographically, the pyloric canal is elongated, narrow, and somewhat unyielding. This distinctive roentgenographic appearance need not be present, however, and a proportion of patients will show a picture consistent with duodenal ulcer deformity or cicatricial pyloric stenosis, even when an ulcer cannot be demonstrated at subsequent operation [181]. The most frequent complications are the fluid and electrolyte disturbances commonly associated with other forms of pyloric stenosis. Bleeding has been reported in the absence of ulceration but is quite uncommon; perforation is even more rare [111].

In some instances the pyloric deformity cannot be differentiated preoperatively from chronic ulcer disease or infiltrative carcinoma. For this reason, and because nonsurgical treatment is not effective, an operation should be advised when this diagnosis is entertained in adults. At exploration, a nodular or generalized thickening of the pylorus is apparent with fibrous constriction of the lumen. The treatment of choice is pyloroplasty [95, 120, 145].

POSTOPERATIVE GASTRIC ATONY

The stomach may not recover emptying function postoperatively after either a resection or a drainage procedure [155]. Vagotomy, in particular, is thought to play a causative role [144]. In a typical instance, oral feeding is begun on the sixth postoperative day and is followed one or two days later by vomiting of undigested food without bile. Roentgenographic investigation shows a dilated stomach and failure of contrast material to leave the stomach. The apparent obstruction often appears to be complete since no contrast material enters the small intestine; in a few instances, a trickle of contrast medium can be seen to leave the stomach. Despite the roentgenographic appearance, there is no mechanical obstruction to gastric emptying in this disorder. The problem is an abnormality in coordination of gastric muscular contraction, is not related to electrolyte or other disturbance, and eventually remits spontaneously in most instances. The objectives in clinical management are to confirm the absence of mechanical obstruction, maintain nutritional status, and attempt to improve gastric emptying while awaiting the expected recovery of function.

Parenteral nutrition should be instituted when the diagnosis is suspected. Endoscopic confirmation of the open gastric outlet should be obtained after the tenth postoperative day. Administration of metoclopramide or bethanechol chloride (Urecholine) should be tried; both drugs should be tested, since a patient may respond to one but not the other. If drug therapy succeeds, oral feedings may be resumed. If not, parenteral nutrition should be continued. The disorder usually disappears after three or four weeks, but may persist as long as three months. Reoperation and reresection, formerly advised as treatment for this condition, are not advisable. Unless near-total gastrectomy is accomplished, there is no evidence that reoperation and any lesser resection procedure influences the course of postoperative gastric atony.

Dilatation and Rupture of the Stomach

ACUTE DILATATION OF THE STOMACH

Fifty years ago acute gastric dilatation was commonly listed as a cause of death. Now it is rarely so listed, probably because gastric distention is promptly treated today by nasogastric suction. Acute dilatation of the stomach is seen most often after upper abdominal operations, but it can occur in any debilitating illness (particularly in the elderly), after starvation, in peritonitis, and after abdominal trauma [160]. It is frequently associated with gastric hemorrhage.

Acute dilatation probably is a variety of segmental ileus; inhibition of an intrinsic motor pacemaker has experimental support [184]. Dilatation often is aggravated by aerophagia in apprehensive or dyspneic patients. Iatrogenic dilatation may be produced by vigorous ventilation of a patient during induction of anesthesia or by administration of nasal oxygen if the oxygen catheter tip is placed well into the hypopharynx. Even with the use of green plastic catheters to identify the route of oxygen administration, the simultaneous administration of nasal oxygen when nasogastric suction also is being employed is a potentially hazardous practice. Transposition of the tube connections, with delivery of oxygen under pressure into the stomach, results in disaster.

Symptoms of acute dilatation may not be specific. Patients usually have hiccups and may complain of heartburn. Frequently, small emeses occur. Symptoms may be more dramatic and may mimic angina pectoris, myocardial infarction, or pulmonary embolus. It is good to remember that shock can occur in acute gastric dilatation caused by interference with caval blood flow [275].

Examination of a patient with acute gastric dilatation shows the upper abdomen to be distended and tympanitic. A succussion splash may be demonstrable. Plain abdominal roentgenograms usually will demonstrate the distended stomach and confirm the clinical impression [164].

The greatest danger of gastric dilatation lies in aspiration of vomitus with resultant pneumonia or even drowning. In the postoperative patient, disruption of suture lines is an additional danger. Occasionally rupture of the intact stomach may occur [204, 335]. Treatment requires prompt passage of a nasogastric tube, institution of gastric suction, and appropriate fluid replacement.

SPONTANEOUS PERFORATION AND RUPTURE

Spontaneous perforation of the stomach is exceedingly rare in adults. It usually occurs in the region of the upper lesser curvature near the esophagogastric junction and is associated with severe vomiting. The sudden vomiting also produces mucosal lacerations in the region of the cardioesophageal junction and results in massive gastrointestinal hemorrhage similar to that seen in the Mallory-Weiss syndrome, but the lacerations are deeper and extend across the cardioesophageal junction. Rupture of the stomach probably is secondary to the transient formation of a closed loop followed by a sudden increase in intraluminal pressure as a consequence of vomiting [159].

The sudden appearance of signs of peritoneal irritation in the epigastrium associated with upper gastrointestinal hemorrhage following an episode of forceful vomiting should immediately lead to a suspicion of gastric rupture. Roentgenograms of the upper abdomen may show free air or air trapped in the lesser sac or dissecting the tissues along the upper lesser curvature. Treatment is immediate exploration and repair of the laceration as outlined below for the management of traumatic perforations.

A related lesion, the Boerhaave syndrome, also is produced by forceful vomiting and results in a rupture limited to the distal esophagus; significant hematemesis is unusual in this lesion, while empyema of the left chest is a regular consequence.

TRAUMATIC GASTRIC PERFORATION

Traumatic perforation of the stomach usually is secondary to a penetrating wound, although blunt external trauma rarely may be the cause [69, 382]. The diagnosis usually is indicated by the history of injury plus the demonstrable entry wound or ecchymosis in a patient presenting with or in whom signs develop of upper abdominal peritonitis. The diagnosis is substantiated by the demonstration of free peritoneal air on physical examination or roentgenogram and by the return of bloody gastric juice from a nasogastric tube. In evaluating wounded patients, one must be aware that gastric wounds rarely exist in isolation and frequently are associated with injury to adjacent structures.

Preoperative resuscitative measures include nasogastric suction, rapid blood replacement, and control of any associated pneumothorax or hemothorax. Operative exploration should be performed as soon as possible through an upper midline incision to control hemorrhage and to minimize leakage of gastric contents. After rapid clearing of blood clot and food from the peritoneal cavity, active bleeding should be controlled and any sucking diaphragmatic wound sutured.

The number and extent of gastric wounds should then be determined. For every wound of entry, a wound of exit must be sought. It is mandatory to enter the lesser sac through the gastrocolic omentum to inspect the posterior gastric wall and the pancreas. Wounds of exit may be particularly difficult to identify high along the posterior greater curvature, where they may be hidden between the leaves of the gastrosplenic omentum.

Lacerations of the stomach should be closed by two-layer inverting suture; purse-string suture of small perforations is undesirable because it does not control the large submucosal vessels. If damage to the stomach is extensive, partial gastrectomy may be required. Drainage may be indicated in specific situations, but generally it is not required for traumatic gastric wounds.

FOREIGN BODIES IN THE STOMACH

Ingested foreign bodies in the stomach may remain as individual objects or aggregate to form a *bezoar*. Individual foreign objects in the stomach may be anything that can traverse the oropharynx (Fig. 21-7). Fantastic collections

Fig. 21-7. Multiple gastric foreign bodies. Pyloric obstruction resulted from impaction in the pylorus of the rubber sink-stopper, which was attached to the end of the long chain in the stomach.

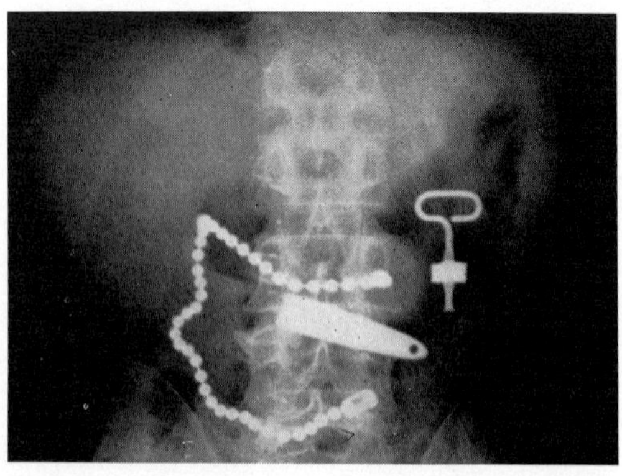

can accumulate, and every hospital seems to have at least one "character" who is seen at intervals with *another* foreign body in his or her stomach.

There is little doubt that a derangement of personality exists in many patients presenting repeatedly with gastric foreign bodies. Ingestion of foreign bodies is also common in the mentally retarded [302]. Devanesan and colleagues [84] reported on a man who, over the course of eleven years in a state hospital, managed to accumulate in his stomach 648 separate objects. The world record for such events seems to be held by a patient from whom 2533 foreign objects were recovered.

Accidental ingestion also occurs, usually as an isolated episode. In certain occupations, however, the practice of holding needles, tacks, or nails in the mouth while working may produce repeated accidental ingestions [311].

While most individual foreign bodies pass the pylorus unaided and ultimately are passed in the stool, sharp objects may penetrate the stomach wall and require endoscopic or surgical removal. Larger objects or accumulations of many objects may produce ulceration with pain, bleeding, or obstruction, and they should be recovered surgically. Needless to say, psychiatric evaluation and aid should be sought for chronic offenders.

BEZOARS AND CONCRETIONS

Bezoars are of diverse types and consist of agglutinated, molded, or matted masses of hair (trichobezoars), vegetable matter (phytobezoars), or combinations of the two (trichophytobezoars). Concretions are rare forms of bezoars made up of precipitated or solidified chemicals that have been ingested purposely or accidentally. The commonest concretion is the shellac-resin mass that occurs with repeated ingestion (for its alcohol content) of furniture polish.

Trichobezoars

Masses of matted hair may completely fill the stomach and form a cast of the organ. Frequently a tail of hair extends through the pylorus and into the duodenum. Occasionally a mass of hair may be carried into the small intestine and result in mechanical small intestinal obstruction, [353] or hair may become lodged in the appendix [105].

Most affected patients are under 30 years of age, and 90 percent are women. These statistics are in keeping with the factors encouraging trichophagy—the presence of long hair accessible to the mouth in girls and the nervous habits more frequently present and more socially acceptable in younger women. Less than 15 percent of patients harboring a trichobezoar exhibit frank mental illness, but psychoneurotic problems are a prominent feature of these patients.

The hairball presents the clinical features of a movable epigastric mass in a patient complaining of abdominal pain, nausea, and vomiting. Weight loss, weakness, and malabsorption occur in a minority of patients.

Complications that can ensue are obstruction (11 percent), ulceration (10 percent), and inanition (8 percent). The symptoms and complications are caused by obstruction of the food pathway and irritation of the mucosa. Anorexia and starvation, which may be associated with trichobezoars, are secondary to the underlying neurosis. Once a diagnosis has been established, removal is mandatory. If the hair mass is small enough, or can be broken up, the possibility of endoscopic removal can be entertained. Often, surgical removal proves necessary.

Phytobezoars

Since the advent of vagotomy and partial gastric resection for peptic ulcer disease, the incidence of phytobezoars has steadily increased. Postgastrectomy bezoars can add considerably to postoperative morbidity [52, 241, 331]. Development of a phytobezoar has also been noted in patients with diabetic gastroparesis [53].

Various vegetable structures, such as leaves, roots, seeds, and fibers, become molded together in a firm mass to form a phytobezoar. The accumulation of yeast cells, *gastric mycosis,* occurs in up to one-third of patients after vagotomy and resection; in some instances, aggregates of yeast may form [285]. About 70 percent of phytobezoars follow the ingestion of persimmons. Because of the frequency of persimmon bezoars, they have been given a separate designation, *diospyrobezoar* [78]. Persimmons contain soluble resins that are converted by gastric juice into a tenacious gum that agglutinates seed and skin fragments of the ingested persimmon. Other forms of phytobezoars are chunks of insoluble and indigestible vegetable material, often of citrus fruit origin, that have been mechanically aggregated into a solid mass [82].

Phytobezoars differ from trichobezoars in that most occur in patients older than 30 years of age, and 75 percent of affected patients are men. Phytobezoars also tend to be smaller than trichobezoars and less often are palpable on abdominal examination. Clinical signs and symptoms of phytobezoars are pain, nausea, and vomiting, present singly or in combination, in three-fourths of patients. A minority of patients report weight loss or weakness or have a demonstrable abdominal mass.

Complications are the same as those listed above for trichobezoars, but the incidence of all complications with the exception of inanition is much higher. Starvation occurs in only 1 percent of these patients, but obstruction and ulceration each occur in about 25 percent.

The initial treatment approach to all but the largest phytobezoars is to disrupt the mass with enzymes or with bicarbonate lavage [75, 76, 279, 319]. Often after initial enzyme treatment, the mass can be broken up by forceps manipulation through an endoscope. The objective is to reduce the bezoar to pieces small enough to pass through the intestine and be eliminated. The addition of metoclopramide to the regimen has been helpful [377]. Surgical removal of a phytobezoar is needed only in unusual situations.

Inflammatory and Infectious Lesions of the Stomach

The common forms of both acute and chronic gastritis are considered elsewhere in this volume. What remains for discussion is a heterogenous collection of curious gastric mucosal afflictions.

ALKALINE (BILE REFLUX) GASTRITIS

Bilious vomiting following gastric resection and gastrojejunostomy may not be caused by only an afferent loop syndrome. The presence of duodenal content in the stomach can induce vomiting [239]. If the bilious vomit is not foul in nature, alkaline reflux gastritis should be suspected [49, 347]. The clinical symptom triad is of epigastric pain, often quite severe, accompanied by bilious vomiting and weight loss.

The onset of alkaline gastritis occurs months to years after an operation for ulcer disease. Roentgenogram of the upper gastrointestinal tract show nothing abnormal. Iron deficiency anemia and hypochlorhydria often are found. The diagnosis is confirmed endoscopically by visualization of free reflux of bile into the stomach in the presence of diffuse gastritis [183, 221].

Lawson [202] demonstrated experimentally that reflux of bile and duodenal content into the stomach resulted in inflammation of gastric mucosa. Du Plessis [93] observed the same sequence of events in patients. Release of gastrin augments bile flow [253] and enhances regurgitation of duodenal contents into the stomach [182]. Teorel [339] postulated that gastric mucosa acts as a semipermeable membrane, in effect a "barrier." This barrier can be functionally "broken" by a number of substances, including bile. The relevant physiology has been reviewed by Ritchie [290] and by Fromm [115].

Treatment with cholestyramine is often effective. This resin serves to chelate bile salts; if fed between meals, it may reduce the degree of gastritis so that symptoms are tolerable or even absent [310]. Surgical therapy should be undertaken in patients who have severe symptoms or who do not respond well to or tolerate cholestyramine therapy.

Simple conversion of a Billroth II anastomosis to a gastroduodenostomy has been helpful in some patients, but it has a high failure rate [2]. Similarly, the Henley-Hedenstedt je-

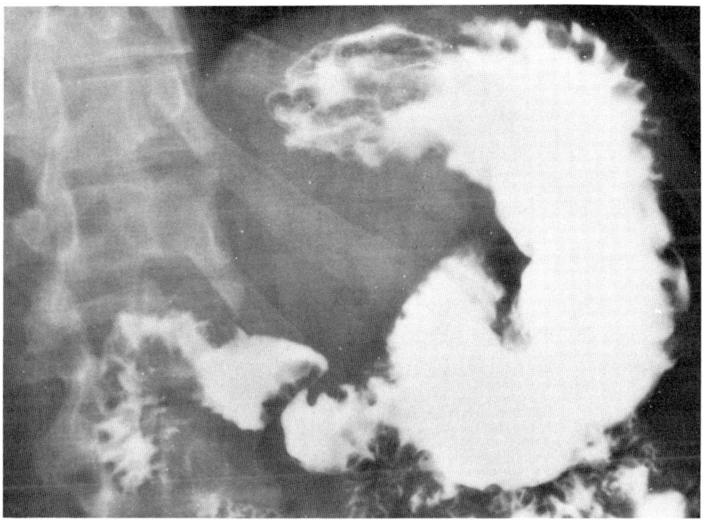

Fig. 21-8. Large folds of hypertrophic gastric mucosa, mainly in the fundus and body of the stomach. These folds are typical of Ménétrier disease.

junal interposition gastroduodenal loop procedure results in improvement in only half the patients so treated [352]. The long (40-cm) Roux-en-Y gastrojejunostomy and the Tanner "19" loop seem to have the best record of success; the conditions of up to 84 percent of patients having these Roux-en-Y procedures have been improved [39, 306]. All these diversionary procedures are potentially ulcerogenic; a complete vagotomy should be accomplished in every instance.

MÉNÉTRIER DISEASE

This entity is characterized by the presence of giant hypertrophic mucosal folds of the stomach, protein-losing gastropathy, and hypoproteinemia. The incidence of Ménétrier disease is said to be increased in families with polyendocrine adenomatosis, but unlike the Zollinger-Ellison syndrome and other endocrine adenoma syndromes, Ménétrier disease is uncommonly associated with peptic ulcer. Evolution of hypertrophic mucosa to atrophic gastritis has been reported [29].

The features that serve to identify patients with Ménétrier disease are as follows:

1. Hypertrophy of the gastric mucosa with giant rugal folds involving the fundus, cardia, and body of the stomach but sparing the antrum (Fig. 21-8)
2. Mucosal hypertrophy consisting of mucus-secreting cells with diminished or absent parietal cells and chief cells
3. Gastric hypersecretion of large volumes containing excess mucus, a greatly increased protein concentration, and low-to-absent acid concentration
4. Systemic hypoproteinemia secondary to the loss of serum proteins from the gastric mucosa [74, 309].

The etiology of Ménétrier disease is unknown, although it appears to be an acquired lesion. The rate of progression of the disease is quite variable, and spontaneous regression has been documented [112]. A unique instance with abrupt onset and a short course followed by complete resolution has been reported. In this instance it seems likely that the clinical symptoms and findings represented an allergic reaction [206].

Although a connection has been suggested in the past between Ménétrier disease and gastric carcinoma, the relationship is probably coincidental [282, 300]. Although patients with minimal-to-moderate symptoms can compensate for their protein loss by increased albumin synthesis and turnover, patients with severe symptoms have life-threatening losses of both albumin and gamma globulin. Nonsurgical therapy in such instances is not effective [180, 186]. Total gastrectomy should be performed, preferably with construction of a jejunal food pouch [7, 309].

CORROSIVE GASTRITIS

This is a severe form of gastric mucosa inflammation caused by accidental or suicidal ingestion of either strong alkali or acid. Caustic (alkaline) chemicals produce liquefaction necrosis of the gastric mucosa. Because normal gastric acidity tends to neutralize caustic agents, their most marked effect is usually in the mouth and esophagus, although gastric burns can also occur. Strong acids tend to spare the esophagus and to cause serious gastric lesions, since they are not neutralized in the stomach and they destroy the mucosa by coagulation. Other chemical agents such as phenol and formalin also tend to destroy the mucosa by coagulation.

Lye is the most common agent that produces corrosive injury of the stomach [9]. The severity of injury depends on the original strength of the agent and its ultimate concentration in the stomach as well as the duration of mucosal contact. All grades of inflammation from simple hyperemia to maceration and perforation may occur. A squamous cell carcinoma following lye-induced corrosive gastritis has been reported [95].

Acute management is directed at removing, diluting, and neutralizing the agent. Neutralization of strong acids can be obtained with common antacids (e.g., milk, aluminum hydroxide, milk of magnesia), while dilute vinegar or citrus fruit juice may be helpful following alkali ingestion.

Removal is best accomplished by aspiration and lavage carried out through a soft, nontraumatic tube. Emesis is not recommended, since it may cause further esophageal damage; but emesis should be induced if evacuation and neutralization are not possible. Some corrosive chemicals such as mercury bichloride are also systemic poisons; if these have been ingested, prompt lavage must be supplemented by antidotes, catharsis, and systemic treatment.

Patients who do not have extensive gastric necrosis should be treated with oral antacids and parenteral steroids and antibiotics. Administration of cortisone or hydrocortisone may prevent scarring [60].

Mucosal damage in corrosive gastritis may be complicated by hemorrhage or perforation. Management beyond that previously outlined should be supportive, using sedation, antibiotics, intravenous fluids, analgesics, and blood transfusion as required. Laparotomy for corrosive perforation of the stomach is necessary only in the rare instance of near-total dissolution of the stomach or esophagus. In such situations, esophagogastrectomy with exteriorization of the proximal esophagus in the neck and tube duodenostomy are usually necessary. Thoracotomy can be avoided—the esophagus can be removed bluntly from the mediastinum. Anastomosis in the acute phase is to be avoided [87]. A feeding jejunostomy should be created. The late sequelae of corrosive gastritis are caused by scarring of the injured stomach wall. Antral or pyloric obstruction may require resection, pyloroplasty, or gastrojejunostomy (Fig. 21-9).

GASTROMALACIA

Gastromalacia is characterized by an acute erosive process involving nearly all the gastric mucosa and associated with a gelatinous softening of the remaining layers of the stomach wall. The erosion and softening may progress to actual dissolution. In contrast to inflammatory forms of gastritis, there is little or no inflammatory response in gastromalacia. This lesion is seen predominantly in patients with acute disorders of the central nervous system and probably is related to Cushing ulcer. If perforation occurs, the resultant defect is so large and the leak so massive that hope for recovery lies only in prompt recognition and operation. Survival of a patient with this lesion has been recorded [26], but the high mortality

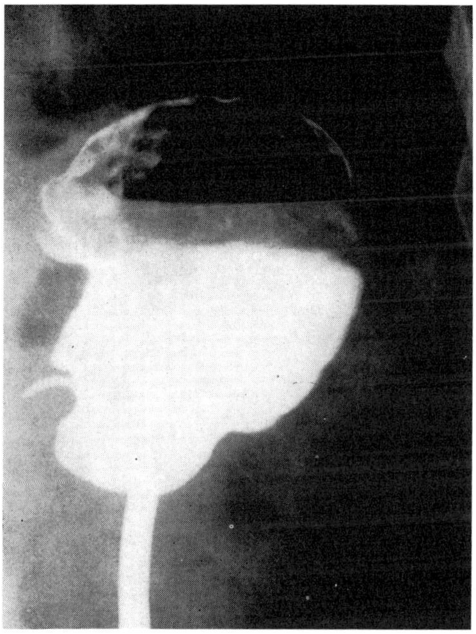

Fig. 21-9. Esophageal and pyloric strictures caused by ingestion of a large volume of lye. The barium used in this examination was introduced through a gastrostomy tube.

of gastromalacia is indicated by the fact that most references in the literature regard it as an agonal process [73].

SUPPURATIVE GASTRITIS

Suppurative (phlegmonous) gastritis is a rare and frequently fatal bacterial infection that produces a spreading intramural cellulitis of the stomach wall. The mode of infection leading to suppurative gastritis remains obscure. Hematogenous dissemination of bacteria has been suggested, but there is no adequate explanation to account for the discrete localization of this infectious process in the wall of the stomach. Direct invasion through the gastric mucosa is another possibility, although ulcers or other mucosal defects usually are not found in affected patients. Hemolytic streptococcus is the most common infecting organism, but many other bacteria, particularly fecal organisms, have been implicated [327].

The rarity of serious infections of the stomach wall is remarkable when one thinks of the number of patients with ulcerated stomach carcinoma and similar lesions and the constant stream of swallowed infective material to which the stomach is exposed. Typically, suppurative gastritis occurs in middle-aged male alcoholics with hypochlorhydria, and it usually complicates a preexisting gastric lesion [100].

There are no pathognomonic signs or symptoms. The patient presents signs of an acute abdomen and septicemia. There is usually sudden onset of nausea, continuous vomiting, and fever and prostration. Abdominal pain and rigidity are present initially in the epigastrium; subsequently, signs of peritonitis become generalized. Fulminant infection and progression to death within a few hours may occur.

A diagnosis of phlegmonous gastritis must be considered in a patient with a history of ethanol intake and a recent bout of gastritis or respiratory infection who presents with acute upper abdominal pain, fever, signs of peritonitis, and purulent ascitic fluid. Definitive treatment appears to be resection or drainage of the stomach combined with large doses of systemic antibiotics [240].

A diagnosis of suppurative gastritis rarely is made preoperatively. Usually the patient's abdomen is explored because there are progressing signs of peritonitis. At exploration the stomach appears discolored; the serosa may be covered with a fibrinopurulent exudate that usually does not extend beyond the cardia or pylorus. If the process involves only a portion of the stomach, a partial gastric resection may be carried out [257]; otherwise, the stomach is best left alone, and the patient should be treated vigorously with systemic antibiotics.

Necrotizing Gastritis

This condition is a variant of phlegmonous suppurative gastritis in which the causative organisms are the fusiform and spirochetal organisms commonly present in the mouth. They produce a primary necrosis and gangrene of the stomach wall rather than an intramural cellulitis or abscess. Successful management requires early recognition, either preoperatively or at laparotomy; prompt institution of intensive antibiotic therapy; and appropriate supportive measures. Successful outcomes have resulted from completely nonsurgical supportive and antibiotic therapy.

Intramural Gastric Abscess

The clinical course of this disorder is similar to that described for suppurative gastritis. The bacteria involved, primarily hemolytic streptococci, also are similar. The abscess typically is located in the submucosa [250]. Segmental or distal gastrectomy is usually required.

GRANULOMATOUS GASTRITIS

Tuberculosis of the stomach is rare. When found, it usually is secondary to active pulmonary tuberculosis. The gastric lesion usually consists of multiple ragged ulcers with undermined edges and caseous bases. Discrete gray tubercles may be visible in or adjacent to the ulcer or, more rarely, may be present alone as a nonulcerative form of mucosal tuberculous infection. Serosal scarring is prominent, and the draining lymph nodes often are caseous.

The diagnosis can be difficult to establish, but it should be considered in any patient with known pulmonary tuberculosis in whom an antral ulcer or deformity develops. Endoscopic examination of the gastric lesion together with biopsy should be carried out. Histological demonstration of a granuloma-containing tubercle bacillus absolutely establishes the diagnosis. In general, gastric tuberculosis is treated with appropriate antibiotic agents. Those patients who have extensive scarring with obstruction should be treated by gastric resection after a preliminary course of antibiotic therapy.

Mycoses and other nontuberculous granulomatous lesions of the stomach are described at intervals in the literature. Recent reports have been of histoplasmosis [260], actinomycosis [235, 350], and sarcoidosis [195]. Candidiasis is an uncommon infection of the stomach; patients who have had a gastric resection appear to be somewhat more predisposed to the development of this lesion [285]. The endoscopic appearance of yeast infections of the gastric mucosa is quite characteristic [277]. Syphilis of the stomach was never very common and is now quite rare [287].

Eosinophilic granuloma is a rare gastric lesion of unknown cause. An eosinophilic infiltration of the stomach wall occurs as either a diffuse or a focal process. This lesion is unrelated to the xanthomatous eosinophilic granuloma of bone. It may be a precursor of lymphoma. When localized, the gastric granuloma forms a polypoid mass that can grow to several centimeters in diameter and can become pedunculated. The most common location is the prepyloric area. Eosinophilic infiltration of the stomach, particularly in focal form, may be associated with symptoms of obstruction, ulceration, or hemorrhage. In either the diffuse or focal form, the disease is easily misinterpreted as carcinoma. Management of this lesion should follow that outlined for adenomas and other benign tumors.

Herpes zoster involving the upper gastrointestinal tract has been thought to be very rare. However, vesicular herpetic lesions can be seen in the esophagus and stomach if sought while skin lesions are present [118, 379].

CROHN DISEASE OF THE STOMACH

Involvement of the stomach by regional enteritis is extremely rare. There is always associated disease elsewhere in the intestine, typically in the distal small intestine and often also in the duodenum. A roentgenographic sign, the so-called ram's horn sign, has been described and is thought to be characteristic of Crohn disease of the stomach [106]. Clinically and roentgenographically, regional enteritis involving the proximal duodenum or distal antrum can mimic peptic ulcer disease. In patients known to have ileal or colonic Crohn disease, however, a disease process involving the antral-duodenal region and appearing to be ulcer disease is more likely to be Crohn disease [47, 108, 345, 378].

EMPHYSEMATOUS GASTRITIS

Air in the gastric wall may have bacterial or nonbacterial causes; each type presents a characteristic roentgenographic appearance

[256]. The nonbacterial syndrome usually results from pyloric obstruction or is associated with rupture of an emphysematous bulla into the esophageal wall, with subsequent dissection of air into the gastric wall. In many respects this is reminiscent of the process involved in pneumatosis cystoides intestinalis of the colon. The gas appears on abdominal roentgenogram as a linear collection outlining the gastric wall; it does not change with alteration of the patient's position, which serves to differentiate intramural from intraluminal gas collections. Linear gas collections that are limited to the fundus suggest that there has been injection of air into the gastric wall during endoscopy. Benign interstitial gastric emphysema is also seen occasionally after lye ingestion [62], accompanying distal obstruction, and in massive intestinal infarction caused by occlusion of the superior mesenteric artery.

In instances of severe bacterial infection of the gastric wall (see Suppurative Gastritis, p. 595), intramural collections of gas may be found. In this situation the gas collections are bubbly and frothy and are irregularly distributed within the thickened wall of the stomach [136]. On extremely rare occasions, the irregular collections of gas and edematous gastric wall may simulate a carcinoma. Angiography will help to differentiate these two entities, since the carcinomas are poorly vascularized, whereas suppurative gastritis shows a hyperactive and dilated circulation [190].

Miscellaneous Gastric Lesions

ANGIODYSPLASIA

Wider use of angiography for diagnosis has led to recognition that vascular malformations are a relatively frequent cause of bleeding. Although most of these lesions occur in the colon, they may be found elsewhere in the gastrointestinal tract and, rarely, in the stomach and duodenum. Aortic valve disease occurs in a disproportionate number of patients with gastroduodenal angiodysplasia [361].

Each lesion consists of a nest of dilated capillaries and venules in the mucosa and submucosa. They tend to bleed abruptly and massively, and cease, often before diagnostic studies can be accomplished. Angiography is the best diagnostic examination; some lesions can be visualized at endoscopy. Surgical treatment is indicated if a lesion causes bleeding. The involved tissue is excised as a wedge with a minimal border of surrounding normal gastric or duodenal wall. Sometimes a partial-thickness wedge excision to include the abnormal submucosal vessels will suffice [207].

DIEULAFOY GASTRIC EROSION

Chronic gastritis predisposes to vascular dysplasia, which leads to thrombosis and necrosis of the arterial wall before rupture and exigent hemorrhage. It seems that the common denominator that triggers this pathological sequence is drug (usually alcohol) abuse. The pathological entity occurs in about 1.3 percent of patients who undergo an operation for massive gastric bleeding [174].

HETEROTOPIC GASTRIC MUCOSA

Gastric mucosa may be located heterotopically anywhere in the gastrointestinal tract, but it is more frequently reported in association with a Meckel diverticulum or with a duplication of the ileum. Gastric mucosa has been reported in the tongue [131]; in the duodenum [166]; in the gallbladder [28, 258]; in the wall of the cystic duct, where it produced obstruction [380]; in the main hepatic duct, where it caused intermittent jaundice [176]; in a rectal polyp [122, 171]; and in a rectal duplication [324].

DORSAL ENTERIC GASTRIC CYSTS

Dorsal enteric cysts are congenital lesions similar in structure to duplications of the intestine except that they are not intimately attached to the muscle of the normal intestine. They can be found in a wide variety of locations. Not infrequently they are situated in the gastrocolic omentum. Gastroenterogenous cysts may ascend into the pleural cavity or mediastinum and on occasion may communicate with a bronchus, producing "peptic bronchitis" [267, 269].

AMYLOIDOSIS
Amyloid rarely involves the stomach wall. When it does, it produces a marked, leathery thickening of the muscularis, together with mucosal ulceration and hemorrhage [222]. When the pylorus is involved, complete obstruction with tumorlike filling defects can occur. The general debility of patients with amyloidosis, together with the widespread disease in the stomach itself, makes resection extremely liable to complications of faulty healing [192].

INTESTINAL HETEROTOPIA IN THE STOMACH
An intestinal type of epithelium may be found in the stomach as a result of persistence of a congenital rest or as the result of faulty regeneration following chronic irritation (intestinal metaplasia). Aberrant intestinal epithelium tends to be found more frequently in patients of advanced age and in those with atrophic gastritis, gastric ulcer, gastric polyps, or carcinoma. The aberrant tissue not only looks like normal small intestine histologically but also can function as an absorptive mucosa [301].

SITUS INVERSUS
Situs inversus can be either limited to the stomach or part of a more generalized mirror-image anatomical configuration. It can create considerable problems of gastroenterological diagnosis. This subject has been reviewed by Lopez-Gallart [216].

Duodenal Trauma

Most patients suffering injuries to the duodenum are between 20 and 40 years of age, and men predominate in a ratio of 7 to 1. Injuries to the duodenum are unique in two additional respects. The first is the desultory nature of the symptoms in many patients, which leads to delay in diagnosis. The second feature, related to the first, is the high mortality. Although mortality has been steadily decreasing over the past four decades, it still is on the order of 30 percent in many reported series.

The development of specialized intensive care units has been associated with a further decrease in mortality [68]. But the high incidence of major injury to organs immediately surrounding the duodenum, coupled with the high complication rate, continues to yield mortalities on the order of 10–15 percent, even in specialized facilities.

PENETRATING TRAUMA
Penetrating wounds are the most common cause of duodenal trauma. Bullet injuries are the most frequent, followed by stab and shotgun injuries. Blunt injuries are increasing in frequency. In 1958 Webb and colleagues [362], reporting from Grady Memorial Hospital, indicated that blunt injuries account for 10 percent of all duodenal injuries treated in that institution. Corley and associates [68], reporting their experience at the Cook County Hospital a decade later, found that the incidence of blunt injury had more than doubled, having risen to 23 percent.

MECHANISM OF BLUNT DUODENAL INJURY
Beyond the duodenal bulb the duodenum is fixed in a retroperitoneal position by the posterior peritoneum and by the attachments of the duodenum to the pancreas. Posteriorly the duodenum is well protected from injury by the spine, the lumbar musculature, and the posterior parts of the lower ribs. Despite its deep and relatively protected location, however, blunt force applied to the anterior abdominal wall, especially if the abdominal musculature is relaxed, can bring about severe injury to the duodenum. Three mechanisms may be involved; blowout perforation of a transiently closed loop, shearing at a point of fixation, or crushing against the skeleton [139, 283].

A closed duodenal loop can be formed transiently between the partially closed pylorus and the duodenojejunal flexure if forces applied to the body cause momentary angulation of the intestine as it emerges under the ligament of Treitz. The loop need not be absolutely closed at either end; all that is required is a constriction of the lumen that restricts transmission of pressure from the duodenum to the proximal or distal intestine. Under such circumstances a sudden rise in pressure within the lumen of the duodenum may lead to a perforation, typically through the anterior or lateral wall in the second portion of the duodenum and less frequently in the third part.

Shearing forces may be applied to the intestine at points of fixation during rapid deceleration. In the duodenum, shearing injuries occur in relation to the ligament of Treitz and involve the fourth portion of the duodenum. Crushing injuries also typically involve the fourth portion of the duodenum, the intestine being trapped between the blunt injuring object and the vertebral column.

ASSOCIATED INJURIES

Injury to adjacent organs commonly accompanies duodenal trauma and may play the most important role in determining the ultimate outcome. The pancreas and liver are the organs most frequently injured in addition to the duodenum, followed by the transverse colon, small intestine, and stomach. All of the aforementioned organs have an incidence of injury in association with duodenal trauma exceeding 25 percent. In addition, injury to the gallbladder and extrahepatic biliary system, the inferior vena cava, and the right ureter and kidney is reasonably frequent, with an incidence on the order of 10–15 percent. Ureteral injury in particular is easily overlooked during exploration of a complicated duodenal injury and should especially be sought by appropriate retroperitoneal dissection [68, 362].

SYMPTOMS AND SIGNS

About a fourth of patients with major duodenal trauma arrive at the hospital in a state of shock that in some is so advanced as to be refractory to administration of large volumes of crystalloid solutions and blood. Most of these patients have a major vascular injury involving the superior mesenteric artery or vein, the portal vein, the inferior vena cava, or the aorta. They require an emergency laparotomy as part of their resuscitation.

A second group of patients comes to the hospital because of a gunshot wound to the abdomen. The symptoms and signs are quite variable, depending on the extent of associated injuries and the degree of peritoneal contamination from the open duodenum. However, since all of these patients require a laparotomy, the pattern of their clinical complaints is of less importance; the diagnosis will be made intraoperatively.

It is the third group of patients that presents the diagnostic problem. Included in this group are most of the patients whose duodenal injury was caused by blunt abdominal trauma, together with a small group of patients who have sustained a stab wound with a small instrument and in whom there is initially little or no evidence of intraperitoneal injury. Symptoms are quite variable and may progress in a very desultory manner; their intensity depends on many factors. The size of the rupture, the nature of the duodenal contents at the time of injury and the subsequent secretory activity, and the nature and degree of associated injuries all act to modify the acuteness and the rate of progression of symptoms. Intramural hematoma without rupture is most insidious, presenting the features of duodenal obstruction rather than those of an acute abdomen.

Rupture of the duodenal bulb into the free peritoneal cavity produces early symptoms and signs of upper abdominal peritonitis. Pain, tenderness, and muscular rigidity, all increased by deep breathing, appear quite promptly and are usually accompanied by diminished bowel sounds. However, unless there is continued leakage of gastric and duodenal contents, the peritoneal signs may not progress much beyond those of an acute abdominal condition.

Retroperitoneal rupture usually produces less striking clinical signs and symptoms and presents the greatest diagnostic difficulty. With retroperitoneal rupture there is often an asymptomatic latent period following the trauma. Epigastric or right upper quadrant pain, nausea and vomiting, and occasionally hematemesis may subsequently develop over a period of several hours. Signs of peritoneal irritation are variable and may be entirely absent, but in the typical case some epigastric or right-sided tenderness and guarding are demonstrable.

As the retroperitoneal extravasation of duodenal juice extends into the right gutter over the kidney and psoas muscle and into the transverse mesocolon and mesentery of the small intestine, more generalized ileus and pain involving the flank and the entire right side may ensue. Pain in the right testicle and extraperitoneal emphysema, which is detectable by rectal examination, is an unusual manifestation of retroperitoneal rupture of the duodenum.

Patients with suspected duodenal trauma should have roentgenological examinations, beginning with plain upright roentgenograms of the abdomen. Although no definite abnormalities may be detected in up to half the patients with blunt injury to the duodenum, obliteration of the right psoas or renal shadows by retroperitoneal fluid or the fracture of a lumbar transverse process on either side should increase the degree of suspicion that significant trauma to the duodenum may be present. In about a third of the patients, retroperitoneal emphysema along the lateral curve of the duodenum is detectable; and in a few patients free intraperitoneal gas may be reflected by larger bubbles in the region of the duodenum or, on occasion, by subdiaphragmatic collections.

An intravenous pyelogram should be obtained in all patients suspected of having duodenal injuries because of the high frequency of associated injuries to the right kidney and ureter. An upper gastrointestinal series with water-soluble contrast medium also may be helpful, particularly in patients in whom there is little clinical evidence of leakage from the duodenum but who have vomiting or other signs suggestive of obstruction. The upper gastrointestinal series may demonstrate an intramural hematoma or the site of rupture.

MANAGEMENT

Patients with penetrating wounds of the abdomen and those with peritoneal signs following blunt injury should undergo laparotomy. Preoperative preparation is directed at restoration of blood volume and assurance of adequate pulmonary and renal function. Parenteral fluids and blood may not resuscitate patients who have sustained major vascular injury in association with the duodenal injury; these patients require an immediate laparotomy for control of their continuing hemorrhage.

In every patient undergoing exploratory laparotomy after abdominal trauma, but particularly in those in whom even the slightest suspicion of duodenal trauma can be entertained, the entire duodenum must be visualized. Since all but the first portion of the duodenum is retroperitoneal, the intestine must be mobilized, using the Kocher maneuver. Exposure of the distal parts of the duodenum requires division of the transverse mesocolon to obtain full visualization of the third part of the duodenum [56]; the beginning of the fourth portion of the duodenum is exposed by dividing the ligament of Treitz. Deliberate examination of the entire duodenum is especially important when more obvious damage, for example a ruptured liver, occupies the surgeon's primary attention intraoperatively.

At exploration, the second portion of the duodenum will most frequently be found to be the site of injury; this part of the duodenum is involved in half of the instances of traumatic duodenal perforation. The third and fourth portions of the duodenum are also frequently involved, although less commonly than the second portion. The third portion will be found to be injured in about one-fourth of the instances of duodenal trauma, and the fourth portion of the duodenum in about one-fifth of all instances. Curiously, the free intraperitoneal portion composing the first part of the duodenum is injured least frequently; it is involved in only 5 percent of all instances.

Lacerations and perforations involving less than half the circumference of the duodenum usually can be managed by debridement and primary closure [248]. The closure should be in two layers. The inner layer may be of any suture material, but the outer seromuscular closure must be made with nonabsorbable suture; otherwise, pancreatic ferments will promptly digest the suture line. Closure preferably should be made in a transverse direction to avoid compromise of the lumen of the duodenum [152]. However, if transverse closure is not feasible because of the direction or extent of the wound, longitudinal closure is permissible [194].

The repair of the duodenal wound can be reinforced by applying a pedicle of omentum externally. If the suture line seems particularly tenuous, it may be good to bring up a loop of small intestine through the base of the transverse mesocolon and to suture the serosal aspect of the loop on top of the closed duodenal wound to reduce the chance of subsequent disruption [27, 83, 237, 337].

Wounds involving more than half the circumference of the duodenum should be repaired by reanastomosis whenever feasible. The anastomosis should be made in two layers, the external layer being approximated with nonabsorbable suture material. If primary restoration of continuity is impossible, the distal end should be carefully oversewn. Vagotomy, limited distal gastric resection, and gastrojejunostomy will restore gastrointestinal continuity [31]. The resulting isolated proximal portion of the duodenum is managed by drainage into a jejunal Roux-en-Y loop attached either to the residual duodenum or directly to the pancreatic and biliary ductal system [32]. Pyloric exclusion and gastrojejunostomy after complex operations such as repair after trauma have been effective [64, 230].

Following primary closure of a major duodenal injury, the lumen of the duodenum should be decompressed by insertion of a tube through the proximal jejunal loop directed retrogradely so that it lies within the lumen of the repaired duodenum. In addition, a gastrostomy should be placed. Both the jejunostomy and the gastrostomy tubes are placed on suction. Finally, a feeding jejunostomy should be inserted into the upper small intestine somewhat distal to the decompressing jejunostomy tube.

For more extensive injuries, no single method of treatment can be recommended categorically. Decisions must be made during the operation, taking into consideration the extent of the pancreaticoduodenal injury, the nature of any associated injuries, and the patient's overall condition. In general, debridement of devitalized tissue, suture closure of the disrupted duodenum, suture of the pancreatic capsule, and adequate drainage will prove satisfactory in most instances [218]. Very occasionally pancreaticoduodenectomy may be required. Extensive devitalization of the duodenum and adjacent pancreas is the only absolute indication for pancreaticoduodenectomy. This procedure should not be resorted to indiscriminately for lesser degrees of injury [316, 369, 385].

Adequate drainage, anticipating the possible postoperative development of a duodenal fistula or a subhepatic abscess, must be established in every instance. Multiple soft Penrose drains should be placed from the lesser sac through the foramen of Winslow and from the entire lateral aspect of the repaired duodenum and the remainder of the subhepatic space and should be brought out through dependent stab wounds in the flank. Provision for an adequately dependent drainage pathway may require mobilization of the hepatic flexure, deflecting it inferiorly to permit the direct passage of drains to the flank. If there has been injury to the common bile duct, T-tube drainage should be established following ductal repair or diversion. However, routine T-tube drainage of the uninjured common bile duct is unnecessary. If the pancreas has been extensively injured, sump suction drains should be placed in addition to the soft rubber drains.

COMPLICATIONS

Complications are frequent following repair of duodenal injuries. Complications to be anticipated are retroperitoneal cellulitis or abscess, peritonitis and intraabdominal abscess, external duodenal fistula, duodenal obstruction, pancreatitis, pancreatic pseudocyst, prolonged postoperative paralytic ileus, and wound dehiscence. In addition, nutritional problems are frequent but should have been anticipated by the placement of a feeding jejunostomy.

Infection occurs in about one-third of the patients. In patients who have had a preceding gastric resection, the problems of infection are complicated by the fact that swallowed microorganisms are no longer killed by the acid milieu of the stomach. A variety of purulent pathogens can be transported to the duodenum, and in the presence of laceration or rupture, they contaminate the retroperitoneal space. Yeo and McNamara [386] have reported on two patients who had clostridial gas gangrene of the retroperitoneum under such circumstances.

A duodenal fistula will develop in about 10 percent of the patients. Duodenal fistula is a particularly distressing complication, since it leads to uncontrolled loss of duodenal contents, wasting, cachexia, and major fluid-electrolyte problems including metabolic alkalosis, hyponatremia, hypokalemia, and dehydration. Activation of pancreatic ferments by the presence of bile and tissue juice leads to the digestion of skin around the margins of the draining fistula. Some duodenal fistulas may close spontaneously [92], whereas others require surgical management.

INTRAMURAL HEMATOMA

This entity may arise spontaneously as a complication of anticoagulation treatment, or it may be a consequence of blunt abdominal trauma. At times the antecedent blunt injury may appear to be trivial, and it is often ignored by the patient until signs of complications develop. Spontaneous intramural hematomas also appear in nontraumatized patients suffering blood dyscrasias.

Traumatic intramural hematoma of the duodenum is seen primarily in young children. It produces a duodenal obstruction, resulting in progressive bilious vomiting that is occasionally associated with abdominal pain and tenderness. Pancreatitis may be associated in traumatic situations, and the signs and symptoms of the pancreatitis soon may obscure the presence of the intramural hematoma. An intramural hematoma of the duodenum developing after peroral suction biopsy has been reported by Toban et al. [343].

The diagnosis may be delayed or totally missed, so any suspicion of duodenal injury demands observation in a hospital. Abdominal tenderness in the epigastrum or right upper quadrant is characteristic, but an epigastric mass is unusual. The fall in hematocrit reading is usually not alarming, typically being on the order of 3–5 percent. Hyperamylasemia occurs in only a few patients.

An exact diagnosis can be established by the history of trauma, the clinical course, and the roentgenological findings. An upper gastrointestinal series will demonstrate partial or complete duodenal obstruction associated with thickening of the mucosal folds—the so-called coiled-spring or stacked-coin signs. Plain roentgenograms of the abdomen may show a gas-filled stomach with extrinsic pressure on the inferior greater curvature by the ovoid duodenal mass. Laboratory data will show a moderate leukocytosis; serum amylase level may be elevated if there is a retroperitoneal leak of pancreatic juices or associated pancreatitis. Associated renal trauma may produce hematuria.

If the presence of the intramural hematoma is noted during laparotomy, the hematoma should be evacuated through a seromuscular incision that does not traverse the submucosa or mucosa. If there is a question of the viability of the traumatized duodenal wall, excision may be required [157]. In patients who have not been operated on and in whom duodenal perforation or any other associated injury requiring laparotomy can be excluded, nonoperative therapy gives as good results as does operation. Oral intake is restricted; nasogastric intubation and suction are instituted when indicated by continued vomiting or gastric distention; and fluids, electrolytes, and nutrients are administered intravenously [116].

Duodenal Obstruction

A number of lesions can produce duodenal obstruction. The older literature abounds with terms such as *duodenal ileus, duodenal stasis, megaduodenum,* and *gastromesenteric ileus,* all of which refer to the presence of duodenal obstruction. Any obstructive lesion can produce duodenal stasis and, if it is persistent, may produce dilatation or megaduodenum. Therefore, duodenal obstruction is best described and understood in terms of its cause and pathological anatomy. The pediatric aspects of certain of these lesions are discussed in Chapter 27.

The causes of duodenal obstruction in adults include the following:

1. Congenital anomalies: malrotation, peritoneal bands, and related lesions; duodenal diverticulum; duodenal diaphragm; duodenal stenosis; duplication and enterogenous cyst; annular pancreas; "true" megaduodenum.
2. Extrinsic lesions: abdominal aneurysm; pancreatic tumors and cysts; mesenteric and retroperitoneal adenopathy and neoplasms; arterial mesenteric obstruction.
3. Intrinsic acquired lesions: ulcer, inflammation, neoplasm; foreign bodies; intramural hematoma; extraluminal diverticulum.

CONGENITAL ANOMALIES

Most congenital anomalies are symptomatic in infancy, but for unknown reasons certain lesions occasionally are silent for years and symptoms of obstruction do not appear until adulthood.

The most prominent symptom produced by this group of lesions is vomiting. The vomitus contains bile if the obstruction is distal to the ampulla of Vater, which is usually the case. More proximal obstruction of the second portion of the duodenum is not rare, however, and in such instances bile is absent from the vomitus. Pain, sometimes colicky in nature, is an inconstant feature of duodenal obstruction.

Dilatation of the duodenum proximal to the obstruction may produce a roentgenographic appearance of a double bubble, even in an adult, but rarely is the upper abdomen appreciably distended on examination. Swallowed small foreign bodies, which normally would pass easily in the feces, may be retained in persons with congenital duodenal obstructions. The appearance on a roentgenogram of such objects should raise a suspicion of partial duodenal obstruction [178].

Pancreatitis may accompany duodenal obstruction [254] and, when present, probably is related to increased secretion pressure caused by entry of the pancreatic duct into the intermittently closed loop formed between the pylorus proximally and the obstructing lesion distally. Upper gastrointestinal bleeding may occur with any of these lesions and rarely may produce a major hemorrhage [86].

Malrotation and Related Lesions

Malrotation of the intestine is accompanied by abnormal or incomplete fixation of the small intestinal mesentery and the colon to the posterior abdominal wall. As a result, unusual mobility of the intestine permits a variety of complications. The embryology of these lesions has been reviewed by Wang and Welch [356] and by Firor and Harris [109]. Malrotation rarely is combined with intrinsic duodenal obstruction [193]. With complete failure of rotation, the duodenum as well as the rest of the intestine is mobile and nonfixed.

Volvulus of the midgut results in obstruction at the duodenojejunal junction because of angular rotation and torsion of the jejunum. More commonly, malrotation is associated with the presence of peritoneal (Ladd) bands that obstruct the distal duodenum. These bands link the malrotated cecum in the left upper abdomen to the right lateral abdominal wall. They cross the fourth part of the duodenum and produce obstruction by compression. Treatment is section of the bands.

Duodenal Diverticula

These lesions may be extraluminal or intraluminal in position. They usually arise near the ampulla of Vater.

Extraluminal diverticula are more common, and they occur with increasing frequency in persons over 50 years of age. The exact cause of these acquired lesions is unclear. But, if it is permissible to extrapolate from what is known of the genesis of diverticula at other intestinal sites, it is probable that duodenal extraluminal diverticula represent the end result of disturbed motility. Typically, they arise from the medial wall of the duodenum in the region of the ampulla and may pass posterior to the pancreas if they become large (see Fig. 21-4).

Extraluminal diverticula usually are asymptomatic and ordinarily need no treatment. Very occasionally a large diverticulum may

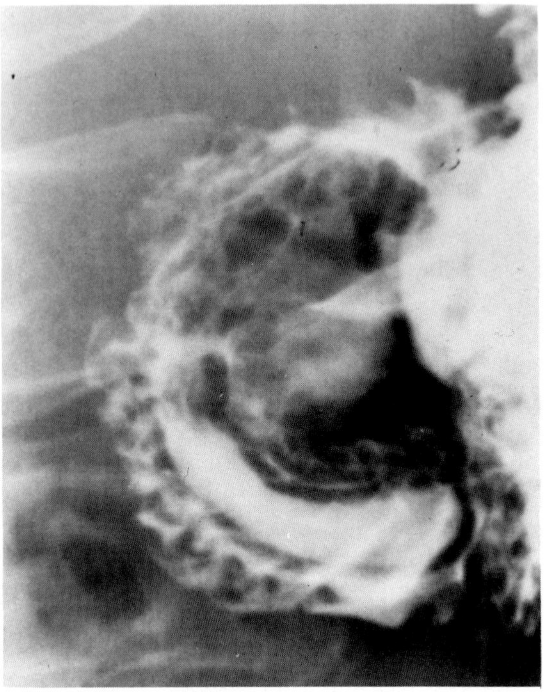

Fig. 21-10. A large intramural duodenal diverticulum filled with barium. The wall of the diverticulum forms a characteristic halo within the lumen of the duodenum. (From Fleming et al. [110], *Mayo Clin. Proc.* 50:244, 1975.)

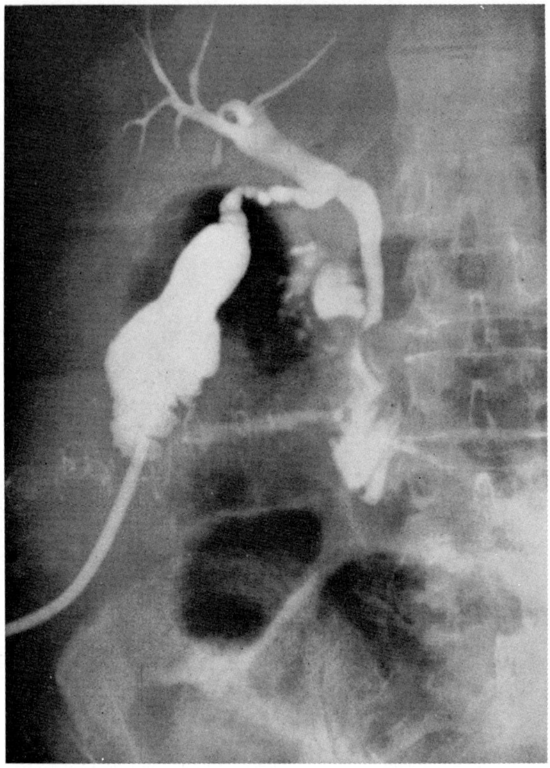

Fig. 21-11. Termination of the common bile duct in the neck of a duodenal diverticulum, fortuitously demonstrated by cholangiography in a patient who had a cholecystostomy for acute cholecystitis.

lead to intermittent symptoms of biliary or pancreatic duct obstruction and, if the patient is sufficiently disabled, may require excision [153, 224]. Even less commonly the diverticulum may be associated with such complications as perforation or bleeding and may require more urgent operative intervention [90, 170]. An excess incidence of recurrent biliary calculi following cholecystectomy also has been attributed to the presence of a periampullary duodenal diverticulum [217].

An intraluminal diverticulum represents a remnant of one of the multiple passages formed during recanalization of the duodenal lumen during early fetal development [142]. This variety of diverticulum appears as a sac within the lumen of the duodenum (Fig. 21-10), usually with an eccentric proximal mouth, arising from the medial wall near the papilla and lined on both sides by duodenal mucosa [110, 333]. A barium meal examination usually shows a central mass filled with barium surrounded by a radiolucent halo formed by the wall of the diverticulum. The common bile duct may terminate in the wall of the sac (Fig. 21-11). Treatment usually is excision with appropriate care to avoid injury to the biliary or pancreatic ducts and attention to the possibility of other associated anomalies [96]. Proximal duodenojejunostomy as a bypass may be required in unusual situations in adults.

Duodenal Diaphragm or Web

These congenital lesions are related to intraluminal diverticula and represent another anomaly of incomplete restoration of the

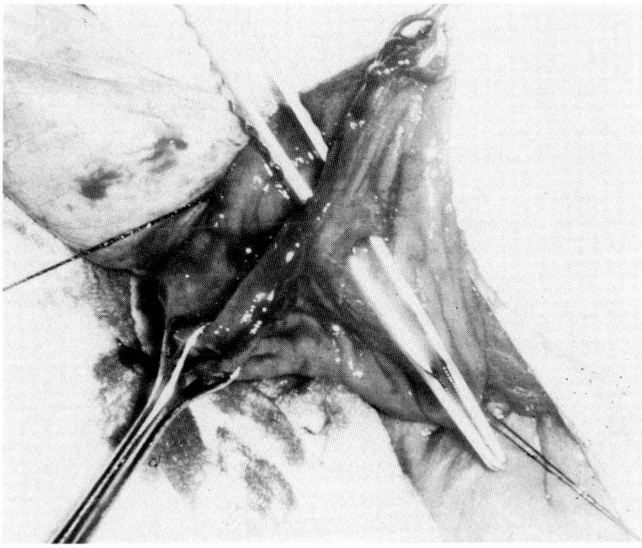

Fig. 21-12. A forceps has been passed through the central orifice of this duodenal diaphragm, which was demonstrated intraoperatively. The diaphragm has been partially transected; section was continued into the central orifice. The common bile duct terminated in the medial wall of the diaphragm adjacent to the central orifice.

gut lumen during embryological development [40]. In instances of duodenal diaphragm, the mucosal plate attaches to the entire circumference of the duodenum rather than just to the posteromedial wall, as is the case in intraluminal diverticulum. The diaphragm usually contains a small central or eccentric port through which intestinal content passes (Fig. 21-12). Continued proximal pressure against the diaphragm may produce elongation, resulting in an intraluminal "wind sock" [203]. Because of the frequent association of the common bile duct with the diaphragm, the safer surgical approach is to bypass the lesion by duodenojejunostomy. In an occasional instance, partial-to-complete excision of the diaphragm may be undertaken [273].

Duodenal Stenosis

These lesions are generally much more symptomatic and therefore are treated in infancy. Rare instances of survival with symptoms to adulthood have been reported [220, 342]. Such patients should be treated by duodenojejunostomy to bypass the obstruction.

Double Pylorus

Most instances of double pylorus are acquired in the course of duodenal ulcer disease [185]. A few instances, distinguished by the presence of muscularis mucosae on both sides of the pyloric septum, seem to be congenital in nature [372]. Symptoms, when present, are caused by duodenal ulcer, and treatment is directed to that disorder.

Duplication and Enterogenous Cyst

These are rare lesions of the duodenum, especially if they remain relatively asymptomatic until adulthood. The symptoms are caused by progressive duodenal obstruction, resulting from gradual distention of the cystic duplication by its mucosal secretions. Surgical management is complicated by hazards of the variant anatomy of the biliary and pancreatic ducts and the presence of a common blood supply to both the functional duodenum and the duplication [2].

The various surgical approaches used in the past have been reviewed by Inouye et al.

[156]. Cystojejunostomy [3] is the preferred method of drainage, although occasionally excision can be accomplished [20]. Duodenojejunostomy is successful only if the cyst is confined to the distal duodenum and, like gastrojejunostomy, is undesirable because the expanding cyst is left in situ. Drainage of the cyst into the duodenum by formation of a distal window in the common cyst-duodenal wall has been applied successfully [117].

Annular Pancreas

This congenital defect arises from an abnormal rotation of the ventral pancreatic duct, resulting in an obstructing ring of pancreatic tissue around the second portion of the duodenum. The pancreatic annulus may cause duodenal obstruction primarily or may represent only partial failure of growth of that segment of the duodenum [101]. This lesion is probably the only congenital anomaly that, if not symptomatic in infancy, does not become symptomatic until after 30 years of age, and then sometimes only as a sequel of pancreatitis [214, 231, 357].

The symptoms reflect the degree of obstruction associated with the annulus. Peptic ulceration is present in about one-fifth of instances, adding the symptoms of ulcer disease to those of duodenal obstruction. Roentgenograms usually show characteristic dilatation of the duodenal bulb above a smooth filling defect of the second part of the duodenum.

A related lesion, *heterotopic pancreas* in the wall of the duodenum, also arises from the dorsal pancreatic primordium [162]. In this disorder the pancreatic rest does not form an encircling ring as in typical instances of annular pancreas, so mechanical obstruction is not usually a clinical feature.

If symptoms of annular pancreas necessitate operative relief of the obstruction, the procedure of choice is a duodenojejunostomy [341]. If the first part of the duodenum is not of adequate dimension or is scarred because of duodenal ulcer disease, vagotomy and gastroenterostomy should be performed. If a gastroenterostomy is chosen, vagotomy must be done, even in the absence of ulcer disease, to forestall development of a stomal ulcer. Excision of the constricting ring is fraught with the dangers of hemorrhage and postoperative fistula and should be avoided. If common duct obstruction coexists, choledochoenterostomy or a cholecystoenterostomy may be required. Pancreaticoduodenectomy may be indicated in the unusual patient with long-standing obstruction that has led to advanced duodenal dilatation and atonicity [329].

Megaduodenum

Typically, enlargement of the duodenum is the secondary result of an obstruction (Fig. 21-13). However, there is a form of "true" megaduodenum that is analogous to megacolon, in that marked duodenal dilatation is present without obstruction. This entity is apparently the result of an abnormality in neuromotor function. Barnett and Wall [19] have described a specimen that on histological examination showed replacement of Auerbach's plexus in

Fig. 21-13. Complete obstruction of the descending duodenum, with resultant megaduodenum, caused by invasive carcinoma of the pancreas.

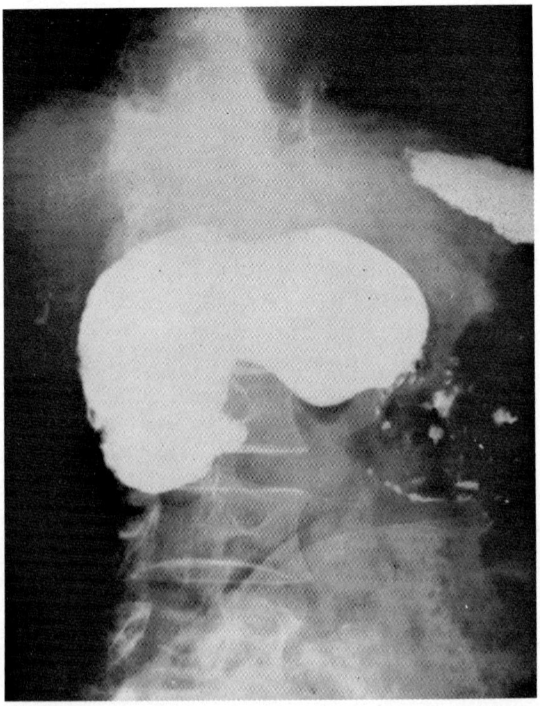

the involved segment with a "profusion of what appears to be sheath cells of a neural type." The functional obstruction caused by this unusual entity is probably best relieved by construction of a proximal duodenojejunostomy.

Megaduodenum may produce secondary effects similar to those of a blind loop or a large diverticulum of proximal small intestine. Bacterial overgrowth, deconjugation of bile salts, malabsorption, and polyneuropathy may be found in varying degrees [198]. Megaduodenum, resulting in a malabsorption syndrome, has also been reported in a patient with Ehlers-Danlos syndrome [148].

EXTRINSIC LESIONS

When an extraduodenal lesion produces obstruction, the mechanism of obstruction is, of course, compression, which may occur at any level of the duodenum. Whenever possible, management is directed at the extrinsic lesion. If removal or reduction in size of the compressing entity is impossible, duodenojejunostomy or vagotomy and gastrojejunostomy, as appropriate, may be done to relieve the obstructive symptoms.

Arteriomesenteric Occlusion

This entity, also known as Wilkie disease, is the result of compression of the fourth portion of the duodenum between the vertebral column and the superior mesenteric vessels (Fig. 21-14). Normally the superior mesenteric vessels ride gently over the horizontal portion of the duodenum. In instances of arteriomesenteric occlusion, loss of the protective pad of fat or abnormal fixation of the small intestinal mesentery is present. Factors that may accentuate the tendency of the superior mesenteric vessels to obstruct the duodenum include acute weight loss, the presence of abnormal mesenteric or peritoneal bands, and an unusually low aortic origin of the superior mesenteric artery [6, 264, 312, 360].

The clinical signs and symptoms are variable, but patients commonly complain of episodic postprandial pain, bloating, eructation, or vomiting. There is a tendency toward duodenal ulceration [15, 34]. If obstruction persists long enough, the malabsorptive complications of megaduodenum may ensue [233]. In a variant of arteriomesenteric obstruction known as the *cast syndrome,* symptoms begin within two weeks of application of a body cast [33].

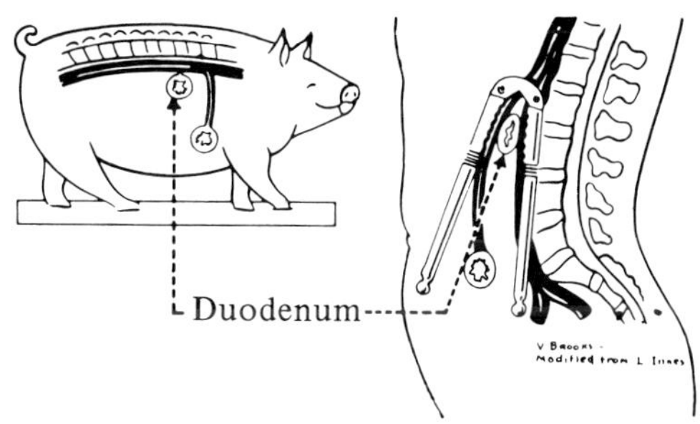

Fig. 21-14. Arteriomesenteric duodenal obstruction. This drawing emphasizes the importance of erect posture (or the supine position) in humans as well as the anatomical relationship of the superior mesenteric artery and duodenum in the genesis of clinical symptoms of obstruction. (From Jones et al. [168].)

Characteristic roentgenographic features include dilatation of the duodenum, but rarely of the stomach, associated with a sharp indentation or cutoff appearance of the duodenum as it passes over the vertebral column. If the roentgenographic findings are not entirely clear, Jones et al. [168] suggest that the patient be tipped backward about 30 degrees from the vertical position so that the superior mesenteric root compresses the duodenum; reverse peristalsis in the proximal dilated duodenum should be demonstrable in this position.

Management initially consists of decompression of the stomach and duodenum by nasogastric suction and feeding of small meals, with the patient in the prone position or knee-chest posture. If the obstruction is caused by application of a body cast and symptoms persist, the cast should be removed; windowing of the cast is not sufficient.

The recent tendency to operate for this lesion is to be deplored [5]. Surgical therapy is indicated only in a persisting obstruction with progressive weight loss and in the presence of unrelenting chronic symptoms. At operation the diagnosis should be confirmed by demonstrating the anatomical deformity and the release of duodenal obstruction following elevation of the mesenteric root. Duodenojejunostomy to bypass the obstruction is the most effective surgical procedure.

Gastrointestinal Hemorrhage from the Duodenum

Duodenal ulcer is, of course, the most common duodenal lesion that produces upper gastrointestinal bleeding. Duodenitis is the second most frequent disorder, but it is much less common than ulcer disease. Both of these entities are discussed elsewhere in this volume.

The following duodenal lesions may on occasion produce gastrointestinal hemorrhage:

1. Arteriovenous malformation [245]
2. Intramural hematoma
3. Delayed traumatic necrosis
4. Heterotopic gastric epithelium
5. Extrinsic diverticula
6. Intrinsic diverticula
7. Duodenal diaphragm
8. Heterotopic pancreas
9. Giardiasis
10. Benign intramural tumors (erode overlying mucosa)
11. Carcinoma of the ampulla of Vater
12. Carcinoma of the pancreas (invades medial wall)
13. Duodenocaval fistula [175]
14. Aortoduodenal fistula [243, 278]
15. Superior mesenteric aneurysm [223]
16. Pancreatic pseudocyst (through the pancreatic duct to the duodenum)
17. Splenic artery aneurysm (erodes into the pancreas)
18. Hemobilia (bleeding originates in the liver but enters the gastrointestinal tract in the duodenum)
19. Regional enteritis
20. Sclerosing mesenteritis (causes ischemia and ulceration)
21. Duodenal biliary fistula
22. Spontaneous enteric fistula

Aortoduodenal fistula produces an exsanguinating hemorrhage that is fatal if not corrected. The most typical clinical pattern is of an initial hemorrhage that stops, followed by an interval of varying duration and then a second and fatal hemorrhage. This lesion should be suspected in any patient who has upper gastrointestinal bleeding and in whom an aortic aneurysm is present or in whom an aortic prosthesis has previously been placed. Not all aortoduodenal fistulas are secondary to the placement of a prosthesis, but when a prosthesis is in place in a bleeding patient, this diagnosis should be first on the list of possibilities. Treatment usually involves excision and replacement of the graft, although a "roof patch" may be appropriate in some instances [42].

Tumors of the Duodenum

Neoplasms of all portions of the small intestine are rare. However, if the relative length of the various segments of intestine is considered, tumors are more common in the duodenum than in the ileum or jejunum. The rarity of duodenal tumors is indicated by the fact that a combined series of more than 110,000 surgical specimens and 16,000 autopsies uncovered only 39 duodenal tumors [146, 149, 280, 291]. Only 13 primary duodenal tumors (9 benign and 4 malignant) were found in the total surgical experience at Columbia University over several years [370].

BENIGN TUMORS OF THE DUODENUM

In a collected series of 367 benign duodenal tumors, adenoma, leiomyoma, and lipoma were the most commonly encountered, each type of tumor accounting for approximately 20 percent of all tumors observed [375]. Fibroma, angioma, and neurogenic tumors are much less frequent [291]. Benign duodenal tumors are of clinical importance because they may produce hemorrhage, pain, or obstruction. They rarely may lead to intussusception [205]. Discovery of a duodenal neoplasm always raises the question of actual or potential malignancy; with rare exceptions, the demonstration of a duodenal filling defect on roentgenographic studies should lead to surgical removal of the lesion.

Adenoma

Duodenal adenomas show no unusual characteristics except for their relative frequency among this total group of unusual tumors. Local excision, with histological verification of the benign nature of the adenoma, is adequate treatment. Adenomas located at the ampulla of Vater are relatively frequent in the Gardner syndrome variant of familial polyposis coli [50, 383] and may degenerate to adenocarcinoma. Waltz and Gerrish [355] reported a unique instance of Peutz-Jeghers syndrome with chronic pancreatitis and common duct obstruction caused by a duodenal polyp around the ampulla of Vater.

Brunner's Gland Hyperplasia and Adenoma

These are the most commonly reported forms of duodenal adenoma (Fig. 21-15). The lesions are not distinguishable from other varieties of mucosal adenoma except by microscopical examination. Because the mucus secreted from Brunner's glands serves to protect duodenal mucosa from acid-peptic ulceration, patients with Brunner's gland hyperplasia or adenoma do not have duodenal ulcers, and these lesions are not a primary cause of gastrointestinal hemorrhage [128].

Fig. 21-15. A large filling defect in the duodenal bulb, typical of Brunner's gland adenoma.

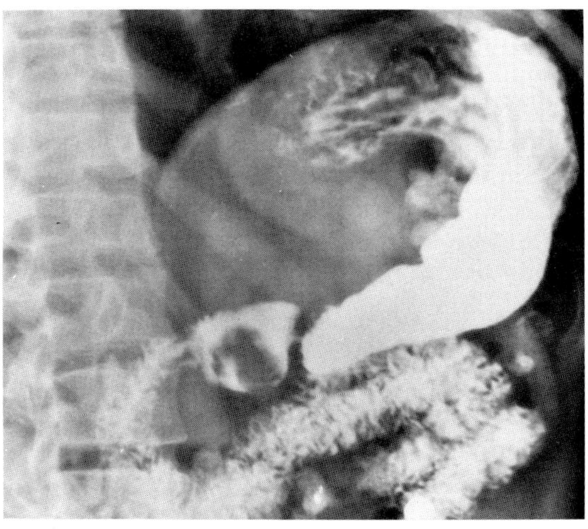

Simple polyps should be excised locally [57, 266]. An occasional unusual case with diffuse nodular hyperplasia of most of the mucosa of the first part of the duodenum may require a bypass by means of gastroenterostomy [177].

Villous Adenoma

Although villous adenomas of the duodenum are rare (41 cases reported in the literature [67, 197, 308]), treatment may be a problem because of the association of villous tumors with invasive adenocarcinoma (27 percent). The symptoms of a duodenal villous tumor may be nonspecific dyspepsia and nausea, but about one-fourth of the patients with these lesions report bleeding, jaundice, or symptoms of duodenal obstruction [308, 317]. Hypokalemia, which is seen in colonic villous tumors, does not occur in the duodenal variety. Hypotonic duodenography and biopsy through a fiberoptic endoscope will help to establish a preoperative diagnosis of villous tumor.

The potential for malignant metaplasia is common to all villous tumors, and cancer is found in about one-third of duodenal villous tumors. Invasive cancer is more common in patients older than 50 years of age, in tumors larger than 4 cm in diameter, and in tumors located in the third and fourth portions of the duodenum.

Treatment of benign lesions is local excision. The entire lesion should be carefully examined by frozen section to exclude, insofar as possible, the presence of invasive carcinoma. Pancreaticoduodenectomy is recommended for tumors that contain invasive carcinoma, as long as the patient does not have metastases, and for tumors in which carcinoma is strongly suspected on clinical grounds and cannot be excluded by histological examination of the locally excised tumor [242].

Lipoma

Lipomas of the duodenum are rare lesions. Most recorded instances have been found incidentally during autopsy examination. These tumors are not clinically unique in any respect. They produce symptoms of pain, obstruction, or hemorrhage, as do other varieties of duodenal neoplasms. The treatment of choice is local excision [94, 263].

Leiomyoma and Leiomyosarcoma

Leiomyomas of the duodenum are very rare lesions, occurring in approximately 1 in 200,000 hospital admissions [179]. Starzl and colleagues [322] collected 61 instances of leiomyosarcoma of the duodenum in 1960. Patients with duodenal leiomyoma commonly present with unexplained melena and anemia. Less commonly symptoms of partial obstruction are present. The most frequent site of leiomyoma is in the second portion of the duodenum. The tumor may grow either into the intestinal lumen or extrinsically and may give rise to sudden and massive hemorrhage.

The origin of leiomyosarcoma and its relationship to leiomyoma continues to be debated. Some believe leiomyosarcomas arise by degeneration of a benign leiomyoma, while others view these lesions as having been malignant from their inception [88]. In any case, leiomyoma, wherever it may be located in the gastrointestinal tract, poses a problem in determination of possible malignancy. The problem is compounded in the duodenum, however, since an uncertain pathological diagnosis cannot easily be compensated for by a more extensive excision.

Radical excision may be required at times, but it should be kept in mind that leiomyosarcoma is not a very aggressive tumor. While structures that are grossly involved in the tumor must, of course, be sacrificed, the wide margins that are typical of operations for adenocarcinoma may not be necessary. "Second-look" operations probably would have real value in the treatment of this lesion.

Depending on the location and extent of the tumor, one may elect local excision, segmental duodenal resection, or pancreaticoduodenectomy. More localized resections are usually feasible in the third and fourth portions of the duodenum. Local excision or segmental resection is also possible in the first portion of the duodenum. If full-thickness resection of the duodenal wall is necessary, difficulty may be encountered in closure, and either a patch or modified gastroduodenostomy may need to be used [169, 201]. Pancreaticoduodenectomy most commonly is necessary in lesions involving the second portion of the duodenum. Lymphatic spread is unusual in leiomyosarcoma; metastases usually occur either by vascular embolization or by direct peritoneal implantation during resection [321].

Aberrant Pancreas

Pancreatic rests may be found in the wall of any portion of the gastrointestinal tract, but 28 percent of such lesions are located in the duodenum [17]. Pancreatic rests are relatively sessile nodules that tend to ulcerate, so generally duodenal ulcer is the diagnosis entertained most strongly preoperatively. Finding a duodenal tumor mass at laparotomy can be disconcerting in such circumstances, but, with histological verification, simple excision serves as treatment [357].

Neurogenic Tumors

These lesions are quite rare and usually asymptomatic, although ulceration of the overlying mucosa may lead to some blood loss. If they become quite large, which is not the usual case, obstructive symptoms, jaundice, or bleeding may supervene. Typically, neurogenic tumors are small lesions, less than 2 cm in diameter, and they present as polypoid and rubbery submucosal nodules. Neurofibromas are most common, followed by neurilemomas, ganglioneuromas, and paraganglioneuromas [373]. The most common clinical association is of duodenal neurofibroma with generalized neurofibromatosis (Recklinghausen's disease).

Primary Carcinoma of the Duodenum

Primary carcinoma of the duodenum, excluding the ampulla of Vater, is a rare lesion. The incidence is approximately 0.01–0.04 percent in necropsy studies [45, 97, 374]. Although the overall incidence is small, the number reported seems to be increasing. Sakker and Ware [302] were able to assemble 126 instances in the decade 1963–1973. Joesting and colleagues [163] reported 104 instances collected from 1937–1977 at one institution. Carcinoma of the duodenum in association with Peutz-Jeghers syndrome has been reported [286], and the regular association of duodenal adenocarcinoma with Gardner's syndrome [307] is now well recognized [383].

Most (59 percent) duodenal carcinomas are located immediately adjacent to the papilla of Vater (periampullary carcinoma); 23 percent are suprapapillary and 18 percent infrapapillary [191]. Patients with infrapapillary tumors tend to be younger than those with carcinoma of the organs adjacent to the duodenum. Although the possibility that duodenal ulcer plays a role in the genesis of duodenal carcinoma has been raised in the past [8, 284], such a possibility can be ignored clinically because of the extreme rarity of carcinoma of the duodenum, particularly of the duodenal bulb, compared with the frequency of duodenal ulcer.

These tumors are histological adenocarcinomas. They exhibit a variety of growth patterns. Most commonly, a bulky, friable, polypoid intraluminal tumor prone to ulceration occurs. Annular constricting lesions also are seen. The clinical signs and symptoms often can be correlated with the location of the cancer. Suprapapillary tumors, for example, characteristically produce symptoms suggesting pyloric obstruction. Infrapapillary tumors are marked by silent gastrointestinal hemorrhage. The periampullary lesions tend to produce obstructive jaundice or pancreatitis [262].

The initial presenting complaints often are nonspecific, but they usually lead to suspicion of gastroduodenal or biliary disease. Abdominal pain of varying severity, bleeding by history or a positive stool guaiac examination, and associated anemia are present in more than 50 percent of the patients. Frequently patients complain of nausea and vomiting, and jaundice is present in about one-third of the patients. Roentgenographic demonstration of a duodenal abnormality that is suggestive of a tumor can be made in more than three-fourths of the patients (Fig. 21-16). Direct endoscopic visualization, using the fiberoptic endoscope and biopsy of the lesion will establish the diagnosis preoperatively. Cytological diagnosis of these tumors is also possible [123].

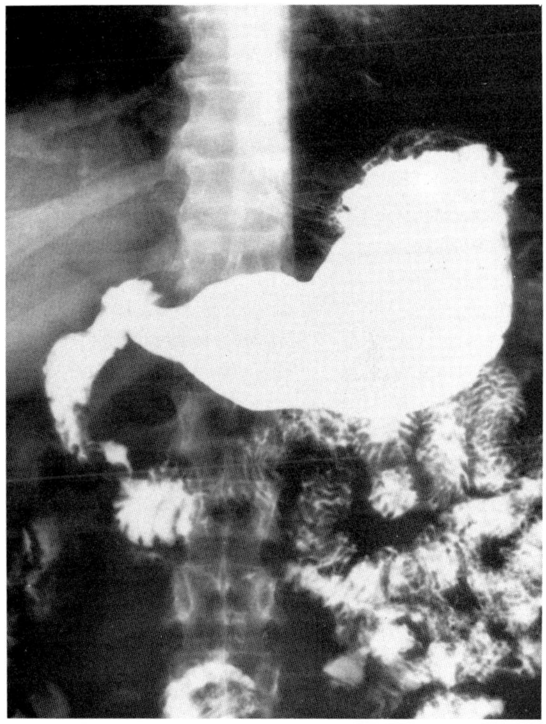

Fig. 21-16. A constricting lesion, with eccentric ulceration in the middle duodenum, which was demonstrated during a diagnostic workup of acute pancreatitis in a man in his middle fifties. The lesion proved to be a primary duodenal adenocarcinoma; the patient had a pancreatoduodenectomy.

The anatomical peculiarities of the duodenopancreatic region contribute to the difficulties of surgical management. The lymphatic drainage of the duodenum is primarily through the anterior and posterior pancreaticoduodenal and gastroduodenal nodes to the hepatic nodes and secondarily to the superior mesenteric chain. This potential lymphatic involvement, when added to invasion of the contiguous biliary and pancreatic ducts, head of the pancreas, and superior mesenteric vessels, poses a formidable technical problem at operation.

Pancreaticoduodenectomy is the treatment of choice for duodenal carcinomas that are confined to the duodenum and the immediately adjacent region of the head of the pancreas [71, 187, 323, 376]. Even with lesser resections, several instances with a long survival have been reported [163], so this tumor may sometimes behave biologically in a desultory manner. This behavior should not encourage lesser resection; rather, it should encourage the performance of pancreaticoduodenectomy even when the tumor has undergone local spread. Most patients, however, demonstrate metastases to regional lymph nodes and to the liver at operation. For these patients radical resection should probably not be undertaken; a bypassing gastrojejunostomy should be constructed instead. A recent report indicates that there may be a place for radiation therapy and for chemotherapy in the management of disseminated duodenal carcinoma [303].

Sarcoma of the Duodenum

Sarcoma is an extremely rare lesion, occurring less than once in 6000 autopsies. Most sarcoma tumors are leiomyosarcomas, which have been discussed previously.

CARCINOID–ISLET CELL TUMORS

These tumors, which have morphological and functional features of both foregut carcinoid and pancreatic islet cell tumors [363, 364], belong to the general group of gastrointestinal tumors derived from neuroectoderm, which are grouped together as polypeptide-secreting "apudomas" [114, 365]. In about half the patients with these lesions, the dominant cell type is the non-beta islet cell associated with gastrin secretion, hypergastrinemia, and the clinical signs and symptoms of the Zollinger-Ellison (Z-E) syndrome [104]. In about half the patients with the Z-E syndrome, that is, in about one-fourth of the patients with carcinoid–islet cell duodenal tumors, other manifestations of the various endocrine polyglandular syndromes also are present.

True serotonin-secreting carcinoids in this tumor group are quite rare; when carcinoidlike cells predominate, most often the tumors are asymptomatic. Ulcerogenic tumors most commonly are isolated lesions located in the submucosa of the second part of the duodenum, proximal to the ampulla of Vater. However, about one-fourth of the patients have lymph node metastases, and about another one-fourth also have a concomitant pancreatic lesion [150].

Local excision of the tumor satisfactorily controls ulcerogenic symptoms or intractable diarrhea in the absence of distant metastases [261]. This is the one circumstance in which a procedure of lesser magnitude than total gastrectomy may be considered in the management of the Z-E syndrome [150].

Local tumor excision combined with antrectomy and vagotomy has also been recommended because patients with Z-E syndrome have parietal cell hyperplasia [150]. Patients must have gastrin levels measured after local resection of a duodenal tumor and must be closely followed, since metastases that were inapparent at the time of the original exploration subsequently may become symptomatic. In patients who have symptoms of Z-E syndrome and whose duodenal tumor is not localized, or in patients whose symptoms recur following resection of the duodenal tumor, total gastrectomy is the treatment of choice, as is true in other instances of the Z-E syndrome.

METASTASES TO THE DUODENUM

Secondary deposits of cancer in the duodenum may be about as frequent as are primary malignant tumors. The clinical features of these "alien cancers," their multiple modes of metastatic spread, and their treatment have been reviewed by Veen and associates [354].

Regional Enteritis

Crohn disease of the duodenum is usually associated with regional enteritis involving the stomach or other gastrointestinal organs. In a 1971 review Wise and colleagues [378] recorded 73 reported instances. Ten further instances were reported by Haggitt and Meissner [134].

The pathology in the duodenum is similar to that of regional enteritis in the more distal in-

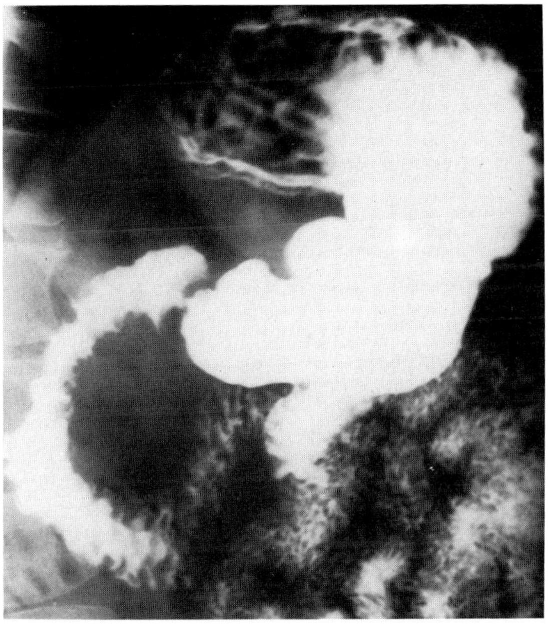

Fig. 21-17. Typical roentgenographic features of regional enteritis involving the duodenum.

testine. Acute, chronic, and obstructive stages may occur. Symptoms vary with the stage of the disease, but they generally consist of intermittent or continuous epigastric and right upper quadrant pain that is aggravated by food and is complicated by fever, nausea, and vomiting in the acute stages (Fig. 21-17). Weakness, weight loss, macrocytic anemia, and steatorrhea develop as the disease progresses, and in the final stages complete obstruction may occur. Clubbing of the fingers is thought to be more frequent if regional enteritis involves the proximal intestine [13].

Surgical treatment of duodenal regional enteritis is complicated by the difficulties of resection related to the regional anatomy. Most instances are best managed by performing a bypass gastrojejunostomy and vagotomy [251, 297].

References

1. Abrams, J. S. Multiple malignant carcinoids of the stomach. *Arch. Surg.* 115:1219, 1980.
2. Ackerman, N. B. Duodenal duplication cysts: Diagnosis and operative management. *Surgery* 76:330, 1974.
3. Adams, T. W. Obstructing enterogenous cyst of the duodenum treated by cystojejunostomy. *Ann. Surg.* 144:902, 1956.
4. Ahnlund, H. O., Pallin, B., Peterhoff, R., and Schonebeck, J. Mycosis of the stomach. *Acta Chir. Scand.* 133:555, 1967.
5. Akin, J. T., Gray, S. W., and Skandalakis, J. E. Vascular compression of the duodenum: Presentation of ten cases and review of the literature. *Surgery* 79:515, 1976.
6. Akin, J. T., Jr., Skandalakis, J. E., and Gray, S. W. The anatomic basis of vascular compression of the duodenum. *Surg. Clin. North Am.* 54:1361, 1974.
7. Albo, R. J., Peters, H. E., and Williams, R. R. Giant hypertrophic gastritis. *Am. J. Surg.* 126:229, 1973.
8. Allen, C. I. Primary carcinoma of the duodenum: Report of 11 cases. *Am. J. Surg.* 40:89, 1938.
9. Allen, R. E., Thoshinsky, M. J., Stallone, R. J., and Hunt, T. K. Corrosive injuries of the stomach. *Arch. Surg.* 100:409, 1970.
10. Allen, W. S. A., and Miller, R. W. S. Glomus tumor of the stomach. *Br. J. Surg.* 48:145, 1960.
11. Alschibaja, T., Putnam, T. C., and Yablin, B. A. Duplication of the stomach simulating hypertrophic pyloric stenosis. *Am. J. Dis. Child.* 127:120, 1974.
12. Anderson, C. B., Weisz, D. D., Rodger, M. R., and Tucker, G. L. Combined pancreaticoduodenal trauma. *Am. J. Surg.* 125:530, 1973.
13. Anderson, D. O., Mullinger, M. A., and Bogoch, A. Regional enteritis involving the duodenum, with clubbing of the fingers and steatorrhea. *Gastroenterology* 32:917, 1957.
14. Anderson, J. R., Lee, D., Naysmith, A., and Busuttil, A. Gastric pseudolymphoma. *Br. J. Surg.* 67:672, 1980.
15. Anderson, W. C., Vivit, R., Kirsh, I. E., and Greenley, H. B. Arterial mesenteric duodenal compression syndrome: Its association with peptic ulcer. *Am. J. Surg.* 125:681, 1973.
16. Armstrong, C. P., King, P. M., Dixon, J. M., and Macleod, I. B. The clinical significance of heterotopic pancreas in the gastrointestinal tract. *Br. J. Surg.* 68:384, 1981.
17. Barbosa, J. J. de C., Dockerty, M. B., and Waugh, J. M. Pancreatic heterotopia: A review of literature and report of 41 authenti-

cated surgical cases, of which 25 are clinically significant. *Surg. Gynecol. Obstet.* 82:527, 1946.
18. Bar-Maor, J. A., Nissen, S., and Nevo, S. Pyloric atresia: A hereditary congenital anomaly with autosomal recessive transmission. *J. Med. Genet.* 9:70, 1972.
19. Barnett, W. O., and Wall, L. Megaduodenum resulting from absence of the parasympathetic ganglion cells in Auerbach's plexus. *Ann. Surg.* 141:527, 1955.
20. Baroody, W. G., Innes, R., and Harrison, H. N. Enterogenous cyst of the duodenum. *Gastroenterology* 30:523, 1956.
21. Barrocas, A., Fontenelle, L. J., and Williams, M. J. Gastric heterotopic pancreas: A case report and review of literature. *Am. Surg.* 39:361, 1973.
22. Bartels, R. J. Duplication of the stomach. *Am. Surg.* 33:747, 1967.
23. Bartholomew, L. G., Dahlin, D. C., and Waugh, J. M. Intestinal polyposis associated with mucocutaneous melanin pigmentation (Peutz-Jeghers syndrome). *Mayo Clin. Proc.* 32:675, 1957.
24. Beard, R. J., Gruebel Lee, E. C., Haysom, A. H., and Melcher, D. H. Non-carcinomatous tumors of the stomach. *Br. J. Surg.* 55:535, 1968.
25. Bedikian, A. Y., Khankhanian, N., Valdivieso, M., et al. Sarcoma of the stomach: Clinicopathologic study of 43 cases. *J. Surg. Oncol.* 13:121, 1980.
26. Bell, L. G., Thomas, E. E., Jr., and Skillicorn, S. A. Gastromalacia: A review and report of one case with recovery. *Ann. Surg.* 143:106, 1956.
27. Bender, H. W., Sebor, J., and Zuidema, G. D. Serosal patch grafting for closure of posterior duodenal defects. *Am. J. Surg.* 115:103, 1968.
28. Bentivegna, S., and Hirschl, S. Heterotopic gastric mucosa in the gallbladder presenting as a symptom-producing tumor: A case report. *Am. J. Gastroenterol.* 57:423, 1972.
29. Berenson, M. M., Sannella, J., and Freston, J. W. Menetrier's disease: Serial morphological, secretory, and serological observations. *Gastroenterology* 70:257, 1976.
30. Berman, J. K., and Ballenger, F. Prepyloric membranous obstruction. *Q. Bull. Ind. Univ. Med. Ctr.* 4:14, 1942.
31. Berne, C. J., Donovan, A. J., and Hagen, W. E. Combined duodenal pancreatic trauma. *Arch. Surg.* 96:712, 1968.
32. Berne, C. J., Donovan, A. J., White, E. J., and Yellin, A. E. Duodenal "diverticulization" for duodenal and pancreatic injury. *Am. J. Surg.* 127:503, 1974.
33. Bisla, R. S., and Louis, H. J. Acute vascular compression of the duodenum following cast application. *Surg. Gynecol. Obstet.* 140:563, 1975.
34. Black, S. Chronic arterial mesenteric duodenal ileus complicated by peptic ulcer: Case report and surgical procedures. *Am. Surg.* 32:619, 1966.
35. Bodily, K. C., Mowlem, A., and Hoffman, J. E. Multiple gastric polyps and parathyroid adenomas. *Am. J. Surg.* 132:118, 1976.
36. Boley, S. J., McKinnon, W. M. P., and Marzulli, V. F. The management of familial gastrointestinal polyposis involving stomach and colon. *Surgery* 50:691, 1961.
37. Bone, G. E., and McClelland, R. N. Management of gastric polyps. *Surg. Gynecol. Obstet.* 142:933, 1976.
38. Bonfield, R. E., Martel, W., and Batsakis, J. G. The significance of small gastric filling defects. *Surg. Gynecol. Obstet.* 127:1231, 1968.
39. Boren, C. H., and Way, L. W. Alkaline reflux gastritis: A reevaluation. *Am. J. Surg.* 140:40, 1980.
40. Boyden, E. A., Cope, J. G., and Bill, A. H., Jr. Anatomy and embryology of congenital intrinsic obstruction of the duodenum. *Am. J. Surg.* 114:190, 1967.
41. Brand, B., and Bernstein, L. H. Emergency gastroscopic polypectomy for control of hemorrhage. *Gastroenterology* 65:956, 1973.
42. Brenner, W. I., Richman, H., and Reed, G. E. Roof patch repair of an aortoduodenal fistula resulting from suture line failure in an aortic prosthesis. *Am. J. Surg.* 127:762, 1974.
43. Brodie, N., Klatzo, M., and Siegman, F. A. Duplication of the stomach associated with bleeding duodenal ulcer. *Arch. Surg.* 80:354, 1960.
44. Brunn, H., and Pearl, F. Diffuse gastric polyposis: Adenopapillomatosis gastrica. *Surg. Gynecol. Obstet.* 43:559, 1926.
45. Burgerman, A., Baggenstoss, A. H., and Cain, J. C. Primary malignant neoplasms of the duodenum, excluding the papilla of Vater. *Gastroenterology* 30:421, 1956.
46. Burgess, J. N., Dockerty, M. B., and ReMine, W. H. Sarcomatous lesions of the stomach. *Ann. Surg.* 173:758, 1971.
47. Burgess, J. N., Legge, D. A., and Judd, E. S.

Surgical treatment of regional enteritis of the stomach and duodenum. *Surg. Gynecol. Obstet.* 132:628, 1971.
48. Burnett, K. R., Keyser, B., Tomasulo, J., and Edwards, K. C. Giant gastric villous adenoma. *Am. J. Gastroenterol.* 74:368, 1980.
49. Bushkin, F. L., Wickbom, G., Deford, J. W., and Woodward, E. R. Postoperative alkaline reflux gastritis. *Surg. Gynecol. Obstet.* 138:933, 1974.
50. Bussey, H. J. R., Veale, A. M. O., and Morson, B. C. Genetics of gastrointestinal polyposis. *Gastroenterology* 74:1325, 1978.
51. Cabre-Fiol, V., Vilardell, F., Sala-Cladera, E., and Mota, A. P. Preoperative cytological diagnosis of gastric leiomyosarcoma. A report of three cases. *Gastroenterology* 68:563, 1975.
52. Cain, G. D., Moore, P., and Patterson, M. Bezoars: A complication of the postgastrectomy state. *Am. J. Dig. Dis.* 13:801, 1968.
53. Canivet, B., Creisson, G., Freychet, P., and Dageville, X. Fibre, diabetes and risk of bezoar. *Lancet* 2:862, 1980.
54. Carney, J. A., Sheps, S. G., Go, V. L. W., and Gordon, H. The triad of gastric leiomyosarcoma, functioning extra-adrenal paraganglioma and pulmonary chondroma. *N. Engl. J. Med.* 296:1517, 1977.
55. Carter, R., Brewer, L. A., and Hinshaw, D. B. Acute gastric volvulus: A study of 25 cases. *Am. J. Surg.* 140:99, 1980.
56. Cattell, R. B., and Braasch, J. W. A technique for the exposure of the third and fourth portions of the duodenum. *Surg. Gynecol. Obstet.* 111:378, 1960.
57. Chato, L. M., Gonzalez, P., and Schmitz, R. L. Polypoid adenomas of Brunner's glands. *Arch. Surg.* 106:667, 1973.
58. Chodack, P., and Hurwitz, A. Lymphangiectasis of the stomach. *Arch. Intern. Med.* 113:225, 1964.
59. Chodoff, R. J., and Sarpour, A. Lymphosarcoma of the stomach: A long-term followup report of two cases of reticulum cell sarcoma. *Am. J. Surg.* 101:521, 1961.
60. Chong, G. C., Beahrs, O. H., and Payne, W. S. Management of corrosive gastritis due to ingested acid. *Mayo Clin. Proc.* 49:861, 1974.
61. Christodoulopoulos, J. B., and Klotz, A. P. Carcinoid syndrome with primary carcinoid tumor of the stomach. *Gastroenterology* 43:429, 1961.
62. Clearfield, H. R., Shin, Y. H., and Schreivman, B. K. Emphysematous gastritis secondary to lye ingestion: Report of a case. *Am. J. Dig. Dis.* 14:195, 1969.
63. Clement, K. W., and Escamilla, H. A. Duplication of the stomach. *J. Natl. Med. Assoc.* 66:282, 1974.
64. Cogbill, T. H., Moore, E. E., Newman, M. M., and Hallgrimson, C. G. Pyloric exclusion in the management of complicated duodenal and pancreatic disease. *Am. Surg.* 50:244, 1984.
65. Colizza, S., Tiso, B., Bracci, F., et al. Cystic lymphangioma of stomach and jejunum: Report of one case. *J. Surg. Oncol.* 17:169, 1981.
66. Contreary, K., Nance, F. C., and Becker, W. F. Primary lymphoma of the gastrointestinal tract. *Ann. Surg.* 191:593, 1980.
67. Cooperman, M., Clausen, K. P., Hecht, C., et al. Villous adenomas of the duodenum. *Gastroenterology* 74:1295, 1978.
68. Corley, R. D., Norcross, W. J., and Shoemaker, W. C. Traumatic injuries to the duodenum: A report of 98 patients. *Ann. Surg.* 181:92, 1975.
69. Courcy, P. A., Soderstrom, C., and Brotman, S. Gastric rupture from blunt trauma: A plea for minimal diagnostics and early surgery. *Am. Surg.* 50:424, 1984.
70. Cox, R., and MacKenzie, D. H. Adenoacanthoma of the pylorus: Report of a case. *Br. J. Surg.* 47:390, 1960.
71. Crane, J. M., Gobbel, W. G., Jr., and Scott, H. W., Jr. Surgical experience with malignant tumors of the ampulla of Vater and duodenum. *Surg. Gynecol. Obstet.* 137:937, 1973.
72. Curry, J. L., and Howland, W. J. Prolapsing pseudopolyp due to redundant gastric mucosa. *Gastroenterology* 46:785, 1964.
73. Dalgaard, J. B. Intracranial infections causing esophagomalacia and gastromalacia. *Gastroenterology* 37:28, 1959.
74. Davis, J. M., Gray, G. F., and Thorbjarnarson, B. Menetrier's disease: A clinicopathologic study of six cases. *Ann. Surg.* 185:456, 1977.
75. Davis, R. C., and Farugui, A. M. A. Endoscopic enzymatic dissolution: Non-surgical therapy for gastric phytobezoars. *J.A.M.A.* 229:1332, 1974.
76. Deal, D. R., Vitale, P., and Raffin, S. B. Dissolution of a postgastrectomy bezoar by cellulase. *Gastroenterology* 64:467, 1973.
77. DeAngelis, V. R. Gastric teratoma in a newborn infant: Total gastrectomy with survival. *Surgery* 66:794, 1969.
78. DeBakey, M. E., and Ochsner, H. Bezoars

and concretions. *Surgery* 4:934, 1938; 5:132, 1939.

79. DeBord, J. R., Majarakis, J. D., and Nyhus, L. M. An unusual case of heterotopic pancreas of the stomach. *Am. J. Surg.* 141:269, 1981.
80. DeCastro, F. J., Olsen, W. R., and Littler, E. R. Gastric leiomyoblastoma in an adolescent. *Am. J. Surg.* 123:614, 1972.
81. Deitel, M. Chronic or recurring organoaxial rotation of the stomach. *Can. J. Surg.* 16:195, 1973.
82. Delio, C. W. Phytobezoars (diospyrobezoars): A clinical pathologic correlation and review of 6 cases. *Arch. Surg.* 82:579, 1961.
83. DeShazo, C. V., Snyder, W. H., Daugherty, C. G., and Crenshaw, C. A. Mucosal pedicle graft of jejunum for large gastroduodenal defects. *Am. J. Surg.* 124:671, 1972.
84. Devanesan, J., Pisani, A., Sharma, P., et al. Metallic foreign bodies in the stomach. *Arch. Surg.* 112:664, 1977.
85. DeVito, R. Miscellaneous Surgical Diseases of the Stomach. In H. N. Harkins and L. M. Nyhus (Eds.), *Surgery of the Stomach and Duodenum* (1st ed.). Boston: Little, Brown, 1962.
86. Dickinson, W. E., Weinberg, S. M., and Vellios, F. Perforating ulcer in a duodenal duplication. *Am. J. Surg.* 122:418, 1971.
87. Di-Costanzo, J., Cano, N., Martin, J., and Noirclerc, M. Surgical approach to corrosive injuries of the stomach. *Br. J. Surg.* 68:879, 1981.
88. Dodds, J. J., and Beahrs, O. H. Leiomyosarcoma of the duodenum. *Am. J. Surg.* 105:245, 1963.
89. Dolan, R. V., ReMine, W. H., and Dockerty, M. B. The fate of heterotopic pancreatic tissue: A study of 212 cases. *Arch. Surg.* 109:762, 1974.
90. Donald, J. W. Major complications of small bowel diverticula. *Ann. Surg.* 190:183, 1979.
91. Dudley, G. S., Miscall, L., and Morse, S. F. Benign tumors of the stomach. *Arch. Surg.* 45:702, 1942.
92. Dudrick, S. J., Wilmore, D. W., Steiger, E., et al. Spontaneous closure of traumatic pancreatoduodenal fistulas with total intravenous nutrition. *J. Trauma* 10:542, 1970.
93. du Plessis, D. J. Gastric mucosal changes after operations on the stomach. *S. Afr. Med. J.* 36:471, 1962.
94. Duthie, H. L., and Forrest, A. P. M. Submucous lipoma of the duodenum. *Br. J. Surg.* 45:201, 1957.
95. Eaton, H., and Tennekoon, G. E. Squamous carcinoma of the stomach following corrosive acid burn. *Br. J. Surg.* 59:382, 1972.
96. Economides, N. G., McBurney, R. P., and Hamilton, F. H. Intraluminal duodenal diverticulum in the adult. *Ann. Surg.* 185:147, 1977.
97. Eger, S. A. Primary malignant disease of the duodenum. *Arch. Surg.* 27:1087, 1933.
98. Eker, R., and Efskind, J. Sarcoma of the stomach. *Acta Chir. Scand.* 3:386, 1956.
99. Eklof, O., Engstedt, L., and Reizenstein, P. Intrinsic factor deficiency, achlorhydria, and malignancy in polyps of the stomach and duodenum. *Acta Med. Scand.* 171:601, 1962.
100. Eley, A., and Richards, H. G. H. A case of localized gastric abscess. *Br. J. Surg.* 47:97, 1959.
101. Elliott, G. B., Kliman, M. R., and Elliott, K. A. Pancreatic annulus: A sign or a cause of duodenal obstruction? *Can. J. Surg.* 11:357, 1968.
102. Elsborg, L., Andersen, D., Myhre-Jensen, O., and Bastrup-Madsen, P. Gastric mucosal polyps in pernicious anaemia. *Scand. J. Gastroenterol.* 12:49, 1977.
103. Eras, P., and Beranbaum, S. L. Gastric diverticula: Congenital and acquired. *Am. J Gastroenterol.* 57:120, 1972.
104. Evans, W. E., Armstrong, R. G., Schulte, W., and Garancis, J. C. Ulcerogenic tumor of the duodenum. *Am. J. Surg.* 124:596, 1972.
105. Falk, V. S. Trichobezoar. *Wis. Med. J.* 78:31, 1979.
106. Farman, J., Faegenburg, D., Dallemand, S., and Chen, C. K. Crohn's disease of the stomach: The "ram's horn" sign. *Am. J. Roentgenol. Radium Ther. Nucl. Med.* 123:242, 1975.
107. Feldman, A. J., Weinberg, M., Raess, D., et al. Gastric carcinoid tumor. *Arch. Surg.* 116:118, 1981.
108. Fielding, J. F., Toye, D. K. M., Beton, D. C., and Cooke, W. T. Crohn's disease of the stomach and duodenum. *Gut* 11:1001, 1970.
109. Firor, H. V., and Harris, V. J. Rotational abnormalities of the gut: Re-emphasis of a neglected facet, isolated incomplete rotation of the duodenum. *Am. J. Rogentgenol. Radium Ther. Nucl. Med.* 120:315, 1974.
110. Fleming, C. R., Newcomer, A. D., Stephens, D. H., and Carlson, H. C. Intraluminal duodenal diverticulum: Report of two cases and review of the literature. *Mayo Clin. Proc.* 50:244, 1975.

111. Fleming, L. B., Horton, J. A. G., and Wagget, J. Spontaneous rupture of the stomach: A rare complication of pyloric stenosis. *Br. J. Surg.* 53:384, 1966.
112. Frank, B. W., and Kern, F., Jr. Menetrier's disease: Spontaneous metamorphosis of giant hypertrophy of the gastric mucosa to atrophic gastritis. *Gastroenterology* 53:953, 1967.
113. French, W. E. Pancreatic tissue in antral wall. *Am. J. Surg.* 114:956, 1967.
114. Friesen, S. R., Hermreck, I. J., and Mantz, F. A., Jr. Glucagon, gastrin and carcinoid tumors of the duodenum, pancreas and stomach: Polypeptide "apudomas" of the foregut. *Am. J. Surg.* 127:90, 1974.
115. Fromm, D. Drug-induced gastric mucosal injury. *World J. Surg.* 5:199, 1981.
116. Fullen, W. D., Selle, J. G., Whitely, D. H., et al. Intramural duodenal hematoma. *Ann. Surg.* 179:549, 1974.
117. Gardner, C. E., Jr., and Hart, D. Enterogenous cysts of the duodenum: Report of a case and review of the literature. *J.A.M.A.* 104:1809, 1935.
118. Gatell-Artigas, J. M., Saumell, C. B., Aused-Faure, R., and Llebaria, C. Herpes zoster of upper gastrointestinal tract. *Lancet* 2:43, 1980.
119. Ghohremani, G. G. Nonobstructive mucosal diaphragms or rings of the gastric antrum in adults. *Am. J. Roentgenol. Radium Ther. Nucl. Med.* 121:236, 1974.
120. Go, T. S., and Morse, W. H. Hypertrophic pyloric stenosis in adults. *Am. J. Gastroenterol.* 60:400, 1973.
121. Golden, T., and Stout, A. P. Smooth muscle tumors of the gastrointestinal tract and retroperitoneal tissues. *Surg. Gynecol. Obstet.* 73:784, 1941.
122. Goldfarb, W. B., and Schaefer, R. Gastric heterotopia in the rectum. *Ann. Surg.* 154:133, 1961.
123. Goldgraber, M. B., Rubin, C. E., and Owens, F. J. The cytologic diagnosis of duodenal sarcoma. *Ann. Intern. Med.* 39:1316, 1953.
124. Goldman, D. S., and Appelman, H. D. Gastric mucosal polyps. *Am. J. Clin. Pathol.* 58:434, 1972.
125. Goldman, R. L., and Friedman, N. B. Neurogenic nature of so-called inflammatory fibroid polyps of the stomach. *Cancer* 20:134, 1967.
126. Gosin, S., and Ballinger, W. F., II. Recurrent volvulus of the stomach. *Am. J. Surg.* 109:642, 1965.
127. Graham, D. Y., Kimbrough, R. C., and Fagan, T. Congenital gastric diverticulum as a cause of massive hemorrhage. *Am. J. Dig. Dis.* 19:174, 1974.
128. Griffith, C. A., and Harkins, H. N. The role of Brunner's glands in the intrinsic resistance of the duodenum to acid-peptic digestion. *Ann. Surg.* 143:160, 1956.
129. Grosfeld, J. L., O'Neill, J. A., Jr., and Clatworthy, H. W., Jr. Enteric duplication in infancy and childhood. *Ann. Surg.* 172:83, 1970.
130. Gruhn, J., Blake, K., and Saracco, T. Gastric heterotopia. *Am. J. Surg.* 100:396, 1960.
131. Gruskin, P., and Landolfe, F. R. Heterotopic gastric mucosa of the tongue. *Arch. Pathol.* 94:184, 1972.
132. Habeshaw, J. A., Hayward, M. J., and McVie, J. G. Extramedullary plasmacytoma of stomach. *Scand. J. Haematol.* 14:57, 1975.
133. Haddad, V., Macon, W. L., and Islami, M. H. Mucosal diaphragms of the gastric antrum in adults. *Surg. Gynecol. Obstet.* 152:227, 1981.
134. Haggitt, R. C., and Meissner, W. A. Crohn's disease of the upper gastrointestinal tract. *Am. J. Clin. Pathol.* 59:613, 1973.
135. Haller, J. A., Jr., and Cahill, J. L. Combined congenital gastric and duodenal obstruction: Pitfalls in diagnosis and management. *Surgery* 63:503, 1968.
136. Harned, R. K., and Melamed, A. Interstitial gastric emphysema: A case report. *Nebr. Med. J.* 59:98, 1974.
137. Hartmann, W. H., and Sherlock, P. Gastroduodenal metastases from carcinoma of the breast: An adrenal steroid-induced phenomenon. *Cancer* 14:426, 1961.
138. Hawkins, M. L., Lowery, C. H., and Mullen, J. T. Gastric duplication. *South. Med. J.* 67:189, 1974.
139. Hawkins, M. L., and Mullen, J. T. Duodenal perforation from blunt abdominal trauma. *J. Trauma* 14:290, 1974.
140. Hay, L. J. Polyps and adenomas of the stomach. *Surgery* 33:446, 1953.
141. Hay, L. J. Surgical management of gastric polyps and adenomas. *Surgery* 39:114, 1956.
142. Heilbrun, N., and Boyden, E. A. Intraluminal duodenal diverticulum. *Radiology* 82:887, 1964.
143. Hershlag, A., Argov, S., and Barzilai, A. Postvagotomy gastric atony: A simple new method of treatment and a survey of the literature. *Curr. Surg.* 36:3, 1979.
144. Hertzer, N. R., and Hoerr, S. O. An interpre-

tive review of lymphoma of the stomach. *Surg. Gynecol. Obstet.* 143:113, 1976.
145. Hiebert, B. W., and Farris, A. M. Hypertrophic pyloric stenosis in the adult: Review of 22 cases. *Am. Surg.* 32:712, 1966.
146. Higgins, D. C., Judd, E. S., and Dockerty, M. B. Surgical aspects of infrapapillary duodenal tumors. *Surgery* 49:149, 1961.
147. Highman, L. M., Fantelli, F. J., and Hermann, R. E. Pseudolymphoma of the stomach. *Arch. Surg.* 116:227, 1981.
148. Hines, C., Jr., and Davis, W. D., Jr. Ehlers-Danlos syndrome with megaduodenum and malabsorption syndrome secondary to bacterial overgrowth: A report of a first case. *Am. J. Med.* 54:539, 1973.
149. Hoffman, D. P., and Grayzel, D. M. Benign tumors of the duodenum. *Am. J. Surg.* 70:394, 1945.
150. Hofmann, J. W., Fox, P. S., and Wilson, S. D. Duodenal wall tumors and the Zollinger-Ellison syndrome: Surgical management. *Arch. Surg.* 107:334, 1973.
151. Huppler, E. G., Priestley, J. T., Morlock, C. G., and Gage, R. P. Diagnosis and results of treatment in gastric polyps. *Surg. Gynecol. Obstet.* 110:309, 1960.
152. Hutchinson, W. B. Duodenotomy. *Am. J. Surg.* 122:777, 1971.
153. Iida, F. Transduodenal diverticulectomy for periampullary diverticula. *World. J. Surg.* 3:103, 1979.
154. Ikeda, T., Senoue, I., Hara, M., et al. Gastric pseudopolyposis: A new clinical manifestation of Type A gastritis. *Am. J. Surg.* 80:82, 1985.
155. Ingram, D. M., and Sheiner, H. J. Postoperative gastric emptying. *Br. J. Surg.* 68:572, 1981.
156. Inouye, W. Y., Farrell, C., Fitts, W. T., Jr., and Tristan, T. A. Duodenal duplication: Case report and literature review. *Ann. Surg.* 162:910, 1965.
157. Janson, K. L., and Stockinger, F. Duodenal hematoma: Critical analysis of recent treatment techniques. *Am. J. Surg.* 129:304, 1975.
158. Javdan, P., Pitman, E. R., and Schwartz, I. S. Gastric xanthelasma: Endoscopic recognition. *Gastroenterology* 67:1006, 1974.
159. Jefferiss, C. D. Spontaneous rupture of the stomach in an adult. *Br. J. Surg.* 59:79, 1972.
160. Jennings, K. P., and Klidjian, A. M. Acute gastric dilatation in anorexia nervosa. *Br. Med. J.* 2:477, 1974.
161. Jensen, F. B. Primary gastric sarcoma. *Acta Chir. Scand.* 133:139, 1967.
162. Jochimsen, P. R., and Lewis, J. W. Symptomatic pancreas relieved by surgical excision. *Surg. Gynecol. Obstet.* 153:49, 1981.
163. Joesting, D. R., Beart, R. W., van Heerden, J. A., and Weiland, L. H. Improving survival in adenocarcinoma of the duodenum. *Am. J. Surg.* 141:228, 1981.
164. Joffe, N. Some unusual roentgenologic findings associated with marked gastric dilation. *Am. J. Roentgenol. Radium Ther. Nucl. Med.* 119:291, 1973.
165. Joffe, N., Goldman, H., and Antonioli, D. A. Transpyloric prolapse of polypoid gastric carcinoma. *Gastroenterology* 72:1326, 1977.
166. Johansen, A., and Hansen, O. H. Macroscopically demonstrable heterotopic gastric mucosa in the duodenum. *Scand. J. Gastroenterol.* 8:59, 1973.
167. Johnson, G. K., Soergel, K. H., Hensley, G. T., et al. Cronkite-Canada syndrome: Gastrointestinal pathophysiology and morphology. *Gastroenterology* 63:140, 1972.
168. Jones, S. A., Carter, R., Smith, L. L., and Joergenson, E. J. Arterial mesenteric duodenal compression. *Am. J. Surg.* 100:262, 1960.
169. Jones, S. A., and Joergenson, E. J. Closure of duodenal wall defects. *Surgery* 53:438, 1963.
170. Jones, T. W., and Merendino, K. A. The perplexing duodenal diverticulum. *Surgery* 48:1068, 1960.
171. Jordan, F. T., Mazzeo, R. J., and Soiderer, M. H. Heterotopic gastric mucosa on the rectum: A rare cause of rectal bleeding. *Arch. Surg.* 118:876, 1983.
172. Jordan, G. L., Bolton, B. F., Heard, J. G., and Waldron, G. W. Sarcomas of the stomach. *Surg. Gynecol. Obstet.* 100:453, 1955.
173. Joseph, J. I., and Lattes, R. Gastric lymphosarcoma: Clinical pathologic analysis of 71 cases and its relation to disseminated lymphosarcoma. *Am. J. Clin. Pathol.* 45:653, 1966.
174. Juler, G. L., Labitzke, H. G., Lamb, R., and Allen, R. The pathogenesis of Dieulafoy's gastric erosion. *Am. J. Gastroenterol.* 79:195, 1984.
175. Justiniani, F. R., Wigoda, L., and Ortega, R. S. Duodenal caval fistula due to toothpick perforation. *J.A.M.A.* 227:788, 1974.
176. Kalman, P. G., Stone, R. M., and Phillips, M. J. Heterotopic gastric tissue of the bile duct. *Surgery* 89:384, 1981.
177. Kaplan, E. L., Dyson, W. L., and Fitts, W. T.,

Jr. Hyperplasia of Brunner's glands of the duodenum. *Surg. Gynecol. Obstet.* 126:371, 1968.

178. Kassner, E. G., Rose, J. S., Kottmeier, P. K., et al. Retention of small foreign objects in the stomach and duodenum. A sign of partial obstruction caused by duodenal anomalies. *Radiology* 114:683, 1975.
179. Kavlie, H., and White, T. T. Leiomyomas of the upper gastrointestinal tract. *Surgery* 71:842, 1972.
180. Keat, E. C. Giant hypertrophic gastritis (Ménétrier's disease) *Proc. R. Soc. Med.* 65:749, 1972.
181. Keet, A. D., and Heydenrych, J. J. Hiatus hernia, pyloric muscle hypertrophy and contracted pyloric segment in adults. *Am. J. Roentgenol. Radium Ther. Nucl. Med.* 113:217, 1971.
182. Keighley, M. R. B., Asquith, P., and Alexander-Williams, J. Postoperative duodenogastric reflux: A cause of gastritis and symptoms. *Gut* 15:336, 1974.
183. Keighley, M. R. B., Asquith, P., and Alexander-Williams, J. Duodenogastric reflux: A cause of gastric mucosal hyperemia and symptoms after operations for peptic ulceration. *Gut* 16:28, 1975.
184. Kelly, K. A., Code, C. F., and Elveback, L. R. Patterns of canine gastric electrical activity. *Am. J. Physiol.* 217:461, 1969.
185. Kelly, M. E., Motashemi, H., and Patel, S. H. Report of a case of double pylorus. *Dig. Dis. Sci.* 24:807, 1979.
186. Kenney, F. D., Dockerty, M. B., and Waugh, J. M. Giant hypertrophy of gastric mucosa: A clinical and pathological study. *Cancer* 7:671, 1954.
187. Kerremans, R. P., Lerut, J., and Penninckx, F. M. Primary malignant duodenal tumors. *Ann. Surg.* 190:179, 1979.
188. Keynes, W. M. Simple and complicated hypertrophic pyloric stenosis in the adult. *Gut* 6:240, 1965.
189. King, R. M., van Heerden, J. A., and Weiland, L. H. The management of gastric polyps. *Surg. Gynecol. Obstet.* 155:846, 1982.
190. Kinkhabwala, M. N., Konradi, H., Farman, J., and Rabinowitz, J. G. Acute emphysematous gastritis: The significance of the angiographic findings. *Radiology* 109:553, 1973.
191. Klinerman, J., Yardumian, K., and Tamaki, H. T. Primary carcinoma of the duodenum. *Ann. Intern. Med.* 32:451, 1950.
192. Klingenberg, P. H. Amyloidosis of gastrointestinal tract simulating gastric carcinoma. *Am. J. Surg.* 96:713, 1958.
193. Knutrud, O., and Eek, S. Combined intrinsic duodenal obstruction and malrotation. *Acta Chir. Scand.* 119:506, 1960.
194. Kraus, M., and Condon, R. E. Technic of duodenotomy. *Surg. Gynecol. Obstet.* 139:417, 1974.
195. Kremer, R. M., and Williams, J. S. Gastric sarcoidosis: A difficult diagnosis. *Am. Surg.* 36:686, 1970.
196. Krone, C. L., and Gelfand, M. D. Gastritis presenting as multiple polyposis of the stomach. *Gastroenterology* 57:703, 1969.
197. Kutin, N. D., Ranson, J. H. C., Gouge, T. H., and Localio, S. A. Villous tumors of the duodenum. *Ann. Surg.* 181:164, 1975.
198. Lapin, R., Kamath, M. L., Engler, J., and Friedman, H. Massive gastrointestinal hemorrhage from duodenal diverticula. *Am. J. Gastroenterol.* 61:185, 1974.
199. Lasser, A., and Koufman, W. B. Adenomyoma of the stomach. *Dig. Dis. Sci.* 22:965, 1977.
200. Lattes, R., and Grassi, C. Carcinoid tumors of the stomach. *Cancer* 9:698, 1956.
201. Lawrence, W., Jr., McNeill, D. D., Jr., Cohen, A., and Terz, J. J. Benign duodenal tumors: Unusual surgical problems. *Ann. Surg.* 172:1015, 1970.
202. Lawson, H. H. Effect of duodenal contents on the gastric mucosa under experimental conditions. *Lancet* 1:469, 1964.
203. Lawson, T. L. Intraluminal duodenal diverticulum: A rare cause of acute pancreatitis. *Am. J. Dig. Dis.* 19:673, 1974.
204. Leigh, T. E. Acute gastric dilatation. *J.A.M.A.* 172:1376, 1960.
205. Lempke, R. E. Intussusception of the duodenum: Report of a case due to Brunner's gland hyperplasia. *Ann. Surg.* 150:160, 1959.
206. Lesser, P. B., Falchuk, K. R., Singer, M., and Isselbacher, A. J. Menetrier's disease: Report of a case with transient and reversible findings. *Gastroenterology* 68:1598, 1975.
207. Lewis, J. W., Mason, E. E., and Jochimsen, P. R. Vascular malformations of the stomach and duodenum. *Surg. Gynecol. Obstet.* 153:225, 1981.
208. Lichstein, A., and Asher, L. M. Benign prolapse of gastric mucosa: Clinical, roentgenologic and gastroscopic study. *J.A.M.A.* 151:720, 1953.

209. Lindberg, B., and Kock, N. G. A family with atypical colonic polyposis and gastric cancer: A three-decade followup. *Cancer* 35:255, 1975.
210. Lindsay, P. C., Ordonex, N., and Raaf, J. H. Gastric leiomyosarcoma: Clinical and pathological review of fifty patients. *J. Surg. Oncol.* 18:399, 1981.
211. Linnemann, M. P., and Johnson, V. W. Ehlers-Danlos syndrome presenting with torsion of stomach. *Proc. R. Soc. Med.* 68:330, 1975.
212. Linos, D. A., Dozois, R. R., Dahlin, D. C., and Bartholomew, L. G. Does Peutz-Jeghers syndrome predispose to gastrointestinal malignancy? A later look. *Arch. Surg.* 116:1182, 1981.
213. Littler, E. R., and Gleibermann, E. Gastritis cystica polyposa (gastric mucosal prolapse at gastroenterostomy site, with cystic and infiltrative epithelial hyperplasia). *Cancer* 29:205, 1972.
214. Lloyd-Jones, W., Mountain, J. C., and Warren, K. W. Annular pancreas in the adult. *Ann. Surg.* 176:163, 1972.
215. Loehr, W., Mujahed, Z., Zahn, F. D., et al. Primary lymphoma of the gastrointestinal tract: A review of 100 cases. *Ann. Surg.* 170:232, 1969.
216. Lopez-Gallart, M. Duodenal ulcer in a patient with gastrointestinal situs inversus and dextrocardia. *Rev. Esp. Enferm. Apar. Dig.* 41:827, 1973.
217. Lotveit, T., Osnes, M., and Larsen, S. Recurrent biliary calculi: Duodenal diverticula as a predisposing factor. *Ann. Surg.* 196:30, 1982.
218. Lucas, C. E., and Ledgerwood, A. M. Factors influencing outcome after blunt duodenal injury. *J. Trauma* 15:839, 1975.
219. MacDonald, J. A. E. Adult hypertrophic pyloric stenosis. *Br. J. Surg.* 60:73, 1973.
220. Mackay, A. G., Elo, D. R., and Reines, H. Congenital duodenal web in an adult. *Am. Surg.* 40:355, 1974.
221. Mackman, S., Lemmer, K. E., and Morrissey, J. F. Postoperative reflux alkali gastritis and esophagitis. *Am. J. Surg.* 121:694, 1971.
222. Macmanus, Q., and Okies, J. E. Amyloidosis of the stomach: Report of an unusual case and review of the literature. *Am. Surg.* 42:607, 1976.
223. Maloney, R. D., Nealon, T. F., and Roberts, A. B. Massive bleeding from a ruptured superior mesenteric artery aneurysm into duodenum. *Arch. Surg.* 111:286, 1976.
224. Manny, J., Muga, M., and Eyal, Z. The continuing clinical enigma of duodenal diverticulum. *Am. J. Surg.* 142:596, 1981.
225. Marangos, G. N. Haemangiopericytoma of the stomach. *Gut* 6:77, 1965.
226. Marer, J. G., Donohoe, J. F., Fennelly, J. J., et al. Extragenital choriocarcinoma in a female presenting as a gastric tumor. *Br. J. Surg.* 57:73, 1970.
227. Marshak, R. H., and Feldman, F. Gastric polyps. *Am. J. Dig. Dis.* 10:909, 1965.
228. Marshall, S. F. Gastric tumors other than carcinoma. *Surg. Clin. North Am.* 35:693, 1955.
229. Marshall, S. F., and Meissner, W. A. Sarcoma of the stomach. *Ann. Surg.* 131:824, 1950.
230. Martin, T. D., Feliciano, D. V., Mattox, K. L., and Jordan, G. L. Severe duodenal injuries: Treatment with pyloric exclusion and gastrojejunostomy. *Arch. Surg.* 118:631, 1983.
231. Mast, W. H., Telle, L. D., and Turek, R. O. Annular pancreas: Errors in diagnosis and treatment of 8 cases. *Am. J. Surg.* 94:80, 1957.
232. Mattingly, S. S., Cibull, M. L., Ram, M. D, Hagihara, P. F., and Griffen, W. O. Pseudolymphoma of the stomach. *Arch. Surg.* 116:25, 1981.
233. Matzen, P., Davidsen, D., and Stenfeldt-Mathisen, M. Megaduodenum: A case with bacterial overgrowth, deconjugation of bile salts, malabsorption, and polyneuropathy. *Scand. J. Gastroenterol.* 9:645, 1974.
234. Mayo, H. W., Jr., McKee, E. E., and Anderson, R. M. Carcinoma arising in reduplications of the stomach (gastrogenous cyst): A case report. *Ann. Surg.* 141:550, 1955.
235. Mazuji, M. K., and Henry, J. S. Gastric actinomycosis: Case report. *Arch. Surg.* 94:292, 1967.
236. McCraken, J. D., and Davenport, O. L. Carcinoid of the stomach with giant duodenal ulcer. *Am. J. Surg.* 110:776, 1965.
237. McInnis, W. D., Aust, J. B., Cruz, A. B., and Root, H. D. Traumatic injuries of the duodenum: A comparison of 1° closure and the jejunal patch. *J. Trauma* 15:847, 1975.
238. Meissner, W. A. Leiomyoma of the stomach. *Arch. Pathol.* 38:207, 1944.
239. Meshkinpour, H., Marks, J. W., Schoenfield, L. J., et al. Reflux gastritis syndrome: Mechanism of symptoms. *Gastroenterology* 79:1283, 1980.
240. Miller, A. I., Smith, B., and Rogers, A.

I. Phlegmonous gastritis. *Gastroenterology* 68:231, 1975.

241. Minami, A. Gastric bezoars after gastrectomy. *Am. J. Surg.* 126:421, 1973.
242. Mir-Madjlessi, S. H., Farmer, R. G., and Hawk, W. A. Villous tumors of the duodenum and jejunum: Report of 4 cases and review of the literature. *Am. J. Dig. Dis.* 18:467, 1973.
243. Mir-Madjlessi, S. H., Sullivan, B. H., Jr., Farmer, R. G., and Beven, E. G. Endoscopic diagnosis of aortoduodenal fistula. *Gastrointest. Endosc.* 19:187, 1973.
244. Monaco, A. P., Roth, S. I., Castleman, B., and Welch, C. E. Adenomatous polyps of the stomach: A clinical and pathologic study of 153 cases. *Cancer* 15:456, 1962.
245. Moore, J. D., Thompson, N. W., Appleman, H. D., and Foley, D. Arteriovenous malformations of the gastrointestinal tract. *Arch. Surg.* 111:381, 1976.
246. Morrissey, K., Cho, E. S., Gray, G. F., Jr., and Thorbjarnarson, B. Muscular tumors of the stomach: Clinical and pathological study of 113 cases. *Ann. Surg.* 178:148, 1973.
247. Morton, J. H., Stabins, F. J., and Morton, J. M. Smooth muscle tumors of the alimentary canal. *Ann. Surg.* 144:487, 1956.
248. Morton, J. R., and Jordan, G. L. Traumatic duodenal injuries. *J. Trauma* 8:127, 1968.
249. Munro, A., and Simpson, J. G. Nodular lymphomoid hyperplasia of the stomach and small intestine with hypogammaglobulinemia. *Br. J. Surg.* 61:953, 1974.
250. Murphy, J. F., Graham, D. Y., Frankel, N. B., and Spjut, H. J. Intramural gastric abscess. *Am. J. Surg.* 131:618, 1976.
251. Murray, J. J., Schoetz, D. J., Jr., Nugent, F. W., et al. Surgical management of Crohn's disease involving the duodenum. *Am. J. Surg.* 147:58, 1984.
252. Nadau, M. R., and Abrams, M. W. Congenital pyloric atresia: A report of three cases and a review of the literature. *Surgery* 69:130, 1971.
253. Nahrwold, D. L., Cooke, A. R., and Grossman, M. I. Choleresis induced by stimulation of the gastric antrum. *Gastroenterology* 52:18, 1967.
254. Nance, F. C., Cocchiara, J., and Kinder, J. L. Acute pancreatitis associated with an intraluminal duodenal diverticulum. *Gastroenterology* 52:544, 1969.
255. Naqvi, M. S., Burrows, L., and Kark, A. E. Lymphoma of the gastrointestinal tract: Prognostic guides based on 162 cases. *Ann. Surg.* 170:221, 1969.
256. Nelson, S. W. Extraluminal gas collections due to diseases of the gastrointestinal tract. *Am. J. Roentgenol. Radium Ther. Nucl. Med.* 115:225, 1972.
257. Nevin, N. C., Eakins, D., Clarke, S. D., and Carson, D. J. L. Acute phlegmonous gastritis. *Br. J. Surg.* 56:268, 1969.
258. Nickerson, W. R., and Boschetti, A. E. Heterotopic gastric mucosa of gallbladder. *Am. J. Surg.* 125:345, 1973.
259. Nissen, S. Duplications of the stomach. *Am. J. Surg.* 100:59, 1960.
260. Nudellman, H. L., and Rakatansky, H. Gastric histoplasmosis. *J.A.M.A.* 195:134, 1966.
261. Oberhelman, H. A., Jr. Excisional therapy for ulcerogenic tumors of the duodenum: Long-term results. *Arch. Surg.* 104:447, 1972.
262. Ochsner, S., and Kleckner, M. S. Primary malignant neoplasms of the duodenum: Discussion based on 17 cases, with emphasis on radiologic diagnosis. *J.A.M.A.* 163:413, 1957.
263. Ochsner, S., and Lynch, R. C. Duodenal lipoma. *Ochsner Clin. Rep.* 3:24, 1957.
264. Ogbuokiri, C. G., Law, E. J., and MacMilllan, B. G. Superior mesenteric artery syndrome in burned children. *Am. J. Surg.* 124:75, 1972.
265. Orlando, R., Pastuszak, W., Preissler, P. L., and Welch, J. P. Gastric lymphoma: A clinicopathologic reappraisal. *Am. J. Surg.* 143:450, 1982.
266. Osborne, R., Toffler, R., and Lowman, R. M. Brunner's gland adenoma of the duodenum. *Am. J. Dig. Dis.* 18:689, 1973.
267. Overton, R. C., Jr., and Overstreet, J. W. Peptic bronchitis: Case report of mediastinal gastrogenic cyst with bronchial communication. *Am. Surg.* 29:64, 1958.
268. Pack, G. T. Unusual tumors of the stomach. *Ann. N.Y. Acad. Sci.* 114:985, 1964.
269. Page, V. S., and Bigelow, J. C. A mediastinal gastric duplication leading to pneumonectomy. *J. Thorac. Cardiovasc. Surg.* 54:291, 1967.
270. Palmer, E. D. Benign intramural tumors of the stomach: A review with special reference to gross pathology. *Medicine* 30:81, 1951.
271. Palmer, E. D. Course in prognosis of sarcoma of the stomach: 21 cases. *Gastroenterology* 33:389, 1957.
272. Palmer, E. D. Gastric diverticula with special reference to subjective manifestations. *Gastroenterology* 35:406, 1958.

273. Parker, H. W., Stewart, E. T., Geenen, J. E., and Hogan, W. J. Double duodenal diaphragms in an adult: Endoscopic, radiographic, and operative findings. *Gastroenterology* 71:663, 1976.
274. Parrish, R. A., Kanavage, C. B., Wells, J. A., and Moretz, W. H. Congenital antral membrane. *Surg. Gynecol. Obstet.* 127:999, 1968.
275. Passi, R. B., Kraft, A. R., and Vasko, J. S. Pathophysiologic mechanisms of shock in acute gastric dilatation. *Surgery* 65:298, 1969.
276. Paulson, D. L. Transthoracic gastric surgery with the report of transthoracic resection of diverticulum of stomach. *J. Thorac. Surg.* 13:518, 1944.
277. Peterhoff, R., and Schonebeck, J. Roentgen and gastrophotographic features of intraluminal gastric mycosis. *Scand. J. Gastroenterol.* 2:301, 1967.
278. Pinkerton, J. A., Jr. Aortoduodenal fistula. *J.A.M.A.* 225:1196, 1973.
279. Pollard, H., and Block, G. Rapid dissolution of phytobezoar by cellulase enzyme. *Am. J. Surg.* 116:933, 1968.
280. Raiford, T. S. Tumors of the small intestine. *Arch. Surg.* 25:122, 1932.
281. Ramsay, G. S. Enterogenous cyst of the stomach simulating hypertrophic pyloric stenosis. *Br. J. Surg.* 44:632, 1957.
282. Raotma, H., Angervall, L., Dahl, I., and Dotevall, G. Clinical and morphological studies of giant hypertrophic gastritis (Menetrier's disease). *Acta Med. Scand.* 195:247, 1974.
283. Rasaretnam, R., and Thavendran, A. Rupture of the retroperitoneal duodenum after blunt abdominal trauma. *Br. J. Surg.* 61:893, 1974.
284. Rabinovitch, J., Anton, J. I., Rabinovitch, P., and Mitchell, N. Primary carcinoma of the infrapapillary portion of the duodenum. *Arch. Surg.* 73:290, 1956.
285. Rehnberg, O., Faxen, A., Haglund, U., et al. Gastric mycosis following gastric resection and vagotomy. *Ann. Surg.* 196:21, 1982.
286. Reid, J. D. Duodenal carcinoma in the Peutz-Jeghers syndrome: Report of a case. *Cancer* 18:970, 1965.
287. Reisman, T. N., Leverett, F. L., Hudson, J. R., and Kalser, M. H. Syphilitic gastropathy. *Am. J. Dig. Dis.* 20:588, 1975.
288. ReMine, W. H. Gastric sarcomas. *Am. J. Surg.* 120:320, 1970.
289. Rigler, L. G., Kaplan, H. S., and Fink, D. I. Pernicious anemia and the early diagnosis of tumors of the stomach. *J.A.M.A.* 128:426, 1945.
290. Ritchie, W. P. Bile acids, the "barrier," and reflux-related clinical disorders of the gastric mucosa. *Surgery* 82:192, 1977.
291. Rivers, L., Silverstein, J., and Tope, J. W. The nine neoplasms of the small intestine. *Int. Abstr. Surg.* 102:1, 1956.
292. Roberts, L. J., Marney, S. R., and Oates, J. A. Blockade of the flush associated with metastatic gastric carcinoid by combined histamine H_1 and H_2 receptor antagonists. *N. Engl. J. Med.* 300:236, 1979.
293. Rooney, D. R. Aberrant pancreatic tissue in the stomach. *Radiology* 73:241, 1959.
294. Rooney, J. A., and Guzanskas, A. C. Submucous lipoma of the stomach. *Am. J. Surg.* 110:967, 1965.
295. Rosato, F. E., and Noto, J. A. Gastric polyps. *Am. J. Surg.* 111:647, 1966.
296. Ross, R., Nichols, P., Wright, W., et al. Asbestos exposure and lymphomas of the gastrointestinal tract and oral cavity. *Lancet* 2:1118, 1982.
297. Ross, T. M., Fazio, V. W., and Farmer, R. G. Long-term results of surgical treatment of Crohn's disease of the duodenum. *Ann. Surg.* 197:399, 1983.
298. Rowling, J. T. Some observations on gastric cysts. *Br. J. Surg.* 46:441, 1959.
299. Roxburgh, R. A. The case for total gastrectomy in multiple polyposis of the stomach. *Gut* 3:224, 1962.
300. Rubin, C. R., and Fink, H. Giant hypertrophy of the gastric mucosa associated with carcinoma of the stomach. *Am. J. Gastroenterol.* 47:379, 1967.
301. Rubin, W. Intestine in the stomach: Transformation of the gastric mucosa into an absorptive tissue. *Gastroenterology* 54:116, 1968.
302. Saiken, L. Foreign bodies in the stomach. *Am. J. Surg.* 97:342, 1959.
303. Sakker, S., and Ware, C. C. Carcinoma of the duodenum: Comparison of surgery radiotherapy and chemotherapy. *Br. J. Surg.* 60:867, 1973.
304. Salmon, P. A. Carcinoma of the distal duodenum. *Arch. Surg.* 108:89, 1974.
305. Sampsel, J. W., and Callaway, F. Gastric carcinoid with ossification. *Am. J. Surg.* 124:108, 1972.
306. Sawyers, J. L., Herrington, J. L., and Buckspan, G. S. Remedial operation for alkaline reflux gastritis and associated postgastrectomy

syndromes. *Arch. Surg.* 115:519, 1980.
307. Schnur, P. L., David, E., Brown, P. W., Jr., et al. Adenocarcinoma of the duodenum and the Gardner syndrome. *J.A.M.A.* 223:1229, 1973.
308. Schulten, M. F., Jr., Oyasu, R., and Beal, J. M. Villous adenoma of the duodenum: A case report and review of the literature. *Am. J. Surg.* 132:90, 1976.
309. Scott, H. W., Jr., Shull, H. J., Law, D. H., IV, et al. Surgical management of Menetrier's disease with protein-losing gastropathy. *Ann. Surg.* 181:765, 1975.
310. Scudamore, H. H., Eckstam, E. E., Fencil, W. J., and Jaramillo, C. A. Bile reflux gastritis: Diagnosis, medical and surgical therapy. *Am. J. Gastroenterol.* 60:9, 1973.
311. Serlin, O., and Wohl, G. T. The surgical implications of unsuspected ingested foreign bodies. *Am. J. Surg.* 99:223, 1960.
312. Shrum, R. C. Duodenal obstruction due to pressure of superior mesenteric vessels. *J.A.M.A.* 148:550, 1952.
313. Skandalakis, J. E., Gray, S. W., and Shepard, D. Smooth muscle tumors of the stomach. *Surg. Gynecol. Obstet.* 110:209, 1960.
314. Skandalakis, J. E., Gray, S. W., Shepard, D., and Bourne, G. H. Leiomyomas and Leiomyosarcomas: A Review of 2525 Cases. In *Smooth Muscle Tumors of the Alimentary Tract.* Springfield, Ill.: Thomas, 1962.
315. Sloop, R. D., and Montague, A. C. Gastric outlet obstruction due to congenital pyloric mucosal membrane. *Ann. Surg.* 165:598, 1967.
316. Smith, A. D., Jr., Woolverton, W. C., Weichert, R. F., III, and Drapanas, T. Operative management of pancreatic and duodenal injuries. *J. Trauma* 11:570, 1971.
317. Sobol, S., and Cooperman, A. M. Villous adenoma of the ampulla of Vater: An unusual case of biliary colic and obstructive jaundice. *Gastroenterology* 75:107, 1978.
318. Sommer, A. W., and Goodrich, W. A. Gastric diverticula. *J.A.M.A.* 153:1424, 1953.
319. Sparberg, M., Nielsen, A., and Andruczak, R. Bezoar following gastrectomy. *Am. J. Dig. Dis.* 13:579, 1968.
320. Spriggs, E. I., and Marxer, O. A. Polyps of the stomach and polypoid gastritis. *Q. J. Med.* 12:1, 1943.
321. Stanley, P. G., and Robinson, F. W. Leiomyosarcoma of the duodenum: Report of two cases and a review of the literature. *Am. Surg.* 36:702, 1970.
322. Starzl, T. E., Bernhard, V. M., and Heneger, G. C. Leiomyosarcoma of the duodenum. *Surg. Gynecol. Obstet.* 110:313, 1960.
323. Stephenson, L. W., Blackstone, E. H., and Aldrete, J. S. Radical resection for periampullary carcinomas. *Arch. Surg.* 112:245, 1977.
324. Stockman, J. M., Young, V. T., and Jenkins, A. L. Duplication of the rectum containing gastric mucosa. *J.A.M.A.* 173:1223, 1960.
325. Stone, D. D., Riddervold, H. O., and Keats, T. E. An unusual case of aberrant pancreas in the stomach: A roentgenographic and gastrophotographic demonstration. *Am. J. Roentgenol. Radium Ther. Nucl. Med.* 113:125, 1971.
326. Stout, A. P. Bizarre smooth muscle tumors of the stomach. *Cancer* 15:400, 1962.
327. Strauss, R. J., Friedman, M., Platt, N., et al. Gangrene of the stomach: A case of acute necrotizing gastritis. *Am. J. Surg.* 135:253, 1978.
328. Stroehlein, J. R., Weiland, L. H., Hoffman, H. N., and Judd, E. S. Untreated gastric pseudolymphoma. *Dig. Dis. Sci.* 22:465, 1977.
329. Strully, L. V., Schwartz, D. N., and Nagaraj, G. S. Pancreaticoduodenectomy in annular pancreas for relief of duodenal obstruction. *Am. J. Dig. Dis.* 20:671, 1975.
330. Swartz, W. T., and Shepard, R. D. Congenital mucosal diaphragm of the pyloric antrum. *J. Ky. Med. Assoc.* 54:149, 1956.
331. Szemes, G. C., and Amberg, J. R. Gastric bezoars after partial gastrectomy. *Radiology* 90:765, 1968.
332. Tan, K. L., and Murugasu, J. J. Congenital pyloric atresia in siblings. *Arch. Surg.* 106:100, 1973.
333. Tandon, V. M., Oesau, H. T., Jr., and Rassa, R. Intraluminal diverticulum of the duodenum. *Ann. Surg.* 178:787, 1973.
334. Tanimura, H., and Furuta, M. Carcinosarcoma of the stomach. *Surg. Gynecol. Obstet.* 110:702, 1967.
335. Tanner, N. C. Acute gastric distention in man and animals. *Proc. R. Soc. Med.* 52:379, 1959.
336. Taylor, T. V., and Torrance, H. B. Hemangiomas of the gastrointestinal tract. *Br. J. Surg.* 61:236, 1974.
337. Taylor, W. H. Isolated open ileal patches. *Arch. Surg.* 100:594, 1970.
338. Tedesco, F. J., Hosty, T. A., and Sumner, H. W. Hereditary hemorrhagic telangiectasia presenting as an unusual gastric lesion. *Gastroenterology* 68:384, 1975.
339. Teorell, T. Electrolyte diffusion in relation to

the acidity regulation of the gastric juice. *Gastroenterology* 9:425, 1947.
340. Thomas, T. V. Herniation of the stomach presenting as a diverticulum. *Postgrad. Med.* 50:67, 1971.
341. Thomford, N. R., Knight, P. R., Pace, W. G., and Madura, J. A. Annular pancreas in the adult: Selection of operation. *Ann. Surg.* 176:159, 1972.
342. Threadgill, F. D., and Hagelstein, A. Duodenal diaphragm in the adult. *Arch. Surg.* 83:878, 1961.
343. Toban, J. J., Jr., Schlang, H. A., and James, D. R. Intramural hematoma of the duodenum associated with peroral small-bowel biopsy. *J.A.M.A.* 198:211, 1966.
344. Tomasulo, J. Gastric polyps: Histologic types and their relationship to gastric carcinoma. *Cancer* 27:1346, 1971.
345. Tootla, F., Lucas, R. J., Bernacki, E. G., and Tabor, H. Gastroduodenal Crohn disease. *Arch. Surg.* 111:855, 1976.
346. Touroff, A. S. W., and Sussman, R. M. Congenital prepyloric membranous obstruction in a premature infant. *Surgery* 8:739, 1940.
347. Toye, D. K. M., and Williams, J. A. Postgastrectomy bile vomiting. *Lancet* 2:524, 1965.
348. Trimble, I. R., and Harkins, G. A. Sarcoma of the stomach. *Surg. Gynecol. Obstet.* 110:437, 1960.
349. Uei, Y., Koketsu, H., Konda, C., and Kimura, K. Cytodiagnosis of HCG-secreting choriocarcinoma of the stomach: Report of a case. *Acta Cytol.* 17:431, 1973.
350. Urdaneta, L. F., Belin, R. P., Cueto, J., and Doberneck, R. C. Intramural gastric actinomycosis. *Surgery* 62:431, 1967.
351. Utsunomiya, J., Maki, T., Iwama, T., et al. Gastric lesion of familial polyposis coli. *Cancer* 34:745, 1974.
352. Van Heerden, J. A., Phillips, S. F., Adson, M. A., and McIlrath, D. C. Postoperative reflux gastritis. *Am. J. Surg.* 129:82, 1975.
353. Vaughan, E. D., Jr., Sawyers, J. L.,and Scott, H. W., Jr. The Rapunzel syndrome: An unusual complication of intestinal bezoar. *Surgery* 63:339, 1968.
354. Veen, H. F., Oscarson, J. E. A., and Malt, R. A. Alien cancers of the duodenum. *Surg. Gynecol. Obstet.* 143:39, 1976.
355. Waltz, R. C., and Gerrish, E. W. Oral pigmentation, duodenal polyps and obstructive pancreatitis: A case report. *Ann. Surg.* 145:595, 1957.
356. Wang, C., and Welch, C. E. Anomalies of intestinal rotation in adolescents and adults. *Surgery* 54:839, 1963.
357. Warren, K. W. The surgical treatment of uncommon lesions of the duodenum. *Surg. Clin. North Am.* 32:877, 1952.
358. Watanabe, A., Nagashima, H., Motoi, M., and Ogawa, K. Familial juvenile polyposis of the stomach. *Gastroenterology* 77:148, 1979.
359. Watson, R. J., and O'Brien, M. T. Gastric pseudolymphoma (lymphofollicular gastritis). *Ann. Surg.* 171:98, 1970.
360. Wayne, E. R., and Burrington, J. D. Duodenal obstruction by the superior mesenteric artery in children. *Surgery* 72:762, 1972.
361. Weaver, G. A., Alpern, H. D., Davis, J. S., et al. Gastrointestinal angiodysplasia associated with aortic valve disease: Part of a spectrum of angiodysplasia of the gut. *Gastroenterology* 77:1, 1979.
362. Webb, H. W., Howard, J. M., Jordan, G. L., and Vowles, K. D. J. Surgical experiences in the treatment of duodenal injuries. *Surg. Gynecol. Obstet.* 106:105, 1958.
363. Weichert, R. F., Roth, L. M., Krementz, E. T., et al. Carcinoid-islet cell tumors of the duodenum: Report of 21 cases. *Ann. Surg.* 121:195, 1971.
364. Weidner, F. A., and Ziter, F. M. H. Carcinoid tumors of the gastrointestinal tract. *J.A.M.A.* 245:1153, 1981.
365. Welbourn, R. B. Current status of the apudomas. *Ann. Surg.* 185:1, 1977.
366. Welbourne, J. K., Ponka, J. L., and Rebuck, J. W. Lymphoma of the stomach. *Arch. Surg.* 90:480, 1965.
367. Welch, C. E. *Polypoid Lesions of the Gastrointestinal Tract.* Philadelphia: Saunders, 1964.
368. Welch, J. P. Smooth muscle tumors of the stomach. *Am. J. Surg.* 130:279, 1975.
369. Werschky, L. R., and Jordan, G. L. Surgical management of traumatic injuries to the pancreas. *Am. J. Surg.* 116:768, 1968.
370. Whipple, A. O. Non-Ulcerative Lesions of the Duodenum. In F. Christopher (Ed.), *Textbook of Surgery* (5th ed.). Philadelphia: Saunders, 1950. Pp. 992–1000.
371. White, J. J., and Morgan, W. W. Improved operative technique for gastric duplication. *Surgery* 67:522, 1970.
372. Williams, R. S., Gilmore, I. T., and Johnson, A. G. Congenital double pylorus: A case report. *Br. J. Surg.* 68:65, 1981.

373. Williams, S. J., Lucas, R. J., and McCaughey, R. S. Paraganglioma of the duodenum: A case report. *Surgery* 87:454, 1980.
374. Willis, R. A. *Pathology of Tumors*. London: Butterworth, 1948. P. 411.
375. Wilson, J. M., Melvin, D. B., Gray, G., and Thorbjarnarson, B. Benign small bowel tumor. *Ann. Surg.* 181:247, 1975.
376. Wilson, S. M., and Block, G. E. Periampullary carcinoma. *Arch. Surg.* 108:539, 1974.
377. Winkler, W. P., and Salek, J. Metoclopramide in the treatment of gastric bezoars. *Am. J. Gastroenterol.* 78:403, 1983.
378. Wise, L., Kyriakos, M., McCown, A., and Ballinger, W. F. Crohn's disease of the duodenum: A report and analysis of 11 new cases. *Am. J. Surg.* 121:184, 1971.
379. Wisloff, F., Bull-Berg, J., Myren, J. Herpes zoster of the stomach. *Lancet* 2:953, 1979.
380. Wittaker, L. D., Lynn, H. B., Dockerty, M. B., and Stickler, G. B. Heterotopic gastric mucosa in the wall of the cystic duct. *Surgery* 62:382, 1967.
381. Woolley, M. M., Gwinn, J. L., and Mares, A. Congenital partial gastric antral obstruction: An elusive cause of abdominal pain and vomiting. *Ann. Surg.* 180:265, 1974.
382. Yajko, R. D., Seydel, F., and Trimble, C. Rupture of the stomach from blunt abdominal trauma. *J. Trauma* 15:177, 1975.
383. Yao, T., Iida, M., Ohsato, K., et al. Duodenal lesions in familial polyposis of the colon. *Gastroenterology* 73:1086, 1977.
384. Yarniss, H., Marshak, R. H., and Friedman, A. I. Gastric polyps. *J.A.M.A.* 148:1088, 1952.
385. Yellin, A., and Rosoff, L. Pancreatoduodenectomy for combined pancreatoduodenal injuries. *Arch. Surg.* 110:1177, 1975.
386. Yeo, C. K., and McNamara, J. Retroperitoneal rupture of duodenum with complicating gas gangrene. *Arch. Surg.* 106:856, 1973.

EDITOR'S COMMENT

Robert Condon has gathered together a marvelous collection of more, and sometimes very much less, common curiosities; one has a tendency—which I am sure Dr. Condon would not mind—to read the chapter to see if there is anything that can be added. Perhaps there could be one addition concerning the Ehlers-Danlos syndrome, which is certainly mentioned in relation to gastric torsion and volvulus and its association with hemorrhage from the upper gastrointestinal tract. There are eight types of the syndrome, and all may be associated with a tendency to bruising. Unless this possibility is borne in mind, patients with less obvious degrees of the syndrome and gastrointestinal hemorrhage may undergo unnecessary and repeated investigations, as happened to one of our patients, before the correct diagnosis is made.

One other curiosity that has been brought to the fore by the use of the drug omeprazole is the development of enterochromaffin-like tumors in the stomach. These may develop in the stomachs of patients with pernicious anemia and have recently been described in toxicological studies in rats (mainly female) given high doses of omeprazole.

C.W.

22

Gastroesophageal Reflux

C. Thomas Bombeck

Although gastroesophageal reflux is not truly a disease of the stomach or duodenum, it is appropriate to consider it in this volume because its surgical treatment requires manipulation of the stomach and may eventually require duodenal diversion. Also, the disease process that results from reflux of gastric content into the esophagus, *reflux esophagitis,* is often misnamed "peptic esophagitis," implying an abnormal secretory state of the stomach or that the resultant esophageal inflammation is caused solely by abnormal contact of the esophagus with gastric secretions. Neither is necessarily true, although both factors may play a role in this disease complex. The proper nomenclature for the process is "reflux esophagitis and its consequences."

Because a hiatal hernia is not essential to the causation of reflux, it is often asked whether it should be repaired at the time that a true antireflux operation is carried out. The answer is that it should be repaired to prevent such complications as entrapment of a Nissen fundoplication within the thorax, but not with the expectation that hernia reduction will contribute to the antireflux properties of the operation.

Definition of Gastroesophageal Reflux

The term *reflux esophagitis* is relatively new in the spectrum of disease. Although the corrosive effect of gastric juice was recognized by Winkelstein in 1935 [137], it was not until 1946 that reflux of gastric content was understood to be the culprit in the production of the syndrome [2]. Reflux esophagitis may be defined as chemical inflammation of the distal esophagus caused by abnormal contact of the esophagus with normal gastric content, or possibly by normal contact of the esophagus with abnormal gastric content. This suggests that the etiology of the process is multifactorial, and evidence is rapidly accumulating to confirm this speculation [52, 104, 135].

All healthy persons experience gastroesophageal reflux [44, 48]. The difference between healthy persons and patients with reflux esophagitis is not in the event of reflux but in its degree or in the composition of the refluxed material. Eructation and vomiting are normal reflux events as well. There is further evidence that the patient may also be unable to clear normally refluxed material from his or her esophagus with the same facility as non-diseased persons [22, 28, 124, 126]. The event central to the production of reflux esophagitis is, however, gastroesophageal reflux.

ETIOLOGY OF REFLUX

The medical literature is replete with reports of one or another mechanism purported to be central in the normal prevention of gastroesophageal reflux. Allison, the father of modern antireflux surgery, asked why it was that when an individual enjoyed a picnic lunch and then bent over to observe his reflection in a stream, he did not observe his lunch to be floating away downstream! He proposed that the loss of the lunch was prevented by the sling mechanism of the esophageal hiatal musculature producing acute angulation in the distal esophagus in the same way that the puborectalis sling angulates the rectum [3]. His operation, the Allison repair for hiatal hernia, was based on this concept but was ineffective in the prevention of reflux.

As for the role of the sliding hiatal hernia, it is now generally agreed that it has little to do with the causation of gastroesophageal reflux [83, 98]. In the first place, a hernia may be demonstrated in most of the patient population older than 50 years of age [138], with an incidence approximating its occurrence in the population of patients with reflux esophagitis. DeMeester et al. [45] observed that the only relationship that can be demonstrated is that in patients with both reflux and a hernia, the larger the hernia, the more severe the reflux is likely to be. My associates and I have confirmed this observation. In the second place, approximately one-third of patients with reflux will not have any evidence of hiatal hernia, confirming that a hernia cannot be essential to the production of reflux [67].

In the years since 1951, 27 other mechanisms have been proposed to account for the normal competence of the gastroesophageal junction. The only one of these that has withstood the test of time is the lower esophageal sphincter (LES) mechanism [61, 70]. It is now generally agreed that the LES is the single most important physiological mechanism in prevention of reflux [51], but this realization was delayed by the inability of anatomical investigators to demonstrate a well-defined muscular structure at the gastroesophageal junction [75]. Anatomists sought a structure that would be analogous to the muscle band found at the pylorus, but despite the fact that the circular muscle at the gastroesophageal junction (GEJ) is somewhat thicker and more bulky than that found elsewhere in the esophagus, it does not correspond to the classical definition of a sphincter [85]. It remained for the elegant and painstaking studies of Liebermann-Meffert et al. [86] to define the anatomy of the gastroesophageal junction.

Using specimens obtained from cadaver kidney donors after the kidneys had been harvested, Liebermann-Meffert et al. dissected and measured all the muscle layers of the stomach and distal esophagus. The results of those studies demonstrated that the LES is a two-component structure, composed of horseshoe- or clasp-shaped muscle fibers clustered on the lesser curvature side of the esophagus and extending above and below the true gastroesophageal junction for approximately 4 cm in each direction, and the condensation of the oblique muscle layer of the stomach, which forms a sling on the greater curvature side of the esophagus (Fig. 22-1). The sling was first described by Thomas Willis in 1731, but its participation in the LES complex was not realized until 1979.

That the sling was important in LES closure was demonstrated by Gahagan [62] and by Vandertoll et al. [131], and the mechanism of its action was described by Samelson et al. [113]. At the time of this writing, the most tenable hypothesis is that the sling acts to protect and reinforce the sphincter action of the clasp fibers. Pettersson et al. [100] suggested that the sphincter is opened from below by tension communicated to it from the gradually distending stomach wall. Samelson et al. [116] confirmed this observation and demonstrated that limitation of distention of the lower end of

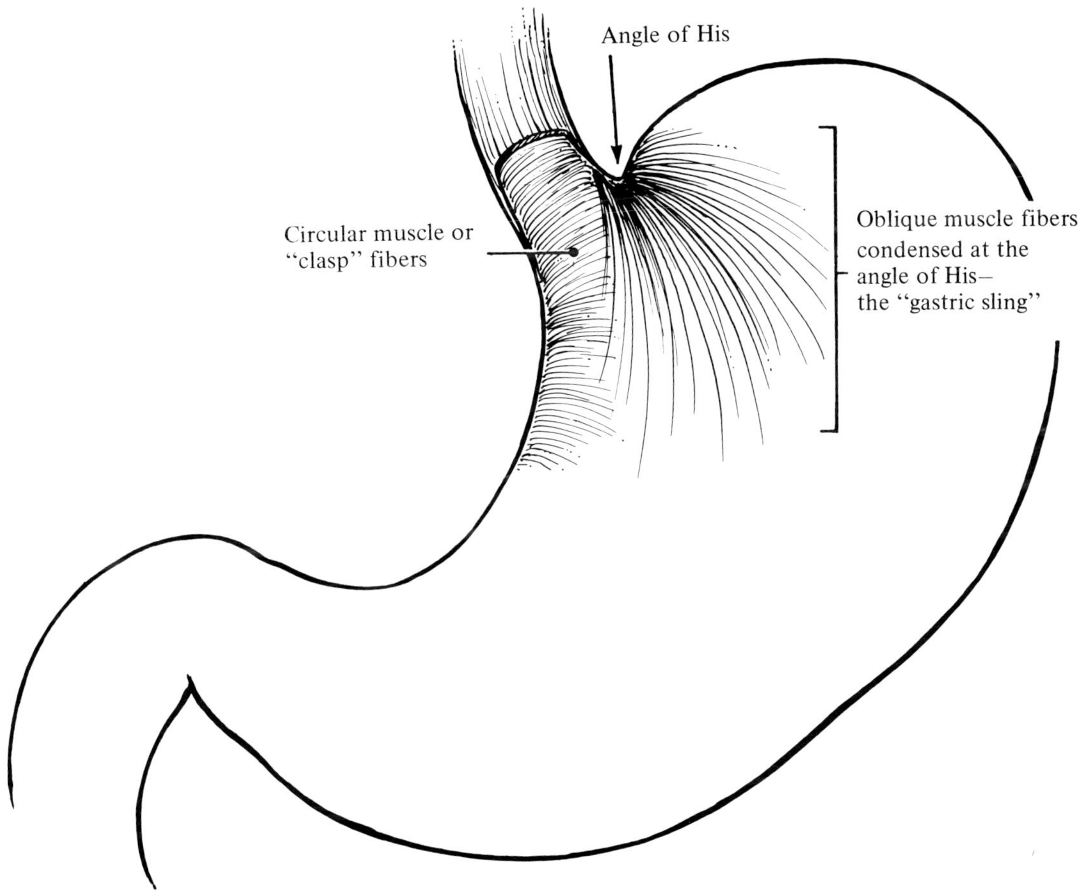

Fig. 22-1. Muscle fiber distribution at the gastroesophageal junction.

the sphincter protected it from being opened from below, an observation first made by Pettersson et al. [101]. The sling is ideally placed to perform this function naturally. Blum and Siewert [22] showed that the musculature of the sling, distinct from that of the remainder of the stomach, responds to the same stimuli as the circular muscle of the lower esophagus, providing both further evidence that the sling is a part of the LES and a rationale for its action: Any stimulus that would cause the circular muscle portion of the LES to contract would also cause the sling to contract to protect and reinforce the circular muscle closure of the distal esophagus. Winans [136] first demonstrated that the contractile force of the LES is asymmetrical, with higher pressures observed in the left and posterior aspects of the LES when simultaneous circumferential pressures are measured throughout the length of the sphincter by drawing a manometric catheter with radial pressure sensing openings at the same level back through its length. This high pressure area of the LES would correspond to the anatomical location of the sling and would thus be the area expected to be the strongest. Finally, Ellis and Olsen [58] and others [7, 125] have repeatedly cautioned that during the performance of a Heller myotomy for achalasia, it is the last few centimeters of the myotomy extending down onto the stomach that are responsible for the most common complication of myotomy—gastroesophageal reflux. It is of course those last few centimeters that would sever the sling.

CAUSES OF LOWER ESOPHAGEAL SPHINCTER FAILURE

LES opening is not to be confused with LES failure. In healthy persons there appears to be a dynamic balance between the normal forces that attempt to open the LES from below and the combined contractile force of the sling and clasp portions of the LES, which tend to keep it closed. That balance may be upset normally, as in the act of eructation, during which the LES is challenged by gastric distention with gas and the individual experiences a feeling of discomfort. He or she may belch spontaneously if the distracting force on the LES is great enough or may initiate the belch by swallowing a bolus of air. When the bolus reaches the LES, carried downward by primary peristalsis, the LES is inhibited, thereby upsetting the balance and allowing the sphincter to be opened by the distention forces in the stomach.

On the other hand, some mechanism may either prevent the LES from developing its normal contractility or increase the gastric challenge to the point that the LES, although otherwise sufficient, can no longer withstand the pressure. The efficiency of closure of the LES may be compromised by inability of the mucosa lining the LES to produce a sufficient "seal" even though the muscular action of the sphincter closes it. Simple mucosal superficial ulceration such as that produced by reflux can produce such damage [115], leading to the hypothesis that reflux esophagitis, at least when mild, may be a self-perpetuating disease. This has also been suggested by Richter and Castell [109], who postulated that the vicious circle may be caused by actual LES damage. Higgs et al. [69] demonstrated that esophagitis damages the LES in the experimental animal.

Intrinsic muscle damage may also compromise the LES. The esophageal defect in scleroderma, or mixed collagen-vascular disease, is well known [38]. Long-standing, severe inflammation may also damage the muscular sphincter. Such a defect is seen in severe esophagitis or in other forms of chemical trauma to the esophagus, such as acute lye burns. Direct trauma can destroy the musculature of the distal esophagus. Trauma may be either accidental, as from a gunshot wound, or intentional, as from a Heller myotomy or pneumatic or hydrostatic dilatation of the esophagus.

An abnormal or unusual hormonal milieu may affect the LES. It is likely that the commonly observed gastroesophageal reflux of pregnancy is caused not by increased abdominal contents of the pregnant woman, but rather by the prolonged increased levels of circulating estrogen in pregnancy. Progesterone has been shown to decrease LES pressures [40].

Medications or drugs may produce gastroesophageal (GE) reflux. All anticholinergic medications both decrease LES pressures and further aggravate reflux by decreasing gastric motility, leading to both gastric stasis and distention, which augments the normal gastric challenge to the LES. Caffeine and nicotine also have this effect [46, 47, 87].

At least theoretically, various peptide-secreting tumors should also inhibit the LES. Many of the peptide hormones exert an action on the LES, either inhibitory or stimulatory, so it is reasonable to assume that those actions accompany the tumor that secretes them in excess. Such an action has been shown only for the non-beta islet-cell tumor of the pancreas associated with the Zollinger-Ellison syndrome. In that disease LES pressures are increased [76].

Dillard and Anderson [49, 50] postulated mechanical embarrassment of the LES by diaphragmatic tension communicated to it through a phrenoesophageal ligament, which was or could be attached to the sphincter in a lower than normal location. In an anatomical investigation in humans, my associates and I [26] confirmed that hypothesis and demonstrated that it could be experimentally duplicated in dogs [25]. Unfortunately, because of both the tenuous nature of the phrenoesophageal membrane and its inaccessibility, this hypothesis could not be confirmed in living persons. Nonetheless, all operations that have been shown to be successful in the treatment of reflux have in common either ablation of tension on the ligament or its destruction.

Gastric challenge to the LES may be increased by anything that either increases intragastric pressure or increases gastric distention. The most common condition that appears to do this is obesity. In addition, any condition inhibiting gastric emptying will have the same effect. Gastroesophageal reflux is a common accompaniment to gastric outlet obstruction from whatever cause, and patients with gastroesophageal reflux have a much higher incidence of delayed gastric emptying than normal, without any anatomical lesion to account for it [89].

In any patient with reflux, it is common to find during an operation one or more of the aforementioned factors. Nonetheless, the single largest group of patients will be found to have no significant contributing factor when thoroughly studied by all the modalities at the physician's disposal. Although difficult to prove, since esophagitis itself decreases sphincter pressure [56, 121], it is likely that LES failure is most commonly idiopathic.

It is an intriguing hypothesis at present to consider that "reflux may be the cause of reflux." It is well known that chemical damage to the lower esophageal mucosa decreases measured LES pressure. Whether this is an actual decrease in contractile strength of the LES or an artifact of the measurement in the presence of mucosal ulceration is not clear [115]. If the former is true, it is reasonable to assume that esophagitis might result from some temporary imbalance in the dynamic relationship between LES strength and the gastric challenge to it, which would then allow pathological reflux to occur. Once the reflux began, mucosal chemical damage would be the necessary consequence. This would decrease the strength of contraction of the LES, allowing reflux to continue even if the initiating cause were removed, thereby establishing a "vicious circle" in which the esophagitis would become self-perpetuating. That this hypothesis is tenable is supported by the often demonstrated fact that patients with mild degrees of esophagitis readily respond to medical or nonoperative therapy and discontinue that therapy without recurrence of the esophagitis. Clearly nothing was done to the LES in those situations, except for reduction or healing of the overlying mucosal inflammation. This hypothesis, which would account for most instances of idiopathic LES failure, is currently under investigation in my laboratories.

PATHOPHYSIOLOGY OF REFLUX ESOPHAGITIS

Although gastroesophageal reflux is the prerequisite for the development of reflux esophagitis, it is not the only requirement. Indeed, healthy persons may reflux for as much as 5 percent of any 24-hour period [44] and do not have esophagitis. For the full-blown syndrome to occur, the following conditions must be present:

1. The patient must reflux in sufficient amounts.
2. The refluxed material must remain in contact with the esophagus.
3. The material must be capable of damaging the esophagus, i.e., capable of producing esophagitis.
4. The esophagus must be susceptible to damage from the refluxed material.

As stated, there must be sufficient reflux episodes to allow enough of the gastric content to enter the esophagus. The episodes must be sufficient not only in number, but in duration as well. DeMeester et al. [44] have shown that the individual with esophagitis not only refluxes more than normal, but the events last longer than normal.

The normal response to contact of the esophagus with low pH gastric content is the institution of a secondary peristaltic wave, which sweeps the esophagus clear of the refluxed material. It has been shown that the individual with esophagitis also has defective clearing of the esophagus, allowing the reflux episode to last longer [28, 81, 126]. It is difficult to distinguish defective clearing of the esophagus from prolonged and continuous reflux, but the point is moot. Either will result in prolongation of contact of the esophagus with the refluxed material. A similar "vicious circle" to that possibly seen with LES failure may pertain here. Reflux esophagitis causes disordered esophageal motility, which causes decreased esophageal clearing, which causes reflux esophagitis [51].

Normal acid-peptic gastric content will produce mild degrees of esophagitis if left in contact with the esophagus for sufficient periods of time. The most pronounced and severe degrees of esophagitis, however, are associated with reflux of a mixture of gastric and duodenal content [63, 64, 112]. The real culprit in the production of esophagitis is most probably bile salt from the duodenum. It has been shown that inhibition of gastric acid secretion results in the alleviation of the symptoms of esophagitis, without improving the severity of the disease process [11, 34, 105, 109]. When all other surgical procedures fail, simple diversion of duodenal content away from the stomach has been shown to be effective as a treatment of esophagitis.

Finally, every experienced esophagologist is familiar with the patient with all the symptoms of chronic regurgitation of gastric content who does not have demonstrable esophagitis. Such patients are rare. For reasons yet unknown, it appears that there is a small number of persons whose esophageal mucosa is impervious to prolonged contact with gastric content. This phenomenon has been called "increased mucosal resistance." These patients remain vulnerable to the other consequences of reflux, such as aspiration lung disease, and can be inconvenienced by the chronic regurgitation that they experience, but esophagitis does not develop. Such patients are sufficiently uncommon that each must be treated individually when encountered, and treatment must be designed to correct the symptoms as found. Rarely, some form of surgical intervention is required.

PATHOLOGY OF REFLUX ESOPHAGITIS

The pathological changes encountered with this disease are subtle. Microscopical observations are not classical, as found in other forms of gastrointestinal ulceration, and may be entirely overlooked by the pathologist unfamiliar with evaluation of esophageal biopsy specimens. Most experienced clinicians rely almost exclusively on gross appearance of the esophagus to diagnose the disease and follow the progress of treatment. For this reason, we have found it helpful to develop a staging system for rating the severity of reflux changes. It is based on the original criteria suggested by Moersch et al. [92].

Microscopical changes range from simple increases in the length of the squamous epithelial papillae with or without neutrophil infiltration in the milder degrees of esophagitis to complete mucosal destruction with acute inflammatory cell infiltration into the muscularis, with varying degrees of circumferential fibrosis. Fibrosis may extend through the wall of the esophagus and involve contiguous structures. All stages of acute and chronic ulceration may be present between these extremes [12, 77]. The columnar-lined esophagus deserves special mention. Most investigators [33, 94] now believe that this is an acquired condition. Paull et al. [99] demonstrated that, as a probable stage of healing of esophagitis, the mucosal lining of the distal esophagus may consist of atrophic fundic cells, including parietal cells; cardiac-type cells; or mostly mucus-secreting cells; or it may demonstrate intestinal metaplasia. The latter is important because of the demonstrated propensity of this condition for malignant degeneration [95]. It has also been demonstrated that chronic peptic ulcer of the esophagus usually occurs in this type of epithelium [107].

The gross classification as employed in our laboratories is as follows:

Stage O. No disease noted. Mucosa of the esophagus is the normal pink-tan color and is not fragile or friable, and the squamocolumnar junction is sharp and well-defined (see Plate 22-1).

Stage I. Mild esophagitis only. Mucosa may be erythematous with mild mucosal edema. The squamocolumnar junction will have lost definition, and, in places, the color change between the esophagus and stomach is not sharp but gradual. The mucosa tends to bleed with mild trauma, such as that produced by endoscope passage. All changes

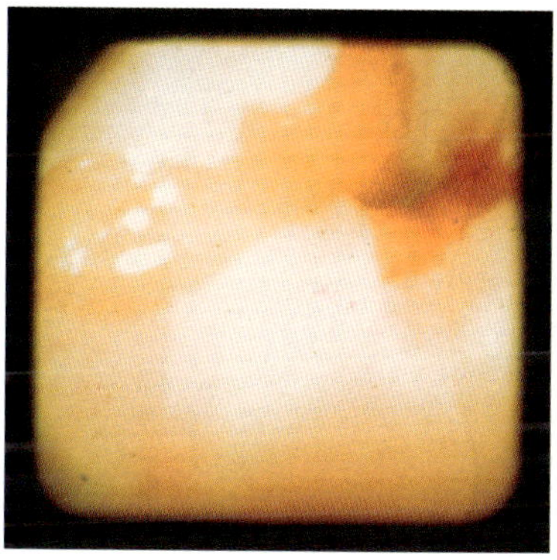

Fig. 22-2. Normal squamocolumnar junction.

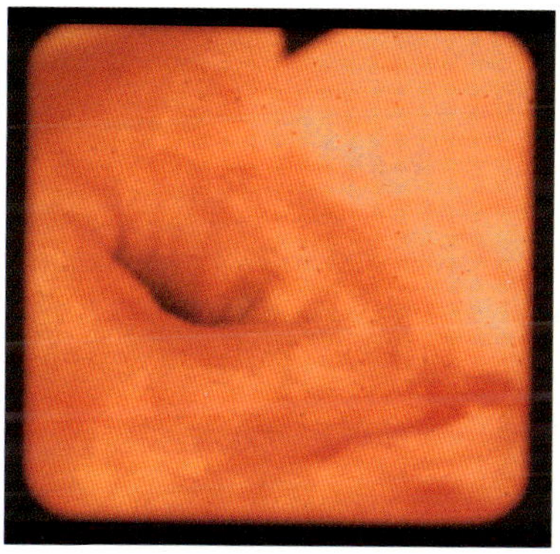

Fig. 22-3. Stage I esophagitis.

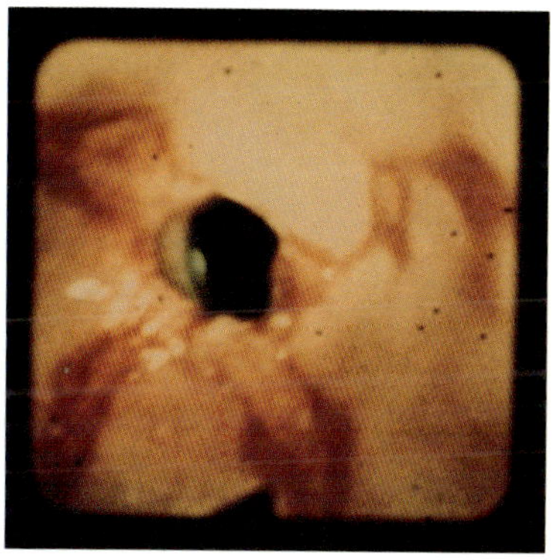

Fig. 22-4. Stage II esophagitis.

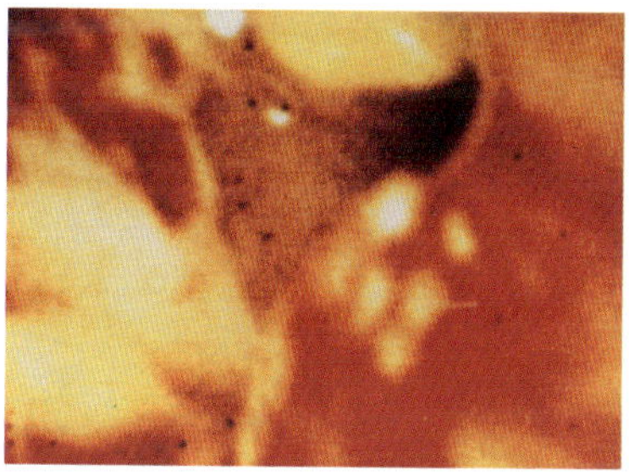

Fig. 22-5. Stage III esophagitis. Note bile-stained reflux.

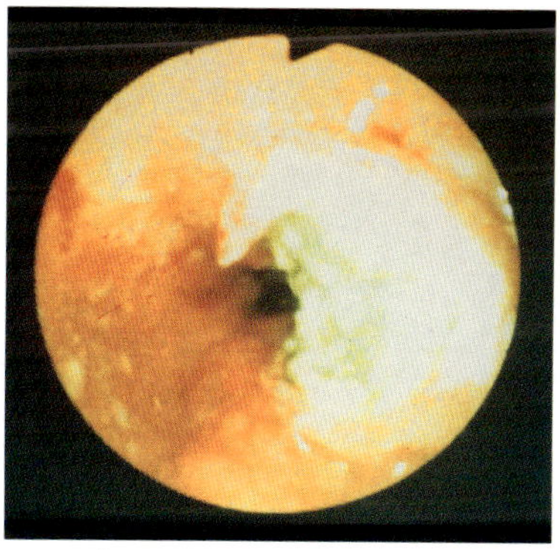

Fig. 22-6. Esophageal candidiasis.

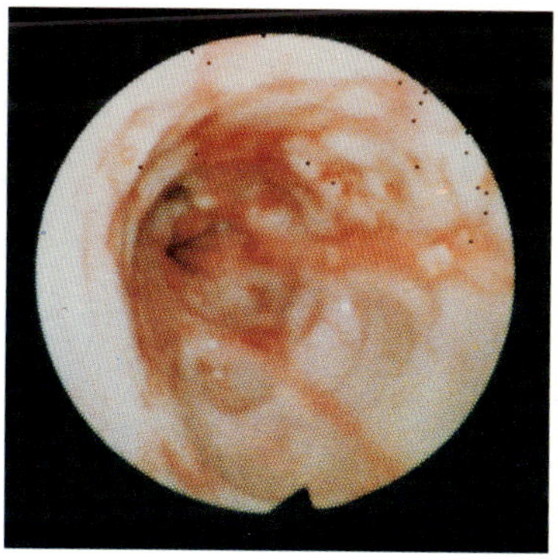

Fig. 22-7. Esophageal stricture with esophagitis.

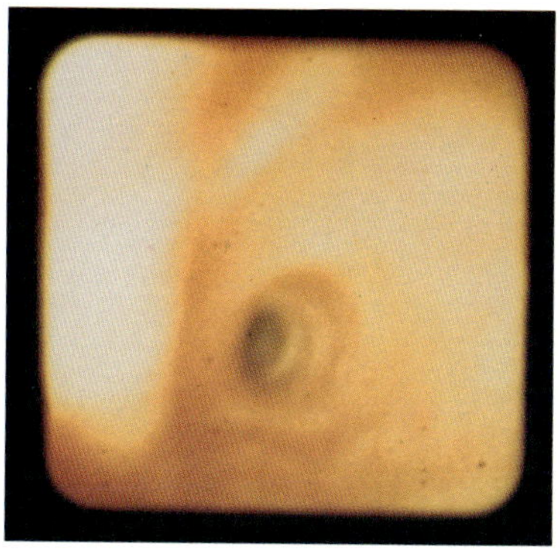

Fig. 22-8. Benign stricture without esophagitis above it.

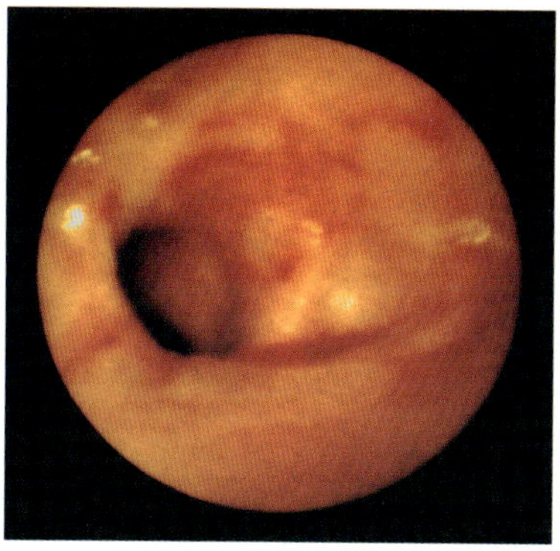

Fig. 22-9. Esophageal ulcer at squamocolumnar junction.

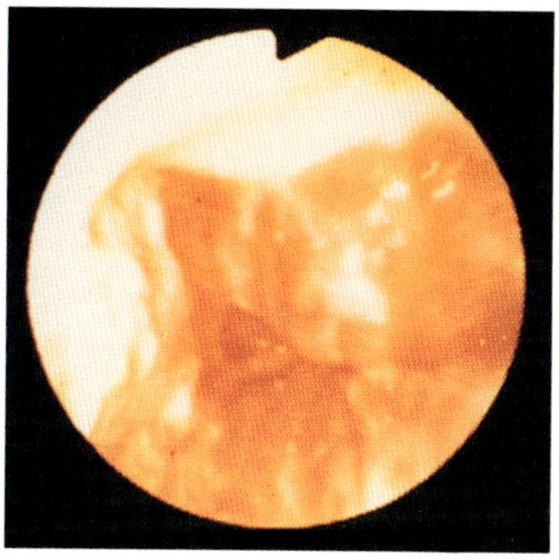

Fig. 22-10. Barrett's esophagus.

are irregular, so areas of normal mucosa are interspersed with areas of change (see Plate 22-1).

Stage II. Moderate esophagitis. All the changes seen in stage I are present but usually more pronounced. In stage II there are linear ulcerations of the mucosa as well. These are acute partial-thickness ulcerations of the esophageal mucosa, extending in a radial manner from the closed LES proximally (see Plate 22-2).

Stage III. Severe or florid esophagitis. All the changes found in earlier stages are present, except they are confluent in the distal esophagus. Squamocolumnar junction definition is lost entirely. Ulcerations are diffuse and too large to be described as "linear" but are still not full-thickness. A fibrinopurulent exudate is frequently present and may form a pseudomembrane. When the exudate is removed or dislodged with the end of the endoscope, the underlying ulcerated mucosa bleeds freely. This stage of the disease is easily confused with acute candidiasis of the esophagus if the pseudomembrane is thick and "cheesy" in character. Adequate differentiation is achieved by removing a segment of the membrane for immediate Gram stain and by assessment of the general condition of the patient. Candidiasis is usually only found in the debilitated or immunosuppressed patient (see Plates 22-3 and 22-4).

Stage IV. Complicated or advanced chronic esophagitis. This stage is characterized by the presence of one of the complications of long-standing, severe esophagitis. These include chronic fibrous stricture, chronic ulcer, and Barrett syndrome. Acute edematous stricture, which can be easily dilated, usually with the endoscope itself, is properly considered a severe form of stage III disease (see Plates 22-5 through 22-8).

We have found it useful to distinguish two types of esophageal stricture, since the degree of stricturing influences the method of treatment. The first, acute edematous stricture, is really not a true stricture at all, although the patient may present with the symptoms of stricture, i.e., dysphagia. This pseudostricture is caused by full-thickness inflammation of the distal esophagus, extending into the muscular layers but without destruction of those layers. The actual mechanical obstruction is produced by marked edema of the mucosa and submucosa, but not by permanent replacement with fibrous tissue. This form of stricture is reversible early in the course of treatment by any means that will correct its underlying cause, although it may require one or more dilations to reverse the dysphagia.

The second type of stricture, the chronic fibrous stricture, is a true fibrous scar of the distal esophagus. The submucosal and at least part of the muscular layers of the esophagus are replaced by fibrous tissue. Dilation of this type of stricture is extremely difficult, and the stricture promptly recurs after dilation. A progressive decrease in the time interval between required dilations in the patient who is undergoing long-term treatment for esophagitis with stricture is a signal that the stricture is undergoing transition from the acute to the chronic stage and an indication for reevaluation of the form of antireflux therapy being used. Fortunately, chronic fibrous stricture is rare, accounting for only a small percentage of strictures diagnosed for the first time. It is most commonly seen as a consequence of chemical trauma to the esophagus, such as a chronic lye stricture.

Barrett esophagus, first described in 1954 as a possible congenital esophageal lesion [8], has now been shown to be almost exclusively a stage of chronic, severe esophagitis [32, 74]. It is most commonly described as "the lower esophagus lined by columnar epithelium" [1]. It actually is produced by columnar metaplasia of the distal esophageal mucosa, although some investigators have suggested that it is an extension of gastric columnar epithelium upward from the stomach. It is frequently associated with a stricture at the upper extent of the metaplastic process, but the stricture is almost always of the acute edematous type. We have observed downward migration of this stricture with successful treatment of the condition. This has been confirmed by others [30].

Diagnosis of Reflux Esophagitis

SIGNS AND SYMPTOMS

The classical symptoms of reflux esophagitis include heartburn (pyrosis) most commonly; followed by nocturnal regurgitation; regurgitation of gastric content on bending, stooping, or other physical exertion; pain on swallowing; and aggravation of symptoms on ingestion of acid foods. The patient may complain of "excessive gas" or chronic flatulence and describes attempts to alleviate the symptoms by swallowing. The symptoms are unreliably relieved by antacids. The condition is more common in women, and obesity of some degree is a common finding.

As in most diseases of the esophagus, the classical symptoms are present only approximately one-third of the time [9]; although they are suggestive, further evaluation is usually required. Dysphagia is not a feature of ordinary reflux esophagitis, and its presence demands prompt endoscopic examination. In no instance is the severity of symptoms a reliable indicator of the severity of the disease process. When the symptoms are classical, however, and when there is no suggestion of esophageal obstruction, a short course of nonsurgical therapy is indicated on the basis of complaints alone. The standard nonoperative measures without supplemental medication except antacids for relief should bring prompt relief of symptoms, at least within one month after they are begun. If nonsurgical intervention does not succeed, further evaluation is required.

ROENTGENOGRAPHIC EXAMINATION

The place of roentgenography in the evaluation of esophageal disease is becoming more and more questionable. At this time, it is still recommended as the first examination to be carried out after the history and physical evaluation, although that recommendation may change in the near future. Certainly if there is any indication of difficulty in swallowing, it must be carried out promptly. If the dysphagia is located high in the chest or in the neck, lateral roentgenograms of the neck must be included as well to rule out pharyngoesophageal diverticulum (Zenker).

Many modifications of the standard roentgenographic techniques have been proposed, but none have survived for more than a few years. The best examination is the simple barium contrast swallow, performed by an experienced fluoroscopist, with the anteroposterior, lateral, and both oblique views obtained for documentation. If there is any suggestion of obstruction, short of complete closure, those views should be followed routinely by a radiopaque bolus swallow to evaluate esophageal patency. An esophageal relaxant, such as glucagon, should be incorporated with the bolus to rule out local areas of diffuse spasm and to confirm that an observed obstruction is truly an anatomical one. That portion of the examination should be reserved until the end because glucagon markedly deranges esophageal motility.

Procedures such as exaggerated Trendelenburg examinations, abdominal bolsters, abdominal compression, or the "water siphonage" test [88] are misleading and cause the patient excessive discomfort. Other interesting procedures, such as the "acid-barium swallow" [55], which was intended to provoke either esophageal pain or an acid-induced motility change, have proved to be without value. Even the cine-esophagogram is of questionable merit; at best, it serves as a permanent record of the fluoroscopy, but a good roentgenologist should be able to capture the pertinent anatomical findings of the fluoroscopy on one of the static roentgenograms. The expense of the cine does not seem to justify the luxury in this time of cost-consciousness in medicine. The same is true of the video esophagogram, which is of even less value because of its poor resolution of mucosal detail.

The primary difficulty with all types of esophageal roentgenographic examinations is the high incidence of false negative results obtained. It is that incidence that has spurred the search for more accurate and sensitive examinations. Positive findings are of considerable value when they can be documented, such as the presence of any constant anatomical abnormality of the esophagus, including all types of obstruction, and the presence of free gastroesophageal reflux with the patient at rest in the supine position. Other efforts to increase the findings of reflux in patients with esophagitis increase the incidence of false positive results as much as they do the incidence of true positive findings. Newer techniques such as the intensified computed tomogram of the esophagus with contrast have not been completely evaluated, and it is unlikely that they will be because of the rapid advances that have been made with endoscopy.

UPPER GASTROINTESTINAL ENDOSCOPY

Upper gastrointestinal endoscopy has become the "gold standard" of the diagnosis of esophageal disease. Fiberoptic instruments, which have been adopted widely by physician and surgeon alike, make this examination so simple, safe, and accurate that it is now an absolutely indispensable part of any complete esophageal evaluation. Its omission in any patient who does not respond promptly to simple therapy for reflux is a serious error. Every physician who treats more than the simplest form of esophageal disease should be able to perform the examination. Certainly every surgeon who operates for esophageal disease should personally look at the lesion before the operation. As a corollary to this, the examination must precede every operation done for esophageal disease so that the proper therapy can be planned. Only in the relatively uncommon situation in which the surgeon is closely associated with a physician-endoscopist who thoroughly documents all findings with adequate photography and biopsy is the surgeon excused from this responsibility.

A variety of instruments from several companies are now available. The differences among them are minor and clearly cater to individual preferences among users rather than the accuracy or safety of the examination. The instrument of choice is one of the smaller caliber, adult, end-viewing endoscopes. These have been called "panendoscopes" since they are the most versatile of all the instruments manufactured. An excellent second instrument for surgical gastroenterologists is a pediatric endoscope. Pediatric endoscopes have the same features as the larger instruments, with limitations as the result of their smaller size, thus requiring smaller biopsy ports, for example. They are especially useful for evaluating esophageal strictures, since the larger endoscope may not pass through the stricture. The pediatric endoscope may also serve as a backup for the larger endoscope when it is out of the hospital or office for repair, another feature shared by all endoscopes! Each endoscope should have its full complement of biopsy instruments, cytological brushes, washing tubes and traps, and irrigation or spray apparatus. An endoscopically passed dilator such as the Eder-Puestow (Key-Med Inc.) is an extremely useful accompaniment for stricture calibration or dilation at the time of endoscopy. Photographic capabilities are desirable for documentation or for following the progress of a lesion, although they are not absolutely essential.

The indications for upper gastrointestinal endoscopy in this situation are simple. Any patient who has any esophageal symptoms other than simple pyrosis, or any patient with pyrosis who does not respond to simple mechanical therapy within one month of the start of treatment, should have an endoscopic examination for verification of the diagnosis.

The procedure is simple [18, 20] and done on an outpatient basis. The patient is prepared by withholding all oral ingesta except water for 12 hours before the examination. At the time of the examination, the patient comes to the endoscopy room either in the physician's office or in the hospital. At the beginning of the examination, an intravenous portal is established with a heparin lock, and local anesthesia is produced with one of the aerosal anesthetic sprays, provided there is no allergy to these agents. Ordinarily sedation is not used unless the patient demands it or seems unduly apprehensive. It is rarely required for second-time or follow-up examinations. When sedation is needed, it is my practice to employ small bolus injections of meperidine through the IV portal. This drug has the advantage that it may be reversed with naloxone at the end of the procedure. As in all invasive procedures of this magnitude, facilities for emergency cardiopulmonary resuscitation should be at hand, although my associates and I have never had to use them in over 10,000 examinations.

The technique of endoscopy is beyond the scope of this volume. An experienced endoscopist should be able to examine the esophagus adequately in 15 minutes and the entirety of the esophagus, stomach, and duodenum in fewer than 30 minutes, including ancillary procedures such as endoscopic photography and limited biopsies. The gross stages of esophagitis observed endoscopically are shown in Figures 22-3 through 22-10.

SPECIALIZED TECHNIQUES

In patients with milder degrees of esophagitis, which usually respond readily to medical therapy, the aforementioned examinations will usually suffice. When symptoms are bizarre or when they persist despite endoscopic healing of esophagitis, further examinations are warranted. In more severe degrees of esophagitis, such as grades 3 or 4, and especially when a surgical procedure is contemplated, some assessment of esophageal motility is indicated. It is also helpful to have an objective measurement of the severity of reflux itself, if for no other reason than to document the results of treatment.

Esophageal Manometry

This is really a collection of examinations during which intraluminal pressures are measured throughout the body of the esophagus, including the LES under resting and stressed conditions and during swallowing. The primary value of these examinations is not in making the diagnosis of reflux, but rather in excluding other entities that may produce symptoms resembling those of reflux and esophagitis and that may persist after adequate treatment for reflux, resulting in unsatisfactory therapeutic results. Diseases such as achalasia, diffuse spasm of the esophagus, esophageal diverticula, and mixed collagen-vascular disease (scleroderma) of the esophagus all may be mistaken for simple reflux esophagitis and may have some component of reflux as part of their disease process. In most instances reflux is a result of the disease, not its cause, and prevention of reflux will only unmask the primary process, not treat it. Adequate diagnosis of the diseases of motility is achieved only by a well-performed esophageal manometric examination. Roentgenological evaluation provides information only when these diseases are far advanced and is not sufficiently discriminatory to distinguish one from another.

The role of manometry in the assessment of LES competence is not clear. The manometric measurement of LES contractile strength does not discriminate between the failing LES and the competent one, except at the extremes of the spectrum of LES contraction [27]. We have postulated that the reason for this discrepancy is that standard manometry does not measure the gastric sling component of the LES and that a decreased or absent sling allows the LES to be opened even when it appears relatively normal on ordinary measurement [113]. Manometry is therefore of value in reflux disease principally for the information it provides about the motility of the body of the esophagus. The assessment of reflux itself is best accomplished by the standard acid reflux test (SART) and by prolonged pH monitoring in the body of the esophagus above the LES.

Standard Acid Reflux Test

Primarily because of the difficulty in differentiation of the normal esophagus from one with reflux on manometry alone, many investigators have adapted the pH reflux test described by Tuttle et al. [130] to refine the results and make the test more discriminatory. The standard acid reflux test (SART) devised by Kantrowitz et al. [79], is one of these refinements. It is based on measurement of intraesophageal pH with an electrode positioned 5 cm above the LES in the patient whose stomach content is guaranteed acid by the prior instillation into the stomach of acidified barium suspension initially, and later, acid alone. Esophageal pH is monitored at rest with the patient in the supine position and then going through a standardized series of maneuvers in a standardized sequence. The whole series is repeated with the patient in each decubitus position and in the 20-degree head-down position. Based on the results of this testing, a reflux "score" is computed for each patient. The scoring method provides a more reliable method for diagnosis of reflux than either manometry or simple pH measurement on withdrawal of an electrode from the stomach across the LES, and it has the advantage that it can be performed in about 15 minutes by supporting personnel with relatively simple equipment. Several studies of the accuracy of this test have been carried out, demonstrating high sensitivity but poor specificity [40].

Twenty-Four Hour pH Monitoring

As a further refinement of SART and as a quantitative method for the measurement of reflux, Johnson and DeMeester [78] proposed the monitoring of intraesophageal pH over a 24-hour period at a point just above the LES, with the patient recording sensations of heartburn and physical activities. pH is recorded on a strip chart recorder, and patient responses are correlated to this permanent record. Although efforts are currently being made to refine this method by incorporation of radiotelemetry or computer recording of results, at present the method requires that the patient be hospitalized for the 24 hours of the test and that he or she be "tethered" to the pH recorders by the measurement leads. In addition, the 24-hour record produced by the test, a minute-to-minute measurement, is voluminous and requires a prolonged and tedious reading to interpret results. Nonetheless, the method is now accepted as the most accurate way to incriminate reflux as a cause of a patient's symptoms. Recent reports of computerization of this method [31, 91] promise to reduce the expense and inconvenience of performing it.

Using this method, several parameters are studied. The number of reflux episodes can be determined and the duration of each measured. Reflux is defined as a measured esophageal pH below 4. The pattern of reflux also is determined with relation to the position of the patient and whether or not the patient has a full stomach, i.e., the relationship to meals. In my laboratories [118] healthy persons without esophageal disease or symptoms reflux less than 5 percent of the time, do so only in the immediately postprandial period, and have reflux episodes of 1 minute or less. Reflux usually occurs in the upright position. Patients with reflux esophagitis reflux more than 5 percent of the time and almost always more than 15 percent of the time. Reflux episodes last longer than 5 minutes and occur in the recumbent position without relation to meals. Patients who reflux in both the recumbent and upright positions generally have the worst degrees of esophagitis. All patterns revert to normal after successful antireflux operations.

Recently we have become aware of a variant of the patient with pathological reflux. These are patients who have reflux material of an abnormally high pH—the alkaline refluxers. These individuals frequently have undergone a surgical procedure that has compromised their antral-pyloric anatomy, allowing duodenogastric reflux. The more severe degrees of esophagitis are usually found in this subgroup.

Esophageal Acid Clearing

For reflux to produce esophagitis, it seems evident that the refluxed material must remain in contact with the esophageal mucosa for a prolonged period of time above normal, since some degree of reflux is a normal event. Booth et al. [28] proposed a test of the ability of the esophagus to clear a challenging acid load. In the test, a bolus of 0.1 N HCl is instilled into the esophagus 10 cm above a pH electrode that is itself positioned above the LES. Esophageal motility is simultaneously recorded. The patient is then instructed to swallow voluntarily, thereby inducing primary peristaltic waves that can be measured. In our laboratories, nondiseased persons clear the esophagus of acid, shown by a rise in esophageal pH to above 4, in six or fewer swallows. The patient with significant reflux esophagitis requires more than 12 swallows, ranging all the way to complete inability to clear. The test is neither as specific nor as accurate as 24-hour pH monitoring. It also suffers from the inability to discriminate between a defective clearance mechanism and a totally incompetent LES. An incompetent LES may masquerade as a defective clearing mechanism, since relaxation of an effective peristaltic wave will immediately allow free reflux of the cleared material back up into the esophagus. (No mechanism exists to keep the cleared material in the stomach.) Nonetheless, the test is an easily performed component of the standard motility examination and occasionally is the most strikingly abnormal component of that examination.

Esophageal and Gastric Scintiscanning
Radioisotopic scintiscanning, using a variety of isotopes, has been adapted to several tests related to gastroesophageal reflux. In the simplest methods, technetium-labeled egg is given to the patient orally, and serial gamma camera scans of the esophagus and stomach are made. This allows semiquantitative estimation of both esophageal and gastric emptying times as well as semiquantification of the amount and severity of reflux if present [60, 72]. A further refinement of these measurements has been proposed by Wolverson et al. [139] in which the patient is given two isotopes, both of which are accumulated by the liver but only one of which is excreted in the bile. Using computerized isotopic subtraction techniques, the amount of isotope excreted into the duodenum is measured and the degree of both duodenogastric and gastroesophageal reflux is determined. At this time the technique is still experimental, requires highly sophisticated and expensive equipment, and takes several hours to perform.

Esophageal Acid Perfusion Test
This test, first introduced in 1958 by Bernstein and Baker [19], remains an important method for the diagnosis of esophagitis in many laboratories [19]. The test is carried out by having the patient sit in a chair with a nasogastric tube placed with its orifice just above the LES. Normal saline solution is dripped through the tube at a rate of 100 drops per minute for 15 minutes. Without informing the patient of the change, 0.1 N HCl is substituted for the saline solution at the same rate. The test is considered positive if the patient's symptoms are duplicated by the change. Benz et al. [17] claimed that this is the most sensitive and accurate of esophageal diagnostic tests. Experience in our laboratories has been disappointing: Only about 50 percent of patients with endoscopically demonstrated esophagitis have a positive test—the same incidence expected by chance. The test has been adopted as part of the motility examination, wherein acid is instilled into the esophagus and its effect on motility observed. Results have been inconsistent.

Many other types of studies have been proposed over the years in attempts to correlate patient symptoms, material refluxed, amount of reflux, and mucosal damage. These have included measurement of transmucosal potential difference, wall thickness, LES resistance to dilatation, LES "squeeze" strength, and other factors. At this time none of these is used clinically, and it would seem that the tests already described are adequate.

Approach to the Patient with Esophagitis

A flow chart outlining the steps in diagnosis and management of the patient with symptoms of gastroesophageal reflux is given in Figure 22-11. Much of the diagnosis of the severity of the disease complex is based on the patient's response to treatment, so diagnostic interventions are timed to provide information when helpful. As a general rule 40–50 percent of patients who are seen for the first time with heartburn of sufficient severity to make them contact a physician respond to simple mechanical measures to reduce reflux; 30 percent require intensive medical therapy, with half of this group requiring some form of ongoing therapy to prevent relapse; and approximately 5 to 10 percent require some form of operation. The remaining 10 percent either have sufficiently severe esophagitis to require immediate, vigorous antireflux therapy—either medical or surgical or both—or have some other disease, possibly including carcinoma.

MEDICAL THERAPY FOR ESOPHAGITIS
The nonsurgical treatment of gastroesophageal reflux has been well summarized by the

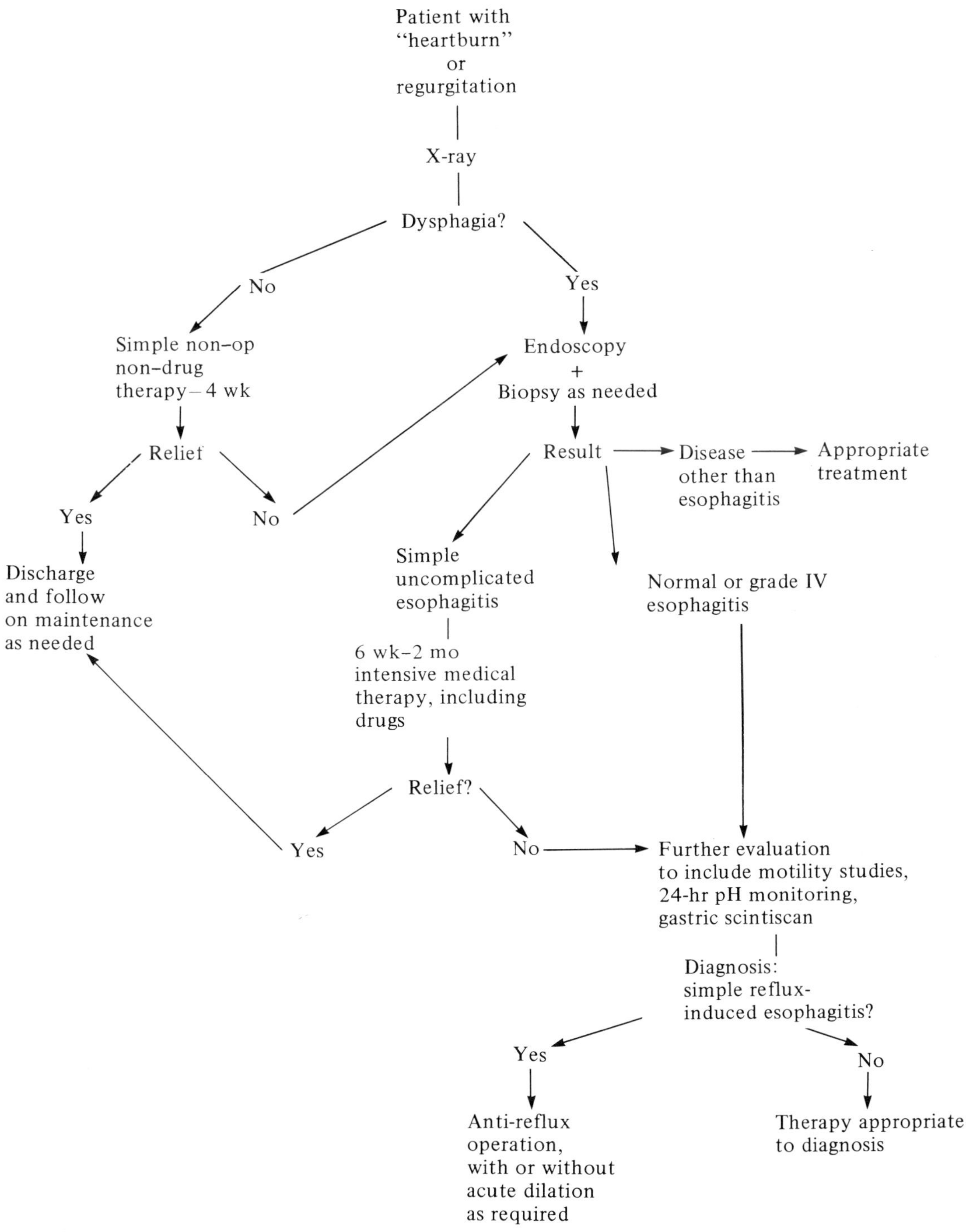

Fig. 22-11. Flowchart outlining the decision process in the approach to the patient with esophagitis.

Castell group [37, 108]. It must be noted that only recently has medical therapy included anything but simple mechanical measures, coupled with antacids mostly for symptomatic relief, to reduce reflux. Because therapy has been largely mechanical, little evidence is available regarding the newer, more powerful, methods of drug therapy, but it is to be expected that as the drugs are used, reflux esophagitis will require surgical intervention even less frequently than it does now.

"Medical" therapy may be divided into five general classes as follows. The classes are ranked in the order of their rigorousness to the patient and generally represent the phases of treatment to be carried out in order. The last—surgical treatment—is included under the heading of medical therapy because it is the internist or generalist who must make the initial decision regarding whether or not the patient requires an operation.

1. Simple mechanical intervention to reduce reflux.
   a. Elevation of the head of the bed on 8-inch blocks. This means blocks placed under the legs of the bed, not extra pillows!
   b. Avoidance of oral ingesta for 3 hours before reclining in the evening, so that the stomach will be empty during sleep.
   c. Avoidance of tight clothing, lifting of heavy objects, and bending or stooping, generally any maneuvers that raise intra-abdominal pressure.
   d. Weight reduction if obese. Even the loss of a few critical pounds often produces dramatic relief of reflux symptoms.
2. Simple modification of dietary and social habits.
   a. Avoidance of foods that aggravate reflux, such as chocolate, alcohol, carminatives, or carbonated beverages.
   b. Avoidance of foods directly irritating to the esophagus. For example, orange juice has a pH of 2.1, cola, 2.5, and fruit-flavored carbonated beverages, 3.5.
   c. Cessation of smoking, especially when reclining. Two cigarettes within 20 minutes will decrease LES pressure by 50 percent.
3. Reduction in gastric acid or acid reflux.
   a. Antacids. Simple antacids produce pain relief, and there is evidence that they increase LES pressures, possibly by antral gastrin release.
   b. Alginate preparations. Sodium alginate in combination with sodium bicarbonate produces a viscid "plug" that floats on the gastric liquid pool and, theoretically, occludes the gastroesophageal junction to prevent reflux. When incorporated with antacids, these preparations may improve mucosal adherence of the antacid. In my laboratories, this combination is little better than antacid alone.
   c. Cimetidine or ranitidine. The H_2-receptor blocking agents do not affect the LES but act only to decrease gastric acid secretion. Evidence that they promote healing of esophagitis is lacking, but they produce relief of heartburn, leading to the suggestion that simple acid reflux is not central to the production of esophagitis but to production of its symptoms.
   d. Anticholinergic agents. These should be avoided. Although they decrease gastric acid secretion, they also decrease LES pressures and prolong gastric emptying times.
4. Agents that increase LES pressure include bethanechol chloride (Urecholine), metoclopramide, and domperidone. All these agents stimulate the LES to contract, thereby improving the antireflux barrier. They also increase the efficiency of esophageal emptying, and the latter two promote gastric emptying. Metoclopramide has a high incidence of central nervous system (CNS) side effects. Domperidone does not cross the blood-brain barrier but is not yet approved for use in the United States. Bethanechol appears to be slightly more effective than the others.
5. Antireflux surgery

SURGICAL INDICATIONS

These are relatively simple when medical therapy fails after an adequate trial. The usual indications of intractability, obstruction, bleeding, or perforation are all included in this statement. In the past, we have defined an adequate trial of medical therapy to mean at least one year of intensive treatment but have now modified that dictum to two months of modern intensive medical treatment, including pharmacological augmentation of the LES. Although there have been no controlled studies on the subject, it has been our general experience in the treatment of more than 900 patients with esophagitis that if the patient is to respond, he or she will do so within two months of the institution of therapy. The questions then arise whether the patient will have a relapse if intensive treatment is stopped and how long the patient is willing to maintain the rigorous discipline necessary for adequate medical treatment should he or she respond to it and be dependent on it. Clearly the indications must be individualized for each patient. There has been one attempt to contrast medical with surgical therapy for esophagitis [13], in which surgical treatment proved superior in terms of alleviation of symptoms. Unfortunately, that study was carried out before the modern era of drug augmentation of the LES, so it is currently meaningless.

Many investigators have attempted to define objective criteria based on the various diagnostic modalities to make a decision for operation. None of these has proved absolute, although some are better than others. They are as follows:

1. LES resting pressure of less than 3 mmHg
2. Failure of the LES to respond to bethanechol chloride (Urecholine)
3. Grade 3 or higher esophagitis

Although patients in these categories are much less likely to respond to nonsurgical treatment, some will, and who they will be is unpredictable.

In the last analysis, in high success rates of all the procedures currently available, the variable complication rates with each procedure, the small though significant mortality, and the difficulty of prolonging nonoperative treatment must all be weighed together.

VAGOTOMY IN THE TREATMENT OF REFLUX DISEASE

From its introduction in the mid-1940s until about 1963 there were multiple recommendations that some form of vagotomy be included as an integral part of antireflux procedures. Although highly selective or parietal cell vagotomy may be incorporated in all the antireflux procedures and is remarkably easy to perform with the exposure necessary for the antireflux procedure, such incorporation is done only if the patient has concomitant peptic ulcer disease. Vagotomy is contraindicated in pure antireflux operations for two reasons: Reflux esophagitis is not a disease of gastric hypersecretion, and vagotomy of any form has complications of its own [132].

SURGICAL PROCEDURES FOR GASTROESOPHAGEAL REFLUX

These procedures may be divided into two general categories—those for simple reflux with esophagitis and those for failures in the first category along with those for esophagitis complicated in some way.

Simple Antireflux Procedures

With one exception, all currently acceptable operations embody some form of fundoplication, i.e., plication of the fundus of the stomach around a variable portion of the circumference of the esophagus. These are the Nissen fundoplication [96], currently the most popular operation in the world; the Belsey Mark IV fundoplication [10]; the Hill posterior gastropexy [71, 111]; and modifications of these [23, 29, 42, 106, 123, 129]. The exception is the recently introduced silicone esophageal prosthesis of Angelchik and Cohen [4]. That prosthesis does not produce any degree of fundoplication but acts to protect the LES from gastric distraction and has led to a whole new concept of how the other procedures may be effective [16, 114]. Samelson and Castell [16, 114] have each advanced a hypothesis for the mechanism of action of the prosthesis. Their hypotheses are similar in that both postulate protection of the LES. Samelson believes the LES is protected by augmentation and reinforcement of the sling mechanism, and Castell believes the mechanism is posterior bolstering of the LES. Samelson et al. also have provided direct evidence that the fundoplication procedures act to limit the effect of gastric wall distraction on the LES, giving the fundoplications and the prosthesis a common mode of action.

Other mechanisms have been proposed to account for the efficacy of the fundoplications. It is of interest that each operation was initially proposed primarily as a treatment of hiatal hernia, and the rationale for each operation was revised as it became apparent that a hernia could recur while the antireflux action of the operation remained intact. The same phenomenon has been observed with the prosthesis: Its initial mechanism was postulated to be hernia reduction; as it became apparent that hernia reduction was not essential for reflux prevention, alternative explanations were sought. In 1967 my colleagues and I coined the term "valvuloplasty" [25] to describe the Nissen fundoplication, only to become aware that if the operation did indeed achieve an adequate one-way valve, allowing ingress into the stomach but preventing retrograde egress, a whole new set of complications ensued, now called the "gas bloat" syndrome because of the individual's inability to belch.

Blum and Siewert [22] then postulated that the fundoplications acted to augment the contractile muscle mass of the LES, since measured LES pressure was raised by the operations. Hill [71] still recommends that this augmentation is necessary and measures it in the operating room as an index of an effective operation. Few others have adopted this practice because of the specialized equipment required and the time added to the operative procedure. Because of concern about the overly effective Nissen procedure, Donahue and I [53] modified the procedure originally described by Nissen and called the modification the *floppy Nissen*. That operation has now widely supplanted the original procedure. In studies of patients with the floppy Nissen (FN), it became evident that the increased LES pressure observed with the standard procedure was not present. Nonetheless, reflux was prevented. This has been observed by many investigators [5, 80, 93]. The modus operandi of the fundoplications now seems to be transfer of the point at which gastric wall distraction acts on the LES from the GEJ, or lower end of the sphincter, to some point higher on the body of the sphincter, thereby allowing the sphincter to act normally without challenge. For this action to occur, the fundoplications must also provide at least minimal sphincteric augmentation, since a nonexistent sphincter cannot act regardless of how well it is protected. For the same reason, the prosthesis must also provide a modicum of LES augmentation, but its method of doing so remains unclear.

Nissen Fundoplication

This operation, modified by Donahue as the FN, is the most widely used procedure in the world for the treatment of simple reflux. In a survey of 1354 recently graduated surgeons taken between 1981 and 1983, 97 percent were found to prefer the Nissen as the operation of first choice for simple reflux [24]. Those surgeons were candidates for the general surgery board examinations and included few thoracic surgeons.

The Nissen fundoplication is based on enfolding the distal 3 cm of the esophagus, immediately above the gastroesophageal junction, in the fundus of the stomach. The enfolding must be loose and pliable or the procedure will produce a one-way valve and prevent normal (belching, vomiting) as well as abnormal reflux. Several points of the operation are critical, and it should not be undertaken by a surgeon who seldom does the operation. The steps of the operation are shown in Figure 22-12.

TECHNIQUE. The patient is placed on the operating table in the supine position, and a rolled bolster is placed under the midback to provide hyperextension. The gastroesophageal junction is approached through a variety of incisions, depending on the practice of the operating surgeon. I use an upper abdominal midline incision, extending from the apex of the left xiphoid-costal angle to or below the umbilicus. The left triangular ligament is divided as far to the right as possible, with care

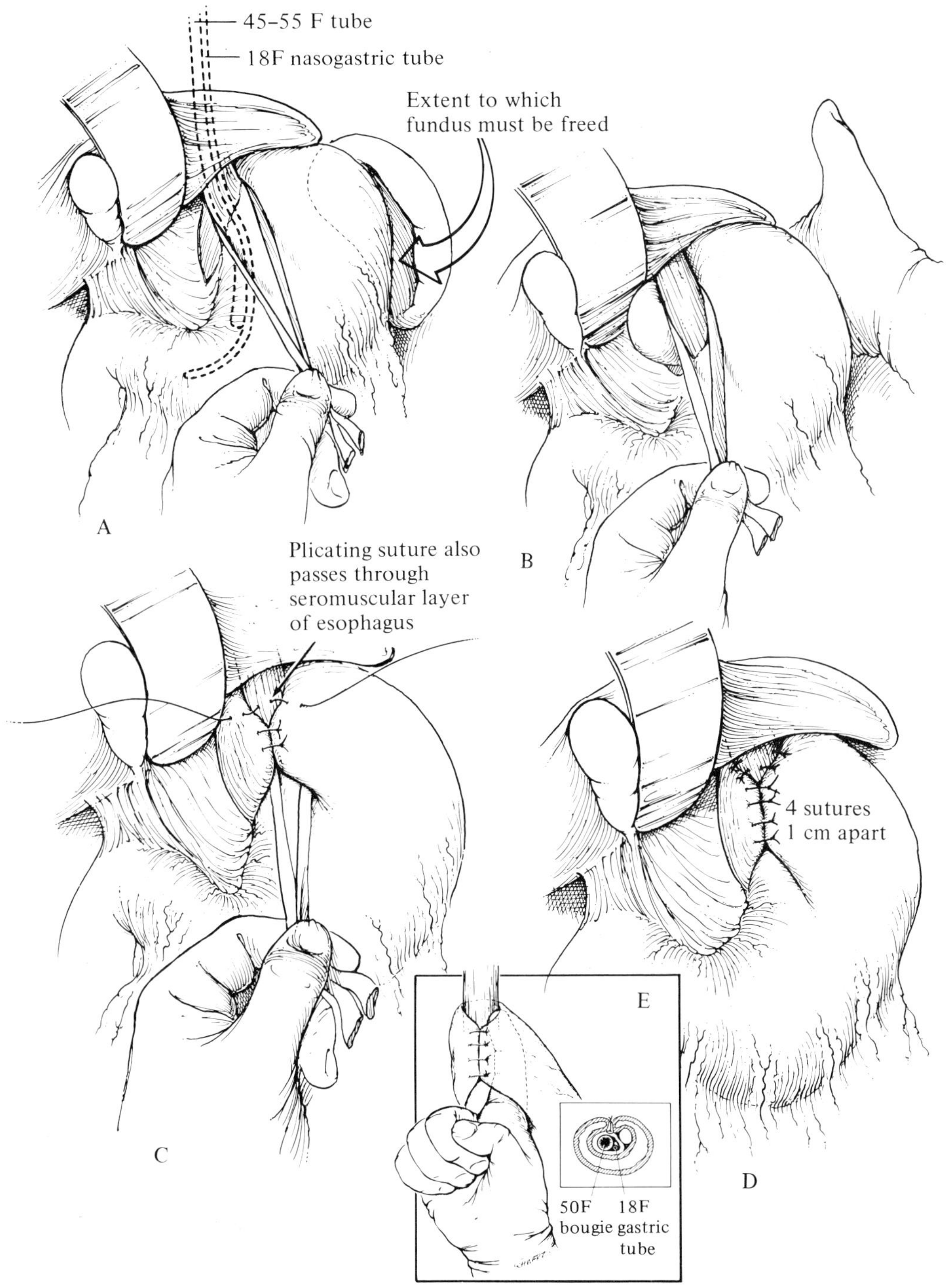

Fig. 22-12. Steps in the floppy Nissen fundoplication. (A) Fundus of stomach freed down to midpoint of short gastric vessel supply. (B) Fundus loosely folded around esophagus. (C) Fundus sewn in place with four sutures, which also anchor it to the esophagus. (D) Completed fundoplication, anchored to esophagus at its upper margin. (E) Cross-section of fundus cuff showing tubes in place.

to avoid the phrenic veins in the medial portions. The left lobe of the liver is reflected to the right to expose the gastroesophageal junction. Further exposure is provided by one of the table-mounted self-retaining retractors to elevate and spread the costal margin further. Extra attention to establishing good exposure at the beginning of the procedure is well worth the time required and the occasional postoperative discomfort of the patient caused by the retracted costal margin. A large-bore tube such as a Ewald tube is placed in the esophagus by the anesthesiologist to serve as a guide to its identification, which is occasionally helpful in the patient with severe periesophagitis. An endoscope is occasionally used instead of the tube in situations in which the anatomy is distorted, as from a prior operation.

The gastroesophageal junction is next dissected free with a combination of sharp and blunt dissection. The vagi are identified and carefully protected. The posterior vagus may be separated from the esophagus, and it is pushed posteriorly, out of harm's way. The anterior vagus is left in situ on the anterior surface of the esophagus. During this process, both the gastrohepatic and gastrophrenic ligaments are divided from the gastroesophageal junction up to the esophageal hiatus, which is formed primarily of fibers of the right diaphragmatic crus. An Amendola retractor is helpful in retracting the gastroesophageal junction to the left to facilitate exposure of the hiatus posteriorly. A half-inch Penrose drain is passed around the esophagus and double-looped around the gastroesophageal junction to keep it from slipping down when traction is applied to it.

If the hiatus is widened, i.e., if the patient has a sliding hiatal hernia, it is closed with two to six sutures of 00 silk posterior to the esophagus to prevent subsequent herniation and entrapment of the fundoplication. This step is carried out at this time because the fundoplication makes exposure more difficult after it is constructed.

The greater curvature of the stomach is then freed, with sufficient short gastric vessels divided to allow complete mobility of the fundus. Failure to free the fundus adequately is probably one of the most serious reasons for subsequent fundoplication disruption. In most patients, freeing the fundus requires division of about half the short gastric vessels. Until this step is completed, great care is exercised not to place traction on the stomach to avoid tearing the splenic capsule. Splenic injury should not occur with this procedure except in highly unusual circumstances.

Traction is then placed on the previously placed Penrose drain, elevating the gastroesophageal junction anteriorly, and the freed fundus of the stomach is folded around the lower esophagus by pushing it posterior to the gastroesophageal junction with the fingers of the surgeon's right hand. We have used a specially modified Babcock clamp for this purpose, but that modification is really not necessary. As the fundus is seen to the right of the esophagus, it is grasped with a large Babcock or Duval clamp and pulled around the gastroesophageal junction. It must come into position freely, without any suggestion of tension or resistance. It may be necessary to free more of the greater curvature at this point to obtain sufficient free fundus.

As soon as the fundus is in place, the floppy fundoplication is constructed. This is done with four 00 silk sutures placed 1 cm apart, beginning at the gastroesophageal junction and extending upward. No plication is done below the gastroesophageal junction since that would not prevent reflux and might lead to postoperative obstruction. In practice, the uppermost sutures are placed first and gently tied as they are placed. Each suture passes through the fundic wall to the left of the esophagus, through the esophageal wall, taking care not to enter the lumen, and through the fundic wall to the right of the esophagus. During placement of the plicating sutures, the surgeon may ensure sufficient "looseness" of the plication by inserting a No. 14 Hegar dilator under the right margin of the cuff. An index finger serves the same purpose. The Ewald tube is left in place during the entire procedure to calibrate the fundoplication internally.

As a final step in the operation, two sutures are placed between the upper edge of the fundoplication and the esophageal wall on each side of the esophagus. The purpose of these sutures, as well as the bites taken in the esophageal wall with the plicating sutures, is to prevent the plication from slipping down onto the body of the stomach. This situation, the "slipped Nissen," is one of the well-recognized complications of this procedure.

The abdomen is then irrigated and closed in a manner dictated by the incision used. No drains are employed. In the postoperative period, nasogastric decompression is maintained until there is absolutely no doubt about the return of normal gastric motility. It is better to err on the side of leaving the tube too long than to chance having the patient vomit, thereby disrupting a fresh fundoplication. If a problem with prolonged postoperative decompression is anticipated in advance, a temporary gastrostomy is put in place during the operation. In the past, my associates and I routinely did a gastrostomy, but recently we have opted for as many as six to seven days of nasogastric decompression.

The essential components of this operation are as follows:

1. Absolutely no tension in any component
2. Fundoplication no more than 3 cm in length
3. Fundoplication carried out with at least a 55F stent
4. Loose plication allowing a No. 14 Hegar dilator to be slipped under it, with the esophageal stent in place

COMPLICATIONS. These relate to three areas: the overly competent fundoplication, the displaced or misplaced plication, and the disrupted plication (failure). In addition, other surgeons have reported a high incidence of splenic injury during the procedure, necrosis or perforation of the fundoplication cuff, and perforation and fistulization from the esophagus itself, from the site of sutures placed in the esophageal wall [6, 35, 36, 103, 120].

The overly competent plication occurs when the original recommendations for the procedure are followed. Patients experience some degree of dysphagia, although this is usually transient. A few have required postoperative dilation. Gas bloat is the most common of these complications, occurring as often as 30 percent of the time. In the last 37 patients we treated with the floppy modification, there has been no incidence of this problem. When gas bloat does occur it usually improves with time, as patients learn to stop swallowing air. In a few instances, the plication cuff may require dilation. When it does only forceful, pneumatic dilation, as for achalasia, will suffice since the cuff must be partially disrupted.

The displaced or misplaced plication is a much more serious problem than the other complications. The cuff may slide down onto the body of the stomach, producing an obstructed gastric fundus. It may even be displaced to the midcorpus, producing a dramatic situation with an obstructed proximal pouch of stomach. This leads to a serious recurrence of reflux, together with symptoms from the obstructed pouch including gastric ulceration. Misplacement is also a severe problem, occurring when the fundoplication herniates into the posterior mediastinum through a hiatus dilated just enough to admit it, or as the result of disruption of the diaphragmatic closure after a transthoracic Nissen procedure and becoming entrapped there. Hiatal compression of the plication may produce lower esophageal obstruction in this situation, or if low enough on the body of the stomach, may actually cause a "closed loop" type of obstruction with the entrapped gastric loculus closed at the top by the fundoplication and at the bottom by hiatal compression. In either of these situations, the only treatment is revision of the operation.

Disruption of the plication is almost the sole reason for its failure. Whereas the hallmark of a successful Nissen fundoplication is dramatic cessation of all symptoms of reflux, usually noted by the patient in the early postoperative period, the hallmark of a disrupted plication is dramatic, usually abrupt and sudden, resumption of the symptoms. If disruption occurs, it usually does so in the first month after the operation. Patients usually give a history of forceful vomiting for some reason as the precipitating event. My group had one patient who noted resumption of symptoms after quickly drinking four pints of a carbonated soft drink in rapid succession during his fourth postoperative week! Patients should be cautioned against such artificial stresses.

The diagnosis of disruption is usually simple. Repeat studies demonstrate recurrent reflux, and endoscopy shows either a partial or absent Nissen "nipple" when the gastroesophageal junction is viewed with the endoscope retroflexed in the stomach [21]. The treatment is restoration of the plication with avoidance of the situation that caused it to disrupt.

Belsey Mark IV Procedure

This operation (Fig. 22-13) is a combined hernia reduction–fundoplication procedure and is carried out through a transthoracic approach. As such it is often favored by those thoracic surgeons who also perform antireflux operations [73, 97]. The principle of its action differs little from that of the Nissen fundoplication save for the additional provision of reduction of a possibly concomitant hiatal hernia with restoration of a length of intra-abdominal esophagus. It also accomplishes a limited fundoplication. Instead of the complete enfolding of the distal esophagus as achieved by the Nissen fundoplication, the Belsey procedure is limited to a two-thirds enfolding of the lower esophagus. This suggests that it is not quite as effective an antireflux procedure as the Nissen, but that it is not as subject to the complications of too complete a valvuloplasty that threaten the Nissen. Both predictions have proved true. Belsey suggests the following for a successful operation [14, 15]:

There are four main criteria:

1. Complete, permanent relief of all symptoms and complications of reflux.
2. The ability to eat normally, drink normally, and lead a normal life without recourse to any further medical or postural treatment.
3. The ability to relieve gas distention of the stomach by belching.
4. The ability to vomit when necessary.

Provided that these four criteria are fulfilled, any technique is acceptable.

TECHNIQUE. The patient is placed in the right lateral position on the operating table. An oblique incision is made over the sixth intercostal space and carried downward and forward as far as the costal margin. Posteriorly, the incision is carried upward along the lateral margin of the erector spinae muscle, 6–8 cm from the midline.

The incision is carried deeply, preserving the latissimus dorsi and serratus anterior muscles for the greater portion of their lengths, and the seventh rib is divided posteriorly. The pleura is opened along the upper margin of the rib. The ribs are spread only to allow adequate exposure of the gastroesophageal junction from above.

The lung is retracted anteriorly and upward, and the inferior pulmonary ligament is divided up to the level of the inferior pulmonary vein. The mediastinal pleura is opened from the diaphragm to the aortic arch. The esophagus is identified and gently freed from its bed with sharp and blunt dissection. This step may be difficult if there is marked periesophagitis. Adequate mobilization of the esophagus from the diaphragm to the aortic arch is essential.

The gastroesophageal junction is mobilized by division of the phrenoesophageal ligament. Traction on the esophagus then brings the gastric peritoneal reflection or hernial sac into view. This is incised, effecting entry into the peritoneal cavity. This incision is carried circumferentially around the gastroesophageal junction to the posterior right aspect, where

Fig. 22-13. Steps in the Belsey Mark IV procedure. (A) The incision. (B) The lung is reflected. (C) The esophagus is isolated and ensnared. (D) The "artery of Belsey" is divided. (E) The hernia (if any) is freed and stomach brought above the diaphragm. (F) Sutures are placed but not tied so that the hiatus can be closed. (G) First row of plicating sutures placed. (H) Plicating sutures are tied, achieving a 180–270 degree fundoplication. (I) The second row of plicating sutures is placed, protecting abdominal contents with a "spoon." (J) Sutures are in place, ready to tie. (K) Sutures are tied, bringing plicating segment below the diaphragm and anchoring it there.

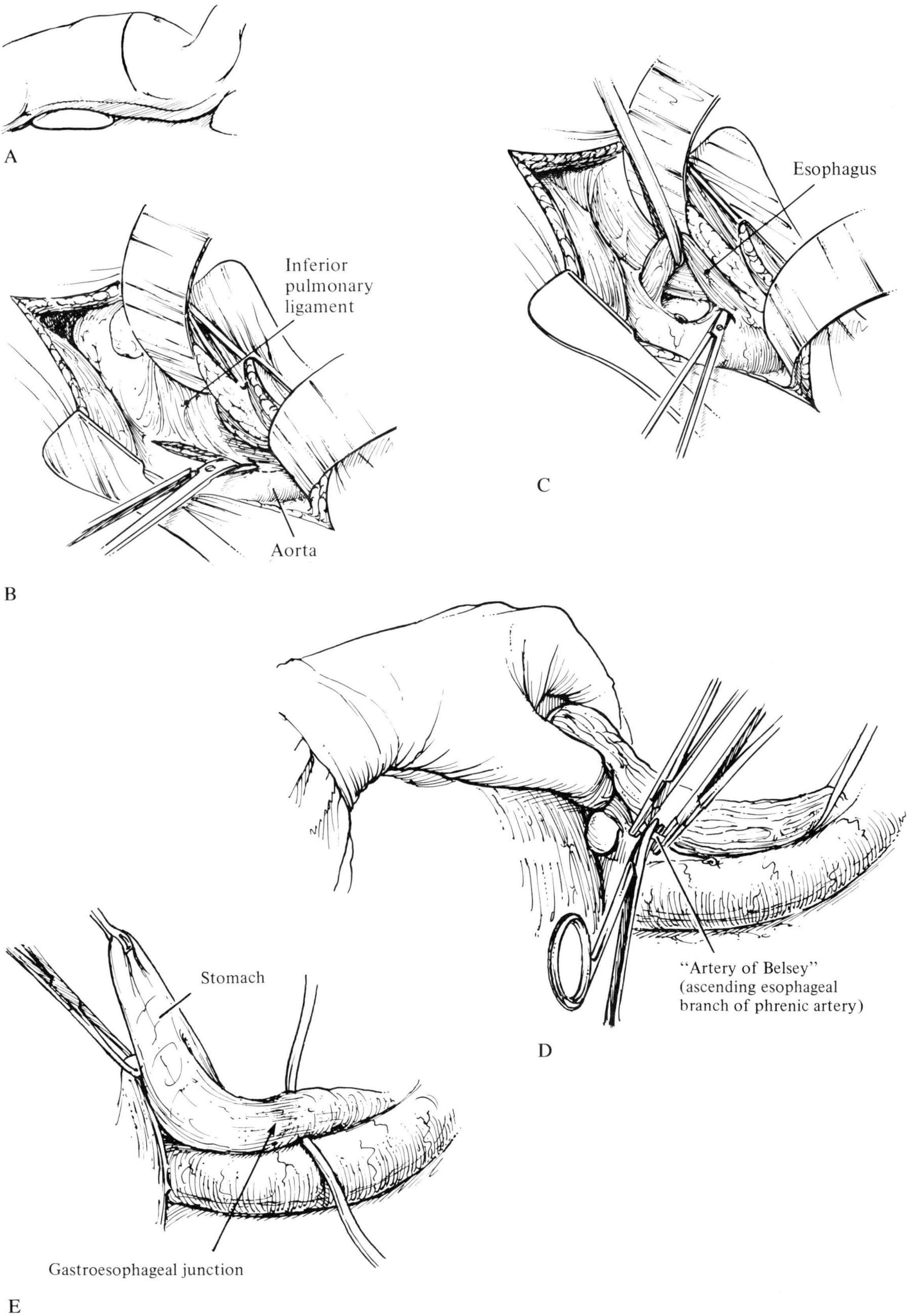
A
Inferior
pulmonary
ligament
Aorta
B
Esophagus
C
"Artery of Belsey"
(ascending esophageal
branch of phrenic artery)
D
Stomach
Gastroesophageal junction
E

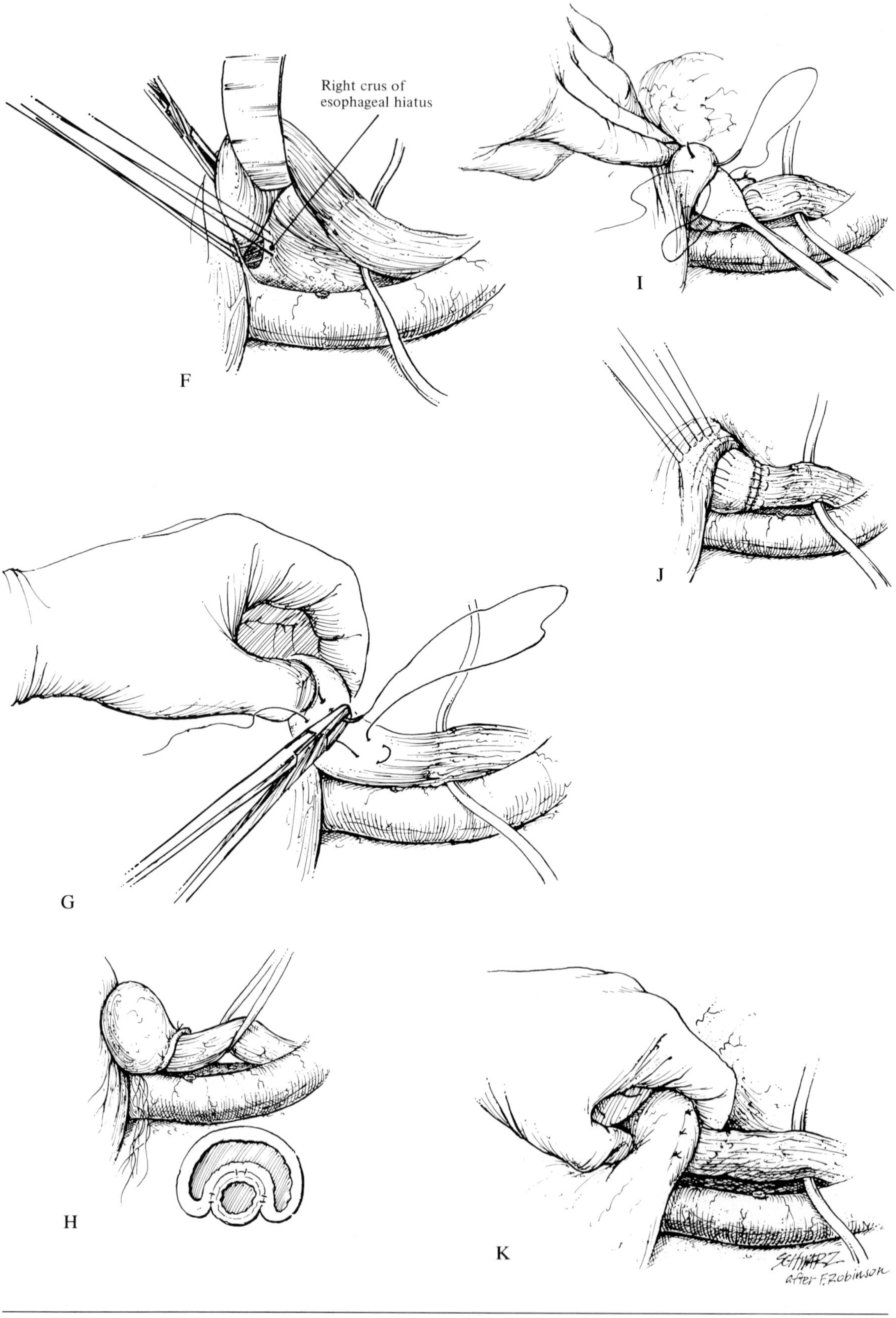
Right crus of
esophageal hiatus
F
I
J
G
H
K
SCHWARZ
after F. Robinson

the leaves separate the greater and lesser sacs. The left index finger is passed around the gastroesophageal junction just above the left gastric artery. The lesser sac is opened, with caution to ligate and divide the "Belsey artery," which is a branch of the left gastric to the inferior phrenic artery. Further mobilization is accomplished by division of several of the uppermost short gastric vessels, a step similar to that taken in the Nissen procedure.

The gastroesophageal junction is cleaned of hernial sac remnants and fat to allow a clear attachment of the fundus of the stomach to the esophagus. The vagi are dissected free of the esophagus and dropped back into the bed of the esophagus. The crura of the hiatus are repaired if a hiatal hernia is present. Stitches apposing the crural arms of the hiatus are placed but not tied until the fundoplication is completed. Three to five sutures are normally required.

The fundoplication is then carried out, with the anterior lateral fundus of the stomach sutured to the distal 3–5 cm of esophagus around two-thirds of its circumference with two rows of sutures. The upper row of sutures also passes through the diaphragm 1–2 cm from the margin of the hiatus, so that when they are tied the fundus is plicated to the esophagus and the gastroesophageal junction is restored to the abdomen. The posterior approximating crural sutures, previously placed, are then tied, closing the hiatus posteriorly around the esophagus. The hiatus is calibrated by insertion of a finger through it posterior to the esophagus. It should not compress the esophagus. Too lax a closure is preferable to too tight a closure.

The incision is closed with appropriate intercostal tubes. Fluids by mouth are permitted on the same day and a full diet resumed as soon as peristalsis returns.

The postoperative complications are those of any thoracotomy, with the long-term complications the same as those of the Nissen fundoplication, although not as pronounced. Results are discussed later in this chapter.

An interesting variation on the Belsey theme has been proposed by Skinner [122]. Using essentially the same approach as in the Belsey, he carries out a transthoracic Nissen fundoplication. In this instance the fundoplication is not sutured to the underside of the diaphragm, as in the Belsey, but is retained in the abdomen by posterior closure of the crural arms of the esophageal hiatus. This procedure has been compared in a prospective randomized manner with the Belsey procedure as described in this chapter and found to be superior to it [43].

"Thoracic" Repair Versus "Abdominal" Repair

A chronically recurring question about the most suitable method for treatment of reflux has been whether the transthoracic repairs are equal, superior, or inferior to the transabdominal repairs. This question seems primarily related to whether gastroesophageal reflux should be treated by thoracic surgeons or by general or abdominal surgeons and is a question of territorial imperatives more than efficacy of the operations. The query becomes meaningless when it is considered that almost any procedure can be carried out by either approach, although only the Nissen lends itself to both with equal facility. The thoracic-versus-abdominal debate is a consideration of approaches to the gastroesophageal junction, not to the actual repairs used.

Hill Posterior Gastropexy

This procedure (Fig. 22-14) accomplishes hernia reduction by a novel step in which the stomach is tethered to the posterior abdominal wall [41]. The operation, as currently performed by Hill, depends on intraoperative calibration of LES augmentation by intraoperative manometry.

TECHNIQUE. The general operative approach is the same as that described for the transabdominal Nissen procedure. The lesser omentum (gastrohepatic ligament) is divided as close to the liver as possible to leave a "bundle" of tissue on the stomach for the later

Fig. 22-13 (continued)

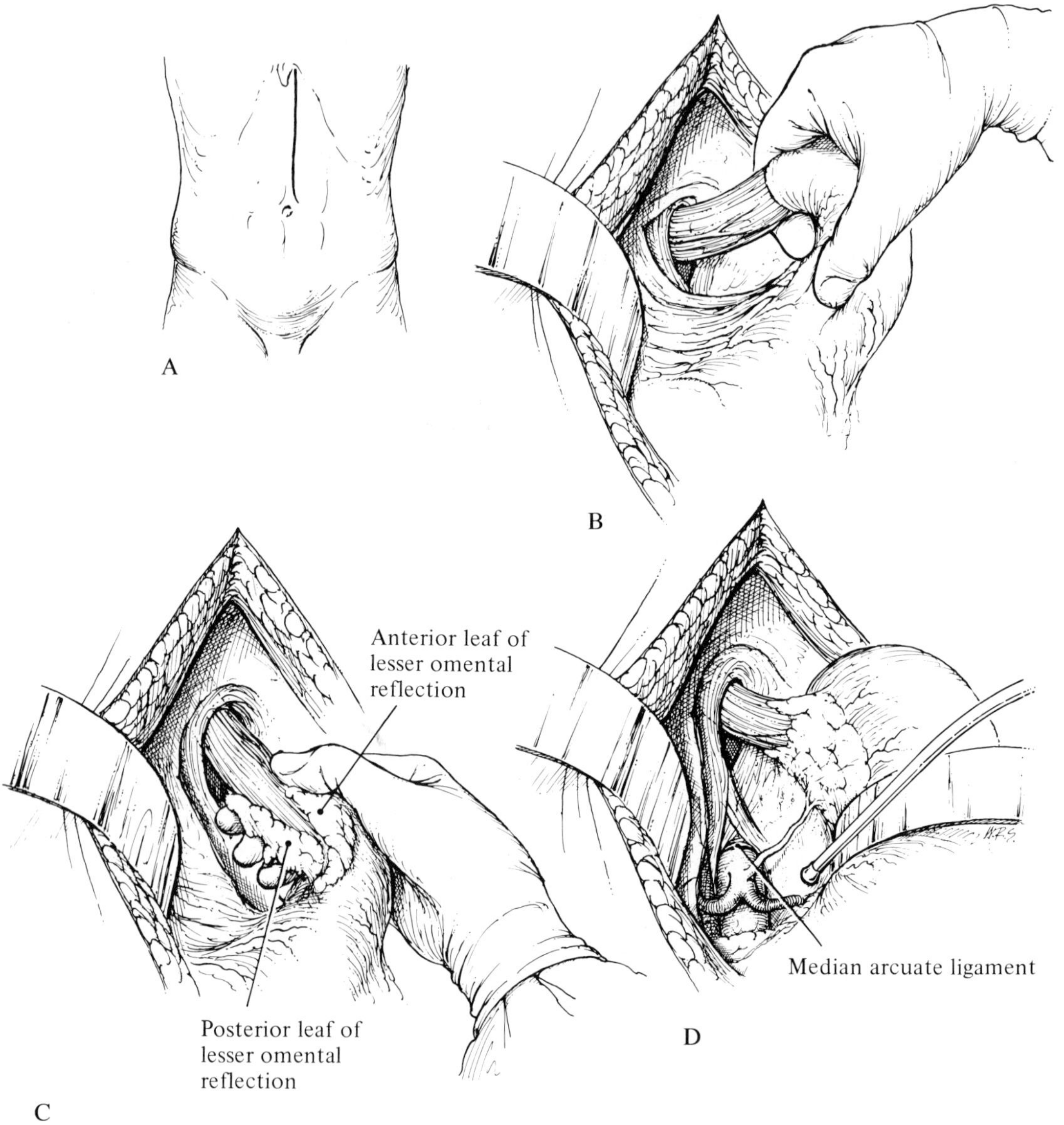

Fig. 22-14. The Hill posterior gastropexy with partial fundoplication. (A) The incision. (B) The esophagus and upper fundus are freed. (C) The fundus is partially plicated. (D) The median arcuate ligament is exposed. (E) The median arcuate ligament is lifted off the aorta and celiac trunk. (F) A cervical dilator is used to protect the celiac trunk and aorta. (G) The combination gastropexy and plicating sutures are placed. (H) The sutures are tied and the esophageal hiatus is closed.

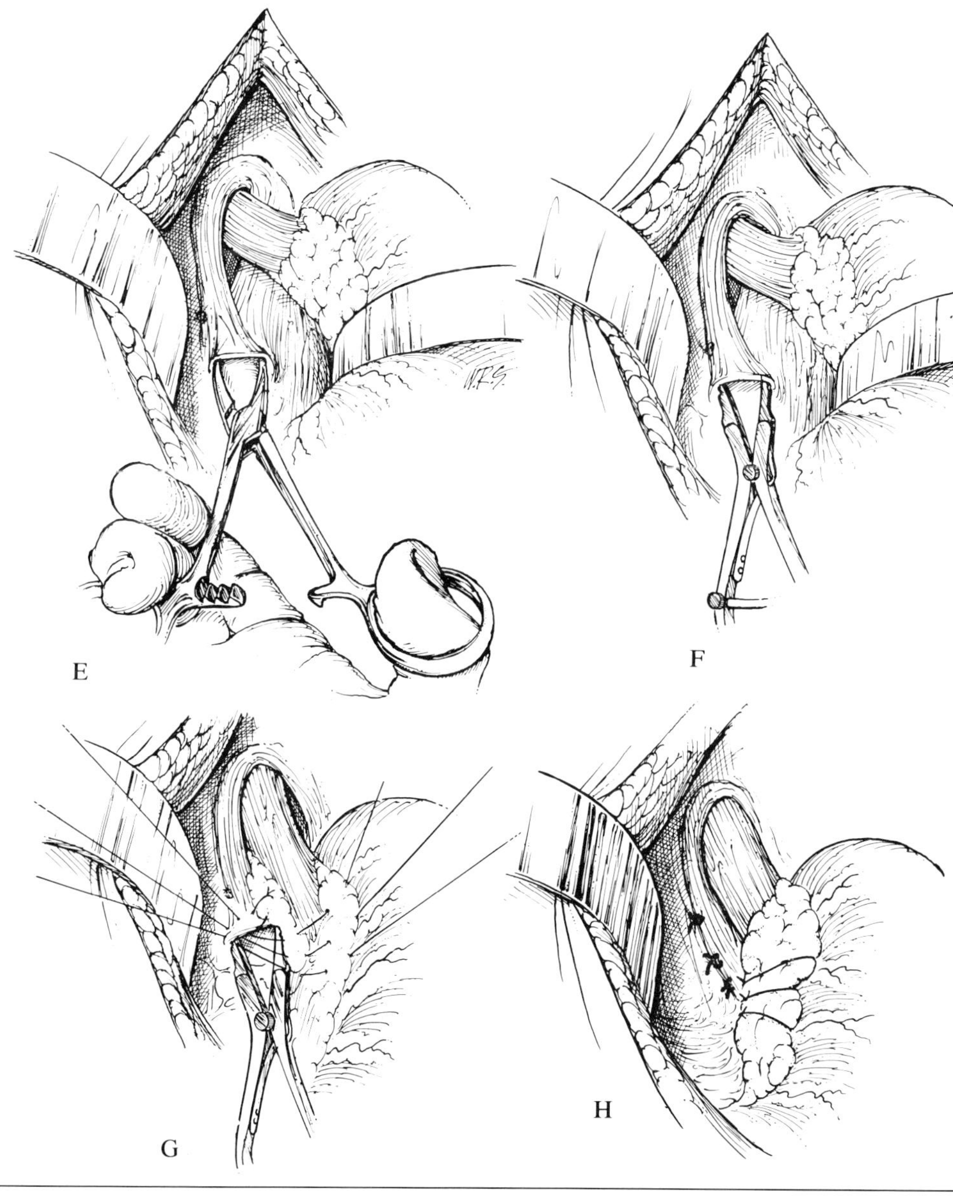

repair. The short gastric vessels are next divided as for a Nissen fundoplication, except that the extent of the division need not be as extensive. The gastroesophageal junction is bluntly encircled and retracted to the patient's left, exposing the crural arms of the esophageal hiatus and both the anterior and posterior reflections of the decussating leaves of the lesser omentum on the stomach. These retract onto the body of the stomach as two bundles of fibroareolar tissue. The vagi are identified and avoided. If peptic ulcer is part of the patient's symptom complex, a highly selective vagotomy may be added at this time. Vagotomy is never part of the treatment for reflux, however.

The stomach is retracted to the left, exposing the preaortic fascia. The aorta and celiac trunk are palpated. The median arcuate ligament lies immediately above the celiac trunk.

It is exposed by careful dissection over the midpoint of the aorta. A Goodell cervical dilator is passed under the free edge of the median arcuate ligament cephalad. This step must be performed gently to avoid damage to either the celiac trunk or the aorta. Numbers of alternative techniques have been described for this step to protect the vessels [133, 134].

The crural arms of the esophageal hiatus are apposed behind the esophagus, as in both the Belsey and the Nissen procedures. The operation continues as described by Russell and Hill [111]:

The stomach is then rotated in a clockwise direction to expose the posterior part of the stomach, thereby clearly displaying the anterior and posterior phrenoesophageal bundles. If the surgeon cannot see the posterior gastric wall, the dissection has been insufficient and the mobilization is incomplete. Once the bundles are clearly demonstrated, they are grasped with special Babcock clamps just above the left gastric artery and on a level with the vagus nerves. Care should be taken not to include the vagus nerves in the clamps. Strong nonabsorbable sutures, either 00 silk or 00 synthetic material, are used. The first suture is placed through the anterior and posterior phrenoesophageal bundles to include the seromuscular layer of the underlying stomach, avoiding the esophagus and vagi. This suture, which does not pass through the preaortic fascia, is designated as the imbricating suture. Four to five additional sutures are then passed beneath the anterior and posterior phrenoesophageal bundles, with the vagus nerve displayed in each instance, and then passed through the MAL [median arcuate ligament] or preaortic fascia. These sutures are passed from the patient's left to the right and are tested, both in the phrenoesophageal bundles and in the median arcuate and preaortic fascia, to make certain that stout tissue is obtained. The top three sutures, including the imbricating sutures, are then tied with single knots so that they can be tightened or loosened as necessary. A clamp is placed on these sutures and the esophageal sphincter pressure is measured by passing the side hole of the modified nasogastric tube through the gastroesophageal sphincter. If the pressure is above 60 mm Hg, the sutures are loosened. If it is below 40 mm Hg, the sutures are tightened. A pressure of 45–50 mm Hg appears to be ideal. After the proper pressure is obtained, all of the sutures are tied and a final pressure measurement is obtained. The barrier is about 3–4 cm long.

The abdomen is irrigated and closed in the standard manner. The nasogastric tube is left in place for three to four days, and when it is removed the patient is advanced to a regular diet as rapidly as can be tolerated.

Postoperative complications are essentially the same as those occurring after the Nissen procedure, except that "gas bloat" does not seem to be as prominent a problem. Woodward et al. [141] recommend this procedure over the Nissen operation on that basis. Contrariwise, Gregorie et al. [65] combine the Nissen fundoplication with posterior gastropexy.

Angelchik Prosthesis

In 1981, during an investigation of the effect of sliding hiatal hernia on LES dynamics, my colleagues and I became aware that simple, mild constriction of the stomach either at or just below the gastroesophageal junction would protect the LES from distraction by increasing gastric wall tension. This protection could be afforded by a simple silk ligature tied loosely around the cardia of the stomach. An operation proposed by Angelchik seems to rely on that principle, although like all other antireflux procedures, it was first proposed as a treatment for hiatal hernia [4]. Benjamin et al. [16] proposed that the device acts as a posterior bolster for the gastroesophageal junction, thereby producing an artificial pressure barrier.

The procedure depends on placement of a silicone polymer prosthesis (Fig. 22-15) around the gastroesophageal junction and securing it in place by tying synthetic polymer "tabs," which are integral parts of the prosthesis. The device is produced by the same technology used for the standard silicone gel breast prostheses, and its construction is similar. It consists of a relatively highly polymerized outer shell of Silastic, which is formed into a doughnut shape and filled by injection with a lesser polymerized Silastic "jelly." The inner filling can leak out of the prosthesis if it is punctured for any reason, and this has been

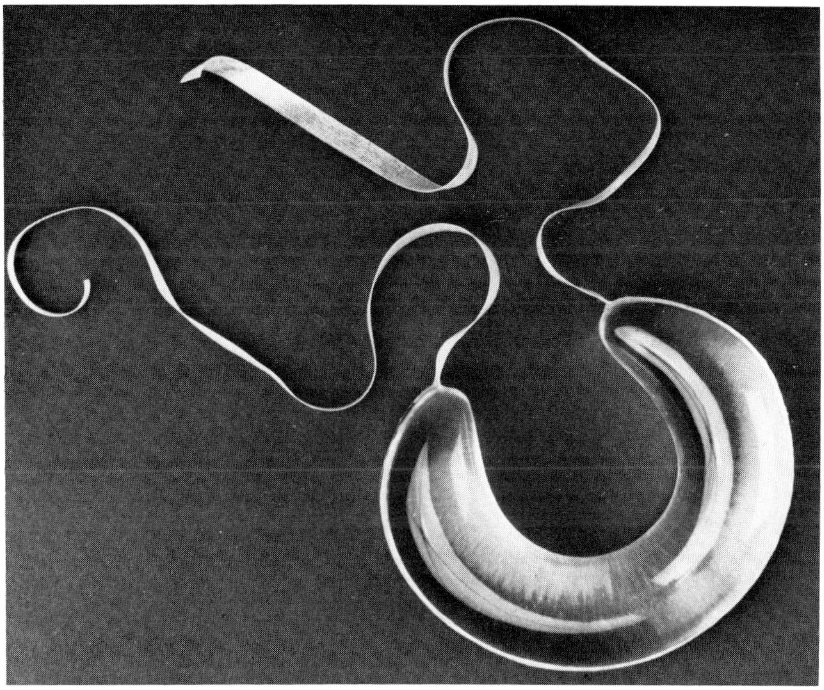

Fig. 22-15. The Angelchik silicone polymer esophageal prosthesis. (Courtesy American-Heyer Schulte, Inc.)

a rare complication of its use. The attachment of the tabs used to tie the prosthesis in place has proved critical. In early models of the device the tabs were avulsed from the ends of the prosthesis, allowing it to be dislodged and to fall into the peritoneal cavity. Current models avoid this problem by using a continuous strip of tab material bonded to the entire outside circumference of the device, with the free ends left long to serve as ties.

TECHNIQUE. The advantage of the prosthetic device is primarily the ease with which it may be put in place (Fig. 22-16). The surgical procedure is usually short, requiring less than an hour of time under anesthesia. The steps for implanting the device are simple and not subject to variations in judgment, as are the fundoplication procedures, so the same degree of experience is not required for this operation. The description of the operation has been contributed by Angelchik [personal communication].

Identification of the esophagus is made easier by inserting a Maloney bougie or a large nasogastric tube. The abdomen is entered through a midline incision extending from the xiphoid to the umbilicus. After a thorough routine exploration of the abdominal cavity, Angelchik and colleagues customarily use the Overholt and Balfour retractors for exposure.

The left lobe of the liver is retracted medially and cephalad without transecting the triangular ligament. The hernia, if present, is reduced intra-abdominally with traction on the stomach. The peritoneum is incised at the esophagocardiac junction. The right index finger dissects behind the esophagus to come around to the right side. (The immobilized esophageal segment should be of sufficient length to permit encirclement by the prosthesis, and more extensive dissection is not recommended or necessary.) A hemostat is used to grasp the end of one of the tie straps of the prosthesis to bring the strap down and around the surgeon's finger. The finger is brought from right to left, bringing the strap with it, and the strap is grasped on the left side. The prosthesis is gently pulled around the esophagus, and the straps are tied anteriorly with at least four knots, with the ends of the prosthesis touching. (A hemostat or any other instrument must not be used to hold the straps closed while tying, because this could damage the straps.) A large hemoclip is placed just outside the knot, and the straps are cut leaving approximately 1 inch in length. The prosthesis fits loosely with a space for one or

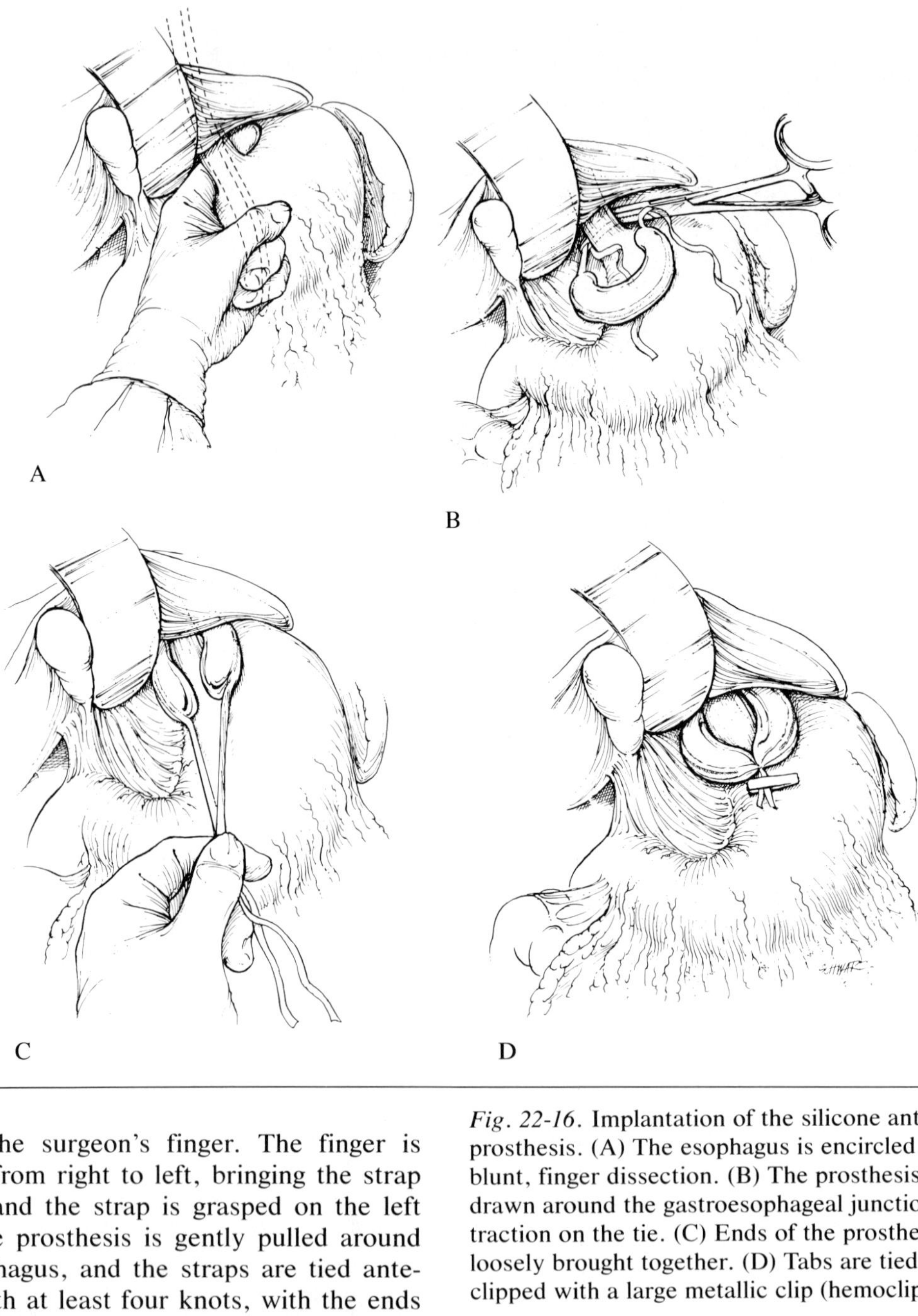

Fig. 22-16. Implantation of the silicone antireflux prosthesis. (A) The esophagus is encircled with blunt, finger dissection. (B) The prosthesis is drawn around the gastroesophageal junction by traction on the tie. (C) Ends of the prosthesis are loosely brought together. (D) Tabs are tied and clipped with a large metallic clip (hemoclip).

two fingers between it and the esophagus. The tie straps should not be sutured to the stomach or diaphragm.

The fibers of the vagus are left undisturbed; usually the left vagus is encircled by the prosthesis while the right remains on the outside. It is not necessary to approximate the crura. If a large hiatal hernia defect exists, we prefer to perform an anterior gastropexy on the way out before closing the abdomen.

At the end of the operation, the nasogastric tube or dilator is removed. The wound is closed in layers as preferred by the surgeon, and no drains are used.

Because the prosthesis has a radiopaque marker, the position of the device can be determined in postoperative roentgenograms. Figure 22-17 shows the prosthesis in place, in sagittal section.

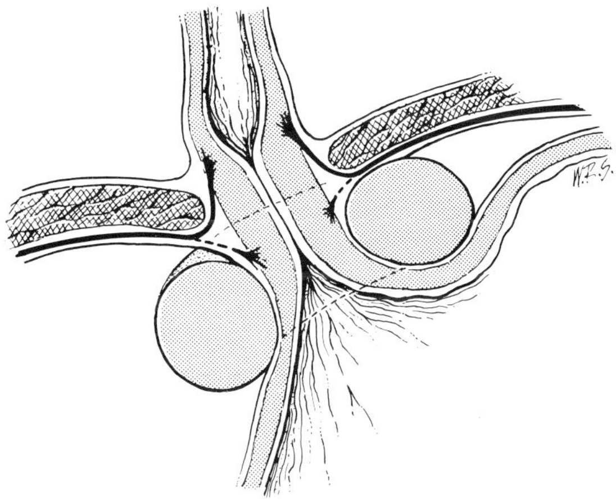

Fig. 22-17. Sagittal section of the esophagus and diaphragm with the prosthesis in place.

At this writing, approximately 15,000 of the devices have been used worldwide. The success rate at prevention of reflux appears to be approximately 90 percent, with the major complication being some degree of postoperative dysphagia in approximately 30 percent of patients. This incidence of dysphagia has necessitated surgical revision of the implant in less than 1 percent of patients. A small number of other complications has been reported, but these problems have attracted much attention because of their spectacular nature. These have included displacement of the prosthesis into the mediastinum, leakage of the device, complete avulsion of the device allowing it to fall through the peritoneal cavity into the pouch of Douglas, and erosion of the device into the stomach. In one instance, a prosthesis was removed at endoscopy. In another, a patient brought the device back to her physician, having passed it in her stool. None of the spectacular complications has resulted in other morbidity or mortality, a somewhat surprising finding in view of the size of gastric perforation that must have been necessary for the prosthesis to have eroded into the stomach [39, 102].

Another potential complication has been addressed by several authors [102]. As is well known with the breast prostheses, which are made of the same material as the Angelchik prosthesis, these devices provoke varying degrees of fibrotic reaction, resulting in some degree of encapsulation. The capsule then produces a fibrotic collar around the gastroesophageal junction. It has been speculated that this might lead to eventual obstruction of the distal esophagus with an external stricture, although this has not yet occurred. It is of interest that in the few patients in whom the prosthesis has been either displaced or surgically removed, leaving the fibrotic reaction behind, the incidence of recurrent reflux has been much lower than expected. I would suggest that this phenomenon is caused by the residual capsule, which in the absence of the prosthesis, might act in the same manner as the device itself, either to limit the effect of gastric wall tension on the LES or to bolster it externally.

RESULTS OF SURGICAL TREATMENT OF SIMPLE ESOPHAGITIS

Although there have been many anecdotal reports of series of patients treated with one of the fundoplications or one of their variants, there have been almost no prospective, randomized studies of these operations in humans. Part of the reason for this lack is the small number of patients who eventually come to surgical treatment in any one center. Another part is the satisfaction that many groups

Table 22-1. Nonrandomized reports: results of antireflux operations

Procedure	Follow-up (months)	No. of patients	Results (%)			
			Excellent	Good	Fair	Poor
Nissen [21, 110]	50	723	83	4	1	10
Belsey [73, 97]	60	1496	60	23	—	6
Hill [41, 111]	54	101	80	10	—	6
Prosth [82, 12, 128]	9	38	84	5	—	5

seem to feel with the particular procedure they prefer. Nonrandomized retrospective studies seem to confirm this impression. Reported results with any of the procedures seem very good, and a large series of patients with nearly 100 percent follow-up information would be required to demonstrate any differences among operations. A sample of the available anecdotal data is shown in Table 22-1.

If "good" or "excellent" results are generally understood to mean complete absence of reflux symptoms without reliance on medical therapy of any kind, all procedures seem to be accompanied by approximately a 90 percent success rate. The increased incidence of complications of the Nissen procedure is approximately offset by the increased efficacy of the procedure compared to the others. Based on the available evidence, therefore, it can only be recommended that the surgeon choose the fundoplication procedure with which he or she is most familiar and confident, and that the surgeon be responsible for ascertaining by careful follow-up study that the results are comparable to those obtained with other procedures.

The prosthetic implant has been reported in four anecdotal series of patients to date and in one randomized series, in which it was compared to the Nissen fundoplication. All series discounted the importance of postoperative dysphagia and reported approximately 90 percent success in reflux control. The comparative study [39] has demonstrated equal efficacy in reflux control with the Nissen. No long-term studies are available to assess the durability of the device, a paramount consideration in any procedure that depends on the continuous integrity of a large, implanted prosthesis. At this time available results support the recommendation that the prosthesis is suitable for the treatment of reflux in patients who would not tolerate one of the fundoplications, and then only when its expected duration of required action did not exceed 7–10 years because of the age or physical status of the patient. In those patients, its use would be an acceptable and perhaps desirable option.

There has been only one truly prospective randomized study of antireflux operations in which the Nissen, Belsey, and Hill procedures have been compared strictly [45]. In that study, the Nissen fundoplication was clearly the most effective procedure, but it succeeded at the risk of destroying the patient's ability to vomit.

TREATMENT OF REFLUX COMPLICATIONS

Esophageal ulcer, bleeding, and Barrett syndrome really represent forms of advanced esophagitis, and unless accompanied by some anatomical alteration such as a stricture require only the antireflux procedure. Savary et al. [117] recommended total or limited esophagectomy for Barrett syndrome because of the recognized premalignant potential of this condition. Other investigators including my group, have noted regression of the columnar lining of the esophagus when reflux is successfully treated either operatively or nonoperatively [30]. Any degree of esophagectomy with its attendant risks therefore seems unwarranted.

Esophageal stricture is a reflux complication that demands treatment. In the first place, it is essential that carcinoma be excluded as a cause of the stricture, regardless of how classical the symptoms of reflux may be. A combination of adequate esophagoscopy with visualization of the esophagus both above and below the stricture, with biopsies, brushings, and washings of the stricture, achieves 99.4 percent accuracy in this differentiation [84]. It is then necessary to determine the nature of the stricture. Very few esophageal strictures produced by reflux esophagitis are caused by complete transmural fibrosis of the esophageal wall [140]. Most produce esophageal obstruction because of the edema associated with acute and chronic inflammatory reaction surrounding the stricture, especially on its gastric side. If this inflammatory reaction can be controlled by successful reflux prevention, the edema will subside and the residual fibrous mucosal stricture can almost always be dilated in one or two sessions with a mercury-filled bougie. Dilation of the stricture at the time of the antireflux procedure may be all that is required [67].

FAILURE OF FUNDOPLICATION

The most common reason for failure of any of the fundoplications is disruption of the plication caused by suture line separation. In such an instance, the surgeon may elect either to repeat the previous operation or to switch to another fundoplication or a different surgical approach. It is common to treat a failed transabdominal fundoplication by a transthoracic Nissen or Belsey procedure, or vice versa.

In a few instances either there may be insufficient stomach because of a prior resection to carry out a fundoplication or the stomach may not be suitable for fundoplication because of previous damage or disease. The stomach may also be so scarred or otherwise damaged from a prior fundoplication attempt that a repeat fundoplication is impossible. In these situations three other options are available: drainage of the stomach by a long-limbed (45-cm) Roux-en-Y duodenal diversion [59, 66], substitution of the LES by interposed jejunum [90], or possibly, implantation of a prosthesis. The last is still an unproved procedure.

Duodenal diversion is an attractive alternative. The degree of esophagitis associated with a failed fundoplication is almost always that associated with duodenogastroesophageal reflux, leading to the conclusion that diversion of duodenal content away from the stomach changes the nature of the refluxed material sufficiently that the residual acid-induced esophagitis will be mild. In many instances the gastric mucosa has been sufficiently damaged either by duodenal reflux or by prior operations that acid secretion is also markedly reduced, alleviating even this minor problem.

Although it is an extremely effective alternative to fundoplication, jejunal interposition requires careful consideration because of the severity and risk of the operation in an already compromised surgical field. It nonetheless may be the only option available and should be used when needed.

As a disease entity, reflux esophagitis was not recognized until the end of World War II. Since that time the diagnosis and treatment of the problem have gone through several phases, based on either the increasing understanding of the anatomy and physiology of the stomach and lower esophagus or the periodic introduction of newer and more powerful diagnostic modalities such as esophageal manometry and fiberoptic endoscopy. At the present time, medicine is possessed of powerful and effective surgical and nonsurgical methods for its recognition and treatment, which are summarized in this chapter. It would be naive to assume that a plateau has been reached if only because of the rapid progress that has been made in the last 10 years. The age of computers is upon us. Computers promise to supply the next quantum jump in the diagnosis of esophageal disease, and the introduction of newer and more effective medications for LES augmentation promises to be the next significant advance in its therapy. It is a fascinating subject and an exciting time.

References

1. Adler, R. H. The lower esophagus lined by columnar epithelium. *J. Thorac. Cardiovasc. Surg.* 45:13, 1963.
2. Allison, P. R. Peptic ulcer of the esophagus. *J. Thorac. Surg.* 15:308, 1946.

3. Allison, P. R. Reflux esophagitis, sliding hiatus hernia and the anatomy of repair. *Surg. Gynecol. Obstet.* 92:419, 1951.
4. Angelchik, J. P., and Cohen, R. A new surgical procedure for the treatment of gastroesophageal reflux and hiatal hernia. *Surg. Gynecol. Obstet.* 148:246, 1979.
5. Bahadorzadeh, K., and Jordan, P. H. Evaluation of the Nissen fundoplication for treatment of hiatal hernia. *Ann. Surg.* 181:402, 1975.
6. Balison, J. R., Macgregor, A. M. C., and Woodward, E. R. Postoperative diaphragmatic herniation following transthoracic fundoplication. *Arch. Surg.* 106:164, 1973.
7. Barrett, N. R. Chronic peptic ulcer of the esophagus and "esophagitis." *Br. J. Surg.* 38:175, 1950.
8. Barrett, N. R. Hiatus hernia: A review of some controversial points. *Br. J. Surg.* 42:231, 1954.
9. Battle, W. S., Nyhus, L. M., and Bombeck, C. T. Gastroesophageal reflux: Diagnosis and treatment. *Ann. Surg.* 177:560, 1973.
10. Baue, A. E., and Belsey, R. H. R. The treatment of sliding hiatus hernia and reflux esophagitis by the Mark IV technique. *Surgery* 62:396, 1967.
11. Behar, J., Brand, D. L., Brown, F. C., et al. Cimetidine in the treatment of symptomatic gastroesophageal reflux: A double blind controlled trial. *Gastroenterology* 74:441, 1978.
12. Behar, J., and Sheahan, D. C. Histologic abnormalities in reflux esophagitis. *Arch. Pathol.* 99:387, 1975.
13. Behar, J., Sheahan, M. B., Biancani, P., et al. Medical and surgical management of reflux esophagitis: A 38 month report on a prospective clinical trial. *N. Engl. J. Med.* 293:263, 1975.
14. Belsey, R. O. Introduction. In *Surgical Techniques Illustrated* Vol 1, no. 2. Boston: Little, Brown, 1976. Pp. 2–5.
15. Belsey, R. O. Surgical treatment of hiatus hernia and reflux esophagitis. *World J. Surg.* 1:421, 1977.
16. Benjamin, S. B., Knuff, T. K., Fink, M., et al. The Angelchik antireflux prosthesis: Effects on the lower esophageal sphincter of primates. *Ann. Surg.* 197:63, 1983.
17. Benz, L. J., Hootkin, L. A., Margulies, S., et al. A comparison of clinical measurements of gastroesophageal reflux. *Gastroenterology* 62:1, 1972.
18. Berci, G. *Endoscopy.* New York: Appleton-Century-Crofts, 1976.
19. Bernstein, L. M., and Baker, L. A. A clinical test for esophagitis. *Gastroenterology* 34:760, 1958.
20. Berry, L. H. Gastrointestinal Pan-endoscopy. Springfield: Thomas, 1974.
21. Bettex, M., and Stillhart, H. Operation for hiatus hernia and cardioesophageal achalasia by fundoplication after Nissen. *Surgery* 55:451, 1964.
22. Blum, A. L., and Siewert, J. R. Reflections upon the lower esophagus. *Surg. Annu.* 11:59, 1979.
23. Boerema, I. Hiatus hernia: Repair by right-sided subhepatic anterior gastropexy. *Surgery* 65:884, 1969.
24. Bombeck, C. T. Unpublished data.
25. Bombeck, C. T., Aoki, T., and Nyhus, L. M. Anatomic etiology and operative treatment of peptic esophagitis: An experimental study. *Ann. Surg.* 165:752, 1967.
26. Bombeck, C. T., Dillard, D. H., and Nyhus, L. M. Muscular anatomy of the gastroesophageal junction and role of the phrenoesophageal ligament: Autopsy study of the sphincter mechanism. *Am. Surg.* 164:643, 1966.
27. Bombeck, C. T., Helfrich, G. B., and Nyhus, L. M. Planning surgery for reflux esophagitis and hiatus hernia. *Surg. Clin. North Am.* 50:29, 1970.
28. Booth, D. J., Demmerer, W. T., and Skinner, D. B. Acid clearing from the distal esophagus. *Arch. Surg.* 96:731, 1968.
29. Boutelier, P., and Jonsell, G. An alternative fundoplicative maneuver for gastroesophageal reflux. *Am. Surg.* 143:260, 1982.
30. Brand, D. L., Yivisaker, J. T., Gelfand, M., and Pope, C. E., II. Regression of columnar esophageal (Barrett's) epithelium after antireflux surgery. *N. Engl. J. Med.* 302:844, 1980.
31. Branicki, F. J., Evans, D. F., Jones, J. A., and Hardcastle, J. D. The assessment of gastroesophageal reflux using a portable radiotelemetry system to monitor oesophageal pH. *Gut* 22:5, 1981.
32. Bremner, C. G. The columnar lined (Barrett's) esophagus. *Surg. Annu.* 9:103, 1977.
33. Bremner, C. G., Lynch, V. P., and Ellis, F. H., Jr. Barrett's esophagus: Congenital or acquired? An experimental study of esophageal mucosal regeneration in the dog. *Surgery* 68:209, 1970.

34. Bright-Asare, P., and El-Bassoussi, M. Cimetidine, metoclopramide, or placebo in the treatment of symptomatic gastroesophageal reflux. *J. Clin. Gastroenterol.* 3:149, 1980.
35. Burnett, H. F., Read, R. C., Morris, W. D., and Campbell, G. S. Management of complications of fundoplication and Barrett's esophagus. *Surgery* 82:521, 1977.
36. Campbell, R., Kennedy, T., and Johnston, G. W. Gastric ulceration after Nissen fundoplication. *Br. J. Surg.* 70:406, 1983.
37. Castell, D. O. Medical therapy of reflux esophagitis. *Ann. Intern. Med.* 93:926, 1980.
38. Cohen, S., Fisher, R., Lipshutz, W., et al. The pathogenesis of esophageal dysfunction in scleroderma and Reynard's disease. *J. Clin. Invest.* 51:2663, 1972.
39. Condon, R. E. More misadventures with the esophageal collar. *Surgery* 93:477, 1983.
40. Cooper, J. D., and Jeejeebhoy, K. N. Gastroesophageal reflux: Medical and surgical management. *Ann. Thorac. Surg.* 31:314, 1981.
41. Csendes, A., and Larrain, A. Effect of posterior gastropexy on gastroesophageal sphincter pressure and symptomatic reflux in patients with hiatal hernia. *Gastroenterology* 63:19, 1972.
42. de Castro, V. A. M., Nyhus, L. M., Gillison, E. W., et al. Posterior gastropexy (Hill) in the treatment of reflux esophagitis: An experimental study in the dog. *Scand. J. Gastroenterol.* [Suppl.] 9:49, 1971.
43. DeMeester, T. R. Results submitted for publication.
44. DeMeester, T. R., Johnson, L. F., and Joseph, G. J. Patterns of gastroesophageal reflux in health and disease. *Ann. Surg.* 184:459, 1976.
45. DeMeester, T. R., Johnson, L. F., and Kent, A. H. Evaluation of current operations for the prevention of gastroesophageal reflux. *Ann. Surg.* 180:511, 1974.
46. Dennish, G. W., and Castell, D. O. Inhibitory effect of smoking on the lower esophageal sphincter. *N. Engl. J. Med.* 284:1136, 1971.
47. Dennish, G. W., and Castell, D. O. Caffeine and the lower esophageal sphincter. *Am. J. Dig. Dis.* 17:993, 1972.
48. Dent, J., Dodds, W. J., Friedman, R. H., et al. Mechanism of gastroesophageal reflux in recumbent, asymptomatic human subjects. *J. Clin. Invest.* 65:256, 1980.
49. Dillard, D. H. Esophageal sphincter and reflux. *Surg. Clin. North Am.* 44:1201, 1964.
50. Dillard, D. H., and Anderson, H. N. A new concept of the mechanism of sphincteric failure in sliding esophageal hiatal hernia. *Surg. Gynecol. Obstet.* 122:1030, 1966.
51. Dodds, W. J., Hogan, W. J., Helm, J. F., and Dent, J. Pathogenesis of reflux esophagitis. *Gastroenterology* 81:376, 1981.
52. Dodds, W. J., Hogan, W. G., and Miller, W. N. Reflux esophagitis. *Am. J. Dig. Dis.* 21:49, 1976.
53. Donahue, P. E., and Bombeck, C. T. The modified Nissen fundoplication: Reflux prevention without gas-bloat. *Chir. Gastroenterol.* 11:15, 1977.
54. Donahue, P. E., Bombeck, C. T., and Nyhus, L. M. Endoscopic findings after Nissen fundoplication simplify evaluation of postoperative symptoms. Presented at Second World Congress of the Collegium Internationale Chirurgie Digestivae, Tokyo, 1982.
55. Donner, M. W., Sibiger, M. L., Hookman, P., and Hendrix, T. L. Acid barium swallows in the radiographic evaluation of clinical esophagitis. *Radiology* 87:220, 1966.
56. Eastwood, G. L., Castell, D. O., and Higgs, R. H. Experimental esophagitis in cats impairs lower esophageal sphincter pressure. *Gastroenterology* 69:146, 1975.
57. Ellis, F. H., Garabedian, M., and Gibb, S. P. Fundoplication for gastroesophageal reflux. *Arch. Surg.* 107:681, 1973.
58. Ellis, F. H., and Olsen, A. M. Achalasia of the esophagus. Philadelphia: Saunders, 1969. Pp. 174–76.
59. Fekete, F., Breil, P., and Gayet, B. The role of total duodenal diversion in the treatment of reflux esophagitis. Presented at the Second International Conference on Diseases of the Esophagus, Chicago, 1983.
60. Fisher, R. S., Malmud, L. S., Roberts, G. S., and Lobis, I. F. Gastroesophageal (GE) scintiscanning to detect and quantitate GE reflux. *Gastroenterology* 70:301, 1976.
61. Fyke, F. E., Jr., Code, C. F., and Schlegel, J. F. The gastroesophageal sphincter in healthy human beings. *Gastroenterology* 86:135, 1956.
62. Gahagan, T. H. The function of the musculature of the esophagus and stomach in the esophagogastric sphincter mechanism. *Surg. Gynecol. Obstet.* 114:293, 1962.
63. Gillison, E. W., de Castro, V. A. M., Nyhus, L. M., et al. The significance of bile in reflux

esophagitis. *Surg. Gynecol. Obstet.* 134:419, 1972.
64. Gillison, W. W., Kusakari, K., Bombeck, C. T., and Nyhus, L. M. The importance of bile in reflux esophagitis and the success in its prevention by surgical means. *Br. J. Surg.* 59:79, 1972.
65. Gregorie, H. B., Jr., Cathcart, R. S., III, and Gregorie, R. J. Surgical treatment of intractable esophagitis. *Ann. Surg.* 199:580, 1984.
66. Herrington, J. L., and Mody, B. Total duodenal diversion for treatment of reflux esophagitis uncontrolled by repeated antireflux procedures. *Ann. Surg.* 183:636, 1976.
67. Herrington, J. L., Wright, R., Edwards, W., and Sawyers, J. Conservative surgical treatment of reflux esophagitis and esophageal stricture. *Ann. Surg.* 181:552, 1975.
68. Hiebert, C. A. The recognition and management of gastroesophageal reflux without hiatal hernia. *World J. Surg.* 1:445, 1977.
69. Higgs, R. H., Castell, D. O., and Eastwood, G. L. Studies on the mechanism of esophagitis induced lower esophageal sphincter hypotension in cats. *Gastroenterology* 71:51, 1976.
70. Hightower, N. C., Jr., Code, C. F., and Maher, F. T. A method for the study of gastrointestinal motor activity in human beings. *Proc. Staff Meeting Mayo Clin.* 24:453, 1949.
71. Hill, L. D. An effective operation for hiatal hernia: An eight-year appraisal. *Ann. Surg.* 166:681, 1967.
72. Hoffman, G. C., and Vansant, J. H. The gastroesophageal scintiscan: Comparison of methods to demonstrate gastroesophageal reflux. *Arch. Surg.* 114:727, 1979.
73. Hughes, R., Carey, J., and Reemtsma, K. Operative internal rupture and Belsey hiatal hernia repair for reflux esophageal stricture. *Ann. Thorac. Surg.* 9:203, 1970.
74. Iascone, C., DeMeester, T. R., Little, A. G., and Skinner, D. B. Barrett's esophagus: Functional assessment, proposed pathogenesis and surgical therapy. *Arch. Surg.* 118:543, 1983.
75. Ingelfinger, F. J. The sphincter that is a sphinx. *N. Engl. J. Med.* 285:1095, 1971.
76. Isenberg, J., Csendes, A., and Walsh, J. H. Resting and pentagastrin stimulated gastroesophageal sphincter pressures in patients with Zollinger-Ellison syndrome. *Gastroenterology* 61:665, 1971.
77. Ismail-Beigi, F., Horton, P. F., and Pope, C. E., II. Histological consequences of gastroesophageal reflux in man. *Gastroenterology* 58:163, 1970.
78. Johnson, L. F., and DeMeester, T. R. Twenty four hour pH monitoring of the distal esophagus: A quantitative measure of gastroesophageal reflux. *Am. J. Gastroenterol.* 62:325, 1974.
79. Kantrowitz, P. A., Corson, J. G., Fleischli, D. J., and Skinner, D. B. Measurement of gastroesophageal reflux. *Gastroenterology* 56:666, 1969.
80. Katz, L. A., Mass, L. C., and Vastola, D. L. Physiological effects of surgical repositioning of the lower esophageal sphincter. *Gastroenterology* 66:720, 1974.
81. Kjellen, G., and Tibbling, L. Influence of body position, dry and water swallows, smoking, and alcohol on esophageal acid clearing. *Scand. J. Gastroenterol.* 13:283, 1978.
82. Kozarek, R. A., Phelps, J. E., Sanowski, R. A., et al. An antireflux prosthesis in the treatment of gastroesophageal reflux. *Ann. Intern. Med.* 98:310, 1983.
83. Kramer, P. Does a sliding hiatus hernia constitute a distinct clinical entity? *Gastroenterology* 57:442, 1969.
84. Larson, G. M., and Bombeck, C. T. Accuracy of endoscopy in esophageal cancer. *Gastrointest. Endosc.* 23:232, 1977.
85. Lendrum, F. C. Anatomic features of the cardiac orifice of the stomach: With special reference to cardiospasm. *Arch. Intern. Med.* 59:474, 1937.
86. Liebermann-Meffert, D., Allgower, M., Schmid, P., and Blum, A. L. Muscular equivalent of the lower esophageal sphincter. *Gastroenterology* 76:31, 1979.
87. Lind, J. T., Crispin, J. S., and McIver, D. K. The effect of atropine on the gastroesophageal sphincter. *Can. J. Physiol. Pharmacol.* 46:233, 1968.
88. Linsmans, J. F. Gastroesophageal reflux elicited while drinking water (water siphonage test): Its clinical correlation with pyrosis. *Am. J. Roentgenol. Radium Ther. Nucl. Med.* 94:325, 1965.
89. McCallum, R. W., Berkowitz, D. M., and Lerner, E. Gastric emptying in patients with gastroesophageal reflux. *Gastroenterology* 80:285, 1981.
90. Merendino, K. A., and Dillard, D. H. The concept of sphincter substitution by an interposed jejunal segment for anatomic and physiologic abnormalities at the esophagogastric junction with special reference to reflux esophagitis,

cardiospasm and esophageal varices. *Ann. Surg.* 142:486, 1955.

91. Miller, J. M., Fannin, S. W., Steiner, P. R., et al. A computerized system for the automatic storage and interpretation of continuous 32 hour esophageal pH records: Outpatient use. Presented at the Second International Conference on Diseases of the Esophagus, Chicago, 1983.
92. Moersch, R. N., Ellis, F. H., and McDonald, J. R. Pathologic changes occurring in severe reflux esophagitis. *Surg. Gynecol. Obstet.* 108:476, 1959.
93. Moran, J. M., Pihl, C. O., and Norton, R. A. The hiatal hernia–reflux complex: Current approaches to correction and evaluation of results. *Am. J. Surg.* 121:403, 1971.
94. Mossberg, S. M. The columnar lined esophagus (Barrett's syndrome): An acquired condition? *Gastroenterology* 50:671, 1966.
95. Naef, A. P., Savary, M., and Ozello, L. Columnar lined lower esophagus; an acquired lesion with malignant predisposition: Report of 140 cases of Barrett's esophagus with 12 adenocarcinomas. *J. Thorac. Cardiovasc. Surg.* 70:826, 1975.
96. Nissen, R. Gastropexy and "fundoplication" in surgical treatment of hiatal hernia. *Am. J. Dig. Dis.* 6:954, 1961.
97. Orringer, M., Skinner, D., and Belsey, R. Long-term results of the Mark IV operation for hiatal hernia and analyses of recurrences and their treatment. *J. Thorac. Cardiovasc. Surg.* 69:25, 1972.
98. Palmer, E. D. The hiatus hernia–esophagitis–esophageal sphincter complex: Twenty year prospective study. *Am. J. Med.* 44:566, 1968.
99. Paull, A., Trier, J. S., Dalton, M. D., et al. The histologic spectrum of Barrett's esophagus. *N. Engl. J. Med.* 295:476, 1976.
100. Pettersson, G. B., Bombeck, C. T., and Nyhus, L. M. The lower esophageal sphincter: Mechanisms of opening and closure. *Surgery* 88:307, 1980.
101. Pettersson, G. B., Bombeck, C. T., and Nyhus, L. M. The influence of hiatal hernia on lower esophageal sphincter function: An experimental study. *Ann. Surg.* 193:214, 1981.
102. Pickleman, J. Disruption and migration of an Angelchik esophageal antireflux prosthesis. *Surgery* 93:467, 1983.
103. Polk, H. C. Fundoplication for reflux esophagitis: Misadventures with the operation of choice. *Ann. Surg.* 183:645, 1976.
104. Pope, C. E., II. Pathophysiology and diagnosis of reflux esophagitis. *Gastroenterology* 70:445, 1976.
105. Powell-Jackson, P., Barkley, H., and Northfield, T. C. Effect of cimetidine in symptomatic gastroesophageal reflux. *Lancet* 2:1068, 1978.
106. Randolph, J., Lilly, J., and Anderson, D. Surgical treatment of gastroesophageal reflux in infants. *Ann. Surg.* 180:479, 1974.
107. Ransom, J. M., Patel, G. K., Clift, S. A., et al. Extended and limited types of Barrett's esophagus in the adult. *Ann. Thorac. Surg.* 33:19, 1982.
108. Richter, J. E., and Castell, D. O. Drugs, foods, and other substances in the cause and treatment of reflux esophagitis. *Med. Clin. North Am.* 65:1223, 1981.
109. Richter, J. E., and Castell, D. O. Gastroesophageal reflux: Pathogenesis, diagnosis, and therapy. *Ann. Intern. Med.* 97:93, 1982.
110. Rosetti, M., and Hell, K. Fundoplication for the treatment of gastroesophageal reflux in hiatal hernia. *World J. Surg.* 1:439, 1977.
111. Russell, C. O. H., and Hill, L. D. Gastroesophageal reflux. *Curr. Probl. Surg.* 20:209, 1983.
112. Salo, J. A., and Kivilaakso, E. The role of bile salts and trypsin in the pathogenesis of experimental alkaline esophagitis. *Surgery* 93:525, 1983.
113. Samelson, S. L., Bombeck, C. T., Abuabara, S. F., et al. The effect of focal mucosal lesions on lower esophageal sphincter function: An experimental study, In press.
114. Samelson, S. L., Bombeck, C. T., and Nyhus, L. M. Lower esophageal sphincter competence: anatomic-physiologic correlation. Presented at 2d International Conference on Diseases of the Esophagus, Chicago, 1983.
115. Samelson, S. L., Bombeck, C. T., and Nyhus, L. M. Successful antireflux procedures: A common mechanism of action. Presented at the European Society for Surgical Research, Athens, May 1983.
116. Samelson, S. L., Bombeck, C. T., Nyhus, L. M., et al. A new concept in the surgical treatment of gastroesophageal reflux. *Ann. Surg.* 197:254, 1983.
117. Savary, M., Miller, G., and Roethlisberber, B. Spezielle Probleme des Endobrachyoesophagus in Reflux Therapie, Berlin: Springer, 1981. Chap. 36.
118. Schlesinger, P., Schmid, B., and Layden, T.

Value of 24 hour esophageal pH monitoring as a clinical test. *Gastroenterology* 84:1301, 1983.
119. Shah, I. K., and Daniel, O. The results of fundoplication for the relief of oesophageal reflux due to hiatus hernia. *Br. J. Surg.* 59:285, 1972.
120. Siewert, J. R., Weiser, H. F., and Blum, A. L. Postoperative syndrome in reflux therapy. Berlin: Springer, 1981. Chap. 44, Pp. 519.
121. Sinar, D. R., Fletcher, J. R., Cordova, C. C., et al. Acute acid induced esophagitis impairs esophageal peristalsis in baboons. *Gastroenterology* 80:1286, 1981.
122. Skinner, D. The Transthoracic Nissen Fundoplication. In *Surgical Techniques Illustrated,* Vol 1, no. 2. Boston: Little, Brown, 1976.
123. Skinner, D., and Belsey, R. Surgical management of esophageal reflux and hiatus hernia. *J. Thorac. Cardiovasc. Surg.* 53:33, 1967.
124. Skinner, D. B., and Booth, D. J. Assessment of distal esophageal function in patients with hiatal hernia and/or gastroesophageal reflux. *Ann. Surg.* 172:627, 1970.
125. Smiddy, F. G., and Atkinson, M. Mechanisms preventing gastroesophageal reflux in the dog. *Br. J. Surg.* 47:680, 1960.
126. Stanciu, C., and Bennett, J. R. Oesophageal acid clearing: One factor in the production of reflux esophagitis. *Gut* 15:852, 1974.
127. Starling, J., Pellett, J., and Belzer, F. Experience with a prosthetic device for the treatment of reflux esophagitis. *Ann. Surg.* 195:686, 1982.
128. Temple, J. G., Bainbridge, E. T., Ellis, D. J., et al. The Angelchik antireflux prosthesis: A U.K. multicentre pilot study. Presented at the Second World Congress of the Collegium Internationale Chirurgie Digestivae, Tokyo, 1982.
129. Thomas, H., Clarke, J., Rayl, J., and Woodward, E. Results of the combined fundic patch–fundoplication operation in the treatment of reflux esophagitis with stricture. *Surg. Gynecol. Obstet.* 135:241, 1972.
130. Tuttle, S. G., Bettarello, A., and Grossman, M. I. Esophageal acid perfusion test and a gastroesophageal reflux test in patients with esophagitis. *Gastroenterology* 38:861, 1960.
131. Vandertoll, D. J., Ellis, H. F., Schlegel, J. F., et al. An experimental study of the role of gastric and esophageal muscle in gastroesophageal competence. *Surg. Gynecol. Obstet.* 122:575, 1966.
132. VanSant, J. H., and Baker, J. W. Complications of vagotomy in the treatment of hiatal hernia. *Ann. Surg.* 183:629, 1976.
133. VanSant, J. H., Baker, J. W., and Ross, D. G. Modification of the Hill technique for repair of hiatal hernia. *Surg. Gynecol. Obstet.* 143:637, 1976.
134. Warshaw, A. L. Simplified isolation of the median arcuate ligament for posterior gastropexy. *Surg. Gynecol. Obstet.* 154:733, 1982.
135. Winans, C. S. Diagnostic evaluation of esophageal function. Presented at the Second International Symposium on the Esophagus, Chicago, 1983.
136. Winans, C. S. Manometric asymmetry of the lower esophageal high pressure zone. *Gastroenterology* 62:830, 1972.
137. Winkelstein, A. Peptic esophagitis: A new clinical entity. *J.A.M.A.* 104:906, 1935.
138. Wolf, B. S., and Guglielmo, J. The roentgen demonstration of minimal hiatus hernia. *Med. Radiogr. Photogr.* 33:90, 1957.
139. Wolverson, R. L., Donovan, I. A., Harding, L. K., et al. A bile reflux provocation test and its use in the investigation of patients with a peptic ulcer diathesis. Presented at the Seventh World Congress of the Collegium Internationale Chirurgie Digestivae, Tokyo, 1982.
140. Woodward, E. R. Surgical treatment of gastroesophageal reflux and its complications. *World J. Surg.* 1:453, 1977.
141. Woodward, E. R., Thomas, H. F., and McAlhany, J. C. Comparison of crural repair and Nissen fundoplication in the treatment of esophageal hiatus hernia with peptic esophagitis. *Ann. Surg.* 173:782, 1971.

23

Stress Ulceration

Wallace P. Ritchie, Jr.

The term *stress ulcer* was introduced by Selye [63] in 1936 to describe all ulcerations of the stomach and duodenum that arise coincident with the general alarm reaction induced by stressful environmental stimuli. Numerous laboratory and clinical studies conducted during the past two decades suggest that this definition is too broad and that the term properly applies only to those multiple, superficial, erosive lesions of the proximal acid-peptic secreting portion of the gastric mucosa (occasionally discovered in association with acute ulcerations of the duodenum as well) that develop as a consequence of massive trauma, extensive thermal injury, or systemic sepsis, i.e., in the setting of severe and unremitting physiological stress. Progression and coalescence of these lesions can result in overt hemorrhage of life-threatening severity, an occurrence known as *acute hemorrhagic gastritis*.

Historical Background

Although stress ulcer disease has only recently been recognized as a distinct clinical entity, the relationship between gastrointestinal bleeding and trauma has been appreciated by military surgeons since antiquity. Celsus is credited with providing a description of this association based on observations of injured Roman legionnaires. Seven centuries later, Treille commented on the exceptional frequency with which multiple gastric erosions were encountered at autopsy in soldiers dying of infected wounds during the Napoleonic campaigns [73]. In the interim, astute civilian physicians also remarked on the relationship and broadened its scope. In the eighteenth century, John Hunter collected and reported several instances of a peculiar "gastromalacia" seen on postmortem examination in patients who had sustained severe head injury. These observations were confirmed by Rokitansky in 1861 (he called the lesions "decubiti of the gastric mucosa") and were later (1932) reconfirmed and extended to include acute duodenal ulcers by Harvey Cushing, who contributed his name to the mucosal defects [11].

The development of acute gastroduodenal ulceration after thermal injury was first described by Swan in 1823, was rediscovered by Dupuytren in 1833, and was finally formalized by Curling in a report of 10 instances published in 1842 [10]. The association between systemic sepsis and acute mucosal disease was first noted considerably later (1875) by Parrott, who described a "pseudomembranous gastritis" in an infant dying of bronchopneumonia. In 1910 Dieulafoy reported several instances of generalized mucosal necrosis involving the entire gastrointestinal tract of patients who had died of pneumonia, appendicitis, or strangulating small intestinal obstruction. He called this condition "exulceratio simplex."

As the capacity to care for the critically ill grew more sophisticated in the years following World War II, it became apparent that these observations were of more than historical interest. Shortly after the introduction of cardiopulmonary bypass, reports of massive postoperative gastrointestinal bleeding began to appear [74]. Between 1966 and 1972, Altemeier et al. [2] were able to identify 54 patients in whom severe gastroduodenal hemorrhage developed in association with polymicrobial sepsis, despite appropriate antibiotic therapy. In 1970 Pruitt et al. [47] reported a 12 percent incidence of clinically significant bleeding from acute gastric or duodenal ulcerations in a large population of burned patients. Others found a similar incidence of hemorrhage following extensive emergent or elective general surgical procedures [19]. With the introduction of fiberoptic endoscopy as a diagnostic tool, it was quickly realized that stress ulceration was responsible for bleeding in most of these instances. Subsequently, the pathological anatomy and natural history of these lesions were identified, the pathophysiology of the disease was clarified, and effective forms of prophylaxis were introduced. The result was that the prevalence and severity of acute hemorrhagic gastritis declined sharply.

Stress Ulcer Defined

Four unique clinicopathological features characterize the gastric mucosal lesions that arise de novo in the critically ill. First, they are acute in onset. Lucas et al. [34] performed serial endoscopies in 42 selected patients undergoing emergent operation for severe traumatic injury. Within hours of the insult, all demonstrated erosions of the proximal gastric mucosa. A similar circumstance was observed by Czaja et al. [12] in patients who underwent endoscopy as early as 5 hours after a major burn. A second feature of stress ulcers is that, in contrast to most chronic peptic ulcerations, they are multiple in more than 90 percent of instances, tending to occur in clusters in the fundus and along the greater curvature of the stomach. Multiplicity is particularly prominent in the presence of systemic sepsis [16].

A third distinctive feature is that the lesions are located primarily in the acid-peptic secreting region of the gastric mucosa. Lucas et al. [34] observed that early erosions were confined exclusively to the proximal half of the stomach. If progression ensued in the face of clinical deterioration, an occasional lesion developed in the antrum; no patient had isolated antral involvement, however, and most patients with severe disease of the gastric body demonstrated antral sparing. A somewhat higher incidence of antral involvement (33 percent) has been reported in patients with major body burns, although always in association with proximal involvement [12]. A final unique feature of stress ulcer disease is that when patients with isolated central nervous system injury are excluded, hypersecretion of gastric acid is not present, even in the face of documented erosions [30]. In a prospective evaluation of 50 trauma patients, Stremple et al. [70] found that acid output was initially low but gradually returned to normal within five days of injury. No differences were apparent between patients who bled and those who did not. Czaja et al. [14] noted that burned patients with gastric disease tended to produce more acid than did those with normal-appearing mucosa, but the levels of acid output reported were well within the range observed in healthy persons.

When these distinctive features are used to characterize stress ulcer disease, it becomes apparent that the acute erosions seen early after massive trauma or major burns conform well to the definition. In contrast, the acute gastric or duodenal ulceration associated with isolated central nervous system trauma probably represents a different pathogenetic entity: Patients sustaining this type of injury, particularly if it is located intracranially, demonstrate high acid output associated with elevated levels of circulating serum gastrin, a consequence, perhaps, of excessive vagal excitation [5, 70]. Furthermore, Cushing's ulcers are most often solitary, occur as frequently in the duodenum as in the stomach, and have a marked tendency to perforate [11]. By the same criteria, it is also inappropriate to classify as a stress ulcer the chronic duodenal or gastric ulcer that is reactivated after injury. Finally, although the drug- or alcohol-induced erosive gastropathies resemble stress ulceration in many respects (indeed, they may share a common pathophysiology, albeit at different ends of the spectrum), they cannot be considered true stress ulcers, because the setting in which they develop is unrelated to any systemic physiological insult and their clinical course is considerably more benign.

Pathological Anatomy and Natural History

In virtually all patients who undergo endoscopy within hours of sustaining severe trauma, the gastric mucosa presents a generally pale appearance, suggesting the presence of ischemia, and demonstrates numerous focal areas of punctate erythematous petechiae. Mucosal disease is confined to the fundus at this time; the remaining body, antrum, and duodenum are spared [12, 34]. On light microscopy the mucosa is edematous and the submucosal vasculature is engorged, but inflammatory infiltration is sparse. More severe injury is apparent on scanning electron micrographs—scattered surface epithelial cells have lost their apical membranes, and, in some areas, whole sheets of surface cells have sloughed to reveal the underlying lamina propria [32, 34]. Gastric secretory volume and acid output are low at this time and remain so for four to five days.

By 24 to 48 hours after injury, the mucosal disease has invariably progressed [32]. Punctate black-based erosions, 1–2 mm in diameter, are apparent throughout the entire gastric corpus. In addition, the mucosa of the duodenum may appear edematous and friable in as many as 50 percent of patients, particularly if the initial insult was thermal in nature [13]. Microscopically, wedge-shaped intramucosal hemorrhages and segmental coagulation necrosis of the superficial layers of the gastric mucous membrane are apparent. Fortunately, the mucosal disease will progress no farther in patients who have been successfully resuscitated at this stage. Indeed, by three to four days after the injury, both macroscopical and microscopical evidence of healing is apparent in more than 90 percent of patients. This process is usually complete within 10–14 days [31].

In the face of continued physiological insult, however, mucosal disease concomitantly worsens. Erosions coalesce and enlarge to form ovoid or, less commonly, linear full-thickness mucosal ulcerations that penetrate deeply into the mucosa and submucosa to expose and disrupt nutrient vessels [32, 34]. In patients with associated duodenitis, a similar progression is observed, which may result in acute duodenal ulcers. These are usually solitary but may on occasion be multiple [13]. At this time gastric secretory volume and acidity typically increase, and gastric content becomes heavily bile-stained and blood-flecked. This circumstance presages the development of clinically overt hemorrhage, which typically occurs between the fifth and tenth day after injury [33].

Progression of the early, universal mucosal disease to the far less common but more devastating problem of acute hemorrhagic gastritis depends on the severity and duration of the underlying physiological stress to which the patient has been and is being subjected. Special risk factors for bleeding from stress ulcer include (but are not limited to) the following: moderate-to-severe systolic hypotension following injury, simultaneous trauma to the abdomen and thorax, large posttraumatic transfusion requirements, development of the adult respiratory distress syndrome, presence of oliguric renal failure, hepatic dysfunction, thermal injury involving more than 35 percent of the body surface area, and, most important, systemic sepsis from any source. In the absence of prophylactic measures, the probability of bleeding in the presence of any single risk factor alone varies from 5 to 15 percent. As the number of risk factors multiplies, the likelihood of hemorrhage also increases dramatically [12, 33, 67].

Pathophysiology

It was once remarked that the stomach, like the city of San Francisco, lives on the brink of disaster. This comment is not entirely facetious: The normal gastric mucosa is constantly exposed to a highly caustic acid and a powerful proteolytic enzyme, both of which exist in enormous concentrations in the gastric lumen with respect to the blood. In most semipermeable epithelial membranes of the body, a concentration gradient of this magnitude would favor massive diffusion of both H^+ and pepsin into the tissue, resulting in the membrane's proteolytic destruction. Clearly this does not occur in the gastric mucosa under ordinary circumstances. The capacity of the stomach to resist autodigestion has been termed *cytoprotection*. Because stress ulcer disease represents a fundamental failure of this capacity, considerable experimental effort has been directed toward defining its characteristics. Several factors have been tentatively identified, although the exact relevance of each to the clinical problem under consideration cannot be stated with certainty. It is tempting to speculate that these factors may act as a series of barriers that undergo progressive recruitment as the magnitude of the "cytotoxic" insult increases.

MUCUS

Interest in the cytoprotective role of the gastric mucosubstances has been rekindled as the result of a more sophisticated understanding of their physical chemistry and structure [1]. Mucus is secreted by surface epithelial cells in the form of a complex glycoprotein that adheres to the mucosal surface. Current evidence suggests that the prostaglandins, with which the gastric mucosa is abundantly supplied, may be intimately involved in this process [4, 27]. The potential importance of gastric mucus to cytoprotection is related to the fact that it is a highly viscous gel, containing numerous lamellae of stagnant, unstirred water, through which molecules of small diameter diffuse at an extremely slow rate. Retardation of diffusion depends on the integrity of the molecular structure of the gel as well as on the absolute thickness of the mucous layer. It has been suggested that this property provides the gastric surface cells with a protective shield against inwardly diffusing luminal H^+ and pepsin [75]. Such a mucous barrier is fragile, however; a variety of topically damaging agents, including aspirin, the bile acids, and even pepsin itself, can alter the structure of mucus, decrease its thickness, or diminish its secretion, with potentially harmful consequences.

HCO_3^-

A related cytoprotective process is the ability of gastric mucosa to secrete alkali into the gastric lumen in the form of HCO_3^- [26]. Although the energetics of this reaction are incompletely defined, it is known that the expenditure of metabolic energy is involved and that the presence of carbonic anhydrase is required. The gastric mucosa contains considerable quantities of this enzyme, particularly in the region of the surface epithelial cells. Luminal alkalinization is stimulated by acetylcholine and the E-type prostaglandins and is inhibited by acetazolamide, aspirin, indomethacin, and the bile salts. Although the absolute amounts of HCO_3^- appearing in the gastric lumen are small regardless of the stimulus, current evidence indicates that a layer of alkali accumulates at the apical membranes of the surface cells, probably because the production of HCO_3^- is closely linked to the secretion of mucus, which prevents outward movement of the ion into the lumen [60]. Bicarbonate produced as a consequence of active secretion of H^- (the "alkaline tide") may also represent an important source of buffer at the intracellular level [65].

GASTRIC MUCOSAL BARRIER

Despite these intriguing findings, the role of endogenous mucus and HCO_3^- secretion in ameliorating or preventing stress ulceration following trauma is problematic at best. In contrast a third factor, the so-called gastric mucosal barrier, may have considerable cytoprotective importance clinically. As originally defined by Davenport [15], this "barrier" was the ability of the gastric mucosa to maintain a high intraluminal pH gradient between the gastric content and the subjacent mucous membrane. Several topical agents, including the bile acids, urea, lysolecithin, alcohol, aspirin, and other nonsteroidal anti-inflammatory compounds, possess the capacity to breach this barrier with the result that large amounts of H^+ diffuse into the mucosa [55]. The precise anatomical locus of the barrier is unknown. It was originally thought that the tight junctions that exist between adjacent surface epithelial cells were responsible for the restricted permeability of the gastric mucosa. It is now clear, however, that many of the topically damaging agents enumerated can produce severe morphological injury without disrupting these structures [24]. Experimental evidence from my laboratory and others suggests that an intact monolayer of surface epithelial cells may be critical to the integrity of the barrier and may even constitute its true anatomical site [40]. That the barrier may be damaged in the clinical setting of stress ulcer disease is suggested by the observations of Gordon et al. [20], who noted that when compared with healthy controls 50 percent of critically ill patients demonstrated significantly greater-than-normal rates of back diffusion of an instilled H^+ load from the intact stomach. Others have been unable to confirm this finding using the lithium flux technique, the validity of which is highly questionable [42, 61].

MICROCIRCULATION

A final cytoprotective factor of importance is related to the gastric microcirculation [54]. When applied topically at low pH, damaging agents such as the bile acids and aspirin induce a significant increase in mucosal blood flow, the magnitude of which is related in a linear manner to the amount of the H^+ lost from the lumen. This response is clearly cytoprotective because, when it alone is blunted, lesions that are indistinguishable from clinical stress ulcers develop in the gastric mucosa. It seems likely that the enhanced mucosal blood flow observed under these circumstances serves to clear or neutralize influxing H^+, thereby maintaining intramucosal pH at near normal levels. Studies from my laboratory suggest that endogenous histamine is not involved in this response; rather, endogenous prostaglandins appear to serve as the principal mediators.

INTRALUMINAL ACID

It is impossible to identify with certainty which of these cytoprotective mechanisms fails in the clinical setting of a massive systemic physiological insult. Nevertheless, near universal agreement exists that at least two factors are indispensable to the genesis and evolution of stress ulcer disease in humans. The first of these is intraluminal acid. A wide variety of animal models have been developed that closely simulate clinical stress ulcer disease; each requires the presence of at least some acid in contact with the mucosa to produce appropriate lesions. It is also clear that the severity of experimental ulcer formation is a significant linear function of the concentration of H^+ in the mucosal bathing solution [56] and that the mucosa is protected from ulceration when its capacity to secrete acid is diminished or when it is in contact with potent intraluminal buffers [65]. Clinical evidence indirectly supports these observations: Mucosal disease begins in the acid-peptic secreting region of the stomach, and measures designed to neutralize intragastric acid are effective in preventing disease progression.

GASTRIC MUCOSAL BLOOD FLOW
A second feature common to all experimental models of stress ulceration is diminished gastric mucosal blood flow. The early pale appearance of the mucosa after injury and the hypotension and hypovolemia that commonly accompany the development of stress ulcers clinically suggest that this factor may be operative in patients as well. Although the precise consequences of ischemia remain to be completely defined, numerous studies demonstrate that decreased flow, however induced, is associated with profound physiological alterations in mucosal function, including an inability to maintain an electrical gradient between lumen and blood [51], inhibition of a variety of active transport processes [58], a reduction in intracellular pO_2 and PD in surface epithelial cells [6], and a decrease in intramucosal pH [28]. When topical agents capable of damaging the barrier (e.g., the bile acids and lysolecithin) are concomitantly applied at low pH, ischemia also induces striking morphological damage to the mucosa [52]. Although the absolute magnitude of H^+ diffusing from lumen to tissue is not increased relative to nonischemic mucosa under these conditions, severe ulcerogenesis results, because no compensatory increase in blood flow occurs. This too may have relevance clinically, since enterogastric reflux commonly precedes the development of overt hemorrhage in patients. Even in the face of hyperdynamic sepsis, a condition in which total organ blood flow may be normal or even increased, experimental evidence indicates that the more superficial layers of the gastric mucosa are relatively underperfused, an effect that may be mediated by endorphin release [45, 48].

Ischemia also directly influences the metabolism of the gastric mucosa. Menguy [38] demonstrated that hemorrhagic shock produces a mucosal energy deficit (decreased levels of ATP) that is far more pronounced in the corpus than in the antrum, probably because of the relatively sparse glycogen stores normally present in the proximal stomach. Prefeeding blunts the severity of this deficit by providing the mucosa with greater energy stores. Others have indirectly corroborated these findings by demonstrating that enhanced nutrition exerts a salutary effect on mucosal injury induced by a variety of topical agents [18]. The relevance of this energy deficit to stress ulcer disease is unclear, however, because it has not been shown that these alterations are either a function of or altered by the concentration of H^+ present in the gastric lumen [64].

pH
In the final analysis it seems likely that the critical determinant of whether or not acute mucosal injury develops is the level of pH in the mucosa itself. A considerable body of experimental evidence provides both direct and indirect support for this statement. Studies from my laboratory clearly indicate that, in dogs, the severe and extensive lesion formation that occurs only in the simultaneous presence of topical H^+, topical bile acid, and mucosal ischemia is invariably associated with severe gastric venous acidosis. Conversely, in the absence of topical acid, H^+ loss from the lumen into the mucosa is negligible, mucosal damage is correspondingly small, and no gastric venous acidosis develops [59]. Similarly, Kivilaakso et al. [28] demonstrated that a significant linear relationship exists between H^+ back diffusion and intramucosal pH in rabbit fundic mucosa exposed to intraluminal acid. Furthermore, during hemorrhagic shock the intramucosal pH falls to levels far below those found in systemic arterial blood. Concomitantly, severe mucosal damage is produced. In contrast, the pH of fundic mucosa exposed to intraluminal buffer during shock falls to a much lesser extent, approximating the decrease in systemic arterial pH observed. Under these conditions, minimal damage is encountered. The same group also reported that, in the dog, fundic intramucosal pH declines only slightly during shock in the presence of intraluminal buffer, decreases to a greater extent when challenged with a high intraluminal H^+ concentration, and is profoundly depressed when bile acids are added to the acidic

bathing solution. Only under this last circumstance are severe and extensive mucosal ulcerations noted. The obverse of the proposition has also been tested. Cheung and Porterfield [7] showed that the systemic administration of alkali in large amounts vitiates the acute mucosal damage induced in shocked dogs by topical acid and bile acid application despite luminal H^+ loss of comparable magnitude in both control and test animals. Similar results were reported in rats by Starlinger et al. [68], who also implicated HCO_3^- as the principal physiological buffer of importance in this response.

The clinical implication of the foregoing analysis is clear: In patients susceptible to the development of bleeding from stress ulcers, if progression of disease is to be avoided efforts must be directed toward controlling intragastric pH, restoring intravascular volume, supporting cardiac output, maintaining normal acid-base balance, and providing adequate nutritional support.

Diagnosis

The diagnosis of acute hemorrhagic gastritis should be entertained whenever a critically ill patient has a painless hemorrhage from the upper gastrointestinal tract. This event is manifested most commonly by hematemesis or by the appearance of either bright red blood or acid hematin in nasogastric aspirate. Rarely, melena or frank hematochesia may be the index sign of active hemorrhage. In a few patients, the bleeding may wax and wane over several days, a pattern that suggests alternate healing and reactivation of the responsible lesions.

The site of hemorrhage is best identified by fiberoptic endoscopy, a procedure that can be performed expeditiously at the bedside once the patient has been resuscitated and stabilized. Premedication should be kept to a minimum in these critically ill patients. Successful localization requires that the gastric lumen be cleared of clotted blood. This can usually be accomplished easily by lavaging the stomach through a large-bore orogastric tube. In most instances, this maneuver not only will clear the stomach of clots but also will arrest the hemorrhage, at least temporarily, thus permitting adequate visualization of the gastric mucosa. Endoscopic identification of the precise source of bleeding can be achieved in more than 90 percent of instances when the procedure is performed by an experienced individual within 48 hours of the onset of hemorrhage [71]. In contrast, the use of barium roentgenography is uniformly disappointing. Although such studies may demonstrate the presence of an appropriate lesion in a few instances, they give no information as to whether or not that lesion is the cause of hemorrhage. With respect to bleeding from stress ulcers in particular, the upper gastrointestinal series is of limited value since the responsible erosions are superficial and small.

On rare occasions the rate of hemorrhage may be so torrential that endoscopic identification of the bleeding site is impossible. Under these conditions, angiographic localization may be required. Complete evaluation of the celiac, left gastric, gastroduodenal, and superior mesenteric arteries is indicated under these circumstances. Bleeding from acute hemorrhagic gastritis is most often visualized with selective left gastric artery injection of contrast, appearing as a local hypervascular blush with intense opacification of the gastric lumen. Multiple discrete points of dye extravasation may also be noted.

Treatment of Established Bleeding

In the presence of clinically significant hemorrhage from stress ulcer disease, the aims of therapy are basically four: first, to resuscitate and stabilize the patient; second, to control the hemorrhage; third, to prevent recurrent bleeding; and fourth, to achieve patient survival. Because acute hemorrhagic gastritis represents an end-organ response to severe underlying illness, it is frequently possible to achieve the first three aims without accomplishing the fourth. This fact serves to emphasize the critical importance of defining all the associated risk factors and of attempting to correct them as expeditiously as possible.

Initial resuscitation of the bleeding patient is well standardized, irrespective of the source of hemorrhage, and ought to precede any diagnostic evaluation. With respect to acute hemorrhagic gastritis specifically, two features of the process require emphasis. First, bleeding and clotting studies should always be obtained, since abnormalities in these factors frequently exist in the clinical setting in which the disease develops and must be corrected before any therapy can be successful. Second, if the patient is receiving nonsteroidal anti-inflammatory compounds by any route for any reason, these should be discontinued because of their demonstrated capacity to promote mucosal injury. Whether this injunction also applies to systemic steroid administration is unclear. On the one hand, Chung et al. [8] reported that, when given chronically to dogs, steroids facilitate alterations in mucosal permeability induced by topically damaging agents. On the other hand, it has been demonstrated in my laboratory that, when given acutely in massive doses, steroids are actually cytoprotective in the face of a standard experimental insult because of their capacity to enhance gastric mucosal blood flow [57]. Based on the latter observation, it has been recommended that steroids not be withheld if the clinical situation dictates their use.

NONSURGICAL THERAPY

Given the importance of acid in the genesis of acute ulceration in the experimental setting, it is not surprising that measures designed to control intragastric pH have been the cornerstone of nonsurgical therapy for stress bleeding. Two general approaches to pH manipulation have been used, either alone or in combination: inhibition of acid secretion at the cellular level, and intraluminal neutralization of acid already secreted [49]. Based on the results of an uncontrolled trial in 49 patients, 31 of whom had typical stress ulcerations, Simonian and Curtis [66] have suggested that intragastric titration with antacids to maintain an intraluminal pH of 7 or greater is effective. Hemorrhage was controlled initially in 27 patients, rebleeding occurred in 3, and continued bleeding required operation in 4. Although prospective evaluation of antacid therapy compared to placebo has not yet been undertaken in this setting, these results seem to represent a superior outcome when considered in the context of historical controls.

Intravenous administration of H_2-receptor blocking agents, both alone and in association with intragastric antacid titration, has also been widely employed for the treatment of established bleeding from stress ulcers. Unfortunately, most of the studies evaluating this form of therapy either have been uncontrolled or have failed to address specifically the effect of the H_2-receptor blockade per se in acute hemorrhagic gastritis. For these reasons, contradictory results have been reported. In a retrospective, nonrandomized study, Dunn et al. [17] noted that 12 of 13 patients with endoscopically documented stress ulcer bleeding, none of whom were helped by other therapeutic measures, stopped bleeding during a short course of intravenous cimetidine. Three patients subsequently rebled, and two required operation. Only one patient died of hemorrhage, but overall mortality was high (69 percent) because of severe underlying multisystemic disease. Similar results were achieved by MacDonald et al. [35], who reported that a short course of metiamide, the progenitor of cimetidine, led to permanent cessation of bleeding in each of nine instances of stress-related hemorrhage.

In contrast, the results of the only double-blind randomized trial of the efficacy of H_2-receptor blockade in acute hemorrhagic gastritis are far less salutary [72]. Hemostasis was achieved within 48 hours in only 5 of 15 actively bleeding patients treated with intravenous cimetidine (1200 mg/day) combined with intragastric antacids (15 ml every 2 hours) and in 4 of 12 patients treated with antacids alone. Furthermore, no differences were apparent between the two groups with respect to endoscopic healing of the responsible erosions, transfusion requirements, or mortalities (40 percent and 33 percent, respectively). Of interest, however, was the observation that oral cimetidine (1 gm/day) again in combination with antacids, was significantly superior to antacids alone in preventing rebleeding in patients who had recently had hemorrhages but were not actively bleeding at the time of entry into the study.

In patients who fail to respond to the maneuvers outlined, the use of selective intra-arterial infusion of vasoconstricting drugs should be considered. While it may seem paradoxical to add an ischemic insult to a disease process in which mucosal hypoperfusion is thought to be a prominent causative factor, the presence of active bleeding dictates a change in therapeutic priorities from prevention of hemorrhage to its control. Most studies addressing the efficacy of this approach have used selective infusion of vasopressin into the left gastric artery, although epinephrine has also been employed. Nusbaum et al. [44] were the first to report successful control of bleeding in two instances of "gastritis" (both probably drug-induced) using this approach. The largest single experience with vasopressin infusion in acute hemorrhagic gastritis per se has been accumulated by Athanasoulis and his colleagues [3]. In 37 patients, at least 27 of whom were bleeding in the setting of major trauma or sepsis, vasopressin in 5% dextrose and water was selectively infused at a rate of 0.2 U/ml/min for 20 minutes. If, at the end of that time, angiography demonstrated that the caliber of the distal arterial tree had been reduced and that previously demonstrated extravasation of contrast medium into the lumen had been eliminated, the infusion was continued for 24 hours. If clinical hemostasis was still evident, the infusion rate was reduced to 0.1 U/ml/min for an additional 36 hours, after which 5% dextrose and water alone were infused for another 24 hours before the catheter was removed. Using this technique, therapeutic success was achieved in 31 of the 37 patients during a period of at least five days.

The results achieved in two prospective randomized trials of selective intra-arterial vasopressin infusion tend to confirm these observations [9, 37]. A total of 89 patients were involved, at least some of whom were bleeding from stress ulcerations. In each trial, vasopressin therapy was significantly superior to conventional treatment in achieving initial hemostasis (44 percent and 71 percent versus 15 percent and 28 percent, respectively). In both studies, however, the nonfatal complication rate of the technique was impressive (30–60 percent), the incidence of rebleeding was high (25–45 percent), and overall in-hospital mortality (approximately 50 percent) did not differ between the patients in the experimental and control groups. Whether this last circumstance was caused by the fact that patients failing conventional therapy were subsequently treated with vasopressin is unclear.

Several other nonoperative approaches to the actively bleeding patient have been advocated, including local gastric hypothermia, intragastric levarterenol, intragastric or intraperitoneal norepinephrine, parenteral vitamin A, and subcutaneous growth hormone. For a variety of reasons, none has achieved widespread popularity. Selective arterial embolization of autologous clot has also been attempted in a small number of patients, with generally disappointing results. Endoscopic therapy using either laser energy or electrocautery to control gastroduodenal hemorrhage is so recent a development that its efficacy is unknown.

OPERATIVE THERAPY

The choice of operation for the patient who fails to respond to nonoperative therapy poses a difficult problem for the surgeon. Based on what is known of the pathophysiology of stress ulceration, it is clear that some procedure designed to control acid secretion is appropriate. It must also be recalled, however, that acute hemorrhagic gastritis is a disease of the gastric mucosa and that bleeding can continue after operation if a significant portion of that membrane is left intact. The essence of the dilemma, therefore, is this: The critically ill patient tolerates extensive resective procedures poorly, yet lesser procedures often fail to control hemorrhage initially and are associated with high rates of rebleeding. The available literature provides little insight into the proper choice because many reports that advocate a specific operation have based that recommendation on results achieved in a nonhomogeneous patient population. Specifically, the studies fail to distinguish the drug- or alcohol-induced hemorrhagic gastropathies from the acute hemorrhagic gastritis that develops in the setting of massive physiological stress. This failing is particularly evident in the early series, many of which indicated that nonresective procedures such as truncal vagotomy and drainage were effective in controlling hemorrhage and preventing rebleeding. While this is true in the few instances of drug- or alcohol-induced bleeding that require the attention of a surgeon, such an approach is inadequate for bleeding from true stress ulceration: It fails to control hemorrhage in 50 to 90 percent of instances, and the rate of rebleeding is high (30–60 percent).

In an attempt to provide insight into this problem, Delaney and Michel [16] in 1977 carefully collated the literature published at that time on surgical therapy for acute hemorrhagic gastritis. Their aim was to assess the results of operation only in instances in which a reasonable presumption could be made that hemorrhage developed in the setting of trauma or sepsis. When analyzed in this way, the outcome following vagus section and drainage was less than satisfactory. The results achieved after partial gastrectomy alone were almost as disappointing: Thirty-six of 72 patients continued to bleed, and rebleeding occurred in 29 of those who experienced initial control. On the other hand, if vagotomy was added to resection, hemorrhage was controlled in a commendable 86 percent of instances, and only 8 of 62 patients had considerable rebleeding. The efficacy of added vagotomy in this setting may be related to an acute redistribution of blood flow away from the mucosa, a circumstance for which some experimental evidence exists.

The observations made in this general review are echoed in a report detailing the experience of a single institution with 52 patients bleeding from stress ulcer disease [25]. Procedures such as suture ligation alone, suture ligation combined with vagotomy and drainage, vagotomy and pyloroplasty, and vagotomy and antrectomy failed to control hemorrhage in 43 to 50 percent of instances. When the extent of proximal resection was increased, however, permanent hemostasis was achieved in 11 of 14 patients. This is not surprising, of course, given the predilection of the disease process to develop in the gastric corpus. Indeed, Menguy et al. [39] advocated the use of near-total gastrectomy for acute hemorrhagic gastritis based on their observation that this procedure provided complete and permanent control of hemorrhage in a small group of patients. Because of the high mortality and permanent morbidity usually associated with its use, most surgeons have not adopted such a radical approach to what is potentially only a transient disease. When faced with a patient with uncontrolled hemorrhage from stress ulceration, the author's personal preference is to perform a truncal vagotomy and a 70–80 percent gastrectomy with oversewing of any discrete bleeding points found in the residual gastric pouch. Reconstruction as a Roux-Y limb has been advocated under these circumstances by some in an effort to prevent enterogastric reflux, which, at least in theory, might contribute to continued mucosal disease. This type of reconstruction has not been our practice.

Gastric devascularization, an alternative approach, has been advocated by Richardson and Aust [50]. In this procedure, the right and left gastric and gastroepiploic arteries are ligated near their origins. The entire blood supply of the stomach is derived thereafter from the short gastric vessels. The rate of rebleeding following this procedure was low (9 percent), and no instances of gastric necrosis were reported. The theoretical advantage of this approach is, of course, that disabling postgastrectomy sequelae are avoided in patients who are fortunate enough to survive the underlying physiological insult.

The most distressing feature of all these reports is the high mortality (30–60 percent) associated with active bleeding from stress ulceration, irrespective of the treatment employed. While most patients who do not live die of the multisystemic failure that precipitated bleeding in the first place, inability to control hemorrhage may be directly responsible for death in as many as 25 percent of instances. This fact not only reemphasizes the importance of correcting the underlying metabolic defects responsible for ongoing stress, but also suggests that the most appropriate treatment for bleeding from stress ulceration is its prevention.

Methods of Prophylaxis in Stress Ulcer Disease

As indicated previously, the presence of intraluminal acid is indispensable to the development of gross and microscopical mucosal injury in virtually all experimental models of stress ulcer disease, irrespective of any associated abnormalities that may be demonstrable. Thus clinical methods of prophylaxis closely mimic the nonoperative treatment of established bleeding. The protocols used to determine efficacy have been more sophisticated, however, and therapeutic outcome has been strikingly different.

The first prospective randomized trial evaluating the use of intraluminal antacids for prophylaxis was carried out by McAlhany et al. [41] in 1976. Forty-eight patients who had sustained more than a 35 percent total body surface burn were randomly assigned to receive or not receive liquid antacids hourly to maintain the pH of gastric aspirate at 7. Six of 24 patients in the no-antacid group had clinically significant upper gastrointestinal hemorrhage, defined as a requirement for three or more transfusions in 24 hours, and one patient's solitary gastric ulcer perforated. In contrast, only one episode of severe bleeding and no instances of perforation were encountered in the antacid group; the differences were highly significant statistically. Those patients with evidence of an impaired mucosal barrier seemed to derive particular benefit from antacid titration. A similar study of 100 critically ill patients admitted to a respiratory-surgical intensive care unit was reported by Hastings et al. [22]. In this study, a more liberal definition of bleeding was employed; in addition to hematemesis, melena, and the appearance of bright red blood in nasogastric aspirate, the presence of strongly guaiac-positive material for 3 consecutive hours during any 12-hour period was considered evidence of active hemorrhage, presumably from stress ulcer disease. Hourly treatment with antacids (Mylanta II, 30–60 ml to maintain $pH > 3.5$) was statistically superior to nasogastric suction alone under these circumstances: Only 2 of the 51 treated patients had bleeding, compared with 12 of the 49 controls. Of interest is the fact that no patient in either group required operation because of hemorrhage. Although these data contrast with the results obtained in a third randomized study, which employed a less rigorous dosage schedule without pH titration [36], they have correctly been interpreted as providing clear evidence that intraluminal instillation of antacids provides effective prophylaxis against acute hemorrhagic gastritis when given appropriately to susceptible patients.

The use of H_2-receptor antagonists as the sole method of prophylaxis is also inherently attractive because of the demonstrated capacity of these agents to inhibit secretion of acid at the parietal cell level. It has also been claimed that they possess a variety of additional virtues that might be of benefit in the setting of massive trauma, including the ability to augment compromised gastric mucosal blood flow, the ability to minimize the release of histamine from preformed mucosal stores, and, in combination with H_1-receptor blockade, the ability to "tighten" the mucosal barrier. These benefits may be more illusory than real, however [53].

Several prospective randomized trials have evaluated the efficacy of H_2-receptor blocking agents in the clinical setting. Unfortunately, markedly contradictory and, on balance, generally disappointing results have been achieved. In two studies, comparisons were made with nasogastric suction only, the end point sought being gastrointestinal hemorrhage. In one of these studies, prophylaxis with intravenous metiamide or cimetidine in the presence of fulminant hepatic failure was effective in 25 of 26 treated patients, whereas 13 of 24 controls bled [36]. In the second study, cimetidine (300 mg IV every 4 hours) was significantly better than placebo in preventing gastric hemorrhage in patients who had sustained a closed head injury, even though the type and frequency of associated gross mucosal abnormalities seen on endoscopy was similar in both groups [21]. On the other hand, a third study was unable to detect any significant difference in the incidence of upper gastrointestinal hemorrhage in cimetidine treated (1000 mg/day) or placebo-treated renal transplant recipients [62]. Although homograft rejection was no more frequent in the patients receiving the active drug, theoretical considerations suggest that H_2-receptor blockade in this setting may have the potential for harm.

If the more subtle end point of pH control is chosen, H_2-receptor blockade does not fare especially well, although in most instances it is still more effective than nasogastric suction alone. With one exception [23] most clinical reports indicate that, when given as a 300-mg bolus every 4 hours, cimetidine fails to maintain intragastric pH above 3.5–4 in 34 to 66 percent of instances despite adequate blood levels and a prolonged circulating half-life [29]. Doses as high as 2400 mg/day may also be inadequate in as many as 25 percent of instances, particularly if the patient demonstrates respiratory distress or systemic sepsis. The reasons for this last circumstance are unclear but may relate to inadequate drug delivery because of impaired gastric mucosal perfusion.

The critical question for the clinician is not whether prophylaxis with cimetidine or antacids is better than no prophylaxis at all, but rather, which form of prophylaxis is most effective. The first randomized comparison of antacid and cimetidine for this purpose was carried out in 75 patients by Priebe et al. [46]. Subsequently, at least three additional well-designed prospective trials, involving a total of 450 patients, have been undertaken to answer this question [43, 69, 76]. None has demonstrated that cimetidine is in any way superior to antacids; one showed equivalence but only in terms of the endoscopic appearance of the gastric mucosa after thermal injury. Clinically significant hemorrhage was not encountered in either arm of this particular study, and other measurements of mucosal function were not evaluated [43]. Although each of the remaining three studies differed in certain respects, several common themes were apparent (Table 23-1). Intragastric instillation of antacid was invariably more effective in maintaining the pH of gastric aspirate at 3.5 or above than was cimetidine, irrespective of dosage. In addition, when cimetidine-resistant patients were "crossed over" to antacids, prompt control of pH was achieved in virtually every instance. Conditions that predisposed to failure of pH control were hypotension, pulmonary insufficiency, and systemic sepsis. Depending on the definition, bleeding was encountered in 2 to 18 percent of the cimetidine-treated patients compared to 0 to 5 percent of the antacid-treated group, differences that were statistically significant in each instance. In the absence of renal failure, complications of both types of therapy were few and usually well tolerated. Untoward effects of antacids include diarrhea, mild metabolic alkalosis, modest hypermagnesemia, and rarely, medication bezoars. Complications of cimetidine therapy were also relatively infrequent: obtundity, mild elevations in serum creatinine, and modest neutropenia. In a few instances it was necessary to alter the dosage schedule because of progressive uremia. The one study that attempted to assess the expense of therapy found that, exclusive of nursing time, cimetidine was more costly to use than antacids [76].

Table 23-1. Comparison of the ability of antacids and cimetidine to control intragastric pH (percentages of patients for whom the specific treatment regimen failed)

	Antacid		Cimetidine	
Author	Low dose	High dose	Low dose	High dose
Pribe et al. [46]	24	3	47	18
Stothert et al. [69]	30	0	66	26
Zinner et al. [76]	15	0	34	—

The report of Zinner et al. [76] provides added insight into the question under consideration, even though it is marginally flawed by the fact that a fixed dose of cimetidine was compared to an adjusted dose of antacid. Because large numbers of patients were studied, including a no-treatment group, the results could be stratified, albeit retrospectively, according to the number of risk factors present in any given patient. When analyzed in this way, it was found that cimetidine and antacids were equally efficacious (and superior to no treatment) in preventing hemorrhage in the less critically ill. As the severity of illness increased, however, the superiority of antacids became clear, while cimetidine proved completely ineffective. In a small subgroup of 23 morbidly ill patients (8 percent of the total number studied), neither regimen was significantly better than lack of treatment, a fact that reemphasizes the need for still better methods of prevention. These might take the form of newer and more potent H_2-receptor antagonists and/or the prostaglandins.

The reasons for the relative failure of cimetidine to provide adequate prophylaxis in these studies are unclear. In part, they may relate to inadequate drug delivery resulting in inadequate control of pH, as already noted. It has been suggested, based on experimental data, that cimetidine fails because, coincident with inhibition of acid secretion, the availability of buffer to the mucosa in the form of the "alkaline tide" is also markedly reduced [65]. This assertion is tangentially supported by the clinical observation of Zinner et al. [76] that, in individuals in whom the pH of gastric content was consistently greater than 4, clinically significant bleeding developed more often in those treated with cimetidine than in those treated with antacids (14 versus 6 percent). A similar circumstance has been noted by Priebe et al. [46]. An additional important implication of the hypothesis that H_2-receptor blockade impairs the buffering capacity of the gastric mucosa is that the combination of cimetidine and antacids may prove to be less effective prophylactically than antacids alone. As yet, however, no such trial has been undertaken.

In sum, it is clear from the available data that intragastric titration with antacids is a more reliable form of prophylaxis against bleeding from stress ulceration than is intravenous cimetidine. The task that remains is to identify those patients in whom current prophylaxis regimens are unnecessary and to develop better forms of prevention for patients in whom current prophylactic regimens are inadequate.

References

1. Allen, A., and Garner, A. Mucus and bicarbonate secretion in the stomach and their possible role in mucosal protection. *Gut* 21:249, 1980.
2. Altemeier, W. A., Fullen, W. D., and McDonough, J. J. Sepsis and gastrointestinal bleeding. *Ann. Surg.* 175:759, 1972.
3. Athanasoulis, C. A., Baum, S., Waltman, A. C., et al. Control of acute gastric mucosal hemorrhage. *N. Engl. J. Med.* 290:597, 1974.
4. Basso, N., Materia, A., Forlini, A., and Jaffe, B. M. Prostaglandin generation in the gastric mucosa of rats with stress ulcer. *Surgery* 94:104, 1983.
5. Bowen, J. C., Fleming, W. H., and Thompson, J. C. Increased gastrin release following penetrating central nervous system injury. *Surgery* 75:720, 1974.
6. Bowen, J. C., and Garg, D. K. Effect of graded mechanical ischemia on oxygen tension and electrical potential in the canine gastric mucosa: A new experimental model. *Gastroenterology* 73:84, 1977.
7. Cheung, L. Y., and Porterfield, G. Protection of gastric mucosa against acute ulceration by intravenous infusion of sodium bicarbonate. *Am. J. Surg.* 137:106, 1979.
8. Chung, R. S. K., Field, M., and Silen, W. Effects of methylprednisolone on hydrogen ion absorption in the canine stomach. *J. Clin. Invest.* 62:262, 1978.
9. Conn, H. O., Ramsby, G. R., Storer, E. H., et al. Intraarterial vasopressin in the treatment of upper gastrointestinal hemorrhage: A prospective controlled clinical trial. *Gastroenterology* 68:211, 1975.
10. Curling, T. B. On acute ulceration of the duodenum in cases of burn. *Med. Chir. Trans.* 25:260, 1842.
11. Cushing, H. Peptic ulcers and the interbrain. *Surg. Gynecol. Obstet.* 55:134, 1932.
12. Czaja, A. J., McAlhany, J. C., and Pruitt, B. A. Acute gastroduodenal disease after thermal injury. *N. Engl. J. Med.* 291:925, 1974.
13. Czaja, A. J., McAlhany, J. C., and Pruitt, B. A.

Acute duodenitis and duodenal ulceration after burns. *J.A.M.A.* 232:621, 1975.
14. Czaja, A. J., McAlhany, J. C., and Pruitt, B. A. Gastric acid secretion and acute gastroduodenal disease after burns. *Arch. Surg.* 111:243, 1976.
15. Davenport, H. W. Gastric mucosal injury by fatty and acetylsalicylic acids. *Gastroenterology* 46:245, 1964.
16. Delaney, J. P., and Michel, H. M. Hemorrhagic Gastritis Following Operation. In J. S. Najarian, and J. P. Delaney (Eds.), *Critical Surgical Care*. Miami: Symposia Specialists, 1977.
17. Dunn, D. H., Fischer, R. G., Silvis, S. E., et al. The treatment of hemorrhagic gastritis with cimetidine. *Surg. Gynecol. Obstet.* 147:737, 1978.
18. Gertner, M. H., Mullen, J. L., Hobbs, C. L., et al. Effects of nutrition on gastric secretion and mucosal ulceration in primates. *Surg. Forum* 29:416, 1978.
19. Goodman, A. A., and Frey, C. F. Massive upper gastrointestinal hemorrhage following surgical operations. *Ann. Surg.* 167:180, 1968.
20. Gordon, J. J., Skillman, J. J., Zervas, N. T., et al. Divergent nature of gastric mucosal permeability and gastric acid secretion in sick patients with general surgical and neurosurgical disease. *Ann. Surg.* 178:285, 1973.
21. Halloran, L. G., Zfass, A. M., Gayle, W. E., et al. Prevention of acute gastrointestinal complications after severe head injury: A controlled trial of cimetidine prophylaxis. *Am. J. Surg.* 139:44, 1980.
22. Hastings, P. R., Skillman, J. J., Bushnell, L. S., et al. Antacid titration in the prevention of acute gastrointestinal bleeding: A controlled, randomized trial in 100 critically ill patients. *N. Engl. J. Med.* 298:1041, 1978.
23. Hermann, V., and Kiminski, D. Evaluation of intragastric pH in acutely ill patients. *Arch. Surg.* 114:511, 1979.
24. Hingston, D. J., and Ito, S. Effect of aspirin and related compounds on the fine structure of mouse gastric mucosa. *Gastroenterology* 6:156, 1971.
25. Hubert, J. P., Jr., Kiernan, P. V., Welch, J. S., et al. The surgical management of bleeding stress ulcers. *Ann. Surg.* 191:672, 1980.
26. Kauffman, G. L., Jr. Gastric bicarbonate secretion. *Brain Res. Bull.* 5:15, 1980.
27. Kauffman, G. L., Jr., Reeve, J. J., and Grossman, M. I. Gastric bicarbonate secretion: Effect of topical and intravenous 16, 16-dimethyl prostaglandin E2. *Am. J. Physiol.* 239:G44, 1980.
28. Kivilaakso, E., Fromm, D., and Silen, W. Relationship between ulceration and intramural pH of gastric mucosa during hemorrhagic shock. *Surgery* 84:70, 1978.
29. Kohler, T. R., Dellinger, E. P., Simonowitx, D. A., et al. Cimetidine pharmacokinetics in trauma patients. *Surg. Forum* 30:12, 1979.
30. Larson, G. M., Koch, S., O'Dorsio, T. M., et al. Gastric response to severe head injury. *Am. J. Surg.* 147:97, 1984.
31. Lev, R., Molot, M. D., MacNamara, J., et al. "Stress" ulcers following war wounds in Vietnam. *Lab. Invest.* 25:491, 1971.
32. Lucas, C. E. Prevention and Treatment of Acute Gastric Erosions and Stress Ulceration. In R. C. Fiddian-Green, and J. G. Turcotte (Eds.), *Gastrointestinal Hemorrhage*. New York: Grune & Stratton, 1980.
33. Lucas, C. E. Stress ulceration: The clinical problem. *World J. Surg.* 5:139, 1981.
34. Lucas, C. E., Sugawa, C., Riddle, J., et al. Natural history and surgical dilemma of "stress" gastric bleeding. *Arch. Surg.* 102:266, 1971.
35. MacDonald, A. S., Steele, B. J., and Bottomley, M. G. Treatment of stress induced upper gastrointestinal hemorrhage with metiamide. *Lancet* 1:68, 1976.
36. MacDougall, B. R. D., Bailey, R. J., and Williams, R. H_2 receptor antagonists and antacids in the prevention of acute gastrointestinal hemorrhage in fulminant hepatic failure. *Lancet* 1:617, 1977.
37. Mallory, A., Schaefer, J. W., Cohen, J. R., et al. Selective intraarterial vasopressin infusion for upper gastrointestinal tract hemorrhage. *Arch. Surg.* 115:30, 1980.
38. Menguy, R. Role of gastric mucosal energy metabolism in the etiology of stress ulceration. *World J. Surg.* 5:175, 1981.
39. Menguy, R., Gadacz, T., and Zajtchuk, R. The surgical management of acute gastric mucosal bleeding. *Arch. Surg.* 99:198, 1969.
40. Moody, F. G., Zalewsky, C. A., and Larsen, K. R. Cytoprotection of the gastric epithelium. *World J. Surg.* 5:153, 1981.
41. McAlhany, J. C., Czaja, A. J., and Pruitt, B. A. Antacid control of complications from acute gastroduodenal disease after burns. *J. Trauma* 16:645, 1976.
42. McAlhany, J. C., Czaja, A. J., Villarreal, Y., et al. The gastric mucosal barrier in thermally in-

jured patients: Correlation with gastroduodenal endoscopy. *Surg. Forum* 25:414, 1974.
43. McElwee, H. P., Sirinek, K. R., and Levine, B. A. Cimetidine affords protection equal to antacids in prevention of stress ulceration following thermal injury. *Surgery* 86:620, 1979.
44. Nusbaum, M., Baum, S., Blakemore, W. S., et al. Clinical experience with selective intraarterial infusion of vasopressin in the control of gastrointestinal bleeding from arterial sources. *Am. J. Surg.* 123:165, 1972.
45. Payne, J. G., and Bowen, J. C. Hypoxia of canine gastric mucosa caused by *Escherichia coli* sepsis is prevented with methylprednisolone therapy. *Gastroenterology* 80:84, 1981.
46. Priebe, H. J., Skillman, J. J., Bushnell, L. S., et al. Antacid versus cimetidine in preventing acute gastrointestinal bleeding: A randomized trial in 75 critically ill patients. *N. Engl. J. Med.* 302:426, 1980.
47. Pruitt, B. A., Foley, F. D., and Moncried, J. A. Curling's ulcer: A clinical pathology study of 323 cases. *Ann. Surg.* 172:523, 1970.
48. Rees, M., Payne, J. G., and Bowen, J. C. Naloxone reverses tissue effects of live *Escherichia coli* sepsis. *Surgery* 91:91, 1982.
49. Richardson, C. T. Pharmacologic basis of peptic ulcer therapy. *Viewpoints Dig. Dis.* 17:1, 1985.
50. Richardson, J. D., and Aust, J. B. Gastric devascularization: A Useful salvage procedure for massive hemorrhagic gastritis. *Ann. Surg.* 185:649, 1977.
51. Ritchie, W. P., Jr. Influence of vasopressin and topical bile salts on the gastric mucosal barrier of the subhuman primate. *Surgery* 75:853, 1974.
52. Ritchie, W. P., Jr. Acute gastric mucosal damage induced by bile salts, acid, and ischemia. *Gastroenterology* 68:699, 1975.
53. Ritchie, W. P., Jr. Histamine and gastric mucosal damage. *Gastroenterology* 75:933, 1978.
54. Ritchie, W. P., Jr. Role of bile acid reflux in acute hemorrhagic gastritis. *World J. Surg.* 5:189, 1981.
55. Ritchie, W. P., Jr. Pathogenesis of acute gastric mucosal injury. *Viewpoints Dig. Dis.* 15:17, 1985.
56. Ritchie, W. P., Jr., and Cherry, K. G., Jr. Influence of H^+ on bile acid induced acute gastric mucosal ulcerogenesis. *Ann. Surg.* 189:637, 1979.
57. Ritchie, W. P., Jr., Cherry, K. J., and Gibb, A. Influence of methylprednisolone sodium succinate on bile acid induced acute gastric mucosal damage. *Surgery* 84:283, 1978.
58. Ritchie, W. P., Jr., and Fischer, R. P. Studies on the pathogenesis of "stress ulcer": Electrical potential difference and ionic fluxes against canine gastric mucosa during hemorrhagic shock. *J. Surg. Res.* 12:173, 1972.
59. Ritchie, W. P., Jr., McRea, D. B., Jr., and Felger, T. S. A-V acid-base balance during acute gastric mucosal ulcerogenesis. *Am. J. Surg.* 139:22, 1980.
60. Ross, I. N., Bahari, H. M. M., and Turnberg, L. A. The pH gradient across mucus adherent to rat fundic mucosa in-vivo and the effect of potential damaging agents. *Gastroenterology* 81:713, 1981.
61. Saik, R. P., and Brown, B. Lithium: Not a Sensitive Indicator of Hydrogen Ion Diffusion. *J. Surg. Res.* 25:163, 1978.
62. Schiessel, R., Starlinger, M., Wolf, A., et al. Failure of cimetidine to prevent gastroduodenal ulceration and bleeding after renal transplantation. *Surgery* 90:456, 1981.
63. Selye, H. A syndrome produced by diverse noxious agents. *Nature* 138:32, 1936.
64. Shorr, L. D., Sirinek, K. R., Page, C. P., and Levine, B. A. The role of glucose in preventing stress gastric mucosal injury. *J. Surg. Res.* 36:384, 1984.
65. Silen, W., Merhav, A., and Simson, J. N. L. The pathophysiology of stress ulcer disease. *World J. Surg.* 5:165, 1981.
66. Simonian, S. J., and Curtis, L. E. Treatment of hemorrhagic gastritis by antacid. *Ann. Surg.* 184:429, 1976.
67. Skillman, J. J., Gould, S. A., Chung, R. S. K., et al. The gastric mucosal barrier: Clinical and experimental studies in critically ill and normal man and in the rabbit. *Ann. Surg.* 172:564, 1970.
68. Starlinger, M., Jakez, R., Matthews, J. B., et al. The relative importance of HCO_3^- and blood flow in the protection of rat gastric mucosa during shock. *Gastroenterology* 81:732, 1981.
69. Stothert, J. C., Jr., Simonowitz, D. A., Dellinger, E. P., et al. Randomized prospective evaluation of cimetidine and antacid control of pH in the critically ill. *Ann. Surg.* 192:169, 1980.
70. Stremple, J. F., Molot, M. D., McNamara, J. J., et al. Post traumatic gastric bleeding: Prospective gastric secretion composition. *Arch. Surg.* 105:177, 1972.
71. Sugawa, C., Werner, M. H., Hayes, D. F., et

al. Early endoscopy: A guide to therapy for acute hemorrhage in the upper gastrointestinal tract. *Arch. Surg.* 107:133, 1973.

72. Teres, J., Bordas, J. M., Rimola, A., et al. Cimetidine in acute gastric mucosa bleeding. *Dig. Dis. Sci.* 25:92, 1980.
73. Wangensteen, O. H. Foreword. In S. Day, B. MacMillan, and W. Altemeier (Eds.), *Curling's Ulcer: an Experiment in Nature.* Springfield, Ill.: Thomas, 1972.
74. Williams, J. F., Morrow, A. G., and Braunwald, E. The incidence and management of "medical" complications following cardiac operations. *Circulation* 32:608, 1965.
75. Williams, S. E., and Turnberg, L. A. Retardation of acid diffusion by pig gastric mucus: A potential role in mucosal protection. *Gastroenterology* 79:299, 1980.
76. Zinner, M. J., Zuidema, G. D., Smith, P. L., et al. The prevention of upper gastrointestinal tract bleeding in patients in an intensive care unit. *Surg. Gynecol. Obstet.* 153:214, 1981.

EDITOR'S COMMENT

The problem of stress ulceration continues to plague the medical-surgical community. The high mortality continues, although the risk has been blunted through better methods of prophylaxis. The risk of operation remains so high, however, that we continue to search for methods of nonoperative therapy.

It has been difficult to determine the real efficacy of endoscopic treatment of upper gastrointestinal tract bleeding sites for several reasons. First, since 80 percent of an unselected group are expected to stop bleeding spontaneously, it is important to focus on individuals who continue to bleed instead of the majority whose bleeding would have stopped spontaneously. Second, it is difficult, if not impossible, to have comparable groups of patients with similar lesions and similar rates of bleeding who can be randomly assigned to different treatment groups.

My colleagues and I (Donahue et al. *Surg. Gynecol. Obstet.* 159:113, 1984) have described the use of a bipolar endoscopic coagulation device in 28 patients with active massive upper gastrointestinal tract hemorrhage; they represented 10 percent of patients with hemorrhage during a one-year period. Endoscopic treatment controlled bleeding initially in 23 of these patients. Another 8 patients with recent hemorrhage who were at high risk for recurrent bleeding (visible vessels) had endoscopic coagulation without subsequent hemorrhage.

Of more importance to this chapter, the bleeding from acute gastric mucosal lesions in 10 of 11 patients was controlled initially. Two of the patients rebled at 48 hours, but only 2 of the entire group needed to have an emergency operation.

Immediate operations were required in 5 of the 28 patients and delayed operations in another 4. Mortality among the patients treated by endoscopic or surgical therapy was comparable (20 percent), but no patient died of hemorrhage. The high mortality in this group of patients is explained by associated illnesses.

Bipolar endoscopic coagulation is as effective as other endoscopic treatments for nonvariceal sources of upper gastrointestinal tract hemorrhage. This modality is relatively inexpensive compared with other devices, is theoretically less complicated, and presents minimal risk to the patient. Because of these considerations, it is a technique that deserves wider application and may become the endoscopic treatment of choice for control of upper gastrointestinal tract hemorrhage. Patients with endoscopic control of upper gastrointestinal tract bleeding avoid perioperative morbidity, have a lower transfusion requirement, and may have a shorter hospital stay than comparable patients who require surgical control of bleeding sites.

L.M.N.

24

Bacteriology of the Stomach and Duodenum

Ronald Lee Nichols

The association between the endogenous intragastric microflora and postoperative wound and intra-abdominal infections after gastroduodenal operations has been clarified during the last decade. Before this time surgeons expressed much uncertainty regarding which patients undergoing gastroduodenal procedures were at risk for postoperative infection, where the infective organisms originated (exogenous versus endogenous), and what, if any, techniques could be employed prophylactically to decrease their numbers. The objectives of this chapter include (1) the definition of intragastric microflora, both qualitatively and quantitatively, in health and various disease states; (2) a discussion of the inhibitory factors that regularly exert an influence on the nature of the intragastric microflora; and (3) the presentation of clinical studies that provide insight into the efficacy of antibiotic prophylaxis in gastroduodenal operations.

Intragastric Bacterial Microflora in Health and Common Disease States

INTRAGASTRIC MICROFLORA IN HEALTH

The stomach in a normal fasting individual contains low concentrations ($< 10^2$) of both aerobic and anaerobic bacteria or none at all. This finding is of interest if one considers the large variety and number of bacteria that transiently enter the stomach in swallowed saliva from the oral pharynx and from small intestinal contents that have refluxed through the pylorus. The primary contribution is made by saliva, with total aerobes and anaerobes numbering between 10^6 and 10^8 bacteria per milliliter of saliva. Higher numbers of these bacteria are present in patients with poor dental hygiene, in whom intraoral overgrowth is commonly observed. The proximal small intestinal contents account for smaller numbers of bacteria, usually in the range of 10^2 to 20^3 bacteria per milliliter of intestinal contents. The common types of aerobes and anaerobes that make up the oral and proximal intestinal microflora are listed in Table 24-1.

Table 24-1. Common aerobes and anaerobes isolated from saliva and proximal intestinal contents

Oral microflora	Proximal intestinal microflora
AEROBES	
Streptococci	*Escherichia coli*
Staphylococci	*Klebsiella* species
Neisseria species	*Enterobacter* species
Hemophilus species	Enterococci
ANAEROBES	
Bacteroides oralis	Peptostreptococci
Bacteroides melaninogenicus	Bifidobacteria
Peptostreptococci	

Table 24-2. Indications for operation

Gastric or duodenal disease	No. of patients
Chronic duodenal ulcer	18
Bleeding duodenal ulcer	12
Obstructing duodenal ulcer	9
Gastric ulcer	6
Gastric carcinoma	4
Total	49

Table 24-3. Microflora of stomach in patients with chronic nonobstructing duodenal ulcer

Microflora	No. of patients
No growth	15
Aerobic growth	3
α-streptococcus, enterococcus (1)	
Klebsiella species, *Candida* species (1)	
α-streptococcus, *Neisseria* species (1)	
Anaerobic growth	0
Mixed (aerobic-anaerobic) growth	0
Total	18

INTRAGASTRIC MICROFLORA IN COMMON DISEASE STATES

In 1975 Smith and I [23] reported on the nature of the gastric microflora in 49 patients undergoing either elective or emergent gastric operations. None of these patients received preoperative or intraoperative oral or parenteral antibiotics, which if given could have been expected to alter the intragastric microflora. The indications for operation are listed in Table 24-2. After the peritoneal cavity was entered, a needle aspiration of the greater curvature of the stomach using an 18-gauge needle and 50-cc syringe was performed in each patient. Manual pressure on the anterior surface of the stomach was often necessary to ensure an adequate sample of gastric contents (2–3 ml). The gastric contents were then taken rapidly to the research microbiological laboratory, where standard qualitative aerobic and anaerobic processing was begun within 15 minutes of arrival.

The results of this study revealed that intragastric bacteria were isolated in 32 of the 49 patients. Surprising at the time of this study was the great variation in isolation that occurred in the various disease states. In the 18 patients who underwent elective operation for chronic nonobstructing duodenal ulcer, the gastric aspirate was sterile in 15 patients (Table 24-3). The remaining three patients demonstrated purely aerobic growth representative of the endogenous aerobes of the oropharynx and proximal intestine. One patient had a *Candida* species isolated in addition to an aerobic coliform.

All 12 patients who underwent emergency surgical procedures for acutely bleeding duodenal ulcer showed bacterial growth (Table 24-4). One patient had purely aerobic growth while three patients had anaerobic growth. The remaining eight patients had mixed aerobic-anaerobic growth. The isolated anaerobes were, in all instances, the penicillin-sensitive oral type. Nine patients underwent semielective operations for obstructing duodenal ulcer. The gastric aspirate was sterile in one, while the remaining eight showed growth (Table 24-5). Five of these patients had purely aerobic growth, including a *Candida* species in

Table 24-4. Microflora of stomach in patients with bleeding duodenal ulcer

Microflora	No. of patients
No growth	0
Aerobic growth	1
Escherichia coli, α-streptococcus, *Neisseria* species (1)	
Anaerobic growth	3
Peptostreptococcus (1)	
Bacteroides oralis, Bacteroides melaninogenicus (2)	
Mixed (aerobic-anaerobic) growth	8
α-streptococcus, *Bacteroides oralis* (2)	
Escherichia coli, Bacteroides oralis, Peptostreptococcus (2)	
α-streptococcus, *Neisseria* species, *Bacteroides oralis, Bacteroides melaninogenicus* (2)	
Klebsiella species, *Bacteroides melaninogenicus* (1)	
Escherichia coli, Klebsiella species, Bifidobacteria (1)	
Total	12

one, while one patient had anaerobic growth and two had mixed aerobic-anaerobic growth. Four patients who underwent gastric resection for carcinoma of the stomach had mixed aerobic and anaerobic bacterial growth isolated from the gastric aspirate (Table 24-6). One patient showed growth of *Bacteroides fragilis,* a penicillin-resistant anaerobe usually found in the distal small intestine and colon. And finally, five of the six patients with gastric ulcer exhibited an intragastric microflora (Table 24-7). One patient had pure aerobic growth, while four patients had mixed aerobic-anaerobic growth.

Postoperative wound infection rates from this study are listed in Table 24-8. The overall wound infection rate was 14 percent. The group of 18 patients with chronic duodenal ulcer had a sparse gastric microflora at the time of operation and had no postoperative wound

Table 24-5. Microflora of stomach in patients with obstructing duodenal ulcer

Microflora	No. of patients
No growth	1
Aerobic growth	5
Candida species (1)	
Enterobacter species (2)	
Klebsiella species, α-streptococcus (2)	
Anaerobic growth	1
Bacteroides oralis, Bacteroides melaninogenicus (1)	
Mixed (aerobic-anaerobic) growth	2
α-streptococcus, *Bacteroides oralis, Peptostreptococcus* (1)	
α-streptococcus, *Neisseria* species, *Bacteroides oralis, Bacteroides melaninogenicus* (1)	
Total	9

Table 24-6. Microflora of stomach in patients with carcinoma of stomach

Microflora	No. of patients
No growth	0
Aerobic growth	0
Anaerobic growth	0
Mixed (aerobic-anaerobic) growth	4
Klebsiella species, *Bacteroides melaninogenicus* (1)	
α-streptococcus, *Neisseria* species, *Bacteroides oralis* (1)	
Neisseria species, *Escherichia coli, Bacteroides fragilis* (1)	
α-streptococcus, *Candida* species, *Bacteroides oralis, Bacteroides melaninogenicus, Peptostreptococcus* (1)	
Total	4

Table 24-7. Microflora of the stomach in patients with gastric ulcer

Microflora	No. of patients
No growth	1
Aerobic growth	1
Klebsiella species, *Escherichia coli*, α-streptococcus (1)	
Anaerobic growth	0
Mixed (aerobic-anaerobic) growth	4
Escherichia coli, *Peptostreptococcus* (1)	
α-streptococcus, *Neisseria* species, *Bacteroides melaninogenicus* (1)	
α-streptococcus, *Peptostreptococcus*, *Bacteroides melaninogenicus* (1)	
Klebsiella species, α-streptococcus, *Bacteroides oralis* (1)	
Total	6

Table 24-8. Postoperative wound infections in patients undergoing gastric operations

Indication for operation	No. infections/ No. patients
Chronic duodenal ulcer	0/18 (0%)
Bleeding duodenal ulcer	4/12 (33%)
Obstructing duodenal ulcer	1/9 (11%)
Gastric ulcer	1/6 (16%)
Carcinoma of stomach	1/4 (25%)
Total	7/49 (14%)

infections. If this group of patients were excluded, there were 7 infections in the remaining 31 patients for an overall 22 percent infection rate. It was apparent from this study that gastric bacterial colonization occurs almost uniformly in patients undergoing operation for bleeding or obstructing duodenal ulcer or for gastric ulcer or malignant tumors (29 of 31 patients). The reason for the gastric colonization in these groups of patients can best be explained by a compromise of the normal inhibitory effects of gastric acid or gastric motility. When present, this gastric microflora is usually equally divided between oral or proximal intestinal aerobes and oral penicillin–sensitive anaerobes. Only one penicillin-resistant anaerobe *(Bacteroides fragilis)* was isolated in our study. These same endogenous gastric microorganisms also contributed to wound sepsis in 6 of 7 patients in this series in whom postoperative infection developed. Based on the results of this study it appeared that the endogenous intragastric microflora was a significant factor in the development of postoperative wound sepsis after gastric resection in those groups of patients with a compromise of their normal gastric antibacterial inhibitory mechanisms.

Inhibitory Factors Preventing Intragastric Bacterial Colonization

The association of the intragastric acid-base balance and the bacterial flora of the stomach, duodenum, and jejunum was stressed by Arnold and Brody [3] as early as 1926. In a series of animal experiments they demonstrated the bacteriostatic action of the gastric acid [2, 3]. Drasar et al. [9] showed that ingested bacteria reside only transiently in the normal stomach but are capable of reducing the local pH to less than 3.0. Franklin and Skoryna [12] found that bacterial species were isolated routinely from stomachs when the pH was above 2.0. Others [4, 6, 15] have also observed that the pH of gastric juice is intimately associated with both the quality and quantity of the microflora found in the stomach and proximal intestine, although the critical intragastric pH necessary to kill bacteria is somewhat variable, usually reported between 1 and 4. Aerobic coliforms are rarely isolated from the normal stomach but are isolated almost uniformly when hypochlorhydria or achlorhydria (pernicious anemia) is present [8, 14]. Frederiksen and colleagues [13] reported that significant bacterial counts were usually found in the proximal intestine when the histamine-stimulated gastric peak acid outputs were between 0 and 5 mEq H^+ per hour (PAO: 0–5) and rarely found that the PAO was above 15 mEq H^+ per hour. Greenlee et al. [16], however, studied bacterial overgrowth in the jejunum after gastric operations for chronic duodenal ulcer and found no definite evidence supporting the importance of gastric acid output in controlling bacterial proliferation of the proximal small intestine. Even in the presence of low acid secretion in some of their patients no bacteria could be isolated, while hypersecretion of acid did not always prevent bacterial growth. Other observers [7, 13, 15] stressed the importance of the inhibitory effect of normal gastric motility and the mechanical cleansing action of small intestinal peristalsis on the microflora of the stomach and proximal small intestine. Dellipiani and Girdwood [8] isolated intestinal coliforms in the stomachs of more than 50 percent of patients with jejunal diverticula and in patients with surgically created blind loops such as gastroenterostomies.

In my study with Smith [23] both gastric acid and normal gastric motility appeared to be important in preventing gastric bacterial colonization. In the group of patients with chronic nonobstructing duodenal ulcer, high acid levels and normal gastric motility were noted preoperatively, few if any gastric bacteria were isolated at the time of operation, and a low postoperative infection rate was observed. In all other groups of patients who had a defect in either gastric acid or motility, intragastric colonization was usually noted. This colonization also resulted in high postoperative infection rates. We reported a retrospective review of 254 consecutive gastroduodenal operations done at the Charity Hospital of Louisiana in New Orleans between 1974 and 1977 [20]. Twenty-two of 30 patients who had postoperative sepsis had compromise of either gastric acidity or motility at the time of the operation.

Muscroft et al. [21] reported on the gastric microflora of 163 patients after gastric operations as well as 72 patients receiving cimetidine therapy for chronic duodenal ulcer disease. They found that the total viable intragastric bacterial count was closely related to the pH of the gastric aspirate and was independent of the cause of the hypochlorhydria. Ninety percent of the gastric aspirates of pH 1–2 were sterile, while 94 percent of those of pH 4–8 contained bacteria.

Postoperative Infection Rates after Gastroduodenal Operations

Prospective studies [18, 23] have defined the relative risk of postoperative infections developing in the various groups of patients undergoing gastric operations. The "low-risk" patients are those who undergo operations for chronic nonobstructing duodenal ulcer. Postoperative infections in this group of patients have been reported to fall in the range of 0–8 percent [18, 20, 23]. Although this indication for operation was common before 1976, modern successful medical therapy with cimetidine has all but eliminated this indication for operation. The only other low-risk group comprises patients operated on for perforated duodenal ulcer. It has long been recognized that the peritonitis encountered at the time of operation for perforated duodenal ulcer is largely chemical and that a bacterial cause is present only if long delays occur before surgical intervention. We recently reported that the lowest infection rate (5.7 percent) following a gastroduodenal operation occurred in this group of patients [20].

"High-risk" patients are those who undergo operations for indications of bleeding or obstructing duodenal or gastric ulcer or malignant tumors. The infection rates in these categories have been reported to fall between 11 and 33 percent [18, 20, 23]. Since the introduction of the histamine H_2-receptor group of drugs for the treatment of chronic nonobstructing ulcer, these disease states associated with a high risk of postoperative sepsis are the usual indications for operation.

Antibiotic Prophylaxis in Gastroduodenal Operations

The authoritative committees that have been assigned the task of making recommendations concerning surgical antibiotic prophylaxis in gastroduodenal operations have, to date, advised their use only in patients undergoing gastric resections for carcinoma [1, 27]. These recommendations have been made with the realization that postoperative wound infections unquestionably cause considerable morbidity and expense [19]. The authors of another review, entitled "Prophylactic antibiotics in surgical procedures," expressed the opinion that the efficacy of antibiotic prophylaxis in gastric operations has not been proved [5]. Nevertheless, the authors of many reports in the surgical literature over the last 15 years have advocated the use of antibiotic prophylaxis in gastric operations [10, 11, 17, 25, 26]. These major differences in attitude undoubtedly arose from a lack of rigidity in scientific design in many of the studies advocating antibiotic prophylaxis.

Unlike antibiotic colonic prophylaxis, in which orally ingested antibiotics have been shown to reduce significantly both the intraluminal bacteria and the postoperative infection rate after elective colonic resection, no studies of gastric operations have been reported using orally administered agents [22]. This is because of the difficulty of using oral antibiotic agents in many of these instances, owing to both the emergent nature of the operations and the failure of local antibiotics to mix adequately with the gastric contents. All studies concerning gastric antibiotic prophylaxis have used parenteral antibiotic agents given appropriately during the perioperative period.

The study designs and results of randomized clinical trials concerning the efficacy of antibiotic prophylaxis in gastroduodenal operations are presented in Table 24-9. The antibiotics used in all but one study were of the cephalosporin group. The prophylactic antibiotics were given during the perioperative period and were generally not continued beyond the first postoperative day. Stone and coworkers [26] demonstrated the lack of efficacy of prophylactic antibiotics started initially during the postoperative period. This faulty timing of administration resulted in postoperative infection rates similar to those of placebo-treated controls ($>$ 15 percent).

Lewis and colleagues [19] were the first to report the value of prophylactic antibiotics in the high-risk patient undergoing a gastroduodenal operation. In their randomized, prospective, nonblind study, prophylactic antibiotics significantly reduced the postoperative infection rate from 26 percent to 0. They included in their high-risk categories all the clinical conditions in which in 1975 we reported gastric bacterial inhibitory factors [23].

My colleagues and I [24] reported on the efficacy of antibiotic prophylaxis in patients undergoing gastroduodenal procedures with an increased risk of postoperative infection, using a randomized, prospective, double-blind design. Between July, 1978 and January, 1980, 43 patients at high risk for postoperative infection were admitted for gastroduodenal operations to the Tulane Surgical Service (Charity Hospital of Louisiana in New Orleans and Tulane Medical Center Hospital). The clinical conditions included gastric ulcer, gastric carcinoma, bleeding duodenal or gastric ulcer, and obstructing duodenal ulcer. Patients were excluded from the study population if they were pregnant, had a history of allergy to penicillin or cephalosporins, were younger than 12 years of age, or had any underlying conditions that would have made evaluation difficult. In addition, any patient who had taken antibiotics during the 72 hours before the operation was not included.

Appropriate patients were randomly assigned to treatment or placebo groups. All medication kits were identical in color and size, and no one having patient contact knew which drug regimen the patients were receiving. "Treatment" patients received a total of 4 gm of cefamandole intravenously, 2 gm 1 hour before operative incision and 1 gm at 4 and 8 hours after the incision. Controls received equal volumes of inert placebo intravenously at the same intervals. The operation performed was necessarily individualized according to the clinical situation. No other antibiotic agents were administered to either group. All patients underwent saline irrigation of the peritoneal cavity and subcutaneous tissue before primary wound closure. All patients were observed daily for signs of infection. If a post-

Table 24-9. Published work advocating prophylactic antibiotics in gastroduodenal operations

Author	Year	Double blind (placebo)	High-risk patients only	No-antibiotic group: No. infections/No. patients	Antibiotic group: No. infections/No. patients	Probability
Feltis and Hamit [11]	1967	No	No	14/64 (22%)	2/40 (5%)	$p > .05$*
Polk and Lopez-Mayor [25]	1969	Yes	No	11/36 (31%)	0/32 (0%)	$p < .001$
Evans and Pollock [10]	1973	No	No	6/30 (20%)	1/33 (3%)	$p > .05$
Griffiths et al. [17]	1976	Yes	No	5/8 (62%)	0/5 (0%)	$p > .05$
Stone et al. [26]	1976	Yes	No	5/23 (22%)	6/73 (8%)	$p > .05$
Lewis et al. [19]	1979	No	Yes	11/42 (26%)	0/41 (0%)	$p < .02$
Nichols et al. [24]	1982	Yes	Yes	7/20 (35%)	1/19 (5%)	$p < .01$

*Difference not significant at $p = .05$.

operative infectious complication was noted, the patient was considered a treatment failure, and subsequent surgical and antibiotic therapy was left to the discretion of the treating physician. A comparison of patient data in the two study groups is listed in Table 24-10.

This study was stopped after the intake of 43 patients because of a significant difference between the two groups. Four of the 43 patients were excluded from analysis: Two patients failed to receive all of the three doses, one patient never began therapy, and one received extended antibiotic therapy. None of these patients had postoperative infectious complications.

Table 24-10. Antibiotic prophylaxis in gastroduodenal operations: comparison of patient data

	Treatment group	Placebo group
Evaluable patients (n)	19	20
Indication for operation		
Gastric cancer	4	4
Gastric ulcer		
Chronic	3	5
Bleeding	2	1
Duodenal ulcer		
Bleeding	6	7
Obstructing	4	3
Demographic features		
Sex		
Male	12	14
Female	7	6
Age (yr)		
Range	39–76	21–78
Under 45	5	6
Over 45	14	14
Preoperative anesthesia risk evaluation		
Good	4	3
Fair	11	12
Poor	4	5

Seven infections were directly attributed to the gastric operation in the 20 patients in the placebo group, whereas there was only one infection in the 19 cefamandole-treated patients (Table 24-11); this difference was statistically significant ($p < .01$).

The seven gastric operation–related infections in the placebo group included four wound infections, two wound infections with associated wound dehiscence, and one instance of abdominal wall clostridial myonecrosis that resulted in death. The single treatment failure was a subhepatic abscess that resulted in the patient's death. There were three nonrelated infections in the placebo group; two urinary tract infections and one instance of pneumonia. In the treated patients there were six nonrelated infections: three urinary tract infections, two instances of pneumonia, and one instance of intravenous catheter–related septicemia. The second death in the placebo group was caused by cardiopulmonary failure without evidence of sepsis.

Initial gastric aspirate for culture was obtained in 35 of the 39 patients studied. Eleven of the specimens were sterile, while the remaining 24 samples revealed growth of one to six different bacterial species similar to those previously reported [23].

In the seven infections related to the operation in the placebo group, four were caused

Table 24-11. Antibiotic prophylaxis in gastroduodenal operations: infectious complications

	Treatment group (n = 19)		Placebo group (n = 20)	
	No.	Percent	No.	Percent
Wound or intra-abdominal infections	1	5	7	35
Unrelated infections (urinary or pulmonary)	6	31	3	15
Deaths	1	5	2	10

by infecting organisms found in the stomach at the time of gastric aspiration. These organisms included α-hemolytic streptococcus, enterococcus, *Streptococcus pneumoniae, Peptococcus,* and *Clostridium perfringens.* Two other patients had organisms similar to those isolated from the gastric aspirate that could have been presented at concentrations too low to be isolated with the techniques used. The cause of subhepatic abscess in the one treatment failure was not ascertained before the patient died or by cultures taken at autopsy.

The nonrelated infections were caused by gram-negative organisms that are the usual causes of nosocomial infections in the study hospitals. Only one of nine patients had an infecting organism that was also isolated from the initial gastric culture.

The results of this study as well as the others discussed in this chapter confirm the efficacy of the use of short-term perioperative antibiotic prophylaxis in patients undergoing gastroduodenal operations for gastric ulcer, bleeding or obstructing duodenal ulcer, or malignant tumors.

References

1. Antimicrobial prophylaxis: Prevention of wound infections and sepsis after surgery. *Med. Lett. Drugs Ther.* 21:73, 1979.
2. Arnold, L. The bacterial flora within the stomach and small intestine. *Am. J. Med. Sci.* 186:471, 1933.
3. Arnold, L., and Brody, L. Bacterial flora and hydrogen ion concentration of the duodenum. *J. Infect. Dis.* 38:249, 1926.
4. Ballinger, W. F., II, Iida, J., Padula, R. T., et al. Bacterial inflammation and denervation atrophy of the small intestine. *Surgery* 57:535, 1965.
5. Berger, S. A., Nagar, H., and Weitzman, S. Prophylactic antibiotics in surgical procedures. *Surg. Gynecol. Obstet.* 146:469, 1978.
6. Broido, P. W., Gorbach, S. L., Condon, R. E., and Nyhus, L. M. Upper intestinal microflora control. *Arch. Surg.* 106:90, 1973.
7. Cregan, J., and Hayward, N. J. The bacterial content of the healthy human small intestine. *Br. Med. J.* 1:1356, 1953.
8. Dellipiani, A. W., and Girdwood, R. H. Bacterial changes in the small intestine in malabsorptive states and in pernicious anaemia. *Clin. Sci.* 26:359, 1964.
9. Drasar, B. S., Shiner, M., and McLeon, G. M. Studies on the intestinal flora. I. The bacterial flora of the gastrointestinal tract in health and achlorhydric persons. *Gastroenterology* 56:71, 1969.
10. Evans, C., and Pollock, A. V. The reduction of surgical wound infections by prophylactic parenteral cephaloridine: A controlled clinical trial. *Br. J. Surg.* 60:434, 1973.
11. Feltis, J. M., Jr., and Hamit, H. F. Use of prophylactic antimicrobial drugs to prevent postoperative wound infections. *Am. J. Surg.* 114:867, 1967.
12. Franklin, M. A., and Skoryna, S. C. Studies on natural gastric flora. I. Bacterial flora of fasting human subjects. *Can. Med. Assoc. J.* 95:1349, 1966.
13. Frederiksen, W., Bruusgaard, A., and Thaysen, E. H. Assessment of the relationship between gastric secretory capacity and jejunal bacteriology. *Scand. J. Gastroenterol.* 8:353, 1973.
14. Giannella, R. A., Broitman, S. A., and Zamcheck, N. Gastric acid barrier to ingested microorganisms in man: Studies in vivo and in vitro. *Gut* 13:251, 1972.
15. Gray, J. D. A., and Shiner, M. Influence of gastric pH on gastric and jejunal flora. *Gut* 8:574, 1967.
16. Greenlee, H. B., Vivt, R., Paez, J., and Dietz, A. Bacterial flora of the jejunum following peptic ulcer surgery. *Arch. Surg.* 102:260, 1971.
17. Griffiths, D. A., Simpson, R. A., Shorey, B. A., et al. Single-dose preoperative antibiotic prophylaxis in gastrointestinal surgery. *Lancet* 2:325, 1976.
18. Lewis, R. T. Wound infection after gastroduodenal operations: A 10 year review. *Can. J. Surg.* 20:435, 1977.
19. Lewis, R. T., Allan, C. M., and Goodall, R. G. Discriminate use of antibiotic prophylaxis in gastroduodenal surgery. *Am. J. Surg.* 138:640, 1979.
20. LoCicero, J., and Nichols, R. L. Sepsis after gastroduodenal operations: Relationship to gastric acid, motility, and endogenous microflora. *South Med. J.* 73:878, 1980.
21. Muscroft, T. J., Deane, S. A., Youngs, D., et al. The microflora of the postoperative stom-

ach. *Br. J. Surg.* 68:560, 1981.
22. Nichols, R. L., Broido, P., Condon, R. E., et al. Effect of preoperative neomycin-erythromycin intestinal preparation on the incidence of infection complications following colon surgery. *Ann. Surg.* 178:453, 1973.
23. Nichols, R. L., and Smith, J. W. Intragastric microbial colonization in common disease states of the stomach and duodenum. *Ann. Surg.* 182:557, 1975.
24. Nichols, R. L., Webb, W. R., Jones, J. W., et al. Efficacy of antibiotic prophylaxis in high risk gastroduodenal operations. *Am. J. Surg.* 143:94, 1982.
25. Polk, H. C., Jr., and Lopez-Mayor, J. F. Postoperative wound infection: A prospective study of determinant factors and prevention. *Surgery* 66:97, 1969.
26. Stone, H. H., Hooper, C. A., Kolb, L. D., et al. Antibiotic prophylaxis in gastric, biliary and colonic surgery. *Ann. Surg.* 184:443, 1976.
27. Veterans Administration Ad Hoc Interdisciplinary Advisory Committee on Antimicrobial Drug Usage. I. Prophylaxis in surgery. *J.A.M.A.* 237:1003, 1977.

EDITOR'S COMMENT

Our understanding of the bacterial milieu of the gastric lumen has been expanded by Dr. Nichols's many studies—of normal as well as abnormal states. The practical information presented in the tables will aid us in our approach to patients.

The effectiveness of cimetidine in altering gastric pH preoperatively suggests that the intragastric bacterial flora might increase significantly, as Dr. Nichols notes. This also was studied by Long et al. (*Arch. Surg.* 118:1413, 1983). In addition to the observation that cimetidine by its effect on pH allowed an increase in numbers of gastric microflora, Long et al. noted that when the administration of cimetidine was stopped at least 6 hours preoperatively, the pH returned to normal and relative gastric sterility was reestablished.

L.M.N.

VI

Gastric Neoplasms

25

Adenocarcinoma of the Stomach

J.W.L. Fielding
J. Alexander-Williams

It is a little over 100 years since Theodor Billroth [12] operated on Theresa Heller for gastric adenocarcinoma. At the laparotomy, a few hazelnut-sized mesenteric lymph nodes were found and resected with the stomach. Microscopically these lymph nodes were involved with a medullary type of cancer. A few months later Mrs. Heller died of recurrent disease. Although this sad story, familiar to the modern surgeon, is still reflective of the presentation and course of gastric cancer in the Western world during the 1980s, there have been some advances during the last 100 years.

Billroth's achievement was to have his patient survive the operation, a rare event 100 years ago for an operation of such magnitude. Perhaps the most important advance of the past century has been to make partial gastrectomy a safe operation. In 1896 the operative mortality from gastrectomy was 54.5 percent [54] compared with 4 percent in the 1960s [71]. This reduction in postoperative mortality has been the result of major improvements in surgical techniques, anesthesia, and supportive care. However, work in Japan during the last 30 years has identified areas in which there might be further improvements in the treatment of gastric cancer. These are early detection and appropriate, safe radical surgical and adjuvant treatment. One purpose of this chapter is to highlight the importance of the early lesion and to draw comparisons between this and the more common advanced disease seen in Europe and the United States. Other purposes will be to examine closely the role of surgical resection, to analyze the reasons for failure after surgical treatment, and to investigate the role of adjuvant therapies.

Importance of the Early Lesion

During the last 30 years Japanese researchers have demonstrated the importance of early detection of gastric carcinomas. Of particular importance is "early gastric cancer," a lesion in which depth of invasion of the primary tumor is limited histologically to the submucosa of the stomach, irrespective of the presence or absence of lymph node metastases [1, 88,

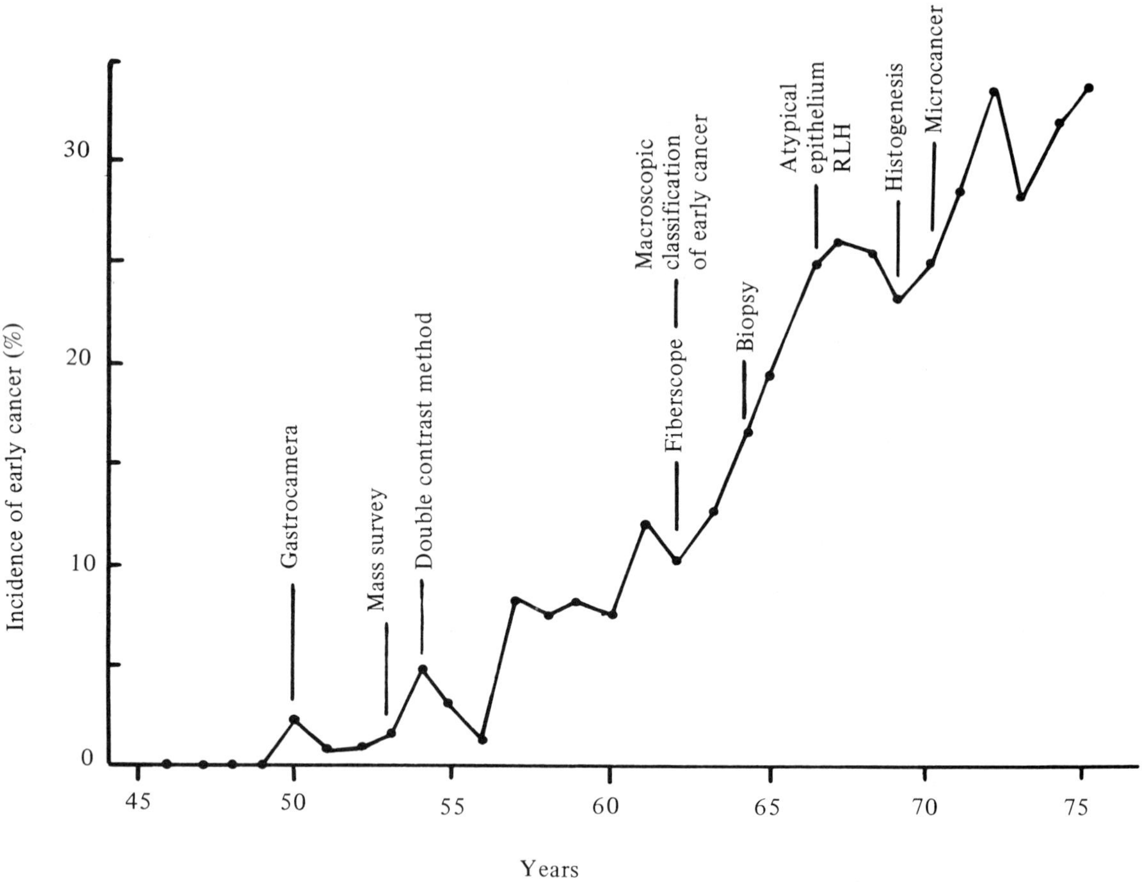

Fig. 25-1. The incidence of early gastric cancer, 1946–1975, Cancer Institute Hospital, Tokyo. (Reprinted by courtesy of Pergamon Press [117].)

107]. The five-year survival rate after surgical resection of this lesion is 90 percent in Japan [72]. Japanese physicians have been able to increase significantly the incidence of detection of early gastric cancer from 1 percent [85] in the period from 1946 to 1950 to 28.1 percent [117] in recent years. This improvement has been effected by developments in diagnostic techniques and institution of mass screening (Fig. 25-1). The Japanese reports stimulated European and American studies, and the effect of the extent of disease on five-year survival rates after gastric resection demonstrates the importance of extent of spread (Table 25-1).

Birmingham Series of "Early" Gastric Cancer

During the decade 1960–1969, a time when endoscopic studies were not readily available, 90 instances of early gastric cancer were identified retrospectively among all instances of gastric adenocarcinoma registered at the Birmingham Cancer Registry [43]. These were lesions in which the depth of penetration was limited to the submucosal layer of the stomach, and none had evidence of lymph node metastases. They were identified from 13,228 gastric adenocarcinomas, of which 3523 were resected. The crude five-year survival rate for all patients was 3.7 percent (age adjusted, 4.7

Table 25-1. Effect of extent of disease on five-year survival after gastric resection in patients from the West Midlands (1960–1969)

	Men			Women		
Extent of spread	No. of patients	Crude 5-year survival rate (%)	Adjusted 5-year survival rate (%)	No. of patients	Crude 5-year survival rate (%)	Adjusted 5-year survival rate (%)
Mucosa	20	60.0	72.3	12	83.3	98.1
Submucosa	39	48.7	61.8	17	64.7	75.7
Muscle	147	33.3	40.3	65	33.8	40.2
Serosa	364	20.1	24.5	227	22.0	26.8
Nodes	1155	5.8	7.1	590	6.9	8.1
Distant metastases	248	1.6	2.0	154	0.6	0.8
Not known	254	13.8	17.3	138	15.9	19.6

Table 25-2. The incidence of "early" gastric cancer at centers in the United Kingdom and in the United States

	Lesions in all patients		Lesions in patients undergoing resection	
Period and place	No. patients	Percent	No. patients	Percent
1960–69 [43] (Birmingham Cancer Registry, U.K.)	90/13,228	0.7	90/3,523	2.6
1960–71 [41] (Llandough Hospital, U.K.)	4/720	0.5	—	—
1970–74 [52] (Columbia University)	—	—	9/109	8.2
1972–77 [41] (Llandough Hospital, U.K.)	10/101	10.0	—	—
1974–79 [64] (Southampton, U.K.)	8/483	1.6	—	—
1977–79 [44] (West Midlands, U.K.)	—	—	5/147	3.4
1975–79 [52] (Columbia University)	—	—	19/104	18.3
1972–82 [21] (University of Virginia)	—	—	5/31	16

percent). The crude five-year survival rate of the 90 patients with early gastric cancers was 57.8 percent (age adjusted, 70.4 percent). In Birmingham, as in Japan, early gastric cancer is associated with a better prognosis. However, the incidence of this lesion is depressingly low. In Birmingham in the 1960s, only 0.7 percent of all gastric cancers were early [44]. Since the 1970s endoscopy has been in routine use in the Western world, and there is evidence that this technique may have effected an increase in the incidence of early gastric cancers in some countries (Table 25-2), although the figures from the West Midlands do not entirely support this. This may be a reflection of the fact that in the West Midlands we had a population-based study, whereas the studies from Llandough, Wales [41] and Columbia University, New York [52], were from centers with a particular interest in gastric cancer; the latter studies may give an indication of what can be achieved through investigation by enthusiastic, motivated staff and may not be representative of other regions. However, the 18.3 percent rate of early gastric cancers (2) achieved in the later quinquennium (1975–1979) of the Columbia University study [52] is the incidence that all physicians should be able to achieve with an awareness of the macroscopical appearance of this lesion (Table 25-2).

The high detection rate of early gastric cancer in Japan is a reflection of the Japanese diagnostic approach to the disease, particularly the mass screening programs. However, there are serious limitations to the concept of mass screening of asymptomatic populations, even in a high-risk country such as Japan. The detection rate is not large; the pickup rate was 1.45 per 1000 screened in 1966 and had decreased to 0.95 by 1978 [60]. This fall in the detection rate may be the result of a decreasing incidence or of the higher detection rate in the early part of the study of quiescent lesions. Another disadvantage of the mass screening is that it is not available to the entire population; only 14 percent of the population in Japan older than 40 years of age was covered by mass screening [62]. These limitations of mass screening of patients without symptoms in a high-incidence country are even more apparent in low-incidence countries. Sherman and Synder [104] investigated 31,895 persons without symptoms in New York and detected only 7 cancers. Therefore, it seems an inappropriate diagnostic approach to gastric cancer for Europe and the United States.

Owen Wangensteen [124] wrote in the preceding edition of this book: "I had the misfortune of having been far too long on the wrong side of the cancer woodpile. Fresh cases were piling in daily, but we failed to recognize them." This situation still pertains today, despite the improved diagnostic techniques of recent years. Physicians must make themselves aware of the groups at risk for gastric cancer and the specific characteristics of early gastric cancer. In this chapter we concentrate on early detection rather than considering the conventional approach in the presentation and diagnosis of gastric cancer.

Early Detection

To define high-risk groups the physician must consider epidemiological factors, predisposing conditions, and precancerous lesions. He or she must also examine the symptoms of gastric cancers, comparing the early with the advanced lesions (Table 25-3).

Table 25-3. Risk factors for gastric cancer

Epidemiological factor
Genetic
Geographical
Occupational
Dietary
Cigarette smoking
Predisposing condition
Pernicious anemia
Postoperative stomachs
Precancerous lesion
Autoimmune gastritis
Environmental gastritis
Dysplasia
Gastric polyps
Patients with symptoms
40 years or more with dyspepsia

EPIDEMIOLOGICAL FACTORS

There are international variations in the incidence of gastric cancer. It is a common lesion in Japan, Chile, and Iceland, but in the United Kingdom only lung, colorectal, and breast cancer are more common. In the United States there has been a dramatic decrease in the incidence of gastric cancer, from 28.8 per 100,000 in 1930 to 13 per 100,000 in 1955 [55]. A decrease has been noted also in Japan and in the United Kingdom. The reasons for this decrease are not clear, however. The variations in incidence suggest that either genetic or environmental factors may be important. Among Japanese migrants to Hawaii, the incidence in the first generation is similar to that in Japan, but the incidence in the second generation is significantly lower although still higher than that of United States whites [56]. This alteration from the incidence in Japan may be attributable to environmental factors, but since the incidence is still not that of the local population, there may still be a genetic influence. Dublin and Marks [37] found among insured persons that those with a family history of gastric cancer had a subsequent gastric cancer mortality about one-third greater than others, and Videbaek and Mosbech [122] reported an incidence of stomach cancer 4 times greater among relatives of 302 cancer patients compared with controls. Further evidence of a possible genetic influence is the higher incidence of gastric cancer among patients of blood group A [6].

The relation between social class and gastric cancer is well established. In the United States, Denmark, and Great Britain, the incidence is higher among those doing physical work than among those in sedentary occupations [55, 114]. The incidence is particularly high in those undertaking heavy work. Stukonis and Doll [114] postulated that heavy workers eat more and therefore are exposed to more carcinogens. Among heavy workers, coal miners have the highest incidence, but for them the important factors may be occupational rather than dietary. Furthermore, there is a lower mortality among farmers, who probably eat as much as miners [30].

The importance of diet in the causation of gastric cancer remains unclear. In the United States the intake of beef, milk, citrus fruits, and green vegetables increased and that of potatoes decreased before and during the time of decline in the incidence of carcinoma [55]. In Japan the striking change in the incidence of gastric cancer has been associated with changes in diet. The consumption of milk products has increased 28-fold from 1949 to 1978, and there is a significant relation between the decline in incidence and the increase in intake of fatty foods, vitamin A, and yellow-green vegetables [60]. The evidence of an association between cigarette smoking and stomach cancer is conflicting; however, Hammond and Horn [58] and Hirayama [60] all reported a positive correlation with cigarette smoking.

PREDISPOSING CONDITIONS

A predisposing condition is a clinical state associated with a significantly increased risk of cancer. Persons with conditions such as pernicious anemia and previous gastric resection have a greater than normal potential for a carcinoma developing.

The risk of carcinoma developing in a patient with pernicious anemia is 3 or 4 times that of the normal population. Those who have had a gastrectomy for a benign condition have a 5.5 percent risk of a carcinoma developing in the gastric stump 10 to 15 years later [35, 109]. In our center evidence has been produced to suggest that there is an increased risk following vagotomy and pyloroplasty [40].

PRECANCEROUS LESIONS

A precancerous lesion is a histopathological epithelial abnormality in which cancer is more likely to occur than in the normal mucosa. The lesions that may be associated with gastric cancer are gastritis, intestinal metaplasia, dysplasia, and gastric polyps. Ménétrier disease has aroused much interest as a possible precancerous lesion; however, it is now thought unlikely that a relationship truly exists [27].

Chronic gastritis is frequently found in association with gastric cancer [48]. Ninety-four percent of superficial cancers are found in areas of gastritis, and carcinomas have been found in as many as 10 percent of patients with chronic gastritis and intestinal metaplasia [31].

Correa [28] has classified chronic gastritis as (1) autoimmune chronic gastritis, (2) hypersecretory chronic gastritis, and (3) environmental chronic gastritis.

Autoimmune chronic gastritis is the classical gastritis associated with pernicious anemia. The lesions involve the body and fundus diffusely, leaving the antrum intact. This type of gastritis increases in prevalence and severity with age and is found more frequently in men than in women. Not all patients with autoimmune gastritis have overt pernicious anemia, but it will develop in a significant proportion [113]. Intestinal metaplasia (Fig. 25-2A) commonly accompanies autoimmune gastritis, and since metaplasia is subject to dysplastic transformation (Fig. 25-2B) and is positively associated with gastric cancer, there is a high risk of malignancy. Characteristically, when cancer develops it is in the body of the stomach.

Hypersecretory chronic gastritis is found in

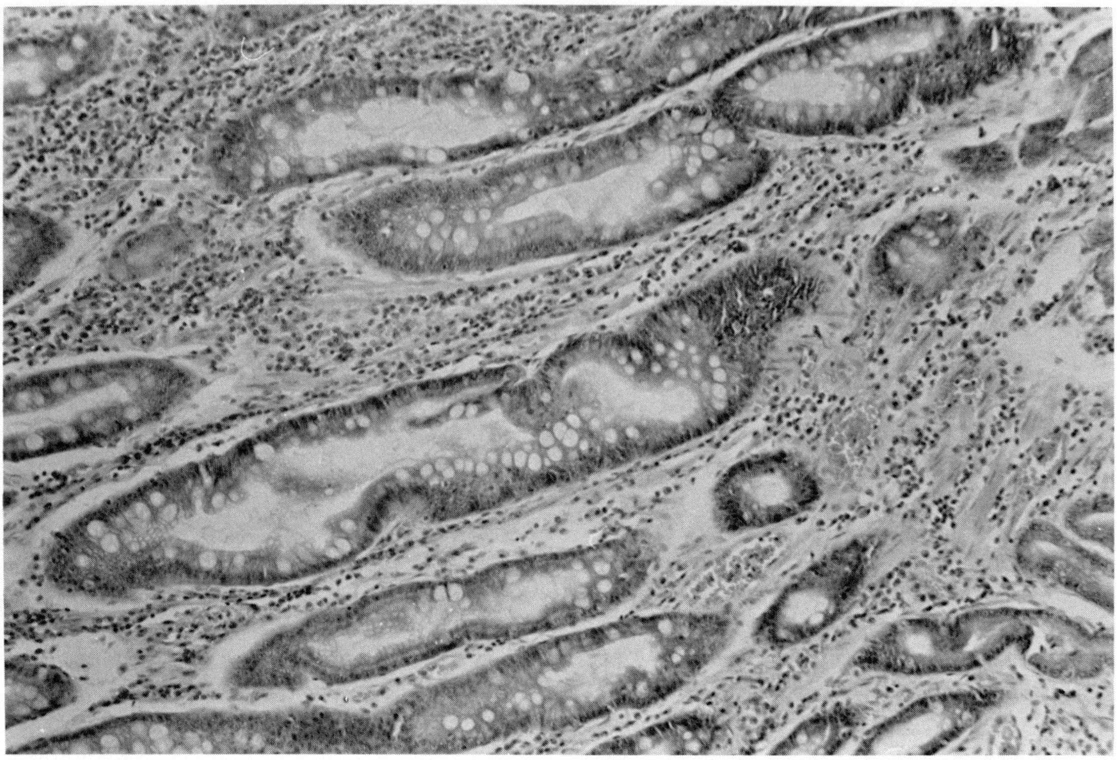

A

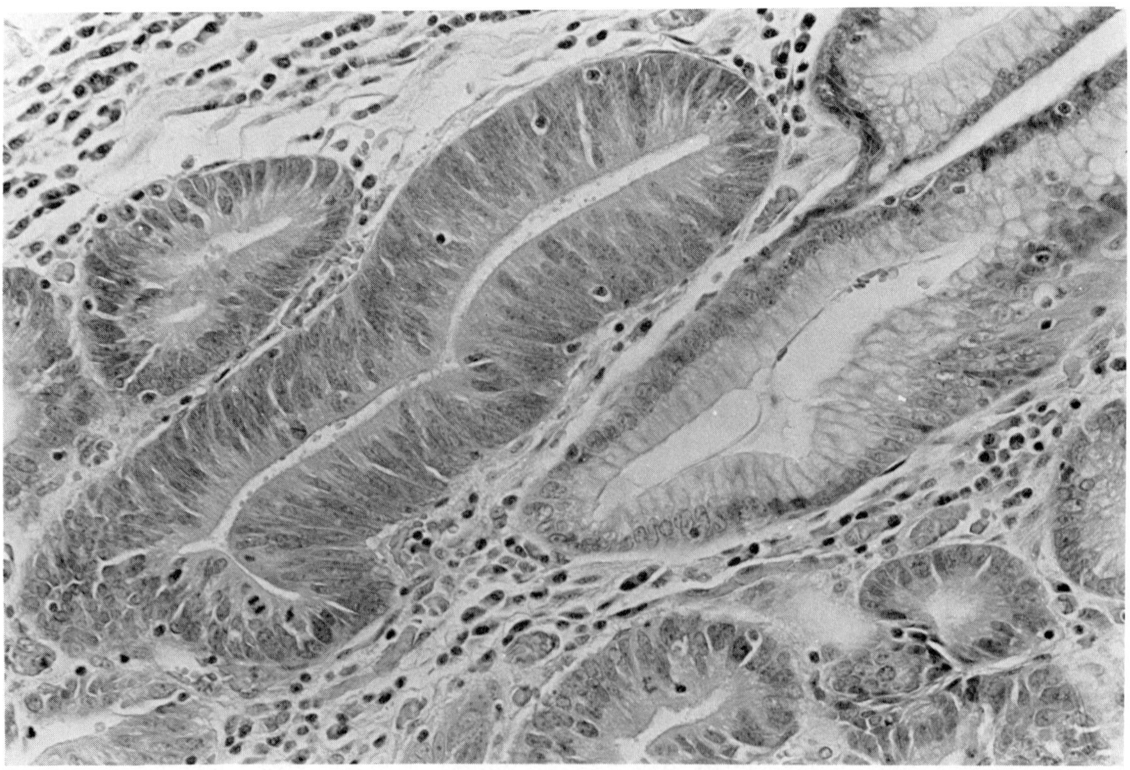

B

Fig. 25-2. Precancerous lesions and adenocarcinomas. (A) Intestinal metaplasia. (B) Dysplasia. (C) Intestinal carcinoma. (D) Diffuse adenocarcinoma. (Courtesy of Dr. H. Thompson, Birmingham General Hospital.)

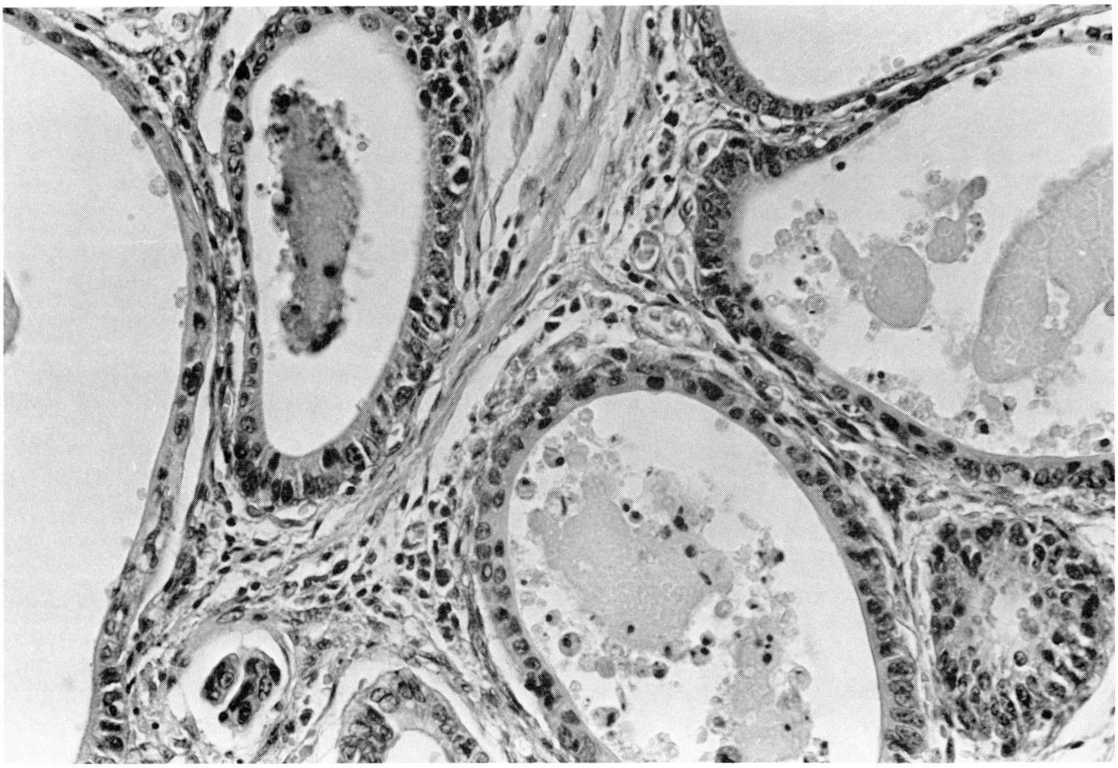

C

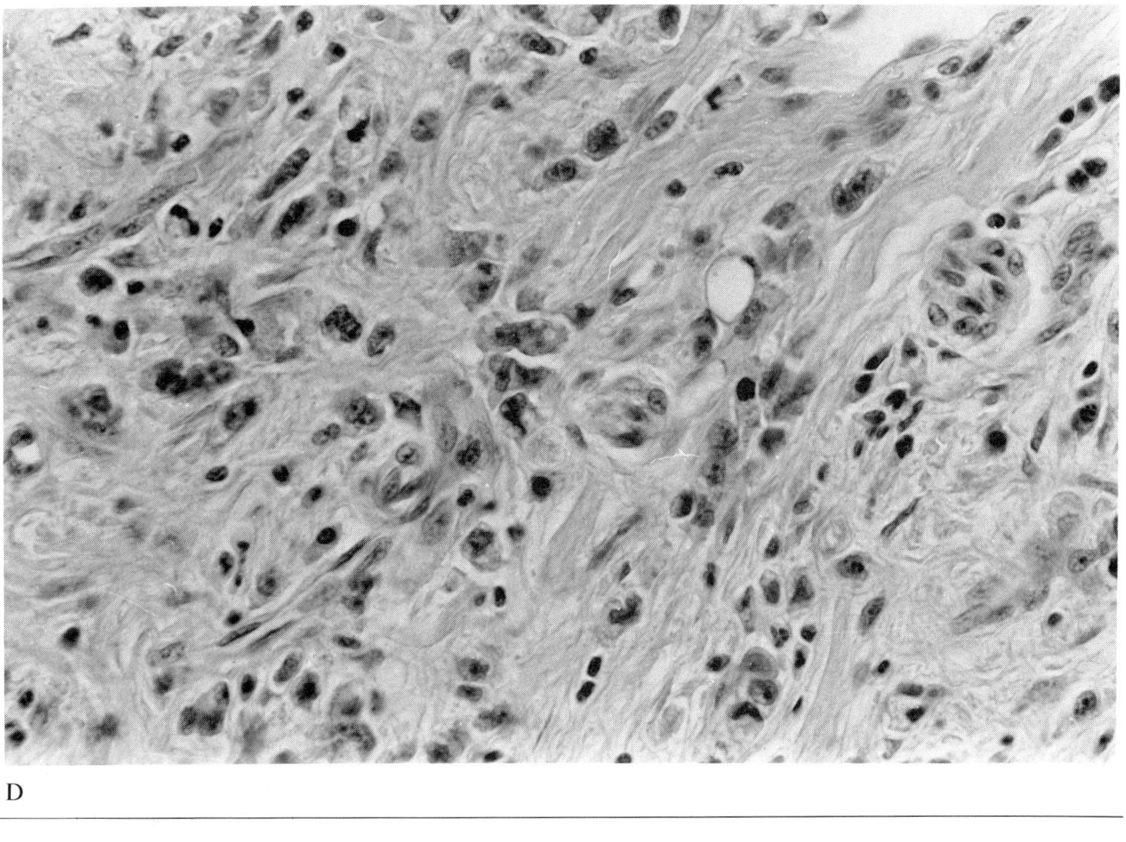

D

association with an ulcer. With a duodenal ulcer the gastritis is confined to the antrum, and with a gastric ulcer it involves the antrum but extends up to and around the ulcer [108, 110]. Histologically there is distortion of the glandular epithelium but no significant intestinal metaplasia or association with malignant change.

Environmental chronic gastritis is prevalent in certain parts of the world. Its geographical distribution coincides with areas of risk of cancers of the intestinal type (Fig. 25-2C). The changes in the gastric mucosa occur early in life. Those of the community in whom gastritis develops have changes identifiable by the ages of 20–25 years [29]. In populations with a low incidence of gastric cancer, environmental chronic gastritis is found in less than 20 percent, but this increases to 70 percent or more in high-incidence areas. This form of gastritis has a characteristic distribution; it is multifocal, involving the antrum and body, with the earlier stages appearing on the lesser curvature below the incisura. Histologically the milder lesions show the characteristic changes of acute gastritis with a dense inflammatory exudate below the lamina propria. As chronicity develops, atrophy of the mucosa occurs because of progressive loss of gastric glands. Subsequent regeneration occurs, and the mucosa is replaced by intestinal-type mucosa. This progression is termed "intestinalization" of the gastric mucosa. Dysplastic changes may then occur and progress to overt malignancy of the intestinal type. The diffuse type of adenocarcinoma is not accompanied by gastritis. The differentiation of gastric carcinoma into intestinal and diffuse types is helpful when related to gastritis and geographical variation; however, the lack of gastritis in diffuse lesions (Fig. 25-2D) makes the relationship unclear. It may be that dysplasia is the important feature, as this can occur in foveolar epithelium as well as in intestinal metaplasia, and it may be the common premalignant mucosal change [87].

Gastric polyps may be classified as focal hyperplasia, hyperplasiagenic polyps, adenomas, and gastric polyposis. The less common adenomas may undergo malignant change, which occurs in 18 to 75 percent [83]. Benign gastric ulcers should not be considered precancerous [17]; the difficulties in interpretation usually occur in establishing an accurate histological diagnosis rather than in identifying a real malignant transformation.

SYMPTOMS

All patients with gastric cancer will have symptoms, and yet the diagnosis is commonly made when the disease is advanced. The difficulty for the physician is to differentiate between the symptoms of benign upper gastrointestinal disorders and those of a malignant tumor. It is important to identify the "symptomatic, at risk" patients, in whom it is essential to establish a precise diagnosis before instituting therapy. This can only be done by studying the clinical features of patients with gastric cancer and the differences between "early" and "advanced" disease.

Men have gastric cancer more commonly than women, in a ratio of 3 : 2; the highest incidence occurs between the ages of 55 and 65 years [18]. Sex and age distribution are the same in both advanced and early gastric cancers [43, 52].

Particularly relevant to the detection of early gastric cancer is an analysis of the first symptoms of the disease. Swynnerton and Trulove [116] studied 371 patients presenting to the Radcliffe Infirmary, Oxford, and Lundh et al. [78] studied 901 patients in a cooperative European study. Table 25-4 presents the type of first symptom that these patients experienced and compares it with the symptoms at the time of hospital treatment of the patients from the West Midlands study with early gastric cancer. Although there is a similarity between the two groups, an evaluation of the precise gastrointestinal symptoms in advanced disease demonstrates that indigestion or upper abdominal pain occurred in 70.6 percent of the patients in the Oxford series [116] and 49.9 percent in the European study [79]. Swynnerton and Truelove [116] made a detailed study of the early dyspeptic symptoms of 251 patients, and in 21.1 percent of these the symptoms were mild (vague abdominal discomfort, fullness, belching, regurgitation),

Table 25-4. Early symptoms of gastric cancer

Symptoms	Radcliffe [116][a] (n = 371)	Europe [79][a] (n = 901)	West Midlands [43] (n = 86)[b]
Gastrointestinal (dyspepsia, vomiting, abdominal pain, epigastric pain, indigestion, dysphagia, hematemesis, melena)	310 (83.6%)	678 (75.2%)	71 (82.5%)
Constitutional (weight loss, anemia, weakness, lassitude, fever)	51 (13.7%)	187 (20.8%)	11 (12.8%)
Other	10 (2.7%)	36 (4.0%)	4 (4.7%)

[a]First symptom.
[b]Symptoms at presentation of "early" gastric cancer; n of 86 includes four patients whose symptoms were not known.

26.3 percent had typical ulcer-type pain, 14.7 percent had pain after meals unrelieved by food or alkalis, 11.6 percent had a long history of vague dyspepsia, 18.7 percent had continuous pain, and 7.6 percent projectile vomiting.

By the time the patient is admitted to the hospital, the clinical features of the advanced lesion have changed from those at the time of the first symptom. The most striking feature is that 78.4 percent of all patients by this time have lost weight [79] compared with only 18.9 percent [43] of patients with early gastric cancers. Similar findings were reported by Green et al. [52] from their direct comparisons of early with advanced lesions. Weight loss was significantly less common in patients with early gastric cancer, and there was a significantly higher incidence of previous peptic ulceration. Two patients with early gastric cancer treated with cimetidine noted marked symptomatic improvement. It is always worth stressing that dyspepsia is a symptom and not a diagnosis and that no patient older than 40 years of age complaining for the first time of dyspepsia should be treated until a definitive diagnosis has been established.

It is apparent that early gastric cancers produce symptoms and that the detection of earlier lesions may be increased by immediate investigation of dyspeptic patients older than 40 years of age. In the Japanese mass screening programs, 50 percent of the patients with early gastric carcinomas had symptoms [62]. The precise nature of the symptoms is often related to the macroscopical type of early gastric cancer (Table 25-5), which is classified as protruded (type I), superficial (type II), and excavated (type III) [88]. In both Green et al.'s [52] and our studies [43] the most common lesion was type III, the one that produces ulcer-type symptoms. Similarly, in Japan type III early gastric cancer was the most common between 1946 and 1955, but since then an increase in the type II lesion and a decrease in type III have been noted, probably the result of screening populations without symptoms [117]. It is likely that the dominant lesion detected by early investigation of symptomatic patients will remain type III. Early lesions are seldom associated with specific signs on physical examination. The presence of a palpable epigastric mass, an enlarged liver, or palpable nodes obviously signifies advanced disease. Thus the absence of physical signs in a patient with symptoms does not exclude a malignant tumor of the stomach. It should be emphasized also that the presence of palpable masses does not indicate inoperability.

Diagnosis and Management

The Japanese roentgenological mass screening programs have investigated gastric cancer in a high-risk environment; it is interesting that many lesions were symptomatic [62]. In Finland the presence of fetal sialoglycoprotein in gastric juice was used in a screening program in which 35 gastric (19 early) cancers were de-

Table 25-5. Incidence of symptoms in patients with early gastric cancer and with type I, type II, and type III lesions (number of patients and percentage)

Symptom	All patients (n = 90)	Macroscopical classification*		
		Type I (n = 18)	Type II (n = 16)	Type III (n = 42)
Epigastric pain	26 (28.9)	1 (5.6)	6 (37.5)	17 (40.5)
Vomiting	21 (23.3)	2 (11.1)	3 (18.8)	14 (33.3)
Other (e.g., malaise, weakness)	21 (23.3)	4 (22.2)	1 (6.3)	5 (11.9)
Abdominal pain	17 (18.9)	3 (16.7)	5 (31.3)	4 (9.5)
Weight loss	17 (18.9)	3 (16.7)	3 (18.8)	5 (11.9)
Anorexia	13 (14.4)	2 (11.1)	2 (12.5)	5 (11.9)
Indigestion	11 (12.2)	1 (5.6)	3 (18.8)	6 (14.3)
Hematemesis, melena	6 (6.6)	4 (22.2)	0	0
Dysphagia	1 (1.1)	0	0	0
Not known from data	4 (4.4)	1 (5.6)	0	3 (7.1)

*Excludes 14 lesions that could not be classified.
Source: Reprinted by courtesy of the *British Medical Journal* [43].

tected in a rural population of 39,706 persons aged 40–70 years [57].

However, the detection rate even from the Japanese and Finnish studies is too small to warrant further large-scale studies; one must consider instead the possible investigation of other high-risk groups without symptoms. Certainly the investigation of patients without symptoms with predisposing conditions is valuable. In an endoscopic study of 80 patients with pernicious anemia, two gastric carcinomas (3 percent) were detected [112]. In addition, 33 had dysplastic changes and only 30 had normal stomachs. In postgastrectomy patients screened endoscopically, 11 (2 percent) of 535 patients had gastric cancers, 5 of which were early [65]. Intestinal metaplasia was present in 48.4 percent and dysplasia in 13.3 percent. One hundred and fifty-seven patients underwent repeat endoscopy after two years, and one additional carcinoma was found. It seems advisable that all patients with pernicious anemia or 15 years after a gastrectomy should undergo endoscopy at 2-year intervals, particularly those with intestinal metaplasia or dysplasia.

What do we do when the diagnosis of a precancerous lesion is established? Gastric polyps, particularly adenomas, should be removed and the patient closely followed by endoscopy. In one study of 6182 patients undergoing polypectomy, 38.6 percent had further polyps; in 6.1 percent this was recurrence, and in the remaining 32.5 percent polyps developed at other sites. These polyps were found 1–7 years after the initial investigation and were not necessarily of the same microscopical type [103]. Because of the high incidence of newly formed polyps, all patients in whom polyps are detected should have regular endoscopic follow-up at yearly intervals. Similar follow-up is advisable in patients found to have either intestinal metaplasia or dysplasia.

Unfortunately, the screening of these high-risk groups is not the whole answer because most patients with gastric cancer do not have precancerous conditions. Only 28 (1.3 percent) of 2130 patients from three series [22, 78, 115, 116] had pernicious anemia, and only 46 (4.5 percent) of the 1026 patients reported from Birmingham had previous gastric operations for benign conditions [40]. Therefore, we must concentrate also on the early investigation of symptoms. The presence of symptoms is the factor common to all patients with gastric carcinoma, except for those with lesions detected in screening programs. The early investigation of dyspeptic patients demonstrates upper gastrointestinal disease and results in a detection rate of gastric carcinomas of from 2 to 8.8 percent [10, 11]. The study of Aste et al. [10] demonstrated a variation in incidence of early gastric cancers of from 7.1 percent to 16.2 percent among the 9000 patients investigated in four regions of Italy. This is certainly a higher incidence than found in our population-based study in the West Midlands and is comparable with the figures produced by other centers (see Table 25-2). In any early diagnosis program it is important to educate the public and general practitioner to reduce the delay time—both patient delay in reporting symptoms and doctor delay in referral to specialist centers. The education of the public should concentrate on groups with higher risk factors, but the general practitioner should refer for immediate diagnosis any new dyspeptic patient older than 40 years of age.

DIAGNOSTIC METHODS

The established methods of investigation of the upper gastrointestinal tract are roentgenography (Fig. 25-3A to D) and fiberoptic endoscopy. These are complementary investigations and should not be considered mutually exclusive.

The only barium meal examination capable of diagnosing early gastric cancer (Fig. 25-3A, B) is a double contrast study, preferably facilitated by induction of hypotonia [105]. Furthermore, the double contrast roentgenogram should be considered technically inadequate if the areae gastricae have not been demonstrated [74]. In a patient with symptoms, a normal, conventional single contrast meal examination can give no grounds for reassurance.

The fiberoptic endoscope permits macroscopical assessment of the gastric mucosa and enables biopsies and direct brush cytologic specimens to be obtained from lesions. After macroscopical assessment of a lesion, at least six to eight biopsy specimens should be obtained [32]. If there is an ulcer, the area of greatest positive yield is its edge. Repeated endoscopy and biopsy may be necessary to establish the diagnosis, especially if there is roentgenographic and endoscopic suspicion of malignancy or if a benign-appearing lesion fails to heal completely or fails to remain healed. In addition, a biopsy should always be done on the healed area on review endoscopy. Accuracy can be further increased by brushing all suspicious lesions for cytological examination. Using roentgenography and endoscopy in combination, the accuracy of diagnosis of gastric cancer is 98 percent [90]. Parenthetically, researchers in Norway [121] have demonstrated that the increased diagnostic accuracy of endoscopic methods has allowed a shift in staging toward less advanced disease.

Other methods of investigation may prove useful in the follow-up study of high-risk patients or as less invasive methods of screening. Elevated levels of enzymes, particularly β-glucuronidase and lactic dehydrogenase, have been found in the gastric juice of patients with gastric cancer [46, 99]. Hakkinen [57] has reported the presence of an oncofetal antigen, fetal sialoglycoprotein, in the gastric juice of patients with cancer. α_1-Acid glycoprotein, an acute phase protein, may be present in the gastric juice of patients with cancer or premalignant lesions [96]. Serological investigations have been explored, particularly carcinoembryonic antigen and α-fetoprotein, but elevated serum levels usually indicate advanced disease [14]. Serum pepsinogen or pepsinogen 1 levels may be altered in patients with cancer or precancerous lesions [13, 92, 111]. Gastric hypochlorhydria may occur in gastric cancer [123]; however, hypochlorhydria is more often a reflection of the size of the carcinoma and certainly would prove an unreliable method of detecting early lesions [84]. None of the markers in either gastric juice or serum is appropriate for the diagnosis of gastric cancer; however, research to detect a marker of early disease or premalignant lesions is of paramount importance and should be pursued actively.

IS EARLY DETECTION WORTHWHILE?

The benefits of early detection of gastric carcinoma are an increase in the incidence of early gastric cancer and improved resectability rates. Theoretically, these should result in an apparent improvement in five-year survival

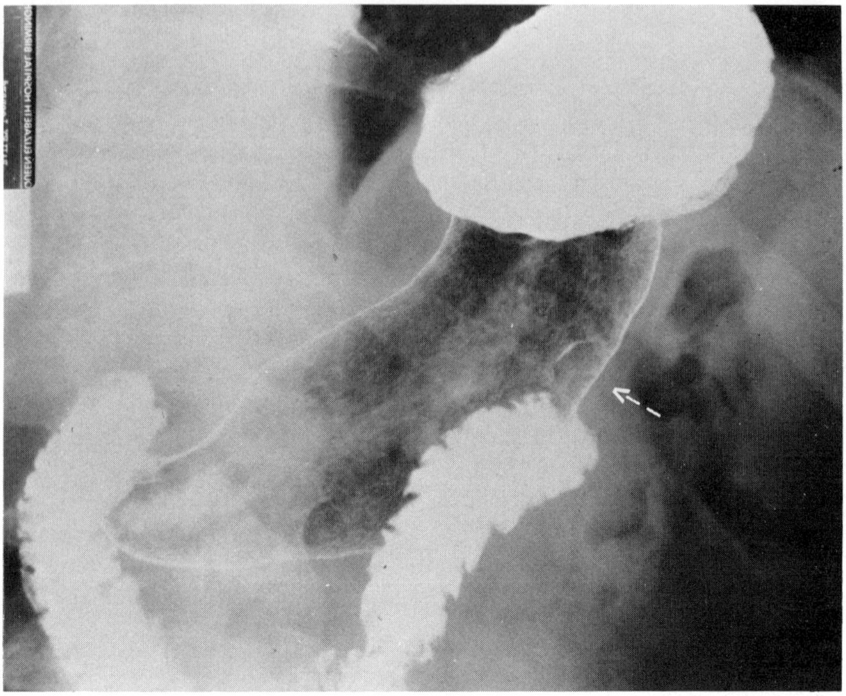

A

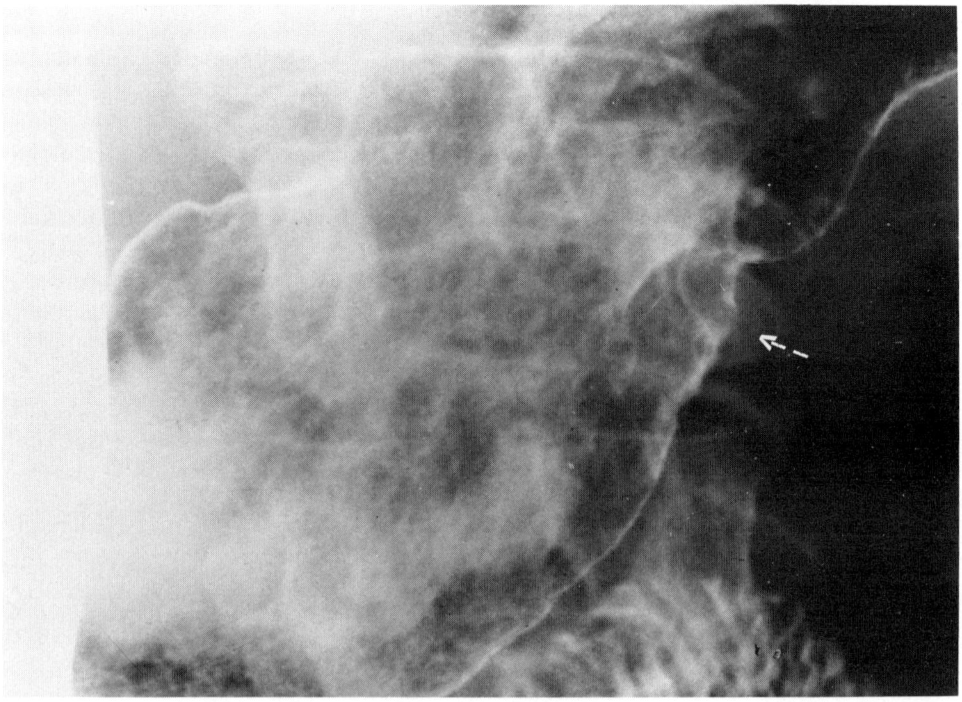

B

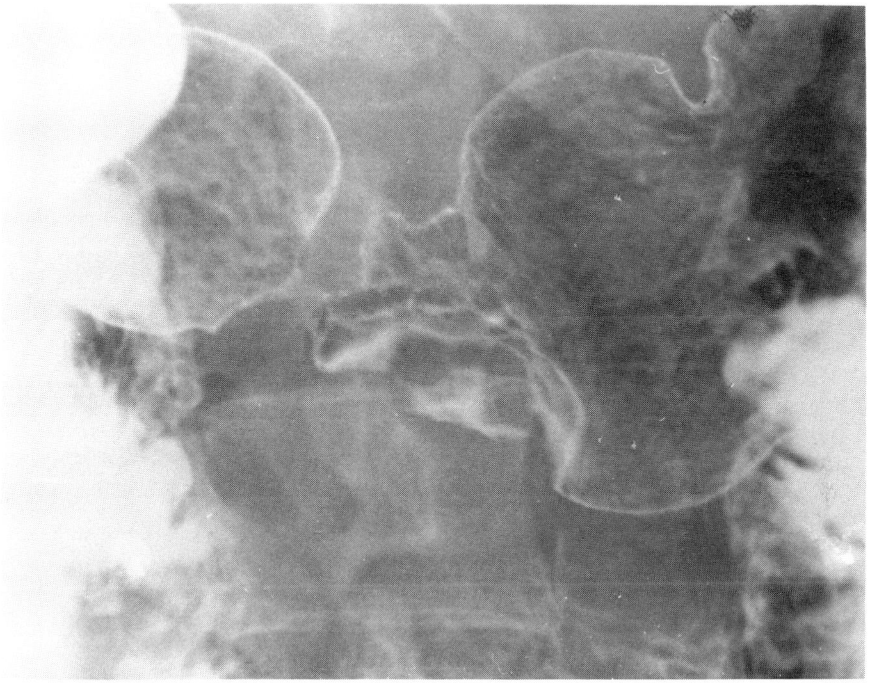

C

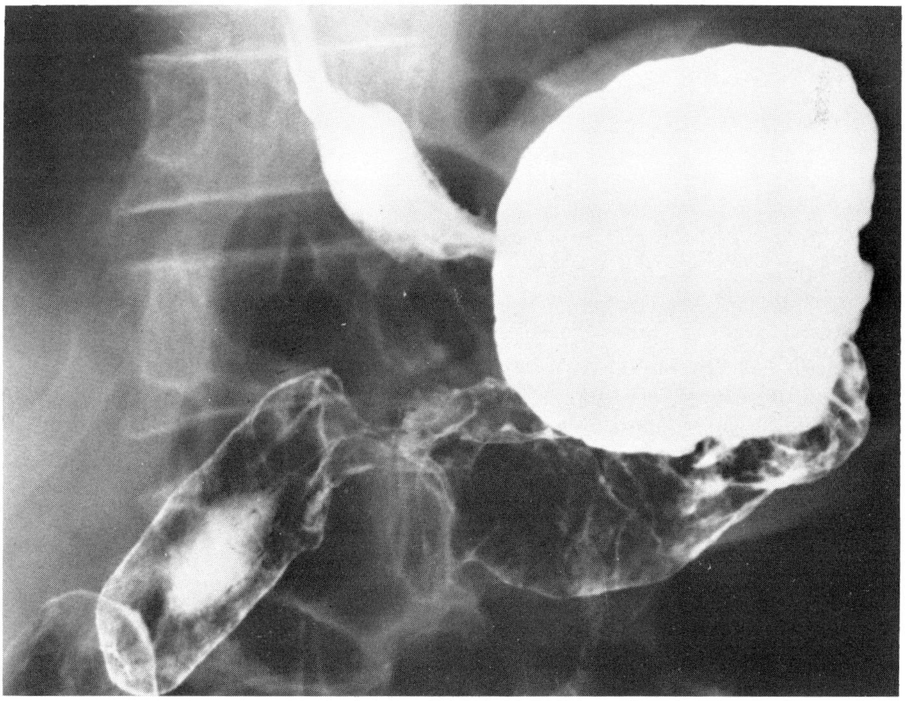

D

Fig. 25-3. Double contrast barium studies demonstrating "early" (A, B) and "advanced" (C, D) gastric adenocarcinomas. (Courtesy of Dr. R. West and Dr. J. Lee, Queen Elizabeth and General Hospitals, Birmingham.)

Table 25-6. Rates and results of an international comparison of the surgical treatment of gastric cancer in Europe, United States, and Japan

Author	Year	Operation rate (%)	Resection rate (%)	Curative resection rate (%)	Overall 5-year survival rate (%)
Europe					
Brookes et al. [17]	1950–1959	63.5	42.5	26.5	4.9
Desmond [33]	1944–1970	—	54.0	18.4	8.0
Svennevig and Nysted [115]	1959–1968	71.3	45.0	32.3	10.0
Inberg et al. [68]	1946–1955	53.9	21.1	17.1	3.7
	1956–1965	62.0	32.1	25.2	6.5
	1966–1972	69.3	45.1	23.6	10.8
United States					
Dupont et al. [38]	1948–1973	76.0	48.0	22.5	7.4
Cady et al. [19]	1940–1949	80.0	—	37.0	7.0
	1957–1966	94.0	58.0	44.0	11.0
Hoerr [63]	1950–1972	96.0	54.6	46.4	15.1
Adashek et al. [5]	1956–1965	71.0	39.0	24.0	8.0
	1966–1975	76.0	51.0	31.0	10.0
Scott et al. [101]	1960–1983	90.0	71.0	42.0	15.0
Japan					
Mine et al. [82]	1955–1963	93.2	63.2	52.3	14.4
Muto et al. [89]	1941–1961	98.7	79.4	—	19.0
Kajitani and Takagi [72]	1946–1970	97.7	—	67.0	33.3
Kajitani and Miwa [71]	1963–1966	94.3	63.4	44.7	16.4

rates. Whether or not this would be a real improvement is difficult to forecast. It might merely reflect earlier treatment, which does not necessarily mean that the natural history of the disease is affected. The Japanese studies have not as yet proved conclusively the long-term benefit of early detection, making allowances for the possible "lead-time" bias. The annual mortalities are lower in screened populations than in unscreened populations [61], and the annual mortalities in the screened populations are lower than the expected rates, although these differences are not yet statistically significant [93].

There are wide international variations in the results of surgical treatment of gastric cancer (Table 25-6). Although the overall results reported from Europe and the United States are similar, they are inferior to those from Japan. The operability rate is higher in Japan, and the most marked improvement in the Japanese statistics in recent years has been in the curative resection rate and in the overall five-year survival rate. Kajitani's figures from the Japanese Cancer Institute [72] demonstrate an increase in the five-year survival rate associated with an increase in the curative resection rate. Most of the results come from personal or individual hospital studies, and it is important to look at larger, population-based studies, which take into account the varying management of cancer in an entire region. Comparing Brookes et al.'s study [17] in the West Midlands in 1965 with Kajitani and Miwa's [71] population-based study of 24,082 patients, the operation, resection, and curative resection rates are all higher in the Japanese study, resulting in an overall five-year survival rate that is 12 percent better in Japan. These increases may simply reflect the stage of disease that is presenting to the surgeon in Japan. Although the surgical resection itself may actually influence prognosis, the data do suggest that earlier detection improves survival rates.

Treatment

An operation is the only effective treatment of adenocarcinoma of the stomach, no patient should be denied its possible benefit. While investigations may give an indication of stage, most patients need a laparotomy. Laparotomy should only be excluded in a terminal stage of disease or if the patient is otherwise unfit for operation. This general principle of operative assessment must be accepted for all patients because the most effective palliation is also achieved by surgical intervention. The aim of the "stage-appropriate" operation for gastric cancer must be to apply a treatment designed for maximal survival time while allowing patients to enjoy an optimal quality of life.

PREOPERATIVE ASSESSMENT

The diagnosis of gastric cancer is established by roentgenography and endoscopy, the latter providing histological confirmation of cancer. Preoperative investigation should include a full hematological and biochemical screen (hemoglobin level, white cell count, erythrocyte sedimentation rate (ESR), urea and electrolyte levels, and liver function tests), chest roentgenogram and assessments of the cardiovascular system. Many patients are malnourished, and hyperalimentation should be considered for them. We have studied the effect of preoperative feeding in patients 15 percent below their ideal body weight [42]. In a controlled trial, malnourished patients received hyperalimentation for three weeks preoperatively; among the 13 patients having total gastrectomies, 3 of the 6 controls (patients not given preoperative hyperalimentation) had an anastomotic dehiscence, compared with none of the 7 patients who did receive hyperalimentation.

Specific preoperative investigations to determine resectability usually prove unreliable. Angiography does not give accurate information related to the size, type, or operability of gastric lesions [39]. Abnormalities in individual liver function tests predict unresectability of the primary lesion in 76–89 percent of instances, and if three or four liver function tests are significantly elevated, radical resection is usually contraindicated [24].

Radioisotopic liver scans have a high percentage of false positive results and are not a reliable method of demonstrating metastatic disease [80]. There is as yet little evidence of the value of computerized axial tomography or ultrasound in assessing the operability of gastric lesions.

PREOPERATIVE PREPARATION

Gastrectomy is a major operation with a significant mortality, particularly in the elderly. The general condition of the patient must be optimum at the time of operation. Particular attention should be paid to nutrition and to the state of the cardiovascular and respiratory systems. Prophylaxis against deep venous thrombosis should be started preoperatively with both subcutaneous heparin (5000 units 3 times a day) and compression stockings.

The role of prophylactic antibiotics in reducing wound infection and anastomotic dehiscence has not been proved conclusively because there have been few controlled studies. The stomach of a normal individual is usually sterile. In patients with either gastric ulcers or carcinomas, however, there is significant colonization of the gastric contents; this is more common when the pH of the stomach is above 4. There was a higher risk of wound sepsis among our patients with a high pH, all of whom had heavily contaminated gastric juice. The most common organisms isolated from gastric juice that were subsequently found in wound infections were *Streptococcus viridans, Streptococcus faecalis, Escherichia coli, Clostridium* species, *Bacteroides* species, *Hemophilus,* and *Staphylococcus albus* [49]. Thus prophylactic broad-spectrum antibiotics should be used, starting preoperatively.

Table 25-7. Lymph node groups for gastric cancer

Site of primary lesion	N1 nodes	N2 nodes
Upper third (Fig. 25-4) (*Left*)	Left cardiac Right cardiac Lesser curvature Greater curvature	Supra-and infrapyloric Left gastric Common hepatic Splenic artery Splenic hilus Celiac axis
Middle third (Fig. 25-4) (*Center*)	Right cardiac Lesser curvature Greater curvature Supra-and infrapyloric	Splenic artery Splenic hilus Left cardiac Left gastric Common hepatic Celiac axis
Lower third (Fig. 25-4) (*Right*)	Lesser curvature Greater curvature Supra- and infrapyloric	Right cardiac Left gastric Common hepatic Celiac axis

N3 nodes: hepatoduodenal ligament, posterior aspect of pancreas, root of mesentery, diaphragmatic, paraesophageal.

N4 nodes: middle colic, para-aortic nodes.

Note: Nodes not common to site groups listed for N1 and N2 nodes have been designated N3 or N4 nodes, depending on site.

PRINCIPLES OF SURGICAL TREATMENT

The most appropriate operation for gastric cancer must be considered in relation to the known pattern of spread of the disease, the known pattern of recurrence following resection, whether the extent of the resection influences long-term survival, the postoperative mortality, and the effects of the reconstructive procedure on long-term morbidity.

Gastrectomy and Lymphadenectomy

In 1932 Carnett and Howell [20] described the mechanism of dissemination from gastric cancers as (1) direct extension into the pancreas, hepatic and splenic pedicles, abdominal wall, esophagus, colon, duodenum, and gallbladder, (2) lymphatic embolization, (3) lymphatic permeation, (4) bloodstream embolism, and (5) transplantation, commonly causing bronchial and ovarian carcinomatosis. Gastric carcinomas may spread by direct extension into the duodenum and esophagus, and it is not true, as was once believed, that the pylorus is the limit of spread. Coller et al. [25] demonstrated microscopic duodenal involvement in 26.4 percent of instances, and this was confirmed in 1949 by Zinniger and Collins [125], who demonstrated that 30 percent of lesions within 5 cm of the pylorus invaded the duodenum. Thus the extent of the gastrectomy must take into account the site of the growth, and in distal lesions the surgeon should remove a significant proportion of duodenum. Similar attention must be paid to lesions at the cardia, achieving at least a 5-cm clearance. Frozen section from the edge of the resected specimen during the operation establishes that microscopical clearance has been achieved.

Lymph node metastases are common. The Japanese Research Society for Gastric Cancer has designated first [N1], second [N2], third [N3], and fourth [N4] tiers of nodes likely to

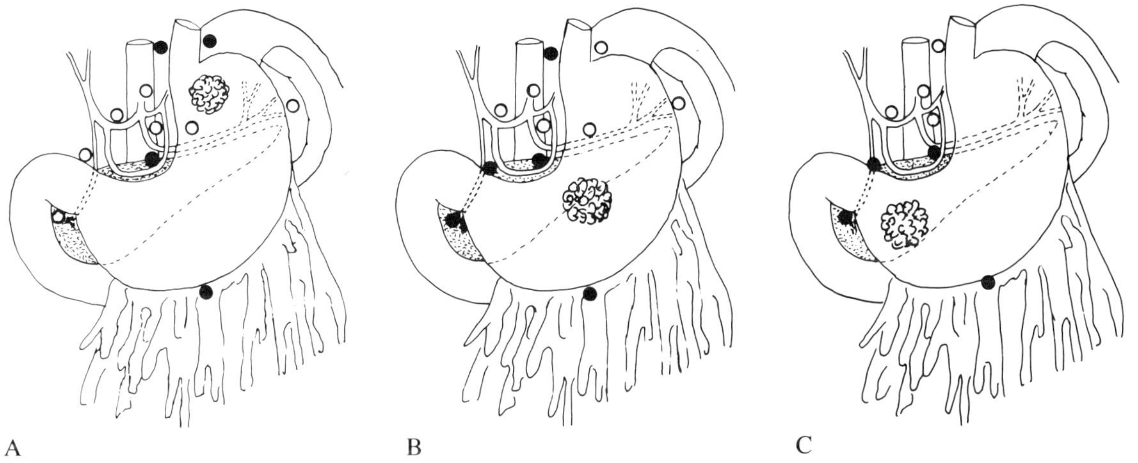

Fig. 25-4. N_1 and N_2 lymph node groups for carcinomas of the upper (*Left*), middle (*Center*) and lower third (*Right*). (An R2 resection of these lesions necessitates removal of these lymph nodes.)

be involved according to the location of the main lesion (Table 25-7, Fig. 25-4). They have defined groups whose involvement indicates increasing advancement of disease [71]. Gastrectomies are defined as R1, R2, and R3 resections according to the extent of lymphadenectomy (e.g., an R1 resection excises N1 nodes). The degree of involvement of these tiers and the extent of surgical lymphadenectomy influence survival. The corrected five-year survival rate for N1 involvement is 38.5 percent, for N2 involvement 22.8 percent, for N3 involvement 11.1 percent, and for N4 involvement 8.5 percent. The corrected five-year survival rate following R0 resections is 26 percent, R1 42.4 percent, R2 49.5 percent, and R3 40 percent. This suggests that an R2 resection is associated with the best survival results and that an R3 resection need be considered only for those with N2 involvement, if the resections can be achieved with an acceptable postoperative mortality. Certainly in Japan the extension of the lymphadenectomy has not been associated with an increase in postoperative mortality.

The observed pattern of recurrence of gastric carcinoma after resection has important implications for surgical therapy. Recurrence occurs in the gastric remnant in 10–15 percent of instances [94], and this has been used as an argument for routine total gastrectomy (total gastrectomy *en principe*). The five-year survival rate following a total gastrectomy *en principe* is 42.1 percent compared to 38.5 percent for subtotal resections for distal lesions. In the Japanese study the five-year survival rate for total gastrectomy was 19.8 percent, for proximal gastrectomy 23.1 percent, and for distal gastrectomy 50.3 percent; the five-year survival rate for distal gastrectomy excising less than four-fifths of the stomach was 52.9 percent, and for gastrectomies excising more than four-fifths of the stomach, it was 45.8 percent. It is true that many of the types of gastrectomies described in the Japanese studies were chosen because of the site and extent of the lesion, so these groups are not strictly comparable. The argument in favor of total gastrectomy to remove a possible site of recurrence is sensible if the postoperative mortality and morbidity rates are the same for all procedures; many times they are not, as is discussed later.

The necessity for the lymphadenectomy in curative operations for gastric cancer is supported by the increased survival rate obtained by R2 resections compared with R1 resections and R0 resections. Further support is gained from the report of 59 patients with apparently benign gastric ulcers removed surgically and subsequently proved by histological examination to be carcinomas [34]. All these patients initially had a nonradical gastrectomy. Twenty-four then had revisional radical operations, and the five-year survival rate in this group was 56 percent. Thirty-five patients had no further resection and a 23 percent five-year survival rate. These results support the concept of wide surgical resection and lymphadenectomy as the treatment of choice for gastric cancer and suggest that surgical resection can influence the natural history of the disease.

A limiting factor to extensive resections is postoperative mortality. Longmire [77] in a review of the literature reported an overall operative mortality of 21 percent for total gastrectomy and believed that this was unacceptably high. Pichylmayr and Mayer's [94] reported mortality was 9.3 percent, and the Japanese mortality after total gastrectomy of 6.2 percent was similar to that of other, less radical gastrectomies [71]. However, Gilbertson [50] noted a large increase in mortality with R3 resections contributing to a reduction in the five-year survival rate from 28 percent to 17 percent. But the operative mortality in Japan was similar for all types of lymphadenectomy [71]. The low mortalities reported are from large series from a small number of surgeons. Thus when a surgeon is not undertaking many gastric operations, his or her postoperative mortality for total gastrectomy is likely to be too high; for such surgeons a subtotal gastrectomy (R2) is the operation of choice. An alternative policy is to centralize the operative management of gastric cancers in centers that can achieve, through experience and expertise, a low mortality even for radical resections.

Principles of Reconstruction

All the features that have been so closely examined in relation to reconstructive procedures for benign disease must be considered in restoring gastrointestinal continuity to the patient with cancer. The reconstructive procedure, if badly conceived, may produce more severe symptoms than does the cancer itself. It is a sad reflection on the surgical art when the patient who had had a curative operation for cancer does not enjoy an optimum quality of life.

Recurrent disease may produce further gastrointestinal complications. This most frequently occurs locally at the site of the previous resection, either in the gastric remnant or in residual nodes [53, 81]. To prevent recurrent disease precipitating intestinal obstruction, it is best to construct a wide stoma at a distance from the site of likely recurrent disease. This is best achieved by a Billroth II anastomosis (Fig. 25-5B). If a Billroth I reconstruction is done, a wide stoma can be achieved by anastomosing the proximal stomach to the duodenum, which has been opened on its inner border (Fig. 25-5A). The incidence of postgastrectomy problems, such as vomiting, diarrhea, dumping, and hematological and nutritional effects, is similar in the classical Billroth I anastomosis and in this modified technique [16]. Bile reflux can occur after a reconstructive procedure for a partial gastrectomy, and its relation to postoperative symptoms is not clear. Bile reflux may be associated with symptoms, but these usually occur when the bile reflux is into the esophagus [8, 120]. Thus there is an argument in favor of reconstructing partial as well as total gastrectomies by a Roux-en-Y technique to provide effective bile diversion (Fig. 25-5C).

The reconstructive procedure following a total gastrectomy is also important. Total gastrectomy is often associated with adverse long-term nutritional effects. The sequelae of this operative procedure are best evaluated after total gastrectomy for the Zollinger-Ellison syndrome, for massive bleeding from the stomach, or for polyposis. Many patients lose weight after total gastrectomy, although this can be corrected by dietary supplementation [3, 15, 102]. Megaloblastic and iron deficiency anemia may also develop in these patients [4].

Malabsorption of fat and protein is common in patients after total gastrectomy, and the absorption of glucose usually shows a pattern of early hyperglycemia and late hypoglycemia [51]. The most significant malnutrition occurs in patients who have severe postgastrectomy

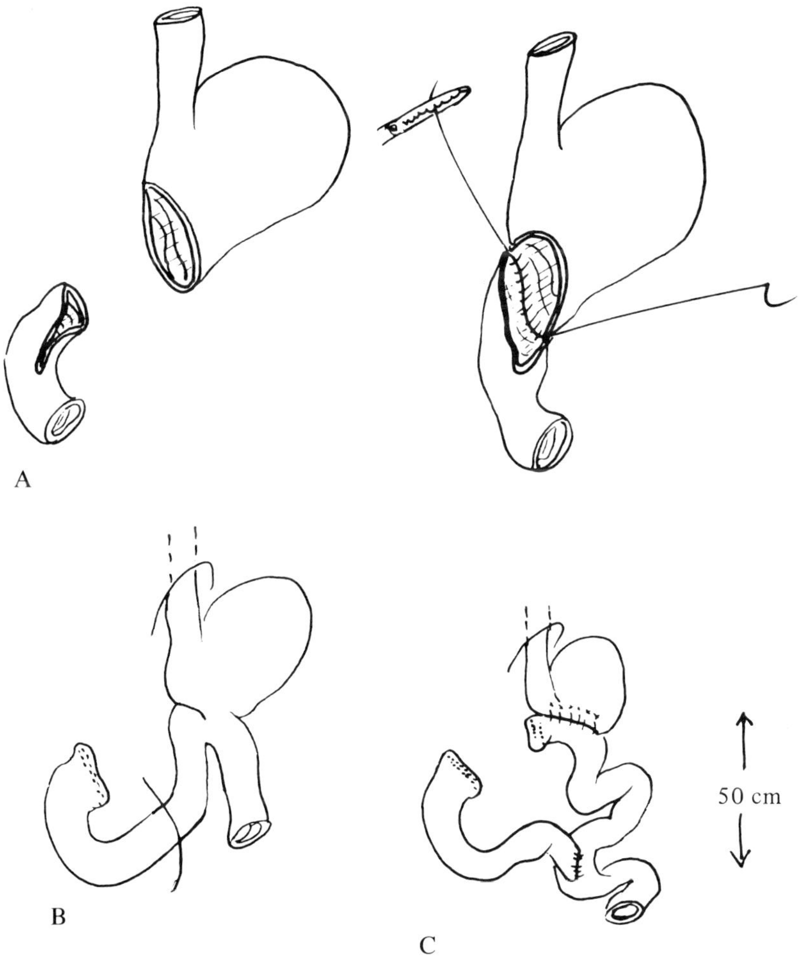

Fig. 25-5. Reconstructive procedures for a partial gastrectomy. (A) Modified Billroth I. (B) Billroth II. (C) Roux-en-Y gastrojejunostomy.

syndromes [7], a fact that indicates the importance of the reconstructive procedure. The construction of gastric pouches and the use of jejunal segments to ensure duodenal passage of food have been used as reconstructive procedures in an attempt to reduce these problems [79], but there is no evidence that they reduce the metabolic consequences.

The most commonly employed reconstructions are the Roux-en-Y, the Henley jejunal interposition, and the omega loop (Fig. 25-6A to D). The incidence of many postgastrectomy syndromes, such as distention, dumping, and diarrhea, is similar for all three methods, occurring in about 20 percent of all patients [66]. In addition, we have found that bile reflux is commonly associated with significant morbidity [36]. Bile reflux was investigated using a technetium 99m HIDA scan (Fig. 25-7). A scan with isotopic activity in the esophageal area correlated well with the presence of endoscopic and microscopical esophagitis. Eight of 10 patients with esophageal reflux were evaluated as Visick grade 3 or 4, in comparison with only 2 patients in Visick grade 3 among 17 patients with no reflux. Reflux was related to the length of the diverting limb. It occurred in Roux-en-Y reconstructions with limbs of 35 cm or less and in 5 of 6 omega loop reconstructions. We were unable to evaluate

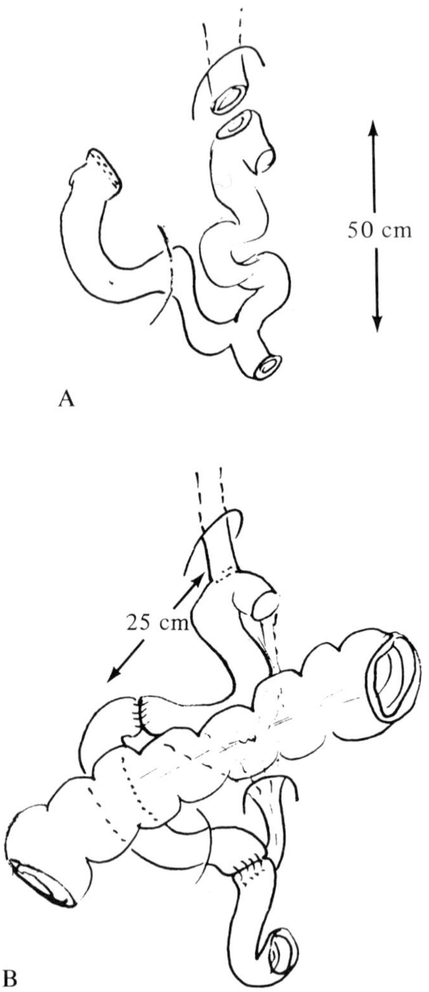

Fig. 25-6. Reconstructive procedures for a total gastrectomy. (A) Roux-en-Y. (B) Henley jejunal interposition. (C) Omega gastrojejunostomy. (D) Lygidakis modification of Roux-en-Y.

the Henley interposition loop [59], but it has been reported to be a satisfactory method of diverting bile if the length of the interposition loop is 25 cm or more [118]. A 50-cm Roux-en-Y reconstruction appears to be the operation of choice because it is simpler to perform than the Henley reconstruction. It has fewer anastomoses and ensures a more certain blood supply at the region of the esophagojejunostomy. Lygidakis [79] described a further development of the Roux-en-Y method of reconstruction (see Fig. 25-6D) and reported improved quality of life with minimal postgastrectomy symptoms.

SURGICAL PROCEDURE

The incision for laparotomy depends on the site of the primary lesion. For lesions of the cardia, for which proximal partial or total gastrectomy might be envisioned, the patient may be placed on his or her right side for an abdominothoracic approach. For the more common lesions of the antrum and body of the stomach, adequate exposure is obtained through the abdomen. At laparotomy the possibility of cure is assessed first. Curative re-

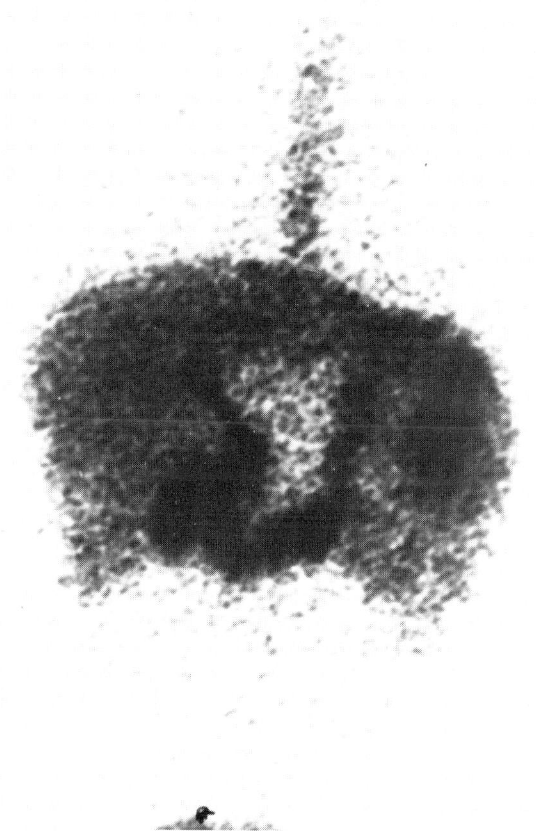

Fig. 25-7. Technetium-labeled HIDA scan demonstrating esophageal reflux of the isotope in a patient with an omega reconstruction.

section should be considered impossible only in the presence of peritoneal seedlings, distant metastases, extension to unresectable adjacent structures, or massive involvement of preaortic lymph nodes. Macroscopical surgical evaluation of lymph nodes adjacent to a gastric tumor is not accurate, and treatment should not be limited because of the presence of palpable nodes.

Radical Gastrectomy

The definitive radical surgical resection must be the equivalent of the R2 resection reported in the Japanese literature. This is a resection that includes the removal of all the N2 tiers of nodes. The precise N1 and N2 nodes vary according to the site of the primary lesion (see Table 25-7 and Fig. 25-4A to C). The two most appropriate operations for gastric cancer are a radical subtotal distal gastrectomy and a total gastrectomy. For the common carcinoma of the lower one-third of the stomach, a subtotal distal gastrectomy will remove the N1 and N2 lymph nodes, although it is necessary to undertake extra dissection to clear the right cardiac, common hepatic, and celiac axis nodes. For lesions of the middle third of the stomach, it may be appropriate to undertake a total gastrectomy, in which case the N1 and N2 nodes should be removed en bloc with the primary lesion. For lesions of the upper third, the most appropriate resection is a total gastrectomy. In all resections at least a 5-cm clearance of the primary lesion should be achieved, and frozen section should be used to confirm microscopical clearance at the resection lines. In addition to the surgical resection, it is important to perform a biopsy on nodes of the N3 and N4 groups so that an accurate staging is obtained; a biopsy should be done on any of the groups of nodes specified in Table 25-7 that are not included in the resection.

The procedure of gastrectomy and lymph node dissection was described by Nakajima and Kajitani [91]. The first step is a detachment of the greater omentum from the transverse colon from left to right. The anterior leaf of the mesocolon is also removed with the omentum. At the inferior margin of the pancreas the right gastroepiploic vessel is ligated with the dissection of lymph nodes along the superior mesenteric vein. The pancreatic capsule—the serous floor of the omental bursa—is removed upward to the common hepatic artery. The gastroduodenal artery is then dissected downward to the right gastroepiploic artery. It is divided and ligated.

The next step includes the detachment of the lesser omentum from the undersurface of the left lobe of the liver upward to the esophageal hiatus, followed by the separation of the anterior leaf of the hepatic duodenal ligament downward to the origin of the right gastric vessels. These vessels are divided and ligated, with removal of the appropriate lymph nodes.

The duodenum is divided, and the distal stomach with the attached omentum is reflected out of the left costal margin of the incision. A portion of duodenal cuff is excised for frozen-section examination. Thereafter the lymph nodes of the hepatoduodenal ligament and those behind the pancreas are dissected en bloc from right to left through the foramen of Winslow, and the dissection is continued to the nodes along the common hepatic artery and those at the root of the celiac artery. The left gastric artery is isolated, divided, and ligated, with removal of appropriate nodes. The lymph nodes along the splenic artery are dissected toward the splenic hilus. If the presence of pancreatic nodal metastases demands it, resection of the pancreas and spleen can be performed for complete clearance. The attachments of the right cardia to the esophageal hiatus are separated, both the vagal nerves are divided, and the lymph nodes of the right cardia are removed, completing the mobilization of the stomach and the lymphadenectomy. Now a partial or total gastrectomy is performed. In a total gastrectomy the spleen is mobilized by dividing the lienorenal ligament; the splenic artery and vein and then the esophagus are divided, and the stomach is removed.

Method of Reconstruction

After a partial gastrectomy, gastrointestinal continuity is restored either by a modification of the Billroth I anastomosis or by a Billroth II anastomosis.

In the modified Billroth I gastrectomy, the whole of the divided end of the stomach is anastomosed end to end to the duodenum. To facilitate this and to obtain a gastroduodenal stoma of 6–8 cm, the incision across the duodenum is extended along the inferomedial border (see Fig. 25-5A). Usually the gastroduodenal anastomosis is performed in two layers. For a Billroth II reconstruction, the duodenal stump is closed in two layers as is the gastrojejunal anastomosis. For a Roux-en-Y reconstruction, the duodenal stump is closed as in a Billroth II gastrectomy, the jejunum is divided 7–10 cm distal to the duodenojejunal flexure, the distal end of the jejunum is closed, and the stomach is anastomosed end to side to this portion of jejunum. The proximal end of jejunum is then anastomosed to the small intestine, 50 cm distal to the gastrojejunal anastomosis (see Fig. 25-5C).

We believe that after a total gastrectomy the best reconstruction is a Roux-en-Y (see Fig. 25-6A). The technique is as described earlier in the chapter, but it is often simple and convenient to use a circular stapling gun for the end-to-side esophagojejunal anastomosis. We have described a modification of the head of the gun to enable it to be inserted without trauma to the esophagus [9].

In a Henley reconstruction, a 25-cm or longer portion of small intestine is dissected starting 10 cm from the duodenojejunal flexure. This is anastomosed in an isoperistaltic manner to the esophagus and duodenum. Small intestinal continuity is reestablished by an end-to-end anastomosis (see Fig. 25-6B).

Postoperative Complications

In addition to the general complications that may be associated with any surgical procedure (e.g., wound sepsis, pneumonia) there are specific complications of gastric resections such as reactionary hemorrhage, and later, dehiscence.

Reactionary hemorrhage is not common if a two-layer suture technique or the circular staple gun is used because both methods have an inner hemostatic layer. However, the principle of the stapling machines is that there are staggered rows that are not totally hemostatic sutures, and great care must be taken to ensure that there is no bleeding. In the event of reactionary hemorrhage, early reoperation is necessary to control the bleeding vessel.

Anastomotic dehiscence is an unusual complication of gastroduodenal or gastrojejunal anastomoses, but it is an important cause of morbidity and mortality following esophagojejunal anastomoses. By using meticulous suture techniques, this complication can be reduced to a minimum.

After total gastrectomy, the patient should be maintained on intravenous fluids or nutrition until the integrity of the esophageal anastomosis has been established on the seventh postoperative day with a water-soluble con-

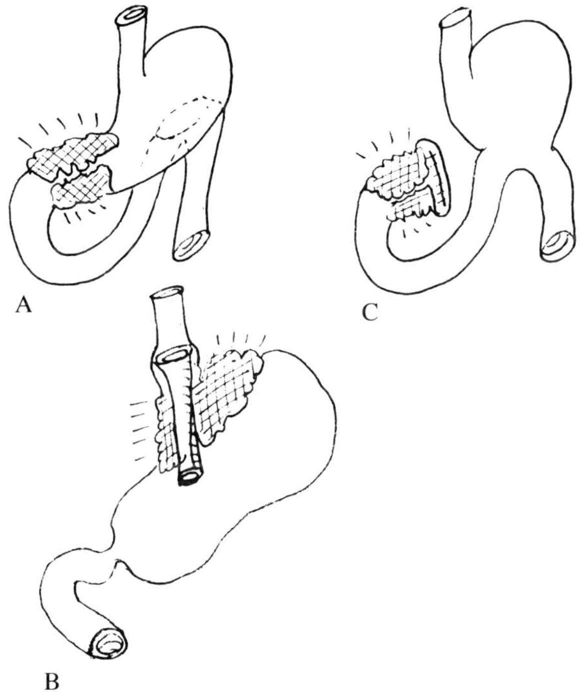

Fig. 25-8. Palliative procedures. (A) Gastroenterostomy. (B) Intubation. (C) Exclusion.

trast roentgenogram. If there is a small leak, parenteral nutrition should be continued until the leak has closed. An anastomotic leak following a total or partial gastrectomy may present as an enterocutaneous fistula, and parenteral nutrition is essential until this closes. Fortunately, it is rare for there to be complete dehiscence; if it does occur, it is often associated with sepsis. The only hope for survival is to isolate the ends of intestine as cutaneous fistulas; for the esophagus this necessitates bringing the cervical esophagus to the surface as an esophagostomy. Long-term parenteral nutrition is needed until the patient is well enough to undergo a second reconstructive operation.

PALLIATIVE SURGICAL TREATMENT

The ideal form of palliative treatment must be determined individually for each patient, after evaluating the symptoms to be palliated and the quality of life afforded by the procedure. The symptoms most commonly requiring palliation are obstruction, hemorrhage, and pain, and the procedures available are bypass (Fig. 25-8A), intubation (Fig. 25-8B), exclusion (Fig. 25-8C), and resection. Pyloric obstruction may be effectively corrected by resection or gastroenterostomy, although in our experience the results of bypass are so disappointing as to make it hardly worth considering. Cardiac obstruction is relieved by resection if feasible, if not, nonoperative endoscopic intubation is preferred to operative intubation. Hemorrhage, if acute, must be treated by resection. In chronic blood loss, however, radiotherapy may be considered [97], although we have no experience with this method.

Pain is a frequent symptom. It may be intermittent, like peptic ulcer pain, or constant and related to extragastric spread of the neoplasm, either locally or distantly. Resection of the carcinoma is effective for ulcer-type pain, but pain related to extragastric extension or metastatic disease is seldom relieved by resection.

Table 25-8. Staging of gastric cancer (TNM-UICC)

Stage	Operation	Pathological features
I	Radical gastrectomy (no macroscopical residual disease)	Muscularis propria normal Serosa normal Nodes normal
II	Radical gastrectomy (no macroscopical residual disease)	Muscularis propria abnormal or serosa abnormal Nodes normal
III	Radical gastrectomy (no macroscopical residual disease)	Nodes abnormal
IV	A. Macroscopical residual disease following palliative resection	Abnormal diagnostic histology
	B. No resection.	Abnormal diagnostic histology

TNM = tumor-node-metastasis; UICC = International Union for the Classification of Cancer.

Symptomatic relief can often be achieved only by analgesics, although occasionally radiotherapy or chemotherapy might help. The best palliation for symptomatic relief follows resection, and the surgeon should always attempt this even if macroscopical disease is left in situ.

PATHOLOGICAL FEATURES

There must be close liaison between the surgeon and pathologist to ensure that the various lymph node groups are defined, labeled, and examined histologically. The precise depth of penetration of the primary lesion should be identified and an indication given of the morphology. The best morphological classification was that described by Lauren [76]. His description of two main histological types, diffuse and intestinal (see Fig. 25-2), relates well to epidemiological findings and prognosis. From these morphological findings and examination of the lymph nodes, a patient's disease can be staged accurately. This is an important feature because it gives an indication of whether the resection has been curative or palliative, of the likely prognosis of the individual patient, and of what residual disease remains. Accurate staging is vital for patients entering controlled trials of adjuvant therapy—first, to facilitate the accurate stratification of trials, and second, to permit the identification of particular groups who might benefit from a particular treatment.

Staging of Gastric Cancer

A staging system helps separate patients into important groups. It should indicate the limits of the surgical resection and the macroscopical clearance achieved. It should account for the important pathological features of the disease. It should be easily understood and applied by the general physician without a special interest and allow further development by physicians with a special interest. In the modern multimodal approach to the management of the patient with cancer, these stages must allow adjuvant therapies to be evaluated in "like" groups.

The early tumor-node-metastasis (TNM) staging systems for gastric cancer were confusing. However, the most recently evolved system [119] is easily understood and should be used routinely (Table 25-8).

The important clinicopathological features of gastric cancer are the resectability and whether the resection is radical or palliative. Pathologically, the important microscopical features are the depth of penetration of the primary tumor and the lymph node involvement (Table 25-1). The efficacy of this system is confirmed in a retrospective study of tumors at the Birmingham Cancer Registry (Fig. 25-9) with respective corrected five-year survival rates of 72.2 percent, 29.4 percent, 9.0 percent, 1.8 percent, and 0.8 percent in stages I, II, III, IVA, and IVB.

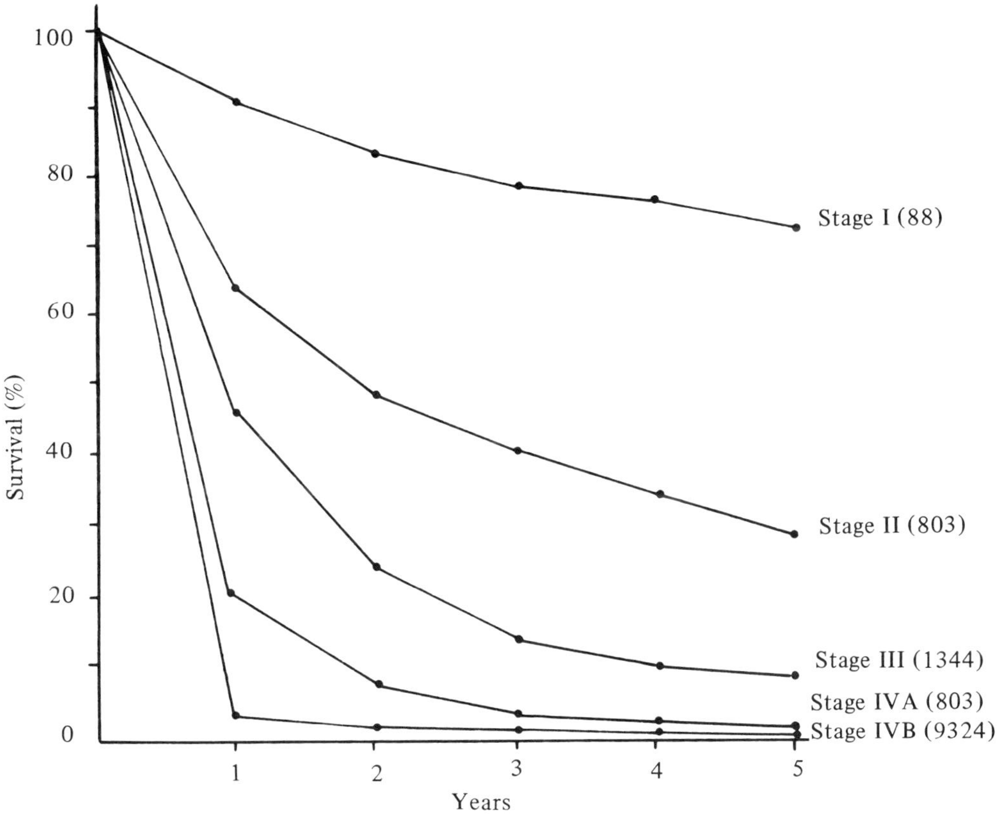

Fig. 25-9. Survival according to stage for gastric adenocarcinomas in the West Midlands (1960–1969). (Figures in parentheses represent number of patients in each group.)

This staging system is easily applied by surgeons and pathologists and provides useful information to oncologists about prognosis and likely residual disease to be treated by adjuvant therapy. It also permits subdivisions of the overall material for comparisons with other series. Each stage may be related to particular features of another stage. For example, the depth of penetration of the primary lesion can be mucosal (m), submucosal (sm), into the muscularis propria (mp), or serosal (s). Thus stage I can be divided into Im and Ism. In stage III it may be important to consider the depth of penetration of the primary lesion, and the stage can be subdivided into stage IIIm, stage IIIsm, stage IIImp, and stage IIIs. The importance of tiers of lymph nodes has been alluded to, and stage III can be subdivided into stages IIIN1, IIIN2, IIIN3, and IIIN4. These examples demonstrate how this system can be used for more detailed assessment of the disease while maintaining its simplicity of comprehension and application for the general physician.

Follow-Up Care of Gastric Cancer Patients

The object of follow-up care in cancer patients is to detect recurrent disease at a sufficiently early stage to allow further treatment and to give moral support to the patient and the family. In addition, postgastrectomy syndromes should be sought; it should never be assumed that the recurrence of the symptoms is related to recurrent disease.

Most patients with gastric cancer will die of recurrent disease within five years of resection [43, 53, 81]. Conventional methods of follow-up care include symptomatic assessment and physical examination. *Symptomatic evaluation is important if recurrence is to be detected at an early stage, and the development of any symptoms in the absence of physical signs should be an indication for upper gastrointestinal investigation.* This investigation should be by endoscopy, since assessment of gastric remnants is difficult roentgenographically. Physical examination will only detect gross recurrent disease, and the chance of curative surgical treatment in this group is remote. However, palliative treatment should always be considered with reference to the patient's symptoms.

In patients with a known precancerous lesion of the gastric mucosa, the only accurate method of detecting gastric remnant recurrence is by regular endoscopic assessment and biopsy.

Nutritional indices must be monitored in the follow-up care of all gastrectomy patients. After total gastrectomy, vitamin B_{12} supplements are necessary. Among the long-term survivors with partial gastrectomy, a considerable proportion will have an iron deficiency anemia and require iron supplements.

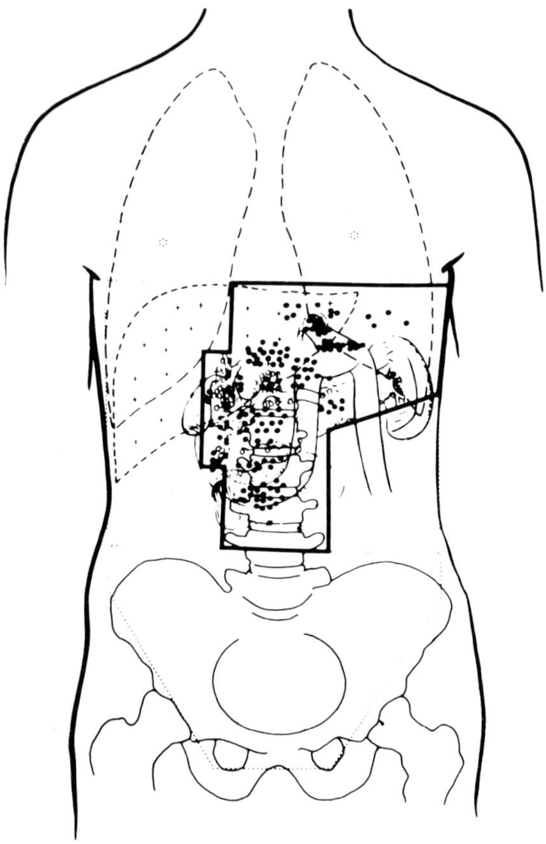

Fig. 25-10. Sites of recurrence after curative resection. (* = lung metastasis; + = liver metastasis; △ = wound implant; ● = local failures in surrounding organs or tissues; ○ = lymph node failures.) (L. L. Gunderson: reproduced with permission of Clinics in Gastroenterology: W. B. Saunders Company Limited [53].)

Reasons for Failure

Recurrent disease following radical resection is caused by the progressive development of micrometastases. The sites of recurrence are both local and distant. The local recurrences may be in the gastric bed, gastric stump, or residual local lymph nodes. Distant metastases may occur at many sites, but they occur most commonly in the liver or peritoneal cavity, and more rarely, in the lungs and bones. In a postmortem study of 92 patients who had previously had curative subtotal gastrectomies, McNeer et al. [81] found some form of local recurrence in 80.5 percent and at distant sites alone in 15.2 percent. Gunderson [53] analyzed the patients in Minnesota who had reoperations. There was evidence of recurrent cancer in 80.4 percent, and the recurrence was only local in 53.7 percent of the group (Fig. 25-10). The high incidence of recurrent disease caused by micrometastases after surgical intervention and the possibility that a more extensive operation might reduce this has already been explored. Radical resection (R_2) may reduce the incidence of local recurrence, but extended radical resections (R_3) are associated with a high postoperative mortality, and the long-term survival rate is not increased. The inability of an operation to eradicate all disease and prevent the development of recurrence highlights the limitations of surgical treatment as a single therapy in the management of gastric cancer. It is clear that adjuvant therapies must be evaluated in an attempt to improve control of this disease.

Nonsurgical Management of Gastric Cancer

Many nonsurgical therapies have been evaluated in patients with gastric cancer, both in the treatment of advanced disease and as an adjuvant to curative resection.

CHEMOTHERAPY IN ADVANCED DISEASE

Cytotoxic agents were evaluated initially as single agents in patients with inoperable disease. The most widely investigated agents and the response rates obtained are illustrated in Table 25-9. In the reported series a "response" is defined as a reduction of at least 50 percent in the size of a measurable lesion. The duration of the response varies from one to five months, and following treatment with a single agent there has been no evidence of significantly increased survival rates in patients with advanced disease.

A combination of cytotoxic agents may be expected to increase response rates. The general principles governing the selection of drugs to be used in combination therapy are (1) the drugs should be active when used alone against the tumor; (2) they should have different modes of action; and (3) the toxic effects of the drug should not be the same, allowing each drug to be used at a maximal therapeutic level [26].

The combinations assessed in the treatment of advanced disease are illustrated in Table 25-9, the best response rate being obtained with fluorouracil (5-FU), doxorubicin hydrochloride (Adriamycin), and mitomycin C (FAM). Some combinations have produced an early improvement in survival rates. Kovach et al. [75] reported a significantly improved survival rate at 18 months when carmustine (nitrosourea BCNU) and 5-FU were used in combination, compared with the survival when 5-FU and BCNU were used singly. However, this difference was not maintained at 28 months. Schien et al. [100] showed significantly improved survival rates in responders treated with FAM compared with nonresponders. A West Midlands study [73] comparing 5-FU and lomustine (methyl CCNU) with a placebo in a randomized, double-blind study of 200 patients demonstrated no benefit in terms of duration of survival. This study also demonstrated the difficulty of giving adequate chemotherapy to ill patients; only 41 percent in the treated group were fit enough to receive both drugs. Among the fitter patients who were able to tolerate the treatment, the median survival time was 25 weeks, compared with 22 weeks for the placebo. Thus there is evidence that gastric carcinomas are sensitive to cytotoxic agents, but in advanced disease there is little to suggest that this affects survival time.

Table 25-9. Cytotoxic agents in advanced gastric cancer

Agent	Response rate (%)
SINGLE AGENTS	
Fluorouracil [26]	22
Mitomycin C [26]	30
Nitrosourea (BCNU) [26]	18
Doxorubicin (Adriamycin) [106]	24
COMBINATION CHEMOTHERAPY	
5-Fluorouracil + methyl-CCNU + doxorubicin (Adriamycin) [106]	36
5-Fluorouracil + methyl-CCNU [106]	40
5-Fluorouracil + BCNU [106]	41
5-Fluorouracil + doxorubicin (Adriamycin) + mitomycin C [100, 106]	43

ADJUVANT CHEMOTHERAPY

Cytotoxic agents should be most effective when the tumor burden is microscopic. A number of adjuvant studies have been undertaken in gastric cancer using single agents and combination chemotherapy. Rake et al. [95]

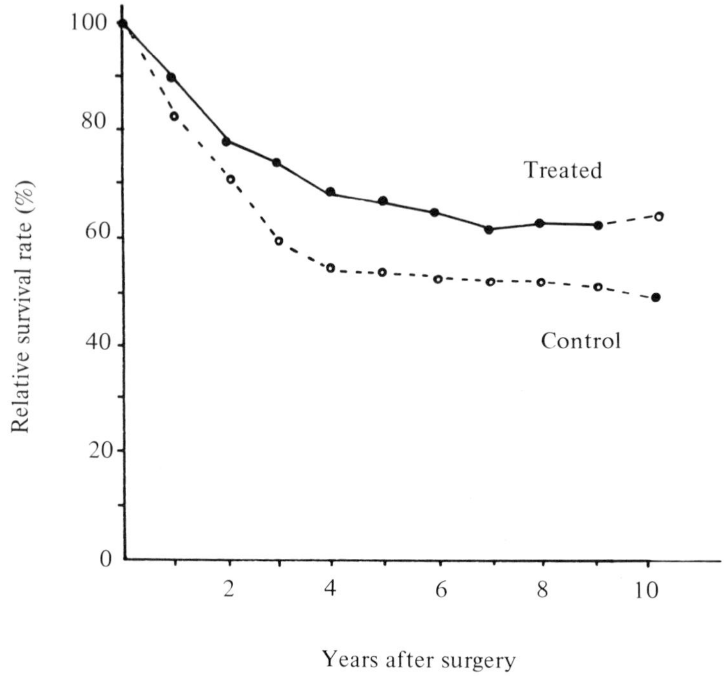

Fig. 25-11. Survival of patients with gastric adenocarcinoma in a controlled trial using mitomycin C in the treated group. (Reprinted by courtesy of the Societé Internationale de Chirurgie [67].)

reported an adjuvant study in 40 patients using 5-FU and mitomycin C after an induction course of 5-FU, vincristine, cyclophosphamide, and methotrexate. They reported a significant difference in median survival time (6 months in the control group and 10 months in the treated group).

Imanaga and Nakazoto [67] reported a controlled study of 2636 patients using mitomycin C twice weekly for five weeks as the active agent and demonstrated an overall improvement of 13.5 percent at 5 years and 10 percent at 10 years in the treated group (Fig. 25-11). In the patient with either nodal or serosal involvement and no residual disease, the five-year survival rate was 45.1 percent in the controls and 78.1 percent in the treated patients. Also in 1977 Franz and Cruz [47] compared patients treated with adjuvant 5-FU with untreated retrospective controls. The one-year survival rate was 73.9 percent in the treated group and 46.7 percent in the untreated group. At two years, however, 47 percent and 40 percent of the patients, respectively, were still alive, and there was no difference at three years. Nakajima and Kajitani [91] demonstrated an improved survival rate with adjuvant mitomycin C after curative surgical treatment in patients with lymph node metastases. In the United Kingdom the British Stomach Cancer Group undertook a multicenter study of mitomycin C and 5-FU with or without an induction course of 5-FU, vincristine, methotrexate, and cyclophosphamide, compared with controls [45, 69]. Four hundred and eleven patients were treated, and early analysis by the life table method demonstrated a 38.1 percent cumulative survival rate at two years following curative surgical treatment—a rate better than that seen in previously reported studies (31.8 percent at two years) following curative operations in the West Midlands [18]. These figures demonstrate the importance of controlled trials and the inadvisability of using retrospective controls. In an interim analysis of this study, the cumulative

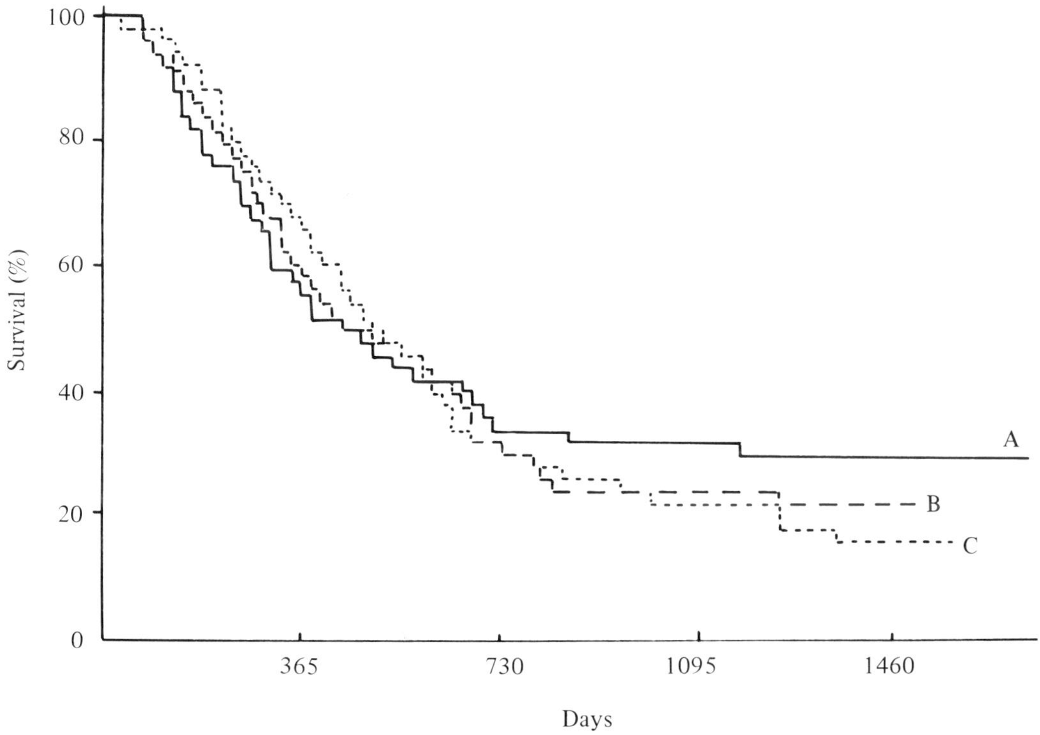

Fig. 25-12. The British Stomach Cancer Group Trial of Adjuvant Chemotherapy: Interim survival analysis of 411 patients: (A) Placebo group; (B) Treatment group: induction course of 5-fluorouracil (5-FU), methotrexate, vincristine, and cyclophosphamide, followed by mitomycin C and 5-FU; (C) 5-FU and mitomycin C.

survival rate at 12 months in the placebo group (A) was 56.3 percent and in the two treatment groups (B and C) was 59.8 percent and 66.5 percent, respectively. However, at two years there was no difference between the groups, and there was no statistically significant difference in the log rank test between the treated and control groups (Fig. 25-12).

The patients entered into this study started treatment at any time during the first three postoperative months. Analysis of the time of the first treatment (Fig. 25-13) demonstrated that the best responses are seen in those who start treatment within the first postoperative month. Although this is not a significant effect, the results achieved by Imanaga and Nakazoto [67] followed the administration of mitomycin C started in the first postoperative week; thus it appears to be important that chemotherapy be started as soon as possible.

While there is no convincing evidence from European and American studies to suggest that chemotherapy should be employed routinely, the fact that responses are obtained and that some studies have shown improved survival rates indicates that this type of treatment must continue to be evaluated in controlled prospective studies.

RADIOTHERAPY

It is pertinent to consider the role of regional radiotherapy because most recurrences of gastric cancer are local or regional, occurring in an area that could be encompassed in a radiotherapy portal (see Fig. 25-10). Radical high-dose irradiation as a primary treatment of gastric cancer is disappointing, and although some responses can be obtained the high doses necessary cannot be tolerated by adjacent critical normal tissues, such as the liver, pancreas, or small intestine. With modern

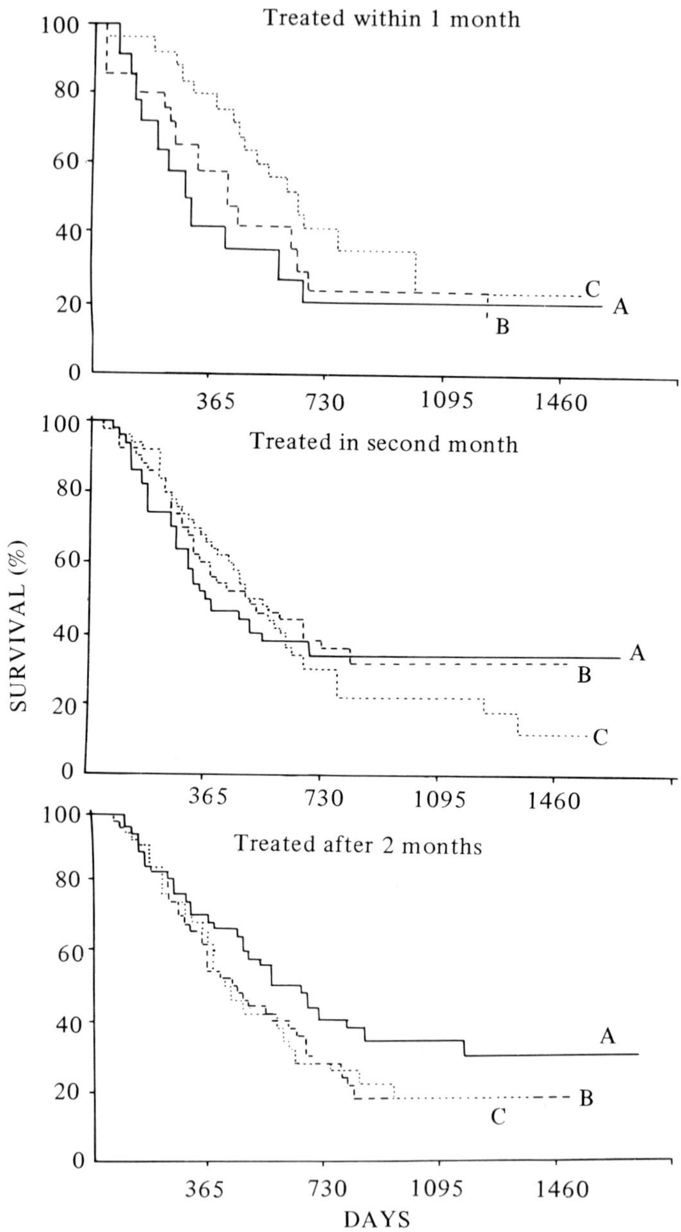

Fig. 25-13. The British Stomach Cancer Group Trial of Adjuvant Chemotherapy: Interim survival analysis of 411 patients, evaluating the effect of treatment beginning within the first, second, and third months after operation.

megavoltage equipment, however, it is possible to administer less radical doses of radiation. Robinson and Cohen [98] demonstrated improved survival rates in patients receiving conventional postoperative irradiation—40 percent survived at two years compared with 20 percent in the group receiving no postoperative irradiation. Catterall et al. [23] used fast neutron irradiation in 29 unselected patients, and among the 19 with a palpable epigastric lesion, produced resolution in 16. Fourteen patients subsequently underwent a postmortem examination, and 10 had no macroscopical evidence of tumor, although all but two had residual microscopical foci of malignant cells. After neutron treatment, however, there was considerable damage to the stomach, and the authors recommended that gastrectomy be performed routinely four to six months after irradiation.

COMBINED MODALITY TREATMENT

Radiotherapy has been evaluated in conjunction with chemotherapy. The combination of radiotherapy and 5-FU produces increased response rates when compared with agents used singly. A prospective study demonstrated significantly improved survival after irradiation and 5-FU (median survival, 13 months) compared to irradiation alone (median survival, 6 months) [86]. It is not clear whether 5-FU was acting as a cytotoxic agent or as a radiosensitizer; in a small study evaluating the radiosensitizer misonidazole given 4 hours before radiotherapy, four of seven patients with gastric cancer had evidence of response to therapy. The best responses were seen in patients with dysphagia, in whom the ability to swallow was restored [79].

Another development in radiotherapy has been in intraoperative treatment, which allows lesions to be exposed directly to radiation and normal sensitive structures to be screened or positioned outside the field. Delivering doses of 2000–4000 rads intraoperatively, Abe [2] reported improved survival in 10 patients after noncurative operations. This method of therapy has so far been limited to small groups of patients, however, and as yet there is no evidence that it produces better results than conventional external beam methods.

The reports of the benefit of radiotherapy in advanced disease demonstrate, nevertheless, that gastric cancer is sensitive to megavoltage radiotherapy, and the British Stomach Cancer Group is exploring the possible role of this method as an adjuvant to curative surgery.

The value of both chemotherapy and radiotherapy in the management of patients with gastric cancer is still limited by their low therapeutic indices. While the surgeon accepts the limitations of curative surgical treatment, it is important to emphasize that the present treatment of gastric cancer remains primarily surgical.

The management of gastric cancer remains a challenging problem. It demands a high degree of clinical suspicion to diagnose the condition at an early stage and a high degree of technical expertise to perform the "stage-appropriate" operation. Much time and thought should be spent in the further management of patients who have undergone "curative" operations, and considerable attention should be given to patients with inoperable disease. The future will probably include adjuvant chemotherapy and radiotherapy, and improvements in the management should be seen during the next decade.

References

1. Abe, S., Ogawa, Y., Nagasue, N., et al. Early gastric cancer: Results in a general hospital in Japan. *World J. Surg.* 8:308, 1984.
2. Abe, M., Takahishi, M., Zabumoto, E., et al. Clinical experience with intraoperative radiotherapy of locally advanced cancers. *Cancer* 45:40, 1980.
3. Adams, J. F. The clinical and metabolic consequences of total gastrectomy. I. Morbidity, weight and nutrition. *Scand. J. Gastroenterol.* 2:137, 1967.
4. Adams, J. F. The clinical and metabolic consequences of total gastrectomy. II. Anemia, metabolism of iron, vitamin B_{12} and folic acid. *Scand. J. Gastroenterol.* 3:145, 1968.

5. Adashek, K., Sangel, J., and Longmire, W. P. Cancer of the stomach: Review of ten year intervals. *Ann. Surg.* 189:6, 1979.
6. Aird, I., Bentall, H. H., and Roberts, J. S. F. A relationship between cancer of the stomach and ABO blood groups. *Br. Med. J.* 1:799, 1953.
7. Alexander-Williams, J. Post gastrectomy problems. *Br. Med. J.* 4:403, 1967.
8. Alexander-Williams, J. Duodenogastric reflux after gastric operations. *Br. J. Surg.* 68:685, 1981.
9. Alexander-Williams, J. To facilitate the insertion of the EEA auto suture head into the oesophagus. *Br. J. Surg.* 69:196, 1982.
10. Aste, H., Amadori, D., Maltoni, G., et al. Early gastric cancer detection in four areas at different gastric cancer death rates. *Acta Endoscop.* 11:123, 1981.
11. Barnes, R. J., Gear, M. W. L., Nicol, A., et al. Study of dyspepsia in a general practice as assessed by endoscopy and radiology. *Br. Med. J.* 4:214, 1974.
12. Billroth, T. Offenses Schreiben and Herrn Dr. L. Wittelshofer. *Wien. Med. Wochenschr.* 31:161, 1881.
13. Bock, O. A. A., Arapakis, G., Witts, L. J., et al. The serum pepsinogen level with special reference to the histology of the gastric mucosa. *Gut* 4:106, 1963.
14. Booth, S. N., King, P. G., Leonard, J. C., et al. Serum carcinoembryonic antigen in clinical disorders. *Gut* 14:794, 1973.
15. Bradley, E. L., Isaacs, J., Hersh, T., et al. Nutritional consequences of total gastrectomy. *Ann. Surg.* 182:415, 1975.
16. Brookes, V. S., Meynell, M. J., Bold, A. M., et al. A review of symptoms, haematology and clinical chemistry following a partial gastrectomy. *Br. J. Surg.* 61:9, 1974.
17. Brookes, V. S., Waterhouse, J. A. H., and Powell, D. J. Carcinoma of the stomach: Ten year survey of results and of factors affecting prognosis. *Br. Med. J.* 1:1577, 1965.
18. Burn, I. A., and Welbourn, R. B. Cancer of the stomach. In R. Smith (Ed.), *Gastric Surgery: Surgical Forum.* London: Butterworth, 1975. P. 121.
19. Cady, B., Ramsden, D. A., Stein, A., et al. Gastric cancer. *Am. J. Surg.* 133:423, 1977.
20. Carnett, J. A., and Howell, J. C. A case of coarctation of the aorta and gastric carcinoma with a discussion of the metastases. *Surg. Clin. North Am.* 12:1351, 1932.
21. Carter, K. J., Schaffer, H. A., and Ritchie, W. P., Jr. Early gastric cancer. *Ann. Surg.* 199:604, 1984.
22. Cassell, P., and Robinson, J. O. Cancer of the stomach: A review of 854 patients. *Br. J. Surg.* 63:603, 1976.
23. Catterall, M., Kingston, D., Lawrence, G., et al. The effects of fast neutrons on inoperable carcinoma of the stomach. *Gut* 16:150, 1975.
24. Cederqvist, C., and Nielsen, J. Value of liver function tests in predicting resectability in patients with gastric cancer. *Acta Chir. Scand.* 139:656, 1973.
25. Coller, F. A., Kay, E. B., and McIntyre, R. S. Regional lymphatic metastasis of carcinoma of the stomach. *Arch. Surg.* 43:748, 1941.
26. Comis, R., and Carter, S. A review of chemotherapy in gastric cancer. *Cancer* 34:1576, 1974.
27. Cooper, B. T., and Chadwick, V. S. Menetrier's Disease. In J. H. Baron and F. G. Moody (Eds.), *Gastroenterology, Vol. 1. Foregut.* London: Butterworth, 1981. P. 141.
28. Correa, P. The Epidemiology and Pathogenesis of Chronic Gastritis: Three Etiologic Entities. In L. Van der Reis (Ed.), *Frontiers of Gastrointestinal Research: The Stomach.* Basel: Karger, 1980. P. 98.
29. Correa, P., Cuello, C., Duque, E., et al. Gastric cancer in Columbia. III. The natural history of precursor lesions. *J.N.C.I.* 57:1027, 1976.
30. Craven, J. L., Baum, M., and West, R. R. Variations in gastric cancer mortality in South Wales. *Clin. Oncol.* 5:341, 1979.
31. Crespi, I. M., and Munoz, N. Gastric precancer states in gastric cancer. *Adv. Biosci.* 32:65, 1981.
32. Dekker, W., and Tytgat, G. N. Diagnostic accuracy of fiberendoscopy in the detection of upper intestinal malignancy: A follow up analysis. *Gastroenterology* 73:710, 1977.
33. Desmond, A. M. Radical surgery in treatment of carcinoma of stomach. *Proc. R. Soc. Med.* 69:867, 1976.
34. Desmond, A., Nicholls, J., and Brown, C. Further surgical management of gastric ulcer with unsuspected malignant change. *Ann. R. Coll. Surg. Engl.* 57:101, 1975.
35. Domellof, L., and Janunger, K. G. The risk of gastric carcinoma after partial gastrectomy. *Am. J. Surg.* 134:49, 1977.
36. Donovan, I. A., Fielding, J. W. L., Bradby, H., et al. Bile diversion after total gastrec-

tomy. *Br. J. Surg.* 69:389, 1982.
37. Dublin, L. I., and Marks, H. H. The inheritance of longevity: A study based on life insurance records. *Proc. Assoc. Life Insurance Directors Am.* 28:89, 1941.
38. Dupont, J. B., Lee Rillens, J., Burton, G. R., et al. Adenocarcinoma of the stomach: Review of 1,497 cases. *Cancer* 41:941, 1978.
39. Efsen, F., and Fischerman, K. Angiography in gastric tumours. *Acta Radiol.* [*Diagn.*] 15:193, 1974.
40. Ellis, D. J., Kingston, R. D., Brookes, V. S., et al. Gastric carcinoma and previous peptic ulceration. *Br. J. Surg.* 66:117, 1979.
41. Evans, D. M. D., Craven, J. L., Murphy, F., et al. Comparison of "early gastric cancer" in Britain and Japan. *Gut* 19:1, 1978.
42. Fabricus, P., Hawker, P., and Dykes, P. Reduction of anastomotic leakage after total gastrectomy by pre-operative feeding. Presented at the World Congress of Gastroenterology, Stockholm, 1982.
43. Fielding, J. W. L., Ellis, D. J., Jones, B. G., et al. Natural history of "early" gastric cancer: Results of a ten year regional survey. *Br. Med. J.* 281:965, 1980.
44. Fielding, J. W. L., Ellis, D. J., Jones, B. G., et al. Early Gastric Cancer in the United Kingdom. In Y. van Maercke, E. van Moerr, and P. Pelckhams (Eds.), *Stomach Diseases.* Amsterdam: Excerpta Medica, 1981. P. 268.
45. Fielding, J. W. L., Fagg, S. L., Jones, B. G., et al. An interim report of a prospective, randomised, controlled study of adjuvant chemotherapy in operable gastric cancer: British Stomach Cancer Group. *World J. Surg.* 7:390, 1983.
46. Figus, A. I. Gastroenterological Welfare Centre and Early Gastric Cancer in Hungary. In E. Grundmann, H. Grunze, and S. Witte (Eds.), *Early Gastric Cancer: Current Status of Diagnosis.* Berlin: Springer, 1974. P. 185.
47. Franz, J. L., and Cruz, A. B. The treatment of gastric cancer with combined surgical dissection and chemotherapy. *J. Surg. Oncol.* 9:131, 1977.
48. Freisen, G., Dockerty, M., and Remine, M. D. Superficial carcinoma of the stomach. *Surgery* 51:300, 1962.
49. Gatehouse, D., Dimock, F., Burdon, D. W., et al. Prediction of wound sepsis following gastric operations. *Br. J. Surg.* 65:551, 1978.
50. Gilbertson, V. A. Results of treatment of stomach cancer. *Cancer* 23:1305, 1969.
51. Goebell, H. Pathophysiological Consequences of Total Gastrectomy. In C. Herfarth and P. Schlag (Eds.), *Gastric Cancer.* Berlin: Springer, 1979.
52. Green, P., O'Toole, K., Weinberg, L., et al. Early gastric cancer. *Gastroenterology* 81:247, 1981.
53. Gunderson, L. Radiation therapy: Results and future possibilities. *Clin. Gastroenterol.* 5:743, 1976.
54. Haberkant, H. Ueber die bis erzielten unmittebran und wetteren erfolge der verschiedene operatione am magen. *Arch. Klin. Chir.* 51:484, 1896.
55. Haenszel, W. Variation of incidence and mortality from stomach cancer with particular reference to the United States. *J.N.C.I.* 21:213, 1958.
56. Haenszel, W., and Kurihara, M. Studies of Japanese migrants. 1. Mortality from cancer and other diseases among Japanese in the United States. *J.N.C.I.* 40:43, 1968.
57. Hakkinen, I. Application of serum and gastric juice tumour markers to early diagnosis and screening of gastric cancer. *Adv. Biosci.* 32:85, 1981.
58. Hammond, E. C., and Horn, D. The relationship between human smoking habits and death rates. *J.A.M.A.* 155:1316, 1954.
59. Henley, F. A. Gastrectomy with replacement: A preliminary communication. *Br. J. Surg.* 40:118, 1952.
60. Hirayama, T. Changing patterns in the incidence of gastric cancer. *Adv. Biosci.* 32:1, 1981.
61. Hirayama, T. Methods and results (cost effectiveness) of gastric cancer screening. *Adv. Biosci.* 32: , 1981.
62. Hisamichi, S., Nuzaki, K., Kitagana, M., et al. Evaluation of mass screening programme for stomach cancer. *Tohuku J. Exp. Med.* 118 (suppl.):69, 1976.
63. Hoerr, S. O. Prognosis for carcinoma of the stomach. *Surg. Gynecol. Obstet.* 137:204, 1973.
64. Holdstock, G., and Bruce, S. Endoscopy and gastric cancer. *Gut* 22:673, 1981.
65. Huibregtse, K. Endoscopic screening for malignancy in the gastric remnant. Presented at the Second British Stomach Cancer Group/Smith, Kline, and French International Workshop on Early Gastric Cancer, Chepstow, 1981.
66. Huguier, M., Lancret, J. M., Benard, P. F., et

al. Functional results of different reconstructive procedures after total gastrectomy. *Br. J. Surg.* 63:704, 1976.
67. Imanage, H., and Nakazoto, H. Results of surgery for gastric cancer and the effect of adjuvant mitomycin C in cancer recurrence. *World J. Surg.* 1:213, 1977.
68. Inberg, M. V., Heinonon, R., Rantakokko, V., et al. Surgical treatment of gastric carcinoma. *Arch. Surg.* 110:703, 1975.
69. Jones, B. Design and progress of a multicentre trial of adjuvant chemotherapy in operable gastric cancer. In A. Gerard. (Ed.), *Progress and Perspectives in the Treatment of Gastrointestinal Tumours.* Oxford, England: Pergamon Press, 1981. P. 36.
70. Jones, B. B. G., Fielding, J. W. L., Fagg, S., et al. A pilot study of misonidazole and radiotherapy in upper gastrointestinal malignancy. *Clin. Onocol.* 7:259, 1981.
71. Kajitani, T., and Miwa, K. Treatment results of stomach carcinoma in Japan, 1963–1966. *WHO-CC Monograph.* Tokyo: WHO, 1979, p. 2.
72. Kajitani, T., and Takagi, I. Cancer of the stomach at Cancer Institute Hospital, Tokyo. *Gann Monogr. Cancer Res.* 22:77, 1979.
73. Kingston, R. D., Ellis, D. J., Powell, J., et al. The West Midlands gastric carcinoma chemotherapy trial: Planning and results. *Clin. Oncol.* 4:55, 1978.
74. Kogo, M., Nakata, H., Kiyonara, H., et al. Minute mucosal patterns in gastric carcinoma. *Radiology* 120:199, 1976.
75. Kovach, J., Moertel, C., Schjutt, A., et al. A controlled study of 1,3-bis-(2 chloroethyl)-1-nitrosourea and 5-fluorouracil therapy for advanced gastric cancer and pancreatic cancer. *Cancer* 33:563, 1974.
76. Lauren, P. The two main histological types of gastric carcinoma: Diffuse and so-called intestinal type carcinoma. *Acta Pathol. Microbiol. Scand.* 64:31, 1965.
77. Longmire, W. P., Jr., Total gastrectomy for carcinoma of the stomach. *Surg. Gynecol. Obstet.* 84:21, 1947.
78. Lundh, G., Burn, J. I., Kolig, G., et al. A cooperative international study of gastric cancer. *Ann. R. Coll. Surg. Engl.* 54:219, 1974.
79. Lygidakis, N. M. Total gastrectomy for gastric carcinoma: A retrospective study of different procedures and assessment of a new technique of gastric reconstruction. *Br. J. Surg.* 68:649, 1981.
80. Machida, K., Watari, T., Hayashi, S., et al. Clinical significance of pre-operative liver scintography in gastric cancer. *Am. J. Gastroenterol.* 68:296, 1977.
81. McNeer, G., Vandenberg, H., Down, F. Y., et al. A critical evaluation of subtotal gastrectomy for cure of cancer of the stomach. *Ann. Surg.* 134:2, 1951.
82. Mine, M., Majima, S., Harada, M., et al. End results of gastrectomy for gastric cancer. *Surgery* 68:753, 1970.
83. Ming, E. C. The adenoma-carcinoma sequence in the stomach and colon. II. Malignant potential of gastric polyps. *Gastrointest. Radiol.* 1:121, 1976.
84. Misaki, F., and Kawai, K. Acid secretion in different stages of gastric carcinoma. *Gut* 22:877A, 1981.
85. Miwa, K. Cancer of the stomach in Japan. *Gann Monogr. Cancer Res.* 22:61, 1979.
86. Moertel, C. G., Childs, D. S., Reitemeier, R. J., et al. Combined 5-fluourouracil and supervoltage radiation therapy of locally unresectable gastrointestinal cancer. *Lancet* 2:865, 1969.
87. Morson, B. C., Sobin, L. H., Grundmann, E., et al. Precancerous conditions and epithelial dysplasia in the stomach. *J. Clin. Pathol.* 33:711, 1980.
88. Murakami, T. Early cancer of the stomach. *World J. Surg.* 3:685, 1979.
89. Muto, M., Maki, T., Majima, S., et al. Improvement in the end results of surgical treatment of gastric cancer. *Surgery* 63:229, 1968.
90. Nagao, F., and Takahishi, M. D. Diagnosis of advanced gastric cancer. *World J. Surg.* 3:693, 1979.
91. Nakajima, T., and Kajitani, T. Surgical treatment of gastric cancer with special reference to lymph node dissection. In M. Friedman, M. Ogawa, and D. Kisner (Eds.), *Diagnosis and Treatment of Upper Gastrointestinal Tumours.* Amsterdam: Excerpta Medica, 1981. P. 207.
92. Nomura, A. M. Y., Stemmermann, G. N., and Samloff, I. M. Serum pepsinogen I as a predictor of stomach cancer. *Ann. Intern. Med.* 93:537, 1980.
93. Oshima, A., Sakagami, F., Hawai, A., et al. Evaluation of a mass screening programme for gastric cancer. In T. Hirayama (Ed.), *Epidemiology of Stomach Cancer.* Tokyo: WHO, 1977. P. 35.
94. Pichlmayr, R., and Meyer, H. J. Patterns of recurrence in relation to therapeutic strategy.

Adv. Biosci. 32:171, 1981.

95. Rake, M., Mallinson, B., Cocking, J., et al. Assessment of the value of cytotoxic therapy in treatment of carcinoma of the stomach. *Gut* 17:832, 1976.
96. Rapp, W., Heim, M., Mikulicz-Radecki, J. G. V., et al. X_1-acid glycoprotein in gastric cancer juice. *Klin. Wochenschr.* 53:139, 1975.
97. Remine, W. H. Preoperative assessment and palliative surgery. *Adv. Biosci.* 32:123, 1981.
98. Robinson, E., and Cohen, Y. The combination of surgery, radiotherapy and chemotherapy in the treatment of gastric cancer. *Recent Results Cancer Res.* 32:177, 1977.
99. Rogers, K., Roberts, G. M., and Williams, G. T. Gastric juice enzymes: An aid in the diagnosis of gastric cancer. *Lancet* 1:1124, 1981.
100. Schien, P. S., Coffey, R., and Smith, F. P. Chemotherapy and combined modality treatment of gastric cancer. *Adv. Biosci.* 32:139, 1981.
101. Scott, H. W., Jr., Adkins, R. B., and Sawyers, J. L. Results of an aggressive surgical approach to gastric carcinoma during a twenty-three-year period. *Surgery* 97:55, 1985.
102. Seifert, R. R., and Way, L. W. Total gastrectomy. *Am. J. Surg.* 135:348, 1978.
103. Seifert, E. High risk groups: Gastric polyps. Presented at 2nd British Society of Gastroenterology/Smith Kline and French International Workshop on Early Gastric Cancer, Chepstow, 1981.
104. Sherman, R. S., and Synder, R. E. Roentgenologic surveys for gastric neoplasms. *J.A.M.A.* 174:949, 1960.
105. Shirakabe, H. X-ray diagnosis of early gastric cancer. *Gann Monogr. Cancer Res.* 11:105, 1971.
106. Smith, F. P., Cambareri, R. J., Killen, J. Y., et al. Gastrointestinal cancer. In H. Pinedo (Ed.), *Cancer Chemotherapy: The EORTC Cancer Chemotherapy Annual 1.* Amsterdam: Excerpta Medica, 1980. P. 284.
107. Sogo, J., Kobayashi, K., Saito, J., et al. The role of lymphadenectomy in curative surgery for gastric cancer. *World J. Surg.* 3:701, 1979.
108. Stadelmann, O., Elster, K., Stolte, M., et al. The peptic gastric ulcer: Histographic and functional investigations. *Scand. J. Gastroenterol.* 6:613, 1971.
109. Stalsberg, H., and Taksdal, S. Stomach cancer following gastric surgery for benign surgical conditions. *Lancet* 2:1175, 1971.
110. Stemmerman, G., Haenszel, W., and Locke, F. Epidemiologic pathology of gastric ulcer and gastric carcinoma among Japanese in Hawaii. *JNCI* 58:13, 1977.
111. Stemmerman, G. N., Samloff, I.M., Nomura, A., et al. Serum pepsinogen I and gastrin in relation to extent and location of intestinal metaplasia in the surgically resected stomach. *Dig. Dis. Sci.* 25:680, 1980.
112. Stockbrugger, R. W., Menon, G. G., Beilby, J. O. W., et al. Endoscopic screening in patients with pernicious anaemia. Presented at the 2nd British Gastroenterology Society/Smith, Kline and French International Workshop on Early Gastric Cancer, Chepstow, 1981.
113. Strickland, R. G., and Mackay, I. R. A reappraisal of the nature and significance of chronic atrophic gastritis. *Am. J. Dig. Dis.* 18:426, 1973.
114. Stukonis, M., and Doll, R. Gastric cancer in man and physical activity at work. *Int. J. Cancer* 4:248, 1969.
115. Svennevig, J. L., and Nysted, A. Carcinoma of the stomach. *Acta Chir. Scand.* 142:78, 1976.
116. Swynnerton, B. G., and Truelove, S. C. Carcinoma of the stomach *Br. Med. J.* 1:287, 1952.
117. Takagi, K. The incidence of early gastric cancer since the advent of endoscopy. *Adv. Biosci.* 32:159, 1981.
118. Tonelli, F., Corazziari, E., and Spirelli, F. Evaluation of alkaline reflux after total gastrectomy in Henley and Roux-en-Y reconstructive procedures. *World J. Surg.* 233, 1978.
119. TNM Classification of Malignant Tumours, 3rd Ed. Geneva: UICC International Union Against Cancer, 1978.
120. Toye, D. K. M., and Alexander-Williams, J. Postgastrectomy bile vomiting. *Lancet* 2:524, 1965.
121. Viste, A., Søreide, O., and Glattre, E. Stomach cancer: Major trends in incidence during introduction of gastroscopy service in Norway. *Scand. J. Gastroenterol.* 20:99, 1985.
122. Videbaek, A., and Mosbech, J. The aetiology of gastric carcinoma elucidated by a study of 302 pedigrees. *Acta Med. Scand.* 149:137, 1954.
123. Wangensteen, O. H. *Cancer of the Esophagus and Stomach.* New York: American Cancer Society, 1951.
124. Wangensteen, O. H., and Wangensteen, S. D. History of gastric surgery: glimpses into its early and more recent past. In L. M. Nyhus

and C. Wastell (Eds.), *Surgery of the Stomach and Duodenum,* 3rd Edition. Boston: Little, Brown, 1977.

125. Zinniger, M., and Collins, W. Extension of carcinoma of the stomach into the duodenum and esophagus. *Ann. Surg.* 130:557, 1949.

EDITOR'S COMMENT

Fielding and Alexander-Williams give considerable attention to the Japanese and Birmingham experiences with early gastric cancer. Surgeons in the United States have not highlighted early gastric cancer in their studies. Fortunately, Carter and colleagues at the University of Virginia have reviewed their experience, giving some insight into the problem (*Ann. Surg.* 199:604, 1984). Although Carter et al. reported small numbers of patients, the median five-year survival rate for early gastric cancer was 100 percent. The prognosis was thus excellent, even in the presence of lymph node metastasis—an observation similar to that made in Japan. Carter et al. admitted an inability to make the diagnosis of early gastric cancer preoperatively and therefore urge an aggressive approach to all patients with resectable gastric neoplasms.

Gastric cancer developing in the gastric stump years after partial gastrectomy is the subject of considerable controversy. Clark et al. (*Br. J. Surg.* 72:591, 1985) have given guidelines for an approach to this subset of patients:

> In man the length of exposure to the putative carcinogen is of the order of 15 years or more after partial gastrectomy. During this period many patients will have died from other diseases, notably carcinoma of the lung, chronic respiratory disease and ischaemic heart disease—all smoking-related. However, if endoscopic screening is to be performed then we suggest that it should be reserved for those patients under 70 years treated by gastric surgery 15 or more years previously, and for those under 55 treated by gastric surgery 10 years previously. Patients who develop mild symptoms 5 or more years following previous gastric surgery will require normal gastrointestinal evaluation, which must include endoscopy.

L.M.N.

26

Nonepithelial Tumors of the Stomach and Duodenum

John E. Skandalakis
Stephen W. Gray
Bobby C. Brown
John D. Mullins

The stomach and duodenum are subject to a variety of neoplasms, many of which also occur elsewhere in the body. These neoplasms may be divided generally into those derived from epithelial cells and those of nonepithelial origin. In this chapter we consider only the latter.

We have excluded adenocarcinoma and pancreatic ectopia, and in addition, we have considered melanomas, choriocarcinomas, and carcinoid tumors to be of epithelial origin or at least of epithelial ancestry. Finally, we have excluded the questionable entity of carcinosarcoma, which has at least one epithelial forebear.

We are left with a few not uncommon tumors, benign and malignant, and a larger number of varieties that are only rarely seen and even more rarely reported. We are responsible for our terminology and readily admit that there are other terms and, indeed, other systems of classification that might have been used.

Few of these neoplasms can be specifically diagnosed by roentgenogram or even by eye during an operation. Most require microscopical examination at least, and often more sophisticated procedures are needed.

The symptoms of gastric neoplasms are rarely useful in specific diagnosis. Hemorrhage, pain, nausea and vomiting, palpable mass, and weight loss occur in various degrees, depending on the location of the tumor more than on its histological characteristics [45]. An exogastric tumor presents as a palpable mass; bleeding may be minimal. An endogastric tumor of the same size may produce symptoms of obstruction if it is in the distal stomach or the duodenum but most frequently causes bleeding ranging from occult to uncontrollable. Frequently even a large endoscopic tumor is not palpable.

Benign Tumors

Among numerous types of benign gastric tumors, only one, leiomyoma, is frequently encountered. Most of the others are clinical curiosities without specific symptoms, distin-

Table 26-1. Incidence of benign tumors in the stomach and duodenum

Benign tumors	Sex and age most affected	Incidence in stomach
Leiomyoma	30–70 years Sexes equal	Most common benign gastric tumor
Glomus tumor (glomangioma)	Adults Sexes equal	About 30 instances known
Fibroma	40–70 years Sexes equal	Uncommon
Rhabdomyoma	Any age? Sexes equal	2 instances known
Reactive lymphoid hyperplasia (pseudolymphoma)	Adults Males 3:1	Rare?
Neurogenic tumors	Adults	
Schwannoma	Sexes equal	About 189 instances known
Neurofibroma		About 29 instances known
Hemangioma	Adults Sexes equal?	< 50 instances known
Lipoma	Adults Sexes equal	> 160 instances known
Granular cell tumor (granular cell myoblastoma)	Adults Female 2:1	< 12 instances known
Gastric teratoma	Infancy Males	About 35 instances known

guishable only by their histological characteristics (Tables 26-1, 26-2).

LEIOMYOMA

Giovanni Battista Morgagni [59] first described a gastric smooth muscle tumor. It was located on the posterior wall of the body of the stomach of a 70-year-old woman who died of pneumonitis. The tumor was exogastric, 3 by 4 inches in size, and weighed 1 pound. The first successful removal of a leiomyoma was by von Erlach in 1895 [23]. Chaffin [15] assembled and evaluated all the published reports up to 1938. We [78, 81] reviewed data on 535 instances published from 1938 to 1959. We have treated 17 benign and 9 malignant smooth muscle tumors in Atlanta hospitals in 18 years [80].

Leiomyomas, of smooth muscle origin, have been reported to make up from 55 to 60 percent of all benign gastric tumors [62]. This is an underestimate, for Meissner [57] reported finding leiomyomas in 46 percent of autopsies in Boston. Most were small and of no clinical importance. Perhaps we all harbor such silent microscopic "tumors"!

About 75 percent of gastric leiomyomas are found in patients between 30 and 70 years of age, evenly divided between men and women. More leiomyomas are found in the stomach than any other part of the alimentary tract. No predilection for a specific part of the stomach can be observed (Fig. 26-1). With increasing size, more leiomyomas bulge into the gastric lumen (endogastric) than protrude from the serosal surface (exogastric) (Fig. 26-2).

Only 67 leiomyomas of the duodenum have been reported from 1938 to 1959 [78]. Most were in the first two parts, only seven occurring in the third or fourth portions (Fig. 26-3). Few bulged into the lumen; most were intramural or serosal.

There are no pathognomonic symptoms of gastric leiomyomas. In more than half of 225 affected patients, hemorrhage (melena or hematemesis) was present. Other, less frequent

Table 26-2. Benign tumors of the stomach and duodenum: symptoms, diagnosis, treatment

Benign tumors	Symptoms	Diagnostic methods and characteristics	Treatment
Leiomyoma	Hemorrhage, pain, palpable mass	Histologic studies at biopsy or operation	Excision, or wedge or sleeve resection; segmental resection of duodenum
Glomus tumor (glomangioma)	Hematemesis or melena; symptoms of obstruction or ulcer; asymptomatic in some patients	Histologic studies at biopsy or operation	Local excision or conservative resection
Fibroma	Hemorrhage, pain, mass	Encapsulated, usually in antrum; resembles leiomyoma	Excision
Rhabdomyoma	None related to tumor	Striated muscle at biopsy	Excision or conservative resection
Reactive lymphoid hyperplasia (pseudolymphoma)	Pain, melena, weight loss, ulcer	Presence of inflammatory cells other than mature lymphocytes; local nodes without signs of sarcoma	Resection to control bleeding if necessary
Neurogenic tumors Schwannoma Neurofibroma	May be associated with von Recklinghausen disease; bleeding, pain, or discomfort, palpable mass	Histologic studies at biopsy or operation	Wide excision
Hemangioma	Hemorrhage, ulcerlike symptoms	May be secondary to systemic disease	Resection
Lipoma	Bleeding, ulcerlike pain; most are symptomatic	Histologic studies at biopsy; resembles leiomyoma on roentgenogram; sometimes radiolucent	Wide excision or subtotal gastrectomy
Granular cell tumor (granular cell myoblastoma)	Gastric discomfort	Submucosal, may become a polyp; may be multiple; histologic studies at biopsy	Subtotal gastrectomy
Gastric teratoma	Dystocia; respiratory embarrassment, distention, hemorrhage	Calcifications at roentgenogram	Excision of tumor; partial or total gastrectomy

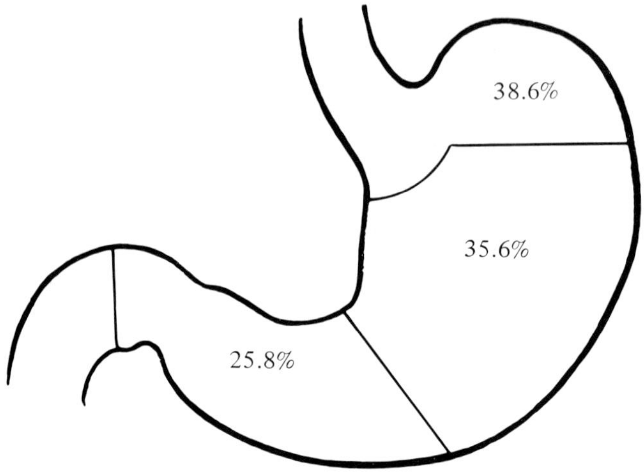

Fig. 26-1. Regions of the stomach in which 184 gastric leiomyomas occurred. No region is immune. (From Skandalakis and Gray, *Smooth Muscle Tumors of the Alimentary Tract,* 1962. Courtesy of Charles C Thomas, Publisher, Springfield, Illinois.)

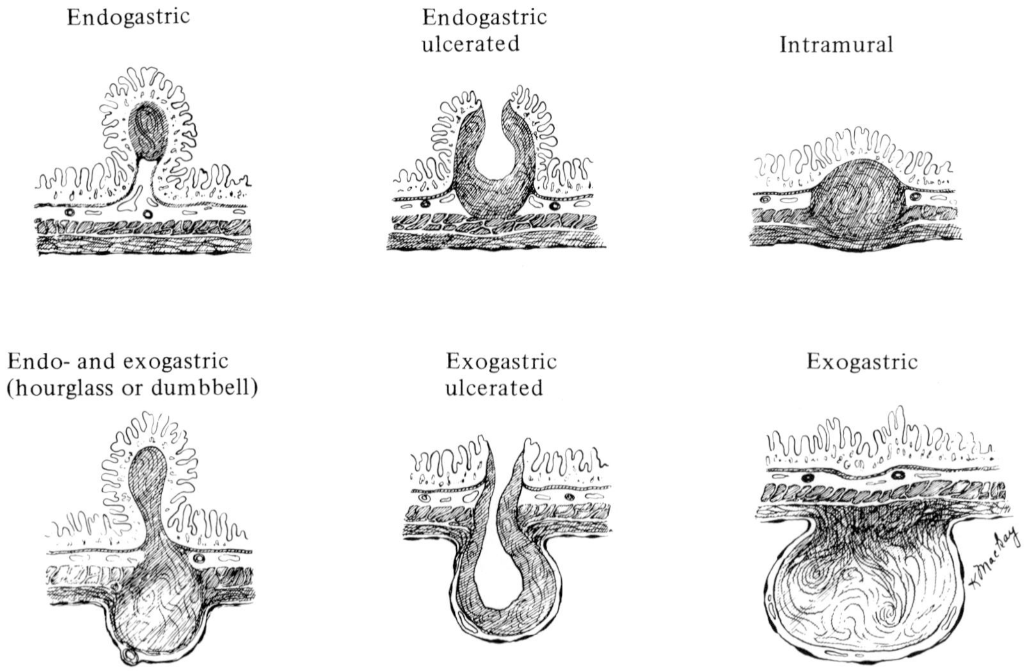

Fig. 26-2. Typical forms assumed by gastric smooth muscle tumors. Most intramural tumors eventually will become endogastric or exogastric. (From Skandalakis and Gray, *Smooth Muscle Tumors of the Alimentary Tract,* 1962. Courtesy of Charles C Thomas, Publisher, Springfield, Illinois.)

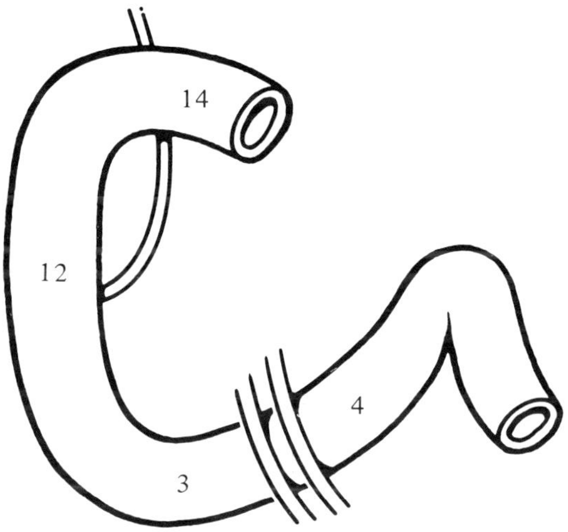

Fig. 26-3. Sites of 33 leiomyomas of the duodenum. Most are found in the first or second portions.

Table 26-3. Surgical procedures for gastric leiomyomas with related mortality in 222 operations

Procedure	No. of operations	Postoperative mortality
Enucleation	6	1[a]
Pedicle cut	7	—
Simple excision	98	3[a]
Wedge or sleeve resection	13	—
Billroth I or II	8	—
Subtotal gastrectomy	71	4
Total gastrectomy	15	1
Biopsy only	4	1[b]
Total	222	10

[a]Death with recurrence of tumor.
[b]Death from perforation.

symptoms were pain or discomfort, palpable mass, weight loss, weakness, and peptic ulcer syndrome. Five percent had no symptoms [78].

Duration of symptoms is of little use in diagnosis. Many tumors of considerable size are silent. In some patients mild symptoms exist for 25 years or more, while in others a single acute episode ends in immediate surgical intervention. Remission and recurrence of one or more symptoms are common.

On microscopical examination, the muscle fibers are arranged in whorls or in palisades. There is usually a thin pseudocapsule present. Pain may be the result of contraction of the smooth muscle of the tumor. This has been reported for tumors of the arrectores pilorum of the skin [25], and contraction of uterine myomas has been seen in vitro [38].

The typical gastric leiomyoma produces a mobile, well-defined, rounded filling defect in the barium-filled stomach. The mucosal folds end sharply at the edge of the tumor. A niche at the apex usually denotes ulceration. There appears to be little disturbance of peristalsis and no evidence of local constriction or spasm as is often seen with benign gastric ulceration. None of these signs is specific for gastric leiomyoma.

The use of gastroscopy dates from 1942 [75]. Leiomyomas appear as smooth, sharply limited tumors in which the overlying mucosal folds are stretched and effaced (Schindler sign). Again, there are no gross characteristics on which to base an unequivocal diagnosis.

For a symptomatic gastric leiomyoma, the treatment of choice is surgical removal of the tumors. Neither total gastrectomy on the one hand nor exploratory laparotomy with a simple biopsy on the other is recommended. Simple excision (not enucleation) or a wedge or sleeve resection is usually adequate (Table 26-3).

When the surgeon is dealing with a giant leiomyoma, subtotal gastrectomy should be considered, especially if the pathologist has any doubt of its benign nature based on frozen sections. Recurrence of the tumor is possible but rare.

An adequate kocherization of the duodenum will help the surgeon greatly. For a lesion proximal or distal to the papilla of Vater, a segmental resection is required. For a lesion close to the ampulla, enucleation or in situ preservation and reimplantation of the ampulla is the procedure of choice.

The surgeon must remember that the pathologist's diagnosis from a frozen section may not be correct. If malignancy is suspected, pancreatoduodenectomy is the procedure indicated. We do not recommend it for unequivocally benign lesions. The mortality from duodenal leiomyomas is similar to that from gastric leiomyoma (Table 26-4).

GLOMUS TUMOR (GLOMANGIOMA)

Gastric glomus tumors are derived from specialized smooth muscle associated with arteriovenous shunts. They are usually found in the gastric antrum, with a protruding surface that frequently ulcerates and bleeds. The tumor is clinically and roentgenologically indistinguishable from an ulcer or other neoplasm.

Only 29 gastric glomus tumors have been reported from their discovery in 1948 up to 1976 [3]. Among these 29 instances 14 were associated with ulcer symptoms and 12 with upper gastrointestinal bleeding, and 10 tumors were found incidentally during clinical evaluation or an abdominal operation.

Glomus tumors appear to be a form of smooth muscle tumor that includes leiomyomas and pericytomas [2, 21, 61]. The relation between glomus tumors and pericyte tumors has been questioned by Toker [90].

A glomus tumor consists of cleftlike vascular channels surrounded by glomus cells in a fine reticular fiber net. The entire tumor is encapsulated with connective tissue and hypertrophied smooth muscle.

A biopsy or operating room frozen section is necessary for differential diagnosis. No recurrences or metastases of gastric glomus tumors have been reported. Surgical removal results in cure in most instances.

FIBROMA

Fibromas, also called inflammatory polyps and eosinophilic granulomas, are spindle cell tumors clinically and often pathologically difficult or impossible to distinguish from leiomyomas or neurogenic tumors [26]. They are usually infiltrated by eosinophils, plasma cells, and lymphocytes.

The symptoms of pain, nausea, vomiting, hemorrhage, and palpable mass are nonspecific. Obstruction is related more strongly to

Table 26-4. Mortality from gastric and duodenal leiomyomas

Relative time of death	Gastric leiomyomas (n = 225)	Duodenal leiomyomas (n = 45)
Died without operation (including discovery at autopsy)	43	6
Died immediately postoperatively	9	3
Died more than 1 year postoperatively	3	—
Total	55 (24%)	9 (20%)

the location of the tumor than to its histological makeup. Many fibromas are asymptomatic and discovered only incidentally.

Fibromas grow slowly but occasionally reach several kilograms in weight [62]. Treatment is by excision or conservative resection.

PRIMARY RHABDOMYOMA OF THE STOMACH

While gastric smooth muscle tumors are not uncommon, striated muscle tumors are rare. A possibly unique example was found incidentally in the stomach of a patient whose death was caused by a villous adenocarcinoma of the rectum [91]. The rhabdomyoma was partially encapsulated in the submucosa of the posterior wall of the cardia. No other instances have been reported in large series of collected reports of gastric tumors [62, 83]. In the reported instance no symptoms could be assigned to the stomach lesion. Treatment would be excision or conservative resection.

REACTIVE LYMPHOID HYPERPLASIA (GASTRIC PSEUDOLYMPHOMA OR PSEUDOTUMOR)

It is well known that malignant lymphoma of the stomach has a better overall prognosis than does gastric adenocarcinoma, but early reports of prolonged survival of patients with gastric lymphomas undergoing minimal treatment or none prompted reexamination of these instances. Of 131 instances reviewed, 42 were found not to be malignant lesions but benign proliferations of inflammatory lymphoid tissue [82]. Following this work, the concept of pseudolymphoma, pseudotumor, or reactive lymphoid hyperplasia was developed. Many clinical and pathological symptoms of this lesion are identical with those of true gastric lymphomas, but most authors today consider them to be a nonneoplastic or perhaps a late stage of benign peptic ulcer disease of the stomach.

About 70 instances have been reported [55]. Morphological criteria for separating these benign lymphoid proliferations from their malignant counterparts consist of the presence of inflammatory cells, including plasma cells and neutrophils; evidence of old peptic ulceration; and especially, the presence of germinal centers. Also important is the presence of a benign hyperplasia of regional lymph nodes [55] and a long history of symptoms [33]. Recently immunological criteria that separate benign from malignant proliferations have been developed for identification of lymphocytes [60]. Careful examination using morphological criteria alone also usually succeeds in identifying them. In long follow-up studies of patients with tumors classified as benign, later development of a true lymphoma has been extremely rare, essentially limited to a single instance [93]. This patient is thought to have had a malignant disease that developed independently in the stomach that could not be ascribed to degeneration of the preexisting benign tumor. Despite the benign nature of the disease, many patients require gastric resection because of complications of the basic underlying ulcerative disease, such as uncontrolled bleeding, pyloric outlet stenosis, and perforation. Radiation therapy is not indicated in patients with this lesion.

TUMORS OF NEURAL ORIGIN

Benign gastric neurogenic tumors are chiefly schwannomas (neurilemomas) and neurofibromas. About 189 instances of gastric schwannoma have been reported [94]. These tumors, usually intramural, frequently ulcerate and bleed. Several very large gastric schwannomas have been reported, one weighing 6000 gm [63], and one, 15,572 gm [42].

There are no roentgenographic or endoscopic criteria for diagnosis. Treatment is by wide excision.

Neurofibromas of the stomach may be isolated tumors [34] or may be associated with systemic neurofibromatosis chiefly affecting the skin (von Recklinghausen disease) [72]. The bones and central nervous system may be involved. Many such gastric tumors of this type are overlooked because of the more dramatic nature of the associated lesions. The disease has been considered to be familial, with autosomal dominance and variable expression, occurring in about 1 in 3000 births [49].

Twenty-four instances of isolated gastric neurofibromas and five instances with associated systemic disease were collected up to 1962 [63]. Neurofibromas have been associated with malignant schwannoma [17], carcinoid tumors [5], and adenocarcinoma [39]. There is a tendency for neurofibromas to undergo malignant degeneration in older patients [48].

Solitary neurofibromas of the stomach may arise from the myenteric plexus (Auerbach) or, less frequently, from the submucosal plexus (Meissner) and may project inwardly, outwardly, or both. Solitary tumors are usually encapsulated; in neurofibromatosis, lesions are less well encapsulated.

Epigastric discomfort and bleeding are the chief symptoms. Gastric bleeding in patients with cutaneous neurofibromatosis should always suggest a gastric neurofibroma. Selective arteriography of the celiac and superior mesenteric artery should be performed immediately [71]. Wide excision is the treatment of choice.

HEMANGIOMA

Gastric hemangiomas are rare lesions involving the stomach only but may be secondary to systemic hereditary hemorrhagic telangiectasia (Rendu-Osler-Weber syndrome). Fewer than 50 reports were in the literature by 1967 [8].

There are two views of the origin of hemangiomas. One is that they develop before birth and represent hamartomas rather than true neoplasms [8]. The other view is that they are neoplastic, developing from the normal vasculature of the affected organ [89]. We cannot resolve this problem here.

Thyssen [89] has argued that hemangiomas are more common than has been thought. He suggests that many idiopathic instances of upper gastrointestinal bleeding, stopped without recourse to operation or as a result of partial resection of the stomach for unidentified causes of bleeding (blind cases), are in fact examples of small hemangiomas that have healed spontaneously. While most gastric hemangiomas are smaller than 0.5 cm in diameter, one lesion involving most of the stomach wall was a mass resembling a human placenta [43].

Hemangiomas are usually asymptomatic, but there is a tendency for surface ulceration to produce ulcerlike pain. Bleeding may become acute and life-threatening. Roentgenographic diagnosis is possible when calcified phleboliths can be demonstrated. Endoscopy can often distinguish hemangioma from secondary, highly vascular granulation tissue at the base of an ulcer. Resection of the lesion results in cure without recurrence.

LIPOMA

While fatty tumors are extremely common in soft tissues, they are unusual in the stomach. About 160 instances were reported by 1965 [92]. Undoubtedly many isolated instances are not reported [35].

Benign gastric lipomas are usually in the posterior wall of the pylorus and may produce mechanical obstruction. Most arise from the submucosa and bulge into the lumen of the stomach, but subserosal lipomas are known. In general, the incidence of lipomas increases with obesity of the patient.

Many lipomas are asymptomatic and are found only incidentally to other complaints. Most remain smaller than 10 cm in diameter.

Grossly, lipomas are composed of yellow fat with well-defined margins but are not encapsulated; they may be recognized by the surgeon in the operating room. Local excision is sufficient if malignancy can be ruled out. If there is doubt, subtotal gastrectomy, omentectomy, and splenectomy should be performed.

Lipomas from the duodenal submucosa eventually become pedunculated in the lumen with bleeding and obstruction; those from the serosal surface of the duodenum may be asymptomatic [68]. Treatment is by wide excision or conservative resection (partial or subtotal gastrectomy).

GRANULAR CELL TUMORS

These rare tumors, originally called granular cell myoblastomas, are of unknown histogenesis. They have been reported in many body tissues and organs, but more than half are found in the tongue or in the skin and subcutaneous tissues. Few are in the viscera; about half a dozen have been reported in the stomach [86].

These tumors are virtually asymptomatic except for mild epigastric discomfort and vomiting. The tumors are small, less than 2.5 cm; discrete, but not encapsulated; and fixed to the mucosa. The overlying mucosa is usually intact, without bleeding or ulceration. In two patients multiple tumors were found, all on the greater curvature [76].

Granular cell tumors elsewhere than the stomach may recur after excision, and in at least one patient there were metastases [71]. Radiation therapy is of no use in primary treatment. The treatment of choice is subtotal gastrectomy.

GASTRIC TERATOMA

These rare lesions, of which fewer than 35 have been reported in the world literature [54], are usually discovered in infancy, although three instances in adults are known [29]. All have been in males.

The posterior wall of the stomach is the most frequent site. The tumors are usually exogastric and range from 100 to 1000 gm in weight. In most instances calcification is present. Curiously there is no relation between the age of the patient and the size of the teratoma. Those from adults are among the smallest.

These embyronal tumors have been divided

into dermoid cysts, containing ectodermal and mesodermal elements, and teratomas, containing endodermal tissues as well. Because these large tumors can rarely be thoroughly examined by histological sectioning, it is difficult to confirm the absence of a tissue. We suggest dropping the term *dermoid cyst*. Tissues of teratomas are often "reminiscent and suggestive of adult tissues, yet unlike any specific tissues they might seem to resemble" [67].

The symptoms depend on the location of the tumor. They are usually abdominal distention, vomiting, nausea, and melena. An epigastric mass may be palpable. All reported gastric teratomas have been benign. Excision of the tumor, partial gastrectomy, or in a few instances, total gastrectomy is required.

Malignant Tumors

Only two of the malignant gastric tumors are at all common—non-Hodgkin lymphoma and leiomyosarcoma (Table 26-5). As with benign tumors, clinical diagnosis is difficult and, for some lesions, impossible (Table 26-6).

LEIOMYOSARCOMA

The line between benign and malignant smooth muscle tumors is difficult to draw. Whorls and palisades of cells are more evident in malignant smooth muscle tumors and they are usually without a capsule. The histological criteria for malignancy are still those of Evans [25]:

1. Increased cell size
2. Increased irregularity of cell size and shape
3. Lack of complete cell differentiation
4. Presence of short, plump cells with oval nuclei
5. Presence of cells with hyperchromic and multiple nuclei with variable staining reactions
6. Presence of mitotic figures, some of which are atypical

Unfortunately, metastases have been associated with tumors showing none of the char-

Table 26-5. Incidence of malignant tumors in the stomach and duodenum

Malignant tumors	Sex and age most affected	Incidence in stomach
Leiomyosarcoma	Adults Male 1.7:1	Second most common malignant gastric tumor
Leiomyoblastoma	?	Uncommon
Hemangiopericytoma	Adults Sexes equal	About 20 instances known
Rhabdomyosarcoma	Any age Sexes equal	6 instances in stomach
Lymphoma (Hodgkin)	Male adults	Occurs only secondary to systemic disease late in course
Lymphoma (non-Hodgkin)	Male adults	Most common malignant gastric tumor
Plasmacytoma	Male adults	70 instances
Granulocytic sarcoma	?	1 instance in stomach
Kaposi sarcoma	Young male adults	Rare, secondary to skin disease; ethnic distribution; probably infectious
Malignant schwannoma	Adults	Rare, usually associated with von Recklinghausen disease; 6 solitary instances in GI tract
Ganglioneuroblastoma	Adults	About 7 instances
Liposarcoma	?	About 12 instances

Table 26-6. Malignant tumors of the stomach and duodenum: symptoms, diagnosis, treatment

Malignant tumors	Symptoms	Diagnostic methods and characteristics	Metastases	Treatment
Leiomyosarcoma	Hemorrhage, pain, palpable mass, weight loss	Those of benign leiomyoma; histologic studies at operation	Omental and mesenteric nodes, liver, lung, other abdominal organs	Subtotal gastrectomy
Leiomyoblastoma	Those of leiomyoma	Round or polygonal cells predominant over spindle cells	Mesenteric lymph nodes	Resection
Hemangiopericytoma	Epigastric mass Ulcerlike bleeding; slow growth	Polyp in antrum; histologic studies at operation	Rare; about 15% from extragastric sites	Resection
Rhabdomyosarcoma	Painless, mobile mass	Presence of striated muscle fibers	Rapid, invasive growth; metastasis to lungs, lymph nodes	Early resection; prognosis poor owing to rapid growth
Lymphoma (Hodgkin)	Hemorrhage; other symptoms of disseminated disease	Presence of Reed-Sternberg cells	All lymphoid tissue of stomach or duodenum	Resection if stomach is the only organ affected (stage I)
Lymphoma (non-Hodgkin)	Abdominal pain, weight loss, nausea and vomiting; insidious onset	Mucosal hypertrophy with mass and ulcer; spread of lesion into duodenal cap or into esophagus	Peripheral lymph nodes, lungs, liver, brain	Wide resection, radiotherapy, chemotherapy

Plasmacytoma	Obstruction, occult bleeding	Multicentric lesions; monoclonal tumor with single immunoglobulin type only	Recurrence after surgery; disseminated disease	Resection, radiation, and chemotherapy
Granulocytic sarcoma	Pain, chronic intestinal obstruction; mass and weight loss	Histochemical studies	Eventual fatal myeloid leukemia	Palliative resection only; prognosis poor
Kaposi sarcoma	Skin disease; hemorrhage from upper GI tract	Skin lesions precede visceral involvement	Disseminated from skin	Palliative resection for control of bleeding
Malignant schwannoma	Those of benign schwannoma; often asymptomatic	Associated with von Recklinghausen disease; similar to those of leiomyosarcoma	Invasive, multiple lesions	Wide resection when possible
Ganglioneuroblastoma	Melena, palpable mass, pain	Presence of neuroblasts	Liver	Resection
Liposarcoma	Hemorrhage and pain	Immature fat cells	Possible, but rare	Resection

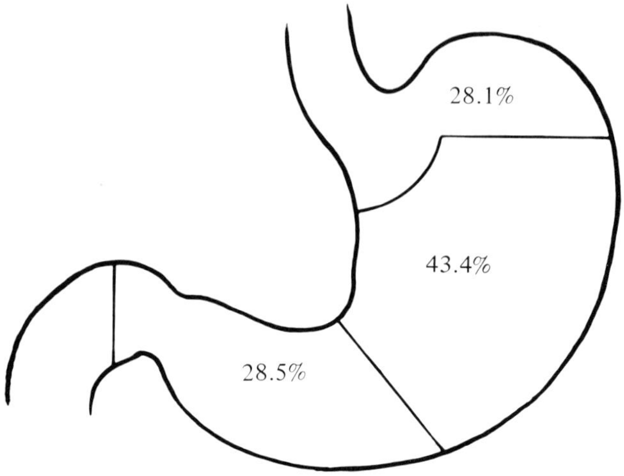

Fig. 26-4. Regions of the stomach in which 140 gastric leiomyosarcomas occurred. This number does not include 12 patients in whom the entire stomach was involved and the site of origin could not be determined. (From Skandalakis and Gray, 1962. Courtesy of Charles C Thomas, Publisher, Springfield, Illinois.)

acteristics listed on p. 735, and one-fourth to one-third of tumors judged malignant have not metastasized. Reports of borderline lesions are rare [73, 79, 81]. Whether this is due to a tendency among pathologists to call doubtful lesions malignant for safety or whether there is no malignant transformation of benign tumors has not yet been settled. New criteria of malignancy are needed.

Among malignant tumors of the stomach, leiomyosarcomas are second only to lymphomas in frequency. From 1938 to 1959, 535 gastric leiomyomas and 260 leiomyosarcomas were reported in the world literature [79], a ratio of 2 : 1. In the duodenum the ratio was 1.2 : 1, similar to that in the jejunum and ileum [72, 73]. Most of the malignant forms are found in patients between the ages of 30 and 70 years, and unlike the benign form, they affect almost twice as many men as women. Their distribution in the stomach is similar to that of leiomyomas (Fig. 26-4).

Duodenal leiomyosarcomas are more common in the second and third portions (Fig. 26-5), and more bulge outward than into the lumen. No symptoms distinguish malignant from benign gastric smooth muscle tumors. Melena or hematemesis is present in just over one-half of patients. The second most common symptom, pain, is present in just under one-half. Neither position in the gastric wall

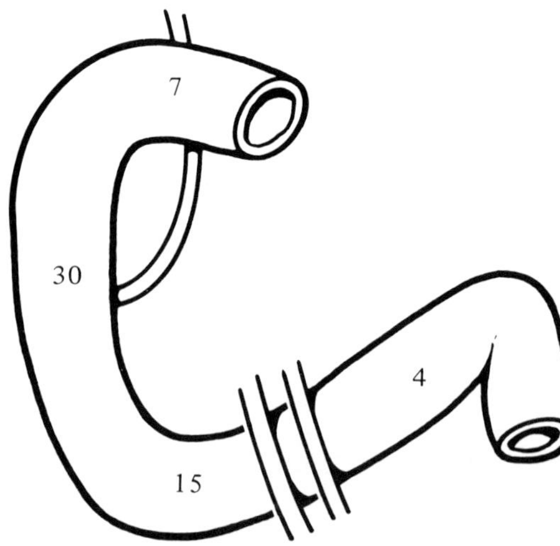

Fig. 26-5. Sites of 56 leiomyosarcomas of the duodenum. Most are found in the second and third portions. Compare with Fig. 26-3.

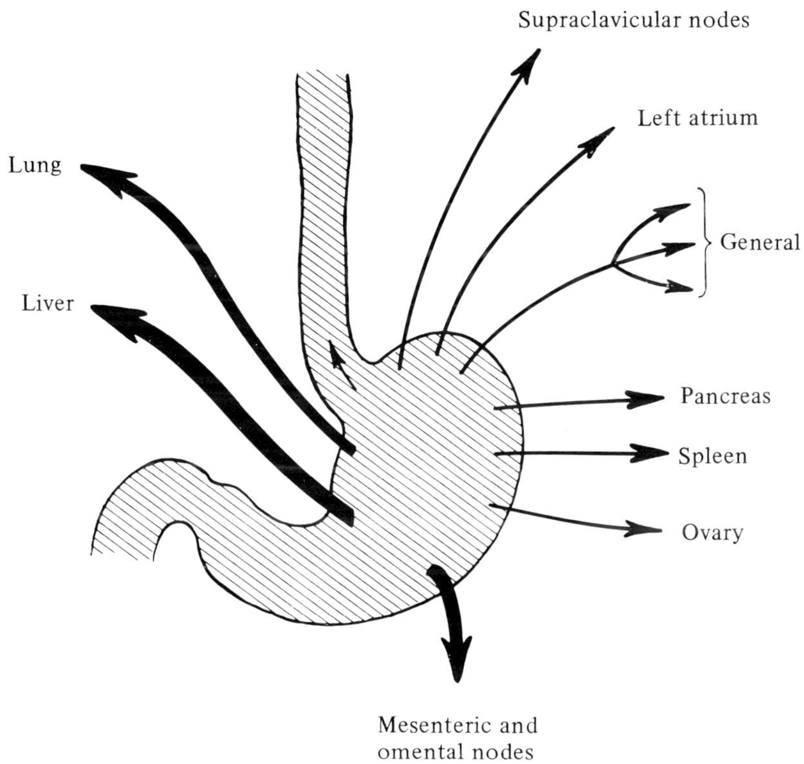

Fig. 26-6. Sites of metastases of 45 malignant smooth muscle tumors of the stomach. More tumors in the proximal stomach metastasized than did those in the distal stomach. Width of *arrows* reflects frequency. (From Skandalakis and Gray, *Smooth Muscle Tumors of the Alimentary Tract,* 1962. Courtesy of Charles C Thomas, Publisher, Springfield, Illinois.)

nor location in the stomach is diagnostic, although more benign than malignant tumors are endogastric, and hence ulcers are more frequent [81].

When metastases from gastric tumors are present, they are, in order of frequency, to liver, mesenteric and omental lymph nodes, and lung. Metastases to pancreas, spleen, ovary, heart, and supraclavicular nodes have all been reported [79] (Fig. 26-6). There are fewer metastases to the lung and more to the distal intestine from duodenal tumors than from gastric tumors (Fig. 26-7).

Gastric leiomyosarcoma should be treated in the same manner as carcinoma. Subtotal gastrectomy is the treatment of choice. Total gastrectomy should be reserved for extensive smooth muscle tumors involving the entire stomach. Distant metastases should not deter the surgeon from performing the planned operation, since leiomyosarcomas grow slowly and the patient may survive many years [78] (Table 26-7). The most recent series have a five-year survival rate of 30–50 percent [44].

The location of a suspected leiomyosarcoma (or any other tumor) in the duodenum requires a special procedure. The second, third, and fourth positions of the duodenum should be explored carefully for small benign or malignant smooth muscle tumors. The following steps will help: (1) performance of a good kocherization by incision of the parietal peritoneum; (2) incision of the transverse mesocolon through the gastrocolic omentum to examine the third portion; (3) further incision of the gastrocolic omentum, reflection of the right colon, and division of the parietal fold

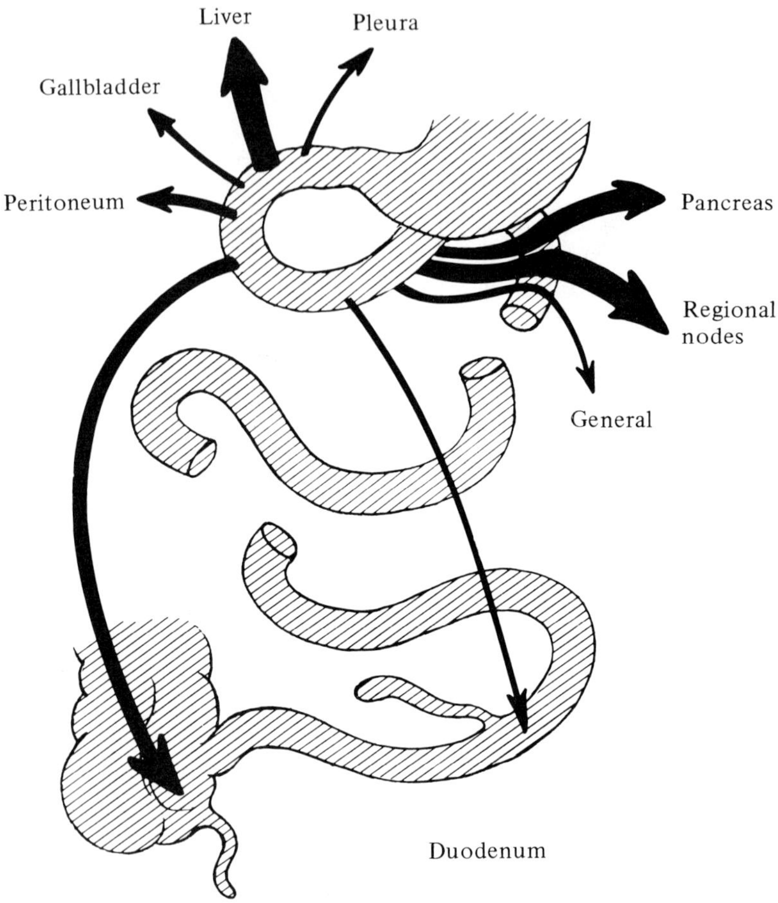

Fig. 26-7. Sites of metastases of 22 malignant smooth muscle tumors of the duodenum. Width of *arrows* reflects frequency. (From Skandalakis and Gray, *Smooth Muscle Tumors of the Alimentary Tract,* 1962. Courtesy of Charles C Thomas, Publisher, Springfield, Illinois.)

inferior to the paraduodenal fossa. Finally, the ligament of Treitz is divided to allow visualization and palpation of the distal duodenum.

LEIOMYOBLASTOMA

First described in 1960 [53], this tumor was named by Stout [83]. It is the "bizarre leiomyoma" of Kay and Still [43]. The tumor contains the spindle cells expected in a leiomyoma as well as polygonal "epithelioid" cells. The relation of this tumor to glomus tumors and pericytomas has been suggested [3, 61, 73].

The coincidental occurrence of a gastric "epithelioid leiomyosarcoma," functional extra-adrenal paraganglioma, and pulmonary chondroma in young female patients has been described by Carney [12]. He considers that the tumors are related, based on the improbability of the simultaneous appearance of such rare tumors.

Leiomyoblastomas are rare-to-common, depending on the bias of the pathologist. DeBray and Martin [18] collected 142 instances from 1960 to 1972. There are no diagnostic symptoms. Recurrence of metastasis may be found in about 10 percent of affected patients [1]. Subtotal gastrectomy is the proper treatment. If metastasis is discovered during an operation or in the postoperative period, combination chemotherapy is indicated [16].

Table 26-7. Mortality from gastric and duodenal leiomyosarcoma

Relative time of death	Gastric leiomyosarcomas (n = 197)	Duodenal leiomyosarcomas (n = 67)
Died without operation (including discovery at autopsy)	27	12
Died immediately postoperatively	16	8
Died less than 1 year postoperatively	16	8
Died more than 1 year postoperatively	7	3
Total	66 (33.5%)	31 (46.3%)

HEMANGIOPERICYTOMA

Reports of primary gastric hemangiopericytoma are few; only about 20 instances have been described. Enzinger and Smith [22] found no gastric tumors among 106 reports of hemangiopericytoma submitted for consultation to the Armed Forces Institute of Pathology. These tumors are thought to be derived from pericytes surrounding some capillaries. These are cells capable of differentiating into smooth muscle cells as well as a variety of connective tissue cell types [69]. The tumors may blend into leiomyoblastomas.

Gastric pericytomas arise in the wall of the stomach and grow slowly, often without visible mitoses. One such tumor in the omentum had been present for 60 years [84]. In another patient, metastases appeared 13 years after complete local removal of the tumor [56]. Pericytomas may become large and produce a palpable mass. Surface ulceration, especially of endogastric tumors, may result in bleeding.

Pericytomas should be treated as potentially malignant. About 15 percent of nongastric hemangiopericytomas eventually metastasize [22]. In several patients, one or more recurrences after surgical treatment have been reported. The treatment of choice is wide resection.

RHABDOMYOSARCOMA

Malignant striated muscle tumors of the stomach are as rare as benign striated tumors. The origin of these striated muscle tumors in organs derived from the primitive foregut is entirely obscure.

Templeton and Heslin [88] reported such a lesion in a three-year-old boy. Both the tumor and the age of the patient when discovered were unusual [51]. There was a tremendous increase in size of the tumor between its discovery and the autopsy six weeks later. Cobalt therapy was ineffective. At autopsy, the entire stomach was found to be involved. The mass extended to the second portions of the duodenum, the left lateral lobe of the liver, the diaphragm, and the pancreas. The only metastasis was to a cervical lymph node. Such rapid growth has been reported in rhabdomyosarcomas elsewhere in the body [28].

If resection of the tumor appears feasible, there should be no delay. "Surgery is a relative emergency" [51].

LYMPHOMA

Lymphoma accounts for about 3 percent of gastric neoplasms, a distant second to gastric carcinoma. While carcinoma has declined in frequency in the last three decades, no such change in lymphoma can be seen. Many exogenous etiologic factors have been implicated in gastric carcinoma, and control of these factors has been cited as a possible cause of the decreasing incidence. No exogenous factors have been identified for lymphoma; hence no potentially preventive measures can be recommended.

DeVita and Hellman [19] listed a number of diseases of chromosomal origin that predispose to lymphoma: Klinefelter's syndrome (XXY); Wiskott-Aldrich syndrome; Swiss type agammaglobulinemia; common variable immunodeficiency syndromes (X-linked recessive); and ataxia-telangiectasia (chromosome 14 anomalies). Other predisposing conditions are receipt of kidney transplant (immunosuppressive therapy), acquired hypogammaglobulinemia, Sjögren's syndrome, rheumatoid arthritis, and systemic lupus erythematosus.

Lymphoma may involve almost any area of the stomach, but the lesser curvature and the anterior and posterior walls are most frequently affected. About one-half of the lymphomas of the gastrointestinal tract occur in the stomach [9].

Diagnosis is often delayed until the tumor becomes very large. Lymphomas more than 10 cm in diameter tend to be multicentric and are not uncommon. They usually develop into a convoluted exophytic mass covered by mucosa, but they may also assume a diffuse, infiltrating pattern similar to the linitis plastica ("leather bottle stomach"). They may also present as giant, hypertrophic rugae with ulceration throughout the mucosa. The histopathology of these tumors is varied, and pathologists recognize a number of separate disease entities. We have discussed the so-called histiocytic lymphomas in the adult gastrointestinal tract in a collective review. [46].

The most obvious division of lymphomas, the one agreed on by almost all workers, is that of Hodgkin disease and non-Hodgkin lymphomas. Hodgkin disease is characterized by the presence of lymphocytes, eosinophils, atypical reticulum cells, and numerous giant mononucleate Hodgkin cells and giant multinucleate Reed-Sternberg cells. The lesion may be primary or diffuse. If the lesion is primary to the stomach or duodenum and no other organs are affected (stage 1), resection should be performed. If the disease is more widespread, resection will not be curative [74]. It usually affects lymph nodes, but it may involve lymphoid tissue of the wall of the gastrointestinal tract. One-third to one-half of the patients with disseminated Hodgkin disease may eventually have gastric lesions, but primary gastric Hodgkin disease is rare or nonexistent [7].

Most gastric lymphomas belong to the non-Hodgkin group. A widely used classification of non-Hodgkin lymphomas is that of Rappaport [66]. It is based on the architecture of the tumor (nodular or diffuse), cytologic factors (lymphocytic or histiocytic), and degree of differentiation. In general, nodular and well-differentiated tumors have the best prognosis.

Lukes and Collins [50] related non-Hodgkin lymphomas to B- or T-lymphocytes and no-marker "null" cells [27, 85]. Some are the "histiocytic" tumors of Rappaport. True histiocytic neoplasms are very rare and should not be considered lymphomas [46]. A third system of classification is that of Lennert and colleagues [47] of Kiel, West Germany. This system separates high-grade and low-grade malignant groups.

Patients with gastric lymphoma complain of epigastric pain, weight loss, and anorexia. This is in contrast to the nausea, vomiting, and hematemesis or melena of gastric carcinoma.

Preoperative diagnosis of malignant gastric lymphoma is difficult. Hodgkin disease is almost impossible to distinguish roentgenologically from gastric carcinoma [58]. Non-Hodgkin lymphomas are usually much larger than carcinomas. Multiple lesions, common in lymphomas, are rare in carcinomas. Destruction of the mucosa and its folds with narrowing of the gastric lumen is usual in gastric carcinoma but not in lymphoma. Because the mucosa over the lymphoma is usually intact, endoscopic biopsy often shows normal or equivocal findings [36]. Gastric perforation through the tumor is possible [24].

Primary gastric lymphomas may be cured by complete resection, so the full extent of the lesion must be determined. Several frozen sections of the proximal and distal edges of the specimen are necessary for this. The tumor extended into the esophagus or duodenum in about one-third of the 81 patients reported on by Hricak and colleagues [36]. Extension to peripheral lymph nodes or metastases to lung, liver, and brain may have occurred by the time the gastric tumor is recognized. Staging of the disease by the Ann Arbor system [11] helps determine the prognosis and treatment for non-Hodgkin lymphomas (Table 26-8).

Prognosis is better for gastric lesions than for intestinal lesions. An early stage (I_E or II_E) or a small lesion (less than 10 cm) carries a

Table 26-8. Ann Arbor staging system

Ann Arbor Stage	Treatment
I_E (disease limited to stomach)	Wide resection with radiotherapy
II_E (disease in stomach and regional nodes)	Wide resection, radiotherapy, and chemotherapy
III_E (disease in stomach, regional nodes, and sites above diaphragm)	Palliative resection only, chemotherapy, and local radiotherapy
IV (widely disseminated disease)	Palliative resection only, chemotherapy, and local radiotherapy

E = extralymphatic spread.
Source: Carbone et al. [11].

good prognosis. The paper of Brady and Asbell [9] should be consulted for a discussion of the factors affecting the prognosis and treatment of malignant lymphomas. Treatment of non-Hodgkin lymphoma is a combination of an operation, radiation, and chemotherapy.

PLASMACYTOMA OF THE STOMACH

A gastric plasmacytoma is a rare malignant neoplasm, with fewer than 70 reports in the world literature. It has been defined by Scott and colleagues [77] as a "monoclonal proliferation of cells forming a single immunoglobulin type with displacement of cells forming other types of immunoglobulins." Patients with this lesion present with epigastric pain, anorexia, weight loss, and weakness. Distal, obstructive lesions in the pylorus may produce nausea and vomiting. Occult gastrointestinal bleeding is not unusual, but melena and massive bleeding rarely occur. This lesion is most common in men in the fourth and fifth decades of life. Gastric plasmacytomas are characteristically intramural, with thinning or occasional ulceration of the overlying mucosa; multicentric lesions are known [30].

It is important to identify these lesions correctly and to differentiate true neoplastic lesions from so-called plasma cell granulomas, which are reactive rather than neoplastic. This can be difficult on morphological grounds alone, but some immunological techniques using immunofluorescence or immunoperoxidase [77] are extremely helpful in distinguishing benign from malignant lesions.

Specific laboratory tests for medullary myeloma are characteristically negative in patients with extramedullary plasmacytoma, including negative dysglobulinemia, Bence-Jones proteins in the urine, bone marrow smears, and bone survey roentgenograms [6]. Even though many of these lesions are technically resectable, prognosis is poor; up to 50 percent of patients die within two years of recurrences or disseminated disease. Recommended treatment includes resection, irradiation, and chemotherapy. Complete remission of symptoms and disappearance of the tumors following chemotherapy has been reported [65]. An indefinite follow-up period with frequent checks for dysglobulinemia is recommended for patients with extramedullary plasmacytomas [30].

GRANULOCYTIC SARCOMA OF THE STOMACH

Occasionally granulocytic leukemia is preceded by a solid tumor manifestation of the disease, namely, granulocytic sarcoma or chloroma, so-called because of its greenish color on cut section. The tumor most frequently involves bones, but two instances have been reported with initial involvement of the stomach and small intestine [10]. Symptoms were epigastric pain, chronic intestinal obstruction, weight loss, and abdominal mass. Surgical excision removes the tumor but does not cure the disease. Overt granulocytic leukemia invariably develops.

KAPOSI SARCOMA

Kaposi sarcoma, first described in 1872 [41], is a peculiar pigmented and multiple neoplastic process primarily involving the skin of the lower extremities but affecting the viscera in approximately 10 percent of patients. The skin lesions are reddish to reddish-brown, often becoming purple or darker in color. These lesions begin as multiple maculae that enlarge and become nodular. Affected viscera include the stomach [70], intestinal tract, lung, liver, lymph nodes, spleen, and bone marrow. When the lesions involve the stomach, as they did in one of Kaposi's patients [41], they frequently ulcerate and produce almost uncontrollable upper gastrointestinal bleeding. Palliative surgical treatment may be indicated to control this complication, but primary treatment is radiotherapy. While indolent in its overall course, with patients living 8 to 10 years after diagnosis, visceral involvement heralds an accelerated course of the disease with poorer prognosis [4].

Until recently the disease has been considered rare, with ethnic and geographical limits. Most affected patients were from southeastern Europe, northern Italy, and central and southern Africa [96].

In 1981 Hymes and associates [37] reported 8 instances of Kaposi sarcoma in young homosexual men in New York City, and the Centers for Disease Control recognized 54 instances between January, 1976 and July, 1981 [13]. The total reached 684 instances of Kaposi sarcoma or serious opportunistic infection by October, 1982. The mortality reached 42.4 percent. Instances were concentrated in, but not limited to, New York and California [31]. Most but by no means all patients were white homosexual men between 25 and 49 years of age [13]. Among heterosexual patients many were intravenous drug abusers. The disease has been identified in hemophiliac and Haitian refugees also. This is in striking contrast to the African and European form of the disease, in which most patients are older and many are female [20].

Kaposi sarcoma is associated with *Pneumocystis carinii* pneumonia [14], Hodgkin disease, and non-Hodgkin lymphoma [52]. One-third of the 90 patients with Kaposi sarcoma at Memorial Sloan-Kettering Cancer Center had two or three concurrent malignant tumors [20]. Both the sarcoma and the pneumonia are the result of a generalized breakdown of the immune response—the acquired immune deficiency syndrome (AIDS)—possibly transmitted by blood, body secretions, or transfusions. Haverkos and Curran [31] discussed four hypothetical causal factors in AIDS: (1) cytomegalovirus, (2) use of nitrite inhalants, (3) immune overload by multiple infections, and (4) a new, unidentified virus or other agent.

MALIGNANT SCHWANNOMA

These tumors are difficult to distinguish from other spindle cell tumors such as leiomyosarcomas. At least three such lesions have been found in the stomach and two in the duodenum [17]. Demonstrable origin from a nerve, a site favored by benign schwannomas, and the absence of myofibrils after phosphotungstic acid stains, are the best criteria for diagnosis. The patient reported on by Croker and Greenstein [17] had concomitant von Recklinghausen disease. The gastric tumor had invaded the liver, and tumor nodules extended along the duodenum and jejunum.

GANGLIONEUROBLASTOMA

A ganglioneuroma is composed of mature autonomic ganglion cells; a ganglioneuroblastoma, the malignant counterpart, contains some neuroblasts [87]. Only seven instances of the latter have been reported in the stomach. Melena, abdominal mass, and epigastric pain are the symptoms. A gastric ulcer may be present.

Ganglioneuromas do not metastasize. They appear in younger patients and are cured by resection. Ganglioneuroblastomas appear in older patients, may metastasize, and have a poor prognosis after resection.

LIPOSARCOMA

These are among the rarest of gastric tumors, fewer than a dozen having been reported. They may grossly resemble benign lipomas, correctly identified only on microscopical examination. No pattern of clinical behavior can be described. In one patient the endogastric tumor had reached a size of 10 by 10 cm without being palpable [32]. Liposarcomas are invasive, are not sharply demarcated, and contain lipoblasts in all stages of differentiation. Ulceration of the mucosa over the tumor produces pain, and uncontrolled bleeding may demand surgical intervention.

Subtotal gastric resection is usually adequate. In one instance, only a biopsy was taken. The patient died without excision of the tumor. Metastasis is rare but probably cannot be ruled out.

Treatment of Nonepithelial Tumors

CHEMOTHERAPY

The gastrointestinal tract is a common site of lymphomas and plasmacytomas; chemotherapy is usually indicated for the diffuse forms of the disease and not for the primary lesion.

Because of the risk of distant metastases in patients with high-grade sarcomas, adjuvant therapy may be useful after local treatment. Studies are ongoing, but adjuvant chemotherapy cannot yet be regarded as conventional treatment. On the other hand, about one-third of patients with disseminated sarcoma respond to cyclophosphamide (Cytoxan), doxorubicin hydrochloride (Adriamycin), or decarbazine (DTIC) [64].

RADIOTHERAPY

The radiotherapy for most nonepithelial tumors of the stomach and duodenum is similar to that for adenocarcinoma therapy: 4000–5000 rads if there is known microscopical residual disease. Nonresectable duodenal sarcoma may be palliated by irradiation, and an occasional histological type will respond to fairly high dosages [40].

Radiation therapy and resection alone appear to be equally effective in controlling stage I lymphoma. Both forms of therapy together are better than either alone for stage II disease. Among 81 patients with stage I and II tumors, 68 percent who failed to respond had recurrence outside the primary field, and 60 percent had metastases outside the abdomen [95].

SURGICAL TREATMENT

The surgical treatment of these tumors ranges from simple excision to total gastrectomy, and occasionally, to superradical procedures that may include removal of the spleen, transverse colon, and greater and lesser omenta. The procedure used in any patient is governed by the answers to the following questions:

1. Is the tumor benign or malignant?
2. How large is it, and where is it?
3. Is it endogastric, exogastric, or intramural?
4. Is it fixed to neighboring structures?
5. Are any lymph nodes involved?
6. Is there evidence of metastasis?

The answers to these questions must be evaluated against the known natural history of the specific tumor and the age and general condition of the patient. In addition, the surgeon must be familiar with the anatomical basis of gastric and duodenal surgery, the physiology that may be changed by the operation, and the pathological changes that may take place as a result of surgical treatment in its absence.

Benign Tumors

If the tumor is benign and small, excisional biopsy, not enucleation or simple biopsy, is the proper procedure. Enucleation, however, should be considered if the tumor lies close to the papilla of Vater or if the age and condition of the patient do not permit a more radical operation. At the other extreme is the giant, ulcerated leiomyoma that, even though benign, dictates a proximal or distal subtotal gastrectomy.

Malignant Tumors

STOMACH. Embryologically, anatomically, and pathologically, the treatment of choice of malignant tumors of the stomach ought to be total gastrectomy with removal of the abdominal esophagus and the proximal duodenum. If the tumor has spread, the spleen, greater and lesser omenta, and transverse colon should be sacrificed. The morbidity and mortality, postoperative complications, and survival rates, however, dictate less radical procedures.

Most surgeons today use a 75–80 percent subtotal, proximal, or distal gastrectomy. The omenta and gastrocolic ligament should be removed. The spleen must be sacrificed with proximal gastric resection but should be saved if possible with distal gastric resection.

The blood supply of the proximal gastric pouch depends on three sources: (1) the ascending branch of the left gastric artery, (2) the short gastric arteries, and (3) the posterior gastric artery, if present. If the spleen is removed, the short gastric arteries must be sacrificed. Every effort should be made to avoid the ascending branches of the left gastric arteries. Adhesions of the posterior gastric wall must not be cut, as such "adhesions" may contain the posterior gastric artery.

In summary, proximal or distal subtotal gastrectomy is the treatment of choice for malignant nonepithelial tumors of the stomach. With proximal gastrectomy, a complementary pyloroplasty is necessary for good gastric emptying. The reconstruction procedure should always (if any procedure can be recommended "always") be a Billroth II anastomosis, modified to the liking of the surgeon.

For unresectable lesions, clips should be placed to help the roentgenologist locate the area to be irradiated. Palliative bypass procedures may be used for huge unresectable tumors of the duodenum, but not for tumors of the stomach.

DUODENUM. When the diagnosis of a malignant tumor of the duodenum is established, and if the age and general condition of the patient permit, the procedure of choice is pancreatoduodenectomy. If the lesion is small and proximal to the ampulla of Vater, however, segmental resection with antrectomy is advisable. For a lesion close to the ampulla, pancreatoduodenectomy should be performed. For a lesion distal to the ampulla, segmental resection will suffice.

The surgeon should remember the blood supply of the duodenum and head of the pancreas and must not ligate the superior and inferior pancreatoduodenal arteries. Such a ligation will produce duodenal ischemia and necrosis. The surgeon should remember that in 10 percent of instances the patient has only one pancreatic duct, the accessory duct (of Santorini). Ligation of this duct would be catastrophic. The duct of Santorini is always located just beneath the gastroduodenal artery.

References

1. Abramson, D. J. Leiomyoblastomas of the stomach. *Surg. Gynecol. Obstet.* 136:118, 1973.
2. Almagro, U. A., Schulte, W. J., Norback, D. H., and Turcotte, J. K. Glomus tumor of the stomach. *Am. J. Clin. Pathol.* 74:415, 1981.
3. Appelman, H. D., and Helwig, E. B. Gastric epithelial leiomyoma and leiomyosarcoma (leiomyoblastoma). *Cancer* 38:708, 1976.
4. Balthazar, E. J., and Richman, A. Kaposi's sarcoma of the stomach. *Am. J. Gastroenterol.* 67:375, 1977.
5. Barber, P. V. Carcinoid tumor of the ampulla of Vater associated with cutaneous neurofibromatous. *Postgard. Med. J.* 52:514, 1976.
6. Barzilai, A., Toledano, C., BenAriz, J., et al. Plasmacytoma of the gastrointestinal tract. *World J. Surg.* 1:267, 1977.
7. Bockus, H. C. (Ed.). *Gastroenterology* (3rd ed.), Vol. 1. Philadelphia: Saunders, 1974.
8. Bongiovi, J. J., and Duffy, J. L. Gastric hemangioma associated with upper gastrointestinal bleeding. *Arch. Surg.* 95:93, 1967.
9. Brady, L. W., and Asbell, S. O. Malignant lymphoma of the gastrointestinal tract. *Radiology* 137:291, 1980.
10. Brugo, E. A., Marshall, R. B., Riberi, A. M., and Pautasso, D. E. Preleukemic granulocytic sarcomas of the gastrointestinal tract. *Am. J. Clin. Pathol.* 68:616, 1977.
11. Carbone, P. P., Kaplan, H. S., Musshoff, K., et al. Report of the Committee on Hodgkin's Disease Staging Classification. *Cancer Res.* 31:1860, 1971.
12. Carney, J. A. The triad of gastric epithelioid leiomyosarcoma, functioning extra-adrenal paraganglioma, and pulmonary chondroma. *Surg. Rounds* 6:32, 1983.
13. Centers for Disease Control. Follow-up on Kaposi's sarcoma and *Pneumocystis* pneumonia. *Morbid. Mortal. Weekly Rep.* 30:409, 1981.
14. Centers for Disease Control. A cluster of Kaposi's sarcoma and *Pneumocystis carinii* pneumonia among homosexual male residents of Los Angeles and Orange Counties, California. *Morbid. Mortal. Weekly Rep.* 31:305, 1982.
15. Chaffin, L. Smooth muscle tumors of the stomach: Review of the literature with report of a case (leiomyosarcoma) *Western J. Surg.* 46:513, 1938.
16. Chaudhuri, P. K., Nyhus, L. M., and Das Gupta, T. K. Sarcoma of the Stomach. In S. I. Schwartz and H. Ellis (Eds.), *Maingot's Abdominal Operations* (8th ed.). Norwalk, Con-

necticut: Appleton-Century-Crofts, 1985.
17. Croker, J. R., and Greenstein, R. J. Malignant schwannoma of the stomach in a patient with von Recklinghausen's disease. *Histopathology* 3:79, 1979.
18. DeBray, C., and Martin, E. Benign Gastric Tumors. In H. L. Bockus (Ed.), *Gastroenterology* Philadelphia: Saunders, 1974.
19. DeVita, V. T., Jr., and Hellman, S. Hodgkin's Disease and the Non-Hodgkin's Lymphomas. In V.T. DeVita, S. Hellman, and S. A. Rosenberg (Eds.), *Cancer, Principles and Practice of Oncology*. Philadelphia: Lippincott, 1982.
20. DiGiovanna, J. J., and Safai, B. Kaposi's sarcoma. *Am. J. Med.* 71:779, 1981.
21. Eimoto, T., Miyake, M., and Sasaki, T. Vascular leiomyoblastoma of the stomach. *Acta Pathol. Jpn.* 29:277, 1979.
22. Enzinger, F. M., and Smith, B. H. Hemangiopericytoma: An analysis of 106 cases. *Hum. Pathol.* 7:61, 1976.
23. von Erlach. Uber ein Myom des Magens und ein Myofibrom der Nierenkapfel. *Wien. Klin. Wochenschr.* 8:272, 1895.
24. Espinosa, M. H., and Salcedo, W. G. Primary gastric lymphoma presenting as gastric perforation: A case report and review of literature. *Abdom. Surg.* 25:10, 1983.
25. Evans, R. W. *Histological Appearances of Tumors*. Edinburgh: Livingstone, 1956.
26. Fayemi, A. O., and Toker, C. Gastrointestinal fibroma. *Am. J. Gastroenterol.* 62:250, 1974.
27. Foucar, K., McKenna, R. W., Frizzera, G., and Brunning, R. D. Incidence and patterns of bone marrow and blood involvement by lymphoma in relationship to the Lukes-Collins classification. *Blood* 54:1417, 1979.
28. Gordon-Taylor, G. On sarcoma of muscles and connective-tissue spaces of limbs. *Br. J. Surg.* 28:1, 1941.
29. Gray, S. W., Johnson, H. C., Jr., and Skandalakis, J. E. Gastric teratoma in an adult: With a review of the literature. *South. Med. J.* 57:1346, 1964.
30. Hara, H., Yamane, T., and Yamashita, K. Extramedullary plasmacytoma of the gastrointestinal tract in a renal transplant recipient. *Acta Pathol. Jpn.* 29:661, 1979.
31. Haverkos, H. W., and Curran, J. W. The current outbreak of Kaposi's sarcoma and opportunistic infections. *CA* 32:330, 1982.
32. Hawkins, P. E., and Terrell, G. K. Liposarcoma of the stomach. *J.A.M.A.* 191:154, 1965.
33. Highman, L. M., Fantelli, F. J., and Hermann, R. E. Pseudolymphoma of the stomach. *Arch. Surg.* 116:227, 1981.
34. Hoare, A. M., and Elkington, S. G. Gastric lesions in generalized neurofibromatosis. *Br. J. Surg.* 63:449, 1976.
35. Hohf, R. P., Engel, K. L., and Capos, N. J. Liposarcoma of the stomach. *Ann. Surg.* 142:1029, 1955.
36. Hricak, H., Thoeni, R. F., Margulis, A. R., et al. Extension of gastric lymphoma into the esophagus and duodenum. *Radiology* 135:309, 1980.
37. Hymes, K. B., Greene, J. B., Marcus, A., et al. Kaposi's sarcoma in homosexual men: A report of eight cases. *Lancet* 2:598, 1981.
38. Ingelman-Sundberg, A., Lindgren, L., Ryden, G., and Sandberg, F. The spontaneous motility of uterine fibromyomata and their responses to pharmacological stimuli. *Acta Obstet. Gynecol. Scand.* 36:263, 1957.
39. Jenkins, D. H. R., and Gill. W. A case of carcinoma of the colon in association with neurofibromatosis. *Br. J. Surg.* 59:322, 1972.
40. Jones, N. E. Personal communication, 1982.
41. Kaposi, M. Idiopathic multiple pigmented sarcoma of the skin. *Arch. Dermatol. Syphilis* 4:265, 1872. Translated in *CA* 32:342, 1982.
42. Katz, L. D., Creech, J. L., and Makk, L. Giant retroperitoneal sarcoma of nerve sheath origin. *South. Med. J.* 67:349, 1974.
43. Kay, S., and Still, W. J. S. A comparative electron microscopic study of a leiomyosarcoma and bizarre leiomyoma (leiomyoblastoma) of the stomach. *Am. J. Clin. Pathol.* 52:403, 1969.
44. Kerekes, E. S. Gastric hemangioma: A case report. *Radiology* 82:468, 1964.
45. Kieffer, R. W., McSwain, B., and Adkins, R. B. Sarcoma of the gastrointestinal tract. *Am. Surg.* 48:167, 1982.
46. Lee, J. R., Gray, S. W., Brown, B. C., and Skandalakis, J. E. Diffuse "histiocytic" lymphomas of the adult gastrointestinal tract. *Surg. Gynecol. Obstet.* 157:286, 1983.
47. Lennert, K., Mohri, N., Stein, H., and Kaiserling, E. The histopathology of malignant lymphoma. *Br. J. Haematol.* 31:193, 1975.
48. Levy, D., and Khatib, R. Intestinal neurofibromatosis with malignant degeneration. *Dis. Colon Rectum* 3:140, 1960.
49. Lukash, W. M., Morgan, R. I., Sennert, C. O., and Nielson, O. F. Gastrointestinal neoplasms in von Recklinghausen's disease. *Arch. Surg.* 92:905, 1968.
50. Lukes, R. J., and Collins, R. D. A functional

approach to the classification of malignant lymphoma. *Recent Results Cancer Res.* 46:18, 1974.
51. Mahour, G. H., Isaacs, H., Jr., and Chang, L. Primary malignant tumors of the stomach in children. *J. Pediatr. Surg.* 15:603, 1980.
52. Mann, S. G. Kaposi's sarcoma: Experience with ten cases. *Am. J. Roentgenol.* 121:793, 1974.
53. Martin, J. F., Bazin, P., Feroldi, J., and Cabanne, F. Tumeurs myoides intramurales de l'estomac: Considerations microscopiques a propos de 6 cas. *Arch. Anat. Pathol.* 5:484, 1960.
54. Matias, I. C., and Huang, Y. C. Gastric teratoma in infancy: Report of a case and review of world literature. *Ann. Surg.* 178:631, 1973.
55. Mattingly, S. S., Cibull, M. L., Ram, M. D., et al. Pseudolymphoma of the stomach. *Arch. Surg.* 116:25, 1981.
56. McCormack, K. J., and Gallivan, W. F. Hemangiopericytoma. *Cancer* 7:595, 1954.
57. Meissner, W. A. Leiomyoma of stomach. *Arch. Pathol.* 38:207, 1944.
58. Menuck, L. S. Gastric lymphoma: A radiologic diagnosis. *Gastrointest. Radiol.* 1:157, 1976.
59. Morgagni, G. B. *The Seats and Causes of Diseases.* Translated by Benjamin Alexander. London 1769, Vol 1, Letter XIX, Article 58. New York: Hafner, 1960.
60. Mori, S., Mohri, N., and Shimamine, T. Reactive lymphoid hyperplasia of the stomach. *Acta Pathol. Jpn.* 30:671, 1980.
61. Osamura, R. Y., Watanabe, K., Yoneyama, K., and Hayashi, T. Glomus tumor of the stomach: Light and electron microscopic study with literature review of related tumors. *Acta Pathol. Jpn.* 27:533, 1977.
62. Palmer, E. D. Benign intramural tumors of the stomach: A review with special reference to gross pathology. *Medicine* 30:81, 1951.
63. Perea, V. D., and Gregory, L. J. Neurofibromatosis of the stomach. *J.A.M.A.* 182:259, 1962.
64. Peroutka, K. Personal communication, 1982.
65. Preud'homme, J. L., Galian, A., Danon, F., et al. Extramedullary plasmacytoma with gastric and lymph node involvement: An immunological study. *Cancer* 46:1753, 1980.
66. Rappaport, H. *Atlas of Tumor Pathology.* Sect. 3, Fasc. 8, Tumor pathology of the hematopoietic system. A.F.I.P., Washington, D. C., 1966.
67. Ravitch, M. M., and McGoon, D. C. Chapter 13. In I. M. Ariel and G. T. Pack (Eds.), *Cancer and Allied Diseases of Infancy and Childhood.* Boston: Little, Brown, 1960.
68. Reddy, R. R., Schuman, B. M., and Priest, R. J. Duodenal polyps: Diagnosis and management. *J. Clin. Gastroenterol.* 3:139, 1981.
69. Rhodin, J. A. G. Ultrastructure of mammalian venous capillaries, venules, and small collecting veins. *J. Ultrastruct. Res.* 25:452, 1968.
70. Richey, L. E., Jr., and Cooley, R. N. Kaposi's sarcoma: The radiographic manifestations of involvement of the stomach. *Gastroenterology* 44:195, 1963.
71. Ross, R. C., Miller, T. R., and Foote, F. W., Jr. Malignant granular cell myoblastoma. *Cancer* 5:112, 1952.
72. Rutgeerts, P., Hendrickx, H., Geboes, K., et al. Involvement of the upper digestive tract by systemic neurofibromatosis. *Gastrointest. Endosc.* 27:22, 1981.
73. Salazar, H., and Totten, R. S. Leiomyoblastoma of the stomach: An ultrastructural study. *Cancer* 25:176, 1970.
74. Schamaun, M. Surgical Treatment in Hodgkin's Disease. In *Progress in Lymphology. Proceeding of International Symposium on Lymphology,* Zurich, Switzerland, July 19–23, 1966. Stuttgart: Thieme, 1967.
75. Schindler, R., and Letendre, P. Analysis of relationship of surgery and gastroscopy in 95 cases of gastric tumor. *Surg. Gynecol. Obstet.* 75:547, 1942.
76. Schwartz, D. T., and Gaetz, H. P. Multiple granular cell myoblastomas of the stomach. *Am. J. Clin. Pathol.* 44:453, 1965.
77. Scott, F. E. T., Path, F. R. C., Dupont, P. A., and Webb, J. Plasmacytoma of the stomach: Diagnosis with the aid of the immunoperoxidase technique. *Cancer* 41:675, 1978.
78. Skandalakis, J. E., and Gray, S. W. *Smooth Muscle Tumors of the Alimentary Tract.* Springfield, Ill. Thomas, 1962.
79. Skandalakis, J. E., and Gray, S. W. Smooth muscle tumors of the small intestine. *Am. J. Gastroenterol.* 42:172, 1964.
80. Skandalakis, J. E., Gray, S. W., and Shepard, D. Leiomyoma and leiomyosarcoma of the stomach. *South. Med. J.* 53:540, 1960.
81. Skandalakis, J. E., Gray, S. W., and Shepard, D. Smooth muscle tumors of the stomach. *Surg. Gynecol. Obstet.* 110:209, 1960.
82. Smith, J. L., and Helwig, E. B. Malignant lymphoma of the stomach: Its diagnosis and biological behavior. *Am. J. Pathol.* 34:553, 1958.

83. Stout, A. P. Bizarre smooth muscle tumors of the stomach. *Cancer* 15:400, 1962.
84. Stout, A. P., and Cassell, C. Hemangiopericytoma of the omentum. *Surgery* 13:578, 1943.
85. Strauahen, J. A., Young, R. C., DeVita, V. T., et al. Clinical relevance of the histopathological subclassification of diffuse "histiocytic" lymphoma. *N. Engl. J. Med.* 299:1382, 1978.
86. Strong, E. W., McDivitt, R. W., and Brasfield, R. D. Granular cell myoblastoma. *Cancer* 25:415, 1970.
87. Tapp, E. Ganglioneuroblastoma of the stomach. *J. Pathol. Bacteriol.* 88:79, 1964.
88. Templeton, A. W., and Heslin, D. J. Primary rhabdomyosarcoma of the stomach and esophagus. *Am. J. Roentgenol.* 86:896, 1961.
89. Thyssen, J. Haemangioma of the stomach: A cause of ulcer and of gastric haemorrhage. *Acta Chir. Scand.* 343:227, 1965.
90. Toker, C. Glomangioma: An ultrastructural study. *Cancer* 23:487, 1969.
91. Tuazon, R. Rhabdomyoma of the stomach. *Am. J. Clin. Pathol.* 52:37, 1969.
92. Turkington, R. W. Gastric lymphoma: Report of a case and review of the literature. *Am. J. Dig. Dis.* 10:719, 1965.
93. Valdes-Dapena, A., Affolter, H., and Vilardell, F. The gradient of malignancy in lymphoid lesions of the stomach. *Gastroenterology* 50:382, 1966.
94. Warren, K. W., and Wiltmann, C. J. Neurilemoma of the stomach appearing as an abdominal mass. *Lahey Clin. Bull.* 17:96, 1968.
95. Weingrad, D., Drosse, F., Sherlock, P., et al. Primary gastrointestinal lymphoma. A 3 year review. *Cancer* 49:1258, 1982.
96. White, J. A. M., and King, M. H. Kaposi's sarcoma presenting with abdominal symptoms. *Gastroenterology* 46:197, 1964.

VII

Pediatric Diseases of the Stomach and Duodenum

27

Pediatric Diseases of the Stomach and Duodenum

Lewis Spitz

PART I
The Stomach

Congenital Gastric Outlet Obstructions

HISTORICAL NOTES

The first descriptions of pyloric atresia are attributed to Wuensche in 1875 [195] and Neale in 1884 [117]. In 1937 Bennett [15] reported on a four-day-old infant operated on for pyloric stenosis who died 36 hours postoperatively. Necropsy revealed a complete prepyloric diaphragm. The first report of a successful surgical correction was by Touroff and Sussman in 1940 [178], who excised a prepyloric diaphragm in a five-day-old female infant. Since that time there have been sporadic case reports and various reviews of the literature [10, 12, 30, 63, 64].

PATHOLOGY

Gerber and Aberdeen [63] proposed the most acceptable classification of congenital gastric outlet obstructions:

1. Pyloric
   a. Membrane
   b. Atresia
2. Antral (1 cm or more proximal to the pylorus)
   a. Membrane
   b. Atresia

Antral or prepyloric diaphragms are more common than pyloric obstructions [92]. The diaphragms are commonly perforated, resulting in a partial obstruction with consequent diagnostic difficulties. The membrane consists of mucosa and submucosa without an intervening muscular layer.

CLINICAL FEATURES

The clinical presentation depends on whether the obstruction is complete or incomplete. In complete obstructions (atresias, nonperforated diaphragm) vomiting of nonbilious gastric contents is evident from birth. There may be moderate upper abdominal distention, and vigorous gastric peristaltic waves may be visible in the left hypochondrium. Polyhydramnios, frequently associated with congenital high intestinal obstructions, may have been present during the last trimester of pregnancy.

With incomplete obstructions (perforated diaphragm), presentation most commonly occurs in the neonatal period or in early infancy. Occasionally the diagnosis is not appreciated until adult life [124]. Recurrent vomiting of nonbilious material is a constant presenting symptom. The vomiting is often forceful and in early infancy is frequently attributed to pyloric stenosis. Older children and adults complain of early satiety and fullness associated with episodes of nausea and vomiting.

INVESTIGATIONS

In newborn infants with a complete obstruction, the plain abdominal roentgenogram shows a dilated gas-filled stomach with no air passing into the distal intestine. Vigorous gastric contraction waves may be seen. In such situations there is no justification for further investigations or the use of radiopaque contrast material. With incomplete obstructions the plain abdominal roentgenogram is of little diagnostic value. Barium contrast studies may reveal a thin, sharp, transverse filling defect approximately 1–2 cm proximal to the pyloric canal. Delayed gastric emptying is usually present. Upper gastrointestinal fiberoptic endoscopy should be carried out to confirm the diagnosis. Characteristic features consist of visualization of the antral membrane, which contains a central aperture through which the pylorus can be seen. The surface of the membrane appears identical to the adjacent gastric mucosa, and there is no evidence of inflammation or scarring [13].

ASSOCIATED ANOMALIES

A familial occurrence has been noted in the literature [8, 30, 53, 120]. A significant proportion (28 percent) of associated anomalies (particularly congenital cardiac malformations) was noted by Bell et al. [12]. The association of pyloric atresia with epidermolysis bullosa [8, 53, 97] is invariably fatal.

TREATMENT

Atresias

A bypass procedure, gastroduodenostomy should be possible in all instances. Gastrojejunostomy is a procedure to be avoided because there is an unacceptably high incidence of stomal ulcers.

Membrane-Diaphragm

It is mandatory to confirm the diagnosis endoscopically before proceeding. Identification of the diaphragm during an operation may be difficult. A useful maneuver is to pass a Foley catheter into the duodenum, inflate the balloon, and gently withdraw the catheter. A gastrotomy is centered at the site of arrest of the catheter. The diaphragm is excised and the mucosal defect sutured [13]. The gastrotomy may be closed transversely as a pyloroplasty if an adequate gastric outlet is otherwise not feasible.

At the Hospital for Sick Children, London, two infants with pyloric atresia have been seen over the past decade. Both infants died. One had associated epidermolysis bullosa, and the other, multiple additional gastrointestinal anomalies.

Spontaneous Perforation of the Stomach in Infancy

HISTORICAL NOTES

Perforation or rupture of the stomach in the neonatal period has been observed with increasing frequency since the original description of this entity by von Siebold in 1826 [186]. More than a century later, Stern reported one of the earliest attempts at surgical intervention, but it was not until 1950 that closure of a neonatal gastric perforation was successfully performed [102].

ETIOLOGY

The etiology and pathogenesis of the condition remain obscure. Before 1943 most instances were attributed to acute peptic ulceration. Evidence to substantiate this hypothesis was provided by Miller [114], who showed high levels of gastric acid secretion in the first 48 hours of life.

In 1943 Herbut [78] postulated a congenital muscular deficiency as the basic cause. The histological finding of a muscular deficit at the edge of the perforation lent support to this theory, which received general acceptance. Shaw et al. [152], in experimental studies on puppies and stillborn infants, produced evidence to refute Herbut's theory. They showed that potential weak points between interlacing muscle bundles were normal anatomical features of the neonatal stomach [96]. Rupture may occur when distention is sufficient to force apart the muscle bundles. The histological features of muscle absence at the edge of the perforation are nonspecific findings, more likely the result of retraction than agenesis.

Gastric ischemia as the major predisposing factor to rupture has generally been adopted as the favored theory. Touloukian [177] was able to demonstrate significant perinatal complications predisposing to asphyxia in all six of his patients as well as in 69 percent of patient reports collected from the literature. Five of the six patients and 41 percent of patients reviewed showed histopathological evidence of gastric ischemia as manifested by mucosal hemorrhage, ulceration, or necrosis. Pneumatic rupture caused by incoordination and immaturity of the vomiting mechanism has recently been postulated as the more logical theory [79, 81, 149].

Other factors, such as gastric outlet obstruction, mechanical trauma from nasogastric or gastrostomy tubes, and septicemia, have also been implicated in the pathogenesis of the condition.

CLINICAL FEATURES

Most instances of spontaneous perforation occur on the second to fifth day of life [84, 86, 151]. Approximately two-thirds of instances occur in premature infants [126]. The clinical course of the condition is remarkably constant. The first evidence of impending difficulty is usually a decreased intake of milk. Respiratory distress often associated with cyanosis then supervenes. Abdominal distention occurs either concomitantly or some hours later, increases rapidly, and further aggravates the respiratory embarrassment.

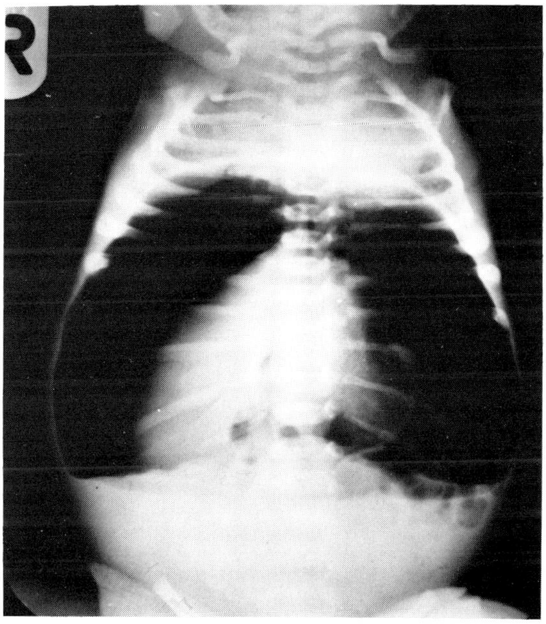

Fig. 27-1. Erect abdominal roentgenogram in a 4-day-old infant with massive abdominal distention and severe respiratory distress, showing a large amount of free intraperitoneal gas (tension pneumoperitoneum).

The presence of edema or erythema of the anterior abdominal wall signifies delayed diagnosis and is associated with an increased mortality. Hypothermia has similar prognostic implications.

INVESTIGATIONS

The erect abdominal roentgenogram usually leads to diagnosis (Fig. 27-1). Pneumoperitoneum with or without evidence of free fluid is invariably present, indicating a gastrointestinal perforation. The absence of a gastric air-fluid level and a paucity of gas in the intestine are more specific signs of a gastric perforation [127].

TREATMENT

Once the diagnosis has been established, urgent resuscitation is required in preparation for surgical intervention. Hypovolemia is corrected by intravenous administration of plasma, 20 ml/kg body weight, as rapidly as possible. Broad-spectrum antibiotic chemotherapy (gentamicin, penicillin, and metronidazole) is given by the intravenous route. Hypothermia is corrected and body temperature maintained. When there are signs of respiratory embarrassment, needle aspiration of the peritoneal cavity may be a life-saving maneuver. In all instances nasogastric decompression is essential in preventing further abdominal distention. Resuscitation should be prompt and should not be unduly prolonged.

Abdominal exploration is carried out by a transverse upper abdominal muscle-cutting incision. The perforation, which in most instances is located at or near the greater curvature of the stomach, is identified [84]. The edges of the defect should be trimmed to excise any ischemic tissue, and the defect is closed in two layers with chromic catgut. Silk sutures should be avoided, especially on the mucosal surface, because they may form a nidus for future peptic ulceration. A tube gastrostomy with or without a transpyloric jejunal feeding tube greatly facilitates the postoperative care.

The postoperative management consists of withholding oral or gastrostomy feedings for at least five days, during which nutrients are administered either by the transpyloric tube or parenterally.

At the Hospital for Sick Children, London, eight infants with spontaneous perforation of the stomach were seen in the 14-year period 1964–1978 [135]. Seven of the eight infants were premature and all were less than four days old. Five of the infants survived surgical closure of the rupture.

Volvulus of the Stomach

HISTORICAL NOTES

The first reported instance of gastric volvulus in a child was in 1902 by Dujon [51]. Before this Berti [19] in 1866 had reported the necropsy finding of a volvulus in a 60-year-old woman. Cole and Dickinson [39] reviewed the world literature in 1971 and could trace only 44 instances in infants and children. Wastell and Ellis [187] found 206 instances, mainly in adults, in an extensive review of the literature to 1971.

CLASSIFICATION

Volvulus occurs when the stomach undergoes a rotation that results in complete obstruction of its lumen. Two types are recognized [158]:

1. *Mesenterioaxial.* Rotation occurs around a vertical axis, which is at right angles to a line joining the pylorus and the cardia (common variety).
2. *Organoaxial.* Rotation occurs around an axis at right angles to a line connecting the gastric cardia and pylorus.

CLINICAL FEATURES

The most constant symptom of gastric volvulus is vomiting or retching, which may or may not be productive. The classical diagnostic triad of Borchardt [25], consisting of (1) nonproductive retching, (2) acute localized gastric distention and pain, and (3) inability to have a nasogastric tube passed into the stomach, is of limited value in this age group.

INVESTIGATIONS

The plain erect abdominal roentgenogram shows a distended stomach often containing two fluid levels, one in the fundus, which is inferior, and the other in the antrum, which is superior [198]. If barium can be made to pass through the esophagogastric junction, a contrast meal will confirm the upside-down position of the stomach. The contrast will outline a beaklike narrowing of the distal stomach with twisting of the gastric mucosal folds.

ASSOCIATED ANOMALIES

There is a high incidence of associated diaphragmatic defects in children with gastric volvulus. In 43 patients reviewed by Cole and Dickinson [39], 28 (65 percent) had either eventration or hernia of the left diaphragm.

This diaphragmatic anomaly is even more frequent in infants less than 12 months of age (81 percent). Malrotation is also frequently present.

TREATMENT

Acute gastric volvulus constitutes a surgical emergency. Prolonged or vigorous attempts at nasogastric decompression should be avoided because perforation of the distal esophagus may occur. At laparotomy, gastric decompression by needle aspiration may be necessary before any manipulation [4]. A careful search is made for any diaphragmatic defect. Fixation of the stomach may be effected either to the anterior abdominal wall (anterior gastropexy) or under the surface of the diaphragm [143]. Recurrence following fixation has been reported.

Swallowed Foreign Bodies in Children

Most ingested foreign bodies causing problems do so in the esophagus (20–30 percent). Once the foreign object has entered the stomach, uneventful passage through the intestinal tract can be expected in more than 90 percent of instances. The levels at which progress may be impeded are the pylorus, duodenum, ileocecal region, and sites of developmental anomalies, such as stenoses and diverticula [164]. The indications for surgical removal of a foreign body in the stomach are danger of perforation and failure of progression.

Perforation may result from the ingestion of a long, slender object with sharp ends, such as a hairpin, needle, pencil, or open safety pin. The danger is especially severe in children younger than two years of age. The development of abdominal pain or tenderness or gastrointestinal bleeding in such a patient under observation constitutes an indication for surgical treatment.

To evaluate progression, a minimum period of two to three weeks of observation before an operation is recommended. Investigations for a possible cause of failure of progression, for example, pyloric stenosis [109] should precede attempts at removal of the foreign object.

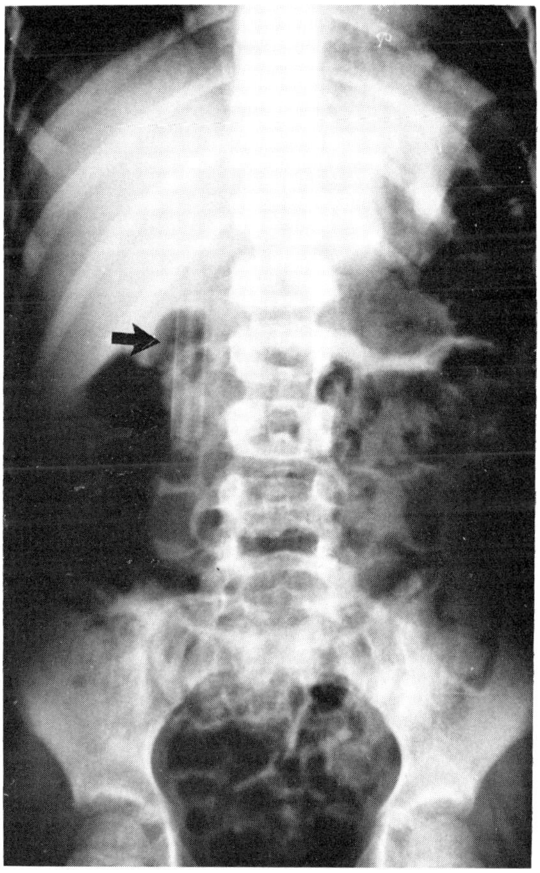

Fig. 27-2. Plain abdominal roentgenogram showing the outline of a 6-cm section of a pencil impacted within the second part of the duodenum in a 2-year-old child.

GENERAL MANAGEMENT

Most ingested foreign objects are amenable to extraction with a flexible gastroscope. Should this maneuver fail or the facilities be lacking, surgical removal through a gastrotomy or duodenotomy should be performed. It is essential to confirm the position of the foreign body by roentgenogram immediately before the operation (Fig. 27-2). An occlusion clamp placed across the pylorus will prevent the object from slipping into the duodenum during the surgical manipulations.

TRICHOBEZOAR

This unusual foreign object consists of a concretion of hair and food particles that forms a cast in the stomach. Other bezoars consist of vegetable matter (phytobezoar) or milk (lactobezoar). Most patients are female and many are mentally retarded or emotionally disturbed [76].

Clinical Features

Presenting symptoms include abdominal pain, vomiting, anorexia, and loss of weight. A history of ingestion of hair may or may not be obtained, and baldness or thinning of the hair may not be evident. A firm, nontender, freely mobile epigastric mass is usually palpable.

Complications

Intestinal obstruction, hemorrhage, ulceration [41], perforation, and peritonitis have all been documented. An unusual complication is the so-called Rapunzel syndrome, in which a long tail of hair passes from the main bezoar through the duodenum and into the jejunum. Tension from peristalsis produces an accordion effect, resulting in intestinal obstruction or perforation from intestinal necrosis [183].

Investigations

A plain abdominal roentgenogram may reveal an intragastric foreign object outlined by surrounding gas (Fig. 27-3). An upper gastrointestinal contrast study will confirm the diagnosis and may also provide information about associated gastric ulceration and extension of the bezoar into the upper small intestine. Endoscopy will clarify the diagnosis when doubt still exists.

Management

In uncomplicated bezoars little preoperative preparation is required. Gentle saline gastric lavage will evacuate the stomach of some malodorous retained secretions. Prophylactic broad-spectrum antibiotic therapy may be of value in preventing wound infection. Chronic anemia and hypoproteinemia should be corrected preoperatively. Urgent resuscitation is required for small intestinal obstruction or perforation.

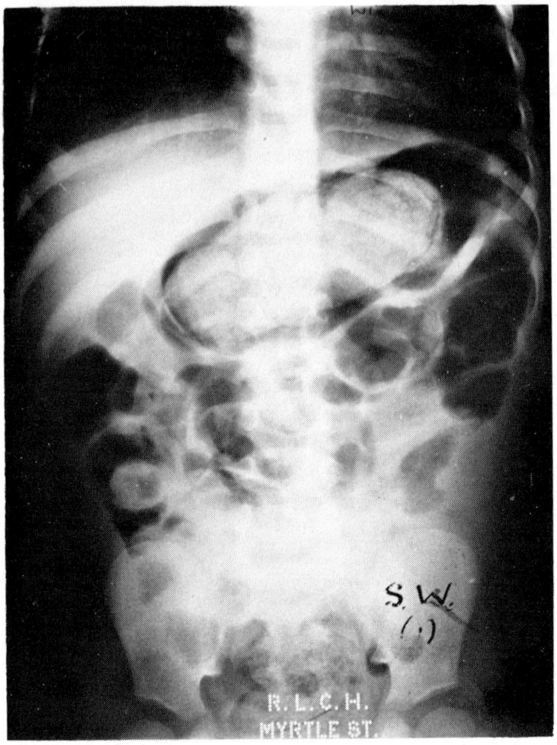

Fig. 27-3. Plain abdominal roentgenogram of a 6-year-old girl presenting with anorexia, weight loss, and anemia showing a large intragastric filling defect (trichobezoar).

The trichobezoar is removed through a generous gastrotomy (Fig. 27-4). Extensions into the small intestine may also be extracted through the gastrotomy or, when difficulties are encountered, through one or more enterotomy incisions. Lactobezoars generally respond to conservative measures, including cessation of feedings, gastric lavage, and dietary changes [72].

Infantile Hypertrophic Pyloric Stenosis

HISTORICAL NOTES

The first report of an infant with pyloric stenosis is attributed to Fabricus Hildanus, a German pediatrician, who in 1646 described the successful treatment of a six-month-old infant using thickened feedings. The accounts of Blair in 1717, Weber in 1758, and Armstrong

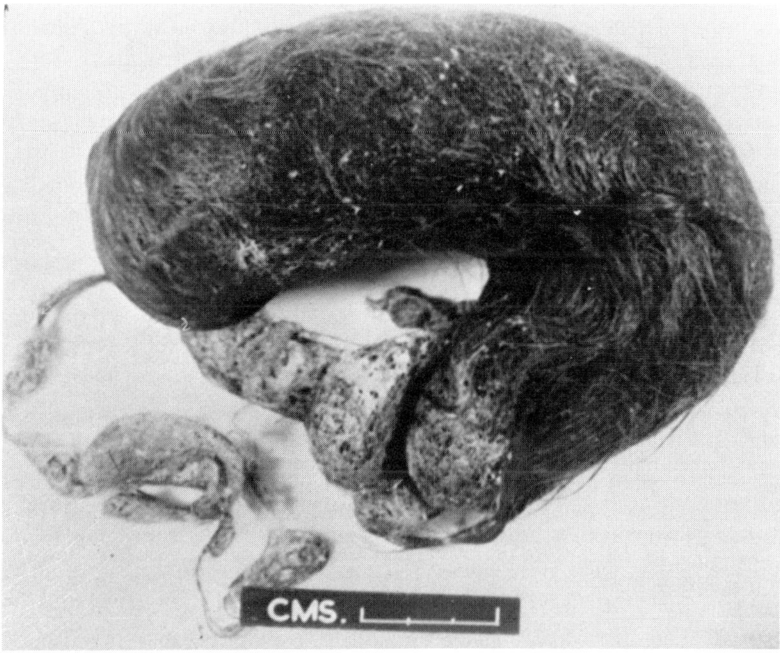

Fig. 27-4. Photograph of the trichobezoar after surgical removal through a gastrotomy.

in 1777 were undoubtedly genuine descriptions of the condition. Beardsley in 1788 was the first American to document a case of infantile pyloric stenosis. The accurate pathological and clinical description in two infants by Harold Hirschsprung in 1888 heralded renewed interest in the condition, which up to that time remained largely undiagnosed and for which little or no treatment was offered. Thereafter rapid progress followed in both the diagnosis and treatment of pyloric stenosis. Finkelstein in 1896 was the first to describe the palpable pyloric tumor.

The preferred method of treatment during this period was medical, including a variety of measures designed to overcome the "pyloric spasm." These included gastric lavage, antispasmodic drugs, diet, and applications of local heat; the mortality was as high as 80 percent. The first successful surgical procedure was carried out in 1898 by Löbker, who performed an anterior gastroenterostomy on a ten-week-old infant. Nicoll in 1899 attempted the Loreta procedure of pyloric divulsion through an open gastrotomy but later abandoned this procedure in favor of the "V–Y pyloroplasty." Braun in 1900 introduced the Heineke-Mikulicz pyloroplasty in infants with pyloric stenosis. This procedure proved to be difficult because the sutures cut through the thickened pyloric muscle. Fredet in 1908 and Ramstedt in 1912 were the innovators of the current surgical procedure of submucous pyloromyotomy. This procedure constituted one of the major advances in pediatric surgery in the past century, and the technical details of the procedure have remained virtually unchanged since. The history of pyloric stenosis is admirably described by Mack [107] and by Ravitch [133].

INCIDENCE

In general, the incidence of pyloric stenosis among Caucasians is 2 to 3 instances per 1000 live births [163]. The incidence is much lower among the black races of America and Africa [95, 153]. Males are affected 4 times as frequently as females, and there is believed to be an increased incidence among first-born infants. The latter statement has been the subject of some dispute [82].

INHERITANCE

A strong familial pattern of inheritance for pyloric stenosis is firmly established [35]. The incidence among sons of male index patients is 5.5 percent and among daughters 2.4 percent, whereas for female index patients the figures are much more striking: 18.9 percent for sons and 7 percent for daughters. These proportions are 10, 25, 40, and 70 times the incidence for the same sex in the general population [37]. Although the number of grandchildren of patients is still small, indications are that the high risk to relatives of female index patients is even more marked in the second generation [38]. Pyloric stenosis has been reported in three [36], four [61], five, [16] and even seven [55] siblings in the same family. Its concurrence has also been documented in numerous sets of twins, uniovular as well as binovular [106, 112] as well as in triplets [165].

ETIOLOGY

Although the precise cause of the condition remains obscure, both hereditary and environmental factors undoubtedly play a role [46]. The genetic pattern of inheritance has been discussed, and the racial and sexual factors have been alluded to in the section on incidence. Blood group has been implicated, with a relatively low incidence in infants with group A blood compared with groups B and O [44]. A seasonal variation in incidence has been noted, with a preponderance of instances in autumn and spring. Maternal stress as a causative factor remains purely speculative.

Numerous theories related to the pathogenesis of pyloric stenosis have been postulated. These vary from muscular imbalances [80, 103] and mechanical trauma of the ingested milk curds causing mucosal edema of the pyloric region [104] to abnormalities of the myenteric nerve plexus [14, 36]. Friesen et al. [59, 60] postulated an immaturity of the myenteric ganglion cells as the primary causative factor, whereas others [1, 11, 118, 168] ascribe the changes seen in the myenteric ganglion cell plexuses to secondary degeneration.

The role of gastrin in the genesis of hypertrophic pyloric stenosis has recently received much attention. Dodge [45] successfully induced hypertrophic pyloric stenosis in puppies by prolonged perinatal administration of pentagastrin. He further implicated maternal stress as the primary factor mediated by increases in the release of the hormone gastrin [47]. The role of gastrin in the etiology of pyloric stenosis remains unresolved despite numerous reports on the subject. Immunoreactive gastric levels have been found to be either normal [75, 87, 140] or raised [169]. The latter authors concluded that the raised serum gastrin levels were largely caused by antral distention secondary to the pyloric obstruction and could not be directly implicated in the causation of the condition. Werlin et al. [190] measured serum gastrin levels in umbilical cord blood of infants in whom pyloric stenosis subsequently developed and found no difference when compared with control specimens. The current consensus is that gastrin plays little or no role in the causation of infantile pyloric stenosis.

PATHOLOGY

The pyloric canal is thickened and elongated and the external surface has a shiny grayish appearance. The consistency of the pylorus is firm-rubbery. The muscular layers of the body of the stomach are thickened because of work hypertrophy, and the lumen is usually dilated to a greater or lesser extent. It is generally accepted that the increase in volume of the pyloric musculature is caused by a true hypertrophy, i.e., an increase in the size of the muscle cell rather than an increase in the number of cells. The increase in volume of pyloric muscle within the confines of the rigid serosal layer is responsible for the firm consistency of the "tumor."

CLINICAL FEATURES

Symptomatology

The average age at onset of symptoms is 3.5 weeks. Ten percent of patients begin vomiting in the first week of life, although in many of these infants the vomiting is not initially projectile. In rare instances, infants have been noted to present with their first symptoms occurring as late as 4, 6, or even 9 months of age [137]. Classically, the vomiting is projectile in nature and occurs 10–20 minutes after a feed. The vomitus contains milk but never any bile. In the late stages of the condition, i.e., in the neglected patient, decompensation occurs and the stomach becomes flaccid and grossly dilated. Vomiting is now regurgitant in type and may occur only once or twice every 24 hours. The presence of blood in the vomitus either in the form of "coffee grounds" or a speckling with bright red blood has been noted in 10–17.5 percent of patients [48, 166]. Although the bleeding is often attributed to stasis gastritis, a prospective endoscopic study of these patients has revealed the cause of the bleeding to be superficial ulcerative esophagitis. Gastric mucosal biopsy in these patients did not show evidence of an acute gastric mucosal lesion [167]. As a result of the persistent vomiting, the infant fails to thrive, bowel movements are infrequent, and constipation develops.

Physical Examination

Although vomiting may have been present for some time, only 10–15 percent of infants are clinically dehydrated on admission. The features of dehydration (depressed fontanelle, sunken eyes, and dry skin and mucous membranes) only become manifest when more than 5 percent of total body water has been lost. Jaundice has been noted on admission in 2–3 percent of patients. The hyperbilirubinemia is largely of the unconjugated type, and it resolves rapidly after relief of the pyloric obstruction. The jaundice has been variously ascribed to obstruction of the common bile duct by the pyloric tumor, increased intra-abdominal pressure causing a reduction in hepatic blood flow from the portal vein, dehydration, hypoglycemia, breast feeding, and prematurity. Hypergastrinemia has also been implicated. An absolute decrease in hepatic glucuronyl-transferase activity has been shown to exist in association with pyloric stenosis [194]. This may be caused by a reduction in caloric intake. Another explanation involves an increase in the enterohepatic circulation of bilirubin. A relative deficiency in the bacterial colonization of the alimentary tract results in an increase in the activity of the deconjugating enzyme β-glucuronidase. This enzyme converts conjugated bilirubin to unconjugated bilirubin, which is readily absorbed in the distal small intestine. The immature liver is incapable of metabolizing the excessive bilirubin load, and the infant becomes clinically jaundiced.

The abdominal examination is best conducted during a test feeding in a warm, comfortable environment. The baby's abdomen should be completely exposed. While the infant is taking the food, waves of gastric peristalsis may become visible. These waves first appear beneath the left costal margin, extend across the epigastrium, and fade out just to the right of the midline. With experience and patience on the part of physicians, more than 90 percent of pyloric "tumors" should be palpable. The clinician should be comfortably seated on the left side of the infant with the fingers of the left hand resting gently on the abdomen in the region of the right hypochondrium. Palpation is carried out during the early stages of a small feeding. A full stomach tends to overlie and obscure the mass. A second opportunity to palpate the tumor occurs immediately after a projectile vomit. The tumor is characteristically olive-shaped and firm and lies deep in the upper abdomen beneath the edge of the liver. Once the presence of a pyloric tumor has been confirmed, further investigations to establish the diagnosis are unnecessary.

Metabolic Disturbances

These are present to a greater or lesser extent in most infants with pyloric stenosis and consist of a metabolic alkalosis in combination with hypochloremic, hypokalemic dehydration. In the early stages, the kidneys are able to compensate by resorbing hydrogen and chloride ions in exchange for sodium, potassium, and bicarbonate ions. As the body stores of sodium and potassium become depleted, these ions are selectively retained, while hydrogen is excreted into the urine, further aggravating the alkalotic state and producing a paradoxical aciduria.

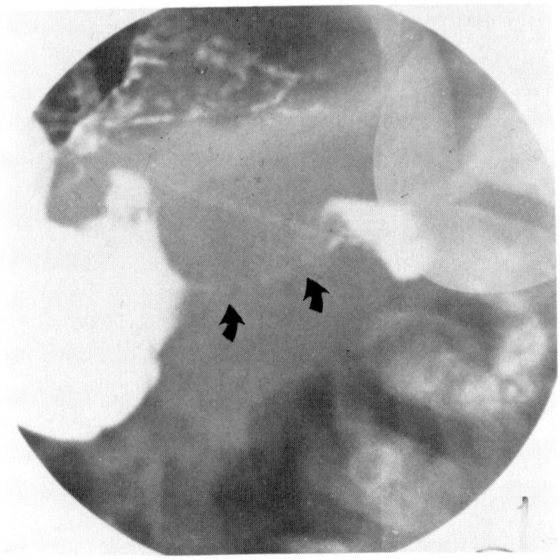

Fig. 27-5. Barium contrast study of the gastric outlet in a 5-week-old infant with projectile vomiting. The pyloric canal is narrow and elongated, and gastric emptying is prolonged.

Roentgenological Examination

This is required only in infants in whom a pyloric mass cannot be palpated, i.e., less than 10 percent of patients. The plain abdominal roentgenogram shows a distended stomach, with or without an air-fluid level, and a paucity of gas beyond the pylorus [139].

The features on barium meal examination [154, 155] characteristic for pyloric stenosis are (Fig. 27-5):

1. "String sign" of the narrow elongated pyloric canal, which is convex upward
2. A "double track" in the pyloric canal caused by infolding of the mucosa
3. The presence of gastric hyperperistalsis on fluoroscopy
4. A "mushroom" effect of the duodenal cap caused by indentation by the pyloric mass

These roentgenographic features may persist for several months after successful relief of the pyloric obstruction and should not in isolation be regarded as an indication for reoperation in the occasional infant whose vomiting persists postoperatively. Ultrasonography has also been used as an ancillary diagnostic investigation (Fig. 27-6).

Real-Time Ultrasonography

Tunell and Wilson [181] have performed real-time ultrasonography on 100 patients with vomiting. When pyloric muscle length was specifically studied, a diagnostic accuracy of 97.8 percent was noted in patients with pyloric stenosis.

Differential Diagnosis

In the absence of a palpable pyloric tumor, the following conditions should be considered:

1. Feeding problems—usually overfeeding
2. Incompetence of the lower esophageal sphincter
3. Generalized infections, such as urinary tract infection, pneumonia, meningitis
4. Adrenal hyperplasia

MANAGEMENT

Preoperative Preparation

The surgical correction of pyloric obstruction is NEVER an emergency, and time spent in rehydrating the infant and correcting the metabolic and acid-base homeostasis is rewarded by simplification of the postoperative course. It may take as long as 48 or 72 hours before the serum biochemistry returns to normal values. In the interim, gentle saline gastric lavages should be performed to evacuate milk curds and residue from the stomach. Oral feedings with milk should be omitted.

The preoperative preparation of the moderate or severely dehydrated infant consists of intravenous administration of an isotonic solution of sodium chloride or plasma in a volume of 20 ml/kg over 1 hour. Once urine flow has been established, 0.45% sodium chloride in 2.5% dextrose with the addition of potassium chloride (10 mmol/500 ml) is given at the rate of 60–120 ml/kg (depending on the state of hydration) over the subsequent 8 hours. Thereafter fluids are administered at a rate of 150 ml/kg/24 hr until rehydration is complete.

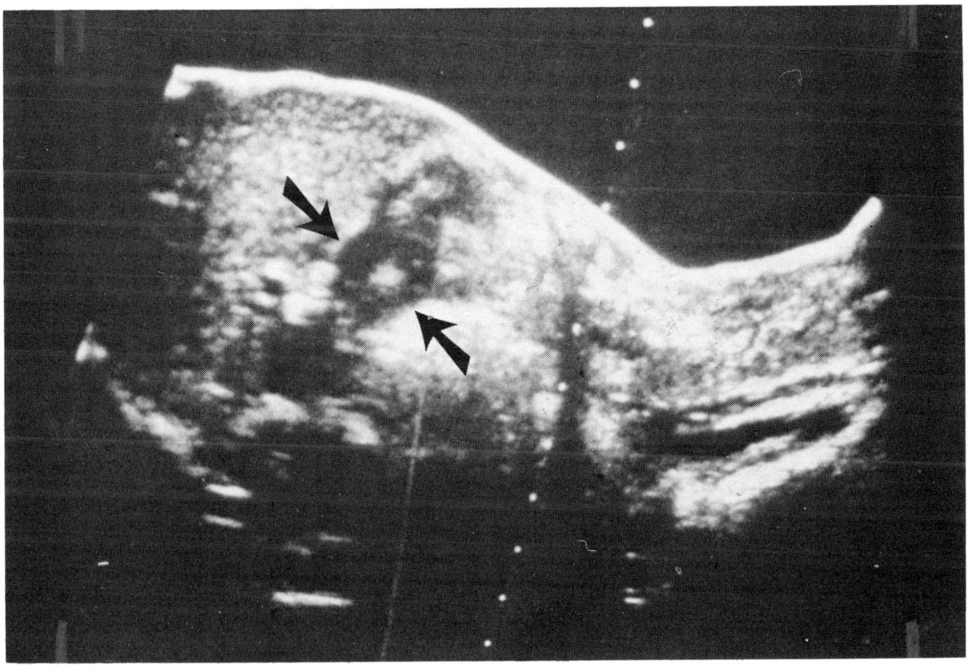

Fig. 27-6. Ultrasonic scan showing the hypertrophied pyloric "tumor" with a central aperture in an infant with pyloric stenosis.

Anesthesia

Although local anesthesia has been successfully used, it is recommended that when an acceptable standard of pediatric expertise exists, general endotracheal anesthesia be used. It is important to ensure that the stomach is empty before the induction of anesthesia. A nasogastric tube is passed and remains in situ during the procedure.

Surgical Procedure

The approach to pyloromyotomy is by a transverse skin crease incision sited in the upper right hypochondrium overlying the anterior surface of the liver (Fig. 27-7). The muscle fibers may be either sectioned transversely in the line of the incision or split in the direction of the muscle fibers as a "gridiron" procedure. The latter method has the advantage of being less prone to dehiscence. The liver is retracted superiorly and the body of the stomach identified. No attempt should be made to deliver the pyloric tumor at this stage because such a maneuver will only result in serosal tears and hemorrhage. The greater curvature of the stomach should be delivered into the incision; the surgeon by gentle traction on the greater curvature in a to-and-fro rocking maneuver delivers the pyloric tumor. A longitudinal incision is made on the anterior surface of the pyloric tumor in the relatively avascular midzone. The incision extends from the pyloric vein of Mayo (marking the pyloroduodenal junction) to the antral region of the stomach. The proximal limit of the incision should extend just beyond the obviously involved pyloric tumor. The incision into the pyloric tumor is split down to the mucosal lining by a blunt instrument (MacDonald dissector, back of the scalpel handle, artery forceps). The shiny mucosal layer is exposed throughout the length of the incision, with particular care exercised in dividing the circular pyloric muscles at the pyloroduodenal junction. The deeper fibers in this region tend to invaginate into the duodenal bulb, exposing the duodenal mucosa to possible trauma unless care is exercised at

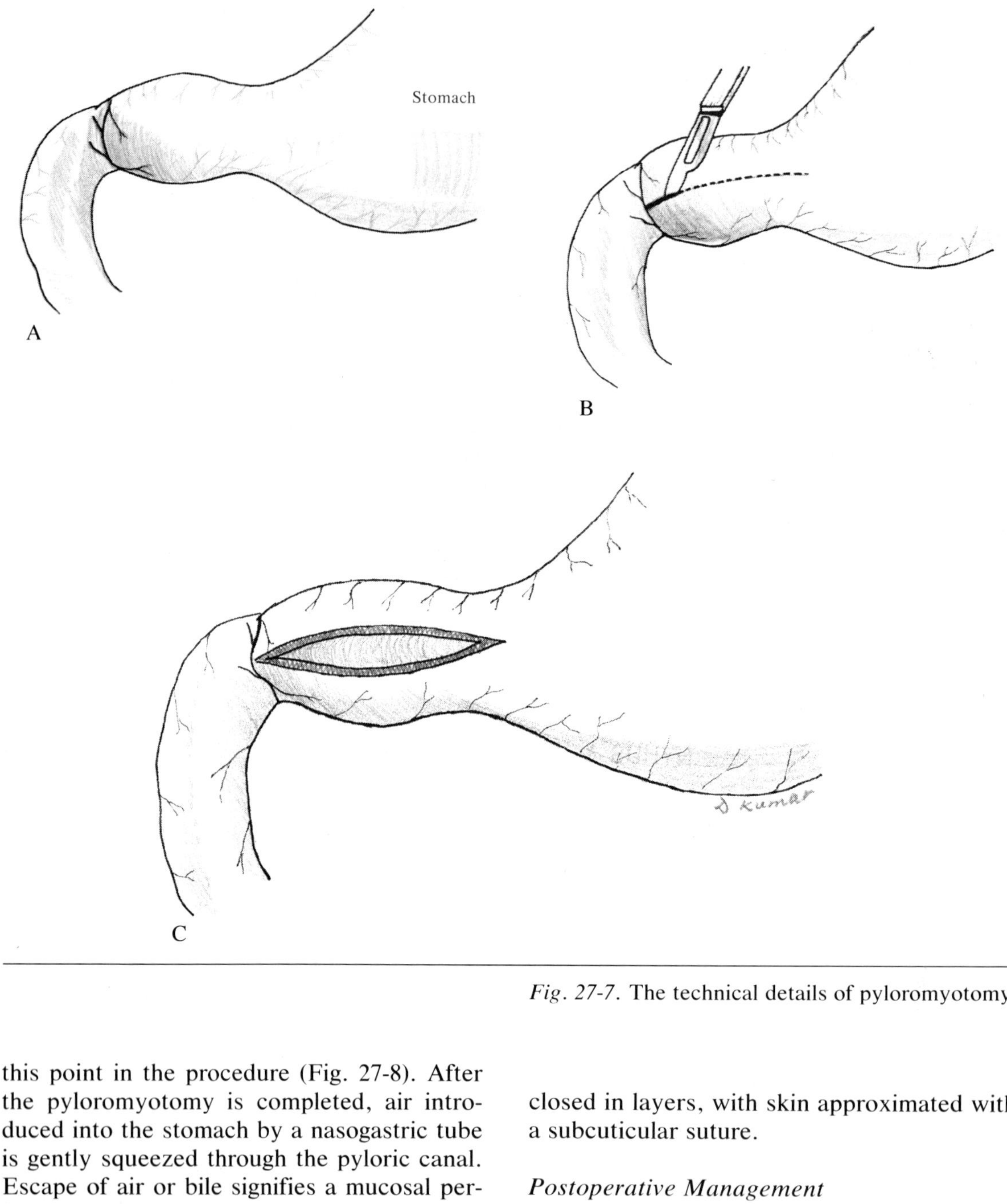

Fig. 27-7. The technical details of pyloromyotomy.

this point in the procedure (Fig. 27-8). After the pyloromyotomy is completed, air introduced into the stomach by a nasogastric tube is gently squeezed through the pyloric canal. Escape of air or bile signifies a mucosal perforation, which should be sealed with 4-0 chromic catgut suture. Suturing omentum over the perforation is unnecessary.

Hemorrhage from the pyloric incision is invariably caused by venous congestion, which is relieved as soon as the pylorus is returned to the peritoneal cavity. The incision is now closed in layers, with skin approximated with a subcuticular suture.

Postoperative Management

Unless a perforation of the mucosa has occurred, the nasogastric tube is removed as soon as the infant has recovered from the anesthesia. Numerous postoperative feeding regimens have been employed, varying from beginning feedings within 4 hours of the operation, to withholding food for 24 hours. It

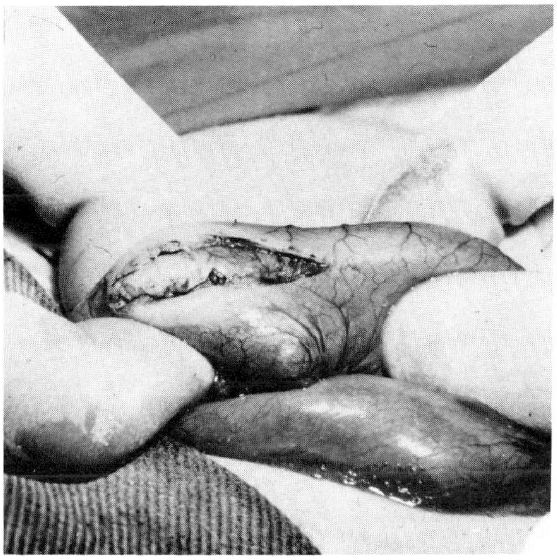

Fig. 27-8. Operative view of the pylorus after pyloromyotomy showing the split hypertrophied pyloric muscle and the underlying mucosa. Note the generous length of the incision.

has been clearly shown that gastric peristalsis is abolished for up to 24 hours postoperatively [144]. The incidence of postoperative vomiting, which is as high as 86 percent in some series, is significantly reduced by withholding food for at least 12 hours. A policy that has been successfully employed includes propping the infant in a feeding chair at an angle of 60 degrees to the horizontal 6 hours after the operation to discourage gastroesophageal reflux and introducing feeds 12 hours postoperatively according to the regimen that is outlined in Table 27-1. The feeding program progresses rapidly through the stages as feeds are tolerated. In most instances the infant is on full feeds and ready for discharge 48–72 hours postoperatively.

The mortality for the surgical treatment of pyloric stenosis is extremely low—well under 1 percent [17, 128]. Wound dehiscence and infection unfortunately are not so rare, particularly in the malnourished infant [67].

Medical Treatment

Since the introduction of pyloromyotomy medical treatment of infantile pyloric stenosis

Table 27-1. Postoperative feeding schedule for infants treated for pyloric stenosis

Stage	Volume (ml)	Feed	Intervals
I	15–30	Glucose-saline	3 hr
II	30	Half-strength milk	3 hr
III	60	Half-strength milk	3 hr
IV	90	Full-strength milk	4 hr

has been all but abandoned in favor of the more definite, simpler, and more effective surgical approach. Medical treatment, which consists of graduated feeding, gastric lavage, and administration of antispasmodics (atropine, scopolamine), has the distinct disadvantages of being unreliable and requiring prolonged hospitalization with meticulous nursing care to prevent vomiting and dehydration.

Duplications of the Stomach

Duplication of the stomach comprises between 2 and 4 percent of all alimentary tract duplications. A review by Bartels [9] in 1967 revealed 55 recorded instances of gastric duplication. During the subsequent decade there have been additional reports in the English literature [129, 192].

Criteria for the diagnosis of a duplication are a hollow structure with a smooth muscle wall lined by a mucous membrane similar to some part of the alimentary canal and attached to and sharing a common blood supply with a part of the alimentary tract [123]. Theories of origin of duplications include the split notochord syndrome and the mucosal disorder syndrome resulting from either defective vacuolization or the formation of diverticula [182]. Duplications involving the stomach are invariably cystic in nature. Most (65 percent) involve the greater curvature of the stomach. Duplications of the pylorus are extremely rare [71].

Clinical presentation consists of a palpable abdominal mass (66 percent), vomiting (64 percent), weight loss or failure to thrive (34

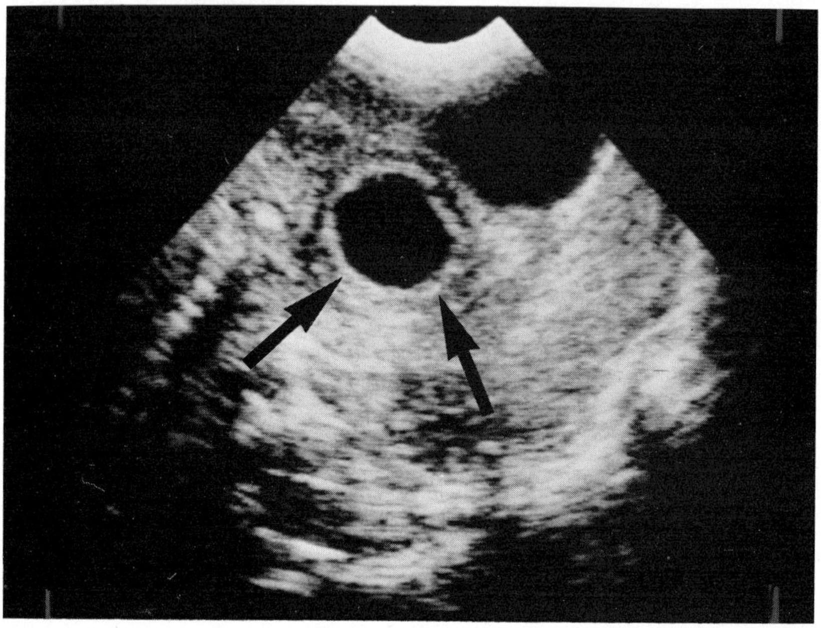

Fig. 27-9. Ultrasonic scan of a gastric duplication cyst showing the thick-walled cystic lesion in the region of the greater curvature of the stomach.

percent), abdominal pain (30 percent), anemia (30 percent), and gastrointestinal hemorrhage (30 percent) [129]. Symptoms generally begin within the first few months of life, but odd instances have been discovered in later life. Kremer [98] stressed the degree of inflammation associated with gastric duplications caused by inadequate drainage of acid-pepsin secretions. The inflammatory reaction is undoubtedly responsible for complications such as ulceration or perforation.

The diagnosis is established on barium contrast examination, which may show an extrinsic filling defect at the site of attachment of the duplication or by abdominal ultrasonic scan, which shows a thick-walled cystic mass in the region of the stomach (Fig. 27-9).

The treatment of gastric duplications is surgical. Because most gastric duplications occur on the greater curvature of the stomach, simple excision, including when necessary the adjacent gastric wall, is the treatment of choice. Duplications in the antrum and pylorus may be removed by careful extramucosal dissection, thereby avoiding opening the lumen of the stomach. In the occasional extensive duplication, internal drainage of the cyst into the stomach (cystogastrostomy) should be performed in preference to extensive gastric resections.

Tumors of the Stomach

Tumors of the stomach are uncommon in the pediatric age group and are usually described in case reports only, with an occasional review of the literature. The following tumors have been reported:

Benign tumors:
- Carcinoid
- Hemangioma
- Lymphangioma
- Neurofibroma
- Lipoma
- Eosinophilic granuloma

- Inflammatory and adenomatous polyps
- Ectopic pancreatic tissue
- Leiomyoma
- Teratoma

Malignant tumors:
- Carcinoma
- Leiomyosarcoma
- Lymphoma

Teratomas are the most common of the benign tumors. Nevertheless, only slightly more than 50 instances have been documented in the literature [110, 116]. With one exception, the patients have been boys [131].

Most of the tumors occur in infants younger than one year of age, and the most common presenting feature is an abdominal mass. Other symptoms include gastrointestinal hemorrhage and vomiting. Any part of the stomach may be involved.

A plain roentgenogram reveals a soft tissue mass with irregular areas of calcification. Surgical treatment consists of excision, which may have to include an adjacent part of the stomach. Extensive resections should be avoided. The prognosis following complete excision is excellent.

Three infants with gastric teratomas have been treated at the Hospital for Sick Children, London. All three were boys, and in each instance resection of the tumor was possible, including a segment of adjacent stomach wall [6] (Fig. 27-10).

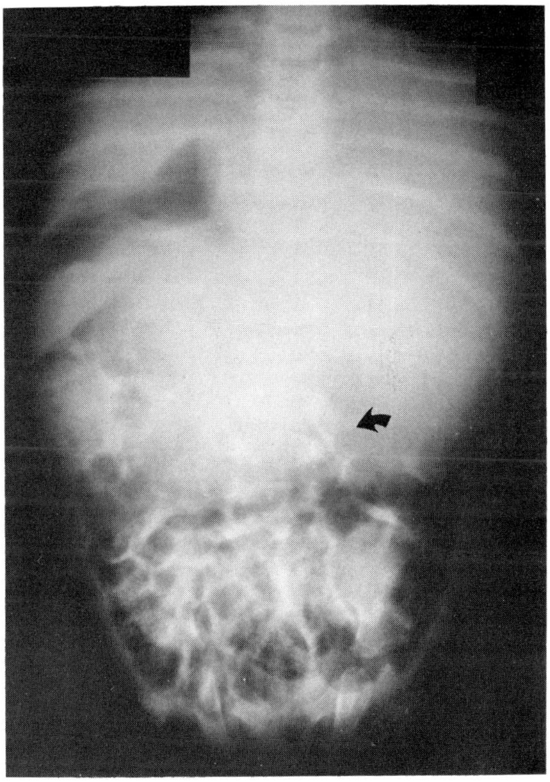

Fig. 27-10. Plain abdominal roentgenogram in a 2-month-old infant with a gastric teratoma showing the upward and medial displacement of the stomach and the large soft-tissue mass with irregular calcification.

Smooth muscle tumors are even rarer. By 1973 Wurlitzer et al. [196] were able to collect only 34 reports in the world literature. Twenty of the tumors were malignant and 14 benign. The most common presenting symptom was hematemesis, melena, or iron deficiency anemia, which occurred in 86 percent of the patients. Barium meal study reveals either a polypoid filling defect or an ulcerating lesion. Metastases or unusual local extension occurred in 10 of the 16 malignant tumors for which accurate descriptions were available. Histopathological diagnosis was frequently inaccurate in determining whether the tumor was benign or malignant. Treatment is by wide local resection or subtotal gastrectomy. When one of these procedures was carried out, 8 of 9 pediatric patients were alive one year postoperatively.

Carcinoma of the stomach in a child has been reported only occasionally [24, 89]. McNeer [111] reviewed the literature concerning all gastric malignant tumors in patients younger than 30 years of age from 1878 to 1940. He found 501 patients, of whom only 19 (3.8 percent) were younger than 15 years of age. The clinical features are similar to those seen in older persons, but presentation may be somewhat delayed [111]. Anaplastic infiltrative adenocarcinoma of the linitis plastica morphologic type is extremely rare [23].

PART II
The Duodenum

Congenital Duodenal Obstructions

Historical Notes

The first recorded report of an infant with duodenal atresia was by Calder in 1733 [34]. In 1862 von Ecker [185] documented annular pancreas for the first time. The first child to survive congenital duodenal obstruction was reported on in 1905 [184]; that child had annular pancreas. Survival from duodenal atresia was noted in two separate reports in 1916 by Ernst [54] and Weeks [188]. Ladd [100] in 1933 presented a series of eight children with intrinsic duodenal obstructions, five of whom survived surgical correction. The first child with extrinsic duodenal obstruction to survive surgical treatment was reported on in 1919 [121].

Classification

Congenital duodenal obstruction may be divided into two categories: (1) intrinsic obstructions, which include duodenal atresia and stenosis, duodenal diaphragm, and annular pancreas, and (2) extrinsic obstructions, which include intestinal malrotation with bands, with or without midgut volvulus.

INTRINSIC DUODENAL OBSTRUCTION

Incidence

The estimated incidence generally quoted in the literature ranges from 1 : 10,000 to 1 : 40,000 births. More recently, however, much higher incidence rates have been determined, such as 1 : 7500 [66], 1 : 6000 [85], and 1 : 4000 [174]. Although familial incidence is not a feature of duodenal atresia, the occurrence of the condition in two, three, and even four siblings has been recorded [57, 83, 138, 197]. A relatively high incidence of twins has also been noted [85, 136].

Anatomy of the Lesion

The various types of anomaly are shown diagrammatically (Fig. 27-11). Of the 503 instances compiled from a review of the members of the surgical section of the American Academy of Pediatrics throughout the 10-year period 1957–1967 [57], 48.7 percent were atresias, in one-fourth of which there was complete separation of the two segments; 41 percent had a diaphragmatic type of obstruction; and 10 percent had duodenal stenosis. Duodenal webs occur in less than 10 percent of instances. Distention of the web produces a classical "wind-sock" deformity [21], in which the duodenum distal to the site of attachment of the web is gradually dilated by its persistent distention and prolapse. In these instances the level of the obstruction appears to be much more distal than is actually the case. Annular pancreas in the absence of an underlying duodenal narrowing is extremely rare. The second part of the duodenum around the entry of the ampulla of Vater is by far the most commonly affected area—the site in 86 of 108 instances in the Liverpool series [85]. In that series 43 percent of the obstructions were located in the preampullary segment of the duodenum, which corresponds closely with the series from the Hospital for Sick Children, London [197], but is considerably higher than the 30 percent rate of preampullary obstructions in the American Academy review and the 21 percent seen by Madden and McCann [108].

Embryology

The vascular catastrophe theory is generally accepted in the pathogenesis of intestinal atresia. In intrinsic duodenal obstructions, in which there is a high incidence of associated malformations, this theory would appear to be untenable. Tandler [173] proposed a failure of recanalization after a temporary solid state as the embryological explanation for duodenal atresia. He had observed epithelial occlusion of the duodenum during the sixth and seventh weeks of intrauterine life. Lynn and Espinas [105] found evidence of duodenal occlusion in 20 of 68 human embryos examined between 5 and 8 weeks' gestational age. Boyden [26, 146] made the most extensive embryological study of the duodenum. He demonstrated that vacuoles develop in the duodenum as the occluding epithelium begins to break up. At the 15-mm stage these vacuoles coalesce to form two

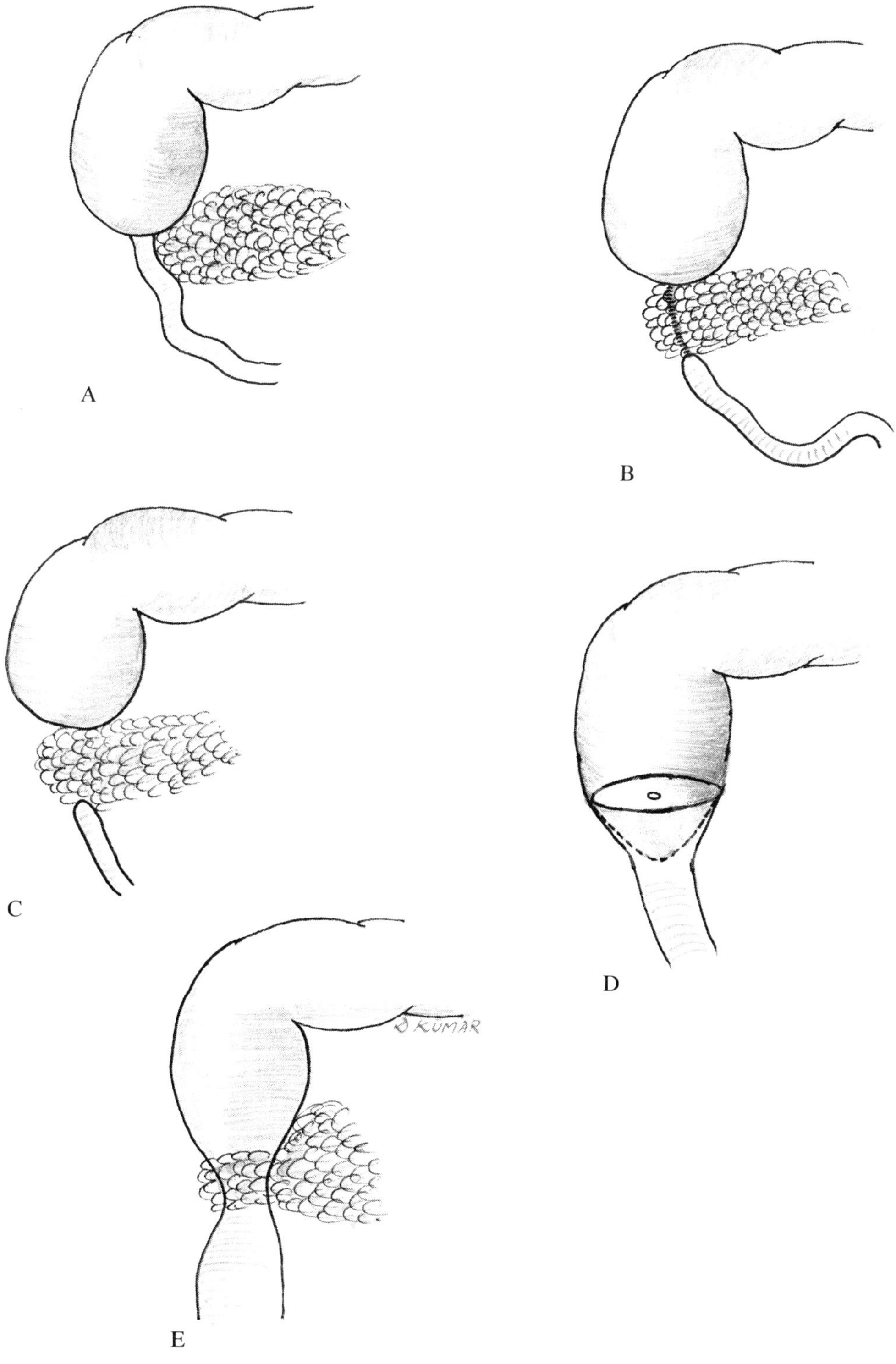

Fig. 27-11. Congenital intrinsic duodenal obstructions. (A) Membranous atresia. (B) Atresia with fibrous connection. (C) Atresia with loss of continuity. (D) Duodenal web showing "wind-sock" deformity. (E) Duodenal stenosis with apparent annular pancreas.

channels, into each of which separately drains a division of the hepatopancreatic duct. This state is transitory, and as fusion of the two vacuoles occurs the lumen of the duodenum is reestablished. Failure of the final stage of fusion results in an atresia or stenosis at the level of the papilla of Vater. Branching of the common bile duct with separate entry into the proximal and distal duodenal segments has been accurately documented in the literature [26, 66, 91].

Clinical Presentation

The incidence of polyhydramnios during the third trimester of pregnancy varies from 30 to 50 percent [57, 85]. Elevated amniotic α-fetoprotein levels have been recorded in duodenal atresia [189]. Prematurity is common in infants with intrinsic, in contrast to extrinsic, duodenal obstructions. The incidence in the larger series is about 50 percent [57, 85, 125, 142]. Dehydration, weight loss, and disturbance of acid-base equilibrium develop when the diagnosis is delayed.

VOMITING. This usually commences within a few hours of birth, although its onset, even in complete atresia, may be delayed for up to 48 hours [85]. In a third of the patients, i.e., those with supra-ampullary atresias, the vomitus is clear, whereas in the remainder it is heavily bile-stained. Bile-stained vomiting in any newborn infant should be regarded as pathological. It implies mechanical intestinal obstruction unless an alternative diagnosis can be made.

ABDOMINAL DISTENTION. Because the obstruction is high in the alimentary tract and most of the proximal accumulated material is evacuated in the vomitus, there is little or no evidence of abdominal distention.

VISIBLE PERISTALSIS. In an attempt to overcome the obstruction, gastric hyperperistaltic waves may be visible in the left upper abdomen. This has been noted in about 15 percent of patients.

MECONIUM. In more than 50 percent of the patients, meconium is passed preoperatively [57, 142]. In general the meconium stools are smaller and drier than normal.

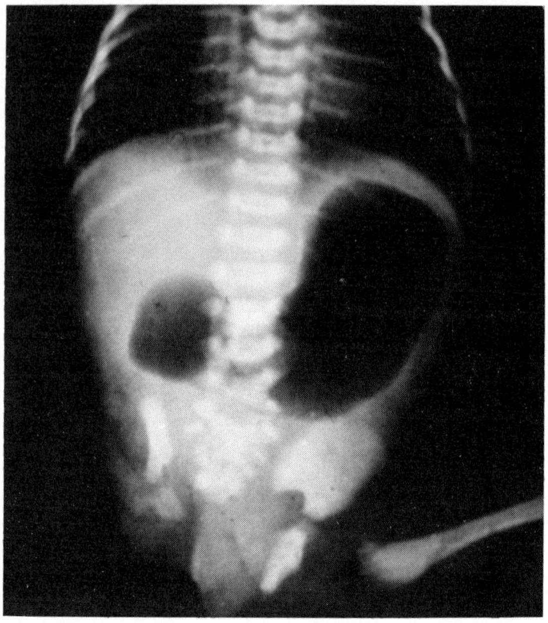

Fig. 27-12. Abdominal roentgenogram in an infant with duodenal atresia showing the typical "double-bubble" appearance.

JAUNDICE. Thirty percent of infants manifest jaundice on admission, but in most instances the hyperbilirubinemia is of the unconjugated type. Obstructive jaundice (conjugated hyperbilirubinemia) is invariably associated with a biliary tract anomaly unless it develops as a consequence of prolonged parenteral nutrition.

Diagnosis

The plain erect abdominal roentgenogram classically shows a "double-bubble" appearance in complete duodenal obstructions. A large air-fluid level is present in the stomach and a smaller one in the duodenum (Fig. 27-12). The appearance of air in the distal intestine is indicative of a stenotic type of obstruction, but small amounts of distal gas may be seen even in complete atresias. The assumption is that air has passed into the distal intestine via a bifid biliary tract [5, 66, 90]. In instances in which the plain abdominal roentgenogram is equivocal, air introduced into the stomach by a nasogastric tube may provide the diagnosis.

In patients with incomplete duodenal obstruction, contrast roentgenography should be carried out. The upper gastrointestinal contrast study should be performed only by an experienced roentgenologist who takes particular care to avoid aspiration of the radiopaque material while at the same time accurately details the anatomy of the lesion.

Associated Anomalies

The incidence of additional congenital abnormalities in conjunction with intrinsic duodenal obstruction ranges from 48 percent [57] to 70 percent [197]. The high frequency of Down syndrome (about 30 percent) in association with duodenal atresia or stenosis demands accurate preoperative assessment and full parental consultation before beginning surgical correction [65]. One-third of patients have incomplete rotation of the midgut in association with intrinsic duodenal obstruction. Because there is a definite potential for the malrotation to undergo volvulus, undue delay in instituting surgical treatment should be avoided. The frequency of associated anomalies is listed in Table 27-2.

Table 27-2. Anomalies associated with intrinsic duodenal obstruction

Anomaly	Incidence (%)
Down syndrome (mongolism)	30
Incomplete rotation of the midgut	30
Congenital cardiac disease	20
Genitourinary anomalies	10
Esophageal atresia	8
Anorectal malformations	7
Skeletal anomalies	6

Treatment

TRANSPORT. Operations on newborn infants are best carried out in specialized centers with a concentration of experienced surgeons. Particular care must be taken during transportation of infants with duodenal obstructions to prevent aspiration pneumonia. The infant is transferred in a portable incubator with a nasogastric tube of adequate size (No. 8F) in position. The stomach is evacuated of its contents at regular intervals to prevent vomiting.

PREOPERATIVE PREPARATION. Infants presenting within the first 24 hours of life are generally in a satisfactory condition. Correction of dehydration and acid-base imbalance is required for infants in whom the diagnosis has been delayed.

OPERATIVE PROCEDURE. With the exception of the duodenal web, the procedure of choice for correction of intrinsic duodenal obstructions is a bypass procedure. The proximity of the biliary and pancreatic systems makes more direct procedures hazardous. Of the bypass procedures, duodenoduodenostomy is the most physiological (Fig. 27-13). Duodenojejunostomy is reserved for high duodenal atresias with a long gap between the segments. Gastrojejunostomy is mentioned only to be condemned because there is an unacceptably high incidence of stomal ulceration and afferent loop syndrome.

The duodenoduodenostomy is performed through a right upper quadrant transverse muscle-cutting incision. The hepatic flexure of the colon is mobilized and the duodenum is widely exposed. Intestinal malrotation is corrected by the standard Ladd procedure (see the section, Extrinsic Duodenal Obstructions). The duodenum is mobilized by a Kocher maneuver. The proximal segment of the duodenum is grossly dilated and the muscle wall hypertrophied. The distal duodenum is thin and collapsed ("unused"). The adjacent walls of the proximal and distal duodenal segments are approximated over a distance of 1.5–2 cm with interrupted seromuscular sutures (4-0 or 5-0 gauge). Two parallel incisions approximately 1.5–2 cm long are made in the proximal and distal duodenum directly adjacent to the previously inserted seromuscular sutures. A side-to-side anastomosis is performed using interrupted 4-0 or 5-0 sutures (silk or polyglycolic acid sutures). A transanastomotic tube is valuable to provide postoperative nutrition without having to resort to parenteral feeding. A thin polymeric silicone (Silastic) tube is introduced into the stomach by a Stamm gastrostomy and is manipulated through the anastomosis into the proximal je-

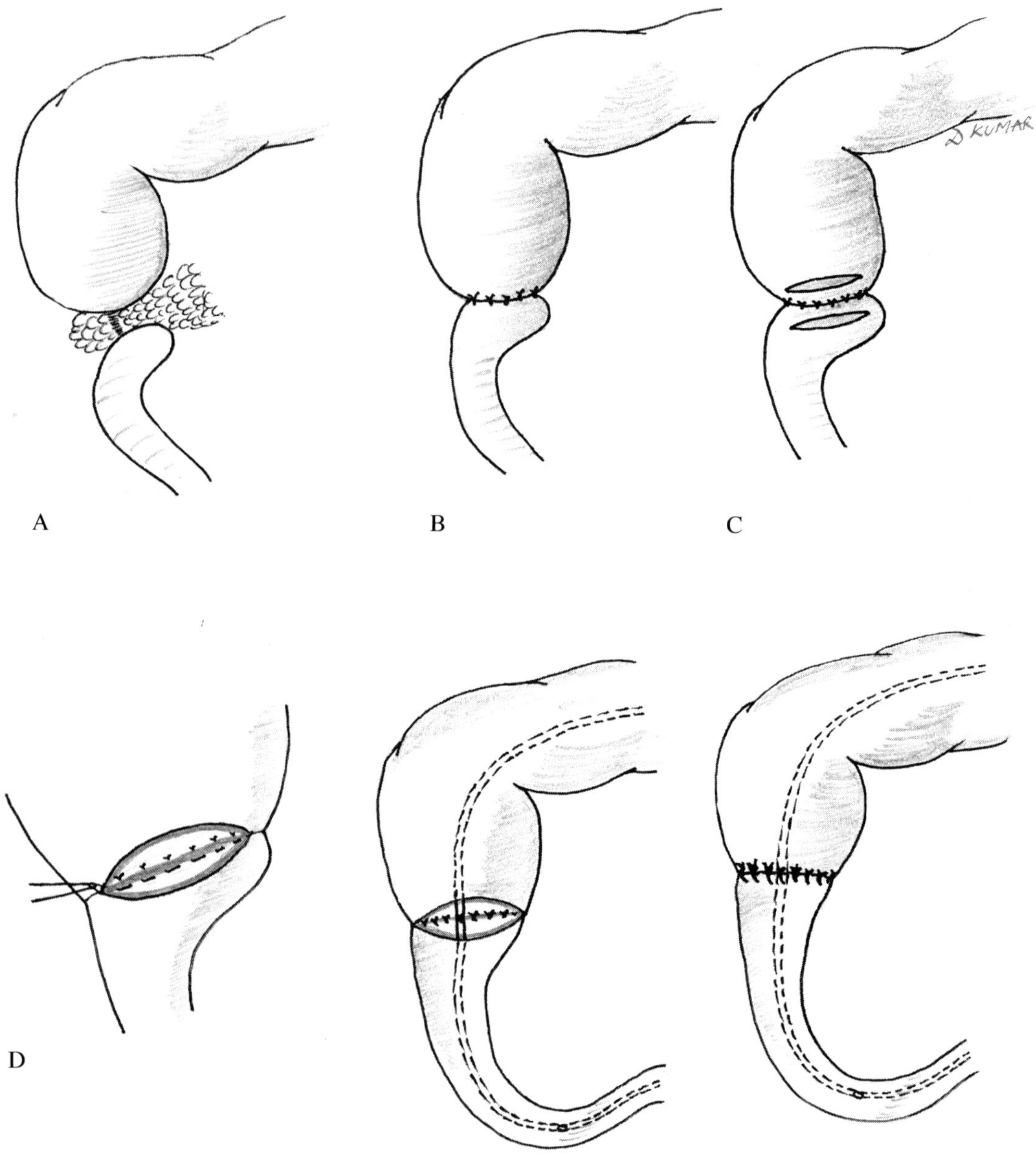

Fig. 27-13. Duodenoduodenostomy. Technical details of the procedure, including the use of a transanastomotic feeding tube.

junum. Passing the tube through the duodenum is a difficult procedure and is best performed before completing the anterior part of the anastomosis. The duodenoduodenostomy is completed by inserting a few anterior seromuscular sutures.

Duodenal webs or diaphragms are best approached by a longitudinal lateral duodenotomy at the level of attachment of the membrane. The membrane is excised only after the ampulla of Vater has been identified. The raw edges of the membrane following excision are oversewn with 4-0 or 5-0 polyglycolic acid sutures.

Before the abdomen is closed, it is essential to exclude additional intestinal anomalies, particularly distal atresias.

POSTOPERATIVE CARE. Fluid and electrolyte homeostasis is kept up by maintenance intravenous fluid administration supplemented by replacement of nasogastric or gastrostomy aspirate. Characteristically there is a prolonged period of duodenal ileus caused by impaired peristalsis of the hypertrophied and dilated proximal duodenum and by anastomotic edema. During this phase, in which food obviously cannot be tolerated, feedings may be introduced into the distal intestine by the transanastomotic tube. Alternatively, parenteral nutrition may be required. The use of a transanastomotic tube is not without complications. Perforation of the jejunum [197], disruption of the anastomosis [85], and retraction of the tube into the stomach have been described.

Results of Treatment

Mortality in intrinsic duodenal obstruction is directly related to the degree of prematurity and the extent of additional congenital anomalies. Traditionally, mortalities are expressed according to risk groups [197].

Group A. Birth weight 2.5 kg with no serious abnormality

Group B. Birth weight 2–2.5 kg with no serious abnormality, and birth weight 2.5 kg with serious abnormality

Group C. Birth weight 2 kg, and birth weight 2–2.5 kg with serious abnormality

Table 27-3. Mortality for intrinsic duodenal obstruction

Author	Year	No. of patients	Mortality (%)
Reid [136]	1973	164	56
Girvan and Stephens [65]	1974	120	33
Perrelli and Wilkinson [125]	1975	51	25.5
Stauffer and Irving [170]	1977	85	38.5
Brown [31]*	1982	98	33

*Hospital for Sick Children, London, 1965–1980.

In 1966 Young and Wilkinson [197] reported the following mortalities in 99 infants with intrinsic duodenal obstruction:

Group A. 14 percent mortality
Group B. 37 percent mortality
Group C. 83 percent mortality

Eight years later a further review from the Hospital for Sick Children, London, revealed the following statistics [125]:

Group A. 4 percent mortality
Group B. 33.3 percent mortality
Group C. 57 percent mortality

Overall it was clearly demonstrated that mortality is directly related to the presence of an associated severe abnormality. When such an anomaly was present, the mortality was between 80 and 90 percent during the entire 23-year period of the study [31, 125]. The overall mortalities for intrinsic duodenal obstructions in the more recent large series in the literature are cited in Table 27-3.

The mortality and complication rate for infants with Down syndrome was significantly raised—43 percent compared with 26 percent [85]. This is directly related to the increased incidence of congenital cardiac malformations in Down syndrome and to these infants' increased susceptibility to overwhelming infection.

EXTRINSIC DUODENAL OBSTRUCTIONS (MALROTATION)

Extrinsic duodenal obstructions account for 30–40 percent of all congenital duodenal obstructions. By far most instances are caused by intestinal malrotation. Duodenal duplications are uncommon and are discussed under a separate heading. Malrotation refers to any interference with the process of orderly fetal rotation of the midgut and the normal fixation of the mesenteries [33].

Historical Notes

The embryological anatomy of normal intestinal development, which provides an explanation of malrotation, is based on the classical studies of Frazer and Robbins [58] in 1915 and Dott [50] in 1923. In 1936 William Ladd [101] published his classical article on malrotation in which he emphasized the importance of dividing the bands that cross over the duodenum and of placing the cecum in the left upper quadrant. This work formed the basis for modern surgical treatment of malrotation.

Embryological Notes

Stage I. Between the fourth and tenth weeks of intrauterine life, growth of the developing fetal intestine proceeds at a rate more rapid than that of the enveloping coelomic cavity. The intestine, particularly the midgut loop, which extends from the proximal jejunum to the midtransverse colon (which is supplied by the superior mesenteric artery) is forced into a physiological hernia within the umbilical cord.

Stage II. From the tenth week the intestines migrate back into the peritoneal cavity. The small intestine returns first and lies mainly on the left side of the abdomen. The cecocolic loop returns last. It initially enters the abdomen in the left lower quadrant but rapidly rotates through 270 degrees in a counterclockwise direction to assume its final position in the right iliac fossa by the twelfth week. Simultaneously the duodenojejunal loop also undergoes a 270-degree counterclockwise rotation, coming to rest behind and to the left of the superior mesenteric vessels.

Stage III. The final stage consists of fusion of various parts of the mesentery with the posterior parietal peritoneum, resulting in fixation of the duodenojejunal junction to the left of the midline and the cecum in the right iliac fossa.

Errors of Intestinal Rotation

These are most conveniently classified according to the stage during which arrest of normal development occurred [68–70].

Stage I. Arrest at this stage will result in an exomphalos. The intestines have failed to return into the abdominal cavity.

Stage II. Errors of intestinal rotation beginning at Stage II are as follows:

1. *Nonrotation.* Failure of rotation following reentry of the midgut loop into the peritoneal cavity leaves the major part of the colon on the left side of the abdomen, the cecum suspended in the midline, and the small intestine to the right.
2. *Incomplete rotation.* The cecum lies in the right hypochondrium anterior to the second part of the duodenum. Ladd bands pass from the cecum across the second part of the duodenum to the posterior and lateral abdominal wall (Fig. 27-14).
3. *Reversed rotation.* The final 180-degree rotation takes place in a clockwise direction so the colon comes to lie posterior to the duodenum and the superior mesenteric vessels.
4. *Hyperrotation.* The normal 270-degree counterclockwise rotation fails to arrest with the cecum in the right iliac fossa. The rotation continues through 450 degrees, and the cecum comes to lie in the region of the splenic flexure of the colon.
5. *Encapsulated small intestine.* The small intestine lies within an avascular sac, the lining of the extraembryonic coelom, which reentered the abdomen with the intestine instead of remaining in the base of the umbilical cord [122].

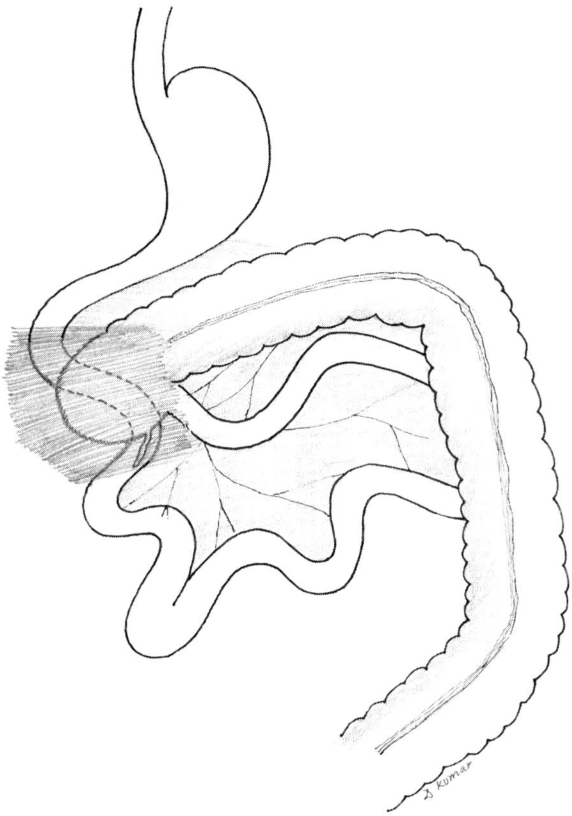

Fig. 27-14. Incomplete rotation. This is the most common form of malrotation. The cecum lies in a subhepatic position in close contact with the duodenum. The entire midgut loop is suspended on a short mesentery.

Stage III. There are three errors to consider at Stage III.

1. *Undescended cecum.* This feature is present in 6 percent of normal individuals [68].
2. *Inverted Cecum.*
3. *Mobile cecum.* This occurs as a result of incomplete fixation of the ascending colon. In about 10 percent of adults the cecum is freely mobile [160].

Associated Anomalies

Malrotation occurs virtually as a standard additional malformation in the following congenital anomalies:

Exomphalos and gastroschisis
Posterolateral diaphragmatic hernia (Bochdalek)
Prune-belly syndrome

It is commonly associated with intrinsic duodenal obstruction (atresia and stenosis) and has been found in conjunction with esophageal atresia [29], anorectal agenesis, Hirschsprung disease [28, 42, 77, 94], biliary atresia [56], and urinary tract anomalies [52]. The incidence of associated anomalies with malrotation is from 10 to 20 percent [71].

Clinical Features

NEONATAL PERIOD. Bile-tinged vomiting is invariably the presenting symptom in this age group. Initially the bilious vomiting may occur intermittently, but this should not delay urgent investigation of the cause of the vomiting. The importance of bilious vomiting, particularly in the neonatal period, cannot be overstated. The cause of the bile-stained vomiting should be considered to be mechanical unless an alternative diagnosis is firmly established. Abdominal distention is usually restricted to the upper abdomen because most of the proximal intestinal content is evacuated in the vomitus.

The risk of volvulus occurring is reported to be between 45 and 65 percent [171, 179]. The onset of volvulus is heralded by the passage of dark blood per rectum and the presence of abdominal distention. The presence of a bloody stool in an infant with acute intestinal obstruction indicates intestine with a compromised blood supply and demands urgent resuscitation and prompt surgical treatment. Midgut volvulus is almost, but not exclusively, confined to infants in the first month of life.

OLDER INFANCY AND CHILDHOOD. A wide spectrum of clinical symptoms has been ascribed to malrotation in the older child. The most common symptom is intermittent or cyclic vomiting, which on occasion may be bile-tinged. Recurrent abdominal pain occurs in 1 in 10 school-age children, and in more than 90 percent of instances no organic lesion can be demonstrated. When the bouts of recurrent abdominal pain are associated with

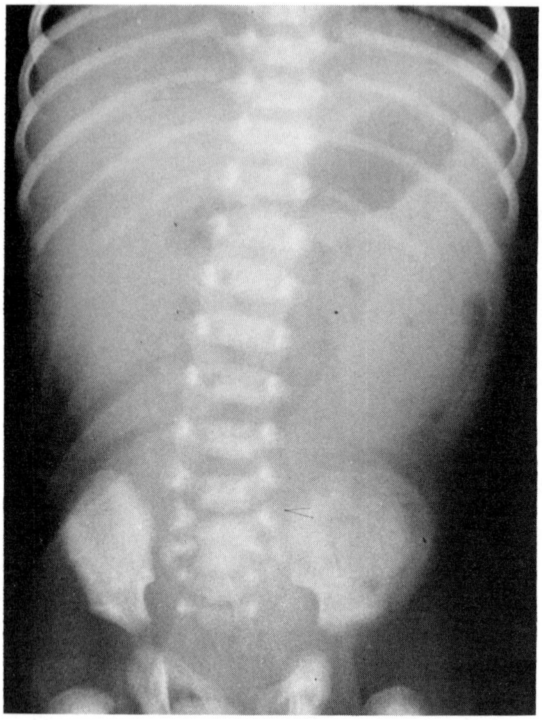

Fig. 27-15. Plain abdominal roentgenogram in an infant with malrotation and volvulus demonstrating the typical "gasless" abdomen.

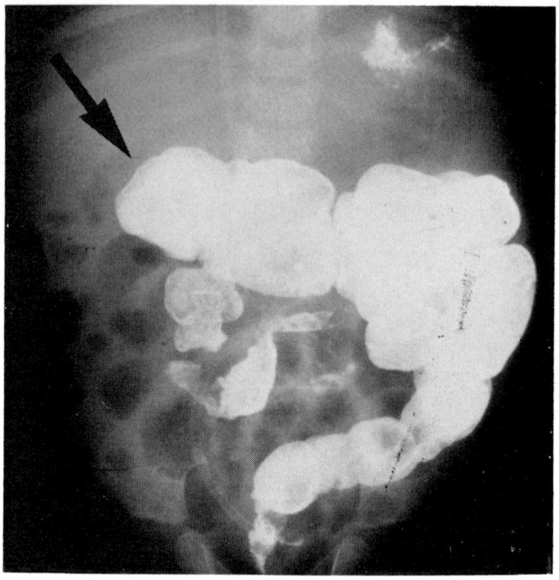

Fig. 27-16. Barium enema from an infant with malrotation showing the centrally placed cecum in the upper abdomen.

bilious vomiting, investigation to exclude a malrotation should be undertaken [3, 88]. Sporadic instances of malabsorption caused by malrotation have been described [171].

Radiological Diagnosis

The plain erect and supine abdominal roentgenograms are of greatest diagnostic assistance in infants with volvulus complicating the malrotation. The significant features are (1) a dilated stomach and first and second part of the duodenum, producing a "double-bubble" appearance on the erect study [172], and (2) a relatively small amount of gas in the intestine distal to the dilated duodenum, giving rise to the so-called gasless abdomen appearance (Fig. 27-15).

When in addition to the aforementioned features on the plain abdominal roentgenogram there are clinical signs of shock, bloody diarrhea, and abdominal distention, contrast studies are superfluous to the diagnosis of midgut volvulus, and urgent resuscitation with emergency laparotomy is the best course of action.

Although the barium enema theoretically should be of value in revealing the position of the misplaced cecum, reflux of contrast into the terminal ileum frequently obscures the precise anatomical position of the cecum. In addition, the significance of a high, mobile cecum is difficult to assess. It is estimated that there is an approximately 10 percent incidence of incompletely attached cecums [20, 93]. Despite these limitations, barium enema examination is the preferred method of investigation by many roentgenologists [18, 159, 161] (Fig. 27-16).

Upper gastrointestinal contrast studies have been advocated as providing more reliable information for the diagnosis of malrotation [42, 56, 157]. The three cardinal signs that should be carefully sought are (Fig. 27-17):

1. Incomplete duodenal obstruction, usually in the third part of the duodenum

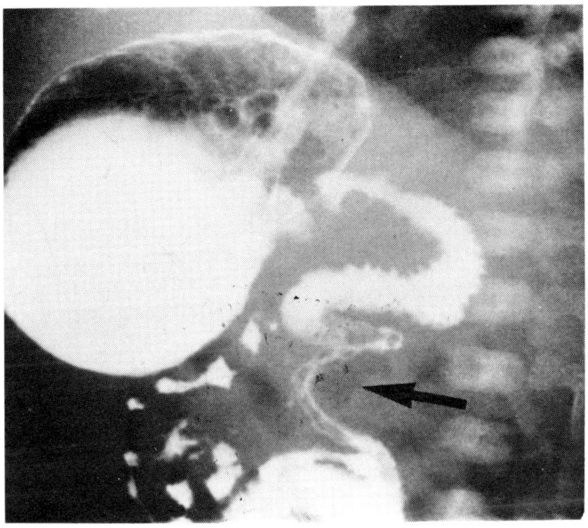

Fig. 27-17. Barium meal and follow-up examination revealing the "twisted coil" appearance of the nonrotated duodenal loop.

2. Abnormal position of the duodenojejunal flexure
3. Abnormal position of the proximal jejunal loops to the right of the midline

Treatment

The operation for malrotation in infancy is generally a surgical emergency. When volvulus has clinically occurred, a brief (1–2 hour) period of intensive resuscitation with intravenous infusion of plasma (20 ml/kg) and nasogastric decompression should be carried out. The infant's temperature should be maintained at as near normothermic levels as possible. In the clinically stable infant without volvulus, operation should be undertaken as soon as possible to prevent this complication, which may result in massive intestinal necrosis.

The procedure is carried out through a right supraumbilical transverse muscle-cutting incision. All the intestine is delivered out of the incision, and any volvulus of the midgut is untwisted, usually in a counterclockwise direction. In infants with massive necrosis of the midgut caused by volvulus, only areas of obvious gangrene of the intestine following reduction of the volvulus should be resected. A second-look laparotomy 24 hours later may reveal relatively healthy intestine, which at the first laparotomy appeared nonviable.

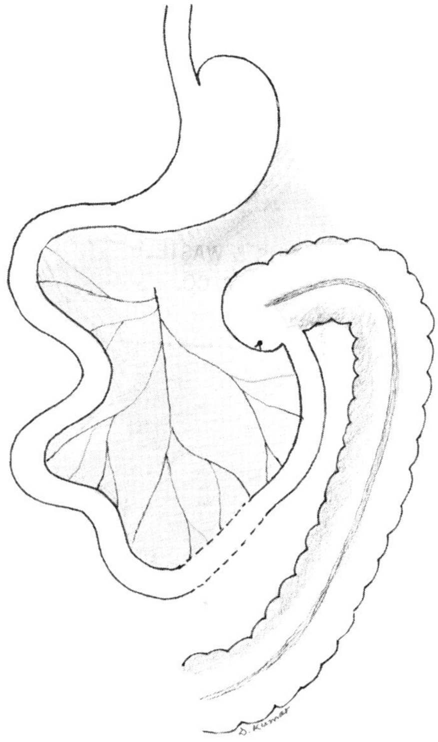

Fig. 27-18. Diagrammatic appearance of the intestine following Ladd's procedure for malrotation. The duodenal loop is straightened and the cecum is placed in the left hypochondrium. Note the wide-based mesentery in which the midgut is suspended.

In the most common variety of malrotation in which volvulus has not occurred, the cecum is located in the right hypochondrium or in the midabdomen. Bands (Ladd signs) that cross from the right colon to the right upper quadrant of the abdomen are lyzed. Adhesions between the cecum and the duodenum are divided, and the duodenal loop is straightened as far as possible. Fibrous tissue within the root of the small intestinal mesentery is divided, and the mesenteric attachment to the posterior abdominal wall is widened.

The small intestine is placed in the right side of the peritoneal cavity and the large intestine in the left side with the cecum in the left upper quadrant (Fig. 27-18). Appendectomy may be performed if the general condition of the patient permits. Some authors advocate fixation of the duodenum to the right kidney and of the cecum to the left abdominal wall [20, 27]. This is claimed to prevent recurrent volvulus. Before the abdomen is closed, the intestine, particularly the duodenum, should be checked for associated intrinsic lesions.

Duodenal Duplications

Duodenal duplications, like gastric duplications, are relatively rare, comprising only about 5 percent of intestinal duplications [73]. The criteria for diagnosis has been set out in the section on gastric duplications. Most duodenal duplications are cystic and are sited on the concave (pancreatic) surface of the first or second part of the duodenum. The serosa surrounds both cyst and adjacent duodenum and they often share a common muscular layer [162]. Only 13 percent of duodenal duplications have an ectopic gastric mucosal lining [175]. The mucosal lining is most frequently duodenal in type.

The clinical presentation is dominated by symptoms and signs of incomplete duodenal obstruction [150]. A cystic mass may be palpable deep in the right upper quadrant of the abdomen. The signs and symptoms and mode of presentation within the first few months of life mimic those of hypertrophic pyloric stenosis. Other features include melena and jaundice.

The diagnosis is made on upper gastrointestinal contrast roentgenography. The barium study shows an intramural mass in the duodenum with partial obstruction to the duodenal lumen.

Treatment is surgical, but because of the proximity of the biliary and pancreatic ducts, complete excision is rarely feasible. Most cystic duodenal duplications are best treated by excising the common wall between the cyst and the adjacent duodenum [62].

It is essential to identify precisely the course of the biliary and pancreatic ducts in relation to the common wall before any part is excised. Suturing the duodenum to the cyst wall ensures hemostasis and keeps the window patent [162].

Peptic Ulceration

Peptic ulceration is a relatively uncommon condition in children. Table 27-4 gives an indication of the frequency with which primary ulcers are encountered in some of the major pediatric surgical centers.

SECONDARY PEPTIC ULCERS

These are encountered more frequently than primary ulcers, particularly in infants. They are acute ulcers that occur in association with another serious medical condition and generally present with a complication such as hemorrhage or perforation. These ulcers are mostly shallow and multiple and occur predominantly in the parietal-cell area of the gastric mucosa, but occasionally appear in the antrum and duodenum [49].

Secondary peptic ulcers may be found in association with the following etiological factors:

1. *Stress ulcers*. These follow severe trauma, septicemia, or hemorrhage.
2. *Burns* (Curling ulcer). These ulcers are usually located in the duodenum and develop two or more weeks after the burn injury. The incidence is between 7 and 9 percent in children with major burns [43, 148].
3. *Central nervous system disorders* (Cushing ulcer). The association was first described by Rokitansky in 1882 and later reviewed by Cushing in 1932. The central nervous system disorders most frequently implicated include cerebral tumors, trauma, and meningitis.
4. *Salicylate ingestion*. Salicylate inhibits the synthesis of mucopolysaccharides, which results in defective gastric mucous production. The lesions are usually multiple, superficial, and associated with hemorrhagic gastritis.
5. *Corticosteroid administration*. The ulcers occur as a result of increased acid secretion

Table 27-4. Frequency of primary peptic ulcer on children

Location of institution	Author	No. of years	No. of patients	Instances per year
Philadelphia	Rosenlund and Koop [141]	20	17	0.85
Boston	Schuster and Gross [145]	32	28	0.88
Toronto	Seagram, Stephens, and Cumming [147]	20	35	1.75
Chicago	Ramos, Kirsner, and Palmer [132]	22	28	1.27
London	Kumar and Spitz [99]	30	30	1.00
Adelaide (Australia)	Williams and Ahmed [193]	11	24	2.18

in the presence of impaired mucosal healing [40].

In patients presenting with hemorrhage, the diagnosis may be confirmed by early upper gastrointestinal fiberoptic endoscopy. The shallow nature of the ulceration does not lend itself to roentgenological diagnosis by contrast studies.

Treatment consists of aggressive medical management with blood replacement, iced saline gastric lavage, and intragastrically administered antacids. The value of H_2-receptor inhibitors such as cimetidine remains controversial. The indications for surgical intervention are uncontrolled hemorrhage or perforation. The surgical procedure of choice is vagotomy and pyloroplasty, combined, when indicated, with oversewing of bleeding vessels [141, 147]. A more aggressive approach of partial gastrectomy with or without vagotomy has recently been recommended as affording maximum protection against recurrent bleeding [115]. Massive gastric resections should be avoided because of the adverse long-term complications.

PRIMARY PEPTIC ULCERS

These ulcers, which occur in the absence of other major medical illness and of which the cause remains uncertain, are predominantly located in the duodenum. A positive family history of peptic ulceration is found in more than 30 percent of instances [119, 147, 180].

For a diagnosis of chronic peptic ulcer to be made it is necessary that the ulcer crater be demonstrated unequivocally either at endoscopy or on barium contrast roentgenography. Lesser roentgenographic features, such as irritability of the duodenal cap, spasm, or duodenitis, are inadequate to establish a diagnosis of peptic ulceration [156]. Boys are affected more commonly than girls in a ratio of 3 : 1 [99, 119, 176] to 4 : 1 [147].

The clinical presentation of primary peptic ulcers varies according to the age group in which the patient falls [22]. For the sake of convenience four groups are identified:

1. *Birth to two weeks.* Although most of the ulcers in this group are stress ulcers, a proportion do occur in otherwise healthy infants [176]. There is no sex difference nor does duodenal ulcer predominate over gastric ulcer. There are no premonitory symptoms or signs, and the first indication of the presence of an ulcer is either hemorrhage, which may be massive, or perforation, or both. The mortality is high because of the acute, often catastrophic, presentation and the delay in instituting surgical treatment.
2. *Three weeks to two years.* These children present with vague gastrointestinal symptoms, such as poor feeding, frequent vomiting (often containing small amounts of altered blood), melena, or nonspecific abdominal pain (which is poorly localized and unrelated to feeding). Once again presentation usually follows the occurrence of complications, principally perforation or hemorrhage.
3. *Two to nine years.* Pain begins to assume a

more prominent place among the symptoms. It is, however, vague and poorly localized, nocturnal, and often relieved by vomiting; however, it does not respond dramatically to food. Complications in children younger than six years of age are mainly hemorrhage, while in those older than six perforation and obstruction occur more frequently. Duodenal ulcers predominate.

4. *Over nine years*. Chronic ulcers in this age group are being diagnosed increasingly. Boys predominate, and the ulcers occur almost exclusively in the duodenum. The symptoms closely resemble the adult pattern of presentation.

DIAGNOSIS

Roentgenographic examination by barium meal requires the demonstration of an ulcer crater or an unequivocal deformity of the duodenal cap before an ulcer can be diagnosed. As stated previously, lesser signs such as spasm or irritability of the duodenal cap are unreliable. Barium studies are of limited value in bleeding ulcers. Fiberoptic endoscopy as a diagnostic investigation is far more reliable for the diagnosis of chronic duodenal ulcers, and especially, of bleeding ulcers [2, 32]. It is our policy to perform an upper gastrointestinal fiberoptic investigation of all infants and children presenting with hematemesis or melena within 24 to 48 hours of admission to the hospital. Gastric acid analysis and serum gastric assays are of doubtful diagnostic value in this age group. From the relatively few controlled studies of gastric acid secretion, it would appear that, as in adults, elevated levels of acid secretion do occur in children with duodenal ulcers, but the elevation is not sufficiently great or sufficiently consistent to be of diagnostic or prognostic value [49].

TREATMENT

Conservative treatment should be carried out in all instances except those in which there is a catastrophic complication, such as perforation or massive uncontrollable hemorrhage. The basic medical therapy consists of the administration of regular antacids, avoidance of foods known to aggravate the pain (e.g., fried foods, spices), and use of cimetidine (a histamine H_2-receptor antagonist) in a dosage of 20–40 mg/kg/day in four divided doses. Rigid dietary restrictions have little effect on the healing of ulcers in children.

Although most primary peptic ulcers heal rapidly with conservative measures, a significant proportion recur once cimetidine is withdrawn [119]. Puri et al. [130] showed a 78 percent incidence of symptoms persisting into adult life when ulcers were treated conservatively in childhood. This is in accord with other series in the literature [7, 74, 113, 191]. When surgical treatment is required for intractable symptoms, vagotomy with pyloroplasty is the procedure of choice [134, 147].

References

1. Alaroutu, H. The histopathologic changes in the myenteric plexus of the pylorus in hypertrophic pyloric stenosis in infants. *Acta Pediatr.* 45 [Suppl.] 107, 1956.
2. Ament, M. E., and Christie, D. L. Upper gastrointestinal fiberoptic endoscopy in pediatric patients. *Gastroenterology* 72:1244, 1977.
3. Andrassy, R. J., and Mahour, G. H. Malrotation of the midgut in infants and children: A 25-year review. *Arch. Surg.* 116:158, 1981.
4. Asch, M. J., and Sherman, N. J. Gastric volvulus in children: Report of two cases. *J. Pediatr. Surg.* 12:1059, 1977.
5. Astley, R. Duodenal atresia with gas below the obstruction. *Br. J. Radiol.* 42:351, 1969.
6. Atwell, J. D., Claireaux, A. E., and Nixon, H. H. Teratoma of the stomach in the newborn. *J. Pediatr. Surg.* 2:197, 1967.
7. Baida, M., McIntyre, J. A., and Deitel, M. Peptic ulcer in children and adolescents. *Arch. Surg.* 99:15, 1969.
8. Bar-Maor, J. A., Nissan, S., and Nevo, S. Pyloric atresia: A hereditary congenital anomaly with autosomal recessive transmission. *J. Med. Genet.* 9:70, 1972.
9. Bartels, R. J. Duplication of the stomach: Case report and review of the literature. *Am. Surg.* 33:747, 1967.
10. Becker, J. M., Schneider, K. M., and Fisher, A. E. Pyloric atresia. *Arch. Surg.* 87:413, 1963.
11. Belding, H. H., and Kernohan, J. W. A mor-

phology study of the myenteric plexus and musculature of the pylorus with special reference to changes in hypertrophic pyloric stenosis. *Surg. Gynecol. Obstet.* 97:323, 1953.
12. Bell, M. J., Ternberg, J. L., Keating, J. P., et al. Prepyloric gastric antral web: A puzzling epidemic. *J. Pediatr. Surg.* 13:307, 1978.
13. Bell, M. J., Ternberg, J. L., McAlister, W., et al. Antral diaphragm: A cause of gastric outlet obstruction in infants and children. *J. Pediatr.* 90:196, 1977.
14. Bendix, R. M., and Mechles, H. Hypertrophic pyloric stenosis: A follow-up study. *J.A.M.A.* 135:331, 1947.
15. Bennett, R. J., Jr. Atresia of the pylorus. *Am. J. Dig. Dis.* 4:4, 1937.
16. Benson, C. D. Infantile pyloric stenosis. *Prog. Pediatr. Surg.* 1:63, 1970.
17. Benson, C. D., and Hight, D. W. Hypertrophic Pyloric Stenosis. In K. J. Welch (Ed.), *Complications of Pediatric Surgery: Prevention and Management*. Philadelphia: Saunders, 1982. P. 276.
18. Berdon, W. E., Baker, D. H., Bull, S., and Santulli, T. V. Midgut malrotation and volvulus: Which films are most helpful? *Radiology* 96:375, 1970.
19. Berti, A. Singolare attortigliamento dell'esofago col duodeno sequito da rapida morte. *Gazz Med. Ital.* 9:139, 1866.
20. Bill, A. H. Malrotation of the Intestine. In M. M. Ravitch, K. J. Welch, C. D. Benson, E. Aberdeen, and J. G. Randolph, (Eds.), *Pediatric Surgery* (3d ed.). Chicago: Year Book, 1979. P. 912.
21. Bill, A. H., and Pope, W. H. Congenital duodenal diaphragm. *Surgery* 35:486, 1954.
22. Bird, C. E., Limper, M. A., and Mayer, J. M. Surgery in peptic ulceration of the stomach and duodenum in infants and children. *Ann. Surg.* 114:526, 1941.
23. Black, R. E. Linitis plastica in a child. *J. Pediatr. Surg.* 20:86, 1985.
24. Blomerus, J. M. Primary carcinoma of the stomach in a child: Review of the literature and case report. *S. Afr. Med. J.* 51:43, 1967.
25. Borchardt, M. Zur pathologie und therapy des magenvolvulus. *Arch. Klin. Chir.* 74:243, 1904.
26. Boyden, E. A., Cope, J. G., and Bill, A. H. Anatomy and embryology of congenital intrinsic obstruction of the duodenum. *Am. J. Surg.* 114:190, 1967.
27. Brennom, W. S., and Bill, A. H. Prophylactic fixation of the intestine for midgut non-rotation. *Surg. Gynecol. Obstet.* 138:181, 1974.
28. Brereton, R. J., Cudmore, R. E., and Carty, H. Hirschsprung's disease with intestinal malrotation: A dangerous combination. *Z. Kinderchir.* 29:176, 1980.
29. Brereton, R. J., Zachary, R. B., and Spitz, L. Preventable death in oesophageal atresia. *Arch. Dis. Child.* 53:276, 1978.
30. Bronsther, B., Nadeau, M. R., and Abrams, M. W. Congenital pyloric atresia: A report of three cases and a review of the literature. *Surgery* 69:130, 1971.
31. Brown, S. Personal communication, 1982.
32. Cadrenel, S., Rodesh, P., Pecters, J. P., and Cremer, M. Fiberendoscopy of the gastrointestinal tract in children. *Am. J. Dis. Child.* 131:41, 1977.
33. Caffey, J. *Pediatric X-ray Diagnosis* (7th ed.). Chicago: Year Book, 1978. P. 738.
34. Calder, J. Two examples of children born with preternatural conformations of the gut. *Med. Essays Observ.* (Edinb.) 1:203, 1733.
35. Cameron, A. L. Familial occurrence of congenital hypertrophic pyloric stenosis: Report of cases in siblings and a cousin and review of the literature. *Arch. Surg.* 70:873, 1955.
36. Cameron, H. C. Vomiting due to obstruction from neuro-muscular inco-ordination. *Br. Med. J.* 1:815, 1925.
37. Carter, C. O., and Evans, K. A. Inheritance of congenital pyloric stenosis. *J. Med. Genet.* 6:233, 1969.
38. Carter, C. O., Evans, K., and Warren, J. The grandchildren of patients with pyloric stenosis. *J. Med. Genet.* 17:411, 1980.
39. Cole, B. C., and Dickinson, S. J. Acute volvulus of the stomach in infants and children. *Surgery* 70:707, 1971.
40. Cushman, P. Glucocorticoids and the gastrointestinal tract: Current status. *Gut* 11:534, 1970.
41. DeBakey, M., and Ochner, A. Bezoars and concretions: A comprehensive review of the literature with an analysis of 303 collected cases and a presentation of 8 additional cases. *Surgery* 4:934, 1938; 5:132, 1939.
42. de Bruyn, R., Hall, C. M., and Spitz, L. Hirschsprung's disease and malrotation of the midgut: An uncommon association. *Br. J. Radiol.,* In press.
43. Dimick, A. Sixth National Burn Seminar. Gastrointestinal ulceration: Bleeding in children. *J. Trauma* 7:119, 1967.

44. Dodge, J. A. Blood groups and congenital hypertrophic pyloric stenosis. *Br. Med. J.* 4:781, 1967.
45. Dodge, J. A. Production of duodenal ulcers and hypertrophic pyloric stenosis by administration of pentagastrin to pregnant and newborn dogs. *Nature* 225:284, 1970.
46. Dodge, J. A. Infantile pyloric stenosis: A multifactorial condition. *G.I. Tract Birth Defects* 8:15, 1972.
47. Dodge, J. A. A Fresh Look at Pyloric Stenosis. In Apley (Ed.), *Modern Trends in Paediatrics*. London: Butterworth, 1974. P. 229.
48. Dodge, J. A. Infantile hypertrophic pyloric stenosis in Belfast 1957–1969. *Arch. Dis. Child.* 50:171, 1975.
49. Dodge, J. A. The Stomach. In C. M. Anderson, and V. Burke, (Eds.), *Paediatric Gastroenterology*. Oxford: Blackwell, 1975. P. 102.
50. Dott, N. M. Anomalies of intestinal rotation. *Br. J. Surg.* 11:251, 1923.
51. Dujon, M. Volvulus de l'estomac. Laparotomie Exploratrice. Relation d'autopsie. *Congres Français de Chirurgia,* 1902. P. 464.
52. Ehrenpreis, T., Ericsson, N. O., and Livaditis, A. Anomalies of the urinary tract in patients with Hirschsprung's disease. *Z. Kinderchir.* 8:89, 1970.
53. El-Shafie, M., Stidham, G. L., Klippel, C. H., et al. Pyloric atresia and epidermolysis bullosa lethalis: A lethal combination in two premature newborn siblings. *J. Pediatr. Surg.* 14:446, 1979.
54. Ernst, N. P. A case of congenital atresia of the duodenum treated successfully by operation. *Br. Med. J.* 1:644, 1916.
55. Fenwick, T. Familial hypertrophic pyloric stenosis. *Br. Med. J.* 2:12, 1953.
56. Filston, H. C., and Kirks, D. R. Malrotation: The ubiquitous anomaly. *J. Pediatr. Surg.* 16:614, 1981.
57. Fonkalsrud, E. W., de Lorimer, A. A., and Hays, D. M. Congenital atresia and stenosis of the duodenum. *Pediatrics* 43:79, 1969.
58. Frazer, J. E., and Robbins, R. H. On facts concerned in causing rotation of the intestine in man. *J. Anat.* 50:75, 1915.
59. Friesen, S. R., Boley, J. A., and Miller, D. R. The myenteric plexus of the pylorus: Its early normal development and its changes in hypertrophic pyloric stenosis. *Surgery* 39:21, 1956.
60. Friesen, S. R., and Pearce, A. G. E. Pathogenesis of congenital pyloric stenosis: Histochemical analyses of pyloric ganglion cells. *Surgery* 53:604, 1963.
61. Gailey, A. A. H. Congenital hypertrophic pyloric stenosis: Report of four cases in brothers. *Br. Med. J.* 1:100, 1948.
62. Gardner, C. E., and Hart, D. Enterogenous cysts in the duodenum. *J.A.M.A.* 104:1809, 1935.
63. Gerber, B. D., and Aberdeen, S. D. Prepyloric diaphragm: An unusual abnormality. *Arch. Surg.* 90:472, 1965.
64. Ghent, C. N., and Denton, M. D. Mucosal diaphragm of the gastric antrum: A case report and review of the literature. *Can. J. Surg.* 17:274, 1974.
65. Girvan, D. P., and Stephens, S. Congenital intrinsic duodenal obstruction: A 20-year review of its surgical management and consequences. *J. Pediatr. Surg.* 9:833, 1974.
66. Gourevitch, A. Duodenal atresia in the newborn. *Ann. R. Coll. Surg. Engl.* 48:141, 1971.
67. Gray, D. W., Gear, M. W., and Stevens, D. W. The result of Ramstedt's operation: Room for complacency? *Ann. R. Coll. Surg. Engl.* 66:280, 1984.
68. Gray, S. W., and Skandalakis, J. E. *Embryology for Surgeons: The Embryological Basis for the Treatment of Congenital Defects.* Philadelphia: Saunders, 1972. P. 135.
69. Grob, M. *Über Lagenabnormalien des Magendarm tracktes infolge Störungen der foctalen Darmdrehung.* Basle: Beno Schwabe, 1953.
70. Grob, M. *Lehrbuch der Kinderchirurgie.* Stuttgart: Thieme, 1957.
71. Grosfeld, J. L., Boles, E. T., and Reiner, C. Duplication of pylorus in the newborn: A rare cause of gastric outlet obstruction. *J. Pediatr. Surg.* 5:365, 1970.
72. Grosfeld, J. L., Schreiner, R. L., Franken, E. A., et al. The changing pattern of gastrointestinal bezoars in infants and children. *Surgery* 88:425, 1980.
73. Gross, R. E., Holcolm, G. W., and Farber, S. Duplications of the alimentary tract. *Pediatrics* 9:449, 1952.
74. Habbick, B. F., Melrose, A. G., and Grant, J. C. Duodenal ulcer in childhood: A study of predisposing factors. *Arch. Dis. Child.* 43:23, 1968.
75. Hambourg, M. A., Mignon, M., Ricour, C., et al. Serum gastrin levels in hypertrophic pyloric stenosis in infancy. *Arch. Dis. Child.* 54:208, 1979.

76. Harris, V., and Hanley, G. Unusual features and complications of bezoars in children. *Am. J. Roentgenol.* 123:742, 1975.
77. Hassinger, D. D., Mulvihill, J. J., and Chandler, J. B. Aarskog's syndrome with Hirschsprung's disease, midgut malrotation and dental anomalies. *J. Med. Genet.* 17:235, 1980.
78. Herbut, P. A. Congenital defect in musculature with rupture in newborn infant. *Arch. Pathol.* 36:91, 1943.
79. Holgersen, L. O. The etiology of spontaneous gastric perforation of the newborn: A reevaluation. *J. Pediatr. Surg.* 16:608, 1981.
80. Horton, B. T. Pyloric musculature, with special reference to pyloric block. *Am. J. Anat.* 41:197, 1928.
81. Houck, W. S., and Griffin, J. A. Spontaneous linear tears of the stomach in the newborn infant. *Ann. Surg.* 193:763, 1981.
82. Huguenard, J. R., and Sharples, G. E. Incidence of congenital pyloric stenosis within sibships. *J. Pediatr.* 81:45, 1972.
83. Hyde, J. S. Congenital duodenal atresia in four sibs. *J.A.M.A.* 191:51, 1965.
84. Inouye, W. Y., and Evans, G. Neonatal gastric perforations: A report of six cases and a review of 143 cases. *Arch. Surg.* 88:471, 1964.
85. Irving, I. M., and Rickham, P. P. Duodenal Atresia and Stenosis: Annular Pancreas. In P. P. Rickham, J. Lister, and I. M. Irving, (Eds.), *Neonatal Surgery* (2d. ed.). London: Butterworth, 1978. Pp. 359.
86. James, A. E., Heller, R. M., and White, J. J., et al. Spontaneous rupture of the stomach in the newborn: Clinical and experimental evaluation. *Pediatr. Res.* 10:79, 1976.
87. Janik, J. S., Akbar, A. M., Burrington, J. D., and Burke, G. The role of gastrin in congenital hypertrophic pyloric stenosis. *J. Pediatr. Surg.* 13:151, 1978.
88. Janik, J. S., and Ein, S. H. Normal intestinal rotation with non-fixation: A cause of chronic abdominal pain. *J. Pediatr. Surg.* 14:670, 1979.
89. Johnston, D. P., van Heerden, J. A., Lynn, H. B., and Motto, J. D. Carcinoma of the stomach in a 10 year old boy. *J. Pediatr. Surg.* 10:151, 1975.
90. Jona, J. Z., and Belin, R. P. Duodenal anomalies and the ampulla of Vater. *Surg. Gynecol. Obstet.* 143:565, 1976.
91. Katz, K. Atresie des duodenums mit Verdoppelung des Ductus choledochus und pancreaticus. *Virchow. Arch.* [*Pathol. Anat.*] 378:290, 1930.
92. Keramidas, D. C. Congenital incomplete prepyloric diaphragm in infants and children. *Surgery* 75:690, 1974.
93. Kieswetter, W. B., and Smith, J. W. Malrotation of the midgut in infancy and childhood. *Arch. Surg.* 77:483, 1958.
94. Kilcoyne, R. F., and Taybi, H. T. Conditions associated with congenital megacolon. *Am. J. Roentgenol.* 108:615, 1970.
95. Klein, A., and Cremin, B. S. Racial significance in pyloric stenosis. *S. Afr. Med. J.* 44:1131, 1970.
96. Kneiszl, F. Some data on the aetiology of gastric rupture in the newborn. *Biol. Neonate* 4:201, 1962.
97. Korber, J. S., and Glasson, M. J. Pyloric atresia associated with epidermolysis bullosa. *J. Pediatr.* 90:600, 1977.
98. Kremer, R. M., Lepoff, R. B., and Izant, R. J. Duplications of the stomach. *J. Pediatr. Surg.* 5:360, 1970.
99. Kumar, D., and Spitz, L. Peptic ulceration in infants and children: 30 years' experience. *Surg. Gynecol. Obstet.* 159: 63, 1984.
100. Ladd, W. E. Congenital obstruction of the small intestine. *J.A.M.A.* 101:1453, 1933.
101. Ladd, W. E. Surgical diseases of the alimentary tract in infants. *N. Engl. J. Med.* 215:705, 1936.
102. Leger, J. L., Ricard, M., Leonard, C., and Piette, J. Ulcère gastrique perfore chez un nouveau né avec survie. *Union Med. Can.* 79:1277, 1950.
103. Lehmann, W. Neuere Anschauungen über die sog. kongenitale pylorusstenose. *Zeitschr. Kinderh.* 50:691, 1930.
104. Lynn, H. B. The mechanism of pyloric stenosis and its relationship to pre-operative preparation. *Arch. Surg.* 81:453, 1960.
105. Lynn, H. B., and Espinas, E. E. Intestinal atresia: An attempt to relate location to embryonic processes. *Arch. Surg.* 79:357, 1959.
106. MacMahon, B., and McKeown, T. Infantile hypertrophic pyloric stenosis: Data on 81 pairs of twins. *Acta Genet. Med. Gemellol.* 4:320, 1955.
107. Mack, H. C. A. A history of hypertrophic pyloric stenosis and its treatment. *Bull. Hist. Med.* 12:465, 1942.
108. Madden, J. L., and McCann, W. J. Congenital diaphragmatic occlusion of the duodenum, with a report of three cases. *Int. Abstr. Surg.* 103:1, 1956.
109. Mandell, G. A., Rosenberg, H. K., and

Schnauffer, L. Prolonged retention of foreign bodies in the stomach. *Pediatrics* 60:460, 1977.
110. Matais, I. C., and Huang, Y. C. Gastric teratoma in infancy: Report of a case and review of world literature. *Ann. Surg.* 178:631, 1973.
111. McNeer, G. Cancer of the stomach in the young. *Am. J. Roentgenol.* 45:537, 1941.
112. Metrakos, J. D. Congenital hypertrophic pyloric stenosis in twins. *Arch. Dis. Child.* 28:351, 1953.
113. Michener, W. M., Kennedy, R. L. J., and Dushane, J. W. Duodenal ulcer in childhood. *Am. J. Dis. Child.* 100:814, 1960.
114. Miller, R. A. Gastric acidity during the first year of life. *Arch. Dis. Child.* 16:22, 1941.
115. Morden, R. S., Schullinger, J. N., Mollitt, D. L., and Santulli, T. U. Operative management of stress ulcers in children. *Ann. Surg.* 196:18, 1982.
116. Nandy, A. K., Sengupta, P., Chatterjee, S. K., and Sarker, S. K. Teratoma of the stomach. *J. Pediatr. Surg.* 9:563, 1974.
117. Neale, A. J. Case of malformation of the stomach. *Lancet* 1:1057, 1884.
118. Neilsen, O. S. Congenital pyloric stenosis as a factor predisposing to the ulcer syndrome. *Acta Paediatr. Scand.* 43:432, 1954.
119. Nord, K. S., Rossi, T. M., and Lebenthal, E. Peptic ulcer in children: The predominance of gastric ulcers. *Am. J. Gastroenterol.* 75:153, 1981.
120. Olsen, L., and Grotte, G. Congenital pyloric atresia: Report of a familial occurrence. *J. Pediatr. Surg.* 2:181, 1976.
121. Ombredanne, L. Volvulus total de l'intestin en evolution chronique. *Bull. Mem. Soc. Chir. Paris* 45:688, 1919.
122. Papez, J. W. A rare intestinal anomaly of embryonic origin. *Anat. Rec.* 54:197, 1932.
123. Parker, B. A. C., Guthrie, J., France, N. E., and Atwell, J. D. Gastric duplications in infancy. *J. Pediatr. Surg.* 7:294, 1972.
124. Parrish, R. A., Kanavage, C. B., Wells, J. A., and Moretz, W. H. Congenital antral membrane. *Surg. Gynecol Obstet.* 127:999, 1968.
125. Perrelli, L., and Wilkinson, A. W. Mortality in neonatal duodenal obstruction. *J. R. Coll. Surg. Edinb.* 20:365, 1975.
126. Persanlidis, D. Neonatal gastric perforation. *J. Mount Sinai Hosp.* 31:97, 1964.
127. Pochaczensky, R., and Bryla, D. New roentgenographic signs of neonatal gastric perforation. *Radiology* 102:145, 1972.
128. Pollock, W. F., Norris, W. J., and Gordon, H. E. The management of hypertrophic pyloric stenosis at the Los Angeles Children's Hospital: A review of 1422 cases. *Am. J. Surg.* 94:335, 1957.
129. Pruksapong, C., Donovan, R. J., Pnit, A., and Heldrich, F. J. Gastric duplication. *J. Pediatr. Surg.* 14:83, 1979.
130. Puri, P., Boyd, E., Blake, N., and Guiney, E. J. Duodenal ulcer in childhood: A continuing disease in adult life. *J. Pediatr. Surg.* 13:525, 1978.
131. Purvis, J. M., Miller, R. C., and Blumenthal, B. I. Gastric teratoma: First reported case in a female. *J. Pediatr. Surg.* 14:86, 1979.
132. Ramos, A. R., Kirsner, J. B., and Palmer, W. L. Peptic ulcer in children. *Am. J. Dis. Child.* 99:135, 1960.
133. Ravitch, M. M. The story of pyloric stenosis. *Surgery* 48:1117, 1960.
134. Ravitch, M. M., and Duremda, G. D. Operative treatment of chronic duodenal ulcer in childhood. *Ann. Surg.* 171:641, 1970.
135. Rees, B. I. Idiopathic gastric perforation in the neonate. *Z. Kinderchir.* 31:191, 1980.
136. Reid, I. S. Intrinsic duodenal lesions: Clinical features. *Aust. N.Z. J. Surg.* 43:158, 1973.
137. Rendle-Short, J., and Zachary, R. B. Congenital pyloric stenosis in older babies. *Arch. Dis. Child.* 30:70, 1955.
138. Richardson, W. R., and Martin, L. W. Pitfalls in the management of the incomplete duodenal diaphragm. *J. Pediatr. Surg.* 4:303, 1969.
139. Riggs, W., and Long, L. The value of the plain film radiogram in pyloric stenosis. *Am. J. Roentgenol.* 112:77, 1971.
140. Rodgers, I. M., Drainer, I. K., Moore, M. R., and Buchanan, K. D. Plasma gastrin in congenital hypertrophic pyloric stenosis: A hypothesis disproved. *Arch. Dis. Child.* 50:467, 1975.
141. Rosenlund, M. L., and Koop, C. E. Duodenal ulcer in childhood. *Pediatrics* 45:283, 1970.
142. Salonen, I. S. Congenital duodenal obstruction. *Acta Paediatr. Scand.* Suppl. 272, 1978.
143. Sawaguchi, S., Ohkawa, H., Kenomotsu, H., Akiyawa, H., Nakajo, T., and Kitamura, T. Idiopathic gastric volvulus in infancy and childhood. *Z. Kinderchir.* 32:218, 1981.
144. Scharli, A. F., and Leditschke, J. F. Gastric motility after pyloromyotomy in infants: A reappraisal of postoperative feeding. *Surgery* 64:1133, 1968.
145. Schuster, S. R., and Gross, R. E. Peptic ulcer

disease in childhood. *Am. J. Surg.* 105:324, 1963.
146. Schwegler, R. A., and Boyden, E. A. The development of the pars intestinalis of the common bile duct in the lumen fetus with special reference to the origin of the ampulla of Vater and the sphincter of Oddi. *Anat. Rec.* 67:441, 1937.
147. Seagram, C. G. F., Stephens, C. A., and Cumming, W. A. Peptic ulceration at the Hospital for Sick Children, Toronto, during the 20-year period 1949–1969. *J. Pediatr. Surg.* 8:407, 1973.
148. Sewitt, S. Duodenal and gastric ulceration after burning. *Br. J. Surg.* 54:32, 1967.
149. Shaker, I. J., Schaefer, J. A., James, A. E., and White, J. J. Aerophagia: a mechanism for spontaneous rupture of the stomach in the newborn. *Am. Surg.* 39:616, 1973.
150. Shallow, T. A., and Wagner, F. B. Enterogenous cysts of the duodenum. *Surgery* 21:532, 1947.
151. Shashikumar, V. L., Bassuk, A., Pilling, G. P., and Cresson, S. L. Spontaneous gastric rupture in the newborn: A clinical review of nineteen cases. *Ann. Surg.* 182:22, 1975.
152. Shaw, A., Blanc, W. A., Santulli, T. W., and Kaiser, G. Spontaneous rupture of the stomach in the newborn: A clinical and experimental study. *Surgery* 58:561, 1965.
153. Shim, W. K. T., Campbell, A., and Wright, S. W. Pyloric stenosis in the racial groups of Hawaii. *J. Pediatr.* 76:89, 1970.
154. Shofner, C. E., Kalman, E. H., and Coin, C. G. The diagnosis of hypertrophic pyloric stenosis. *Am. J. Roentgenol.* 91:796, 1964.
155. Shuman, F. I., Darling, D. B., and Fisher, J. H. The radiographic diagnosis of congenital hypertrophic pyloric stenosis. *J. Pediatr.* 71:70, 1967.
156. Sieber, W. K. The Stomach. In T. M. Holder and K. W. Ashcraft (Eds.), *Pediatric Surgery*. Philadelphia: Saunders, 1980. P. 325.
157. Simpson, A. J., Leonides, J. C., Krasna, I. H., Becker, J. M., and Schneider, K. M. Roentgen diagnosis of midgut malrotation: Value of upper gastrointestinal radiographic study. *J. Pediatr. Surg.* 7:243, 1972.
158. Singleton, A. C. Chronic gastric volvulus. *Radiology* 34:53, 1940.
159. Singleton, E. B. Radiologic evaluation of intestinal obstruction in the newborn. *Radiol. Clin. North Am.* 1:571, 1963.
160. Skandalakis, J. E. Contribution to the study of the pathogenesis of treatment of volvulus of the cecum. Dissertation, Athens, 1949.
161. Soderlund, S. Anomalies of midgut rotation and fixation: Clinical aspects based on 62 cases in childhood. *Acta Paediatr.* [Suppl. 135]225, 1962.
162. Soper, R. T., and Selka, A. C. Duplication cyst of the duodenum: Case report and discussion. *Surgery* 68:562, 1970.
163. Spicer, R. D. Infantile hypertrophic pyloric stenosis: A review. *Br. J. Surg.* 69:128, 1982.
164. Spitz, L. Management of ingested foreign bodies in childhood. *Br. Med. J.* 4:469, 1971.
165. Spitz, L. Congenital hypertrophic pyloric stenosis in triplets. *Arch. Dis. Child.* 49:325, 1974.
166. Spitz, L. Vomiting after pyloromyotomy for infantile hypertrophic pyloric stenosis. *Arch. Dis. Child.* 54:886, 1979.
167. Spitz, L., and Batcup, G. Haematemesis in infantile hypertrophic pyloric stenosis: The source of the bleeding. *Br. J. Surg.* 66:827, 1979.
168. Spitz, L., and Kaufmann, J. C. E. The neuropathological changes in congenital hypertrophic pyloric stenosis. *S. Afr. J. Surg.* 13:239, 1975.
169. Spitz, L., and Zail, S. S. Serum gastrin levels in congenital hypertrophic pyloric stenosis. *J. Pediatr. Surg.* 11:33, 1976.
170. Stauffer, U. G., and Irving, I. Duodenal atresia and stenosis: Long-term results. *Prog. Pediatr. Surg.* 10:49, 1977.
171. Steward, D. R., Colodny, A. L., and Daggett, W. C. Malrotation of the bowel in infants and children: A 15-year review. *Surgery* 79:716, 1976.
172. Tan, W. H. Incomplete rotation of the midgut in the newborn: A clinical and radiologic investigation of 54 patients. *Med. Radiogr. Photogr.* 57:31, 1981.
173. Tandler, J. Zur Entwicklungsgeschichte des menschlichen duodenum in fruhen Embryonalstadien. *Morphol. Jahrb.* 29:187, 1900.
174. Thomas, M. P. Quoted by H. B. Lynn. Duodenal Obstruction: Atresia, Stenosis and Annular Pancreas. In M. M. Ravitch, K. J. Welch, C. D. Benson, et al. (Eds.), *Pediatric Surgery* (3d ed.). Chicago: Year Book, 1979. P. 903.
175. Thompson, N. W., and Labour, S. S. Duplication of the duodenum in the adult. *Arch. Surg.* 94:301, 1967.
176. Thomson, N. B., and Jewitt, T. C. Peptic

ulcers in infancy and childhood. *J.A.M.A.* 189:539, 1964.
177. Touloukian, R. J. Gastric ischaemia: The primary factor in neonatal perforation. *Clin. Pediatr.* 12:219, 1973.
178. Touroff, A. S. W., and Sussman, R. M. Congenital prepyloric membranous obstruction in a premature infant. *Surgery* 8:739, 1940.
179. Tryfonas, G., and Young, D. G. Extrinsic duodenal obstruction in infants and children. *Br. J. Surg.* 62:125, 1975.
180. Tudor, R. B. Peptic ulceration in childhood. *Pediatr. Clin. North Am.* 14:109, 1967.
181. Tunell, W. P., and Wilson, D. A. Pyloric stenosis: Diagnosis by real-time sonography, the pyloric muscle length method. *J. Pediatr. Surg.* 19:795, 1984.
182. Vaage, S., and Knutrud, O. Congenital duplications of the alimentary tract with special reference to their embryogenesis. *Prog. Pediatr. Surg.* 7:103, 1974.
183. Vaughan, E. D., Sawyers, J. L., and Scott, W. H. The Rapunzel syndrome: An unusual complication of intestinal bezoar. *Surgery* 63:339, 1968.
184. Vidal, E. Quelque cas de chirurgie pancreatique. *Assoc. Franc. Chir.* 18:739, 1905.
185. von Ecker, A. Bildungsfahler des Pancreas und des Herzens *Z. Artzl. Med.* 14:354, 1862.
186. Von Siebold, A. E. Brand in der Kleiner Curvatur des Magens eines atrophischen Kindes. *J. Geburtsch. Frauenzimmer Kinderbr.* 5:3, 1826.
187. Wastell, C., and Ellis, H. Volvulus of the stomach: A review with a report of 8 cases. *Br. J. Surg.* 58:557, 1971.
188. Porter, L., and Carter W. E. *Management of the Sick Infant.* St. Louis: Mosby, 1922. Pp. 211–12.
189. Weinberg, A. G., Milunski, A., and Harrod, M. J. Elevated amniotic-fluid fetoprotein and duodenal atresia. *Lancet* 1:496, 1975.
190. Werlin, S. L., Grand, R. J., and Drum, D. E. Congenital hypertrophic pyloric stenosis: The role of gastrin re-evaluated. *Pediatrics* 61:883, 1978.
191. White, A., Carachi, R., and Young, D. G. Duodenal ulceration presenting in childhood: Long-term follow-up. *J. Pediatr. Surg.* 19:6, 1984.
192. Wieczorek, R. L., Seidman, I., Ranson, J. H. C., and Ruoff, M. Congenital duplication of the stomach: Case report and review of the literature. *Am. J. Gastroenterol.* 79:597, 1984.
193. Williams, R. S., and Ahmed, S. Peptic ulcer in childhood. *Aust. Paediatr. J.* 13:299, 1977.
194. Woolley, M. M., Felsher, B. F., Asch, J., et al. Jaundice, hypertrophic pyloric stenosis and hepatic glucuronyl transferase. *J. Pediatr. Surg.* 9:359, 1974.
195. Wuensche, R. Ein Falle von angeboren Verschluss des Pylorus. *Zeitschr. Kinderh.* 8:367, 1875.
196. Wurlitzer, F. P., Mores, A. J., Isaacs, H., Landing, B. H., and Woolley, M. M. Smooth muscle tumours of the stomach in childhood and adolescence. *J. Pediatr. Surg.* 8:421, 1973.
197. Young, D. G., and Wilkinson, A. W. Mortality in neonatal duodenal obstruction. *Lancet* 2:18, 1966.
198. Ziprkowski, M. N., and Teele, R. L. Gastric volvulus in childhood. *Am. J. Roentgenol.* 132:921, 1979.

VIII

Miscellaneous Techniques

28

Stapling in Esophageal and Gastric Surgery

Jameson L. Chassin

The use of stapling devices in a gastric anastomosis goes back to 1924, when von Petz introduced an instrument that placed two rows of B-shaped staples. The next significant advance in the evolution of stapling instruments came with the development of a series of devices at the Institute of Experimental Surgical Apparatus and Instruments in the Soviet Union. Gritsman [12] claimed that using these instruments in 1663 gastric procedures resulted in a reduction in mortality. Ravitch and associates [17] introduced the Russian stapling devices in the United States. In 1967 the United States Surgical Corporation manufactured improved versions of the Russian devices, using disposable cartridges containing up to 33 staples each, obviating the need to reload each device with staples by hand [22]. Since that time the use of stapling in anastomoses of the esophagus and gastrointestinal tract has grown at an explosive rate. This chapter discusses the methods of stapling in esophageal and gastric surgery that I have found both useful and safe.

Physiology of Stapling

Perhaps the most important features of the stapled intestinal anastomosis is the fact that the double row of staples in the B configuration allows blood vessels of substantial size to pass through the staple lines, as demonstrated by the silicone rubber injection technique of Smith et al. [20]. This phenomenon is evident in the operating room when the surgeon observes blood oozing from an everted gastric or intestinal staple line. Stapling devices have the capacity to approximate tissues with precision and with minimal trauma while preserving tissue viability beyond the line of staples. With the end-to-end (EEA) device the inverted cuff of tissue measures no more than 3–4 mm, much less than in the usual sutured end-to-end anastomosis.

Most surgeons have readily accepted the EEA stapling device because it reproduces the inverting anastomosis with which they have long been familiar. Many surgeons, however, hesitate to believe that anastomoses that are in part everting also are safe. Experimental studies by Ravitch and associates [16], as well as a number of studies comparing the complication rates of partially everting stapled gastrointestinal tract anastomoses with sutured anastomoses in humans [6, 14, 18], showed that healing of the anastomoses was equally successful in both groups.

General Precautions

Like sewing techniques, stapling is characterized by pitfalls and danger points that are unique to the method. If serious complications are to be avoided, the surgeon must pay close attention to the precautions necessary to prevent them just as in learning to sew. Most important in this list of precautions is recognition of the condition of the tissues to be anastomosed. Tissues not fit to sew should not be stapled. There are no data to support the concept that in the presence of rampant peritoneal sepsis a stapled anastomosis will heal better than one that is sutured. Similarly, when the wall of the stomach is so thick that compressing it with the TA-90 stapling device will tear the serosa, stapling is contraindicated. When the 4.8-mm staple is fired, it compresses tissues to a thickness of 2.0 mm. If this degree of compression produces necrosis, staples should not be used. The 3.5-mm staple compresses to a thickness of 1.5 mm and is indicated when the stomach is not at all thickened by hypertrophy or disease. Whenever the gastric wall is thickened, the 4.8-mm cartridge should be used. It is especially important to evaluate the thickness of a duodenal stump before closing it with staples during a Billroth II gastrectomy. It is equally important to be certain that the blood supply of the stomach, for example, is adequate before performing an esophagogastric anastomosis.

Although rare, mechanical failure may follow the application of any stapling device. For this reason, after firing a stapling device the staple line should be closely inspected. The B formation must be in the proper configuration. The full thickness of the tissue must be included in the staple line with no gaps. The staple line is gently manipulated to ensure that the staples are holding securely. Excessive bleeding must be watched for. One of the few instances in which bleeding of a serious nature may occur is in the GIA staple line during the Billroth II gastrectomy. If bleeding occurs, it is corrected either with careful application of the electrocautery or by oversewing of the blood vessels with fine atraumatic suture material.

The surgeon must be careful when using the stapled anastomosis to avoid allowing any tension to be applied to the anastomosis. It is my clinical impression that linear tension on a stapled anastomosis is perhaps more dangerous than the same degree of tension when sutures are used. For this reason one must be certain, in esophagogastric anastomoses, to suture the gastric pouch to the mediastinal pleura or the prevertebral fascia in the neck after a cervical esophagogastrostomy. Occasionally a stapling device is injured by wear and tear or damage. When damage is suspected, it is simple to check the instrument by test-firing a cartridge of staples across several thicknesses of latex drain. If all the staples have not closed into the proper B configuration, the instrument should be sent back to the dealer for calibration. Alternatively, disposable instruments may be used, but these cost about 50 percent more than cartridges. A detailed discussion of all the pitfalls and precautions related to stapling is beyond the scope of this chapter and may be found elsewhere [5, 7].

Esophagogastrostomy

Many authors in the past 15 years have reported mortalities from 10 to 34 percent subsequent to esophagectomy or esophagogastrectomy. Wilson and associates [25] found a range of reported anastomotic leak rates between 5 and 21 percent following esophagectomy. About half the patients who experience an esophagogastric anastomotic leak in the thorax die of this complication. That serious leaks following sutured esophagogastric anastomoses are not inevitable is demonstrated by four reports in which there were no fatal leaks subsequent to esophagectomy or esophagogastrectomy [1, 2, 3, 9]. Reports of esophagogastric anastomoses constructed with the EEA method have been relatively few. Graham et al. [11] reported one fatal leak and one stricture in 18 esophagogastrostomies following resection for tumor, but among 70 esophagoesophageal stapled anastomoses for esophageal varices there were 2 leaks and 10 strictures. West and associates [24] reported no leaks after 27 stapled esophagogastric anastomoses, although there were five postoperative strictures, four of which followed the use of the 25-mm EEA cartridge. Each stricture responded successfully to dilation. Fekete and associates [8] reported one fatal leak after 30 esophagogastrostomies as well as three asymptomatic leaks noted on routine contrast roentgenographic examination of the anastomoses. Hopkins and colleagues [13] had only one nonfatal leak after 60 stapled anastomoses. All the authors cited in this section use the U.S. Surgical Corporation EEA device to construct the anastomosis. In 1978 I [4] reported a method of anastomosing esophagus to stomach using the GIA and TA-55 devices. My colleagues and I have now performed this anastomosis in 38 patients with no deaths and no anastomotic leaks..Each patient underwent a Hypaque contrast roentgenographic study of the anastomosis on the seventh postoperative day. The roentgenograms showed no leaks.

The GIA anastomosis has several advantages. It is not necessary to dilate the esophagus as it is with the EEA device. Because the diameter of the anastomosis is large, no patient had strictures except for one who experienced tumor recurrence in the mediastinum that encroached on the lumen of the anastomosis. In addition, as each staple line is inserted there is direct visibility, allowing the surgeon to inspect each staple after it has been fired. Because the instruments are less bulky than the EEA stapler, they fit into the body cavities more easily. Also, it is not necessary to make a second gastrotomy for the introduction of the stapler, as must be done with the EEA stapler. A disadvantage of the GIA technique is the necessity to have a 6-cm overlap of esophagus over the gastric pouch; only 3–4 cm is advised for an end-to-side anastomosis with the EEA stapler. In either situation an end-to-side is safer than an end-to-end anastomosis [3]. Also, there is less tendency for gastroesophageal reflux with a true end-to-side anastomosis. If a patient has a tumor of the proximal stomach but requires more than a 50 percent gastrectomy, anastomosing the esophagus end to end to a relatively small remnant of antrum is likely to be followed by severe and painful esophagitis caused by the continuous reflux of bile. In these situations it is preferable to perform a total gastrectomy with a Roux-en-Y esophagojejunostomy.

For tumors near the esophagogastric junction, I agree with Akiyama [1] that a left thoracoabdominal incision through the sixth (or seventh) interspace is ideal. If a circumferential rather than a radial incision is made in the diaphragm, there will be no damage to the phrenic nerves. Some patients have invasion of the proximal esophagus of as much as 10 cm. It is a simple matter to mobilize the esophagus behind the aorta in instances in which a supra-aortic anastomosis is necessary. For this step, division of the sixth (and rarely, the fifth) rib posteriorly may be necessary. This exposure will make either suturing or stapling the anastomosis simple. For midesophageal lesions, a midline laparotomy plus a right thoracotomy is the procedure of choice. A sutured or stapled anastomosis may be constructed at the apex of the right chest or in the neck, as preferred by the surgeon. With proper technique of sewing or stapling and good gastric blood supply, the incidence of anastomotic leak should be rare; it should not be necessary to perform the anastomosis in the neck simply to avoid the catastrophic results of an intrathoracic leak. It may prove helpful in the right chest if the surgeon uses the EEA device with a *curved shaft* when exposure is limited.

When an esophagogastric anastomosis is to be constructed in the neck, it is often difficult to use the stapling devices because of the small field of exposure, unless the chest is open and the EEA device can be passed through a gastrotomy made in the chest with the tip of the device emerging in the neck. One of the smaller sized cartridges is needed in such a situation because of the limited diameter of the thoracic inlet. In general I prefer to suture the esophagogastrostomy in the neck. Owing to the superficial location of the organs, the anastomosis is generally simple to sew and more difficult to staple.

The GIA esophagogastric anastomosis is described and illustrated in Figure 28-1 and the EEA anastomosis in Figure 28-2. Further details concerning the GIA technique are presented by Chassin [4, 5] and by Ravitch and Steichen [18].

PITFALLS AND PRECAUTIONS IN THE STAPLED ESOPHAGOGASTROSTOMY

The EEA stapler must not be passed through another gastric staple line because its circular blade is not designed to cut through metal. Consequently, in some instances after the EEA is fired it will not be possible to disengage the device because the TA-90 staple line has become entwined in the circular staple line. Forceful efforts at disengaging the EEA anvil will seriously damage the anastomosis. It is sometimes possible to divide the offending staple through the gastrotomy incision. The surgeon should aim to place the esophagogastric anastomosis *at least* 3 cm away from the TA-90 staple line.

Forceful dilation of the esophagus to make it admit the EEA cartridge may rupture the mucosa and submucosa. If this laceration has not been witnessed by the surgeon, postoperative leakage may occur away from the staple line. If the esophagus is torn, the surgeon should excise the damaged esophagus and revert to a sutured anastomosis or use the GIA technique, which does not require any esophageal dilation. Although it is possible to use the 25-mm EEA cartridge, it should be remembered that the capacity of this cartridge must not be exceeded by a large volume of thickened esophagus. In other words, when the esophageal pursestring suture is passed through an esophagus that is both narrow and thickened, the volume of this tissue may exceed the capacity of the cartridge. In this situation, when the tissues are compressed by closing the cartridge some of the thickened esophagus will be extruded between the inverted layers of tissue, as illustrated in Figure 28-3. Since the extruded tissue is devitalized, leakage is likely to occur postoperatively. Tissue extrusion of this type can sometimes be seen through careful observation of the area of the anastomosis as the wing nut is tightened on the EEA device.

Another point of interest with respect to using the small EEA-25 cartridge is the high incidence of postoperative strictures in these anastomoses, as noted by West and associates [24]. Although the internal diameter of the EEA-25 anastomosis is only 15 mm, the staples generally will be extruded into the lumen over a period of time. In the absence of a small leak that causes fibrosis, therefore, the narrow anastomosis will enlarge spontaneously. Otherwise, postoperative dilation will be necessary.

The surgeon must be certain to include all the layers (i.e., both the muscular layer and the mucosa) in the pursestring suture to achieve a proper stapled anastomosis.

After any stapled esophagogastric anastomosis, several hundred milliliters of a methylene blue solution should be instilled through the nasogastric tube to test the integrity of the anastomosis in the operating room. Any minor leaks are corrected with sutures.

Stapled Esophagojejunostomy, Roux-Y, Following Total Gastrectomy

An excellent method of constructing an end-to-side esophagojejunostomy after total gastrectomy, using the EEA stapler, is depicted in Figure 28-4. The jejunum and esophagus will generally admit the EEA-28 cartridge. Efforts at gentle dilation of these two organs may be carried out by digital manipulation. The diameters of the jejunum and esophagus may then be gauged by gently inserting a U.S. Surgical Corporation 25, 28, or 31 sizer. The cartridge should fit loosely in the jejunum. Otherwise it is possible to trap both walls of the descending limb of jejunum in the staple line.

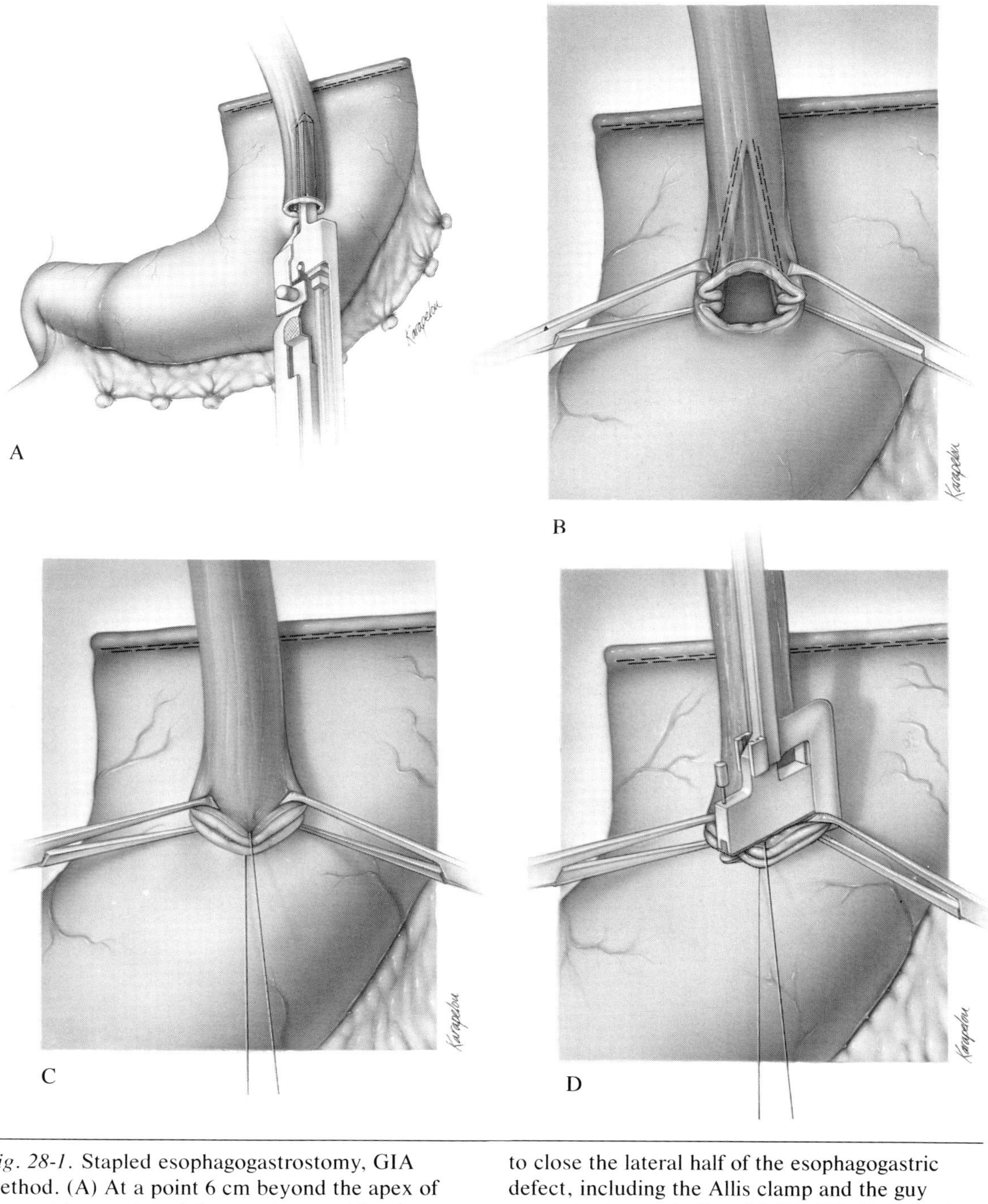

Fig. 28-1. Stapled esophagogastrostomy, GIA method. (A) At a point 6 cm beyond the apex of the gastric pouch, a 1.5-cm stab wound has been made. The GIA stapler has been inserted, one fork into the gastric pouch and one fork into the open lumen of the esophagus, both to a depth of 3 cm. (B) The GIA device has been fired, creating the posterior portion of the anastomosis between the esophagus and the anterior wall of the gastric pouch. Allis clamps have been attached to the right- and left-hand terminations of the GIA staple line. (C) A guy suture has been placed through the midpoints of the remaining defect. The defect is temporarily obliterated by applying traction to the guy suture. (D) A TA-55 device has been applied to close the lateral half of the esophagogastric defect, including the Allis clamp and the guy suture in the staple line. (E) The TA-55 device has been fired, and the redundant esophageal and gastric tissue is being excised, leaving the guy suture intact. (F) The TA-55 stapler is now applied to the medial aspect of the esophagogastric defect, enclosing both the Allis clamps and the guy suture. The TA-55 stapler will now be fired and the redundant tissues excised, flush with the stapler. (G) Appearance of the completed end-to-side anastomosis between the esophagus and anterior wall of the gastric pouch. (From J. L. Chassin, *Am. J. Surg.* 136:399, 1978, with permission.)

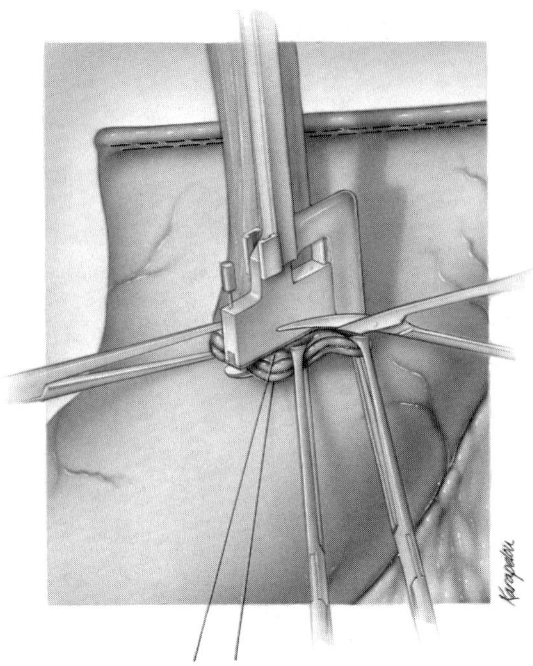

E

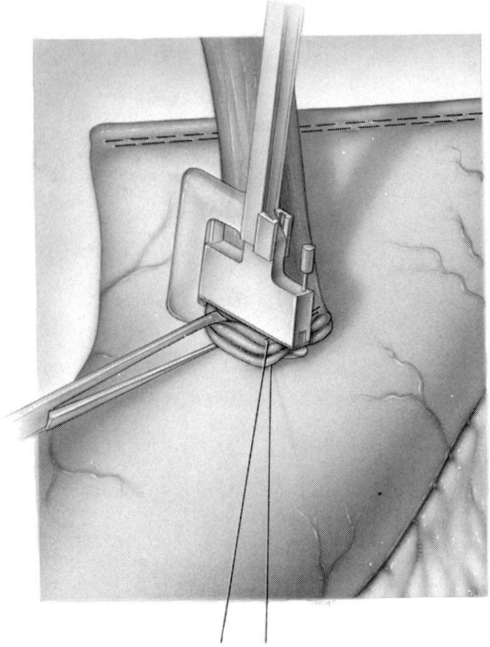

F

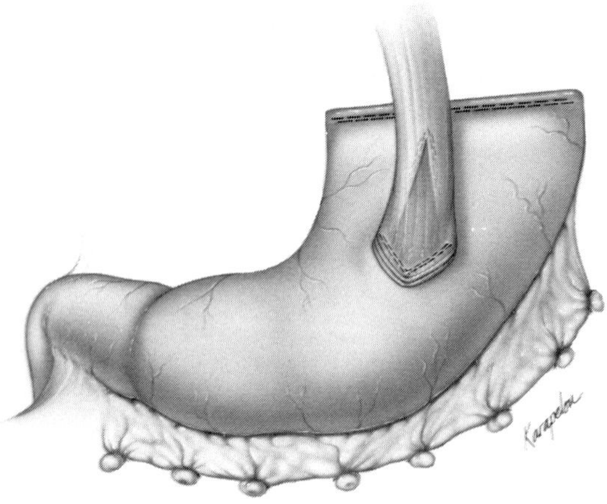

G

Fig. 28-1 (*continued*)

Fig. 28-2. Stapled esophagogastrostomy, end-to-end-anastomosis (EEA) method. (A) The TA-90 has been fired twice and the stomach is being divided between the two staple lines. (B) A 3-cm gastrotomy has been made. I prefer to use electrocautery. The EEA stapler without the anvil has been inserted into the gastrotomy. The mechanical purse-string device is shown applied to the point at which the EEA rod will exit. I prefer to insert the purse-string suture of 00 Prolene (polypropylene) manually. (C) A stab wound has been made to allow the EEA rod to exit. This should be at least 3 cm from the stapled edge of the gastric pouch. Now attach the anvil to the rod. (D) The anterior wall of the esophagus, including the mucosa, has been transected. The purse-string instrument is shown, but I prefer to insert the purse-string manually.

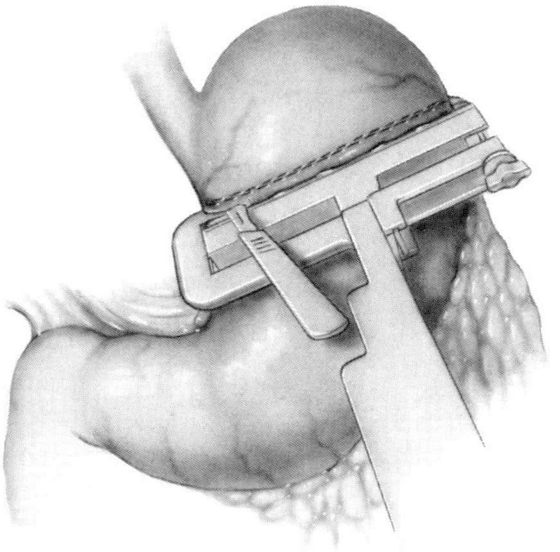

A

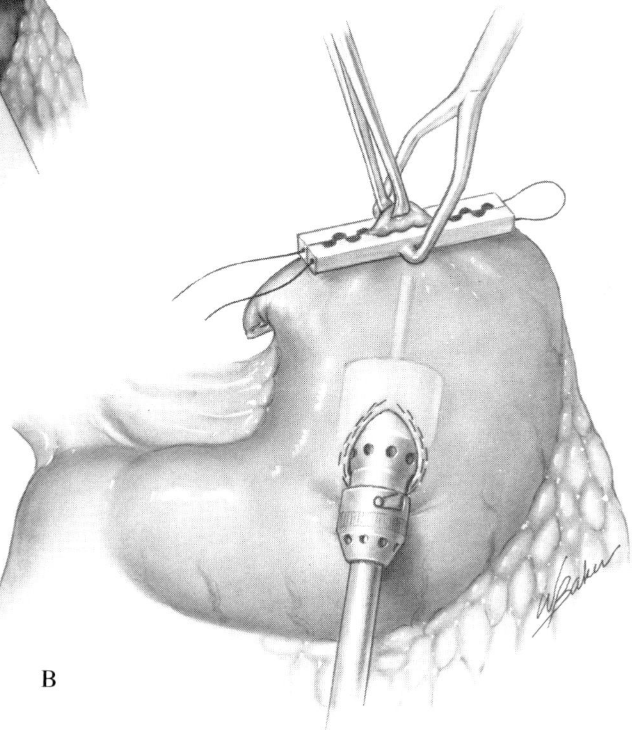

B

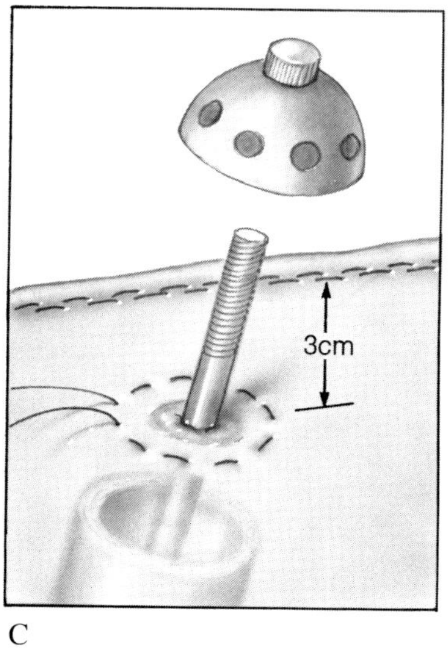

C

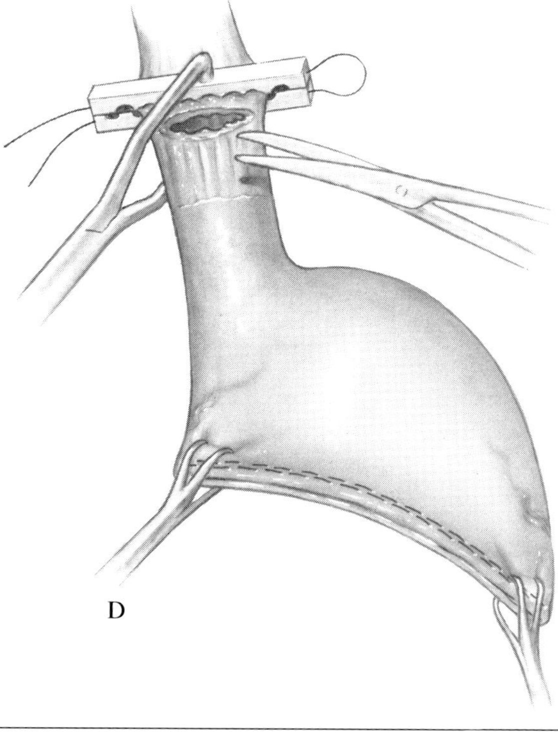

D

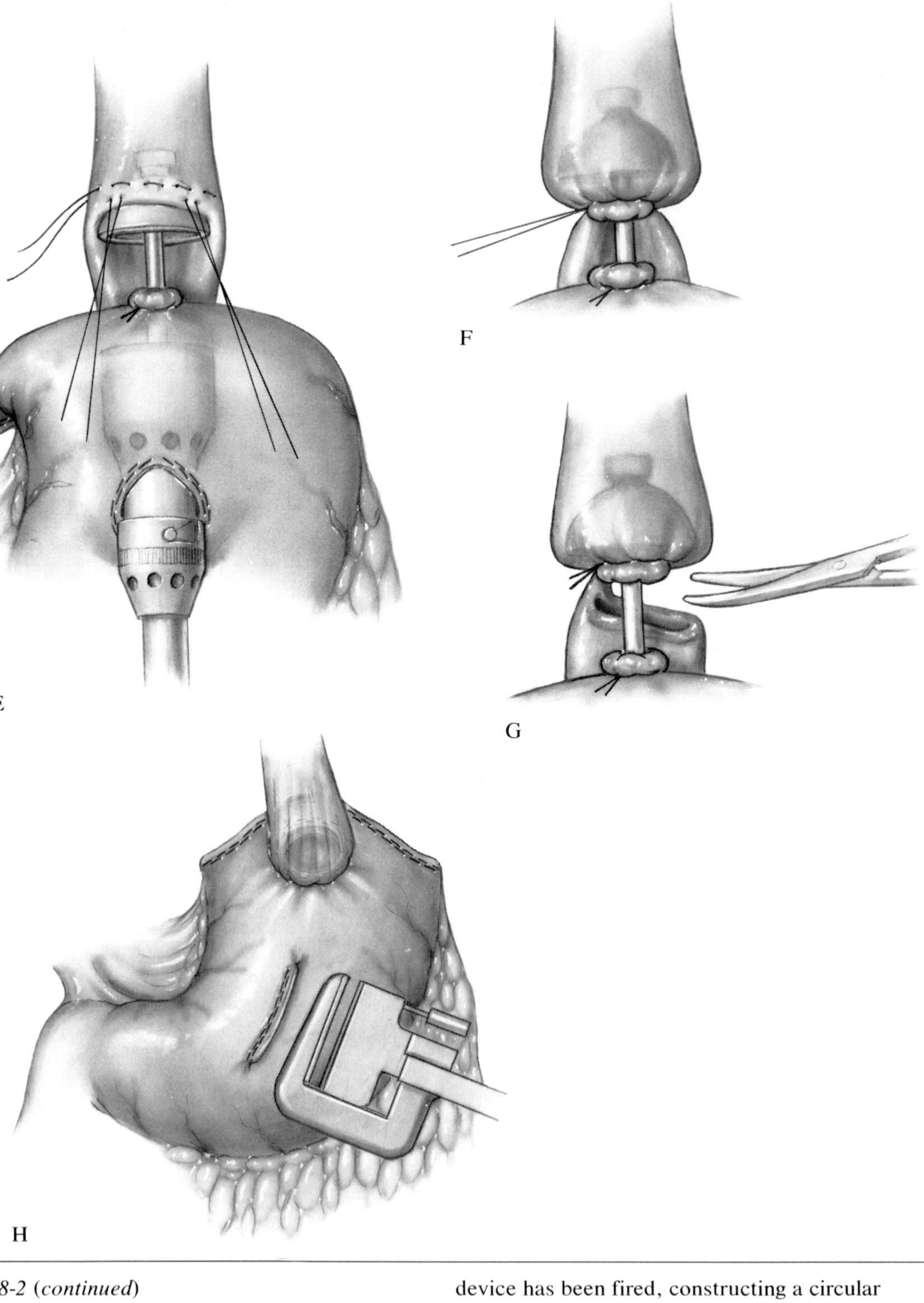

Fig. 28-2 (*continued*)
(E) The anvil has been gently inserted into the esophagus. (F) The purse-strings on the esophagus and on the gastric pouch have been tied. (G) The posterior wall of the esophagus has been divided close to the purse-string suture. (H) The EEA device has been fired, constructing a circular inverting esophagogastric anastomosis. The gastrotomy incision has been closed by a single application of the TA-55 device. Reprinted with permission of U.S. Surgical Corporation © USSC 1974, 1975, 1980. All rights reserved.

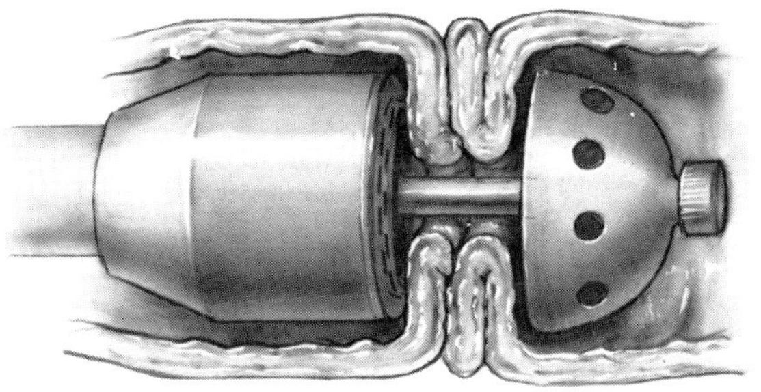

Fig. 28-3. The bulk of tissue, being compressed by the EEA, exceeds the capacity of the cartridge, and the excess tissue is extruded between the two seromuscular coats being coapted by the stapler. Reprinted with permission of U.S. Surgical Corporation © USSC 1974, 1975, 1980. All rights reserved.

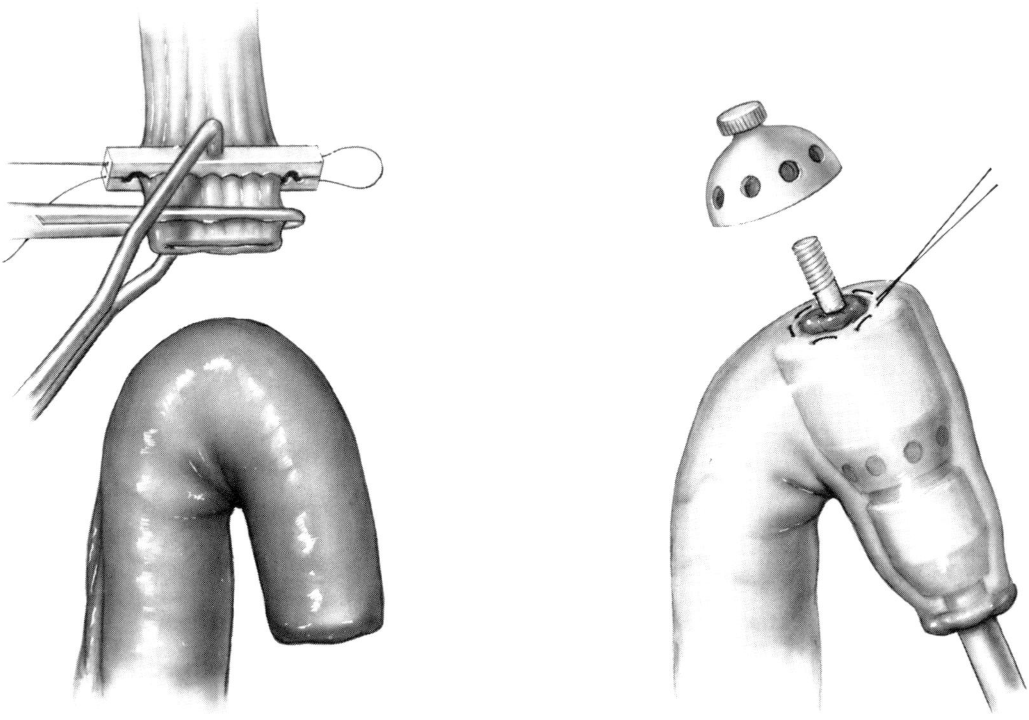

A B

Fig. 28-4. Stapled esophagojejunostomy, Roux-en-Y, following total gastrectomy. (A) A purse-string has been inserted into the lower esophagus. Then the excess esophagus is amputated beyond the purse-string. (B) The EEA device without an anvil has been inserted into the open end of the jejunum. A stab wound has been made on the antimesenteric border of jejunum and a purse-string suture inserted. The anvil will now be attached to the EEA rod.

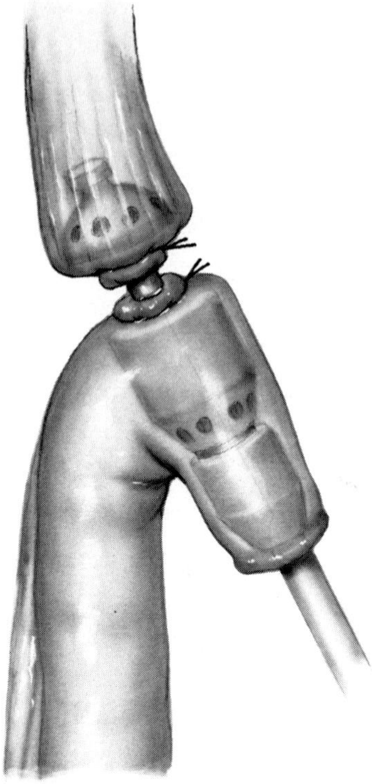

C

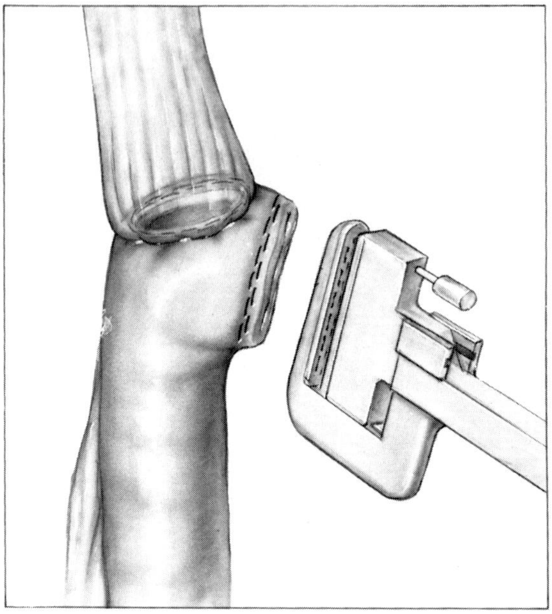

D

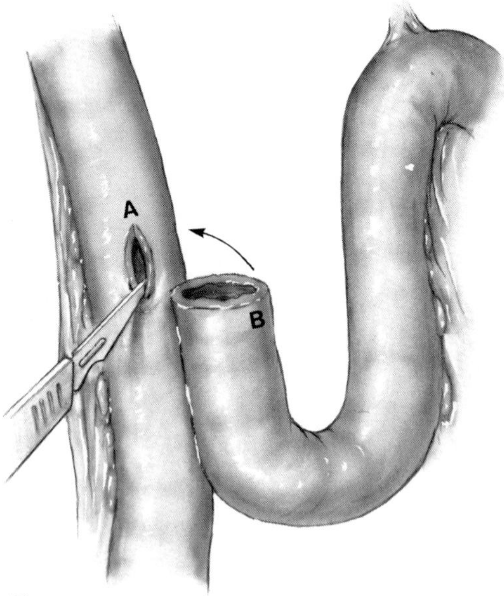

E

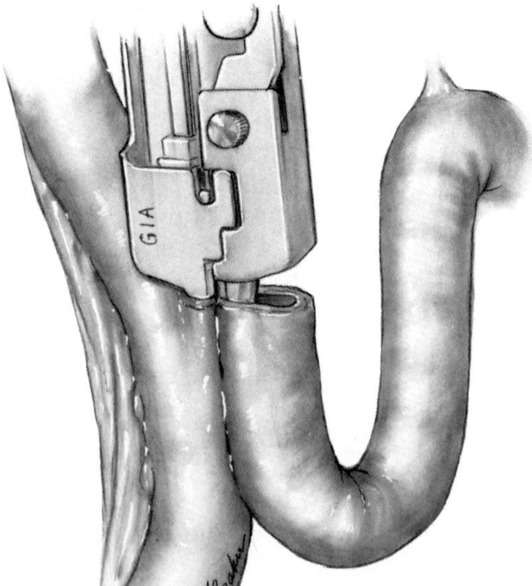

F

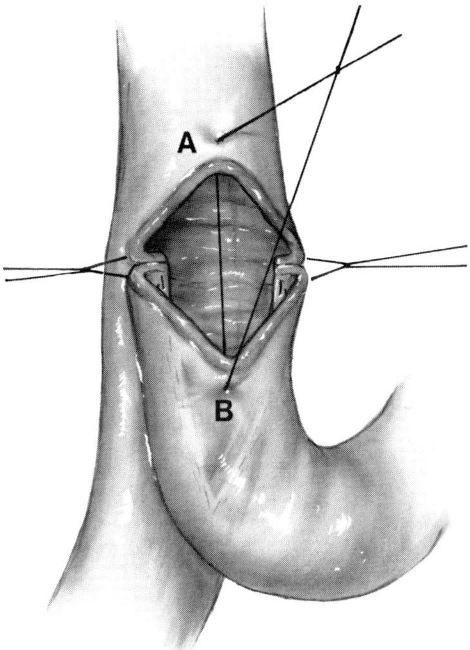

G

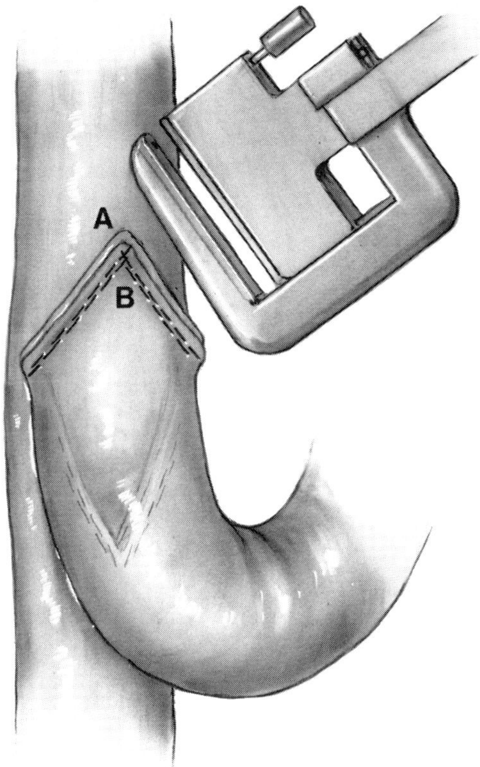

H

Fig. 28-4 (continued)
(C) Both purse-string sutures have been tied. The EEA device will now be closed and fired. (D) A TA-55 stapler has been placed across the jejunum about 1 cm proximal to the completed anastomosis, and a layer of staples has been fired, closing the end of jejunum, mucosa to mucosa. (E) The Roux-en-Y jejunojejunostomy is constructed 60 cm below the esophagojejunostomy. A 1.5-cm stab wound is made on the antimesenteric border of the descending limb of jejunum. Point A on the distal jejunum will eventually be approximated to point B on the proximal jejunum. (F) A GIA device is inserted, one fork into the stab wound of distal jejunum and the other fork into the open end of proximal jejunum. The stapler is activated, creating a side-to-side stapled anastomosis. (G) A stay suture is inserted, catching the left termination of the GIA staple line. A second stay suture catches the right-hand end of the GIA staple line and a third stay suture penetrates points A and B. Each stay suture contains the full thickness of intestine. The anterior portion of the anastomosis is accomplished by triangulation with two applications of the TA-55 stapler, one on the right and one on the left. (H) The large size of the resulting anastomosis is evident. Reprinted with permission of U.S. Surgical Corporation © USSC 1974, 1975, 1980. All rights reserved.

This can completely obstruct the continuity between the esophagus and the descending jejunum. After disengaging the EEA cartridge from the anastomosis, the surgeon should insert his or her index finger to be certain there is complete continuity between the esophagus and the descending limb of jejunum before proceeding to step D in Figure 28-4. In constructing the end-to-side esophagojejunostomy, I have found that the EEA technique is preferable to the GIA method.

The jejunum is sutured to the crux of the diaphragm or to the mediastinal pleura so that there will be no tension on the stapled anastomosis postoperatively.

A number of methods have been described for the construction of substitute gastric pouches by means of stapling after total gastrectomy [21]. Since there are no data demonstrating their superiority over a simple Roux-en-Y esophagojejunostomy, these techniques are omitted from this chapter.

Another operation in which stapling is of great value is the replacement or bypass of the esophagus with a segment of colon. I prefer the left colon, based on the left colic artery. The commonly voiced objection to this procedure is that it is a long operation because it requires three anastomoses, one colocolonic, one cologastric, and one esophagocolonic. When stapling techniques are used the colocolostomy and the cologastrostomy can be completed in 2 or 3 minutes. If exposure in the neck is not sufficient to admit stapling devices, the esophagocolonic anastomosis may be sutured by hand, and the entire colon replacement operation will not take longer than a gastric pullup with esophagogastrostomy in the neck.

The stapling device can also be used for the amputation of a Zenker diverticulum of the esophagus.

Billroth II Gastrectomy

If the duodenal stump is not excessively fibrotic, it is safe to close it by applying the TA-55 stapling device. If the duodenum is of normal thickness, the 3.5-mm stapler should be used. After the device has been fired, the everted mucosa is lightly electrocoagulated. It is not necessary to invert the staple line. This stapled closure has been demonstrated to be as safe as the sutured inverted duodenal closure [6, 14, 19].

In performing the gastrojejunostomy (Fig. 28-6D) the surgeon must be sure to make the stab wound for the GIA device 3 cm behind the TA-90 staple line to preserve the blood supply of the strip of stomach between the two staple lines. After firing the GIA stapler, the surgeon checks carefully for any bleeding along the mucosal surface of this anastomosis since arterial bleeding can occur from the gastric wall. In this situation the bleeding is controlled either with cautious electrocoagulation or by inserting hemostatic sutures of 5-0 Vicryl across the mucosal side of the anastomosis. In closing the stab wound (Fig. 28-6E), both the right-hand and left-hand terminations

Billroth I Gastroduodenostomy

When the duodenal stump is relatively healthy and large enough to admit the EEA cartridge, a stapled gastroduodenal anastomosis may be constructed efficiently with the EEA device. I prefer to perform this anastomosis by the technique described in Figure 28-5 because it offers the opportunity to inspect the mucosal surface of the anastomosis by direct vision through the open end of the stomach. If there are any deformed staples or there is any bleeding, corrective action is simplified. After ascertaining that the anastomosis is perfect, the stomach is closed 3 cm distal to the gastroduodenostomy using the TA-90 stapler and removing the gastric remnant. I prefer to electrocoagulate the everted mucosa lightly before removing the TA-90. One must next check for bleeding. It is not necessary, with the gastroduodenostomy or the esophagogastrostomy, to invert the TA-90 staple line with sutures.

Fig. 28-5. Billroth I stapled gastrectomy. (A) A purse-string suture has been placed in the duodenal stump. The EEA stapler without an anvil has been inserted into the open end of the antrum and emerges from a stab wound through the posterior gastric wall. A purse-string suture has been inserted and tied around this stab wound. The anvil will now be attached to the EEA rod. (B) The anvil has been inserted into the duodenal stump and the duodenal purse-string has been tied. (C) The EEA device has been activated, completing the gastroduodenal anastomosis. (D) A TA-90 stapler has been applied to close the stomach at a point 2–3 cm beyond the anastomosis. The TA-90 is closed and fired, and the specimen is being detached by an incision flush with the TA-90. (E) The gastroduodenal anastomosis is shown, together with the mucosa-to-mucosa closure of the gastric pouch. Reprinted with permission of U.S. Surgical Corporation © USSC 1974, 1975, 1980. All rights reserved.

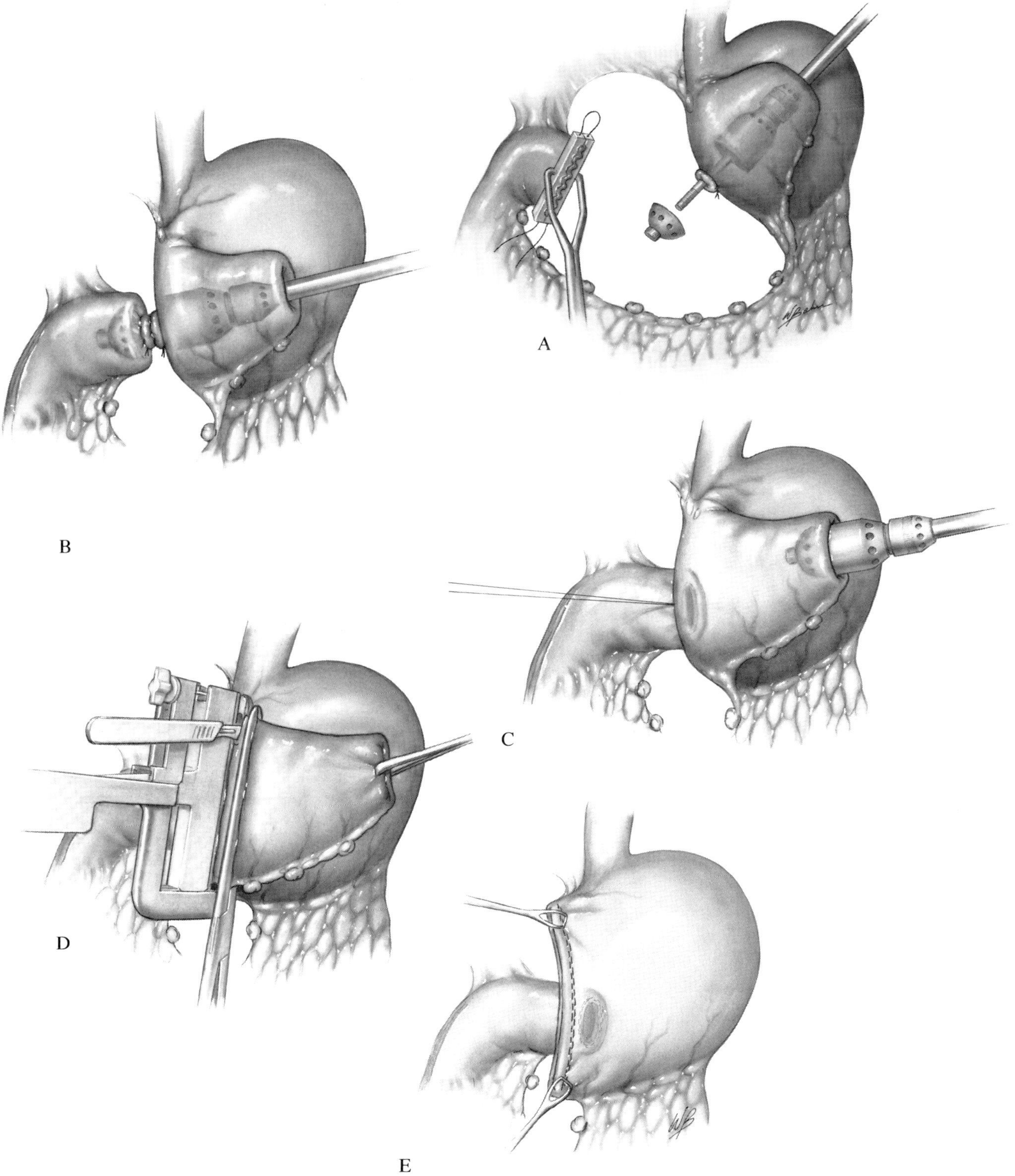
A
B
C
D
E

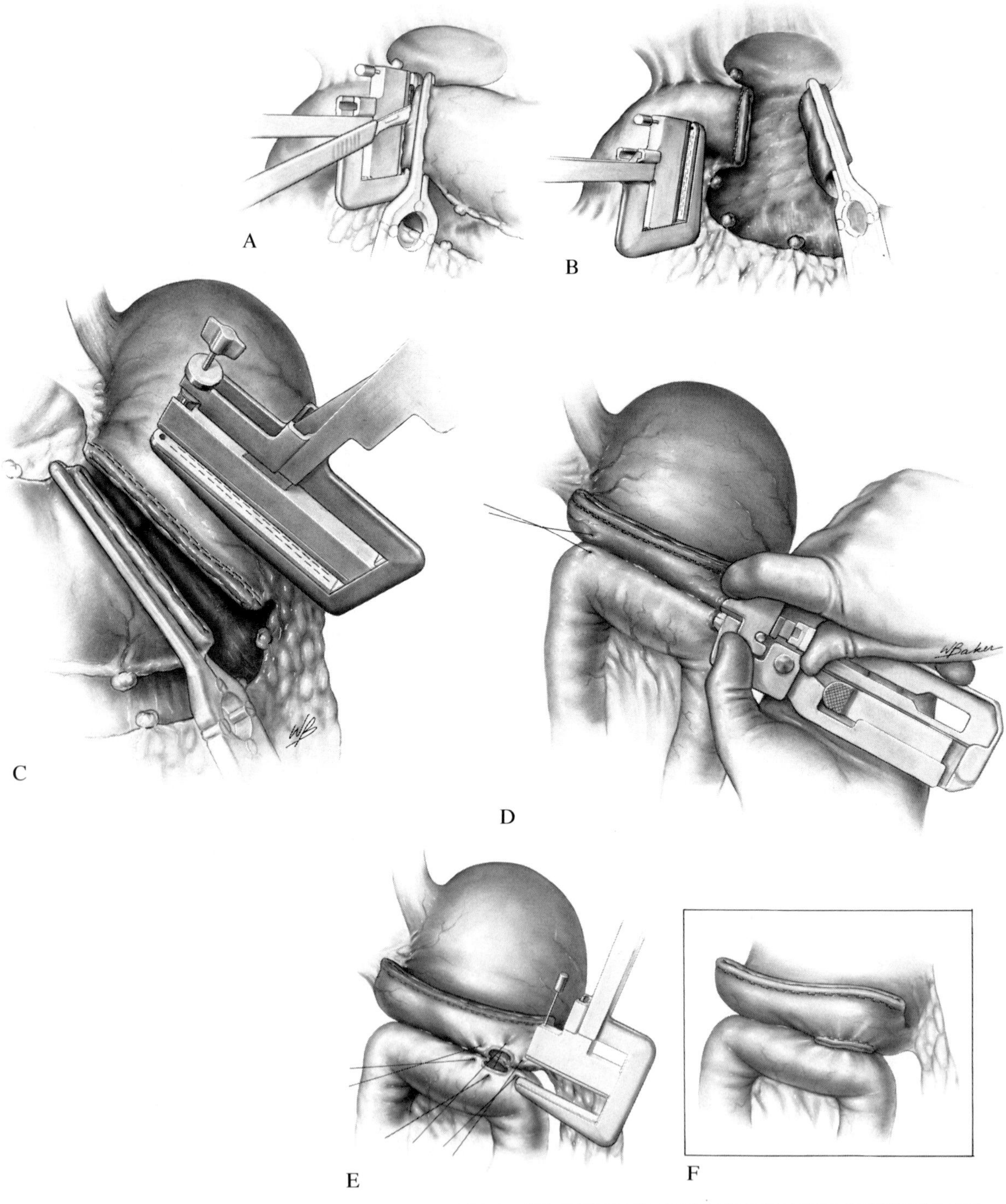
A
B
C
D
E
F

of the GIA staple line must be included in the stay sutures so that when the TA-55 is applied it will close the defect without any gaps. All staple lines should be checked carefully before the next step in the operation is begun.

Pyloroplasty

A Heineke-Mikulicz pyloroplasty may be constructed rapidly and efficiently using the stapling technique (Fig. 28-7). Because of the thickness of the pylorus, a 4.8-mm cartridge will generally be necessary. All the layers of the stomach and duodenum must be incorporated into the staple line. To accomplish this it is advisable to place Allis clamps at intervals of about 1.5 cm along the entire line of tissue to be enclosed in the stapling device. Otherwise, as the wing nut on the stapler is tightened some portion of the tissue may pull away from the device before the firing of the staples.

Fig. 28-6. Billroth II gastrectomy. (A) After the duodenum has been mobilized, a TA-55 stapler is applied and fired. The duodenum is divided flush with the stapler. (B) The completed duodenal closure is shown. (C) The stomach has been transected after having been closed by an application of the TA-90 stapler. (D) A stab wound has been made on the posterior wall of the gastric pouch, 3 cm behind the TA-90 staple line. A second stab wound has been made on the antimesenteric border of the proximal jejunum, and the GIA device has been inserted, one fork into the stomach and one fork into the jejunum. The device is being fired. Then a single seromuscular suture is placed, approximating stomach and jejunum at the termination of the GIA staple line. (E) The GIA device has been removed. The gastrojejunal staple line has been inspected and stay sutures are inserted. The TA-55 will be applied, making certain that it crosses both the right and the left terminations of the GIA staple line. (F) Completion of the anastomosis after the stab wound has been closed by the TA-55 stapler. Reprinted with permission of U.S. Surgical Corporation © USSC 1974, 1975, 1980. All rights reserved.

Local Excision of Gastric Lesion with Stapled Closure

Occasionally it is necessary to perform local excision of a small gastric lesion. If the lesion can be mobilized as shown in Figure 28-8, the surgeon simply applies a TA-90 stapler, fires it, and excises the lesion.

Modified Sugiura Operation for Esophageal Varices

In a simplification of the Sugiura [23] operation, Ginsberg and associates [10] use a left thoracoabdominal incision through the seventh interspace, open the diaphragm circumferentially, perform a splenectomy, and devascularize the proximal half of the stomach and lower esophagus with a highly selective vagotomy. The esophageal devascularization extends to the inferior pulmonary vein but preserves all the longitudinal veins. The EEA stapler is inserted through a gastrotomy into the lower esophagus (Fig. 28-9). A heavy chromic catgut suture is tied around the esophagus, and the EEA stapler is fired, automatically excising a circle of esophagus and reanastomosing the organ end to end. The EEA-25 cartridge is usually required, although a larger cartridge is used if the lumen of the esophagus is large enough. Ginsberg et al. [10] created a loose Nissen type of fundoplication around the lower esophagus, encircling the anastomosis. Otherwise, indications for the use of the EEA stapling device for transection and reanastomosis have been found to be limited [15].

A number of studies have demonstrated that stapling techniques for creation of esophageal and gastric anastomoses are safe, provided the surgeon learns the pitfalls and danger points of each method. When done by an experienced surgeon, stapling an anastomosis saves time—a factor helpful in the care of high-risk and critically ill patients. In such patients the advantage of expediting the operation far outweighs the increased cost of using staples.

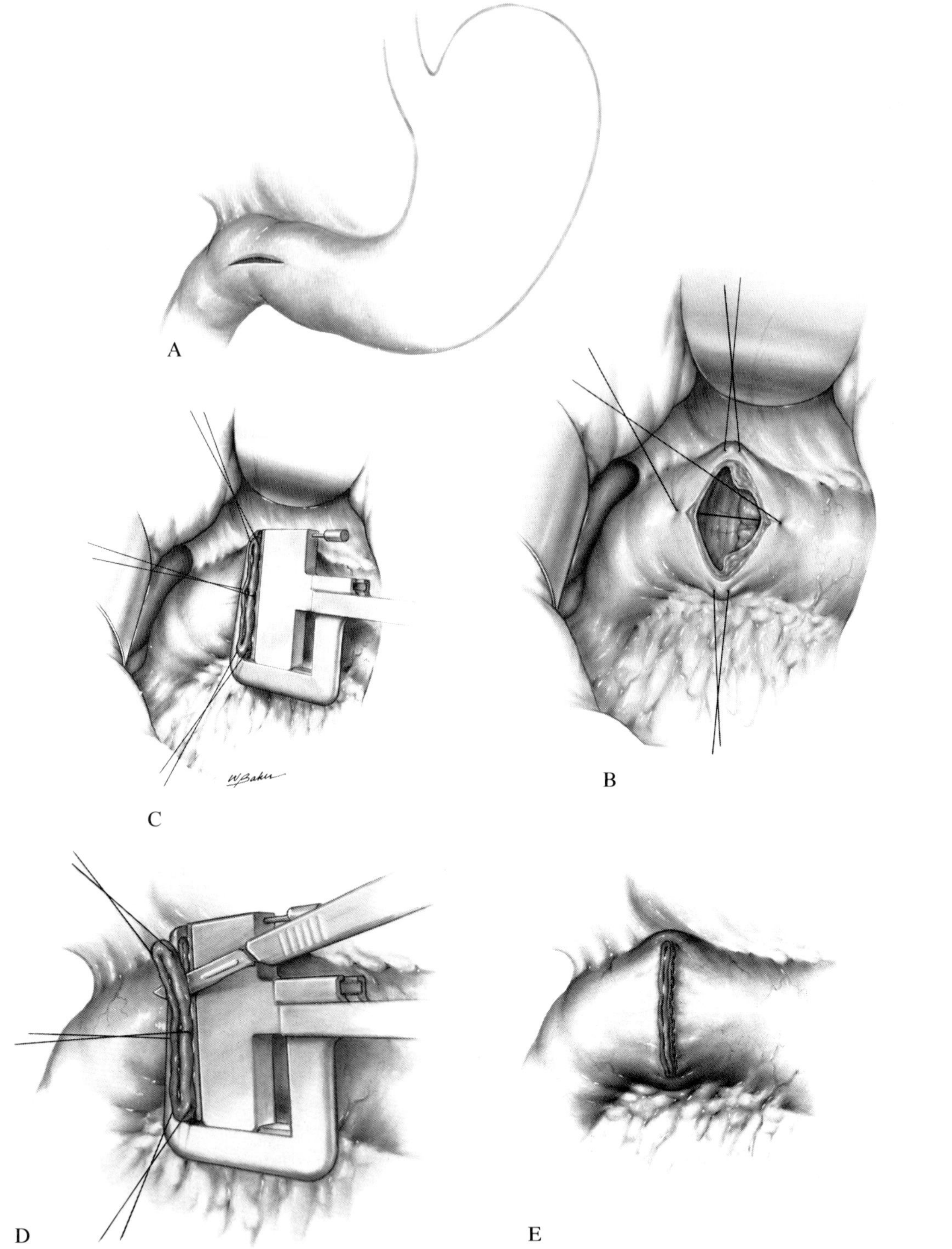

Fig. 28-7. Heineke-Mikulicz pyloroplasty. (A) A 5-cm incision along the anterior wall of antrum and duodenum has been made with its center at the pylorus. (B) Guy sutures have been placed at the midpoints of the incision as well as at the proximal and distal extremities of the incision. (C) A TA-90 stapler has been applied to close the incision in a transverse direction. (D) After the TA-90 has been fired, the surplus tissue is excised. (E) Appearance of the everted pyloroplasty. Reprinted with permission of U.S. Surgical Corporation

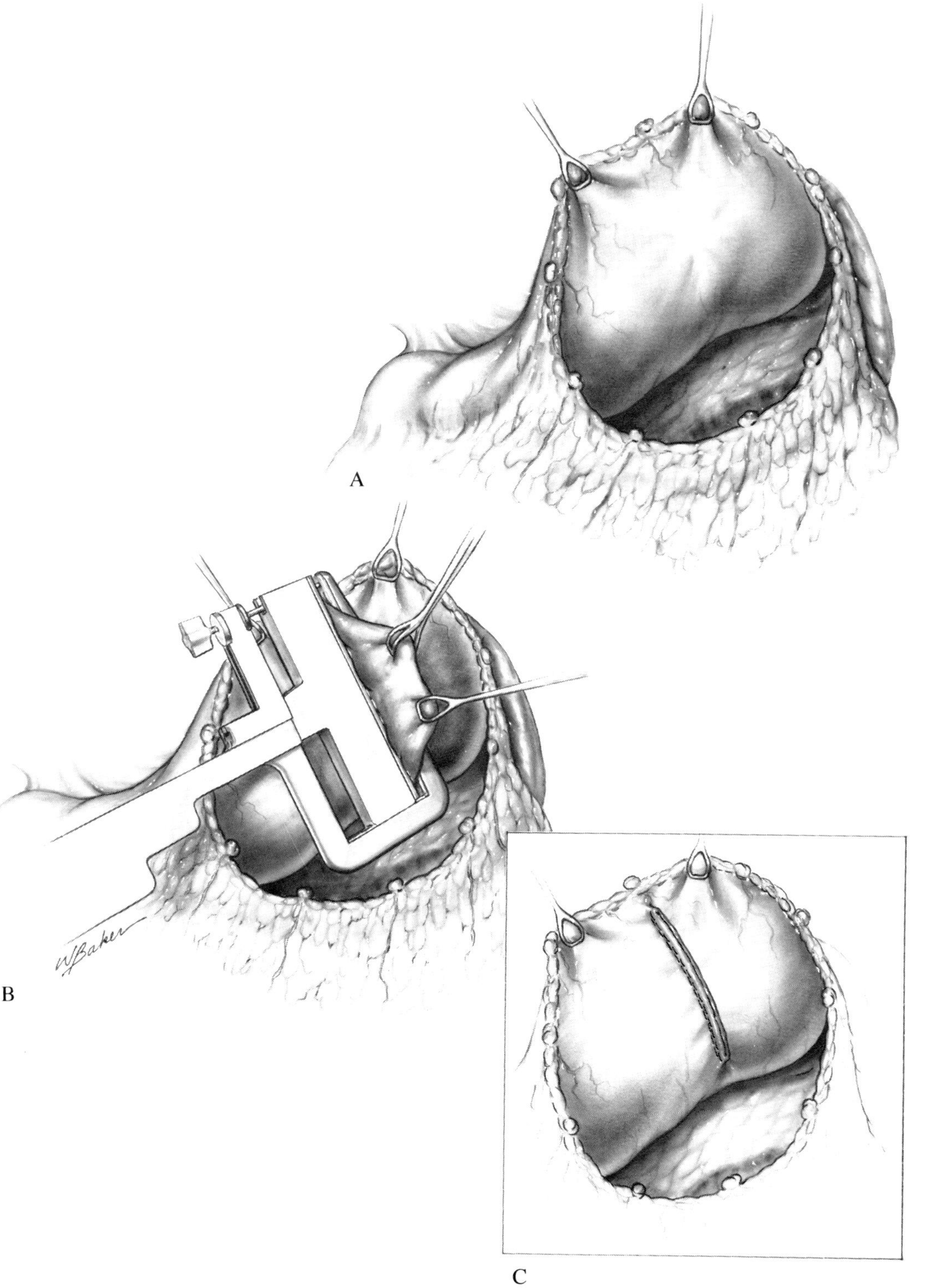

Fig. 28-8. Excision of gastric lesion. (A) Exposure of a benign lesion. (B) The lesion is grasped in Babcock clamps, and a TA-90 stapler has been applied transversely, closed, and fired. The specimen will be removed by applying a scalpel along the stapling device. (C) Appearance of the completed gastric closure. Reprinted with permission of U.S. Surgical Corporation © USSC 1974, 1975, 1980. All rights reserved.

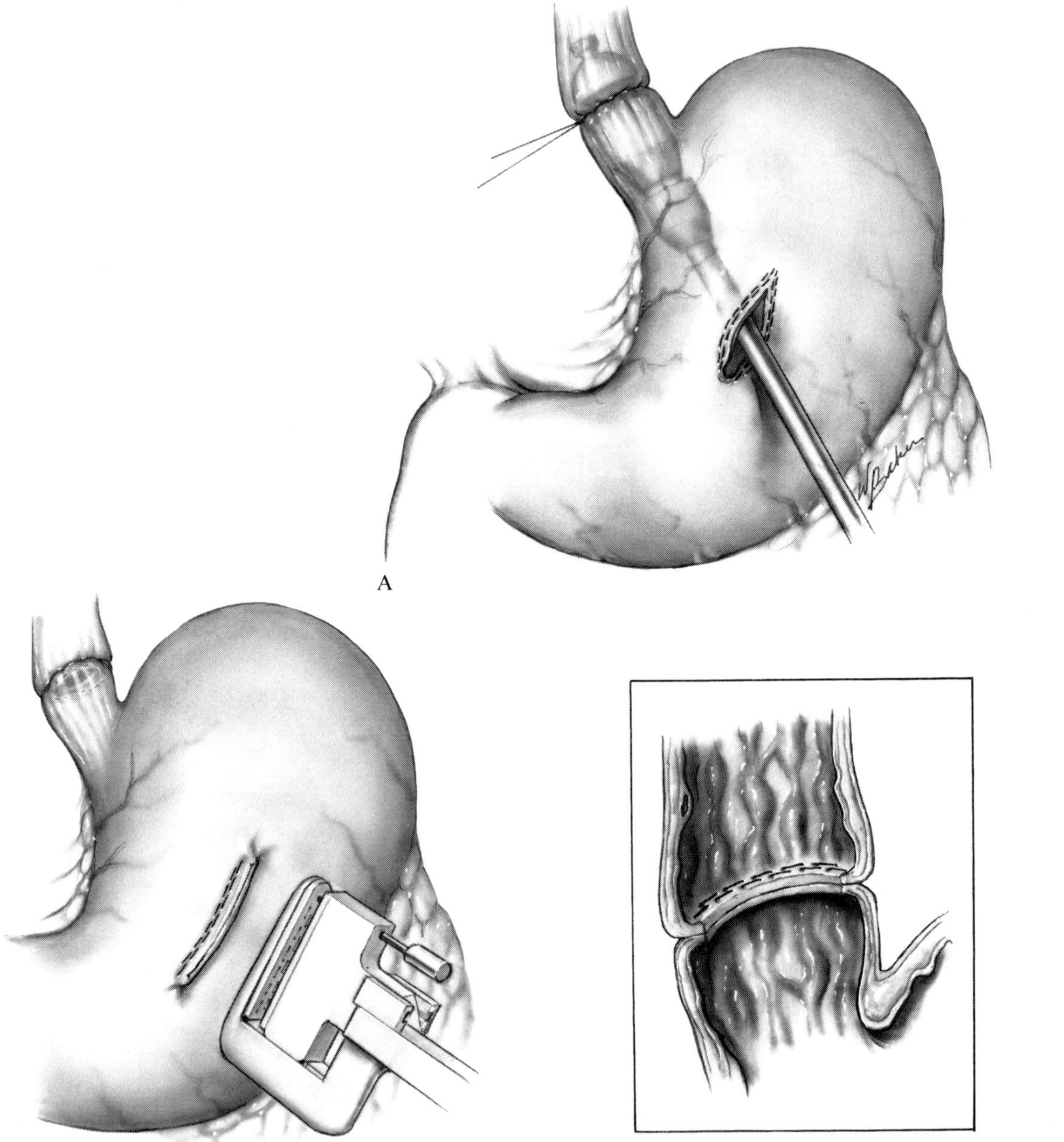

A

B

C

Fig. 28-9. Interruption of esophageal varices. (A) A gastrotomy has been made on the anterior wall of the stomach, and the diameter of the esophagus has been approximated by passing sizers. An EEA-25 or EEA-28 cartridge is inserted through the gastrotomy into the lower esophagus. The wing nut is then rotated to open the space between the anvil and the cartridge. A heavy ligature is passed around the esophagus and is tied so that a ring of esophagus is tightly approximated to the EEA rod. The tails of the ligature are cut. The EEA is closed and fired, excising a complete ring of esophagus and completing an end-to-end anastomosis. The EEA is opened, disengaged, and removed. (B) The gastrotomy incision has been closed by means of a TA-55 stapler. (C) Internal view of the anastomosis. Reprinted with permission of U.S. Surgical Corporation © USSC 1974, 1975, 1980. All rights reserved.

References

1. Akiyama, H. Surgery for carcinoma of the esophagus. *Curr. Probl. Surg.* 17:56, 1980.
2. Carey, J. S., Plested, W. G., and Hughes, R. K. Esophagogastrectomy: Superiority of the combined abdominal–right thoracic approach (Lewis operation). *Ann. Thorac. Surg.* 14:59, 1972.
3. Chassin, J. L. Esophagogastrectomy: Data favoring end-to-side anastomosis. *Ann. Surg.* 188:22, 1978.
4. Chassin, J. L. Stapling technique for esophagogastrostomy after esophagogastric resection. *Am. J. Surg.* 136:399, 1978.
5. Chassin, J. L. *Operative Strategy in General Surgery: An Expositive Atlas,* Vol. I, New York: Springer, 1980.
6. Chassin, J. L., Rifkind, K. M., Sussman, B., et al. The stapled gastrointestinal tract anastomosis: Incidence of postoperative complications compared with the sutured anastomosis. *Ann. Surg.* 188:689, 1978.
7. Chassin, J. L., Rifkind, K. M., and Turner, J. W. Errors and pitfalls in stapling gastrointestinal tract anastomoses. *Surg. Clin. North Am.* 64:441, 1984.
8. Fekete, F., Breil, P. H., Ronsse, H., et al. EEA stapler and omental graft in esophagogastrectomy: Experience with 30 intrathoracic anastomoses for cancer. *Ann. Surg.* 193:825, 1981.
9. Fisher, R. D., Brawley, R. K., and Kieffer, R. F. Esophagogastrectomy in the treatment of carcinoma of the distal two-thirds of the esophagus. *Ann. Thorac. Surg.* 14:658, 1972.
10. Ginsberg, R. J., Waters, P. F., Zeldin, R. A., et al. A modified Sugiura procedure. *Ann. Thorac. Surg.* 34:258, 1982.
11. Graham, H. K., Johnston, G. W., McKelvey, S. T. D., and Kennedy, T. L. Five years' experience in stapling the oesophagus and rectum. *Br. J. Surg.* 68:697, 1981.
12. Gritsman, J. J. Mechanical suture by Soviet apparatus in gastric resection: Use in 4,000 operations. *Surgery* 59:663, 1966.
13. Hopkins, R. A., Alexander, J. C., and Postlethwait, R. W. Stapled esophagogastric anastomosis. *Am. J. Surg.* 147:283, 1984.
14. Lowdon, I. M. R., Gear, M. W. L., and Kilby, J. O. Stapling instruments in upper gastrointestinal surgery: A retrospective study of 362 cases. *Br. J. Surg.* 69:333, 1982.
15. Mucha, P., Jr., and van Heerden, J. A. EEA stapling for control of acute variceal hemorrhage. *Am. J. Surg.* 148:399, 1984.
16. Ravitch, M. M., Brolin, R., Kolter, J., and Yap, S. Studies in the healing of intestinal anastomoses. *World J. Surg.* 5:627, 1981.
17. Ravitch, M. M., Lane, R., Cornell, W. P., Rivarola, A., and McEnany, T. Closure of duodenal, gastric and intestinal stumps with wire staples: Experimental and clinical studies. *Ann. Surg.* 163:573, 1966.
18. Ravitch, M. M., and Steichen, F. M. Technics of staple suturing in the gastrointestinal tract. *Ann. Surg.* 175:815, 1972.
19. Scher, K. S., Scott-Conner, C., and Ong, W. T. A comparison of stapled and sutured anastomoses in gastric operations. *Surg. Gynecol. Obstet.* 154:548, 1982.
20. Smith, C. R., Cokelet, G. R., Adams, J. T., and Schwartz, S. I. Vascularity of gastrointestinal staple lines demonstrated with silicone rubber injection. *Am. J. Surg.* 142:563, 1981.
21. Steichen, F., and Ravitch, M. M. Mechanical sutures in esophageal surgery. *Ann. Surg.* 191:373, 1980.
22. Steichen, F. M., and Ravitch, M. M. Contemporary stapling instruments and basic mechanical suture techniques. *Surg. Clin. North Am.* 64:425, 1984.
23. Sugiura, M., and Futagawa, S. A new technique for treating esophageal varices. *J. Thorac. Cardiovasc. Surg.* 66:677, 1980.
24. West, P., Marbarger, J., Martz, M., and Roper, C. Esophagogastrostomy with the EEA stapler. *Ann. Surg.* 193:76, 1981.
25. Wilson, S. E., Stone, R., Scully, M., Ozeran, L., and Benfield, J. R. Modern management of anastomotic leak after esophagogastrectomy. *Am. J. Surg.* 144:95, 1982.

29

Gastric Reduction for Obesity

Edward E. Mason

Extreme obesity has long been considered a sign of inadequate willpower, and it is generally recognized to be intractable to dietary control [1]. Although many related problems such as diabetes are diagnosed and frequently treated, physicians have been reluctant to accept obesity per se as a disease. In the past, diets were provided for overweight patients with gallstones, hernias, and other conditions requiring elective operations, and these patients were told to return for an operation only after they had lost a specified amount of weight. Because the prescribed weight loss was never achieved, many patients never returned unless their condition produced a crisis.

In 1954 Kremen, Linner, and Nelson [21] reported a study of the deleterious effects of small intestinal bypass on protein digestion and absorption in dogs and mentioned the first use of intestinal bypass in treating an obese woman. Payne and DeWind [33] popularized the use of intestinal bypass in 1969. Although this operation offers at best an exchange of the short bowel syndrome, with its many hazards, for the morbidity of obesity, many morbidly obese patients saw it as an opportunity to begin a new life. The frequency of operations for obesity increased exponentially. Morbid obesity became a recognizable disease only after an effective treatment had been provided. Rejection, shame, depression, and seclusion were replaced by acceptance, hope, and an aggressive demand for treatment.

Criteria for an Acceptable Operation

Initially only extreme obesity justified surgical treatment, and the operation had to be reversible. The first bypass operations of Payne and DeWind were planned as temporary, to be used under close observation as a means of reducing weight but not to maintain weight reduction. Other criteria evolved; present-day bariatric operations must be effective, safe, free of side effects, and reversible although intended to be permanent. Intestinal bypass frequently failed to satisfy all of these criteria. Some patients were well served, but for too

many there appeared to be no margin of safety between weight control and complications.

Gastric bypass, introduced in 1966, was used exclusively at the University of Iowa for 10 years before physicians in other centers became interested in the procedure [31]. To operate in the upper abdomen of a huge patient is indeed a formidable undertaking. The new gastric operation would probably never have been accepted had not intestinal bypass been so fraught with complications that the affected patients were becoming too numerous to care for. Despite complications, however, there was no turning back. Morbid obesity had been recognized as a disease that required attention, and a better operation was needed. In 1976 Hornberger [20] as well as Hermreck et al. [19] reported the first two series of patients treated with gastric bypass outside the University of Iowa. They observed that the procedure was no more difficult technically than intestinal bypass. In 1977 Alden [2] reported a modification with anterior gastroenterostomy and stapling-in-continuity that required little more than an hour to complete. With this procedure the race was on to develop and test many modifications of gastric reduction operations for obesity, and this race continues today.

Specifications for an Effective Gastric Reduction Operation

Specifications for effective gastric reduction operations have been evolving since 1977. Intake limitation requires elimination of the reservoir function of the stomach, but does not require bypass of any part of the digestive tract. In fact, the least interference with normal digestion and absorption should result from some form of gastroplasty that allows the ingested food to traverse the lower stomach, duodenum, and all of the intestine. Optimum results follow creation of (1) an upper gastric pouch volume of less than 25 ml, measured at a pressure of 70 cm of saline solution above the cricoid process when the patient is in a horizontal position; (2) a secure partition between upper and lower stomach segments; and (3) an outlet from the small pouch that has an inside diameter of 12 mm and that will neither narrow nor dilate.

Monitoring, Quality Control, Evaluation, and Audit

Although gastric reduction operations are analogues of resections, they have different objectives. The technical details are also new. The stomach, a muscular pump with tremendous capacity, requires rigid compartmentalization and drainage by a technique that will permanently control bulimia and snacking without producing obstruction. Metal and plastic materials must make the healed partition and stoma permanent without causing infection, perforation, fistula, or excessive scarring, and without producing irreversible change. Intraoperative measurement of volume, pressure, and stomal size must be performed with strict attention to detail, and compliance with specifications should be recorded using the checklist approach common to any high-quality procedure. Lack of attention to these simple intraoperative requirements will result in an unwarranted failure rate and the need for a difficult revisional operation. Indeed, the lack of information about the original operation may even delay a surgeon's recognition of what is wrong and what needs to be done to make the operation effective. Successful weight loss with minimal suffering to the patient requires that surgeons undertaking these operations learn from their own patients and from the experiences of others. Continuity of care helps to tie cause to effect. Excellent record-keeping is essential to provide the rationale for corrections in technique that may be required to reach the safe, effective, and easily tolerated restriction of eating necessary for weight control.

Indications for Surgical Treatment

Almost all patients operated on have failed in repeated attempts to diet. Many have joined

organizations such as TOPS and Weight Watchers. Many have taken appetite suppressant medications and undergone hypnosis or instruction in behavioral modification. In spite of these efforts, often undertaken with the greatest sincerity, the overwhelming majority of patients either fail to lose weight or regain as much or more than they lost.

No patients should be required to develop a complication of morbid obesity before effective treatment is provided. Although diabetes, hypertension, hypoventilation, ruptured intervertebral disc, degenerative arthritis, stasis leg ulcers, giant hernia, gallstones, and other conditions induced or aggravated by obesity add to the urgency for treatment, it would be better to reduce weight before the symptoms appear.

While the risk of morbid obesity is difficult to quantify, it is, nonetheless, real. Drenick et al. [9] found an excessive mortality of from 1.85 to 12-fold, depending on age, in men whose average weight was 143.5 kg. The greatest percentage of increased risk was found in patients between the ages of 24 and 35 years, but increasing age also produced a steady increase in risk. In Drenick's study each of 200 men were followed for an average of 7.5 years, during which time 50 died. We can improve this risk with an effective surgical procedure that has 0.4 percent operative mortality.

Often when patients are reminded that major operations carry a risk of death, they respond that life is not worth living at their current weight. Surgical treatment should be used early enough to prevent the acceleration of degenerative changes that contribute to increased risk of premature death in the obese. Among patients older than 50 years of age who underwent gastric bypass between 1966 and 1970, late deaths caused by coronary artery disease, cancer, and other chronic conditions occurred in 10 percent. For these patients surgical treatment of obesity should have been used at a younger age [15, 18].

Gastric Bypass

Billroth II gastrectomy at one time was the recommended surgical treatment of peptic ulcer. An unwanted side effect of Billroth II gastrectomy for ulcer was poor maintenance of body weight. This previously unwanted side effect became the focus of attention for enhancement in gastric bypass. Some patients, however, managed to maintain an excessive weight after both Billroth II and gastric bypass. Therefore, certain specifications had to be defined to ensure weight control (Fig. 29-1).

More complete details of the evolution of gastric reduction operations are available elsewhere [29]. Briefly, initial concern with gastric bypass was related to its configuration as an exclusion operation. Antral exclusion alone is ulcerogenic, but by excluding acid-secreting mucosa with the antrum, autoregulation is preserved. Along with preserving acid suppression of antral gastrin, gastric bypass obviates stimulation of acid by food. As a result, gastric bypass, when sufficiently extensive to control weight, also decreases acid secretion. Hence stomal ulceration is infrequent unless the obese patient also has an ulcer diathesis from vagal overactivity. The usefulness of near-total gastric exclusion in peptic ulcer has not been tested, but a 60–85 percent exclusion is not effective.

Success in weight control with these operations requires an understanding of the mechanisms at work. If there is an underlying predisposition toward dumping and an ample gastroenterostomy, then dumping, a common cause of asthenia in patients with loss of pyloric muscle control of gastric emptying following gastrectomy, may contribute to a voluntarily reduced intake and change in type of food ingested. More than half of the patients do not have dumping symptoms, and even in patients with such symptoms the effects are usually mild and decrease with time. For a predictable reduction in intake to result in all patients, it is necessary to take the approach of controlling emptying at an appropriately slow rate. This is accomplished by construct-

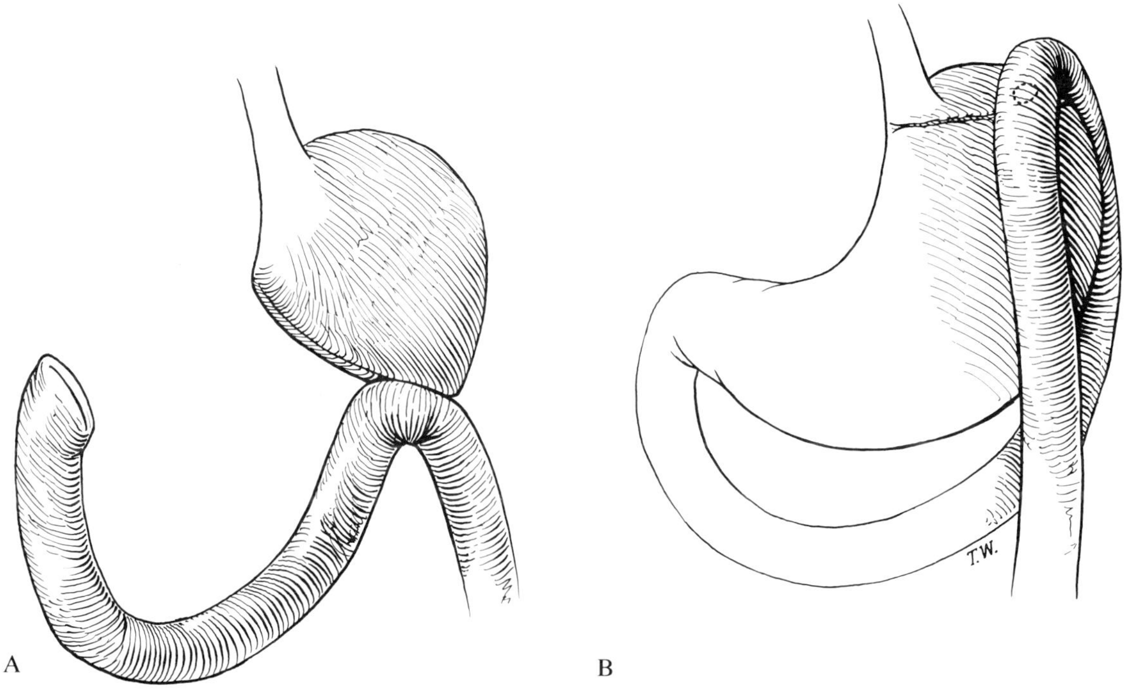

Fig. 29-1. A 60% Billroth II gastrectomy for ulcer (A), and gastric bypass for obesity (B). The gastric bypass has a measured, upper pouch volume of 25 ml or less with a 12-mm diameter stoma. (From Mason, E. E., Gastric reduction for obesity. In L. M. Nyhus and R. J. Baker (Eds.), *Mastery of Surgery*. Boston: Little, Brown, 1984.)

ing a stoma of 10–12 mm in diameter. At the same time dumping symptoms are avoided.

SMALL STOMA

The small stomal size has become a critical issue. If it is too small, obstruction can become a problem, although endoscopic balloon dilation of outlet stenosis has been successful [26]. Not only should the stoma be made appropriately narrow, but some additional technique should be used during the initial operation to prevent later dilatation as the patient attempts to force more food through the area. Unfortunately, the addition of foreign material such as a Marlex mesh collar to an area of anastomosis, combined with potential contamination from transection of stomach and intestine, increases the risk of infection. To date there is no satisfactory solution to this problem in gastric bypass. Results of experimental studies suggest that Marlex mesh sutured to itself does prevent dilatation of the stoma without increasing the incidence of complications [5].

UPPER SEGMENT VOLUME

Another intraoperative measurement that is critical to quality control involves the volume of the upper segment. For 50 years surgeons used gastrectomy for the treatment of peptic ulcer knowing that the size of the resection was important in the incidence of stomal ulcer. Yet they could never think of a way to measure volume accurately. Alder and Terry [3] measured volume in the upper segment during gastric bypass simply by injecting saline solution through the nasogastric tube. I added a manometer and learned that a water pressure of 70 cm can greatly increase the reliability of the volume measurement (Fig. 29-2). Coincident to learning the importance of measuring under a constant pressure, the optimum volumes were reduced from 100 to 60

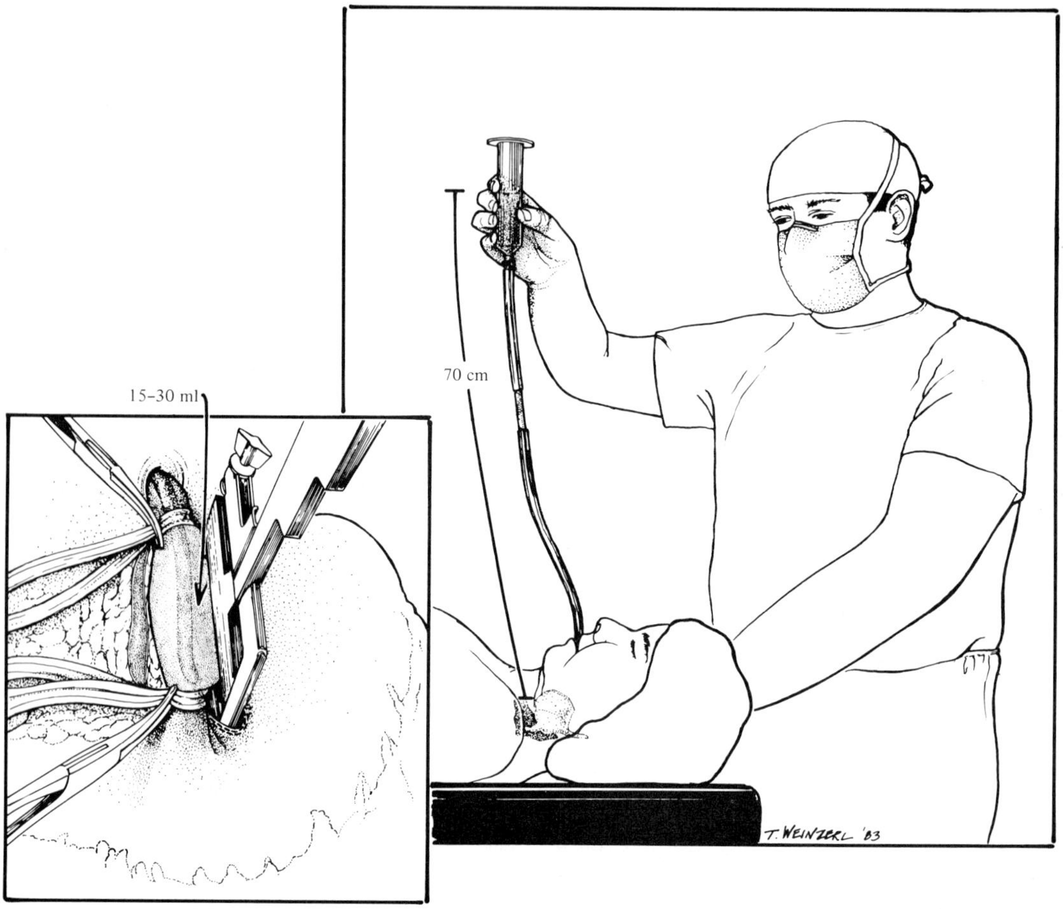

Fig. 29-2. Intraoperative measurement of volume, performed using an open syringe barrel attached to an Ewald tube. The tube openings are in the upper pouch and the esophagus is occluded by temporary placement of a Penrose drain. The stomach is loosely clamped with the TA-90 stapling instrument. (From Mason, E. E., Gastric reduction for obesity. In L. M. Nyhus and R. J. Baker (Eds.), *Mastery of Surgery*. Boston: Little, Brown, 1984.)

ml and finally to 14 ml. We also learned that a small stoma could not compensate for a large volume because such a configuration not only caused frequent vomiting but at the same time allowed the patient to carry a reservoir of digesting food that was slowly but continuously passing through the stoma, thereby sustaining an excessive body weight.

The technique of volume measurement must be simple so that it can be performed by a circulating nurse or anesthesiologist without requiring excessive time searching for special equipment. Otherwise this important measurement may not be performed and recorded routinely. An open barrel of a 60-ml syringe attached to an Ewald tube is filled with saline solution and held high while the surgeon and assistant milk the gastric pouch and tubing to eliminate any air that might be present. The tube is then held below the level of the cricoid process. The stomach pouch should empty. A Penrose drain placed around the esophagus is used as a temporary snare to prevent reflux. After a zero-pressure reading, the syringe barrel is elevated so that the meniscus is 70 cm

above the level of the cricoid process. The use of a 70-cm suture or some other previously measured device facilitates the positioning of the syringe barrel. The volume that runs in under gravity at this level can then be recorded. Of course, the end of the Ewald tube must be placed so that all the holes are below the cardia. Eight ml should be added to the measured volume to account for the space taken up by tubing within the pouch.

STAPLES
Alden [2] introduced stapling-in-continuity in 1977. This technique and other simplifications made gastric bypass easier to perform but also introduced a new problem that required attention to prevent failure of weight control and the need for repeat operations. The staples had a tendency to pull through, allowing the partition to open up. Double stapling with four instead of two rows of staples creates a secure partition in most patients and seems to be safe as long as the interval between rows is narrow. If there is an opening between the staple rows that allows the mucosal secretions to escape into the lumen, there is less scarring and less security. A narrow, closed space causes necrosis of the mucosa and replacement with scar tissue. Too wide an interval between the two applications of staples introduces the risk of perforation in the closed space. Two mm is recommended.

ROUX-EN-Y GASTROENTEROSTOMY
To prevent the occasional development of bile gastritis or bile esophagitis after a loop gastroenterostomy, another modification in gastric bypass has been introduced. This consists in using Roux-en-Y gastroenterostomy in which the jejunum is divided 15 cm aborally from the ligament of Treitz (Fig. 29-3). A 40-cm segment of jejunum is then positioned between the gastroenterostomy and the enteroenterostomy. The latter should be made with the afferent or duodenal limb behind the long limb and with the anastomosis on the left side of the long limb and its mesentery. This prevents peristalsis in the short limb from kinking and obstructing the enteroenterostomy. During the first year following the operation pa-

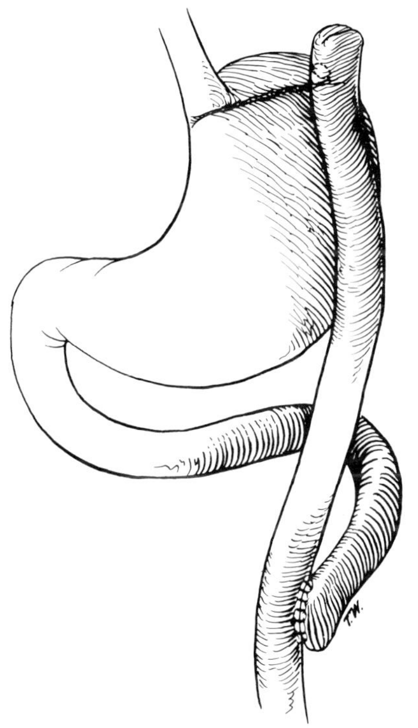

Fig. 29-3. Gastric bypass with a Roux-en-Y gastroenterostomy. (From Mason, E. E., Gastric reduction for obesity. In L. M. Nyhus and R. J. Baker (Eds.), *Mastery of Surgery*. Boston: Little, Brown, 1984.)

tients with loop and Roux-en-Y gastroenterostomies show about the same weight loss patterns. In later years weight loss is somewhat better with the Roux-en-Y anastomosis, because there is less room for a neostomach with only one limb, since bile and pancreatic juice mix less well with ingested food, and perhaps because the stimulation of digestive juices by duodenal hormones is reduced even more in a Roux limb than in a loop of jejunum.

Both procedures have advantages and disadvantages. The loop gastroenterostomy allows retrograde endoscopic examination through the afferent duodenal limb and into the excluded stomach. The Roux-en-Y anastomosis makes the care of any leak around the upper pouch easier and safer by diverting bile and pancreatic juice. The major disadvantage of a Roux-en-Y reconstruction is the increased

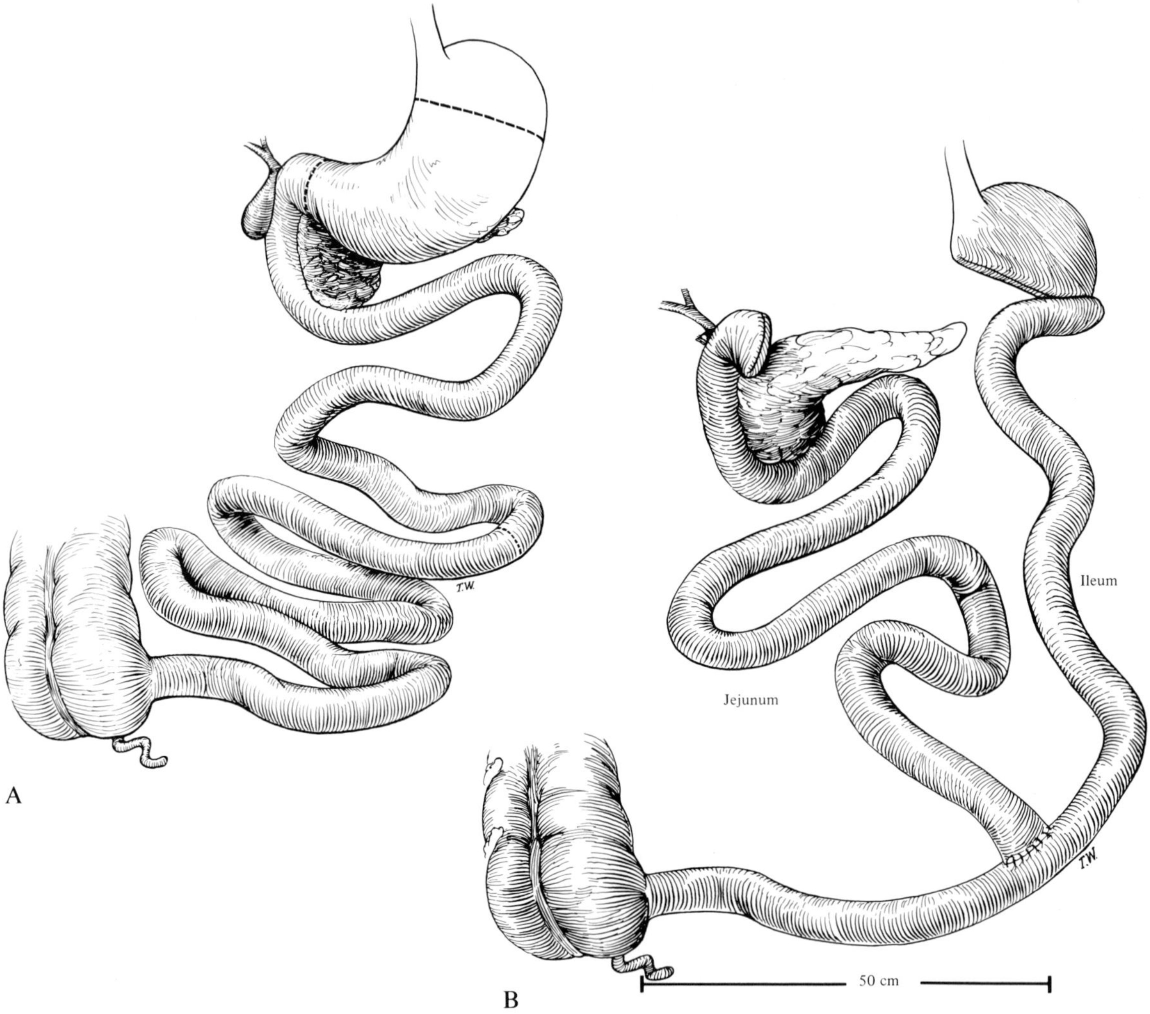

Fig. 29-4. Preparation for pancreatobiliojejunal bypass. Dashed lines indicate sites where transection will be carried out (A). Completed procedure, including 60% gastrectomy and cholecystectomy (B). (From Mason, E. E., Gastric reduction for obesity. In L. M. Nyhus and R. J. Baker (Eds.), *Mastery of Surgery*. Boston: Little, Brown, 1984.)

complexity of the operation. Nevertheless, it is one of the most effective procedures for extreme obesity. With time none of these operations will be completely satisfactory in all patients unless some mechanism is included to prevent dilatation of the outlet of the small fundic segment.

PANCREATOBILIOJEJUNAL BYPASS

Scopinaro [35] uses an even more radical Roux-en-Y type of anastomosis to treat obesity; he divides the small intestine in its midportion and performs an anastomosis of jejunum to ileum at a point 50 cm orad to the ileocecal valve. Because this is a Mann-Williamson type of preparation, which stimulates gastrin and gastric secretion, Scopinaro adds a 60 percent distal gastrectomy (Fig. 29-4). To prevent gallstone formation, a prophylactic cholecystectomy is also performed. A food stream, a pancreatobiliojejunal stream, and a common channel of only 50 ml of terminal

ileum where food and digestive juices can mix are constructed.

This operation is a combination of intestinal and gastric bypass. It differs from other forms of intestinal bypass in that it does not leave any of the intestine without flowing contents, which should decrease the tendency for bacterial overgrowth and resultant problems of liver failure, renal stones, or bypass enteritis. The tendency toward wastage of protein remains, however, and the operation is not completely reversible because of the removal of 60 percent of the stomach. The possibility of additional late and unforeseen complications exists because the anatomy and physiology are so different from normal. Such an operation might be considered in the occasional patient who has the combined problems of obesity and hyperlipidemia. I have treated one such patient in this way with temporary success. An attempt to use gastric bypass rather than resection in the initial operation was followed by stomal ulceration. This necessitated removal of the excluded stomach, which made the final procedure conform to that recommended by Scopinaro.

COMPLICATIONS

Perforation

Certain risks of gastric bypass are shared with the forms of gastroplasty that have a greater curvature stoma [6]. The most serious is perforation. The nasogastric tube must make two sharp turns to be threaded through the stoma. If for any reason the end of the tube presses against the wall of the upper gastric segment for more than 36 hours it can erode the wall of the stomach, causing subsequent shoulder pain, tachycardia, increased abdominal and pelvic pain, the urge to void and defecate, or vaginal pain. These symptoms progress rapidly to signs of circulatory insufficiency and collapse. The most common incorrect diagnoses include pulmonary embolism, atelectasis, and pneumonia. In some patients a correct diagnosis of perforation comes too late to prevent overwhelming peritonitis. A quick diagnosis and a prompt corrective operation influence the prognosis more than any other factor. An early correct diagnosis may be difficult to establish, however, except by another operation.

Another cause of perforation and circulatory failure is acute gastric dilatation of the afferent limb and excluded stomach. This is more likely to occur if the holes in the nasogastric tube are in the efferent limb so the afferent limb and distal stomach are pumped full of swallowed air. This condition may be recognized by supine and upright roentgenograms of the upper abdomen when the distended distal stomach is filled with air. If the excluded segment is distended with fluid, however, a roentgenographic diagnosis may not be possible, nor will injection of contrast medium through the nasogastric tube into the efferent limb demonstrate a leak in the excluded stomach. A normal Hypaque upper gastrointestinal examination is common and does not exclude a diagnosis of perforation or acute gastric dilatation. Fluroscopic manipulation of the nasogastric tube may allow decompression and, if perforation has not occurred, obviates an operation. Usually a prompt operation is essential to decompress the excluded stomach with a gastrostomy. Any perforation should be closed. Nonviable stomach must be resected and the area well drained.

Wound Infection

The wound infection rate, twice as high as that following gastric operations on persons of normal weight, warrants treatment with prophylactic oral and systemic antibiotics beginning 2 hours before the operation and continuing for 24 hours afterward. Gentle handling of tissues, protection against drying of subcutaneous fat, care in draping, and avoidance of hematomas, seromas, devascularization of fatty tissue, and breaks in technique all assume heightened importance in operations on the obese.

Calcium and Iron Malabsorption

Bypass of the duodenum can cause eventual decreased iron and calcium absorption. Occasionally patients need oral iron medications. Pregnancy or abnormal loss of blood from menses, hemorrhoids, or operations such

as panniculectomy without complete replacement of blood loss often makes active correction by oral or parenteral iron medication necessary. A few patients have had their repair converted to a gastrogastrostomy to restore iron absorption and to correct chronic iron deficiency anemia. As yet, osteoporosis has not been observed, but there has not been any systematic study of the problem.

Carcinoma of the Stomach

After gastroenterostomy stomach cancer traditionally has been more common in the fundic segment, probably because increased permeability to carcinogens in the diet follows backwash gastritis. This hazard arises more frequently in countries in which stomach cancer is common and probably will be an infrequent occurrence in the United States. Any signs or symptoms of gastritis or esophagitis should be studied with endoscopy and treated before neoplastic changes occur. It has been difficult to determine the exact state of the mucosa in the bypassed stomach. Flickinger et al. [14] have demonstrated that retrograde duodenogastroscopy is feasible. Their observations suggest that endoscopic gastritis

is rare in the proximal gastric pouch but common in the distal gastric segment and may be related to the presence of bile. Although the gastric mucosa is histologically normal in half of the gastric bypass patients, acute and chronic gastritis, regenerative changes, and intestinal metaplasia may develop in either or both segments.

Stomal Ulcer

Stomal ulcer was so common after antral exclusion and gastroenterostomy in patients with duodenal ulcer that exclusion operations gained an early and deserved avoidance. My early laboratory experiments with Ito [31] showed that when the stomach is divided at a high level, acid secretion is suppressed. An exclusion of enough stomach to produce weight control will also depress gastrin-mediated secretion in response to a standard meal. Before the advent of upper pouch volume measurement, some of our gastric transections were too low, and consequently we observed a 3 percent incidence of stomal ulcer following gastric bypass. A patient with vagal overactivity and duodenal ulcer is likely to have a stomal ulcer even with a high transection. Such a patient needs an extensive gastrectomy if both the ulcer diathesis and the obesity are to be treated. The reconstruction should meet the criteria of an adequate operation for obesity.

If a stomal ulcer necessitates revision of gastric bypass, the antrum may not have been adequately suppressed because the transection was too low. If a gastroenterostomy is used in the reconstruction, therefore, the excluded stomach may also need to be removed. Another approach is to reconstruct the stomach with a gastrogastrostomy after removal of the excess upper pouch. This allows any acid secretion from the upper segment to inhibit the antrum.

REVISION

Most revisions of gastric bypass are required because of failure of the initial operation to control weight. The implications of failing to measure volume during the first operation become evident when this measurement is first made during a revision procedure. The surgeon often discovers a pouch of more than 500 ml in volume. The volume before and after reduction of the size of the upper pouch must be entered in the operative record.

The surgeon must decide what type of reconstruction to use. Although a gastrogastrostomy without reinforcement is the simplest procedure to perform, this is almost certain to fail in controlling weight. A Marlex collar can be placed, but with the extensive dissection and chance for contamination from an open anastomosis and the resection of part of the upper pouch, such a step carries a considerable risk of infection and erosion. Eroding Marlex must be removed, which leads to ultimate failure of weight control and the need for even more surgical procedures. Reconstruction by vertical banded gastroplasty is now the procedure of choice.

Each type of gastric reduction operation I have used so far has a measurable failure rate. The inadequate operations require revisions

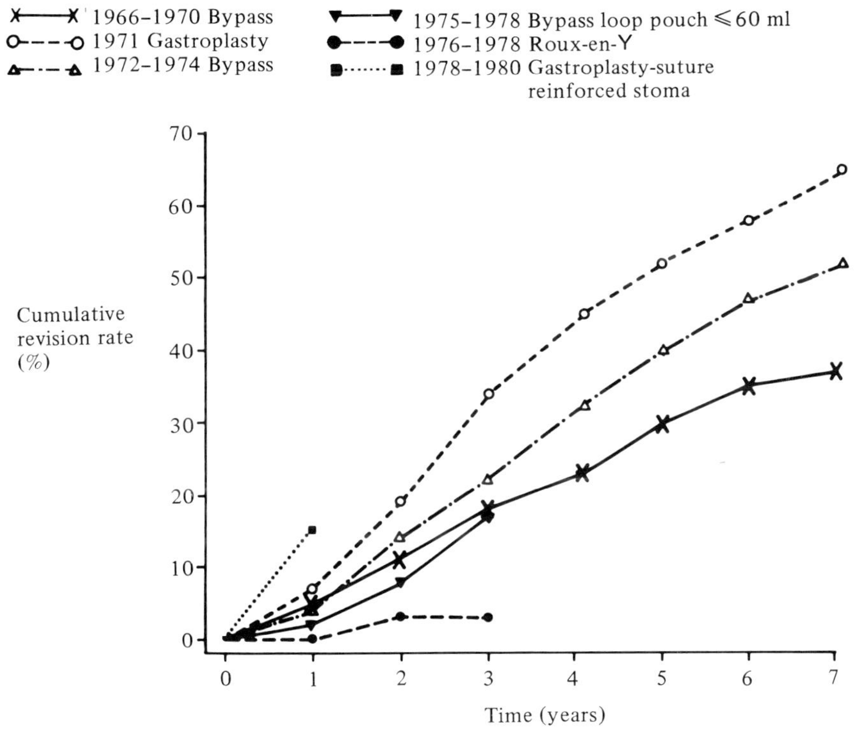

Fig. 29-5. Varying revision rates given in cumulative percentage over time for the various procedures done from 1966 to 1980. (From Mason, E. E., Gastric reduction for obesity. In L. M. Nyhus and R. J. Baker (Eds.), *Mastery of Surgery*. Boston: Little, Brown, 1984.)

so often, usually beginning the first year, that they are quickly abandoned. Effective operations yield a lower, yet persistent, rate of revision (Fig. 29-5). Even at a rate of only 5 percent per year, after 10 years half of the patients will have had revisions. It is urgent, therefore, to find a technique of gastric reduction that will satisfy all the criteria of an effective operation. Gastric bypass with a Roux-en-Y gastroenterostomy is an effective operation [13], but it is rather complicated and offers no satisfactory way to keep the stoma from dilating. Furthermore, bypass of the stomach and duodenum is not necessary to limit food intake. For these and other reasons, gastroplasty has been developed in the search for a simpler and safer procedure.

Gastroplasty

In theory a small-volume upper gastric segment and a small stoma should be sufficient to retard the ingestion of food. Bypass seems both unnecessary and complex. With this in mind, in 1971 Printen and I first used gastroplasty in preference to gastric bypass [34]. In less than a year, gastric bypass was again adopted because gastroplasty was not providing the desired weight control. In retrospect, failure to measure volume intraoperatively and to provide some mechanism to prevent dilatation of the stoma caused the inadequate degree of weight control.

In 1977 Gomez [16] resurrected gastroplasty and added a Mersilene mesh collar around the channel. His attempt to band the channel to prevent its dilatation was frustrated by obstruction, and he fell under the impression that the Mersilene caused fibrosis and stricture. Gomez therefore turned to a running 000

polypropylene (Prolene) seromuscular suture to create a ridge of gastric wall around an indwelling bougie. Although this provided an accurately sized channel, tissue trauma caused early edema and obstruction in some patients. With time, however, the suture would migrate into the lumen and allow the stoma to dilate. Gomez used this method until the middle of 1981.

In the meantime, Kroyer [23] returned to the use of Marlex mesh for reinforcement of the greater curvature stoma in gastroplasty. He also observed early obstruction in several patients but found that instead of concentric narrowing there was kinking of the stoma when the Marlex became adherent to tissues high under the diaphragm. He was able to restore an adequate lumen merely by taking down the adhesion.

Kroyer resolved this problem by suturing the stomach to parietal peritoneum near the left costal margin, thus maintaining the staple line, which had been placed across the stomach, in an observed transverse position on closure of the abdominal incision. He is now following several hundred patients who have had the operation. Grace [17] has also used Marlex mesh to reinforce a greater curvature stoma. In more than two years he had only one true stricture among approximately 65 patients.

At The University of Iowa we used transverse gastroplasty with a running, Prolene-reinforced stoma for about 30 months. Toward the middle of 1980, however, my colleagues, Lewis and Printen, returned to the use of a Roux-en-Y gastric bypass, and I began to modify gastroplasty further to see if some of the remaining problems could be eliminated. Like Gomez, we also had been observing too many early obstructions, and later in their course too many of the patients lost their Prolene suture and began to gain weight.

Because of its simplicity, another type of stapling, introduced at Ohio State University [11], was rapidly adopted by many surgeons. The procedure consisted in removing three staples from the middle of a TA-90 cartridge and applying the stapler once. This tended to crush mucosa in the area of the stoma and would occasionally lead to stricture and obstruction. In addition, staples could cut through at either side of the channel. The early failure rate reached 50 percent, and the surgeons at Ohio State University soon began reporting a series of modifications. These included such things as keeping patients on a liquid diet for several months, using two sets of staples, and reinforcing with sutures. Finally, in early 1981 this operation was abandoned in favor of one developed by Laws, to be described later.

Vertical stapling, undertaken by a number of surgeons, represents another change that made the operation easier but not necessarily more effective. Tretbar [37] was the first to report this modification. He created a narrow pouch much like an extension of the esophagus along the lesser curvature and also rather similar in configuration to a Collis [7] gastroplasty. Tretbar did not attempt to reinforce the outlet. Fabito [12], however, used this approach but added the running Prolene suture, as did Eckhout [10].

Laws and Piantadosi [25] compared Roux-en-Y gastric bypass with the gastric partitioning of Pace et al. [32]. They found much better weight loss with the former but were unwilling to continue dealing with the complexity of a Roux-en-Y gastric bypass. They began using a modification of vertical gastroplasty, which instead of the running seromuscular suture used by Fabito and Eckhout involved a double strand of 00 polypropylene, threaded through a Silastic (silicone rubber) ring [24]. A 32F Hurst dilator was used to calibrate the stoma. They stapled the stomach in continuity and anchored the suture threaded through Silastic by transfixion at the lower end of the staple line. By the time Laws presented the series at a bariatric surgery colloquium held in June, 1981, the Silastic encased suture had cut through into the lumen in one patient. Laws does use interrupted sutures to fold stomach over the Silastic ring, so that if early erosion occurs it does not produce a free perforation. Kridelbaugh [22] used this technique in four patients but abandoned it because the Silastic eroded into the lumen in one patient.

In 1980 I made two changes in my use of gastroplasty. First, I decided to divide the

stomach as we had done in 1971, leaving a channel of undivided tissue at the greater curvature to be used for the outlet. The purpose was twofold: (1) to provide a channel that would be traumatized as little as possible, and (2) to allow the application of some reinforcement that would not be sutured or stapled to the stomach wall and should therefore be less likely to migrate into the lumen. Before long I began applying two sets of staples and opening a window between these near the greater curvature. Finally, I decided to move the window and channel to the lesser curvature to create what I call a vertical banded gastroplasty, to be described later.

A number of different materials were used for reinforcement, including fascia, which stretched and did not allow the required stomal diameter; Dacron-reinforced Silastic, which did not allow ingrowth of fibroblasts and remained as a foreign body surrounded by fluid and liable to infection; and a Prolene tie, which tended to migrate into the lumen. Marlex mesh seemed the best material, provided it could be maintained free of contamination until it became incorporated into the outer wall of the stomach by ingrowth of fibroblasts.

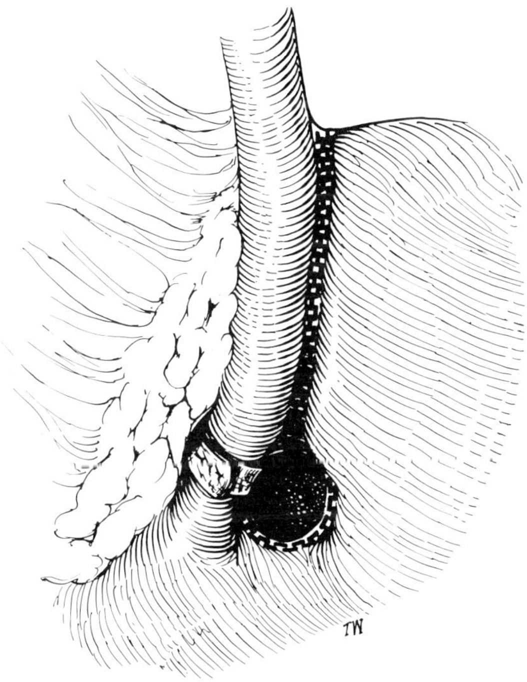

Fig. 29-6. Vertical banded gastroplasty featuring a vertically oriented lesser curvature pouch with a volume of 50 ml or less measured at a pressure of 50 cm of saline solution. The outlet is reinforced with a Marlex mesh collar. A stapled window allows double stapling of the partition without trauma to the stomal mucosa and reinforcement of the stoma without suturing to the stomal wall. (From Mason, E. E., Gastric reduction for obesity. In L. M. Nyhus and R. J. Baker (Eds.), *Mastery of Surgery*. Boston: Little, Brown, 1984.)

Vertical Banded Gastroplasty

Vertical banded gastroplasty (Fig. 29-6) was introduced in November, 1980, at The University of Iowa [30]. Doherty [8] observed one of these operations in February, 1981, and soon began using it in a series of patients at St. Francis Hospital in San Francisco. An increasing number of other surgeons are now using this method, which incorporates all the advantages and, as far as we can tell, avoids the disadvantages of other procedures. Although further follow-up study is needed, the first five years' experience is encouraging. The Marlex collar provides a means of maintaining an outlet of constant diameter for an indefinite period of time. It is anticipated, therefore, that the operation will have a negligible revision rate, but a lifetime of follow-up care is needed to be sure.

The usual midline vertical incision exposes the lesser curvature of the stomach. An opening in the avascular area of the lesser omentum allows the surgeon to grasp the lesser curvature with his or her fingers in the lesser sac. The surgeon places a Penrose drain around the esophagus and makes a small opening adjacent to the stomach just above the crow's-foot of the vagus nerve or 9 cm below the esophagogastric angle.

With a 32F Ewald tube along the lesser curvature on the inside of the stomach and the anvil of the EEA stapler on the posterior surface adjacent to the Ewald tube but outside the stomach, a trochar (from a wound evacuation drainage set) is thrust through both walls

of the stomach and brought out the opening in the lesser omentum. The trochar is followed with an attached piece of tubing, which is in turn attached to the shaft of the EEA. Thus a stapled window 25 mm in diameter can be accurately positioned adjacent to the stomal site with minimal risk of contamination. The stomach wall should not be stretched—rather it should envelop the Ewald tube loosely.

A 24F plastic tube (Argyle chest tube) is threaded through the window, the lesser sac, and the esophagogastric angle and used to guide a TA-90 stapler into place. The surgeon can now occlude both ends of the proposed vertical lesser curvature pouch with volume measurement as described earlier. If the volume is less than 25 ml or greater than 50 ml it can be adjusted by pulling the stomach through the clamp of the loosened TA-90 stapler. Most pouches are about 30 ml in volume measured at 50 cm of pressure. After stapling, the plastic tube is reapplied to the toe of the TA-90 so that the stapler can be backed out, reloaded, and repositioned to fire a second set of staples a few millimeters from the site of the first set.

Finally, the surgeon places a Marlex collar 1.5 cm wide around the stoma, through the window, and through the small opening in the gastrohepatic omentum next to the lesser curvature. To provide an exact 5.0-cm circumference, the surgeon measures and marks the collar where it is sewn to itself. Two additional sutures are used to secure the overlapping end. No suture should be allowed to penetrate the stomach wall. The exact 5.0-cm circumference of the restraining Marlex collar is the most important means of calibrating the stoma. A 7-cm length of Marlex is used to allow adequate overlap for sewing. The Ewald tube is passed through the lumen to ensure that an adequate opening is present. The stomach between the window and lesser curvature should not be folded but should be sufficiently ample to fill the collar. In this way, stomach wall thickness will be adequate to protect against erosion of the Marlex into the lumen. A nasogastric tube is not now used. Finally, greater omentum should be sewn over the Marlex and to the lesser omentum.

This operation requires almost no interruption of gastric blood vessels. It avoids entering the area of the spleen because the fundus is not mobilized. As with all other abdominal operations, care should be taken to avoid tearing the splenic capsule by not placing too much traction on the transverse colon or omentum, as described by Lord and Gourevitch [27]. The entire area of interest in vertical banded gastroplasty lies directly beneath the incision. Correct pouch volume measured at an adequate pressure, a secure partition, a stoma that is exactly constructed by measurement inside and out, and a collar to prevent stretching are all important features of the procedure. Finally, there is minimal trauma to the area and minimal chance for contamination.

After four years of use in 680 patients, 131 patients with vertical banded gastroplasty followed for more than three years constituted a 90 percent follow-up rate. The 109 patients with a 5-cm circumference collar averaged a weight reduction of 43 kg, or 66 percent of excess weight. Patients between 100 pounds over and 225 percent of ideal weight showed an average weight loss of 38 kg, or 69 percent of excess weight. For patients whose initial weight was over 225 percent of ideal, the average weight loss at three years was 56 kg or 47 percent of excess weight. These heavier patients lost more weight but leveled off at a weight that was still well above ideal. For these patients a greater restriction in eating was needed, and a 4.5-cm collar was subsequently used.

Calculated on an actuarial basis, using all available data, the revision rate for vertical banded gastroplasty with a 5-cm collar is 1.5 percent per year. This is the lowest rate observed for any gastric reduction operation used over the last 19 years. A few patients broke their staple line and required restapling. A few of the earlier patients stretched their pouch enough to require a reduction in pouch volume. This problem was solved subsequently by reducing the size of the pouch at the first operation so that it now averages 14 ml, measured at 70 cm of water pressure. A few patients had their 5- or 5.5-cm collar changed to a 4.5-cm collar because of inade-

quate weight loss. To date there have been no erosions of the mesh into the lumen after either the initial operation or after one of these collar changes.

Vertical banded gastroplasty promises to be the ideal gastric reduction operation for morbid obesity.

Summary

Gastric reduction operations for obesity have evolved over the 20 years since their introduction from an empirical analogue of subtotal gastrectomy to a very concise procedure designed specifically for the morbidly obese patient. An estimated thirty thousand of these various procedures are performed yearly. Because of the many variations, it is essential that surgeons keep detailed records and attempt to follow all patients closely [4, 28, 36]. Another decade is required before we can be sure we have reached an ideal surgical treatment of morbid obesity. Perhaps a better understanding of the basic cause of obesity and a more direct and effective medical and psychological approach will preclude the need for such invasive treatment in the not too distant future. In the meantime there is a great deal of work to be done by surgeons who are well trained and truly interested in these procedures and patients.

References

1. Adibi, S. A., and Stanko, R. T. Perspectives on gastrointestinal surgery for treatment of morbid obesity: The lesson learned. *Gastroenterology* 87:1381, 1984.
2. Alden, J. F. Gastric and jejunoileal bypass: A comparison in the treatment of morbid obesity. *Arch. Surg.* 112:799, 1977.
3. Alder, R. L., and Terry, B. E. Measurement and standardization of the gastric pouch in gastric bypass. *Surg. Gynecol. Obstet.* 144:762, 1977.
4. Amaral, J. F., Thompson, W. R., Caldwell, M. D., et al. Prospective metabolic evaluation of 150 consecutive patients who underwent gastric exclusion. *Am. J. Surg.* 147:468, 1984.
5. Brolin, R. E. Laboratory evaluation of four techniques of stapled gastroplasty. *Surgery* 97:66, 1985.
6. Buckwalter, J. A., and Herbst, C. A. Perioperative complications of gastric restrictive operations. *Am. J. Surg.* 146:613, 1983.
7. Collis, J. L. An operation in hiatus hernia with short esophagus. *Thorax* 12:181, 1957.
8. Doherty, C. San Francisco. Personal communication.
9. Drenick, E. J., Bale, G. S., Seltzer, F., and Johnson, D. G. Excessive mortality and causes of death in morbidly obese men. *J.A.M.A.* 243:443, 1980.
10. Eckhout, G. V. Surgery for morbid obesity: Comparison of gastric bypass with vertically stapled gastroplasty, In press.
11. Elliott, J. More help for the morbidly obese: Gastric stapling (news item). *J.A.M.A.* 240:1941, 1978.
12. Fabito, D. C. St. Louis. Personal communication, 1984.
13. Flickinger, E. G., Pories, W. J., Meelheim, H. D., et al. The Greenville gastric bypass: Progress report at 3 years. *Ann. Surg.* 199:555, 1984.
14. Flickinger, E. G., Sinar, D. R., Pories, W. J., et al. The bypassed stomach. *Am. J. Surg.* 149:151, 1985.
15. Gleysteen, J. J., and Barboniak, J. J. Improvement in heart disease risk factors after gastric bypass. *Arch. Surg.* 118:681, 1982.
16. Gomez, C. A. Gastroplasty in the surgical treatment of obesity. *Am. J. Clin. Nutr.* 33:406, 1980.
17. Grace, D. M. London, Ont. Personal communication, 1984.
18. Herbst, C. A., Hughes, T. A., Gwynne, J. T., and Buckwalter, J. A. Gastric bariatric operation in insulin-treated adults. *Surgery* 95:209, 1984.
19. Hermreck, A. S., Jewell, W. R., and Hardin, C. A. Gastric bypass for morbid obesity: Results and complications. *Surgery* 80:498, 1976.
20. Hornberger, H. R. Gastric bypass. *Am. J. Surg.* 131:414, 1976.
21. Kremen, A. N., Linner, J. H., and Nelson, C. H. Experimental evaluation of the nutritional importance of proximal and distal small intestine. *Ann. Surg.* 140:439, 1954.
22. Kridelbaugh, W. W. Albuquerque. Personal communication, August, 1981.
23. Kroyer, J. M. Long Beach, California. Personal communication.

24. Laws, H. L. Standardized gastroplasty orifice. *Am. J. Surg.* 141:393, 1981.
25. Laws, H. L., and Piantadosi, S. Superior gastric reduction procedure for morbid obesity: A prospective randomized trial. *Ann. Surg.* 193:334, 1981.
26. Lineaweaver, W., Ryckman, F., Hawkins, I., et al. Endoscopic balloon dilation of outlet stenosis after gastric bypass. *Am. Surg.* 51:194, 1985.
27. Lord, M. D., and Gourevitch, A. The peritoneal anatomy of the spleen, with special reference to the operation of partial gastrectomy. *Br. J. Surg.* 52:202, 1965.
28. MacLean, L. D., Rhode, B. M., and Shizgal, H. M. Nutrition following gastric operations for morbid obesity. *Ann. Surg.* 198:347, 1983.
29. Mason, E. E. *Surgical Treatment of Obesity.* Philadelphia: Saunders, 1981.
30. Mason, E. E. Vertical banded gastroplasty for obesity. *Arch. Surg.* 117:701, 1982.
31. Mason, E. E., and Ito, C. Gastric bypass in obesity. *Surg. Clin. North Am.* 47:1345, 1967.
32. Pace, W. G., Martin, E. W., Jr., Titirick, T., Fabri, P. J., and Carey, L. C. Gastric partitioning for morbid obesity. *Ann. Surg.* 190:392, 1979.
33. Payne, J. H., and DeWind, L. T. Surgical treatment of obesity. *Am. J. Surg.* 118:141, 1969.
34. Printen, K. J., and Mason, E. E. Gastric surgery for relief of morbid obesity. *Arch. Surg.* 106:428, 1973.
35. Scopinaro, N., Gianetta, E., Civalleri, D., et al. Two years of clinical experience with bilio-pancreatic bypass for obesity. *Am. J. Clin. Nutr.* 33:506, 1980.
36. Smith, L. B., Fricke, F. J., and Graney, A. S. Results and complications of gastric partitioning. *Am. J. Surg.* 146:815, 1983.
37. Tretbar, L. L. Gastric plication vs. fundic exclusion (vertical stapling). Presented at Bariatric Workshop, May 25, 1979, Iowa City.

SPECIAL COMMENT
Truncal Vagotomy: A Regulatory Approach in Obesity Surgery

John G. Kral

Classification of Obesity Surgery

The crucial difference between gastric resection or vagotomy for treatment of ulcer symptoms and any of the more than 20 variant procedures (Table 29-1) for morbid obesity is that ulcer symptoms have an identifiable, curable cause, that is, the ulcer, whereas in obesity there rarely is any detectable cause of the symptom. Furthermore, the most important etiologic factor, eating, is for most people pleasurable; thus eating easily acquires a stigma of immorality if done in "excess," irrespective of how "excess" is defined, which creates controversy over the justification for the treatment.

The two most common procedures in obesity surgery—intestinal bypass and gastric restriction—work principally in different ways. The intestinal procedures permit unlimited ingestion, although in fact food intake is decreased by as yet poorly understood mechanisms [3]. The gastric procedures work much as jaw wiring by imposing a strict limitation on intake, a "chastity belt." A completely different approach based on studies of experimental obesity has been used in the *regulatory* procedures, such as stereotaxic ablation of the putative feeding center, truncal vagotomy without drainage, and ileal interposition [4]. These procedures work by reducing or abolishing the "physiological hunger" drive. Both the restrictive and the regulatory procedures, however, can easily be overridden by "psychological hunger." Consumption of high-caloric liquid or semisolid food or repeated overdistention of pouch and stoma can lead to ultimate failure of weight loss.

Truncal Vagotomy in Morbid Obesity

Vagotomy has been shown to reduce over weight in several species, including humans.

Table 29-1. Surgical methods for treating obesity

I. Physical methods
   A. Lipectomy
   B. Jaw wiring
   C. Intestinal procedures
      1. Resection
      2. Bypass
         a. Jejunocolic
         b. Jejunoileal
            (1) End-side
            (2) End-end
            (3) Biliointestinal
         c. Biliopancreaticojejunal
         d. Duodenoileal
   D. Gastric procedures
      1. Resection
      2. Bypass
         a. Gastrojejunostomy (loop)
         b. Gastrojejunostomy (Roux-Y)
      3. Reduction
         a. Gastroplasty
         b. Partition
         c. Gastrogastrostomy
         d. Vertical stapling
         e. Plication
         f. Netting
      4. Intragastric balloon
   E. Intra-abdominal balloon

II. Regulatory methods
   A. Stereotaxic destruction of neural "hunger" system
   B. Truncal vagotomy
   C. Intestinal bypass
   D. Ileal interposition
   E. Duodenoileal bypass

Various mechanisms may be involved, such as motility, digestion, hunger sensations, and peptide release, to name a few. In an attempt to analyze the reasons for success or failure of weight loss after truncal vagotomy, a series of physiological and psychological studies has been performed [5]. The mean weight loss in 14 successful patients with a mean weight of 129 kg before truncal vagotomy was 30 kg. Just as important, 7 similar patients failed to lose weight. The 21 patients, aged 19–45 years, had no previous history of gastroduodenal disease. Truncal vagotomy without drainage was performed after extensive screening procedures. During a follow-up period of 2.5–5 years, none of the patients had asymptomatic or symptomatic ulcer disease or any other serious complications of the operation. Episodes of diarrhea occurred in 5 of the patients, one of whom experienced a prolonged period of diarrhea, which subsided spontaneously after eight months.

Expected reductions in gastric acid output and glucose-stimulated insulin-release were found in all patients. Furthermore, diminished caloric intake, altered nutrient selection with changed preference and taste acuity for sweetness, as well as reduced hunger ratings were registered.

Critical for the interpretation of the findings and evaluation of this treatment modality, just as in duodenal ulcer disease, is the assessment of completeness of vagotomy. Moreover, the question of vagus nerve regeneration is important for such an evaluation over the long term. Clinical tests of completeness of vagotomy and their shortcomings are discussed elsewhere in this book. In this context it is necessary to point out that insulin hypoglycemia and modified sham feeding are particularly difficult to standardize and interpret in morbidly obese humans.

Interest in behavioral and metabolic effects of vagal nerve function has generated new approaches for assessing completeness of vagotomy [6]. Alterations in feeding patterns—between-meal intervals, meal size, composition of food selection, fluid intake—as well as changes in release of gastrointestinal polypeptides including insulin (e.g., changes in diurnal rhythm and the magnitude of response to defined stimuli after vagotomy) seem to be sensitive indicators of residual vagal function.

New histochemical techniques based on axonal flow and uptake of fluorescing substances, used together with conventional electron microscopy and morphology, are being used to investigate the occurrence of vagal nerve fiber regeneration after complete vagotomy [6]. Findings of vagal regeneration in rats [2] need to be confirmed in other species, and if present, new techniques must be developed to counteract such regeneration.

Implications for Obesity Operations

The experience with truncal vagotomy in morbid obesity indicates that some patients are not helped by the procedure. Similar failure of physical methods, specifically gastric restrictive procedures, are usually attributed to technical flaws such as failure of the pouch or stoma to withstand distention. An alternative interpretation may be entertained. Inability to select patients who are able to modify their behavior sufficiently to prevent repeated distention might be a more important determinant of failure rates.

A certain percentage of morbidly obese patients can decide on their own that they are not appropriate candidates for gastric restrictive operations. Another subgroup of patients seem to be unable to make such a decision on their own, yet will be poor candidates for such procedures. Methods are badly needed to identify these patients. In view of the malignant nature of their condition, patients excluded from the restrictive operations should be offered different procedures. With improved postoperative management and patient cooperation, it is possible that a modified intestinal bypass such as biliointestinal bypass [1] or duodenoileal bypass might be considered in selected instances. Recent data imply that truncal vagotomy potentiates weight loss after vertical banded gastroplasty. Given the complexity of the regulatory mechanisms of food intake, it is highly unlikely that a single method will evolve that can be used with equal success in all morbidly obese patients.

Awareness of the multifactorial etiology of obesity should lead to differentiation in treatment. Appropriate methods of patient selection based on the classifications of obesity with analysis of etiological factors need to be developed to individualize treatment and assign patients to optimal treatment modalities. Obesity surgery should be limited to investigational institutions until more data have accumulated.

Comment References

1. Eriksson, F. Biliointestinal bypass. *Int. J. Obesity* 5:437, 1981.
2. Joffe, S. N., Crocket, A., and Doyle, D. Morphological and functional evidence of reinnervation of the gastric parietal cell mass following a parietal cell vagotomy. *Am. J. Surg.* 143:80, 1982.
3. Koopmans, H. S., and Sclafani, A. Control of body weight by lower gut signals. *Int. J. Obesity* 5:491, 1981.
4. Kral, J. G. Surgical Therapy. In M. R. C. Greenwood (Ed.), *Obesity: Contemporary Issues in Nutrition*. New York: Churchill Livingstone, 1983.
5. Kral, J. G. Behavioral effects of vagotomy in humans. *J. Auton. Nerv. Sys.* 9:273, 1983.
6. Kral, J., Powley, T., and Brooks, C. (Eds.). *Vagal Nerve Function: Behavioral and Methodological Considerations*. Amsterdam: Elsevier, 1983.

30

Ancillary Procedures and Miscellaneous Techniques for Operations on the Stomach and Duodenum

John E. Jesseph
Jerry M. Jesseph

We present here a compilation of techniques with which all general surgeons should be familiar: some for continued application, some for historical perspective, but most for an overall understanding of how the stomach and duodenum can be approached safely and effectively.

Ancillary Procedures

This section deals with the essentials of most of the lesser operative procedures employed in treating gastric and duodenal diseases, especially those techniques that are adjuvant or complementary to other manipulations. Some have ultimate purposes not directly related to the stomach and duodenum (e.g., feeding gastrostomy), while others constitute essential parts of composite procedures used in the treatment of gastroduodenal lesions (e.g., pyloroplasty). A thorough study of these techniques almost amounts to a review of the rise and development of abdominal surgery, so vital has been their role. The conception, evolution, and adoption of these methods have been largely a product of applied laboratory and clinical research in vexing problems of gastrointestinal physiology and pathology. What today seems simple and obvious once seemed an insurmountable hurdle. To realize how difficult the establishment of simple techniques can be, one has only to recall that the now elementary matter of end-to-end intestinal anastomosis defied successful accomplishment for nearly 50 years.

All the methods and techniques to be discussed here should be thoroughly familiar to the abdominal surgeon, not because any one technique will be frequently employed, but because each has peculiar virtues, and when properly employed, each offers particular advantages over other methods. To achieve clarity and avoid tedium, many minute technical details have been omitted; most of these fundamental considerations are described in detail elsewhere in this book.

GASTROTOMY

It is frequently necessary to open the stomach for inspection—for biopsy or removal of a known lesion, to search for sources of bleeding, or to remove foreign bodies. The stomach is so large and has such a plentiful blood supply that incisions may be made in any portion and extended almost at will. Figure 30-1 illustrates the line of incision for a generous gastrotomy.

It should be noted that the pylorus is completely avoided when the incision is made in this manner; therefore, the possibility of pyloroplasty is not forfeited. One can explore the entire stomach through this sort of incision, from the gastroesophageal junction to the pylorus. Closure of gastrotomy incisions carries almost no risk of reducing the lumen, so they may be closed in their original line. A two-layer technique is preferred, using a seromuscular layer of nonabsorbable suture material. In the absence of local disease or undue trauma, these incisions will heal promptly. Unless there is obstruction of the gastrointestinal tract distal to the gastrotomy site or some other procedure has been performed on the stomach, postoperative decompression of the stomach is usually not necessary. However, oral feeding should be deferred for a period of 48–72 hours or until effective peristalsis returns.

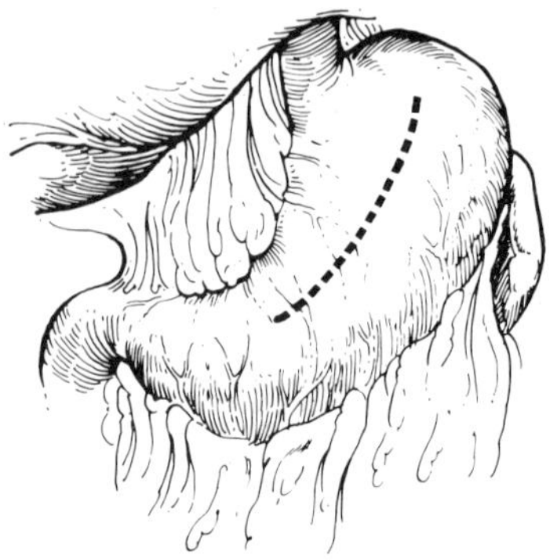

Fig. 30-1. Gastrotomy. The gastric incision (dashed line) will allow exploration of the entire stomach and lower esophagus. The pylorus and proximal duodenum should be inspected through a pyloroplasty incision. This method leaves options open for vagotomy and pyloroplasty or gastric resection as indicated.

DUODENOTOMY

Duodenotomy is commonly employed as an adjuvant to common bile duct exploration for visualization and manipulation of the ampullary sphincter, but it is often useful in removing foreign bodies and is occasionally necessary to discover a source of hemorrhage. The incisions are usually longitudinal in the anterior or lateral aspects of the duodenum. They should be placed near the area of interest and should be kept as short as possible (Fig. 30-2). A Kocher maneuver greatly facilitates duodenotomy and should always be done. Traction sutures placed at either side of the incision help in visualizing the lumen.

Closure of the longitudinal incision is usually done opposite to the line of incision, in keeping with the general principle of longitudinal incision and transverse closure. The validity of this concept was questioned by Longmire [67], who advocates closure of the duodenum in the line of incision. In his experience there have been no fistulas or duodenal strictures. Again, a watertight two-layer closure is preferred, with care taken to avoid inverting too large a mass of tissue. It has been amply shown that careful atraumatic closure will in most instances result in uncomplicated healing, because the vascularity of the duodenum favors prompt agglutination and early union. A soft rubber Penrose drain should be placed near the duodenotomy but should not actually lie against it. Postoperative decompression of the stomach is advisable, either by gastrostomy or by nasogastric suction. Menguy [75] proposed that transverse duodenotomy with transverse closure is a more anatomically correct procedure. He presented a series of 45 patients without morbidity. Work by Kraus and Condon [61] in the laboratory favors longitudinal duodenotomy, with transverse closure preferred but with longitudinal closure acceptable. However it is done, the closure requires great care. A leak in this area can have disastrous results.

GASTROSTOMY

The operation of gastrostomy is one of the oldest in abdominal surgery and one of the most useful. The first gastrostomies were done by

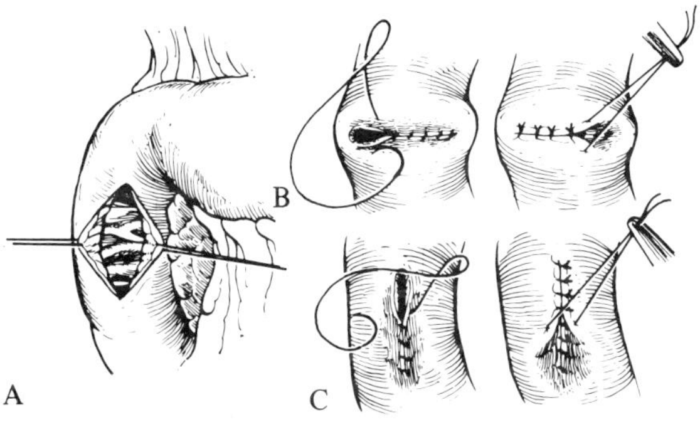

Fig. 30-2. Steps in performing duodenotomy. (A) Longitudinal incision. (B) Two-layer transverse closure. (C) Two-layer longitudinal closure. If the closure is done carefully, the duodenal opening will heal promptly and uneventfully.

Sedillot in 1839 and in 1853 [110], but both patients died. Since the first successful gastrostomy was performed by Verneuil [123], the technique has become widely accepted. Staton performed the first successful gastrostomy in the United States [127].

A great many types of gastrostomy have been devised, some for specific purposes, others as technical modifications of older methods [52]. The stomach is normally large and vascular and possesses "extra" tissue for manipulation. It is therefore easy to make almost any sort of pedicled flap or other arrangement desired. Many of the early techniques were devised to avoid the most common complications of gastrostomy—infection and leakage. Improved techniques, better general care, stapling devices, and antibiotics have helped to control these problems; currently we find that the simplest form of gastrostomy is usually best. Furthermore, the development of more radical, one-stage excisions of esophageal and gastric lesions has decreased the need for prolonged gastric intubation.

Gastrostomy has classically been used as a means of feeding a patient who is unable to swallow either because of an obstructive process in or above the stomach or because of extensive brain damage. Temporary tube gastrostomy has come into increasing use as a means of postoperative decompression. Many authors, including Farris and Smith [24], have pointed out the advantages of this technique over nasogastric intubation, and recognition of the immediate and late complications of nasogastric tubes has accentuated the virtues of temporary gastrostomy. The advantages are improved respiratory care, greater mobility, and vastly improved patient comfort [10, 22, 23, 67, 117, 138].

There are several important general considerations concerning gastrostomy that should be reviewed as a basis for selection of the technique to be used in any patient. Whether the gastrostomy is to be temporary or permanent is the most important single factor, since simple procedures suitable for a few days' decompression after laparotomy are often wholly unsuitable for weeks or months of feeding. Likewise, the patient's condition and habitus are important. In a relatively thin individual, simple tube gastrostomy can be rapidly performed with local anesthesia, whereas the more complex type of permanent gastrostomy usually requires general anesthesia and a full surgical team.

Gastrostomies can be divided into two groups—those lined with serosa and those lined with mucosa. Most temporary tube gastrostomies are lined with serosa, whereas permanent gastrostomies are lined with mucosa. The distinction is most important in anticipation of termination of the need for gastrostomy. A tract lined with serosa closes promptly and permanently once the tube that maintains the tract is removed. A second operation is usually required to terminate a gastrostomy lined with mucosa, as it would be with any other exteriorization of a portion of the gastrointestinal tract. There are other important differences between these two general types that will be pointed out in later descriptions.

Temporary Gastrostomy

STAMM GASTROSTOMY. This technique [115] is the simplest of all methods and probably the most widely used today. It forms a serosa-lined tract into the stomach and is therefore temporary. It can be quickly performed, even in elderly or debilitated patients, and it is easily terminated. It is commonly used for postoperative decompression; for short-term feeding in patients undergoing staged resections of the mouth, pharynx, esophagus, or stomach; as an aid to retrograde esophageal dilation; and for palliative feeding of patients with unresectable malignant neoplasms of the esophagus or stomach, either terminally or during the obstructive phase of irradiation therapy.

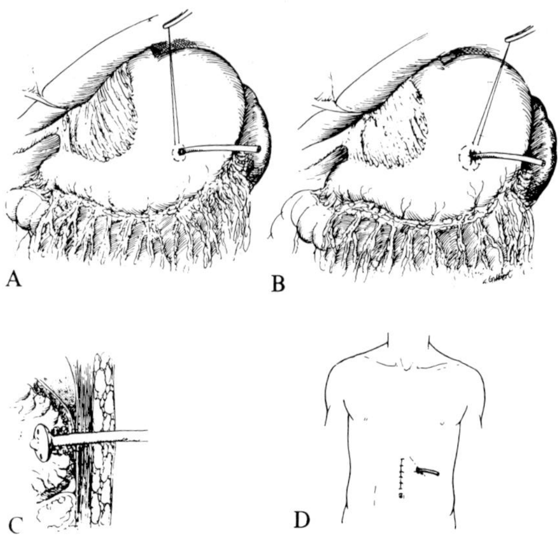

Fig. 30-3. Stamm gastrostomy. (A, B) The mushroom catheter is retained within the stomach by two concentric purse-string sutures. (C, D) The catheter is brought through a stab wound, and the anterior stomach wall is sutured to the peritoneum nearby so that solid fusion takes place, preventing leakage into the peritoneal cavity.

Aside from the advantages of being quickly and easily established, this gastrostomy leaves the stomach relatively normal in contour and volume; therefore, subsequent gastric or upper abdominal operations are not seriously hampered. Its only sequel is a single adhesion of gastric serosa to anterior peritoneum.

Figure 30-3 portrays the steps involved in performing a Stamm gastrostomy. When a gastrostomy is used for postoperative decompression, a Foley or similar catheter is certainly preferable to other types, since a tube with a large lumen can be used with a much smaller risk of becoming misplaced or slipping out of the stomach altogether. Even when used for feeding, a catheter with some form of enlarged end seems advisable so that the frequent manipulations of feeding will not dislodge it. The small intestine can be easily intubated for feeding with a smaller caliber tube through the gastrostomy, decreasing the risk of esophageal reflux and aspiration [106].

Several technical points need emphasis. It is important that the tube be brought through the abdominal wall by way of a small stab wound at a distance of at least several centimeters from the primary incision. Although a recent study showed no increase in complications when the tube was brought through the primary incision [134], many of the early and current complications of Stamm gastrostomy are no doubt caused by the presence of the tube (a foreign body) in the abdominal incision.

The procedure can be done under local anesthesia using a midline, transverse, subcostal, or paramedian incision. Obese or uncooperative patients may require general anesthesia.

Two or three concentric pursestring sutures of silk or other nonabsorbable material (000 or 00) are placed about the gastrostomy site (near the greater curvature at its most dependent part), and the catheter is introduced through a stab wound at the center. The sutures are then drawn up individually, beginning with the most central ones, and are tied and the ends cut. After the catheter has been drawn through the stab wound, traction is applied to approximate the anterior wall of the stomach to the peritoneum, where it is secured with several nonabsorbable sutures. Clearly the exit for the tube must be located where the stomach will not exert traction on these sutures.

When gastrostomy is used for postoperative decompression, it is not necessary to apply suction to the tube. If the tube used is at least No. 18F or No. 20F, it will drain adequately into a dependent container. From 10 to 20 ml of sterile saline solution or water should be flushed into the tube 2 or 3 times daily to prevent clogging. When the patient regains peristalsis, the tube can be clamped and left in place until oral intake is ensured, and then it can simply be withdrawn. In elderly or debilitated patients, or when healing is delayed, it is wise to leave the tube in place for at least a week so that there is no chance of dehiscence of the adhesion between the stomach and the peritoneum, with intraperitoneal leakage of gastric contents. Similarly, tube feeding or other nutrients should not be introduced through the tube for the first two or three days, and certainly not before the danger of gastric dilatation is past.

Regardless of the duration of the gastrostomy, the tract will close promptly after the tube is removed, usually within two or three days. Gastric retention caused by either distal obstruction or ileus tends to cause prolonged drainage, but this should be recognized as a contraindication to removing the tube. The problem of delayed gastric emptying after vagotomy and pyloroplasty for duodenal ulcer is to be expected if preoperative duodenal obstruction with a large, boggy stomach was present. In these situations a soft rubber Levin tube inserted through the stomach wall and through the lumen of the duodenum and into the proximal jejunum is quite helpful. The gastric aspirates are merely reinserted into this tube, thereby simplifying the problems of fluid and electrolyte balance. This second tube is brought through a second stab wound in the abdominal wall.

Many complications have been noted following simple tube gastrostomy, and deaths have resulted [13, 100, 107, 111, 134]. Most common of all is leakage about the tube with excoriation of the skin. This occurs chiefly in conditions of debilitation with poor healing and after prolonged use of the tube for feeding, as in unresectable esophageal carcinoma. To lessen these complications, a gastrostomy lined with mucosa should be used. Infection and partial or complete wound dehiscence can be almost entirely avoided by using a separate stab wound for tube exit. This combined with the use of an appropriate size of stainless steel wire for repair of the fascial layers of the primary incision will largely eliminate these problems. Other complications are aspiration, intragastric bleeding, peritonitis, and pyloric or duodenal obstruction from tube migration.

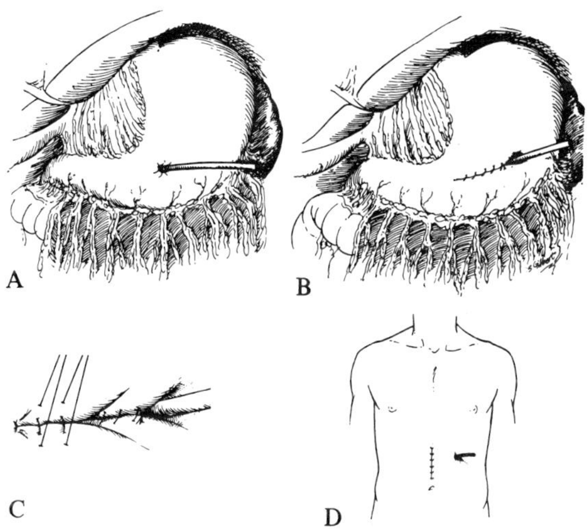

Fig. 30-4. Witzel gastrostomy. After the catheter is placed within the stomach and the single purse-string suture is tied, the anterior stomach wall is closed over the distal portion of the catheter to form a serosal tunnel (A, B). A second inversion of the stomach wall is advisable, using interrupted sutures (C). The catheter is brought out through a separate stab wound (D), and the primary incision is closed.

If the gastrostomy tube is accidentally withdrawn in the first two days, immediate reoperation is recommended to replace the tube. Attempts to replace it through the original tract usually result only in pushing the stomach away from the abdominal wall, increasing the leakage and resultant peritonitis.

The Stamm gastrostomy is certainly the most versatile and useful of all the gastrostomies and can have advantages over nasogastric intubation for postoperative decompression in many patients. In children, tube gastrostomy does not prevent gastroesophageal reflux. It is necessary to perform a "protective antireflux operation" in children referred for feeding gastrostomy [53].

WITZEL GASTROSTOMY. Originally described by Witzel in 1891 [142], this form of serosa-lined temporary gastrostomy was designed to minimize regurgitation and leakage along the tube tract. Figure 30-4 shows the essential steps in the technique. A straight catheter should be used, since it makes later removal through the long serosal tunnel easier. The catheter is retained in the stomach by a single pursestring suture about the stab wound in the distal stomach; then the serosa is plicated over the tube for 4–8 cm proximally in the long axis of the stomach. Here, as in the Stamm gastrostomy, it is important to use a separate stab wound for the exit of the tube and to attach the stomach wall to the peritoneum at this point and also at two or three other points along the serosal tunnel.

Details of postoperative care are essentially identical with those described for the Stamm gastrostomy. It has been stated that the Witzel gastrostomy is less prone to leakage than the Stamm, but because it forms a serosa-lined tract and is intended for temporary use, this advantage is doubted. In general, the technique has little if any advantage over the Stamm method and has the disadvantage of requiring a longer operating time and of producing greater gastric deformity. A modification of tube gastrostomy using features of both the Stamm and Witzel procedures was introduced by Sanders [107]. Through a small serosal incision, he introduces a curved hemostat and forms a subserosal tunnel that accommodates a Foley catheter. He makes no attempt to suture the stomach to the anterior abdominal wall.

T-TUBE GASTROSTOMY. The use of a large T tube for gastrostomy (Fig. 30-5) has been recommended by Santiago-Delpin [108]. The advantages listed include more adequate gastric decompression with the double-ended tube, which is said to be independent of the patient's position. The surgical technique is identical to the Stamm procedure, with the only real innovation being the size and configuration of the tube.

PERCUTANEOUS GASTROSTOMY. Some interest has arisen in the percutaneous establishment of a gastrostomy [94]. We have no experience with this technique and can only comment that, although it may have application in selected situations, as with all "blind" procedures it carries the attendant risks of bleeding and perforation (see Editor's Comment).

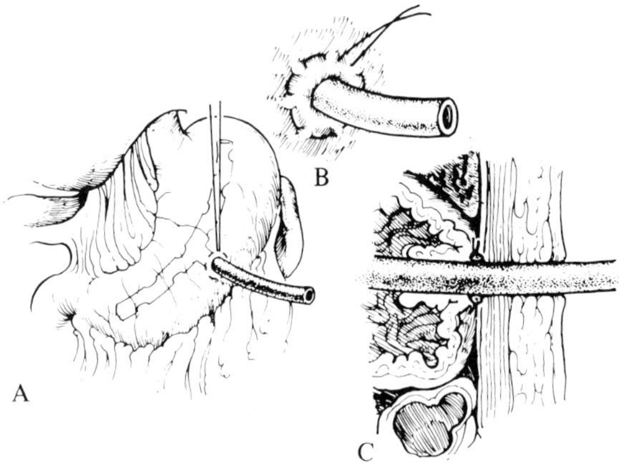

Fig. 30-5. T-tube gastrostomy. (A) The T tube is in place. The tube size should be at least No. 24F, and there should be 10–12 holes in the tube about 1.5 cm apart. (B) Purse-string fixation and mucosal inversion. (C) The stomach is fixed to the anterior abdominal wall in the usual manner.

Permanent Gastrostomy

DEPAGE-JANEWAY GASTROSTOMY. This technique is the prototype of mucosa-lined gastrostomies and is probably the most commonly used of the permanent methods. Originally described by Depage in 1901 [18], the technique was slightly modified by Janeway in 1913 [49] and is the basis for the more complex tubovalvular methods to be described later in the chapter.

This method is probably the best one available for feeding patients with proximal obstructions, such as patients with unresectable esophageal or high gastric cancer. Because it is lined with mucosa, this gastrostomy will not close spontaneously and therefore does not require continuous intubation. The fistula can be used for retrograde intragastric or esophageal manipulations as well.

The operative features of the technique are shown in Figure 30-6. A full-thickness flap of the stomach wall is raised from its anterior wall. While the flap may be oriented in any axis of the stomach, it is generally better to base the flap on the greater curvature, since blood supply is more reliable and the final tube can be brought more easily to the skin surface.

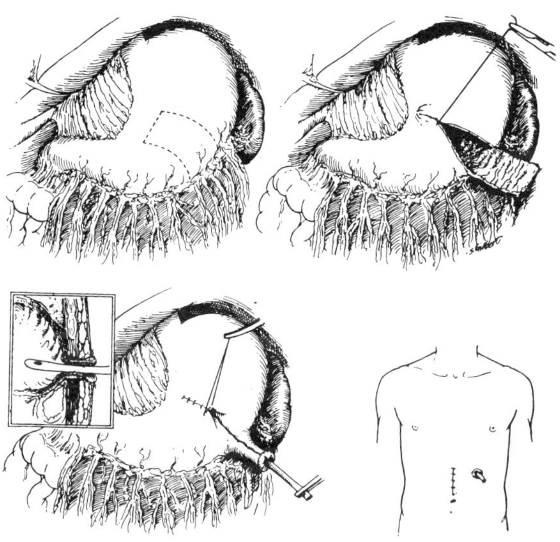

Fig. 30-6. Depage-Janeway gastrostomy. As shown, the flap of stomach wall is converted into a tube by a two-layer closure. A straight or mushroom catheter makes formation of the tube simpler. The tube is brought through a full-thickness excised tract, and its mucosa is sutured to the skin. To prevent retraction, the serosa at the base of the tube is sutured to the peritoneum.

Closure of the gastric defect and formation of the tube are accomplished by two- or three-layer closure, as shown. The inner layers may be continuous, with atraumatic sutures of 000 or 4-0 chromic catgut.

The final layer must be of interrupted nonabsorbable suture using the Lembert, Cushing, or Halsted methods. The tube is formed over a catheter so that it will be uniform throughout and because the added stiffness makes manipulation of the stomach tube easier. The catheter should be 14F–18F. A Foley catheter is sometimes advantageous, as it provides a ball-valve at the gastric orifice of the tube, preventing reflux.

The gastric tube is usually led out through a separate incision and fixed to the peritoneum by a few fine, nonabsorbable sutures. The mucosa of the tube is everted slightly and attached to the skin margins by interrupted catgut sutures. The point of exit should be higher on the abdominal wall (more cephalad) than the gastric opening of the tube to minimize reflux when the patient is sitting or standing.

A simpler and faster way of forming the gastric tube is by using a stapling device [137]. By virtue of its speed and versatility, stapling is, no doubt, the method of choice at present [50, 104]. The tube, as shown in Figure 30-7 is amputated at its tip, and the rest of the procedure is performed as described in the preceding paragraph.

Postoperatively no special precautions are necessary. After healing of the wound, the original tube can be removed and replaced as necessary. It is sometimes possible to intubate the stomach only for feeding, keeping the orifice of the gastrostomy covered with an appropriate appliance between feedings.

BECK-JIANU GASTROSTOMY. The Beck-Jianu gastrostomy [7, 51] also is a mucosa-lined permanent gastrostomy and has the same indications as the Depage-Janeway method. A somewhat larger lumen can be accomplished, and pureed foods can often be inserted through it. Furthermore, when the gastric tube is angulated upward in the subcutaneous tissues before being brought out through the skin, a sort of valve action is formed at the gastric end of the tube.

As shown in Figure 30-8, the procedure is begun with freeing of the greater curvature, with division of the epiploic branches of the left gastroepiploic artery and vein. Noncrushing clamps are applied parallel to the longitudinal axis of the stomach from the antrum well into the corpus to isolate a tubular segment of the stomach. After isolation of the tube, closure of the stomach and tube is accomplished as in the Depage-Janeway method with inner continuous and outer interrupted sutures or by the use of a stapling device. The tube is exteriorized by tunneling upward over the costal margin in the subcutaneous tissue and by suturing the mucosa to the edges of a 2- to 3-cm stab wound over the low anterior chest wall.

This method has the advantage of permanence, ease in tube feeding, and easy management by the patient. The loss of stomach volume is probably unimportant.

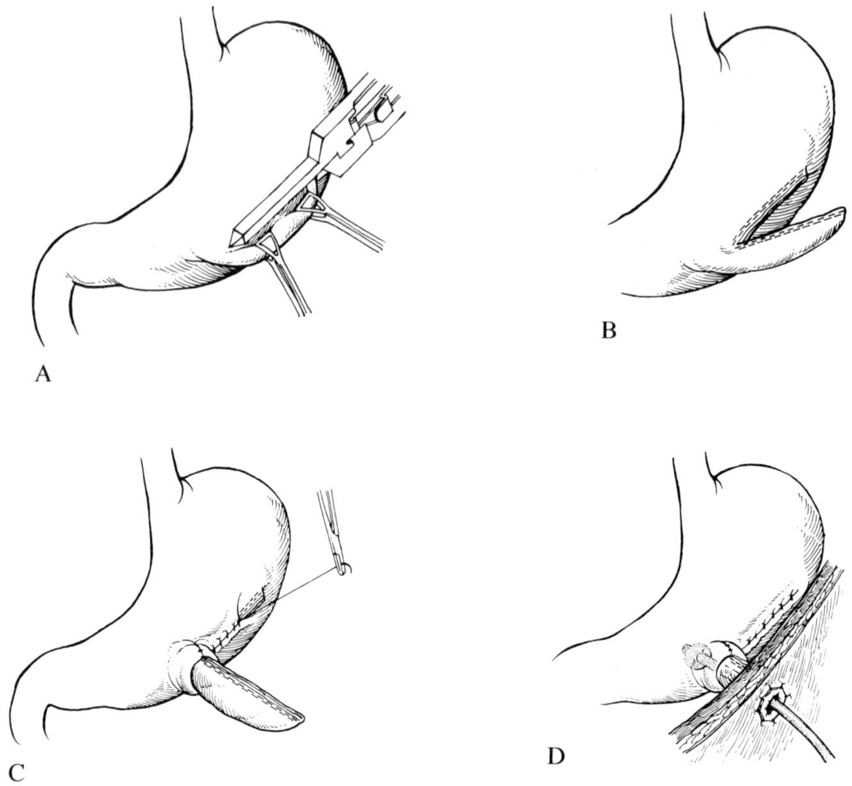

Fig. 30-7. Stapled permanent gastrostomy. This is a variation of the Depage-Janeway technique. A gastric tube is formed (A, B, C) and brought out through a separate incision (D).

PATTON GASTROSTOMY. Another type of permanent gastrostomy was described by Patton in 1955 [88]. He modified the Janeway gastrostomy by making the mucosal incision half as long as the seromuscular incision and by folding the mucosa in on itself to produce a flutter valve. This was designed to allow introduction of a tube for feeding purposes and withdrawal at the completion of the meal. The flutter-valve effect prevents leakage (Fig. 30-9).

SPIVACK (WATSUJI) TUBOVALVULAR GASTROSTOMY. Although this operation is commonly

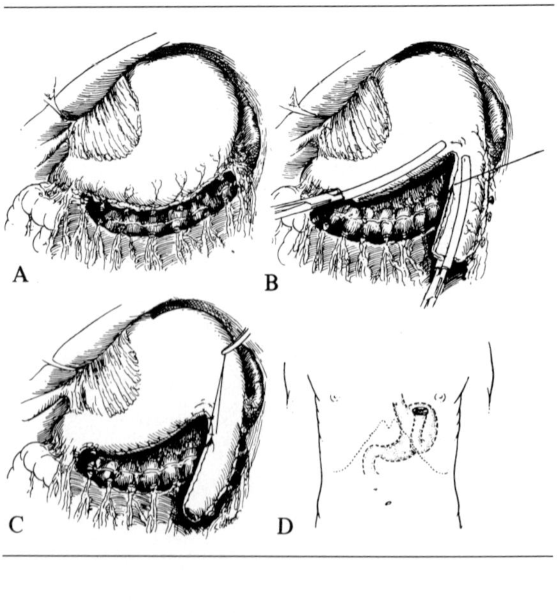

Fig. 30-8. Beck-Jianu gastrostomy. This technique is similar to that of the Depage-Janeway gastrostomy (Fig. 30-7), but it provides a much longer tube that can be brought through an oblique abdominal wall tunnel (A, B, C), forming a valve effect (D). A two-layer closure is used throughout.

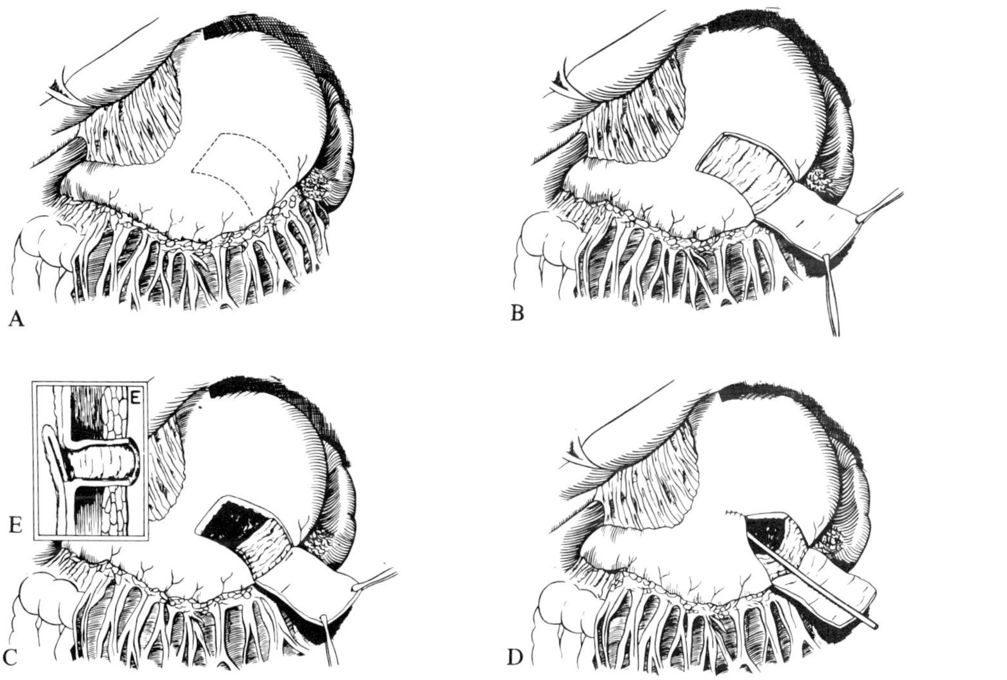

Fig. 30-9. Patton gastrostomy. This differs from the Depage-Janeway gastrostomy in that it includes a mucosal flutter valve. (A) Position of incision. (B) Reflection of seromuscular layer. (C, D, E) Development of mucosal flutter valve.

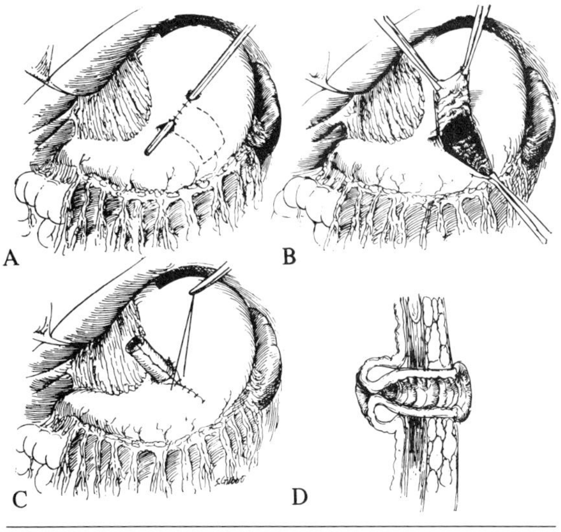

Fig. 30-10. Spivack (Watsuji) gastrostomy. This method forms a true valve at the base of the tube by inverting a roll of stomach wall (A, B, C). After formation of the tube, leakage is prevented by the mucosal "roll" within the stomach lumen. Seromuscular sutures are used to retain the tube within its tract (D), and the mucosal end of the tube is sutured to the skin edge. A soft catheter should be placed through the tube for the first week.

credited to Spivack [114], Thorek [121] demonstrated clearly that priority for the technique belongs to Watsuji [136] of Japan. While interesting, the controversy in no way changes the concept of this modification of the Depage-Janeway tubular gastrostomy. Early experience with reflux leakage stimulated a desire to provide an internal valve mechanism for its prevention.

The steps in formation of the tubovalvular gastrostomy are shown in Figure 30-10. A flap of stomach wall is outlined, but before it is raised the full thickness of the wall across its base is invaginated by a single row of sutures. The flap is then raised so that its "hinge" is the invaginated roll of wall. The tube is formed as in the other methods. Closure approximates the two ends of the roll of stomach wall, forming a collar or "doughnut" of tissue at the gastric opening of the tube that effectively prevents reflux.

The details of operative and postoperative care of the tubovalvular gastrostomy are identical with those of the Depage-Janeway method. The method has the same theoretical and practical advantages and disadvantages as well. Although it requires general anesthesia and at least 1 hour more of full-time operating, it is probably worthwhile in the patient who needs a feeding gastrostomy and who has a prognosis of at least several months of life.

JEJUNAL GASTROSTOMY (TAVEL–NYHUS). In 1906 Tavel [120] described a technique of gastrostomy using a short (7 ½-cm) segment of jejunum interposed between the stomach and the skin. Only a few operations were done, and the method was condemned because of reflux, which nullified the value of the procedure. On the basis of newer concepts of the sphincteric action of jejunal segments of greater length and of their resistance to peptic erosion, as elucidated by Dillard and Merendino [21], Nyhus et al. [84, 85] revived jejunal gastrostomy. By using segments of jejunum from 25 to 35 cm in length, these sets of authors prevented reflux leakage and were able to report satisfactory results in small groups of patients. Subsequent experience with the method has confirmed their confidence in its value.

Jejunal gastrostomy is indicated for the same purposes as any other mucosa-lined permanent gastrostomy. It is probably more truly valvular than the Watsuji-Spivack method, but it is somewhat more difficult to perform. The surgeon must be thoroughly familiar with the requirements of the technique and well versed in the anatomy and blood supply of the jejunum.

Upper abdominal exposure is obtained through a midline or paramedian incision, and the ligament of Treitz is identified. The mesentery of the upper jejunum is carefully inspected using transillumination. If the arterial and venous arcades are found to be continuous, so that blood supply and drainage are ensured, an isolated segment of jejunum is prepared by division of the jejunum 5–15 cm distal to the ligament of Treitz. The straight jejunal arteries and veins are divided, as are both leaves of the peritoneum. Usually two or three vessels must be divided to provide a segment 25–35 cm in length. At the distal point of the segment, only the jejunum is divided, leaving the mesentery intact. This is important because it allows additional communications for venous drainage of the segment.

An incision is made through the transverse mesocolon to the left of the middle colic artery, and the entire isolated segment is brought through it into the supramesocolic space. Using a two-layer technique, the distal end of the segment is anastomosed to the anterior stomach wall, above the midpoint and near the greater curvature. Before the proximal end is exteriorized, a Foley balloon catheter is passed into the stomach through the segment, and the balloon is inflated; the proximal end of the segment is brought to the surface through a stab wound near the left costal margin, and the mucosa is sutured to the skin edges. Full-thickness excision of a "button" of abdominal wall about 2 cm in diameter is preferable, particularly in the obese patient. Intestinal continuity is restored by reanastomosing the jejunum end to end. The opening in the transverse mesocolon should be lightly approximated and tacked to the jejunal loop to prevent herniation of intestine. In addition, it is important to attach the proximal portion of the jejunal segment to the peritoneum for a few centimeters to prevent prolapse of the segment (Fig. 30-11).

Postoperatively the catheter is allowed to drain until peristalsis returns, and then it is used for feeding for another five to seven days. It has been found that about seven to ten days are required for the isolated segment to acquire full propulsive peristalsis. After this period the catheter is withdrawn and used only while feedings are being introduced. The tube need not be passed farther than 5–7.5 cm into the segment, because peristalsis stimulated by food in the segment will cause it to carry the material rapidly into the stomach.

The value of homogenized solid foods in tube feedings should be remembered, especially in the patient who is to be permanently fed by gastrostomy. Whole foods from the kitchen or dining tray can be mixed together in a blender, water added as required, and the

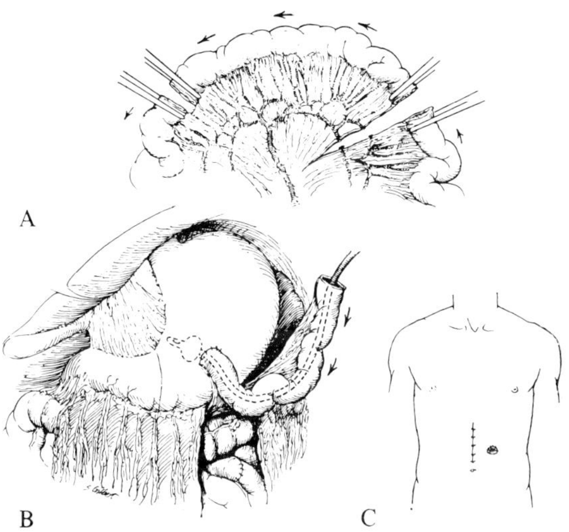

Fig. 30-11. Jejunal gastrostomy. (A) The jejunal segment is prepared by division of the intestine at either end of the 25-cm segment. The venous arcade at the distal end is left intact to assure drainage. The segment is brought through the transverse mesocolon, and the omentum is split up to the greater curvature of the stomach so that the vascular pedicle of the segment is not compromised. The Foley catheter is passed through the segment before the anastomoses are completed (B, C).

whole reduced to a fine suspension that can be easily passed through any gastrostomy. This method enables nutrition to be more easily maintained, since the patient is obviously on a normal, regular diet. The psychological value of such feedings is apparent. In the stuporous or comatose patient close attention to urinary output and skin hydration is necessary, since tube feedings will contain insufficient free water to maintain adequate hydration.

Jejunal gastrostomy has advantages for terminal-care feeding, but it is perhaps of even greater usefulness in patients in whom multiple procedures for reconstruction of the mouth, oropharynx, or cervical esophagus are being done. Such procedures often require months to complete, and the advantage of a completely leakproof gastrostomy is obvious. Patients can care for themselves with ease and need no special equipment or foodstuffs.

This operation has the drawbacks that it demands more skill than other methods, uniformly requires 1½-2 hours of general anesthesia, and carries the risk of two enteric anastomoses as well as of gangrene of the jejunal segment. The last complication is rare when an experienced surgeon performs the operation, but it is often fatal unless promptly recognized. If it is suspected, the patient must undergo an exploratory procedure immediately.

In summary, it should be said that temporary gastrostomy has been enjoying greater application and usefulness, particularly in the management of postoperative patients, while permanent gastrostomy is less often indicated, largely because of improved, definitive methods of cancer therapy.

DUODENOSTOMY (THE DIFFICULT DUODENAL STUMP)

Most external duodenal fistulas result from blowout of a duodenal stump after one of the variations of the Billroth II gastrectomy in which the resection was difficult and closure of the proximal duodenum was insecure. Less commonly, fistula may arise from an anastomotic leak following Billroth I anastomosis. Other causes include penetrating abdominal trauma and surgical accidents. Surgical accidents account for most of the postoperative fistulas, the most common specific causes being operations on the stomach, gallbladder, and bile ducts. Nephrectomy under difficult circumstances may involve clamping or unintentional ligature of a portion of the adjacent duodenal wall, with later necrosis and leakage. The same sort of injury may rarely occur during an operation for retrocecal appendicitis, or damage to the duodenum may be secondary to contiguous cellulitis or to pressure necrosis from inlying tubes or drains.

Whatever the cause, the metabolic effects of external duodenal fistulization can be devastating. The magnitude of the fluid and electrolyte losses and consequent difficulties in management are roughly proportional to the actual size and duration of the fistula itself and to the degree of obstruction distal to the fistula.

The difficult duodenal stump formerly was

estimated to occur in nearly 3 percent of patients after Billroth II gastrectomy [65]. Insecure closure, an edematous or scarred duodenal wall, and fear of damaging the structures of the portal triad all predispose to this accident. Many important technical considerations of this problem were reviewed by Ginzburg in 1954 [33] and more recently by Prigouris and Michas [96].

Catheter duodenostomy has been used with great success by many surgeons [66, 73, 74, 90, 95, 139]. This maneuver is technically simple and may prevent a tragic sequence of fistulization, leakage, hypochloremic alkalosis, inanition, and death. In this technique (Fig. 30-12) a straight urethral catheter is placed in the duodenal lumen and, if the duodenal wall will support a suture, is retained therein by either a pursestring suture of silk or by several interrupted sutures of the same material. The site is covered by omentum, if available, and the tube is exteriorized through a separate stab wound. It is probably advisable to drain the area further by way of a Penrose drain brought out through a second stab wound caudad to the first. Ordinarily suction need not be applied to the duodenostomy catheter, but if after one or two days there is profuse drainage, suction may prevent duodenal distention and ileus and perhaps lessen the obstructive process that perpetuates the leak. Usually the leakage subsides as peristalsis returns, and the catheter can be clamped or removed in 7 to 10 days. If drainage persists beyond this time, frank anatomical obstruction at or beyond the gastroenterostomy site must be suspected and corrected surgically.

Duodenal fistula following gastroduodenal (Billroth I) anastomosis, while less common, usually requires immediate intervention and repair. Since most such anastomoses are made in normal or nearly normal duodenum, with its excellent blood supply, leakage is infrequent. To detect such occurrences some surgeons place a Penrose drain near the anastomosis, but the incidence of leakage probably does not in itself justify routine drainage. Careful attention to the details of the anastomosis and adequate mobilization of the duodenum to prevent tension of the suture line are probably

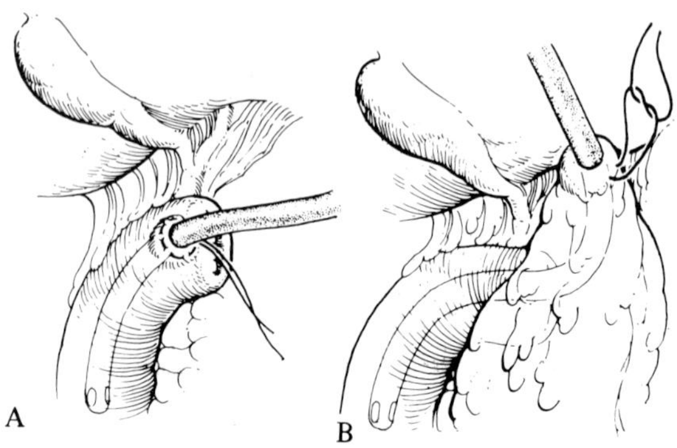

Fig. 30-12. Catheter duodenostomy for the doubtful or frankly inadequate duodenal stump closure (A). The catheter should be at least No. 16F. If available, a large omental tag should be arranged so as to seal the tract around the catheter (B). The tube is brought out of the abdomen through a stab wound separate from the one used to drain the stump closure. Note that the tube enters the side of the duodenum separately from the duodenal closure.

more important factors in the prevention of leaks.

In known or suspected instances in which the duodenal ulcer frankly involves the common bile duct or ampulla of Vater, it is often advisable to identify the common duct by passing a probe through its length. This will facilitate dissection and lessen the chance of injury. The occasional ulcer of the second portion of the duodenum or the massive duodenal ulceration that may occur in association with functioning pancreatic tumors (Zollinger-Ellison syndrome) may make such a maneuver mandatory. On completion of the gastroduodenal portion of the procedure, a T tube should be placed in the duct. If there are gallstones or there is evidence of any degree of cholecystitis, the gallbladder should be removed. Sometimes duodenostomy combined with T-tube drainage of the common duct is the technical salvation of a difficult situation [32] (Fig. 30-13).

Bigg et al. [9] described closure of the duodenal stump by the use of an omental "plug" sutured in place. This procedure was used when the ampulla was noted to be within a few

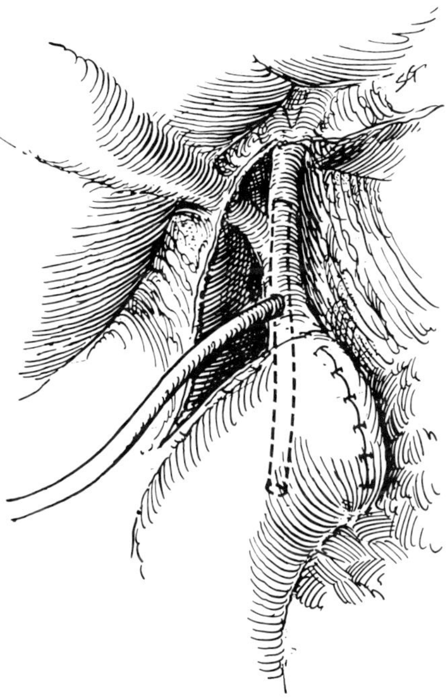

Fig. 30-13. After dissections near the ampulla of Vater or when the common bile duct is explored during an operation for duodenal ulcer, a T tube should be placed in the duct for identification. If needed, catheter duodenostomy may be performed as well.

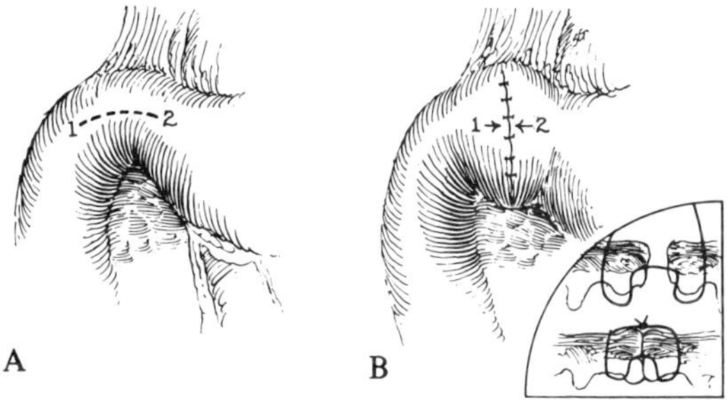

Fig. 30-14. Heineke-Mikulicz pyloroplasty. The longitudinal incision across the pyloric sphincter extends 2.5–3.0 cm into both the stomach and the duodenum. The single layer of nonabsorbable sutures is placed either as Gambee stitches (*inset*) or as simple seromuscular sutures, not including the mucosa. It is important to use only enough sutures for adequate closure and to avoid compromising the duodenal lumen by excessive inversion.

millimeters of the line of transection. If a probe is inserted into the common duct, this technique is rarely needed.

PYLOROPLASTY AND GASTRODUODENOSTOMY

These operations are frequently used in conjunction with other procedures on the stomach, and they generally serve one or both of two purposes—to relieve partial pyloric stenosis caused by active or healed duodenal ulcer, and to facilitate gastric emptying. For example, these procedures are employed to complement vagotomy, or to follow proximal subtotal gastrectomy or hiatal hernia repair [43, 47, 77].

Heineke-Mikulicz Pyloroplasty

This technique of pyloroplasty [76] (Fig. 30-14) is probably the most common method employed at the present time. A longitudinal incision of the pyloric sphincter is extended into the antrum and duodenum, through the full thickness of the wall, for about 2 cm in either viscus. This incision is closed transversely by approximation of its ends, thereby widening the lumen of the pyloric canal. It is usually best to use only a single layer of sutures in this closure, placed as shown in Figure 30-14, since a two-layer closure frequently invaginates so much tissue that the increase of lumen is canceled. This is especially true when there has been narrowing of the entire circumference of the pylorus and proximal duodenum by scarring. When the pylorus is normal and the procedure is done as an ancillary drainage procedure, a two-layer closure is permissible using an inner layer of chromic catgut applied as a continuous Connell suture and an outer layer of interrupted nonabsorbable suture material.

An interesting modification of this technique for use with large bleeding posterosuperior duodenal ulcers has been proposed by Kay and Johnson, whereby the ulcer crater is excluded from the newly formed gastroduodenal channel [56].

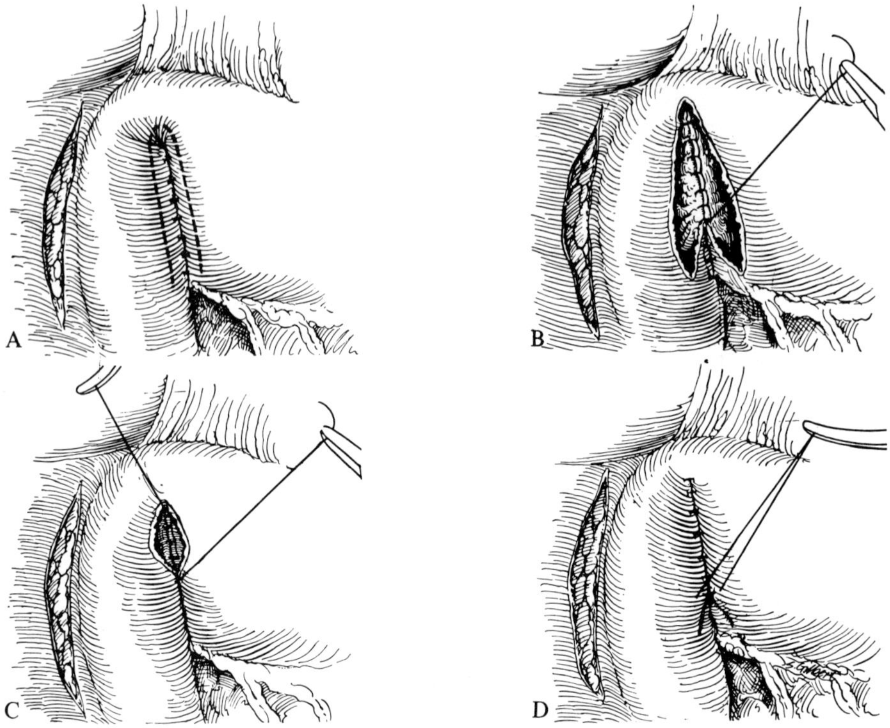

Fig. 30-15. Finney pyloroplasty. After the medial wall of the duodenum has been approximated to the antrum by interrupted sutures, the inverted-U incision is made across the pylorus (A). The mucosa is approximated posteriorly by a continuous locked catgut suture (B) that is continued anteriorly as a Connell suture (C). An anterior row of interrupted sutures completes the procedure (D). Note that the duodenum must be mobilized (Kocher maneuver) before this pyloroplasty can be satisfactorily accomplished.

Finney Pyloroplasty

The Finney pyloroplasty [25, 26] has several advantages over the Heineke-Mikulicz method and is preferred by many surgeons. It amounts to a wide gastroduodenostomy with transection and inclusion of the pyloric sphincter (Fig. 30-15). It provides a much wider stoma than other techniques, is applicable even when there is extensive scarring of the anterosuperior duodenum, and can be more securely closed, since two or even three layers of sutures may be placed. However, unless the second part of the duodenum is normal so that it can be freely mobilized (Kocher maneuver) and brought into opposition with the antrum, this technique should not be used.

After mobilization of the duodenum by lateral peritoneal incision, a single row of seromuscular sutures of 000 or 4-0 silk is placed as a posterior row to approximate the inner curve of the duodenum to the inferior aspect of the antrum and pyloric canal. An incision in the shape of an inverted U is made into the lumen and carried through the pylorus, paralleling the suture line into the duodenum. A posterior continuous chromic catgut suture is used to approximate the inner mucosal edges and is continued upward to close the outer mucosal edges. A final row of silk sutures completes the two-layer closure. The resulting stoma is a good deal larger than the lumen of the duodenum and completely defunctionalizes the pyloric sphincter.

There is a spur of tissue present after construction of a Finney pyloroplasty that may delay gastric emptying in some situations.

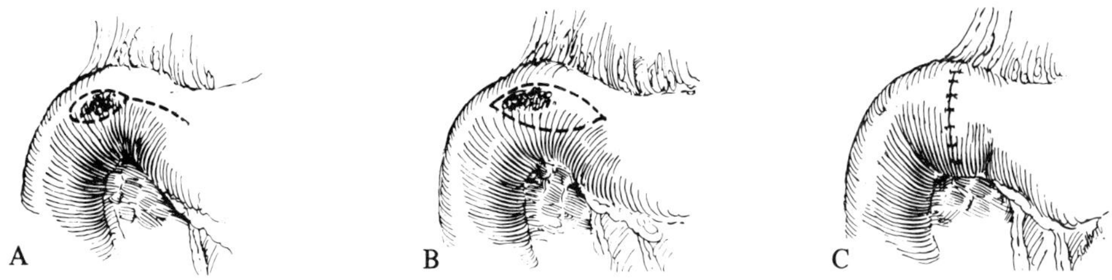

Fig. 30-16. Judd (A) and Horsley (B) pyloroplasties. These techniques were designed for excisional treatment of perforated or cicatrizing anterior duodenal ulcers, but they are not adequate treatment unless they are combined with complete vagotomy. (C) Final closure.

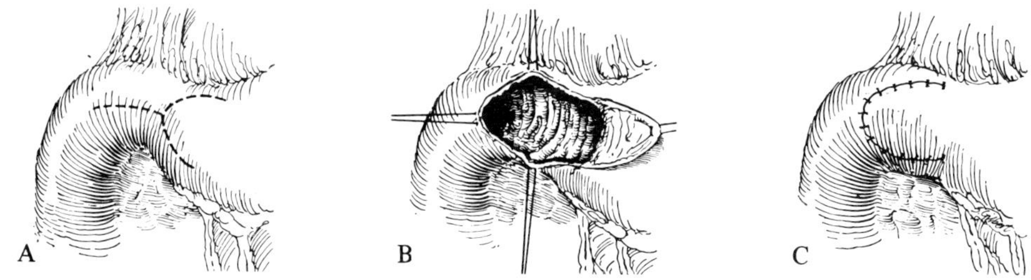

Fig. 30-17. Moschel pyloroplasty. The flap is outlined in the antrum, and the leg of the Y is extended across the pyloric sphincter (A). Advancing the antral flap into the defect thus formed (B) enlarges the duodenal lumen by an amount equal to the width of the flap and produces no "dog-ear" deformity (C). Closure should be performed in two layers.

Howard and Deles [46] modified the classical Finney technique by everting this spur of tissue. They suture the serosal surface of the tissue spur to the greater curvature of the stomach.

Judd and Horsley Pyloroplasties

The Judd [54] and Horsley [45] techniques are only technical variants of the Heineke-Mikulicz pyloroplasty, and since they were originally proposed to include excision of an active or healed duodenal ulcer as definitive treatment, they find little usefulness today. Neither is recommended, although exceptionally a tiny duodenal scar may be better excised during pyloroplasty to facilitate suture of the margins. Figure 30-16 shows the details of these methods.

Moschel Pyloroplasty

The plastic surgical technique of conversion of a Y-shaped incision into a U-shaped closure has been adapted to the pylorus by Moschel et al. [79]. As depicted in Figure 30-17, a flap of antrum is moved into the defect created by longitudinal incision of the sphincter and duodenal wall. Moschel reports excellent results in a small group of patients, and Randolph has found some application of this method in children [98]. This method has the technical advantages of not producing the "dog-ear" deformities of the other methods and of allowing a limited excision of duodenal scar. As in the Finney method, the duodenum must be freely mobilized and closure should be done in two layers. Care must be taken that the antral flap is made short and broad to avoid devascularization of its tip.

Anterior Hemipylorectomy

Another method of draining the stomach is excision of the anterior half of the pylorus with transverse closure. Judd and Nagel [54] introduced this technique for the treatment of marginal ulceration, which was common following the then-popular gastrojejunostomy. Beattie [6] combined this procedure with vagotomy and reported satisfactory results in a series of 115 patients. On the basis of his results, he concluded that this was the operation of choice for duodenal ulcer if technically feasible. Further support for this procedure was given by Holt and Lythgoe [44], who concurred with Beattie that this is the operation of choice. Aust [4] modified the technique by performing an extramucosal anterior hemipylorectomy. The advantage of this is rather doubtful, because it precludes exploration of the duodenum and stomach. Suture-line leakage has not been a problem in any of the reported series. The advantages of this technique are ease of closure and adequate drainage.

Gastroduodenostomy

As a primary method of treatment for duodenal ulcer—particularly the burned-out, cicatricial stenosing variety—the Jaboulay gastroduodenostomy [47] has little current usefulness. It differs from the Finney method in that it is simply a side-to-side technique without division of the pyloric sphincter (Fig. 30-18). Again, the technique requires mobilization of the duodenum. It has the virtue of not requiring complete dissection of the first portion of the duodenum, and therefore it may be easier to perform than the Finney method.

Pylorojejunostomy

Another drainage procedure described by Pecora [91] involves anastomosis of the pylorus to the proximal jejunum. This procedure can be used as an alternative to pyloroplasty, especially in instances in which the pylorus is extremely deformed and scarred, and safe closure by the usual methods of pyloroplasty is not easily accomplished. The procedure involves the usual incision across the pylorus, with excision of an anterior ulcer if indicated.

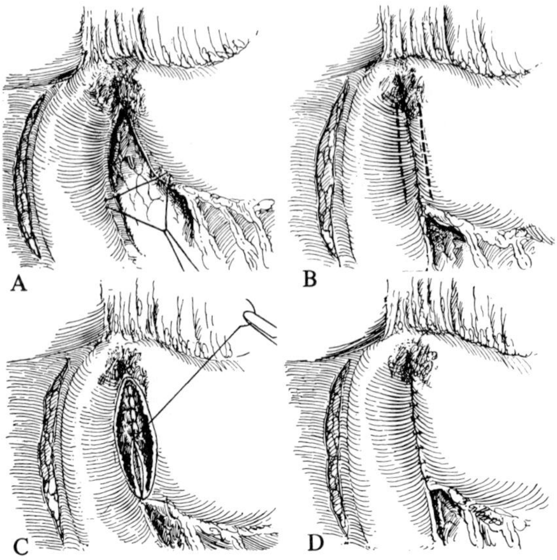

Fig. 30-18. Side-to-side (Jaboulay) gastroduodenostomy differs from the Finney pyloroplasty only in that the incision is not completed superiorly, leaving the pyloric sphincter intact. In instances of severe cicatricial stenosis, side-to-side gastroduodenostomy may be easier to perform. Technical details are essentially identical with those for the Finney method (Fig. 30-15).

A loop of proximal jejunum is brought up in front of the colon, incised in a longitudinal axis on the antimesenteric border, and anastomosed to the pylorus in an isoperistaltic manner (Fig. 30-19). Pylorojejunostomy has physiological and anatomical appeal and therefore may be used as a complementary procedure to vagotomy. It has the obvious drawback of creating a long afferent limb.

DUODENOJEJUNOSTOMY

Certain obstructive processes of the duodenum (superior mesenteric artery syndrome, annular pancreas, and chronic duodenal ileus) may require a bypass procedure. Duodenojejunostomy rather than gastrojejunostomy is the preferred method in these instances, since the former more nearly mimics the normal intestinal continuity.

The third and fourth portions of the duodenum are exposed through an incision in the mesocolon, usually between the right and

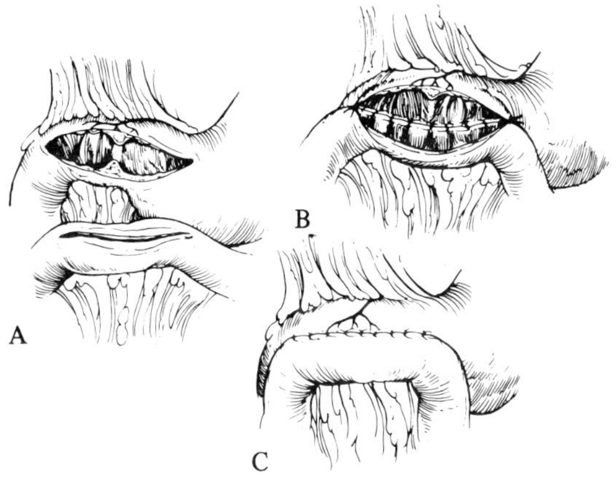

Fig. 30-19. Pylorojejunostomy. The pyloric incision (A) should be about 5 cm unless more exposure is needed for other reasons. The jejunal loop is brought in front of the colon (B) and after longitudinal incision is anastomosed to the pylorus in an isoperistaltic manner (C).

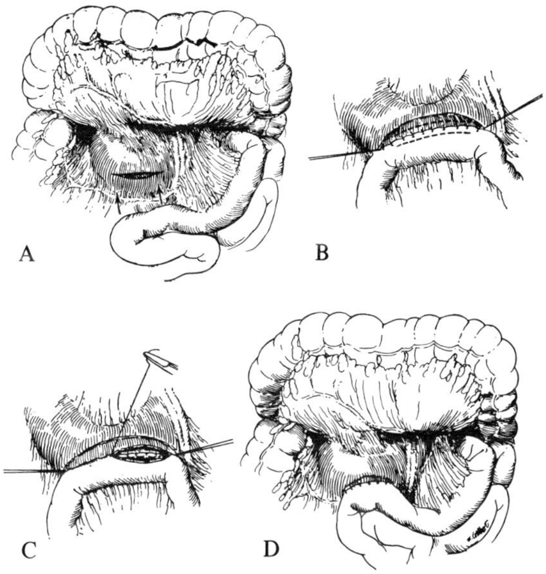

Fig. 30-20. Duodenojejunostomy. The third and fourth portions of the duodenum are exposed beneath the transverse mesocolon (A), and the overlying peritoneum and retroperitoneal areolar tissue are dissected away. The jejunum and duodenum are approximated with interrupted sutures (B), after which both are opened longitudinally. An inner continuous mucosal suture is placed (C), and the anastomosis is completed with an anterior row of interrupted sutures (D).

middle colic arteries (Fig. 30-20). A two-layer side-to-side anastomosis between the duodenum and proximal jejunum is performed, thus eliminating the duodenal-jejunal junction from continuity. Of course the level of the duodenal bypass depends on the entity being treated. The first portion of the duodenum would be involved in instances of annular pancreas and the third portion in the treatment of superior mesenteric artery syndrome or chronic duodenal ileus. Most patients treated by duodenojejunostomy are relieved of their obstructive symptoms, and there is a surprisingly low incidence of postoperative problems.

GASTRIC DIVISION

Gastric division has been recommended in the past as a treatment for bleeding esophageal varices but has found little success. It has been proposed by Randolph et al. [99] as a palliative operation in the critically ill child with esophageal atresia and tracheoesophageal fistula. This is based on the premise that abdominal manipulations are better tolerated than are thoracic procedures in these infants with pulmonary immaturity or compromise [38].

Akiyama and Hiyama [1] used the gastric division concept in esophageal bypass for nonresectable malignant tumors by retrosternal passage and anastomosis of the stomach to the divided cervical esophagus. This procedure also included gastroenterostomy to decompress the bypassed segment and a pyloroplasty.

The use of gastric division for control of morbid obesity is described in Chapter 29.

ESOPHAGEAL REPLACEMENT USING GASTRIC TUBES

The stomach has been used for replacement of the esophagus afflicted with malignant tumors, stricture, or atresia. At times the entire stomach has been mobilized, brought up into the neck, and sutured into place. Various gastric tubes have been constructed for the purpose of esophageal replacement, usually from

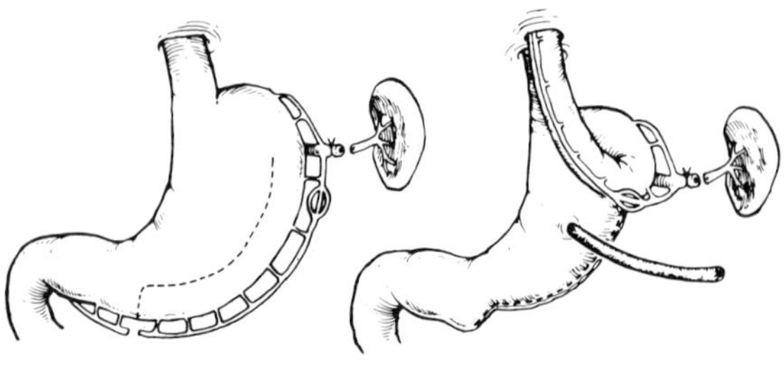

A B

Fig. 30-21. Reversed gastric tube. The tube comprises the entire greater gastric curvature, beginning 5 cm from the pylorus (A). The end product will be about 30 cm long and 2.5 cm in diameter. Note that the blood supply is provided by the left gastroepiploic artery and that splenectomy is performed (B). If a gastrostomy is indicated, it can be placed through the anterior gastric wall.

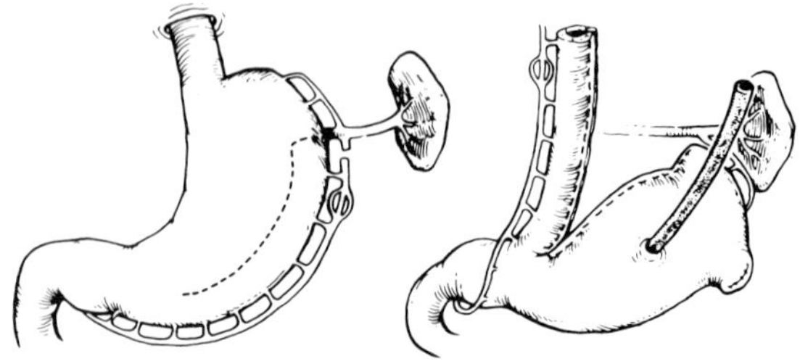

A B

Fig. 30-22. Isoperistaltic gastric tube. (A) The tube is fashioned from the greater curvature and, when used, will twist the stomach in order to obtain full length. If gastrostomy is needed, the posterior wall can be used (B). Note that splenectomy is not necessary.

the greater curvature of the stomach. The most popular type is the reversed gastric tube popularized by Gavriliu and Georgescue [31] and Heimlich [39, 41, 42]. The tube is constructed from the greater curvature and can be anastomosed to the cervical esophagus or pharynx. In principle it is similar to the Beck-Jianu gastrostomy technique (Fig. 30-21).

The reversed gastric tube provides a more physiologically and anatomically correct replacement of the esophagus than does mobilization of the entire stomach into the neck, which removes the reservoir and at times creates the problem of peptic esophagitis. The reversed gastric tube is constructed in the following manner. Just proximal to the pylorus the gastroepiploic vessels are ligated, and an incision is made in the greater curvature. By using a special stapling device or by division and later suturing with a two-layer repair, the surgeon constructs a tube, 2 ½ cm in diameter, from the greater curvature of the stomach, beginning near the pylorus and going up to an area high on the fundus. If the autosuture technique is applied, a second layer of nonabsorbable material is usually used. The gastric tube is drawn upward and can be used either substernally, intrathoracically, or if desired, subcutaneously, to be anastomosed to the cervical esophagus or pharynx. The gastroepiploic vessels accompany the reversed gastric tube, and great care must be exercised not to devascularize the tube. In performing this procedure the splenic vessels are ligated and divided distal to the origin of the gastroepiploic artery, and the spleen is removed. In this manner the tail of the pancreas can be mobilized and elevated, thereby allowing construction of a longer tube.

An isoperistaltic tube has also been described (Fig. 30-22). This is similar to the reversed gastric tube, but it begins on the area of the fundus and is based on the right gastroepiploic artery. Splenectomy is not mandatory in this instance; gastrotomy can accompany the procedure but must be placed in the posterior wall of the stomach. A tube of this type has been used by Heimlich [40] for replacement of the common bile duct, but only in a small number of patients; it has also been used in children with esophageal atresia.

The reversed gastric tube has been used by many surgeons with different indications for esophageal replacement. Some of these indications are chronic peptic esophagitis with stricture and carcinoma of the middle or upper third of the esophagus but not of the lower third; carcinoma of the lower third requires proximal gastrectomy as a portion of the surgical treatment. The reversed gastric tube has also been used extensively for esophageal replacement in small children afflicted with esophageal atresia or caustic injuries. The procedure has been used in children as young as three months of age with good results. The anastomosis must be dilated during the postoperative period, just as it is in other esophageal reconstructive procedures. There is a hazard of stricture at the anastomotic site, and devitalization of the tube itself can occur.

One other indication for a gastric tube has been the creation of a ventriculogastrostomy in the treatment of infantile hydrocephalus [63]. This has been used only as a last resort after the failure of ventriculoperitoneal, ventriculoatrial, and ventriculogallbladder shunts, and it is a promising, ingenious method of ventricular decompression.

GASTROPEXY

Gastropexy (surgical elevation of the ptotic stomach) was proposed and employed many years ago. Several techniques have been described, including pursestring suturing of the lesser omentum and suturing of the stomach to the anterior abdominal wall, methods that employed colonic displacement and gastrojejunostomy, and gastrogastrostomy. Several authors have recently discussed the problem of volvulus of the stomach, both chronic and acute, and have described methods of dealing with this unusual surgical entity. Tanner [119] advocates gastropexy with colonic displacement, and Wastell and Ellis [135] reviewed this subject and expressed a similar opinion. Simple gastropexy or a Stamm-type gastrostomy has been recommended for the problem of volvulus of the stomach in childhood and infancy [12].

Miscellaneous Operations for Gastric and Duodenal Ulcer

In addition to the several "standard" operations currently employed in the surgical treatment of duodenal ulcer, a number of other procedures have been devised. None of these operations is widely used because of recent advances in the medical management of peptic ulcer; however, some of them enjoy greater popularity than others. Unfortunately, their effectiveness has not been proportional to the zeal with which they were first applied. Such a broad front of attack simply confirms the difficulties of management of ulcer disease, our still incomplete knowledge concerning its pathogenesis, and the wide variety of details of individual pathological changes secondary to the ulcerative process in the duodenum. Some operations have been concocted for a particular technical purpose but have failed to fulfill the stringent requirements of time and function. Others have been supplanted because brief trials demonstrated physiological unsuitability. This factor is the key to evaluation of the many operations of the past and present. Accurate understanding of the complex physiological mechanisms of the stomach and duodenum is essential to the design of any procedure calculated to affect those mechanisms.

Some of the operations that have been used—and in some instances continue to be used occasionally—will be described and their results interpreted in the light of current concepts of gastroduodenal physiology. Many are of historic and evolutionary interest only. To minimize confusion, these operations will be considered individually under three general categories: acceptable operations for duodenal ulcer; unacceptable operations for duodenal ulcer; and experimental procedures. In most instances the classification is in agreement with generally accepted surgical opinion.

ACCEPTABLE OPERATIONS

Antral Exclusion with Antral Mucosal Excision

Early in the evolution of gastroduodenal surgery, the proponents of surgical treatment of duodenal ulcer encountered many difficulties in dealing with active, densely adherent, and edematous penetrating ulcers, and the postoperative complications resulting from these encounters led to much anguish and morbidity. Many technical maneuvers were devised in attempts to avoid these problems and leave the ulcer undisturbed yet provide adequate treatment of the ulcerogenic process. Antral

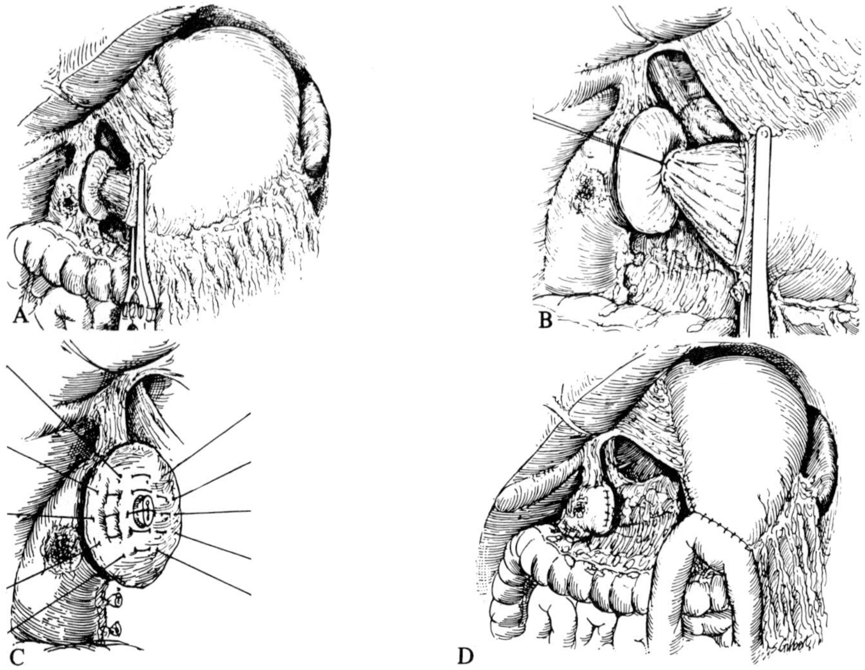

Fig. 30-23. Essential steps in the Bancroft-Plenk operation. (A) The antral seromuscular layer has been reflected to the pylorus. (B) The mucosal tube has been closed by a circular suture. After transection of the mucosa, the seromuscular pouch is closed and obliterated (C) by a series of parallel interrupted sutures. The operation is completed by resection of the distal stomach and antecolic gastrojejunostomy (D).

exclusion (see the section Unacceptable Operations, in this chapter) was originally described as a means by which a difficult ulcer could be excluded from direct gastroduodenal continuity. Early experiences proved that this operation is followed by recurrent ulceration too often for it to be useful.

The method has inherent worth, however, and in 1926 Wilmanns [141] described an operation, involving adequate gastric resection, excision of antral mucosa, and closure of a seromuscular pyloric pouch, that accomplished the objective of exclusion of the ulcer without retaining gastrin-producing antral mucosa. This procedure was modified by Bancroft in 1932 [5] and by Plenk in 1936 [92] and is known by these two names. Many technical modifications of this procedure have been described, most of them designed to prevent the occasional catastrophic blowout of the pyloric pouch [2,97, 129, 143]. The most important technical detail is the preservation of an adequate blood supply to the remaining seromuscular pouch, which requires that the greater and lesser omenta be left intact right up to the point of transection and inversion of the proximal cuff. Of equal importance is hemostasis after excision of the antral mucosa and obliteration of the dead space within the pouch. Figure 30-23 depicts the technique required. After careful pursestring suturing of the sleeve of antral mucosa at the pylorus, the mucosa is excised. A series of parallel catgut sutures is then placed to approximate the denuded muscle surfaces, and a final inverting suture is used to close the stump. This final layer should consist of interrupted nonabsorbable material.

Makkas and Marangos [71] reported a group of 415 patients in whom the Bancroft-Plenk technique was employed, with a mortality of only 2.1 percent and overall good late results in 95 percent. A modification of the technique, using catheter duodenostomy, has been suggested by Harvey [37].

The decision to use the Bancroft technique must be made early in the course of the procedure before the distal antrum has been entirely mobilized. Also, the technique cannot be used after a duodenostomy or pylorotomy, which may be desired for inspection and suture of a bleeding ulcer. The greatest usefulness of the Bancroft-Plenk operation is in treatment of the massively edematous duodenum that is friable and unmanageable.

Partial Longitudinal (Belcher) Gastrectomy

Developed at the Colonel Belcher Hospital in Calgary, Canada, this variation of the Billroth I operation was designed and tested starting in 1952 to overcome several disadvantages of the Billroth II operation [69]. It was hoped that this technique would overcome rapid gastric emptying (dumping), afferent-loop dilatation, and mechanical drag (tension) on the gastric remnant and esophagus. Figure 30-24 depicts the essentials of the technique.

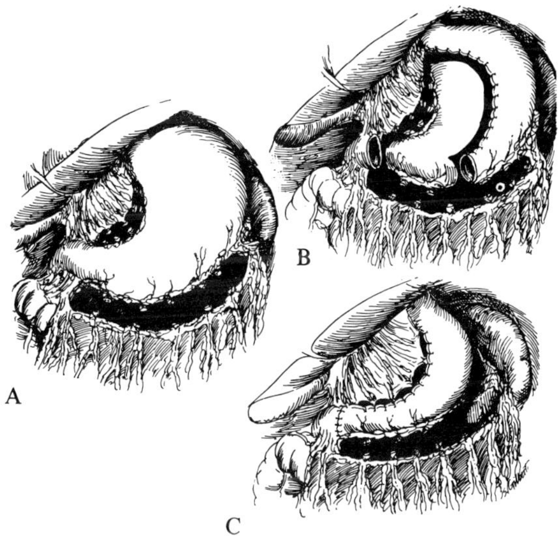

Fig. 30-24. The Belcher gastrectomy. (A, B, C) Successive stages of the resection forming a tubular gastric pouch. Note that the resected portion includes all the antrum.

While the proponents of this procedure provide no objective data, the extent of resection would seem adequate, amounting to 65–75 percent. In addition, the entire antrum is removed. A careful study of 100 consecutive patients has shown satisfactory overall results, with a low (3 percent) incidence of dumping and an acceptable (2 percent) rate of recurrent ulceration [69].

It is claimed that the tubular, elongated gastric pouch delays emptying and thus materially reduces dumping, but the actual depicted configuration varies little from the Schoemaker modification of the Billroth I reconstruction.

UNACCEPTABLE OPERATIONS

A great variety of procedures involving either bypass or resection of some part of the gastroduodenal apparatus has been described, but in only a few procedures has it been possible to prove value. These few have been discussed in earlier sections; the remainder are too numerous for all to be considered. In this section a few operations that have enjoyed great popularity, and may still have adherents, will be discussed. Current concepts of physiology of the stomach and duodenum, together with clinical experience, have proved them to be unacceptable for the surgical treatment of peptic ulcer.

Antral Exclusion with Intact Antral Mucosa

Antral exclusion was originally devised by von Eiselsberg [124] for application to the chronically stenosing or massively penetrating phlegmonous ulcer of the duodenum. The intent of the operation was certainly well conceived, but without knowledge of antral function the procedure was doomed to fail. Stomal ulcers promptly developed in a large percentage of patients, and these ulcers occasionally were more severe than the original ulcer in the duodenum. The technique was soon abandoned.

Recognizing the inherent worth of such a technique and tantalized by the attraction of a procedure that could eliminate the great technical difficulties of resecting some ulcers, many surgeons over the ensuing 35 years attempted to modify antral exclusion so that its

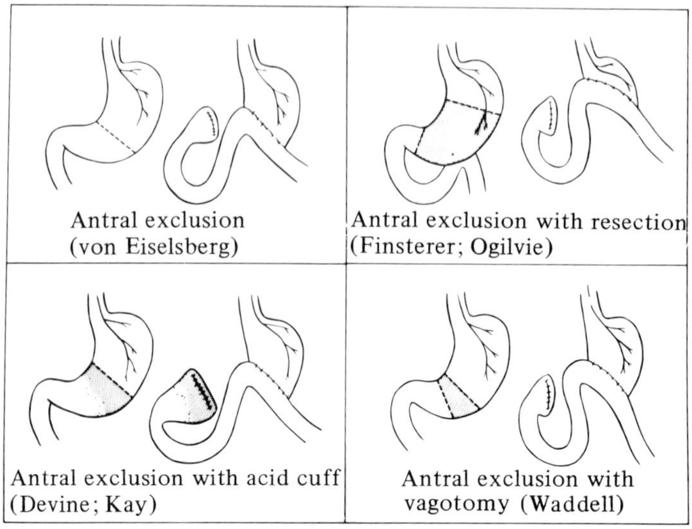

Fig. 30-25. Some currently unacceptable operations for duodenal ulcer. Resected portions of the stomach are indicated by dashed lines. None of the variations of antral exclusion has succeeded in protecting against recurrent ulceration. Similarly, Connell's tubular resection and Wangensteen's modification of it have not met the criteria for an acceptable procedure for duodenal ulcer. (Modified from Nyhus [80].)

technical usefulness would not be outweighed by ulcer recurrence.

Devine [19], Finsterer and Cunha [27], and later, Ogilvie [86] all modified antral exclusion by resection of part of the parietal cell mass, or exclusion of a greater portion thereof (Devine), in an attempt to lower the ulcer recurrence rate. Observation of patients so treated over a period of years showed a prohibitive number of recurrences, however, so the method fell into disfavor [29, 125].

Woodward and Tillmanns [144] pointed out the mechanism of ulcer recurrence following antral exclusion. They demonstrated that the end-isolated antrum, in continuity with the duodenum and not subject to inhibition of activity by an acid environment (and perhaps in fact stimulated by duodenal juice reflux), tended to produce gastric hypersecretion and hyperacidity). The extreme physiological derangement that may result from antral exclusion was well documented by Scobie [109], who noted that excluded gastric antrum simulated the clinical and laboratory findings consistent with the Zollinger-Ellison syndrome. On this basis, Kay [55] performed exclusion leaving a cuff of acid-secreting gastric mucosa in continuity with the antral pouch, thinking this would prevent hyperacidity. Within 26 months he had to report that 8 of 20 patients suffered recurrences with massive stomal ulceration. It should be noted that Devine's operation [20] was quite successful, at least in the early follow-up period, perhaps because his exclusion technique also left acid-forming mucosa attached to the antrum.

The most recent attempt to make exclusion acceptable has been that of Waddell and Bartlett [126]. Waddell performed a small distal resection with antral exclusion and added bilateral truncal vagotomy. After three years of experience, however, 9 jejunal ulcers were noted in a total of 153 patients, an altogether unacceptable rate. Failure of this method has been experimentally confirmed by Root et al. [103].

The modifications of antral exclusion described are shown in Figure 30-25. Nyhus [82] provided a comprehensive review of the role of the antrum in duodenal ulcer surgery and carefully analyzed the several operations just

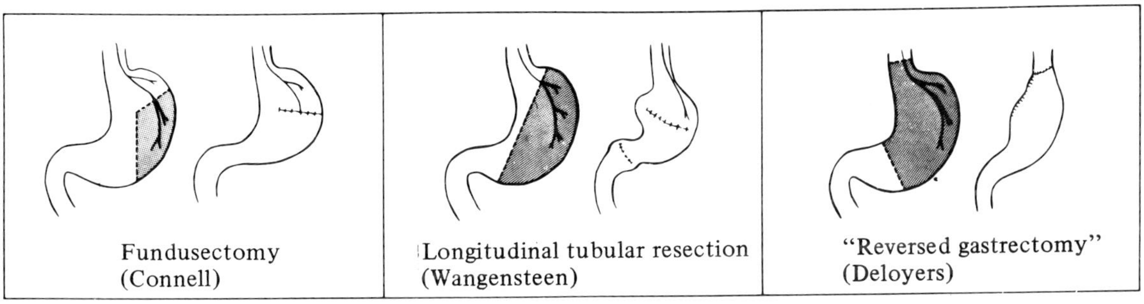

Fig. 30-26. Other procedures for ulcer that have not proved acceptable.

discussed in the light of current knowledge of antral function.

Segmental Gastric Resection

This procedure has been recommended for the treatment of both gastric and duodenal ulcers. Wangensteen [131] was a major supporter of the procedure. As described by him, it involves a 50 percent midgastric resection with a pyloroplasty. Although the recurrence rates quoted by advocates are relatively low, segmental gastric resection is no longer appealing on a physiological basis, since much of the gastric antrum is retained and effective vagotomy by gastric division is questionable. It may be useful in the treatment of some gastric ulcers, however.

Fundusectomy and Longitudinal Tubular Resection with Transverse Gastroplasty

Connell [14, 15], arguing on the basis of the principles of gastroduodenal physiology accepted at the time, was one of the first to propose a resection of fundic acid–secreting gastric mucosa, or fundusectomy (Fig. 30-26), but he did not present clinical data. The procedure never gained wide popularity, nor did it have a strong proponent before Wangensteen [57], largely because of a high rate of ulcer recurrence. The methods of tubular resection and closure (transverse gastroplasty [128, 130]) are shown in Figure 30-26. Wangensteen [131] later indicated that tubular resection with transverse gastroplasty is an unacceptable procedure for duodenal ulcer.

Reports by Pe Thein and Schofield [89], Nyhus et al. [83], and Molina et al. [78] give some indication of the mechanism by which tubular resection fails. Their experimental studies indicate that vagal stimulation can release gastrin from the pyloric antrum. This fact of gastric secretory stimulation would appear sufficient to doom the tubular resection.

Fundusectomy and Esophagoantrostomy

Deloyers [17] suggested resection of the entire body of the stomach with esophagoantrostomy, since removal of all mucosa bearing parietal cells should be a sound physiological approach to the ulcer problem. However, the poor functional results and the considerable technical difficulty inherent in the procedure condemn it for clinical application.

Gastric Devascularization

Somervell [112] demonstrated in both humans and animals that division of all the arteries of both the gastric mesenteries did not produce gangrene of the stomach but tended to reduce acid secretion. When applied to duodenal ulcer in 58 patients, there was relief of symptoms in 51; but in most of these patients gastrojejunostomy was added also. Tanner [118] noted a 20 percent incidence of ulcer recurrence following this operation and abandoned it. Further application is not warranted.

Proximal Duodenectomy with Gastroduodenostomy

MacFee and Sax [68] proposed the excision of the first part of the duodenum (including the pyloric ring) with closure of the duodenal stump and end-to-side von Haberer–Finney gastroduodenostomy. The operation is based on the observation that duodenal ulceration nearly always develops in the first part of the duodenum, and it was speculated that the rapid mixing of the bile and pancreatic juice with acid gastric juice would neutralize the acid present and protect the duodenal mucosa. MacFee and Sax performed this procedure 158 times. After a year or more of follow-up in 116 of the patients, they found 88.8 percent to have good-to-excellent results. The length of the follow-up period and the number of patients are too small to warrant consideration of this procedure as definitive treatment of duodenal ulcer.

EXPERIMENTAL PROCEDURES

Duodenal Reversal

Poth and Gold [93] suggested anatomical reversal of the duodenum to stimulate maximally the inhibitory hormones produced when the duodenum is bathed by acid gastric chyme. They actually perform an anastomosis between the distal duodenum and stomach and the proximal duodenum and jejunum. The procedure has been performed in both animals and humans without vagotomy.

Suprapyloric Antrectomy

Griffith [34] reported his personal series of 40 patients on whom he had performed suprapyloric antrectomy plus selective vagotomy and pyloroplasty (see Chap. 12). He attempted to use this procedure for patients with intractable duodenal ulcer but no significant pyloric obstruction. Results reported to date have been good, with no recurrences and no postoperative dumping syndrome. Maki and co-workers [70] used a similar pylorus-preserving procedure without vagotomy for the treatment of benign gastric lesions.

Mucosal Antrectomy with Vagotomy

An interesting approach has been introduced by Kirk [59]. He excised the antral mucosa after submucosal injection of saline solution and epinephrine in 103 patients [60] as definitive treatment of duodenal ulcer. His results were encouraging; there was not a single recurrent ulcer in a seven-year follow-up period. Kirk believes that removal of other layers of gastric wall is incidental in gastric resection. The procedure can be performed without division of a major gastric blood vessel or manipulation of the duodenum, either in construction of an anastomosis or the fashioning of a stump, and it is therefore safer than conventional partial gastrectomy with reconstruction. The operation is described as simple to perform, and Kirk states that blood loss is minimal. The operation is based on sound physiological principles.

Pyloric and Gastric Preservation with Pancreatoduodenectomy

In an attempt to prevent the dumping syndrome and other postgastrectomy symptoms following the Whipple operation, several groups of investigators have studied the feasibility of preserving the entire stomach, including the pylorus [80, 122]. The operation can be performed with minimal technical difficulty. Furthermore, patients undergoing this modification have fewer postgastrectomy symptoms, increased weight gain, and an improved sense of well-being. Warshaw and Torchiana [132] noted some delay in gastric emptying after pyloric preservation. They recommended placement of a gastrostomy tube in anticipation of a prolonged need for gastric drainage. The gastrostomy tube seemed to reduce a potentially bothersome problem to a well-tolerated minor annoyance. Becker et al. [8] combined mucosal antrectomy with proximal gastric vagotomy in dogs. Their experiments demonstrated complete removal of gastrin-producing antral mucosa without alteration of gastric emptying of solids and liquids.

Surgical Accidents and Errors

This section deals with a few technical errors in surgery of the stomach and duodenum, with emphasis on their prevention, recognition, and correction. Technical errors are made only rarely by the experienced surgeon, yet their occurrence reminds us of our fallibility; only by constant watchfulness can pitfalls be avoided.

GASTROILEOSTOMY

During the period between 1900 and 1935, when gastrojejunostomy alone was frequently used in the treatment of duodenal ulcer, a number of reports appeared concerning the effects of unintentional gastroileostomy. Palumbo et al. [87] found that just over 100 instances were reported in the literature to 1962. It seems certain that this accident must have occurred many more times, but understandably, many instances have not come to light. The clinical syndrome of diarrhea of undigested food, inanition, weight loss, cachexia, and electrolyte disturbances has been well characterized [35, 36, 64, 72, 101, 105]. The intensity and progression of the physiological disturbances seem to be roughly proportional to the proximity of the gastroileal anastomosis to the ileocecal valve. Also, the syndrome is exaggerated after gastrectomy and gastroileostomy, since all gastric outflow must then traverse the short ileal loop. Gastroileostomy without gastric resection produces symptoms that vary from mild, easily tolerated diarrhea to the explosive changes of the full-scale syndrome, depending on the proportion of outflow through the pylorus and duodenum. It has been noted that the healing of a duodenal ulcer may slowly produce obstruction, with increasing shunting of gastric contents into the ileum, gradually increasing the disability.

Experimentally, gastroileostomy has been shown to produce a marked increase in the volume and acidity of secretions from Heidenhain pouches in dogs [116]. The syndrome is reproduced exactly as it is seen in humans. The increased gastric acid secretion probably increases the diarrhea and certainly potentiates ileal ulcerogenesis. The dogs usually die of perforation of ileal ulcers.

In grave situations in which the syndrome has been prolonged and unrecognized, there is usually such severe debility that surgical correction should not be attempted until the patient has undergone extensive rehydration and treatment of electrolyte disturbances. The most damaging and hazardous of these, particularly in the elderly patient, is hypokalemia.

Gastroileostomy should be suspected in any patient who has severe diarrhea, weight loss, and disability following a gastric operation, particularly when the changes begin within a few days after operation. Barium examination of the upper gastrointestinal tract usually establishes the diagnosis. Gastrojejunocolic fistula requires a relatively long free interval for development after gastrectomy and gives a different roentgenographic picture, so differentiation of these two entities is usually easy.

Treatment consists of early operation with reestablishment of normal gastrointestinal continuity.

COMMON BILE DUCT AND MAJOR PANCREATIC DUCT INJURIES

Another unusual but real complication of gastric and duodenal operations is injury to the common bile duct and major pancreatic ducts during gastric resection. White et al. [140] reviewed injuries to the sphincter of Oddi in the course of gastric and duodenal operations. Adding their 6 instances to 65 that appeared in the world literature, they noted that of these 71 instances, 69 occurred during gastric resection for chronic duodenal ulcers. Foley et al. [28] reported on a patient with chronic recurrent pancreatitis caused by injury to the duct of Santorini as a complication of subtotal gastrectomy. Three other instances of common bile duct and major pancreatic injuries were reported by Carpenter and Crandall [11], and six instances of pancreatic injury during gastrectomy were reported by Warren [133]. All authors seem to believe that if the injury is recognized at the operating table and is repaired, morbidity is extremely low, whereas if the injury is missed the outcome will be disastrous. Because of the danger of ductal injury, these authors advocate in many instances using vagotomy and pyloroplasty rather than resection, and they insist that if one is to do a resection in a badly scarred duodenum, a tube should be inserted in the common bile duct so that the surgeon will at all times be aware of the location of the duct. A technique involving closure proximal to the ulcer, as described by Nissen [81], has been advocated by many, as has the use of a catheter duodenostomy. It should be remembered that the position of the ampulla with respect to the pylorus may be changed considerably by the deformity produced by chronic peptic ulceration; therefore, great care should be taken when dissecting the postbulbar region. The mortality and morbidity for postoperative pancreatitis and unrecognized injuries to the biliary tree are extremely high, and it behooves the surgeon to exercise great care when working in this area.

DEVASCULARIZATION OF THE GASTRIC REMNANT

During the course of partial gastrectomy it is possible to devascularize the gastric remnant [48, 102, 113]. This is especially true with large resections; with antrectomy there is a lessened chance. Because of the generally excellent blood supply of the stomach, surgeons have at times been careless and interrupted more of the arterial supply than was necessary, and they have occasionally created the complication of ischemic necrosis of the gastric remnant. The experimental and clinical experience of Kilgore et al. [58] seems to indicate that successive ligation of major vessels increases the incidence of necrosis of the gastric remnant. This is an unusual complication of gastric operations and happens most commonly when a prior splenectomy has been done or when a large resection is undertaken along with truncal vagotomy. Both of these procedures can interrupt the left inferior phrenic supply, the short gastric arteries, and the right and left gastric vessels. Even though these structures are frequently sacrificed, as mentioned, the incidence of necrosis of the gastric remnant is extremely low and should remain an unusual problem with the advent of lesser resections and a better knowledge of the arterial supply of the stomach.

GASTROCOLOSTOMY

Only a few instances of gastrocolostomy appear in the literature, one of which was reported by Landry [64]. Ulceration of the colon is invariable, and in addition to the diarrhea and inanition, there may be occult or massive bleeding. Recognition is easy by barium studies. Treatment is the same as for gastroileostomy: prompt reestablishment of normal continuity.

A simple technique for prevention of these errors was advocated by Deaver [16]. Early in any operation in which gastrojejunostomy is to be employed, the proposed site of the anastomosis should be clearly identified with marking sutures placed in the jejunal wall. Subsequent identification of these sutures eliminates erroneous anastomosis.

TORSION OF THE DUODENAL LOOP

A rare complication of a Kocher maneuver was described by Anderson and Dudley in 1963 [3]. They demonstrated 180-degree clockwise rotation of the duodenum on its horizontal axis in two patients who had undergone antrectomy and vagotomy with Billroth I reconstruction. In one patient persistent postcibal fullness, weight loss, and vomiting necessitated reexploration and restoration of the duodenal loop to its normal position. There was complete remission of all symptoms and no recurrence.

The rarity of this syndrome is apparent when one considers the tremendous number of Kocher maneuvers that have been performed in the 60 years since its introduction. However, torsion of the duodenal loop should be considered in the differential diagnosis of postoperative intermittent high small intestinal obstruction.

POSTGASTRECTOMY HEMORRHAGE

Another avoidable error in operations for duodenal ulcer is failure to control the bleeding site, with resurgence of bleeding following operation. This is most apt to occur after emergency gastrectomies using a Billroth II technique, without removal of the ulcer, or when vagotomy and pyloroplasty are used. During preoperative periods of hypotension, a clot may form in the ulcer base or in the eroded vessel itself, only to be elevated and dislodged by a return of normal blood pressure levels. Prevention of this unfortunate occurrence re-

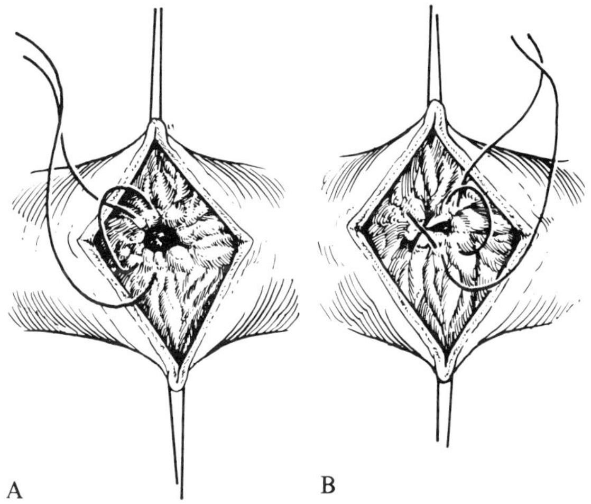

Fig. 30-27. Ligation of bleeding site. (A) Adequate exposure for inspection and (B) placement of nonabsorbable suture material in a figure-of-eight manner will assure against postoperative hemorrhage.

quires only that the general requirements of a good ulcer operation be observed. The ulcer must be removed or excluded and the bleeding must be completely controlled by direct suture of the responsible vessel. Deep bites must be taken in suturing, and nonabsorbable suture material should be used (Fig. 30-27). Failure to observe these requirements has led to a number of unnecessary deaths. Massive bleeding after gastrectomy should be treated by immediate reexploration, not by transfusion and hopeful observation.

References

1. Akiyama, H., and Hiyama, M. A simple esophageal bypass operation by the high gastric division. *Surgery* 75:674, 1974.
2. Allen, A. W., and Welch, C. E. Gastric resection for duodenal ulcer. *Ann. Surg.* 115:530, 1942.
3. Anderson, W. A., and Dudley, H. A. Reversal of the duodenal loop after gastroduodenostomy. *Br. J. Surg.* 50:734, 1963.
4. Aust, J. B. A new technique for pyloroplasty. *Surgery* 53:309, 1963.
5. Bancroft, F. W. A modification of the Devine operation of pyloric exclusion for duodenal ulcer. *Am. J. Surg.* 16:223, 1932.
6. Beattie, A. D. Vagotomy and partial pylorectomy. *Lancet* 1:525, 1950.
7. Beck, C., and Carrel, A. Demonstration of specimens illustrating a method of formation of a prethoracic esophagus. *I.M.J.* 7:463, 1905.
8. Becker, J. M., Kelly, K. A., Haddad, A. C., and Zinsmeister, A. R. Proximal gastric vagotomy and mucosal antrectomy: A possible operative approach to duodenal ulcer. *Surgery* 94:58, 1983.
9. Bigg, R. L., Silver, J. M., and Kram, D. D. Omental closure of the duodenal stump. *Am. J. Surg.* 108:724, 1964.
10. Brunschwig, A. Pezzer catheter gastrostomy. *Am. J. Surg.* 29:384, 1935.
11. Carpenter, J. C., and Crandall, W. B. Common bile duct and major pancreatic duct injuries during operations on the stomach. *Ann. Surg.* 148:66, 1958.
12. Cole, B. C., and Dickinson, J. J. Acute volvulus of the stomach in infants and children. *Surgery* 70:707, 1971.
13. Connar, R. G., and Sealy, W. C. Gastrostomy and its complications. *Ann. Surg.* 143:245, 1956.
14. Connell, F. G. Fundusectomy: A new principle in the treatment of gastric or duodenal ulcer. *Surg. Gynecol. Obstet.* 49:696, 1929.
15. Connell, F. G. Duodenal ulcer: Surgical treatment. *Surg. Gynecol. Obstet.* 62:216, 1936.
16. Deaver, J. M. Gastroileostomy and its prevention. *Surg. Gynecol. Obstet.* 100:621, 1955.
17. Deloyers, L. Description and justification of new curative operation for peptic ulcer "reversed gastrectomy." *Ann. R. Coll. Surg. Engl.* 18:277, 1956.
18. Depage, A. Nouveau procede pour la gastrostomie. *J. Chir. Ann. Soc. Belg. Chir.* 1:715, 1901.
19. Devine, H. B. Basic principles of supreme difficulties in gastric surgery. *Surg. Gynecol. Obstet.* 40:1, 1925.
20. Devine, H. B. Gastric exclusion. *Surg. Gynecol. Obstet.* 47:239, 1928.
21. Dillard, D. H., and Merendino, K. A. New studies in the dog supporting the concept of equal resistance of various levels of intestinal tract to acid-peptic digestion. *Surg. Gynecol. Obstet.* 103:289, 1956.
22. Dorton, H. E. A multipurpose gastrostomy tube. *Surg. Gynecol. Obstet.* 112:122, 1961.

23. Eade, G. G., Metheny, D., and Lundmark, V. O. An evaluation of the practice of routine postoperative nasogastric suction. *Surg. Gynecol. Obstet.* 101:275, 1955.
24. Farris, J. M., and Smith, G. K. An evaluation of temporary gastrostomy. *Ann. Surg.* 144:475, 1956.
25. Finney, J. M. T. A new method of pyloroplasty. *Bull. Johns Hopkins Hosp.* 13:155, 1902.
26. Finney, J. M. T. A new method of gastroduodenostomy, end-to-side; with illustrations. *Trans. South. Surg. Assoc.* 36:576, 1924.
27. Finsterer, H., and Cunha, F. The surgical treatment of duodenal ulcer. *Surg. Gynecol. Obstet.* 52:1099, 1932.
28. Foley, F. E., Kilpatrick, J. T., and Crabtree, S. F. Chronic recurrent pancreatitis due to injury to the duct of Santorini: A complication of subtotal gastrectomy. *Ann. Surg.* 144:87, 1956.
29. Fromme, A. G. E. Oder Palliativresektion beim nicht resezierbaren Ulcus duodeni. *Arch. Klin. Chir.* 196:281, 1939.
30. Gambee, L. P. A single-layer open intestinal anastomosis applicable to the small as well as the large intestine. *West. J. Surg.* 59:1, 1951.
31. Gavriliu, D., and Georgescue, L. Esofagoplastie directa cu material gastric. *Rev. Stiint. Med.* 3:33, 1959.
32. Gingrich, G. W. The use of the T-tube in difficult duodenal stump closures. *Am. Surg.* 25:639, 1959.
33. Ginzburg, L. Management of the difficult duodenal stump: Technical considerations. *Surg. Clin. North Am.* 34:473, 1954.
34. Griffith, C. A. Selective vagotomy plus suprapyloric antrectomy with or without pylorotomy for duodenal ulcer. *Ann. Surg.* 179:516, 1974.
35. Gross, J. B., and Waugh, J. M. The clinical manifestations of gastroileal anastomosis with particular reference to potassium deficiency. *A.M.A. Arch. Intern. Med.* 102:722, 1958.
36. Haas, A., and Ritter, S. A. Gastroileostomy with realignment and recovery. *J. Int. Coll. Surg.* 29:155, 1958.
37. Harvey, H. D. Safety in performing partial gastrectomy for peptic ulcer. *Ann. Surg.* 153:256, 1961.
38. Hays, D. M., Woolley, M. M., and Snyder, W. H. Changing techniques in the management of esophageal atresia. *Arch. Surg.* 92:611, 1966.
39. Heimlich, H. J. The use of a gastric tube to replace the esophagus as performed by Dr. Dan Gavriliu of Bucharest, Rumania. *Surgery* 42:693, 1957.
40. Heimlich, H. J. Bile duct reconstruction with a gastric pedicle tube. *Arch. Surg.* 83:755, 1961.
41. Heimlich, H. J. Esophagoplasty with reversed gastric tube. *Am. J. Surg.* 123:80, 1972.
42. Heimlich, H. J., and Winfield, J. The use of a gastric tube to replace or by-pass the esophagus. *Surgery* 37:549, 1955.
43. Herron, P. W., Thomas, G. I., and Merendino, K. A. An experimental approach to cardiospasm: Appraisal of the Finney pyloroplasty in the prevention of esophagitis following the Heller myotomy. *J. Thorac. Surg.* 34:609, 1957.
44. Holt, R. L., and Lythgoe, J. P. The treatment of chronic duodenal ulcer by vagotomy and anterior pylorectomy. *Br. J. Surg.* 52:27, 1965.
45. Horsley, J. S. *Surgery of Stomach and Small Intestine.* New York: Appleton, 1926. Chap. X.
46. Howard, P. M., and Deles, V. D. A modification of the Finney pyloroplasty in the treatment of duodenal ulcer disease. *Am. J. Surg.* 108:677, 1964.
47. Jaboulay, M. La gastroenterostomie, la jejunoduodenostomie, la resection du pylore. *Arch. Prov. Chir.* (Paris) 1:1, 1892.
48. Jackson, P. P. Ischemic necrosis of the proximal gastric remnant following subtotal gastrectomy. *Ann. Surg.* 150:1071, 1959.
49. Janeway, H. H. Eine neue Gastrostomiemethode. *Munch. Med. Wochenschr.* 60:1705, 1913.
50. Jesseph, J. E., and Fiore, A. C. Gastrostomy. L. M. Nyhus and R. J. Baker (Eds.), *Mastery of Surgery* Boston: Little, Brown, 1984.
51. Jianu, A. Gastrostomie und Oesophagoplastik. *Dtsch. Z. Chir.* 118:383, 1912.
52. Johnston, D. W. B., and Prasad, J. K. A simplified technique for gastrostomy. *Surg. Gynecol. Obstet.* 144:84, 1977.
53. Jolley, S. G., Smith, E. I., and Tunnell, W. P. Protective antireflux operation with feeding gastrostomy: Experience with children. *Ann. Surg.* 201:736, 1985.
54. Judd, E. S., and Nagel, G. W. Excision of ulcer of the duodenum. *Surg. Gynecol. Obstet.* 45:17, 1927.
55. Kay, A. W. The pyloric antrum and peptic ulceration. *Gastroenterologia* 89:282, 1958.
56. Kay, A. W., and Johnson, A. G. The exclusion

pyloroplasty. *Ann. R. Coll. Surg.* 63:277, 1981.

57. Kelly, W. D., Hallgrimsson, S., Egdahl, R., and Wangensteen, O. H. Tubular resection with transverse gastroplasty as a suitable operation for duodenal ulcer. *Surg. Forum* 3:54, 1952.
58. Kilgore, T. L., Turner, M. D., and Hardy, J. D. Clinical and experimental ischemia of the gastric remnant. *Surg. Gynecol. Obstet.* 118:1312, 1964.
59. Kirk, R. M. Mucosal antrectomy in the treatment of peptic ulcer. *Proc. R. Soc. Med.* 59:571, 1966.
60. Kirk, R. M., and Sussman, T. Vagotomy and mucosal antrectomy in the elective treatment of duodenal ulcers. *Am. J. Surg.* 123:323, 1972.
61. Kraus, M., and Condon, R. E. Alternate techniques of duodenotomy. *Surg. Gynecol. Obstet.* 139:417, 1974.
62. Kumar, S. E. Tube gastrostomy: A routine adjunct in major abdominal operations. *Am. Surg.* 51:201, 1985.
63. Lamesch, A. J. Ventriculo gastrostomy by means of gastric tube for the treatment of hydrocephalus: A preliminary report. *J. Pediatr. Surg.* 7:55, 1972.
64. Landry, R. M. Gastroileostomy and gastrocolostomy. *Surgery* 30:528, 1951.
65. Larsen, B. B., and Foreman, R. C. Syndrome of the leaking duodenal stump. *Arch. Surg.* 63:480, 1951.
66. Lippert, K. M., and Coleman, H. V. Duodenostomy in gastric resection for duodenal ulcer. *Am. J. Surg.* 95:781, 1958.
67. Longmire, W. P., Jr. The technique of common duct exploration. *Surg. Gynecol. Obstet.* 117:241, 1963.
68. MacFee, W. F., and Sax, S. D. Proximal duodenectomy with von Haberer–Finney end-to-side gastroduodenal anastomosis for duodenal ulcer. *Ann. Surg.* 161:985, 1965.
69. MacQueen, D. G. The Belcher gastrectomy for peptic ulcer (final report). *Can. Med. Assoc. J.* 78:320, 1958.
70. Maki, T., Shivaton, T., Hatafuku, T., and Sugawara, K. Pylorus-preserving gastrectomy as an improved operation for gastric ulcer. *Surgery* 61:838, 1967.
71. Makkas, M., and Marangos, G. Surgical treatment of non-resectable duodenal ulcer: Antral exclusion operation (Bancroft-Plenk modification). *Br. J. Surg.* 37:206, 1949.
72. Maurer, R. E. Inadvertent gastroileostomy. *Tex. State J. Med.* 60:589, 1964.
73. Mayfield, R. C., and Abramson, P. D. The use of catheter duodenostomy in subtotal gastrectomy. *Am. J. Surg.* 90:998, 1955.
74. McEachern, C. G., Sullivan, R. E., and Arata, J. E. Duodenostomy. *Arch. Surg.* 72:942, 1956.
75. Menguy, R. The technique of duodenotomy with respect to development of lateral cutaneous fistula. *Surg. Gynecol. Obstet.* 121:359, 1965.
76. Mikulicz, J. 1886. Cited in J. Mikulicz, Zur operativen Behandlung des stenosierenden Magengeschwures. *Arch. Klin. Chir.* 37:79, 1888.
77. Millbourn, E. W. Pyloroplasty in subtotal proximal gastrectomy with esophagogastrostomy. *Acta Chir. Scand.* 114:333, 1957.
78. Molina, J. E., Ritchie, W. P., Jr., Edlich, R. F., et al. Release of antral gastrin by electrical stimulation of the vagus. *Surg. Forum* 17:305, 1966.
79. Moschel, D. M., Walske, B. R., and Neumayer, F. A new technique of pyloroplasty. *Surgery* 44:813, 1958.
80. Newman, K. D., Braasch, J. W., Rossi, R. L., and O'Campo-Gonzales, S. Pyloric and gastric preservation with pancreatoduodenostomy. *Am. J. Surg.* 145:152, 1983.
81. Nissen, R. Zur Resektion des tietsitzenden duodenal Geschwurs. *Zentralbl. Chir.* 60:483, 1933.
82. Nyhus, L. M. The role of the antrum in the surgical treatment of peptic ulcer. *Gastroenterology* 38:21, 1960.
83. Nyhus, L. M., Chapman, N. D., DeVito, R. V., and Harkins, H. N. The control of gastrin release: An experimental study illustrating a new concept. *Gastroenterology* 39:582, 1960.
84. Nyhus, L. M., McDade, W. C., Condon, R. E., et al. Further experiences with jejunal gastrostomy. *Arch. Surg.* 83:864, 1961.
85. Nyhus, L. M., Stevenson, J. K., Jones, T. W., et al. Jejunal gastrostomy. *Bull. Soc. Int. Chir.* 17:254, 1958.
86. Ogilvie, W. H. The approach to gastric surgery. *Lancet* 2:295, 1938.
87. Palumbo, P. J., Scudamore, H. H., Gross, J. B., and Ferris, D. O. Inadvertent gastroileostomy. *Gastroenterology* 45:505, 1963.
88. Patton, R. A modified valvular gastrostomy. *Arch. Surg.* 70:859, 1955.
89. Pe Thein, M., and Schofield, B. Release of gastrin from the pyloric antrum following va-

gal stimulation by sham feeding in dogs. *J. Physiol.* 145:14, 1959.
90. Pearson, S. C., MacKenzie, R. J., and Ross, T. The use of catheter duodenostomy in gastric resection for duodenal ulcer. *Am. J. Surg.* 106:194, 1963.
91. Pecora, D. V. Pylorojejunostomy. *Am. Surg.* 33:737, 1967.
92. Plenk, V. A. Zur Technik der Resektion zur Ausschaltung. *Zentralbl. Chir.* 63:3019, 1936.
93. Poth, E., Jr., and Gold, D. Duodenal acidification and peptic ulcer. *Tex. Med.* 65:56, 1969.
94. Preshaw, R. M. A percutaneous method for inserting a feeding gastrostomy tube. *Surg. Gynecol. Obstet.* 152:659, 1981.
95. Priestley, J. T., and Butler, D. B. Technique for management of duodenal stump in certain cases of partial gastrectomy for duodenal ulcer. *Am. J. Surg.* 82:163, 1951.
96. Prigouris, S., and Michas, P. Duodenostomy. *Am. J. Surg.* 138:698, 1979.
97. Qvist, G. A modified Bancroft operation for duodenal ulcer. *Br. J. Surg.* 45:341, 1958.
98. Randolph, J. G., Y-U advancement pyloroplasty. *Ann. Surg.* 181:586, 1975.
99. Randolph, J. G., Tunell, W. P., and Lilly, J. R. Gastric division in the critically ill infant with esophageal atresia and tracheoesophageal fistula. *Surgery* 63:496, 1968.
100. Ripstein, C. B., and Schneider, K. M. An appraisal of temporary gastrostomies and enterostomies. *Am. J. Surg.* 96:90, 1958.
101. Rivers, A. G., and Wilbur, D. L. The syndrome of gastroileostomy and gastroileac ulcer. *Surg. Gynecol. Obstet.* 54:937, 1932.
102. Rodgers, J. B. Infarction of the gastric remnant following subtotal gastrectomy. *Arch. Surg.* 92:917, 1966.
103. Root, H. D., Jenson, C. B., Crisp, N. W., et al. Experimental evaluation of antral exclusion and complemental vagotomy in treatment of duodenal ulcer. *Gastroenterology* 39:602, 1960.
104. Rosado, I. R., and Gilsdorf, R. B. Creating a continent tubeless gastrostomy. *Am. J. Surg.* 146:820, 1983.
105. Rose, T. F. Gastroileostomy. *Med. J. Aust.* 42:353, 1955.
106. Salky, B., Kreel, I., Gelernt, I., and Bauer, J. Nonoperative conversion of tube gastrostomy to feeding jejunostomy. *Am. J. Surg.* 143:387, 1982.
107. Sanders, R. J. A modified technique for tube gastrostomy. *Surg. Gynecol. Obstet.* 120:121, 1965.
108. Santiago-Delpin, E. A. The use of T-tubes for gastrostomy. *Surg. Gynecol. Obstet.* 138:765, 1974.
109. Scobie, B. A. Excluded gastric antrum stimulating the Zollinger-Ellison syndrome. *Gastroenterology* 48:184, 1964.
110. Sedillot, C. E. Observation de gastrostomie. *Gaz. Hop.* 26:160, 1853.
111. Senter, K. L. Complications of temporary tube gastrostomy. *Arch. Surg.* 81:103, 1960.
112. Somervell, T. H. Physiological gastrectomy: The operation of ligature of the arteries of the stomach to relieve hyperacidity and to prevent recurrent ulceration after gastro-enterostomy. *Br. J. Surg.* 33:146, 1945.
113. Spencer, F. C. Ischemic necrosis of remaining stomach following subtotal gastrectomy. *Arch. Surg.* 73:844, 1956.
114. Spivack, J. L. Eine neue Methode der Gastrostomie. *Beitr. Klin. Chir.* 147:308, 1929.
115. Stamm, M. Gastrostomy: A new method. *Med. News* 65:324, 1894.
116. Stevenson, J. K., and Harkins, H. N. Unusual complications from the use of intestinal tubes and drains. *Am. J. Surg.* 91:314, 1956.
117. Stevenson, J. K., Jesseph, J. E., Nyhus, L. M., et al. Heidenhain pouch secretory response as affected by gastroileostomy to the main stomach. *Gastroenterology* 32:262, 1957.
118. Tanner, N. C. Management of peptic ulcer. *Bristol Med. Chir. J.* 63:16, 1946.
119. Tanner, N. C. Chronic and recurrent volvulus of the stomach. *Am. J. Surg.* 115:505, 1968.
120. Tavel, E. Eine neue Methode der Gastrostomie. *Zentralbl. Chir.* 25:634, 1906.
121. Thorek, M. Tubovalvular gastrostomy: History and technique. *J. Mich. Med. Soc.* 44:3, 1945.
122. Traverso, L. W., and Longmire, W. P., Jr. Preservation of the pylorus in pancreaticoduodenectomy: A follow-up evaluation. *Ann. Surg.* 192:306, 1980.
123. Verneuil, M. Observation de gastrostomie pratique avec succes pour retrecissement cicatriciel infranchissable de l'oesophage. *Bull. Acad. Med.* 5:1023, 1876.
124. von Eiselsberg, A. Über Ausschaltung inoperabler Pylorus-strikturen nebst Bemerkungen über die Jejunostomie. *Arch. Klin. Chir.* 50:919, 1895.
125. von Eiselsberg, A. Zur Behandlung des

Ulcus ventriculi et duodeni. *Arch. Klin. Chir.* 114:539, 1920.
126. Waddell, W. R., and Bartlett, M. K. Antral exclusion with vagotomy for duodenal ulcer. I. Acid secretory studies on fifty patients. *Ann. Surg.* 146:3, 1957.
127. Walker, L. G., Jr. L. L. Staton, M. D., and the first successful gastrostomy in America. *Surg. Gynecol. Obstet.* 158:387, 1984.
128. Wangensteen, O. H. Aseptic gastric resection: A method of aseptic anastomosis adaptable to any segment of the alimentary canal (esophagus, stomach, small or large intestine); including preliminary description of subtotal excision of acid-secreting area for ulcer. *Surg. Gynecol. Obstet.* 70:59, 1940.
129. Wangensteen, O. H. Method of closing the pyloro-antral pouch in the antral exclusion operation. *Surgery* 12:731, 1942.
130. Wangensteen, O. H. Evolution and evaluation of an acceptable operation for peptic ulcer (including description of the technic of tubular gastric resection with transverse gastroplasty, and extrapleural sternotomy) for operations in the attic of the abdomen. *Rev. Gastroenterol.* 20:611, 1953.
131. Wangensteen, O. H. Segmental gastric resection: An acceptable operation for peptic ulcer; tubular resection unacceptable. *Surgery* 41:686, 1957.
132. Warshaw, A. L., and Torchiana, D. L. Delayed gastric emptying after pylorus-preserving pancreaticoduodenostomy. *Surg. Gynecol. Obstet.* 160:1, 1985.
133. Warren, K. W. Pancreatic considerations in gastric surgery. *J.A.M.A.* 154:803, 1954.
134. Wasiljew, B. K., Ujiki, G. T., and Beal, J. M. Feeding gastrostomy: Complications and mortality. *Am. J. Surg.* 143:194, 1982.
135. Wastell, C., and Ellis, H. Volvulus of the stomach: A review with a report of 8 cases. *Br. J. Surg.* 58:667, 1971.
136. Watsuji, H. Eine Kombinierte Anwendung des Hackers und Fontanschen Verfahrens bei der Gastrostomie. *Mitt. Med. Gesellsch.* (Tokyo) 13:879, 1899.
137. Webster, M. W., Carey, L. C., and Ravitch, M. M. The permanent gastrostomy. *Arch. Surg.* 110:658, 1975.
138. Welch, C. E. Gastrostomy. *Am. J. Surg.* 101:279, 1961.
139. Welch, C. E., and Radkey, G. V. Method of management of duodenal stump after gastrectomy. *Surg. Gynecol. Obstet.* 98:376, 1954.
140. White, T. T., Sanderson, E. R., and Morgan, A. Injury to the sphincter of Oddi in the course of gastric and duodenal surgery. *Am. J. Surg.* 114:247, 1967.
141. Wilmanns, R. Resectio praepylorica bei Ulcus duodeni. *Zentralbl. Chir.* 53:1874, 1926.
142. Witzel, O. Zur Technik der Magenfistelanlegung. *Zentralbl. Chir.* 18:601, 1891.
143. Wolfson, W. L., and Rothenberg, R. E. The surgical treatment of complicated duodenal ulcer. *Surgery* 3:662, 1938.
144. Woodward, E. R., and Tillmanns, V. C. Mechanism of ulcer recurrence following the antrum exclusion gastrectomy. *Surg. Forum* 6:301, 1955.

EDITOR'S COMMENT

The Beck-Jianu gastrostomy actually should be named the Beck-Carrel gastrostomy, as proposed by Spivak in 1936 [8]. Carl Beck was a professor of surgery at the Chicago College of Physicians and Surgeons at the turn of the century (under lease at that time to the University of Illinois as its College of Medicine). Alexis Carrel visited Dr. Beck and worked with him in the animal laboratory [1]. In 1905 they published a short paper in the *Illinois Medical Journal* [2] that not only mentioned their technique for formation of a gastrostomy, but also laid the experimental background for use of the gastric greater curvature as an esophageal replacement.

A spate of articles has appeared that generally are laudatory regarding percutaneous endoscopic gastrostomy [5–7, 9, 10]. Dozois and Lewis [3] have placed the procedure in proper perspective:

> Because the method is simple, requires little time, and can always be done with use of local anesthesia, it is most attractive in critically ill patients. The procedure should not be used for decompression because of the small size of the catheter that can be placed in such a manner. Moreover, it may not be technically feasible if the anterior wall of the stomach cannot be apposed to the abdominal wall or if the endoscope cannot be introduced into the

stomach because of severe mechanical obstruction of the pharynx or esophagus. Also, in the presence of a fairly high grade stricture, the "rubber bumper" may be dislodged when the mushroom catheter is pulled into the stomach; dislodgment would lead to potential catastrophic consequences if unrecognized. The nonsurgical approach should be considered an advance by all those who treat such patients but should be used only in carefully selected patients. A surgical procedure remains the preferred method of management in patients who require prolonged decompression [3].

I disagree with the Jessephs in their attitude toward the Jaboulay gastroduodenostomy. I have found this technique to enable performance of a duodenal anastomosis well away from the common inflammatory process near the pylorus in patients with advanced duodenal ulcer disease. Contrariwise, there is no question that if the Jaboulay gastroduodenostomy must be taken down at a later date, significant problems can occur [4].

We must report that John Jesseph died after a short illness in 1982. He and I served together as surgical house officers under the late Henry N. Harkins, senior editor of the first and second editions of this book. These were the halcyon days. It was at this time that Jack Jesseph published one of the first, if not *the* first, indictment of serotonin as a prime etiological factor in the dumping syndrome. Because he had spent time with Robert M. Zollinger on the faculty at the medical school of Ohio State University, no one was surprised when in 1971 John Jesseph was chosen to accept the chair in surgery at Indiana University, a chair he filled with distinction until his premature death. Fortunately, his son Jerry, a surgical house officer at Indiana, worked with his father on the text, and thus the fine finished product is before us.

L. M. N.

Comment References

1. Baader, W., and Nyhus, L. M. The life of Carl Beck and an important interval with Alexis Carrel. *Surg. Gynecol. Obstet*, in press.
2. Beck, C., and Carrel, A. Demonstration of specimens illustrating a method of formation of a prethoracic esophagus. *I. M. J.* 7:463, 1905.
3. Dozois, R. R., and Lewis, D. J. Gastrostomy: Scalpel or scope. *Mayo Clin. Proc.* 58:138, 1983.
4. Hoffman, J., Fischer, A., and Jensen, H. -E. Unsuccessful experience with closure of Jaboulay gastroduodenostomies in the treatment of post-vagotomy dumping and diarrhea. *Ann. Surg.* 198:142, 1983.
5. Nyhus, L. M. Editorial comment. *Arch. Surg.* 118:914, 1983.
6. Ponsky, J. L., Gauderer, M. W. L., and Stellato, T. A. Percutaneous endoscopic gastrostomy: Review of 150 cases. *Arch. Surg.* 118:913, 1983.
7. Russell, T. R., Brotman, M., and Norris, F. Percutaneous gastrostomy: A new simplified and cost effective technique. *Am. J. Surg.* 148:132, 1984.
8. Spivak, J. L. *The Surgical Technique of Abdominal Operations*. Chicago: Debour, 1936.
9. Stellato, T. A., Gauderer, M. W. L., and Ponsky, J. L. Percutaneous endoscopic gastrostomy following previous abdominal surgery. *Ann. Surg.* 200:46, 1984.
10. Strodel, W. E., Lemmer, J., Eckhauser, F., et al. Early experience with endoscopic percutaneous gastroscopy. *Arch. Surg.* 118:449, 1983.

Appendixes

A

Vagotomy (Truncal or Selective), Antrectomy, and Gastroduodenostomy for the Treatment of Duodenal Ulcer

Lloyd M. Nyhus

The surgical treatment of complicated duodenal ulcer has undergone marked change since vagotomy was reintroduced by Dragstedt and Owens in 1943. Subtotal gastrectomy alone had been the mainstay operation for the previous half-century, followed by various surgical procedures, including truncal vagotomy, gastroenterostomy, pyloroplasty, 70 percent subtotal gastrectomy, and antrectomy. My experience with the combined operation of truncal vagotomy, antrectomy, and gastroduodenostomy began in the early 1950s. It became apparent that the method of vagotomy could be improved. Therefore, my associates and I modified our technique of vagotomy to the selective method and changed the name of the procedure to the *revised combined operation*. Thus the specific procedure included selective vagotomy, antrectomy (35 percent distal gastrectomy), and gastroduodenostomy (Billroth I anastomosis). This operation has the best record to date of any treatment of duodenal ulcer in terms of ulcer recurrence. The recurrent ulcer rate following this procedure should be no greater than 0.5 percent.

Surgical Technique

The description that follows concerns the technique used on my surgical services. Failure to appreciate technical details is reflected not only in resultant anatomical disturbances such as postoperative suture line leaks, but also in physiological effects, for example, recurrent ulcer from incomplete vagotomy.

My experience in performing the revised combined operation (selective vagotomy plus antrectomy plus gastroduodenostomy) has led to the modification of some steps in the technique.

Surgery is an art and, like all art, it must be developed, not discovered. The technique described is the one that seems to give the best results at the present time. Much of the following surgical technique is applicable to the Billroth II procedure as well as to the Billroth I operation, and of course to my preferred method—the combined operation of selective vagotomy plus antrectomy plus gastroduodenostomy.

General Principles

SUTURES

A variety of sutures is used throughout the operation. Whereas fine silk was used predominantly in the past, the new absorbable and nonabsorbable sutures are now being used. Most vessels are simply ligated, but occasionally transfixion sutures are used. An absorbable suture is used for the inner layer of the anastomosis, essentially as a mucosal stitch with inversion. Seromuscular sutures continue to be of 4-0 or 000 black silk. The abdominal wall closure has changed from silk, to stainless steel wire, to one of several new monofilament synthetic sutures.

OPEN ANASTOMOSIS

I prefer the open to the closed type of anastomosis for several reasons. First, there can be no doubt that bleeding from the anastomosis can be entirely prevented by the use of the open technique with the anastomosis under direct visualization at all times. Second, the size of the anastomotic stoma can be ensured, and the surgeon can be certain that both the anterior and posterior walls are not included in one or more sutures. Third, through the open duodenal stump the ampulla of Vater can be palpated and biliary flow noted; also, the area can be inspected for postbulbar duodenal ulcer and other duodenal abnormalities. I have seen no difficulty arise from soiling of the surgical field with the use of the open technique. The bacterial flora of this portion of the gastrointestinal tract is meager, and adequate protection can be achieved by careful placement of laparotomy pads to protect the remainder of the operative field. An inner mucosal layer of continuous absorbable sutures and an outer serosal layer of interrupted silk sutures complete the anastomosis.

DRAINAGE

If it is suspected that the pancreas has been subjected to undue trauma, a Penrose drain or a double-lumen sump-suction catheter may be placed down to the site of suspected trauma and brought out laterally through the abdominal wall by a stab wound (never through the main incision). Occasionally in obese patients a drain may be placed in the left subphrenic space and in the right anterior infrahepatic space because of the possibility of traumatic fat necrosis.

ADEQUACY OF RESECTION

I adhere inviolably to the dictum that an adequate resection must be done according to the presenting disease before any decision is made to use or not to use any particular type of anastomosis. In fact, this decision is not made until the anastomosis is to be done. If there is any tension whatsoever in attempting to perform a gastroduodenal anastomosis, this method must be abandoned and a modification of the Billroth II procedure used. The anastomosis should not be forced. In general, the resection may be only 35 percent when protected by selective vagotomy.

PROTECTION OF VITAL STRUCTURES

The only way to avoid injury to important structures is to visualize the part of the structure that lies in the field of dissection. The inflammatory reaction and scarring so characteristic of many gastroduodenal lesions may cause distortion of the normal anatomy. This distortion, coupled with the extreme variability in "normal" anatomy, makes dissection in this region extremely hazardous unless good visualization or identification of the vital structures to be preserved is accomplished.

The simple maneuver of intubating the common bile duct in some instances in which the porta hepatis might be involved in ulcer scar or inflammatory reaction is useful. It is important to recognize the possible distortion of normal anatomical configurations of the common bile duct and the pancreatic ducts. Special care should be taken to avoid injury to the common hepatic artery, which sometimes may be retracted near a posterior penetrating duodenal ulcer crater. On the greater curvature side of the pyloric region, the middle colic artery may be so densely adherent to the ulcer scar that it may be easily mistaken for the right gastroepiploic artery.

Caution should be taken against vigorous palpation or traction in the region of the spleen. The splenic vessels, particularly in older persons, are extremely friable and quite easily torn. Moderate traction on the greater curvature of the stomach is sufficient to cause tearing to the splenic vessels or of the splenic substance. When such an accident occurs, an attempt should be made to repair the spleen; however, it may be necessary to proceed with splenectomy. While this is not a catastrophic incident, it may increase the morbidity appreciably and even the mortality.

Following the tenets of good modern surgery—gentle handling of tissues, avoidance of undue traction, and meticulous identification of adjacent structures to be preserved—is essential to a technically satisfactory operation.

AVOIDANCE OF MASS LIGATURES

In dividing the blood supply to the portion of the stomach and duodenum to be resected, it is important that small bites of tissue be ligated. Especially in patients with a large depot of omental fat, there is a tendency, if the vessel ligatures are placed about large quantities of this fat, for the vessels to retract proximal to the ligature and to cause troublesome hematomas or dangerous hemorrhage. Particularly in older individuals, I have been impressed with the increased quantity of fat that surrounds the left gastric vessels high on the lesser curvature. This situation was observed even in thin elderly patients.

REMOVAL OF ULCER

In association with gastric resection, I almost always remove duodenal ulcers for mechanical rather than physiological reasons. Only rarely do I leave a duodenal ulcer in situ. However, I do not hesitate to leave the depths of an ulcer crater in the tissue into which it may have penetrated.

Technical Procedure

Only my preferred technique for the surgical treatment of duodenal ulcer will be described, that is, the combined operation of selective vagotomy plus hemigastrectomy (antrectomy) plus gastroduodenal anastomosis (Table A-1). Variations from this technique, such as procedures for gastric ulcer or radical subtotal resection with omentectomy for carcinoma, are discussed in the chapters on these subjects.

The sequence of performance of the various steps applies to most operations. However, conditions germane to the particular situation may make a somewhat altered sequence more desirable. Description of the technique step-by-step is undertaken merely because it is easier to describe it in this manner. Actually there is a close interdependence of the steps, and it is the integration of all these steps into a smoothly performed surgical procedure that is productive of technical satisfaction.

INCISION

An upper midline abdominal incision is used almost exclusively. This incision is begun in the left xiphocostal angle and is extended down the linea alba to the level of the umbilicus or below if necessary. The incision is usually about 15 cm long. In patients in whom the distance between the costal arch and the um-

Table A-1. Step-by-step outline of the combined procedure for selective vagotomy plus antrectomy plus gastroduodenal anastomosis

1. Incision
2. Abdominal exploration
3. Selective vagotomy
4. Freeing of the greater curvature
5. Mobilization of the duodenum
6. Strauss maneuver for division of the duodenum
7. Division of the gastrohepatic omentum and left gastric vessels
8. Resection
9. Closure of the Schoemaker suture line
10. Anastomosis
11. Wound closure

bilicus is short, I extend the incision inferiorly to one side of the umbilicus. If more room is needed, I excise the xiphoid process. The peritoneum is cut about 2 cm to the left and lateral to the skin and fascial incision, giving a "staggered" effect, so that the under part of the fascial closure is protected by intact peritoneum.

ABDOMINAL EXPLORATION
The surgeon must curtail his or her enthusiasm to attack the gastroduodenal disease for which the operation was performed until he or she has had ample opportunity to explore the entire peritoneal cavity. Unless a general exploration is performed as soon as the peritoneal cavity is entered, this important step is likely to be forgotten. In addition, it is probably better technique to explore the general peritoneal cavity before the gastrointestinal tract is entered to avoid the small but ever-present chance of distributing contaminating debris. Two exceptions to the rule of exploring the general abdominal cavity before beginning the gastric procedure are emergency operations for a bleeding gastroduodenal lesion, in which control of the hemorrhage should take priority, and operations for obvious perforation of a peptic ulcer.

It is only after adequate inspection of the gastroduodenal pathology that the final decision to perform a gastric procedure should be made. This decision should, however, depend on the sum total of information available about the patient and not solely on the findings at the operation. Most often the presence of active ulcer, ulcer scar, or carcinoma of the stomach can be detected by external inspection and palpation. Occasionally a posterior duodenal or a lesser curvature gastric ulcer may be identified by palpating the crater through the anterior wall of the duodenum or stomach. Often, after rapid withdrawal of the palpating finger, the anterior wall of the duodenum or stomach may be observed to remain depressed into the crater by a suction effect.

VAGOTOMY
Since most surgeons are familiar with the technique of *truncal* vagotomy, I will begin the description of how we perform this operation. The modifications used to perform a *selective* vagotomy will then be described so that the difference in technique will stand out.

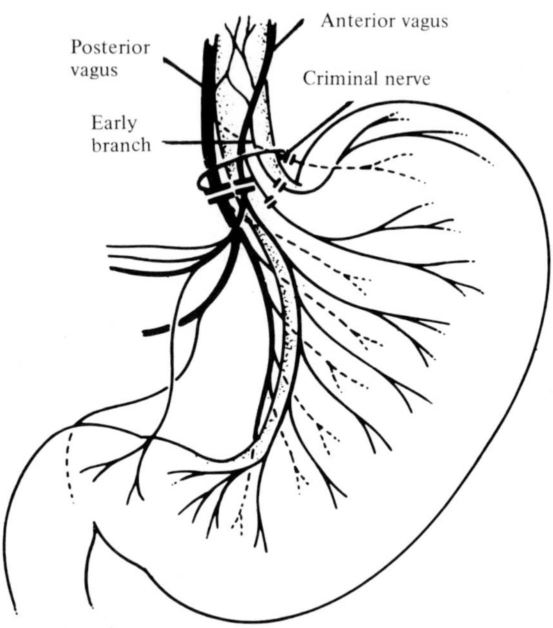

Fig. A-1. In carrying out truncal vagotomy, a careful search must be made for small direct branches, which will be found in a high percentage of instances. Their division can best be ensured by baring the esophagus of all surrounding tissue at the point where the main vagal trunks are divided. This technique results in at least 3–5 cm of esophagus completely bared of adventitial tissue, minimizing the chance of incomplete vagotomy. (From R. M. Zollinger (Ed.). *General Surgery: Current Principles in Practice*. New York: LeJacq, 1979.)

Truncal Vagotomy
This procedure (Fig. A-1) is designed to divide the two main vagal trunks at the esophageal hiatus of the diaphragm. There is a distinct advantage to performing the division of vagal trunks as high as possible, that is, a greater chance of finding the two major trunks before they begin to branch. The disadvantage of this approach is the tendency to stop searching for additional nerve fibers after the two trunks have been found, leading to an increased risk

of missing accessory nerves or direct branches. One must remember that a large number (as high as 30 percent) of patients may have such additional branches and that one major nerve left undivided may account for failure of the operative procedure.

There are specific maneuvers that aid in the intraoperative identification of the vagal trunks and branches. The first of these are exposure and illumination, two aspects of a properly performed procedure that cannot be underestimated. An adequate incision will extend to the xiphisternal junction from below the umbilicus. The use of a mechanical retractor to retract the rib cage cephalad and ventrad is of immense value and makes an operation with one junior assistant not only feasible but pleasant. In addition, the complication of tearing of the splenic capsule, which often occurs early in the operation as the first retractors are placed, is minimized.

For identification of the anterior vagal trunk, inspection of the peritoneal reflection on the lower esophagus will sometimes allow the nerve to be seen. Inspection of the nerves before dissection should not be hurried. Traction on the lesser curvature of the stomach allows palpation of the "violin strings" typical of nerves. This accomplished, incision of the avascular peritoneal reflection, followed by division of any anterior fibers encountered, completes the first part of the operation. All the anterior branches may not have been completely divided, however, and additional steps are recommended, namely, division of all fibroareolar tissue investing the lower esophagus so that a 5-cm-long collar of anterior esophagus is completely denuded.

For identification of the posterior vagus nerve, the distal esophagus is completely mobilized, beginning at the left side of the gastroesophageal junction. One index finger is insinuated into the areolar tissue to the left of the esophagus; palpation of the nasogastric tube helps define the lateral margin of the esophageal lumen. With gentle cephalad-caudad excursions of 1–2 cm, the space to the left of the esophagus is cleared. After palpating the aorta posteriorly, the surgeon moves the same finger in front of the aorta with attention to using a safe, gentle technique. At the right border of the gastroesophageal junction, the finger is pressed against the posterior leaf of the lesser omentum, which is then divided. After isolation of the esophagus, the surgeon's left index finger is placed on the aorta above the celiac axis and behind the stomach. By traction in a caudal direction on the celiac axis, the posterior trunk will be placed on stretch. The posterior trunk may occupy several positions in the retroesophageal tissue. Usually the nerve will be found to the patient's right of the gastroesophageal junction and just anterior to the preaortic fascia. This nerve is divided and ligated as was the anterior nerve.

A careful search for other fibers begins in the process, and all fibroareolar investments of the lower esophagus are carefully divided until a 3- 5-cm area is completely exposed and denuded. Then, gentle traction on the distal esophagus sometimes allows palpation of intramural nerves. When this technique is used, even patients with a plexiform arrangement of the anterior and posterior nerve trunks will have these branches divided.

Selective Vagotomy

This procedure (Fig. A-2) eliminates the division of the hepatic and celiac branches of the vagus nerve. It was developed as an alternative procedure for duodenal ulcer that avoids some of the problems associated with other types of vagotomy, especially truncal vagotomy.

The remarks concerning retraction and illumination are especially relevant in this procedure.

The first portion of the procedure is similar to that for truncal vagotomy, but instead of an incision of the peritoneal reflection at the hiatus, a line of division within the pars flaccida of the lesser omentum is developed, extending across the esophagus to the angle of His. After these steps, all the adventitial tissues anterior to the gastroesophageal junction are divided between clamps. Injury to the esophagus is prevented by using blunt clamps, avoiding rough forceful dissection, and maintaining meticulous hemostasis.

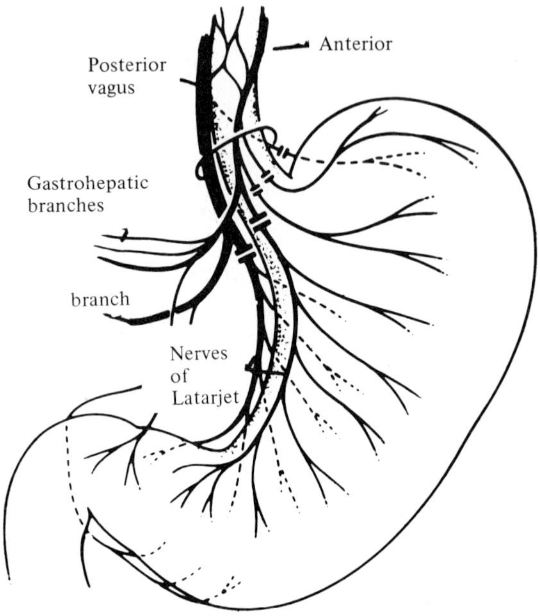

Fig. A-2. Selective vagotomy spares vagal fibers of the hepatic and celiac plexuses. The preferred method of assuring division of all vagal branches to the stomach is to clear the lower 5–6 cm of the esophagus of all surrounding tissues and to section main trunks distal to the hepatic and celiac branches. (From R. M. Zollinger (Ed.). *General Surgery: Current Principles in Practice*. New York: LeJacq, 1979.)

The esophagus is encircled, as the next step, and the posterior trunk is identified. All the tissue between the line of incision in the lesser omentum and the lesser curvature of the stomach is divided between clamps, including the descending branches of the left gastric artery. The lower esophagus must be cleared of all fibroareolar and neural connections for a distance of at least 5 cm proximal to the esophagastric junction.

FREEING OF THE GREATER CURVATURE

The gastrocolic omentum is perforated in an avascular portion by a curved hemostat, thus permitting the lesser peritoneal sac to be entered. Unless pains are taken in the execution of this maneuver, the middle colic vessels may be damaged. To minimize the possibility of such an error, it is recommended that the anterior wall of the stomach and the transverse colon be elevated and gently pulled apart to tense the gastrocolic omentum. It is easier to find a good cleavage plane by entering the gastrocolic omentum at the level of the junction of the lower and middle thirds of the greater curvature of the stomach, or even farther to the left; usually most of the adhesions that tend to obliterate the lesser peritoneal sac are found in the region of the pylorus and lower third of the stomach. At this level, it is easy to identify an avascular area between the main trunk of the gastroepiploic vessels and the colon.

After it is certain that the correct plane has been entered, the defect in the gastrocolic omentum is enlarged superiorly and inferiorly distal to the main gastroepiploic trunk. The avascular portions of the omentum may be divided with scissors without ligation. When vessels have been identified, the omentum is again perforated on the opposite side of the vessel, and ligatures of 4-0 black silk are passed around the vessel. These ligatures are tied, and the vessels are divided between the ligatures. There is a much smaller chance of losing a vessel and having troublesome bleeding and hematoma formation if the ligatures are tied before the vessels are divided. Often these vessels are so fragile that the slightest tension on a clamp will cause tearing. Superiorly, the greater curvature is freed to a point about 14 cm proximal to the pylorus or at a point on the greater curvature perpendicular to the lesser curvature incisura. Transection of the stomach between this point and the mid–lesser curvature (proximal to the gastric incisura) will ensure an antrectomy (approximately a 35 percent distal gastrectomy) (Fig. A-3).

All the freeing of the gastrocolic omentum superior to the point of initial breakthrough is carried out distal to the main gastroepiploic trunk. Inferiorly, the omentum is freed, again distal to the right gastroepiploic trunk, down to a point approximately 5 cm proximal to the pylorus. From this point onward, inferiorly, division of the gastrocolic omentum is carried out between the greater curvature of the stom-

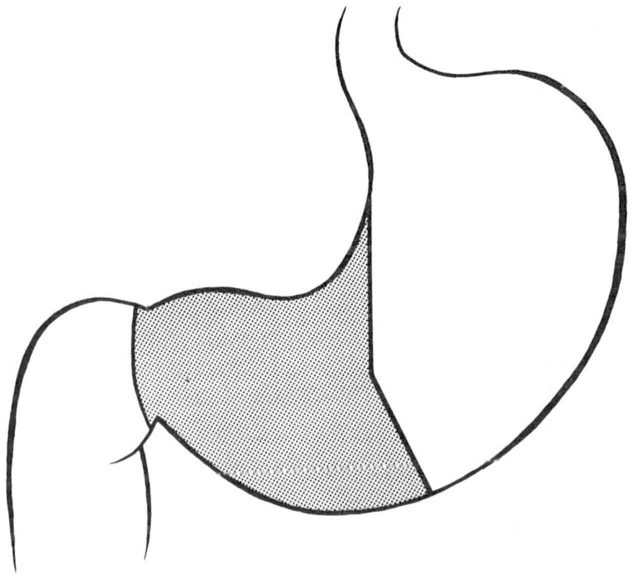

Fig. A-3. Extent of antrectomy (*stippled area*). It should represent a 30–35 percent gastrectomy.

ach and the right gastroepiploic vessel. The main trunk of the right gastroepiploic artery and vein has been transected and ligated previously at about 5 cm proximal to the pylorus. From this point onward, special care must be taken to keep the location of the middle colic vessels constantly in mind.

Approximately at the level of the pylorus, the right gastroepiploic artery at its origin is deep to the line of division of the gastrocolic omentum. Unless the right gastroepiploic vessels are intimately adherent in scar tissue in this region, they can and should be preserved to provide an adequate blood supply to the portion of the gastrocolic omentum that is being left behind. When the right gastroepiploic vessels are intimately adherent, however, and it is impossible to preserve them, they must be sacrificed. Perhaps attempts to protect this vessel represent unnecessary conservatism, but I believe vessels should be preserved when feasible. At this point, any readily accessible adhesions to the posterior gastric wall should be divided to allow greater mobility of the stomach.

MOBILIZATION OF THE DUODENUM

One of the most valuable technical contributions to surgery of the stomach and duodenum is the technique of mobilization of the duodenum originally described by Kocher in 1903.

Duodenal mobilization is one of the two phases of the operation best achieved with the surgeon standing on the left side of the operating table. A laparotomy pack is placed on top of the duodenum, the surgeon pulling the other viscera to the left side of the patient and causing the lateral peritoneal reflection of the duodenum to become taut. The peritoneal reflection can then be plainly seen and incised along the lateral margin of the second portion of the duodenum. By gentle blunt dissection, two fingers can be placed superiorly and inferiorly beneath this layer of peritoneum. By tenting the peritoneum with the fingers, the peritoneum can be incised either with scissors or a scalpel, depending on the preference of the surgeon.

The fascia propria (loose areolar tissue) along the lateral and posterior aspects of the second and third portions of the duodenum is divided by sharp dissection. For the most part this is an avascular plane, although several small bleeding vessels may be encountered.

Mobilization is carried out superiorly and proximally to include the superficial avascular portion of the hepatoduodenal ligament. The duodenum is mobilized distally and inferiorly to the point at which the superior mesenteric vessels cross the third portion of the duodenum. With the duodenum thus mobilized, the second and proximal third portions may be shifted and rotated to the left and superiorly, moving with them the head of the pancreas and the common bile duct. Complete duodenal mobilization should allow visualization of the inferior vena cava. Occasionally the right margin of the aorta can be seen.

The duodenum can usually be mobilized farther than would seem possible. When it appears that the duodenum has been mobilized to its maximal extent, I follow the useful practice of trying again. Usually some additional degree of mobilization can be gained. After complete mobilization of the duodenum, a moist laparotomy pack should be placed beneath the duodenum to elevate it into the more superficial portion of the surgical field. It should be pointed out that maximal mobilization is achieved distal to the head of the pancreas.

Mobilization of the duodenum not only facilitates gastroduodenal anastomosis but also serves two other important functions. It minimizes the chance of injury to the common bile duct by allowing better visualization, and it allows the dissection about the proximal duodenum to be performed in a more superficial part of the surgical field.

After its mobilization, the duodenum is freed, first on its greater curvature (caudal) side and then on its lesser curvature (hepatic) side, with division of the right gastric artery and usually on the supraduodenal artery of Wilkie.

STRAUSS MANEUVER FOR DIVISION OF THE DUODENUM

The proper and safe division of the duodenum is an important and sometimes difficult maneuver, particularly when one is dealing with posterior penetrating duodenal ulcers. I am indebted to the late Alfred A. Strauss and colleagues of the Louis A. Weiss Memorial Hospital, Chicago, for the technique of duodenal division that I use for all duodenal ulcers adherent to the pancreas.

This step is best accomplished when standing at the patient's left side. The maneuver consists in elevating the first portion of the duodenum by a finger placed against the posterior wall of the duodenum just to the right of the head of the pancreas. To conserve all duodenal length possible, no resection clamps are placed on the duodenum before division. The anterior wall of the duodenum distal to the ulcer scar is incised first with a scalpel as close to the pylorus as the duodenal lesion will allow, and the posterior wall is incised under direct vision from the internal to the external side and at a level just distal to any possible posterior wall ulcer disease. By incising the posterior wall from the inside out, one can minimize the danger of injuring the subjacent structures. If the posterior wall is adherent to the pancreas because of a posterior penetrating ulcer, the duodenal mucosa proximal to the line of division is shaved off the adherent area, leaving the outer portion of the duodenal wall adherent to the ulcer scar. When a posterior penetrating ulcer is situated immediately distal to the pylorus, it is usually possible to obtain a satisfactorily mobilized end of the duodenum distal to the line of transection and one that is entirely suitable for end-to-end anastomosis. In brief, the Strauss technique involves a separation of the pylorus from in front and to the left rather than, as is usually done, from behind and to the right.

If the posterior penetrating ulcer lies more distally in the duodenum (beyond approximately 2.5 cm), however, it usually is necessary to leave the posterior wall of the distal duodenal end attached to the posterior penetrating ulcer and to plan a modified closure of the duodenal stump, as will be described. I almost always remove active duodenal ulcers in my resections. However, I occasionally leave active ulcers in situ when they are situated in the more distal parts of the duodenum, and so far I have had no cause to regret doing so.

Under no circumstances must the ulcer crater be excised from the pancreas, as this is a dangerous and unnecessary procedure.

In performing the Strauss maneuver, the following anatomical facts concerning the duodenum are worthy of attention. In hundreds of gastric resections, after cutting across the duodenum just distal to the ulcer (that is, about 2 cm distal to the pylorus), I have regularly felt for the ampulla of Vater. The index finger of the right hand is used and is inserted with the surgeon standing on the left side of the table. The distance to the palpated ampulla is then measured; it averages 5.3 cm from the cut end of the duodenum. Thus the ampulla averages a total of 7.3 cm from the pylorus. Occasionally the opening of the duct of Santorini or a pancreatic lobule may be mistaken for the ampulla. Furthermore, sometimes nothing is palpated; generally, however, palpation seems accurate.

Having identified the exact point at which the common bile duct enters the duodenum, the surgeon can proceed with more assurance that he or she will not interfere with this important ostium. After complete division of the duodenum, a sponge is placed in the distal end and another sponge tied loosely about the proximal end to avoid gross spillage of bile and other contents. As stated before, the final disposition of the duodenal stump is decided on after an adequate resection has been performed.

With the Strauss maneuver, one can remove the duodenal ulcer in most instances. The maneuver has the following advantages. It stops bleeding if present; it removes enough duodenum to ensure that the antrum is out; it eliminates the indeterminate period an unremoved ulcer takes to heal; and it provides a clean duodenum for anastomosis or closure.

DIVISION OF THE GASTROHEPATIC OMENTUM AND LEFT GASTRIC VESSELS

The gastrohepatic omentum is usually a thin layer of peritoneum with a minimal amount of fat, although the latter is somewhat variable. At a distance of 1.5–2 cm from the lesser curvature, no sizable blood vessels are encountered until the level of the left gastric vessels, which are in a separate fold placed more posteriorly. A good portion of the dissection of the gastrohepatic omentum may be carried out without ligatures, and usually it is necessary to ligate only two or three rather small vessels before one reaches the left gastric vessel. This part of the dissection is usually easy, but some difficulty may be encountered when there is thickening, scarring, and inflammatory reaction secondary to a peptic ulcer on the lesser curvature. The hepatic branch of the left vagus nerve lies in this curvature just above the level of the left gastric artery. It should not be cut, although cutting this branch makes no difference if a truncal vagotomy is to be done above this level.

The left gastric artery is the largest artery supplying the stomach, and occasionally division of this vessel gives rise to difficulty. It is usually surrounded by a moderate amount of fat, which is increased in elderly individuals, making it difficult to identify the lesser curvature margin of the stomach. In addition, dissection of this vessel is more hazardous if there is scarring or inflammatory reaction about it secondary to ulceration on the lesser curvature of the stomach.

A word of caution should be interjected at this point concerning the occasional origin of an aberrant left hepatic artery from the left gastric artery. Sometimes this vessel comprises the sole blood supply to the left lobe of the liver, and its sacrifice would almost certainly mean necrosis of the lobe. Therefore, it is worthwhile to examine the configuration of the left gastric artery and its branches carefully and make certain that the vessel is divided distal to any possible aberrant hepatic branch. In patients with benign disease I generally ligate the left gastric artery after it has divided, close to the stomach. This is easier and avoids unnecessary clamping of the celiac branch of the posterior vagus nerve, although, again, if a truncal vagotomy is to be performed, such clamping makes no difference.

RESECTION

The lines of resection of the stomach should now be determined. For duodenal ulcer when selective vagotomy has been performed, 30–

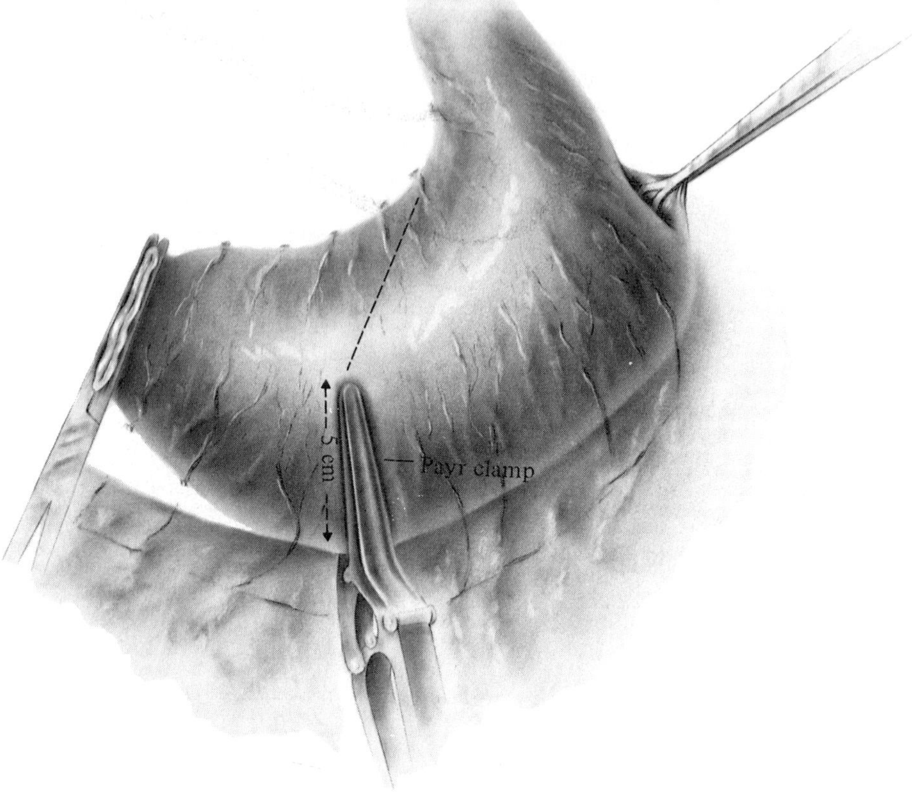

Fig. A-4. Transection of stomach. Placement of a small Payr clamp perpendicular to the greater curvature for a distance of 5 cm across the stomach. To achieve a 30–35 percent distal gastric resection (antrectomy), this Payr clamp is placed approximately 14 cm proximal to the pylorus. The *dashed line* shows the proposed line of excision of the lesser curvature.

35 percent distal resection is sufficient (Fig. A-3). The extent of resection and exact placing of the line of resection are both important. The antrum is higher along the lesser than along the greater curvature. Thus it is important to do a Schoemaker type of tubing of the lesser curvature.

When the site of transection of the stomach has been selected, an Allis clamp is placed on the greater curvature just distal to the selected site. A small Payr clamp is then applied perpendicular to the greater curvature at the selected level and extended across the width of the stomach for a measured distance of 5 cm (Fig. A-4). The clamp is closed and a Carmalt clamp is placed just distal to the Payr clamp and parallel to it. The walls of the stomach between the two clamps are incised with a scalpel to a point just distal to the tip of the Payr clamp (Fig. A-5). The two clamps are separated widely and a von Petz (or other stainless steel clip applicator) sewing clamp is angled up to the lesser curvature side of the stomach approximately 2–3 cm below the esophagogastric junction. A double row of von Petz staples is placed along the line of application of the clamp, and the clamp is removed. The anterior and posterior walls of the stomach are divided between the double row of staples (Fig. A-6). Just before the division of the upper portion of the lesser curvature of the stomach is completed, a 4-0 silk suture is placed in the form of a Lembert suture just above the most superior von Petz clips. With this suture used for traction to prevent the upper portion of the Schoemaker line from springing upward, the

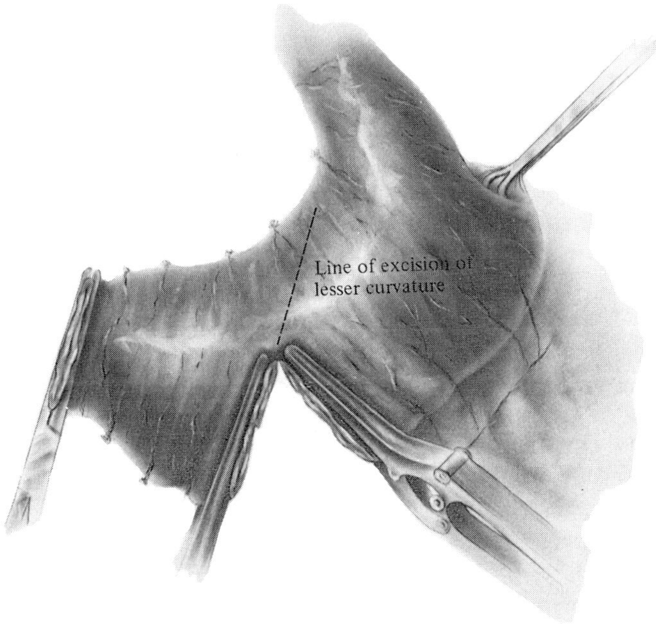

Fig. A-5. A Carmalt clamp is placed parallel to the Payr clamp. Stomach is divided between the two clamps, and a mechanical stapling device is placed along the proposed line of excision of the lesser curvature.

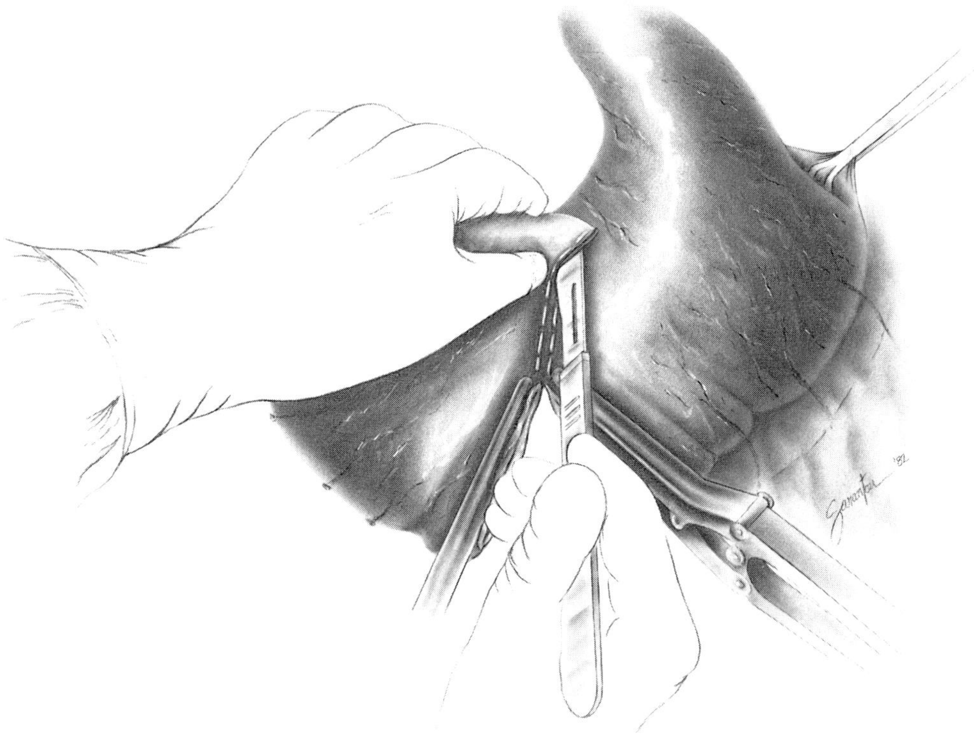

Fig. A-6. Double row of metallic hemostatic staples. Stomach is divided.

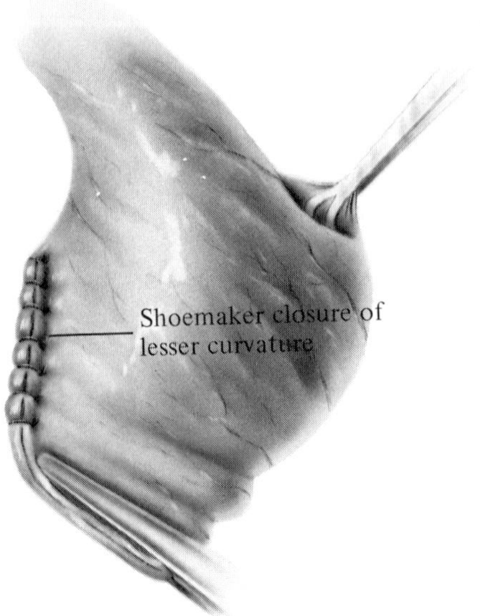

Fig. A-7. The Schoemaker closure of the lesser curvature with interrupted Lembert sutures of 4-0 black silk.

remaining distance between the double row of clips is completely incised and the specimen is discarded from the surgical field. Occasionally a few small vessels will bleed between the von Petz staples. These bleeding points should be clamped and ligated with 4-0 black silk ligatures to achieve complete hemostasis. Otherwise, troublesome hematomas may form and prevent satisfactory closure of the Schoemaker line.

CLOSURE OF THE SCHOEMAKER SUTURE LINE

The clip closure of the Schoemaker suture line is now closed by interrupted 4-0 black silk Lembert sutures placed close enough to obtain continuous serosa-to-serosa approximation. These reinforcing sutures are placed down to a point 1 cm above the tip end of the Payr clamp. This terminal 1 cm is left unsutured until the anastomosis is completed (Fig. A-7).

ANASTOMOSIS

At this point the type of anastomosis must be decided. There are few instances in which a gastroduodenal anastomosis cannot be performed, and usually this anastomosis can be of the end-to-end type. In difficult situations, the scope of the Billroth I anastomosis can be greatly extended by use of the von Haberer–Finney end-to-side anastomosis, particularly when the proximal cut end of the duodenum has to be left attached to the distal margin of a posterior penetrating duodenal ulcer.

The anastomosis should not be forced. If the surgeon believes it is technically difficult to use the duodenum in reestablishing gastrointestinal continuity, a gastrojejunal anastomosis should be performed. If the end-to-end type of anastomosis is decided on, the anastomosis is achieved by means of an outer row of interrupted 4-0 noninverting black silk sutures. The inner row is closed with a continuous 4-0 absorbable suture that includes only the mucosa (Fig. A-8). During the course of the anastomosis, it may be necessary to ligate several bleeding points in the end of the gastric stump.

When the anastomosis is completed, special care is taken to reinforce the critical angle, that is, the point of junction between the Schoemaker suture line and the anastomotic lines. This reinforcement consists in the placement of a 000 black silk pursestring suture, taking a bite of the anterior wall of the stomach, the posterior wall of the stomach, and the wall of the duodenum at the critical angle. When this suture is tied down, there is good serosal apposition of all three components, namely, the anterior gastric wall, the posterior gastric wall, and the wall of the duodenum (Fig. A-9). The completed anastomosis should admit one and one-half to two fingers.

If the end of the duodenum is unsuitable for end-to-end anastomosis, I prefer to use the

Fig. A-9. Completed operation—selective vagotomy, antrectomy, and gastroduodenostomy. *Inset,* infolding of the stomach at the corner of the Schoemaker closure of the lesser curvature and the duodenum at the superior portion of the anastomosis. This suture (usually two bites to the stomach and one or two to the duodenum) protects against an anastomotic leak at this potentially weak part of the closure.

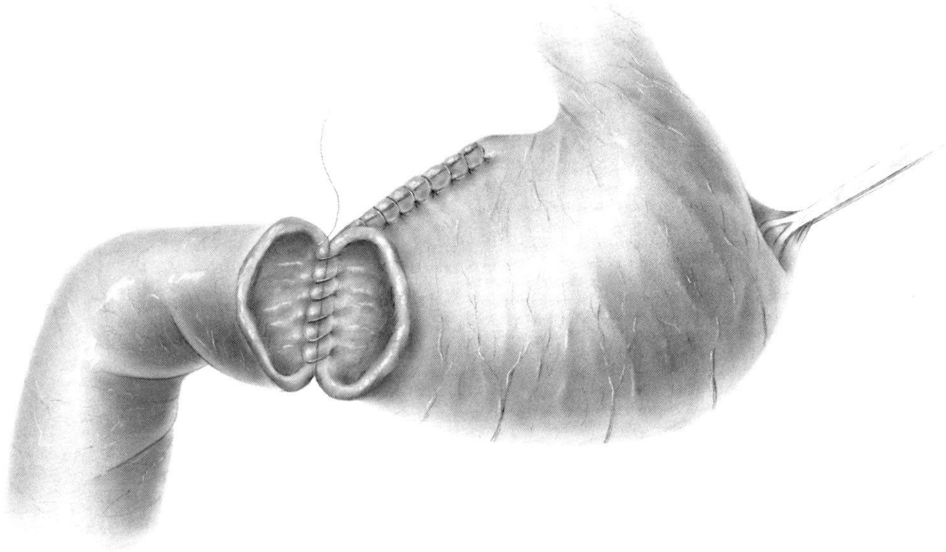

Fig. A-8. The end-to-end anastomosis. The posterior row of interrupted 4-0 black silk seromuscular sutures has been placed. The inner continuous absorbable hemostatic suture (baseball stitch) is seen.

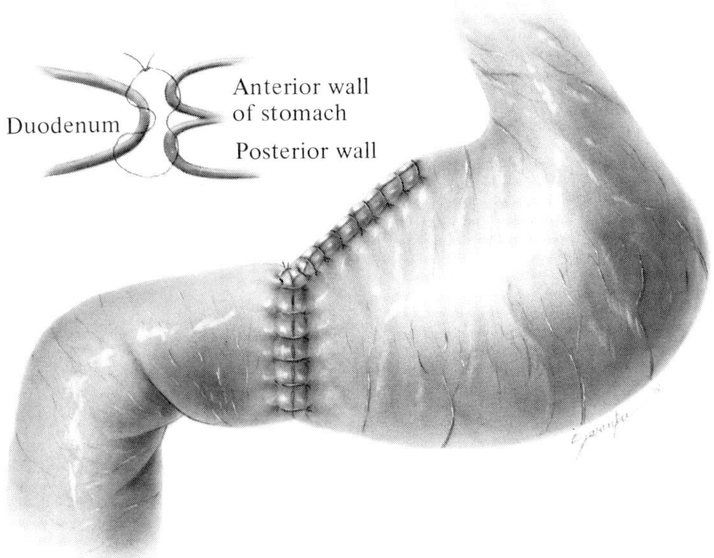

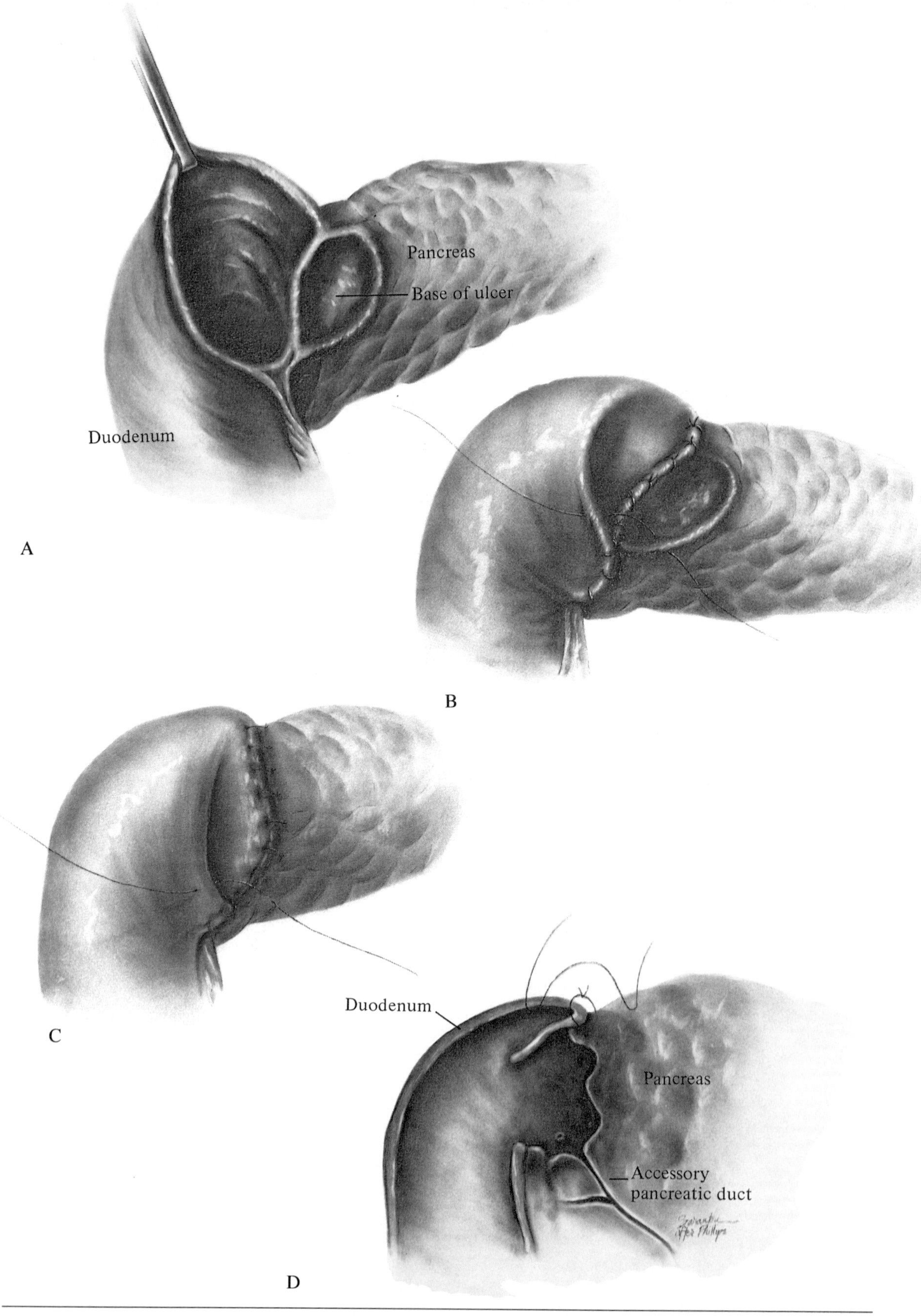
Pancreas
Base of ulcer
Duodenum
A
B
C
Duodenum
Pancreas
Accessory pancreatic duct
D

terminolateral modification of the Billroth I procedure rather than a Billroth II anastomosis. As stated before, the main reason for unsuitability of the end of the duodenum for anastomosis is the presence of a posterior penetrating ulcer. Under these circumstances a modified type of duodenal stump closure is achieved, using the method described by Nissen (Fig. A-10). This method consists in suturing the free anterior wall of the duodenum to the distal margin of the ulcer crater in the pancreas and rolling the anterior wall of the duodenum in such a manner that it covers the ulcer crater.

After the closure of the duodenal stump, an end-to-side gastroduodenal anastomosis is performed just distal to the duodenal stump closure. The resultant anastomosis is the same size as, or slightly larger than, the end-to-end anastomosis. When the end-to-side gastroduodenal anastomosis is used, the ampulla of Vater may be opposite the gastroduodenal stoma.

WOUND CLOSURE

I make no attempt to close the peritoneum and have noted no difficulty or complication arising from this omission. It seems that the ligamentum teres of the liver and the falciform ligament quickly adhere and may form a more anatomical peritoneal closure than would be accomplished by suture. The fascia of the linea alba is closed by interrupted nonabsorbable sutures. No subcutaneous sutures are used, and after closure of the fascia of the linea alba the skin edges are approximated by skin sutures.

Fig. A-10. Closure of the difficult duodenal stump when a terminolateral anastomosis is contemplated (closure after Nissen). (A) The distal duodenum adheres posteriorly to the distal margin of the ulcer bed. (B) The anterior duodenal wall is sutured to the distal margin of the ulcer bed, and a second row of sutures is begun, suturing the anterior wall to the proximal ulcer margin. (C) The second row is completed, and the third and final row is begun, folding the anterior duodenal wall against the capsule proximal to the ulcer. (D) Cross-section showing the omission of the first row of sutures when an accessory pancreatic duct opens into the ulcer bed. This omission allows pancreatic juice to drain into the duodenal lumen.

B

Books on Gastric Surgery

Because we hope that this monograph will be used for reference as well as for study, the editors append a list of 189 books and important theses pertaining to the surgical aspects of the stomach and duodenum. This list supplements the references, chiefly to journals, that appear at the end of the chapters of this book. It is of course impossible to include all books on the subject. Seeking a criterion of selection that would produce a practical list, we decided to limit the listing to those books that are in our combined personal libraries, since we believe they are the best works on the various subjects with which they deal and are available in most medical libraries.

The books are divided into several general categories, and in many instances a comment on the book is added to the listing. The order within each category is chronological.

Anatomy

Michels, N. A. *Blood Supply and Anatomy of the Upper Abdominal Organs with a Descriptive Atlas*. Philadelphia: Lippincott, 1955.

This monograph is limited in scope, but it presents its subject matter in beautiful detail. The stomach and duodenum represent only a small portion of this important contribution.

Oi, M. *The Occurrence of Peptic Ulcers and the Theory of Dual Control Mechanism*. Tokyo, Japan: Nankodo, 1976.

Physiology

The books in this category run the gamut from highly specialized works to Babkin's comprehensive coverage of gastric physiology. Although there is a section on surgical treatment of peptic ulcer in the text by Ivy, Grossman, and Bachrach, the book has been listed in this section because of its excellent section on gastric physiology.

Carlson, A. J. *The Control of Hunger in Health and Disease*. Chicago: University of Chicago Press, 1916.

Babkin, B. P. *Secretory Mechanisms of the Digestive Glands*. New York: Hoeber, 1944.

This is a classical book on the subject.

Ivy, A. C., Grossman, M. I., and Bachrach, W. H. *Peptic Ulcer*. Philadelphia: Blakiston, 1950.

Conway, E. J. *The Biochemistry of Gastric Acid Secretion*. Springfield, Ill.: Thomas, 1953.

James, A. H. *The Physiology of Gastric Digestion*. London: Arnold, 1957.

Smith, A. N. *Surgical Physiology of the Gastrointestinal Tract*. Edinburgh: Royal College of Surgeons of Edinburgh, 1962.

Magee, D. F. *Gastrointestinal Physiology*. Springfield, Ill.: Thomas, 1962.

Grossman, M. I. *Gastrin*. Los Angeles: University of California Press, 1966.

Lick, R. F. *Die Geschichte der Angewandten Magenphysiologie*. Hamburg, Germany: Holst, Materia Medica Nordmark, 1967.

Glass, G. B. J. *Introduction to Gastrointestinal Physiology*. Englewood Cliffs, N. J.: Prentice-Hall, 1968.

Oberhelman, H. A., Jr. *Physiological Principles of Gastric Surgery*. Springfield, Ill.: Thomas, 1968.

Texter, E. C., Jr., Chou, C. -C., Laureta, H. C., and Vantrappen, G. R. *Physiology of the Gastrointestinal Tract*. St. Louis: Mosby, 1968.

Murat, J. *Précis de Chirurgie Expérimentale: Abdominale et Thoracique chez le Chien*. Paris: Masson, 1972.

Sachs, G., Heinz, E., and Ulrich, K. J. *Gastric Secretion*. New York: Academic, 1972.

Jorpes, J. E., and Mutt, V. *Secretin, Cholecystokinin, Pancreozymin and Gastrin*. Berlin: Springer, 1973.

Limbosch, J. M. *Stimulation vagale et gastrinique de la Sécrétion gastrique: Chez le Chien et chez l'Homme*. Brussels: Éditions Arscia, 1973.

Brooks, F. P. *Gastrointestinal Physiology*. New York: Oxford University Press, 1974.

Friedman, M. H. F. *Functions of the Stomach and Intestine*. Baltimore: University Park Press, 1975.

Davenport, H. W. *Physiology of the Digestive Tract* (4th ed.). Chicago: Year Book, 1977.

Johnson, L. R. *Gastrointestinal Physiology*. St. Louis: Mosby, 1977.

Bloom, S. R. *Gut Hormones*. Edinburgh: Churchill Livingstone, 1978.
This volume contains a landmark collection of important papers in this rapidly expanding field of interest.

Brooks, I. P. *Gastrointestinal Pathophysiology* (2d ed.) New York: Oxford University Press, 1978.

Miyoshi, A. *Gut Peptides: Secretion, Function and Clinical Aspects*. Amsterdam: Elsevier–North Holland Biomedical Press, 1978.
A preview of future developments in the understanding of the gut endocrine system is presented.

Johnson, L. R. *Physiology of the Gastrointestinal Tract*. New York: Raven Press, 1981.
This text is outstanding in the detail presented.

Pathology

Few books are presented in this category, but each is a significant contribution.

Stout, A. P. Tumors of the Stomach. In *Atlas of Tumor Pathology*. Washington, D. C.: Armed Forces Institute of Pathology, 1953.

Wangensteen, O. H. *Cancer of the Esophagus and the Stomach*. New York: American Cancer Society, 1956.

Wood, I. J., and Taft, L. I. *Diffuse Lesions of the Stomach*. London: Arnold, 1958.

Fodor, O., Popescu, S., and Urcan, S. *Boala Ulceroasá: Fiziopatologie si patogeneză*. Bucharest: Editura Academiei, 1968.

Diagnosis

Palmer, E. D. *Stomach Disease as Diagnosed by Gastroscopy*. Philadelphia: Lea & Febiger, 1949.

Kalk, H., and Brühl, W. *Leitfaden der Laparoskopie und Gastroskopie*. Stuttgart: Thieme, 1951.
Both of these volumes are highly specialized monographs on gastroscopy.

Palmer, E. D. *Diagnosis of Upper Gastrointestinal Hemorrhage*. Springfield, Ill.: Thomas, 1961.

Berry, L. H. *Gastrointestinal Pan-Endoscopy: Esophagoscopy, Gastroscopy, Bulbar and Postbulbar Duodenoscopy, Procto-Sigmoidoscopy, Colonoscopy and Peritoneoscopy*. Springfield, Ill.: Thomas, 1974.

Berci, G. *Endoscopy*. New York: Appleton-Century-Crofts, 1976.

Gammill, S. L. *A Programmed Introduction to Upper Gastrointestinal Radiology*. Boston: Little, Brown, 1977.

Pearl, R. K. *Gastrointestinal Endoscopy for Surgeons*. Boston: Little, Brown, 1984.

Medical Aspects

Ewald, C. A. *The Diseases of the Stomach*. New York: Appleton, 1892.

Riegel, F. *Diseases of the Stomach*. Philadelphia: Saunders, 1903.

Kemp, R. C. *Diseases of the Stomach, Intestines, and Pancreas*. Philadelphia: Saunders, 1910. *Although not exclusively a book on the stomach, this volume at the time of its publication reflected advanced views on many gastric problems.*

Stockton, C. G. *Diseases of the Stomach*. New York: Appleton, 1914.

Eusterman, G. B., and Balfour, D. C. *The Stomach and Duodenum*. Philadelphia: Saunders, 1935. *This book was co-written by an internist and a surgeon with about equal space given to each sphere of interest. It is probably the best known* nearly *comprehensive clinical work on the stomach published in its time.*

Wolf, S., and Wolff, H. G. *Human Gastric Function* (2d ed.). New York: Oxford University Press, 1947.

Held, I. W., and Goldbloom, A. A. *Peptic Ulcer: Its Diagnosis and Treatment*. Springfield, Ill.: Thomas, 1946.

Smith, L. A., and Rivers, A. B. *Peptic Ulcer: Pain Patterns, Diagnosis, and Medical Treatment*. New York: Appleton-Century-Crofts, 1953.

Boller, R. *Der Magen und seine Krankheiten*. Vienna: Urban & Schwarzenberg, 1954.

Spira, J. J. *Gastroduodenal Ulcer*. London: Butterworth, 1956. *This monograph is related primarily to pathogenesis of ulcer disease. A critique of orthodox treatment is given.*

Albot, G., and Poilleux, F. *La Maladie Ulcéreuse de l'Estomac*. Paris: Masson, 1961.

Hafter, E. *Praktische Gastroenterologie* (2d ed.). Stuttgart: Thieme, 1962.

Sun, D. C. H. *The Management of Peptic Ulcer*. New York: Academy of Sciences, 1962.

Palmer, E. D. *Clinical Gastroenterology* (2d ed.). New York: Hoeber, 1962.

Wolf, S. *The Stomach*. New York: Oxford University Press, 1965.

Sun, D. C. H. *Chemistry and Therapy of Peptic Ulcer*. Springfield, Ill.: Thomas, 1966.

Thompson, C. M., Berkowitz, D., and Polish, E. *The Stomach: Including Related Areas in the Esophagus and Duodenum*. New York: Grune & Stratton, 1967.

Bockus, H. L. *Gastroenterology* (3d ed.), Vol. I. Philadelphia: Saunders, 1974.

Wastell, C., and Lance, P. *Cimetidine*. Edinburgh: Churchill Livingstone, 1978.

Baron, J. H. *Clinical Tests of Gastric Secretion: History, Methodology and Interpretation*. New York: Oxford University Press, 1979.

Rehfeld, J. F., and Amdrup, E. *Gastrins and the Vagus*. London: Academic, 1979.

Porro, G. B., and Bardhan, K. D. *Peptic Ulcer Disease: Advances in Pathogenesis and Treatment*. Verona: Cortina, 1982.

Kral, J. G., Powley, T. L., and Brooks, C. M. *Vagal Nerve Function: Behavioral and Methodological Considerations*. Amsterdam: Elsevier, 1983. *This volume is the report from one of the last Kroc Foundation conferences.*

Surgical: Systems of Surgery

The presentation in many of the books listed here is general. Others give considerable detail, particularly of technique.

Bier, A., Braun, H., and Kümmell, H. *Chirurgische Operationslehre,* Vol. III. Leipzig: Barth, 1923.

Bickham, W. S. *Operative Surgery,* Vol. IV. Philadelphia: Saunders, 1924.

Zenker, R. *Allgemeine und spezielle chirurgische Operationslehre: Die Eingriffe in der Bauchhöhle,* Vol. VII. Berlin: Springer, 1951.

Walters, W. *Lewis' Practice of Surgery,* Vol. VI. Hagerstown, Md.: Prior, 1955.

Nissen, R., and Hess, W. Operationen am Magen und Duodenum. In B. Breitner, L. Zukschwerdt, and H. Kraus (Eds.), *Chirurgische Operationslehre*. Vienna: Urban & Schwarzenberg, 1958.

Quénu, J., and Perrotin, J. *Traité de technique chirurgicale: Parois tube digestif,* Vol. VI. Paris: Masson, 1960.

Baumgartl, F., Kremer, K., and Schreiber, H. W. *Spezielle Chirurgie für die Praxis,* Vol. II. Stuttgart: Thieme, 1969.

Brandt, G., Kunz, H., and Nissen, R. *Intra- und postoperative Zwischenfälle: Ihre Verhutung und Behandlung,* Vol. II. Stuttgart: Thieme, 1971.

Zenker, R., Berchtold, R., and Hamelmann, H. *Allgemeine und spezielle chirurgische Operationslehre,* Vol. VII. *Die Eingriffe in der Bauchhöhle*. Heidelberg: Springer, 1975.

Dudley, H., Pories, W., and Carter, D. *Rob and Smith's Operative Surgery* (4th ed.), Vol. I. London: Butterworth, 1983.

Nyhus, L. M., and Baker, R. J. (Eds.), *Mastery of Surgery*. Boston: Little, Brown, 1984.

Schwartz, S. I., and Ellis, H. *Maingot's Abdominal Operations* (8th ed.). Norwalk, Connecticut: Appleton-Century-Crofts, 1985.

Surgical Theses

The following theses are extremely valuable but somewhat limited in scope.

Bohmansson, G. Studien über die chirurgische Behandlung von Gastroduodenalgeschwüren mit besonderer Berücksichtigung der Operationsanatomie und der postoperativen Digestionphysiologie nebst einem Beitrag zur Frage der chirurgischen Behandlung akuter Ulkusblutungen. *Acta Chir. Scand.* 60: Suppl. VII, 1926.

Schanke, K. The behaviour of gastric and duodenal ulcer. *Acta Chir. Scand.* 94: Suppl. 115, 1946.

Bruusgaard, C. The operative treatment of gastric and duodenal ulcer. *Acta Chir. Scand.* 94: Suppl. 117, 1946.

Fretheim, B. Post-operative hypoproteinemia after gastrectomies. *Acta Chir. Scand.* 96: Suppl. 130, 1947.

Rosenberg, D. *Contribuição para o Tratamento da Ulcera Duodenal Pela Ressecção dos Nervos Vagos.* Thesis: Escola Paulista de Medicina, São Paulo, Brazil, 1949.

Rosenberg, D. *Estudo Anatômico dos Nervos Vagos na Porção Infrabrônquica do Esôfago.* Thesis: Faculty of Medicine, University of São Paulo, Brazil, 1949.

Fitzgerald, O., and Murphy, P. Studies on the physiological chemistry and clinical significance of urease and urea with special reference to the stomach. *Ir. J. Med. Sci.* 292(6th ser.):97, 1950.

Spath, F. *Die chirurgische Therapie des Magenduodenal Ulcus in der Schule von Haberer.* Vienna: Springer, 1950.

Meurling, S. Postcibal symptoms after partial gastrectomy for peptic ulcer. *Acta Soc. Med. Upsal.* Suppl. 3, 1953.

Wallensten, S. Results of the surgical treatment of peptic ulcer by partial gastrectomy according to Billroth I and II methods. *Acta Chir. Scand.* Suppl. 191, 1954.

Viikari, S. J., and Klossner, O. The primary and late results of 1050 partial gastrectomies for chronic gastroduodenal ulcer. *Acta Chir. Scand.* Suppl. 220, 1956.

Norberg, P. B. Results of the surgical treatment of perforated ulcer. *Acta Chir. Scand.* Suppl. 249, 1959.

Borg, I. Gastric flow and acidity before and after Billroth II and Billroth I for gastroduodenal ulcer. *Acta Chir. Scand.* Suppl. 251, 1959.

Bremer, A. Contribution à l'étude des mécanismes de stimulation de la sécrétion acide de l'estomac. *Acta Gastroenterol. Belg.* 22:1959.

Lewin, E. Gastric cancer: A clinical study with reference to total gastrectomy and microscopic grading. *Acta Chir. Scand.* Suppl. 262, 1960.

Aagaard, P. *Studies of Gastric Ulcer.* Copenhagen: Aarhuus Stiftsbogtrykkerie, 1963.

Eklund, A. -E. *Studies on ABO Blood Groups and Blood Group Specific Substances in Gastric Carcinoma.* Stockholm: Svenska Tryckeriaktiebolaget, 1964.

Fenger, H. J. Clinical and experimental studies of dumping disposition. *Acta Chir. Scand.* Suppl. 371, 1967.

Mignon, M. *Le Rôle de la Gastrin dans le Contrôle de la Sécrétion Gastrique de Pepsine.* Thesis: Faculty of Medicine, Paris, 1968.

Rune, S. J. Gastric secretion and ingestion of solid food. *Scand. J. Gastroenterol.* 3:Suppl. 1, 1968.

Semb, L. S. *Studies on Inhibition of Gastric Secretion.* Oslo: Universitetsforlaget, 1968.

Herrington, J. L., Jr. *Remedial Operations for Postgastrectomy Syndromes. Curr. Probl. Surg.* April, 1970.

Linschoten, H. *The Boerema Button for Total Gastrectomy for Carcinoma.* Antwerp: Bussum, 1970.

Burhol, P. G. *Gastric secretion in the chicken. Scand. J. Gastroenterol.* 6:Suppl. 11, 1971.

Kairaluoma, M. I. Experimental gastric ulcer in the Shay rat. I. Pathogenesis of Shay ulcer: Effect of ligation time on ulcer incidence, ulcer index and mortality. *Acta Chir. Scand.* Suppl. 418, 1971.

Varis, K. A family study of chronic gastritis: Histological, immunological and functional aspects. *Scand. J. Gastroenterol.* 6:Suppl. 13, 1971.

Appelqvist, P. Carcinoma of the oesophagus and gastric cardia. *Acta Chir. Scand.* Suppl. 430, 1972.

Friesen, S. R. Zollinger-Ellison syndrome. *Curr. Probl. Surg.* April, 1972.

Herrington, J. L., Jr. Current operations for duodenal ulcer. *Curr. Probl. Surg.* July, 1972.

Kairaluoma, M. I., and Larmi, T. K. I. Experimental gastric ulcer in the Shay rat. II. Healing of gastric ulcers, development of their vascular supply, and effect of vagotomy on healing. *Acta Chir. Scand.* Suppl. 428, 1972.

Flament, J. B. *Les diverticules muqueux de la fenêtre duodenale.* Paris: Impressions C.I.J., 1973.

Moberg, S. *Gastric Emptying and Duodenal Digestion Before and After Partial Gastrectomy and Selective Proximal Vagotomy.* Stockholm: Trycker Balder, 1974.

Frankel, L. A. *Gastric Surgery and the Dumping Syndrome: The "Mirror-Image" Concept.*

Springfield, Ill.: Thomas, 1975.
Geurts, W. J. C. *Hoog selective vagotomie*. Thesis: Rijks University of Utrecht, Netherlands, 1975.
Lundquist, G., and Hedenstedt, S. Jejunal transposition in stomach surgery: Indications and results. *Acta Chir. Scand.* Suppl. 457, 1975.
Schumpelick, V., Farthmann, E., and Schreiber, H. W. Chirurgie des magens. *Med. Welt* 27:2349, 1976.
Specterow, J. *Vagotomia Incompleta E seu Reconhecimento Pelo Teste Endoscopico do Vermelho Congo*. Thesis: Universidade Federal Fluminense, Rio de Janeiro, 1977.
Specterow's thesis is an excellent study of the endoscopic Congo red test for completeness of vagotomy.
Grabner, P. *Studies on the Intestinal Phase of Gastric Secretion*. Thesis: University of Oslo, 1982.
Busman, D. C. *Results of Highly Selective Vagotomy*. Thesis: National University Linburg and Maastricht, 1983.
Stabile, B. E., and Passaro, E., Jr. Duodenal ulcer: A disease in evolution. *Curr. Probl. Surg.* January, 1984.
Thompson, J. C., and Marx, M. Gastrointestinal hormones. *Curr. Probl. Surg.* June, 1984.

Surgical: Abdominal Surgery

The following texts encompass the general area of abdominal surgery, thus including the stomach and duodenum.

Deaver, J. B., and Ashhurst, A. P. C. *Surgery of the Upper Abdomen,* Vol. I. Philadelphia: Blakiston, 1909. (Also 2d ed., 1921).
Moynihan, B. *Abdominal Operations* (3d ed.), Vol. I. Philadelphia: Saunders, 1916.
Juilly, G. H. *Practical Surgery of the Abdomen,* Vol. I. Philadelphia: Davis, 1928.
Bancroft, F. W. *Operative Surgery*. New York: Appleton-Century-Crofts, 1941.
Bancroft, F. W., and Wade, P. A. *Surgical Treatment of the Abdomen*. Philadelphia: Lippincott, 1947.
Shackelford, R. T. *Bickham-Callander Surgery of the Alimentary Tract,* Vol. I. Philadelphia: Saunders, 1955.
Bowers, W. F. *Surgical Gastroenterology* Springfield, Ill.: Thomas, 1960.
Steinberg, M. E. *Gastric Surgery*. New York: Appleton-Century-Crofts, 1963.
White, T. T., and Harrison, R. C. *Reoperative Gastrointestinal Surgery*. Boston: Little, Brown, 1973.
Shackelford, R. T., and Zuidema, G. D. *Surgery of the Alimentary Tract* (2d ed.), Vol. II. Philadelphia: Saunders, 1981.

Surgical: Peptic Ulcer Only

Within the confines of the subject matter selected, excellent coverage is given in all the texts in this category.

Doyen, E. *Traitement Chirurgical des Affections de l'Estomac et du Duodénum*. Paris: Rueff et Cie, 1894.
Heuer, G. J. *The Treatment of Peptic Ulcer*. Philadelphia: Lippincott, 1944.
Both medical and surgical treatments are discussed.
Nissen, R. *Duodenal and Jejunal Peptic Ulcer–Technic of Resection*. New York: Grune & Stratton, 1945.
This monograph has always had a fine reputation for its technical points.
Illingworth, C. F. W. *Peptic Ulcer*. Edinburgh: Livingstone, 1953.
Moore, H. G., Jr., and Harkins, H. N. *The Billroth I Gastric Resection: With Particular Reference to the Surgery of Peptic Ulcer*. Boston: Little, Brown, 1954.
The scope is rather specific and limited.
De Vernejoul, R., Henry, E., and Devin, R. *La Gastrectomie pour Ulcère*. Paris: Masson, 1956.
Many facets of the problem are not discussed in this text, which was not intended to be all-inclusive.
Allen, J. G. *The Physiology and Treatment of Peptic Ulcer*. Chicago: University of Chicago Press, 1959.
An excellent review of benign gastroduodenal disease is provided.
Wells, C., and Kyle, J. *Peptic Ulceration*. Edinburgh: Livingstone, 1960.
Woodward, E. R. *The Postgastrectomy Syndromes*. Springfield, Ill.: Thomas, 1963.
Postlethwait, R. W. *Results of Surgery for Peptic Ulcer*. Philadelphia: Saunders, 1963.
Grassi, G. I. *Resultati della vagotomia nel trattamento dell'ulcera gastroduodenale*. Rome: Edizoni Mediche e Scientifiche, 1965.
Weiss, A. G., and Hollender, L. F. *La vagotomie dans l'ulcère gastro-duodéno-jéjunal*. Paris: Expansion Scientifique Française, 1966.

Cirenei, A., and Speranza, V. *La Terapia chirurgica dell'Ulcera gastrica e dell'Ulcera duodenale*. Padua: Piccin Editore, 1967.

Alexander-Williams, J., and Cox, A. G. *After Vagotomy*. London: Butterworth, 1969.

Alexiu, O., Furtunescu, B., and Păcescu, E. *Les Vagotomies*. Paris: Masson, 1970.

Day, S. B., MacMillan, B. G., and Altemeier, W. A. *Curling's Ulcer: An Experiment of Nature*. Springfield, Ill.: Thomas, 1972.

Holle, F., and Andersson, S. *Vagotomy: Latest Advances*. Heidelberg: Springer, 1974.

Wastell, C. *Chronic Duodenal Ulcer*. London: Butterworth, 1974.

Burge, H., Farthmann, E. H., Grassi, G., Hedenstedt, St. B., Hollender, L. F., Schrieber, H. W., and Tanner, N. C. *Vagotomie: Indikationen, Taktik, Technik, Komplikationen, Ergebnisse, Kommentare*. Stuttgart: Georg Thieme Verlag, 1976.

Menguy, R. *Surgery of Peptic Ulcer*, Vol. XVIII Ser., *Major Problems in Clinical Surgery*. Philadelphia: Sanders, 1976.

Eisenberg, M. M. Physiologic approach to the surgical management of duodenal ulcer. *Curr. Probl. Surg*. 4:3, 1977.

Murakami, T., and Muto, T. *Clinics of Gastric Vagotomy*. Tokyo: Kanehara, 1977.

Klempa, V. I., and Becker, H. D. *Vagus-Gastrin-Magensekretion*. Stuttgart: Georg Thieme Verlag, 1977.

Eisenberg, M. M. *Ulcers*. New York: Random House, 1978.
This is an interesting presentation for the reader who is not in the health professions.

Civalero, L. -A. Selective proximal vagotomy in duodenal ulcer. *Acta Chir. Scand*. Suppl. 491, 1979.

Becker, H. D., and Caspary, W. I. *Postgastrectomy and Postvagotomy Syndromes*. Berlin: Springer, 1980.

Fiddian-Green, R. G., and Turcotte, J. G. *Gastrointestinal Hemorrhage*. New York: Grune & Stratton, 1980.

Carter, D. C. (Ed.), *Peptic Ulcer*. Edinburgh: Churchill Livingstone, 1983.

Surgical: Tumor Only

Wölfler, A. *Ueber die von Herrn Professor Billroth Ausgeführten Resectionen des Carcinomatösen Pylorus*. Vienna: Braumuller, 1881.

Smithies, F., and Ochsner, A. J. *Cancer of the Stomach*. Philadelphia: Saunders, 1916.

Livingstone, E. M., and Pack, G. T. *End-Results in the Treatment of Gastric Cancer*. New York: Hoeber, 1939.

Pack, G. T. *Cancer of the Esophagus and Gastric Cardia*. St. Louis: Mosby, 1949.

Fretheim, B. *Carcinoma Ventriculi Behandlet med Abdominothoracol Total Gastrectomi*. Oslo: Akademisk Trykningssentral-Blindern, 1953.

Señorans, A. J., and Moreno, I. G. *Clínica y Cirugia del Cancer del Estomago*. Buenos Aires: Editorial Medical Brascia, 1954.

Gütgemann, A., and Schreiber, H. W. *Die Chirurgie des Magensarkoms*. Stuttgart: Thieme, 1960.

Massa, J. *Le Petit Cancer de l'Estomac*. Paris: Masson, 1961.

ReMine, W. H., Priestley, J. T., and Berkson, J. *Cancer of the Stomach*. Philadelphia: Saunders, 1964.

Kelsey, J. R., Jr. *Cancer of the Stomach: A Guide for Diagnosis and Treatment*. Springfield, Ill.: Thomas, 1967.

McNeer, G., and Pack, G. T. *Neoplasms of the Stomach*. Philadelphia: Lippincott, 1967.

Surgical: Operative Technique

Maingot, R. *Technique of Gastric Operations*. London: Oxford University Press, 1941.

Nakayama, K. *Anatomy and Techniques of Surgery*. Tokyo: Chugai, Igaku, 1960.

Nakayama, K. *Atlas of Gastrointestinal Surgery*. Tokyo: Igaku Shoin, 1968.

Welch, C. E. *Surgery of the Stomach and Duodenum* (5th ed.). Chicago: Year Book, 1973.

Malt, R. A. (Ed.). Gastrectomies and drainage procedures. *Surg. Tech. Illus*. 1:1, 1976.

Johnson, A. G., and Reynolds, K. W. *Techniques of Vagotomy*. Chicago: Year Book, 1979.

Hollender, L. F., and Marrie, A. *Highly Selective Vagotomy*. Paris: Masson, 1979.

Goffi, F. *Tecnica Cirurgica* (2d ed.). Rio de Janeiro: Livraria Athenen, 1980.

Saik, R. P. *Vagotomy Testing*. Mount Kisco, New York: Futura, 1983.

Surgical: Comprehensive Clinical

Robson, A. W. M., and Moynihan, B. G. A. *Diseases of the Stomach and Their Surgical Treatment*. New York: William Wood, 1901.
This is one of the first truly comprehensive clinical monographs.

Paterson, H. J. *The Surgery of the Stomach: A Handbook of Diagnosis and Treatment* (2d ed.). New York: William Wood, 1914.
Among the many classics listed in this appendix, this must be considered one of the best.

Horsley, J. S. *Surgery of the Stomach and Small Intestine*. New York: Appleton, 1926.
This monograph is not quite as comprehensive as the previous two.

Somervell, T. H. *The Surgery of the Stomach and Duodenum*. Baltimore: Williams & Wilkins, 1948.
This is a good example of comprehensive clinical coverage.

Gueullette, R. *Chirurgie de l'Estomac*. Paris: Masson, 1956.

Oi, M. *Peptic Ulcer: Gastric, Duodenal and Esophageal*. Tokyo: Nankodo, 1957.
Ninety percent of this text is in Japanese. It appears to be extremely comprehensive.

Westhues, H. *Einfachheit und Sicherheit bei Magenund Darmoperationen*. Stuttgart: Thieme, 1961.

Steinberg, M. E. *Gastric Surgery*. New York: Appleton-Century-Crofts, 1963.

Stammers, F. A. R., and Williams, F. A. *Partial Gastrectomy*. London: Butterworth, 1963.

Glassman, J. A. *Stomach Surgery*. Springfield, Ill.: Thomas, 1970.

Smith, R. *Surgical Forum: Gastric Surgery* London: Butterworth, 1975.

Blum, A. L., and Siewert, J. R. *Ulcus-Therapie*. Berlin: Springer-Verlag, 1978.

Holle, F., and Holle, G. E. *Vagotomy and Pyloroplasty: Advances 1975–1980*. Berlin: Springer-Verlag, 1980.
The pioneer of selective proximal vagotomy gives a detailed analysis of his results with more than 2000 patients.

Baron, J. H., Alexander-Williams, J., Allgöwer, M., Müller, C., and Spencer, J. *Vagotomy in Modern Surgical Practice*. London: Butterworth, 1982.

Bunte, H., and Langhams, P. *A Century of Ulcer Surgery: Medical and Surgical Therapy Today*. Munich: Urban & Schwarzenberg, 1984.

Surgical: Comprehensive Clinical and Experimental

Harkins, H. N., and Nyhus, L. M. *Surgery of the Stomach and Duodenum* (1st, 2d eds.). Boston: Little, Brown, 1962, 1969.

Holle, F. *Spezielle Magenchirurgie*. Berlin: Springer, 1968.

Bartelheimer, H., Maurer, H. -J., and Schreiber, H. W. *Magenoperation und Magenoperierter*. Berlin: de Gruyter, 1969.

Nyhus, L. M., and Wastell, C. *Surgery of the Stomach and Duodenum* (3d ed.). Boston: Little, Brown, 1977.

Indexes

Subject Index

Author Index